Easily
confused
drug
names
located
beneath
the header

⚠ High Alert

etoposide (℞)
(e-toe-poe'side)
VePesid, VP-16
etoposide phosphate
Etopophos
Func. class.: Antineoplastic—
miscellaneous
Chem. class.: Semisynthetic podophyllotoxin

Do not confuse:
VePesid/Versed

Action: Inhibits mitotic activity through
metaphase to mitosis; also inhibits cells
from entering mitosis, depresses DNA,
RNA synthesis, cell cycle specific S and
G_2

Uses: Leukemias, testicular cancer, lymphomas, small cell carcinoma of the lung
Unlabeled uses: Lymphomas

DOSAGE AND ROUTES

Testicular cancer
• *Adult:* **IV** 50/100 mg/m²/day × 5 days
given q3-5wk or 200-250 mg/m²/wk, or
125-140 mg/m²/day 3 × wk, q5wk
Small cell carcinoma of the lung

Common unlabeled
uses clearly indicated

[···]/day × 4 days,
[···]/day × 4 days,
[···] day q3-4 wk
50 mg   inj 20 mg/ml; caps

SIDE EFFECTS

CNS: Headache, *fever*, peripheral neurop-
athy, paresthesias, confusion
CV: *Hypotension*, **MI, dysrhythmias**
GI: *Nausea, vomiting, anorexia*, **hepa-
totoxicity**, dyspepsia, diarrhea, constipa-
tion
GU: **Nephrotoxicity**
HEMA: **Thrombocytopenia, leukope-
nia, myelosuppression, anemia**
INTEG: *Rash, alopecia*, phlebitis at IV site,
radiation recall
RESP: **Bronchospasm**, pleural effusion
SYST: **Anaphylaxis**

♣ Canada only

etoposide

Contraindications: Pregnancy (D),
lactation, hypersensitivity, bone marrow
depression, severe renal/hepatic disease,
bacterial infection, viral infection
Precautions: Renal/hepatic disease,
children, gout

PHARMACOKINETICS

Half-life 7 hr, metabolized in liver; excreted in urine; crosses placental barrier

E

INTERACTIONS

Increase: bone marrow depression—
other antineoplastics, radiation
Increase: adverse reactions—live virus
vaccines

NURSING CONSIDERATIONS

Assess:
• CBC, differential, platelet count weekly;
withhold drug if WBC is <1000 or platelet count is <50,000; notify prescriber
• Renal studies: BUN, serum uric acid,
urine CCr, electrolytes before, during therapy
• I&O ratio; rep[ort] [···]
<30 ml/hr; chec[k] [···]
report any signif[···]
• Monitor temp [···] [mean-
ning infection
• Hepatic studies [···]
(bilirubin, AST, A[···]) as needed or
monthly
• Bleeding: hematuria, guaiac stools,
bruising or petechiae, mucosa or orifices
q8h
• Effects of alopecia on body image; discuss feelings about body changes
• Jaundice of skin and sclera, dark urine,
clay-colored stools, itchy skin, abdominal pain, fever, diarrhea
• B/P q15 min during inf, if systolic reading <90 mm Hg, discontinue inf and notify prescriber
• Buccal cavity q8h for dryness, sores or
ulceration, white patches, oral pain,
bleeding, dysphagia
• Local irritation, pain, burning, discoloration at inj site

Nursing considerations
provide guidance
through the nursing
process

Side effects: *italics* = common; **bold** = life-threatening

Formulas for drug calculations

Surface area rule:

$$\text{Child dose} = \frac{\text{Surface area (m}^2)}{1.73 \text{ m}^2} \times \text{Adult dose}$$

Calculating strength of a solution:

Solution Strength: *Desired Solution:*

$$\frac{x}{100} = \frac{\text{Amount of drug desired}}{\text{Amount of finished solution}}$$

Calculating flow rate for IV:

$$\text{Rate of flow} = \frac{\text{Amount of fluid} \times \text{Administration set calibration}}{\text{Running time}}$$

$$\frac{x}{1} = \frac{\text{(ml) (gtt/min)}}{\text{min}}$$

Calculation of medication dosages:

Formula method:

$$\frac{\text{Amount ordered}}{\text{Amount on hand}} \times \text{Vehicle} = \text{Number of tablets, capsules, or amount of liquid}$$

Vehicle is the drug form or amount of liquid containing the dosage. Amounts used in calculation by formula must be in same system.

Ratio—proportion method:

1 tablet:tablet in mg on hand: : x tablet order in mg

        Know or have: :Want to know or order

Multiply means and extremes, divide both sides by known amount to get x. Amounts used in equation must be in same system.

Dimensional analysis method:

$$\text{Order in mg} \times \frac{1 \text{ tablet or capsule}}{\text{What 1 tablet or capsule is in mg}}$$

= Tablets or capsules to be given

If amounts are in different systems:

$$\text{Order in mg} \times \frac{1 \text{ tablet or capsule}}{\text{What 1 tablet or capsule is in g}} \times \frac{1}{1000 \text{ mg}}$$

= Tablets or capsules to be given

Nomogram for calculation of body surface area

Place a straight edge from the patient's height in the left column to the patient's weight in the right column. The point of intersection on the body surface area column indicates the body surface area (BSA). (Reproduced in Behrman RE, Kliegman RM, Jenson HB: *Nelson textbook of pediatrics,* ed 18, Philadelphia, 2007, WB Saunders; Nomogram modified from data of E. Boyd by CD West.)

Alternative (Mosteller's formula):

$$\text{Surface area (m}^2) = \sqrt{\dfrac{\text{Height (cm)} \times \text{Weight (kg)}}{3600}}$$

To access your Online Resources, visit:
http://evolve.elsevier.com/nursingdrugupdates/Skidmore/NDR

Evolve® Online Resources for Skidmore: *Mosby's 2008 Nursing Drug Reference*, offer the following features:

- **Drug Monographs**
  Includes full monographs for drugs new to this edition.

- **FDA Alerts**
  Provides updates on drug recalls, labeling changes, new interactions, and safety warnings.

- **Recently Approved Drugs**
  Offers a table of drugs approved by the FDA after publication of the book, including links to approved product inserts.

- **Drug Name Safety Information**
  Links to organizations and resources involved in reducing medication errors caused by drug name confusion.

- **Selected Prescription Drugs with Potential for Abuse**
  Features a table of drugs that can be addictive or dangerous when misused, provided by the National Institute on Drug Abuse.

- **English-to-Spanish Translation**
  Provides Spanish translations and prounciation for common drug phrases and terms.

http://evolve.elsevier.com/nursingdrugupdates/Skidmore/NDR

2008 *Mosby's* NURSING DRUG REFERENCE

2008 *Mosby's*
NURSING DRUG
REFERENCE

Linda Skidmore-Roth, RN, MSN, NP

Consultant

Littleton, Colorado

Formerly, Nursing Faculty

New Mexico State University
Las Cruces, New Mexico;
El Paso Community College
El Paso, Texas

MOSBY

ELSEVIER

MOSBY
ELSEVIER

11830 Westline Industrial Drive
St. Louis, Missouri 63146

MOSBY'S 2008 NURSING DRUG REFERENCE

ISBN: 978-0-323-04700-5
ISSN: 1044-8470

NOTICE

Knowledge and best practice in this field are constantly changing. As new research and experience broaden our knowledge, changes in practice, treatment and drug therapy may become necessary or appropriate. Readers are advised to check the most current information provided (i) on procedures featured or (ii) by the manufacturer of each product to be administered, to verify the recommended dose or formula, the method and duration of administration, and contraindications. It is the responsibility of the practitioner, relying on their own experience and knowledge of the patient, to make diagnoses, to determine dosages and the best treatment for each individual patient, and to take all appropriate safety precautions. To the fullest extent of the law, neither the Publisher nor the Author assumes any liability for any injury and/or damage to persons or property arising out of or related to any use of the material contained in this book.

The Publisher

ISBN: 978-0-323-04700-5

Executive Publisher: Darlene Como
Managing Editor: Tamara Myers
Senior Developmental Editor: Laura M. Selkirk
Publishing Services Manager: Melissa Lastarria
Senior Project Manager: Joy Moore
Senior Designer: Amy Buxton

Printed in the United States of America

Last digit is the print number:
9 8 7 6 5 4 3 2 1

Working together to grow
libraries in developing countries

www.elsevier.com | www.bookaid.org | www.sabre.org

ELSEVIER   BOOK AID International   Sabre Foundation

Consultants

Victoria Agyekum, RN, MSN
Department Head
Savannah Technical College
Savannah, Georgia

Dana Bartlett, RN, BSN, MSN, MA
Poison Information Specialist
Children's Hospital of Philadelphia
Philadelphia, Pennsylvania

Jennifer Chan, PharmD
Clinical Assistance Professor of
    Pharmacy and Pharmacology
University of Texas Health Science Center
San Antonio, Texas

Amanda Gross, RPh
Pharmacist
University Hospital
Denver, Colorado

Dana H. Hamamura, PharmD
Clinical Pharmacist
University of Colorado Hospital
Denver, Colorado

Joan Knape, RN, BSEd
I Can Do That Services
St. Louis, Missouri

Dorothy Mathers, RN, MSN
Associate Professor
Pennsylvania College of Technology
Williamsport, Pennsylvania

Sandra S. Meeker, RN, MSN
Nursing Professor
Central Texas College
Killeen, Texas

Amy E. Miller, PharmD, BCPS
Assistant Professor of Clinical Pharmacy
Philadelphia College of Pharmacy
University of the Sciences in Philadelphia
Philadelphia, Pennsylvania

Teresa L. Moore, PharmD
Camilla, Georgia

Lisa Nagle, CMA
Program Director–Medical Assisting
Augusta Technical College
Augusta, Georgia

Joshua J. Neumiller, PharmD
Geriatrics Resident/Clinical
    Research Associate
College of Pharmacy
Washington State University
Spokane, Washington

Brenda Condusta Pavill,
    RN, PhD, IBCLC
Associate Professor of Nursing
College Misericordia
Dallas, Pennsylvania

Sarah R. Pool, RN, MS
Nursing Education Specialist
Mayo Clinic
Rochester, Minnesota

Randolph E. Regal,
  BS, PharmD, RPh
Clinical Assistant Professor
College of Pharmacy
University of Michigan Hospital
Ann Arbor, Michigan

Stephen M. Setter, PharmD,
  CDE, CGP, DVM
Associate Professor of Pharmacotherapy
Elder Services/Visiting Nurses
  Association
Washington State University
Spokane, Washington

John J. Smith, EdD
Director–Health Sciences
Corinthian Colleges, Inc.
Santa Ana, California

Travis Sonnett, PharmD
Geriatric Fellow/Clinical Research
  Associate
College of Pharmacy
Washington State University
Spokane, Washington

Patricia R. Teasley, MSN, RN,
  APRN, BC
Professor, Nursing Department
Central Texas College
Killeen, Texas

Preface

Since the first publication of *Mosby's Nursing Drug Reference* in 1988, more than 100 U.S. and Canadian pharmacists and consultants have reviewed the book's content closely. Today, *Mosby's 2008 Nursing Drug Reference* is more up-to-date than ever—with features that make it easy to find critical information fast!

New Facts

This edition features more than 2000 new drug facts, including:
- New drugs and new dosage information
- Newly researched side effects and adverse reactions
- The latest precautions, interactions, and contraindications
- IV therapy updates
- Revised nursing considerations
- Updated patient/family teaching guidelines

New Features
- IV information in a new eye-catching format.
- Twenty-three recent FDA-approved drugs located throughout the book and in Appendix A. Included are monographs for anidulafungin, arformoterol for COPD, conivaptan, darunavir for HIV, dasatinib for leukemia, decitabine, deferasirox, desonide, idursulfase, kunecatechins, lubiprostone, micafungin, nabilone, natalizumab, panitumumab for metastatic colorectal cancer, posaconazole, ranibizumab, ranolazine for angina pectoris, rasagiline, sitagliptin, sunitinib, telbivudine, and varenicline.
- An updated companion CD-ROM that offers complete and printable monographs for 100 of the most commonly prescribed drugs in the United States, numerous patient teaching guides in English and Spanish for these same drugs, hundreds of normal laboratory values, an English-to-Spanish guide for drug phrases and terms, and more than 20 calculators.
- Appendix B, Recent FDA Drug Approvals, lists generic/trade names and uses for four of the most recently approved drugs.
- Two new appendixes—Medications That May Be Inappropriate for Geriatric Patients and Safety in Handling Chemotherapeutic Agents.
- Several combination monographs, including contraceptives and insulins, that have been substantially reorganized.

Organization

This reference is organized into four main sections:
- Drug categories
- Four-color insert
- Individual drug monographs (in alphabetical order by generic name)
- Appendixes (identified by the wide dark blue thumb tabs on the edge)

The guiding principle behind this book is to provide fast, easy access to drug information and nursing considerations. Every detail—from the paper, typeface, cover, binding, use of color, and appendixes—has been carefully chosen with the user in mind.

Color Insert

This insert features 14 detailed, four-color illustrations to help enhance the understanding of the mechanism or site of action for the following select drugs and drug classes:

- ACE inhibitors
- Adrenocortical steroids
- Antidepressants
- Antidiabetic agents
- Antifungal agents
- Antiinfective agents
- Antiplatelet agents
- Antiretroviral agents
- Benzodiazepines
- Diuretics
- Drugs used to treat GERD
- Narcotic agonist-antagonist analgesics
- Narcotic analgesics
- Sympatholytics

Individual Drug Monographs

This book contains monographs for more than 1300 generic and 4500 trade medications. Common trade names are given for all drugs regularly used in the United States and Canada, with drugs available only in Canada identified by a maple leaf ✹.

The following information is provided, whenever possible, for safe, effective administration of each drug:

High-alert status: Identifies high-alert drugs with a label and icon.

"Tall Man" lettering: Uses the capitalization of distinguishing letters to avoid medication errors and is required by the FDA for drug manufacturers.

Pronunciation: Helps the nurse master complex generic names.

℞/otc: Identifies prescription or over-the-counter drugs.

Functional and chemical classifications: Allows the nurse to see similarities and dissimilarities among drugs in the same functional but different chemical classes.

Controlled-substance schedule: Includes schedules for the United States and Canada.

Do not confuse: Presents drug names that might easily be confused, within each appropriate monograph.

Action: Describes pharmacologic properties concisely.

Uses: Lists the conditions the drug is used to treat.

Unlabeled uses: Describes drug uses that may be encountered in practice but are not yet FDA approved.

Dosages and routes: Lists all available and approved dosages and routes for adult, pediatric, and geriatric patients.

Available forms: Includes tablets, capsules, extended-release, injectables (IV, IM, SUBCUT), solutions, creams, ointments, lotions, gels, shampoos, elixirs, suspensions, suppositories, sprays, aerosols, and lozenges.

Side effects: Groups these reactions by alphabetical body system, with common side effects *italicized* and life-threatening reactions in **bold type** for emphasis.

Contraindications: Lists conditions under which the drug absolutely should not be given, including FDA pregnancy safety categories D or X.

Precautions: Lists conditions that require special consideration when the drug is prescribed, including FDA pregnancy safety categories A, B, and C.

Pharmacokinetics: Outlines metabolism, distribution, and elimination.

Interactions: Includes confirmed drug interactions, followed by the drug or nutrient causing that interaction, when applicable.

Drug/herb: Highlights more than 400 potential interactions between herbal products and prescription or OTC drugs.

Drug/food: Identifies many common drug interactions with foods.

Drug/lab test: Identifies how the drug may affect lab test results.

Nursing considerations: Identifies key nursing considerations for each step of the nursing process: Assess, Administer, Perform/Provide, Evaluate, and Teach Patient/Family. Instructions for giving drugs by various routes (e.g., PO, IM, IV) are included, with route subheadings in bold.

Compatibilities: Lists syringe, Y-site, and additive compatibilities and incompatibilities. If no compatibilities are listed for a drug, the necessary compatibility testing has not been done and that compatibility information is unknown. To ensure safety, assume that the drug may not be mixed with other drugs unless specifically stated.

"Nursing Alert" icon ⚠: Highlights a critical consideration.

Treatment of overdose: Provides drugs and treatment for overdoses where appropriate.

Appendixes

Selected new drugs: Includes comprehensive information on 23 key drugs approved by the FDA during the past 12 months.

Recent FDA drug approvals: Summarizes basic information, such as generic name, trade name, and uses, for drugs so recently approved by the FDA that complete information was not yet available when this book went to press.

Ophthalmic, otic, nasal, and topical products: Provides essential information for 135 ophthalmic, otic, nasal, and topical products commonly used today, grouped by chemical drug class.

Vaccines and toxoids: Features an easy-to-use table with generic and trade names, uses, dosages and routes, and contraindications for 32 key vaccines and toxoids.

Antitoxins and antivenins: Provides names, uses, dosages, and contraindications.

Less frequently used antihistamines: Includes names, uses, doses, forms, interactions, and contraindications.

Herbal products: Features basic usage information on more than 47 common herbs and natural supplements.

Combination products: Provides details on the forms and uses of more than 800 combination products.

Look-alike/sound-alike drug names: Includes all current ISMP pairs of generic and trade drug names that are easily confused.

Medications that may be inappropriate for geriatric patients: Features a table of drugs that may increase the risk of drug interactions and adverse effects in older adults.

Drugs metabolized by known P450s: Convenient table provides a quick metabolization reference.

Safety in handling chemotherapeutic agents: Provides basic instruction on handling and preventing undue exposure to chemotherapeutic agents.

High-alert drugs: Lists the 107 drugs in *Mosby's Nursing Drug Reference* that are considered high-alert because of their potential to cause significant harm to patients.

Controlled substance chart: Covers the drug schedules for the United States, with examples.

Immunization schedules for children and adolescents: Convenient, up-to-date reference tables for children and adolescents in the United States.

High-alert Canadian medications: Lists the drugs that the Institute for Safe Medication Practices Canada considers high-alert because of their potential to cause significant harm to patients.

Canadian controlled substance chart: Covers the drug schedules for Canada, with examples.

Canadian recommended immunization schedules for infants and children: Convenient, up-to-date reference table for Canadian patients.

FDA pregnancy categories: Explains the five FDA pregnancy categories.

Weights and equivalents: Provides the conversion for weight and volume among the metric, apothecary, and avoirdupois systems.

Abbreviations: Lists abbreviations alphabetically with their meanings.

Bibliography: Lists key resources used in creating and updating *Mosby's 2008 Nursing Drug Reference*.

I am indebted to the nursing and pharmacology consultants who reviewed the manuscript and thank them for their criticism and encouragement. I would also like to thank Darlene Como, Tamara Myers, and Laura Selkirk, my editors, whose active encouragement and enthusiasm have made this book better than it might otherwise have been. I am likewise grateful to Joy Moore and Graphic World Inc., for the coordination of the production process and assistance with the development of the new edition.

Linda Skidmore-Roth

Contents

Drug categories, 1

Color Insert: Mechanisms and Sites of Action, 53

Individual drugs, 69

Bibliography, 1085

Appendixes, 1087

Index, 1211

ALPHA-ADRENERGIC BLOCKERS

Action: Acts by binding to α-adrenergic receptors, causing dilation of peripheral blood vessels. Lowers peripheral resistance, resulting in decreased blood pressure.

Uses: Used for pheochromocytoma, prevention of tissue necrosis and sloughing associated with extravasation of IV vasopressors.

Side effects: The most common side effects are hypotension, tachycardia, nasal stuffiness, nausea, vomiting, and diarrhea.

Contraindications: Hypersensitive reactions may occur, and allergies should be identified before these products are given. Patients with myocardial infarction, coronary insufficiency, angina, or other evidence of coronary artery disease should not use these products.

Pharmacokinetics: Onset, peak, and duration vary among products.

Interactions: Vasoconstrictive and hypertensive effects of epINEPHrine are antagonized by α-adrenergic blockers.

Possible nursing diagnoses:
• Tissue perfusion, ineffective *[uses]*
• Injury, risk for *[adverse reactions]*
• Sleep pattern, disturbed *[adverse reactions]*

Nursing Considerations

Assess:
• Electrolytes: K, Na, Cl, CO_2
• Weight daily, I&O
• B/P lying, standing before starting treatment, q4h thereafter
• Nausea, vomiting, diarrhea
• Skin turgor, dryness of mucous membranes for hydration status

Administer:
• Starting with low dose, gradually increasing to prevent side effects
• With food or milk for GI symptoms

Evaluate:
• Therapeutic response: decreased B/P, increased peripheral pulses

Teach patient/family:
• To avoid alcoholic beverages
• To report dizziness, palpitations, fainting
• To change position slowly or fainting may occur
• To take drug exactly as prescribed
• To avoid all OTC products (cough, cold, allergy) unless directed by prescriber

Selected Generic Names

phentolamine

ANESTHETICS—GENERAL/LOCAL

Action: Anesthetics (general) act on the CNS to produce tranquilization and sleep before invasive procedures. Anesthetics (local) inhibit conduction of nerve impulses from sensory nerves.

Uses: General anesthetics are used to premedicate for surgery, induction and maintenance in general anesthesia. For local anesthetics, refer to individual product listing for indications.

Side effects: The most common side effects are dystonia, akathisia, flexion of arms, fine tremors, drowsiness, restlessness, and hypotension. Also common are chills, respiratory depression, and laryngospasm.

Contraindications: Persons with CVA, increased intracranial pressure, severe hypertension, cardiac decompensation should not use these products, since severe adverse reactions can occur.

Precautions: Anesthetics (general) should be used with caution in the geriatric, cardiovascular disease (hypotension, bradydysrhythmias), renal disease, hepatic disease, Parkinson's disease, children <2 yr. The precaution for anesthetics (local) is pregnancy.

Pharmacokinetics: Onset, peak, and duration vary widely among products. Most products are metabolized in the liver and excreted in urine.

Interactions: MAOIs, tricyclics, phenothiazines may cause severe hypotension or hypertension when used with local anesthetics. CNS depressants will potentiate general and local anesthetics.

Possible nursing diagnoses:
General:
• Injury, risk for *[adverse reactions]*
• Knowledge, deficient *[teaching]*
Local:
• Acute pain *[uses]*
• Knowledge, deficient *[teaching]*

Nursing Considerations

Assess:
• VS q10min during IV administration, q30min after IM dose

Administer:
• Anticholinergic preoperatively to decrease secretions
• Only with crash cart, resuscitative equipment nearby

Perform/provide:
• Quiet environment for recovery to decrease psychotic symptoms

Evaluate:
• Therapeutic response: maintenance of anesthesia, decreased pain

Selected Generic Names (Injectables Only)

General anesthetics
droperidol
etomidate
fentanyl
fentanyl/droperidol
fentanyl transdermal
midazolam
propofol
thiopental
Local anesthetics
lidocaine
procaine
ropivacaine
tetracaine

ANTACIDS

Action: Antacids are basic compounds that neutralize gastric acidity and decrease the rate of gastric emptying. Products are divided into those containing aluminum, magnesium, calcium, or a combination of these.

Uses: Hyperacidity is decreased by antacids in conditions such as peptic ulcer disease, reflux esophagitis, gastritis, and hiatal hernia.

Side effects: The most common side effect caused by aluminum-containing antacids is constipation, which may lead to fecal impaction and bowel obstruction. Diarrhea occurs often when magnesium products are given. Alkalosis may occur when systemic products are used. Constipation occurs more frequently than laxation with calcium carbonate. The release of CO_2 from carbonate-containing antacids causes belching, abdominal distention, and flatulence. Sodium bicarbonate may act as a systemic antacid and produce systemic electrolyte disturbances and alkalosis. Calcium carbonate and sodium bicarbonate may cause rebound hyperacidity and milk-alkali syndrome. Alkaluria may occur when products are used on a long-term basis, particularly in persons with abnormal renal function.

Contraindications: Sensitivity to aluminum or magnesium products may cause hypersensitive reactions. Aluminum products should not be used by persons sensitive to aluminum; magnesium products should not be used by persons sensitive to magnesium. Check for sensitivity before administering.

Precautions: Magnesium products should be given cautiously to patients with renal insufficiency and during pregnancy and lactation. Sodium content of antacids may be significant; use with caution for patients with hypertension or CHF or those on a low-sodium diet.

Pharmacokinetics: Duration is 20-40 min. If ingested 1 hr after meals, acidity is reduced for at least 3 hr.

Interactions: Drugs whose effects may be increased by some antacids: quinidine, amphetamines, pseudoephedrine, levodopa, valproic acid, dicumarol. Drugs whose effects may be decreased by some antacids: cimetidine, corticosteroids, ranitidine, iron salts, phenothiazines, phenytoin, digoxin, tetracyclines, ketoconazole, salicylates, isoniazid.

Possible nursing diagnoses:
• Chronic pain *[uses]*
• Constipation *[adverse reactions]*
• Diarrhea *[adverse reactions]*

Nursing Considerations
Assess:
• Aggravating and alleviating factors of epigastric pain or hyperacidity; identify the location, duration, and characteristics of epigastric pain
• GI symptoms, including constipation, diarrhea, abdominal pain; if severe abdominal pain with fever occurs, these drugs should not be given
• Renal symptoms, including increasing urinary pH, electrolytes

Administer:
• All products with an 8-oz glass of water to ensure absorption in the stomach
• Another antacid if constipation occurs with aluminum products
• Not to take other drugs within 1-2 hr of antacid administration, since antacids may impair absorption of other drugs

Evaluate:
• The therapeutic effectiveness of the drug; absence of epigastric pain and decreased acidity should occur

Selected Generic Names
aluminum hydroxide
bismuth subsalicylate
calcium carbonate
magaldrate
magnesium oxide
sodium bicarbonate

ANTIANGINALS

Action: The antianginals are divided into the nitrates, calcium channel blockers, and β-adrenergic blockers. The nitrates dilate coronary arteries, causing decreased preload, and dilate systemic arteries, causing decreased afterload. Calcium channel blockers dilate coronary arteries, decrease SA/AV node conduction. β-Adrenergic blockers decrease heart rate so that myocardial O_2 use is decreased. Dipyridamole selectively dilates coronary arteries to increase coronary blood flow.

Uses: Antianginals are used in chronic stable angina pectoris, unstable angina, vasospastic angina. Some (i.e., calcium channel blockers and β-blockers) may be used for dysrhythmias and in hypertension.

Side effects: The most common side effects are postural hypotension, headache, flushing, dizziness, nausea, edema, and drowsiness. Also common are rash, dysrhythmias, and fatigue.

Contraindications: Persons with known hypersensitivity, increased intracranial pressure, or cerebral hemorrhage should not use some of these products.

Precautions: Antianginals should be used with caution in postural hypotension, pregnancy, lactation, children, renal disease, and hepatic injury.

Pharmacokinetics: Onset, peak, and duration vary widely among coronary products. Most products are metabolized in the liver and excreted in urine.

Interactions: Please check individual monographs since interactions vary widely among products.

Possible nursing diagnoses:
• Tissue perfusion, ineffective *[uses]*
• Acute pain *[uses]*
• Injury, risk for *[uses]*
• Knowledge, deficient *[teaching]*
• Cardiac output, decreased *[adverse reactions]*

Nursing Considerations

Assess:
• Orthostatic B/P, pulse

• Pain: duration, time started, activity being performed, character
• Tolerance if taken over long period
• Headache, light-headedness, decreased B/P; may indicate a need for decreased dosage

Perform/provide:
• Storage protected from light, moisture; place in cool environment

Evaluate:
• Therapeutic response: decrease, prevention of anginal pain

Teach patient/family:
• To keep tabs in original container
• Not to use OTC products unless directed by prescriber
• To report bradycardia, dizziness, confusion, depression, fever
• To take pulse at home, advise when to notify prescriber
• To avoid alcohol, smoking, sodium intake
• To comply with weight control, dietary adjustments, modified exercise program
• To carry emergency ID to identify drug that you are taking, allergies
• To make position changes slowly to prevent fainting

Selected Generic Names

Nitrates
amyl nitrite
isosorbide
nitroglycerin
β-Adrenergic blockers
atenolol
dipyridamole
metoprolol
nadolol
propranolol
Calcium channel blockers
amlodipine
bepridil
diltiazem

niCARdipine
NIFEdipine
verapamil
Miscellaneous
ranolazine

ANTICHOLINERGICS

Action: Anticholinergics inhibit the muscarinic actions of acetylcholine at receptor sites in the autonomic nervous system; anticholinergics are also known as antimuscarinic drugs.

Uses: Anticholinergics are used for a variety of conditions: gastrointestinal anticholinergics are used to decrease motility (smooth muscle tone) in the GI, biliary, and urinary tracts and for their ability to decrease gastric secretions (propantheline, glycopyrrolate); decreasing involuntary movements in parkinsonism (benztropine, trihexyphenidyl); bradydysrhythmias (atropine); nausea and vomiting (scopolamine); and as cycloplegic mydriatics (atropine, homatropine, scopolamine, cyclopentolate, tropicamide).

Side effects: The most common side effects are dry mouth, constipation, urinary retention, urinary hesitancy, headache, and dizziness. Also common is paralytic ileus.

Contraindications: Persons with narrow-angle glaucoma, myasthenia gravis, or GI/GU obstruction should not use some of these products.

Precautions: Anticholinergics should be used with caution in patients who are geriatric, pregnant, or lactating or in those with prostatic hypertrophy, CHF, or hypertension; use with caution in presence of high environmental temp.

Pharmacokinetics: Onset, peak, and duration vary widely among products. Most products are metabolized in the liver and excreted in urine.

Interactions: Increased anticholinergic effects may occur when used with MAOIs and tricyclic antidepressants and amantadine. Anticholinergics may cause a decreased effect of phenothiazines and levodopa.

Possible nursing diagnoses:
• Cardiac output, decreased *[uses]*
• Constipation *[adverse reactions]*
• Knowledge, deficient *[teaching]*

Nursing Considerations

Assess:
• I&O ratio; retention commonly causes decreased urinary output
• Urinary hesitancy, retention; palpate bladder if retention occurs
• Constipation; increase fluids, bulk, exercise if this occurs
• For tolerance over long-term therapy, dose may need to be increased or changed
• Mental status: affect, mood, CNS depression, worsening of mental symptoms during early therapy

Administer:
• Parenteral dose with patient recumbent to prevent postural hypotension
• With or after meals to prevent GI upset; may give with fluids other than water
• Parenteral dose slowly; keep in bed for at least 1 hr after dose; monitor vital signs
• After checking dose carefully; even slight overdose can lead to toxicity

Perform/provide:
• Storage at room temp
• Hard candy, frequent drinks, sugarless gum to relieve dry mouth

Evaluate:
• Therapeutic response: decreased secretions, absence of nausea and vomiting

Teach patient/family:
• To avoid driving or other hazardous activities; drowsiness may occur
• To avoid OTC medication: cough, cold preparations with alcohol, antihistamines unless directed by prescriber

Selected Generic Names

atropine
benztropine
biperiden
dicyclomine
glycopyrrolate
hyoscyamine
propantheline
scopolamine (transdermal)
solifenacin
trihexyphenidyl

ANTICOAGULANTS

Action: Anticoagulants interfere with blood clotting by preventing clot formation.

Uses: Anticoagulants are used for deep vein thrombosis, pulmonary emboli, myocardial infarction, open-heart surgery, disseminated intravascular clotting syndrome, atrial fibrillation with embolization, transfusion, and dialysis.

Side effects: The most serious adverse reactions are hemorrhage, agranulocytosis, leukopenia, eosinophilia, and thrombocytopenia, depending on the specific product. The most common side effects are diarrhea, rash, and fever.

Contraindications: Persons with hemophilia and related disorders, leukemia with bleeding, peptic ulcer disease, thrombocytopenic purpura, blood dyscrasias, acute nephritis, and subacute bacterial endocarditis should not use these products.

Precautions: Anticoagulants should be used with caution in alcoholism, geriatric, and pregnancy.

Pharmacokinetics: Onset, peak, and duration vary widely among products. Most products are metabolized in the liver and excreted in urine.

Interactions: Salicylates, steroids, and nonsteroidal antiinflammatories will potentiate the action of anticoagulants. Anticoagulants may cause serious effects; please check individual monographs.

Possible nursing diagnoses:
• Tissue perfusion, ineffective *[uses]*
• Injury, risk for *[side effects]*
• Knowledge, deficient *[teaching]*

Nursing Considerations

Assess:
• Blood studies (Hct, platelets, occult blood in stools) q3mo
• Partial prothrombin time, which should be 1½-2 × control PPT daily, also APTT, ACT
• B/P, watch for increasing signs of hypertension
• Bleeding gums, petechiae, ecchymosis; black, tarry stools; hematuria
• Fever, skin rash, urticaria
• Needed dosage change q1-2wk

Administer:
• At same time each day to maintain steady blood levels
• Do not massage area or aspirate when giving SUBCUT injection; give in abdomen between pelvic bone, rotate sites; do not pull back on plunger; leave in for 10 sec; apply gentle pressure for 1 min

- Without changing needles
- Avoiding all IM injections that may cause bleeding

Perform/provide:
- Storage in tight container

Evaluate:
- Therapeutic response: decrease of deep vein thrombosis

Teach patient/family:
- To avoid OTC preparations that may cause serious drug interactions unless directed by prescriber
- That drug may be held during active bleeding (menstruation), depending on condition
- To use soft-bristle toothbrush to avoid bleeding gums, avoid contact sports, use electric razor
- To carry emergency ID identifying drug taken
- To report any signs of bleeding: gums, under skin, urine, stools

Selected Generic Names

ardeparin
argatroban
dalteparin
danaparoid
desirudin
enoxaparin
fondaparinux
heparin
lepirudin
tinzaparin
warfarin

ANTICONVULSANTS

Action: Anticonvulsants are divided into the barbiturates (p. 28), benzodiazepines (p. 29), hydantoins, succinimides, and miscellaneous products. Barbiturates and benzodiazepines are discussed in separate sections. Hydantoins act by inhibiting the spread of seizure activity in the motor cortex. Succinimides act by inhibiting spike and wave formation; they also decrease amplitude, frequency, duration, and spread of discharge in seizures.

Uses: Hydantoins are used in generalized tonic-clonic seizures, status epilepticus, and psychomotor seizures. Succinimides are used for absence (petit mal) seizures. Barbiturates are used in generalized tonic-clonic and cortical focal seizures.

Side effects: Bone marrow depression is the most life-threatening adverse reaction associated with hydantoins or succinimides. The most common side effects are GI symptoms. Other common side effects for hydantoins are gingival hyperplasia and CNS effects such as nystagmus, ataxia, slurred speech, and mental confusion.

Contraindications: Hypersensitive reactions may occur, and allergies should be identified before these products are given.

Precautions: Persons with renal or hepatic disease should be watched closely.

Pharmacokinetics: Onset, peak, and duration vary widely among products. Most products are metabolized in the liver and excreted in urine, bile, and feces.

Interactions: Decreased effects of estrogens, oral contraceptives (hydantoins).

Possible nursing diagnoses:
- Injury, risk for *[uses]*
- Noncompliance *[teaching]*

• Sleep pattern, disturbed *[adverse reactions]*

Nursing Considerations

Assess:
• Renal studies, including BUN, creatinine, serum uric acid, urine creatinine clearance before and during therapy
• Blood studies: RBC, Hct, Hgb, reticulocyte counts qwk for 4 wk then qmo
• Hepatic studies: AST, ALT, bilirubin, creatinine
• Mental status, including mood, sensorium, affect, behavorial changes; if mental status changes, notify prescriber
• Eye problems, including need for ophthalmic exam before, during, and after treatment (slit lamp, funduscopy, tonometry)
• Allergic reactions, including red, raised rash; if this occurs, drug should be discontinued
• Blood dyscrasia, including fever, sore throat, bruising, rash, jaundice
• Toxicity, including bone marrow depression, nausea, vomiting, ataxia, diplopia, cardiovascular collapse, Stevens-Johnson syndrome

Administer:
• With food, milk to decrease GI symptoms

Perform/provide:
• Good oral hygiene is important for hydantoins

Evaluate:
• Therapeutic response, including decreased seizure activity; document on patient's chart

Teach patient/family:
• To carry emergency ID stating drugs taken, condition, prescriber's name, phone number
• To avoid driving, other activities that require alertness

Selected Generic Names

Hydantoins
fosphenytoin
phenytoin

Succinimides
ethosuximide

Miscellaneous
acetaZOLAMIDE
carbamazepine
clonazepam
diazepam
felbamate
gabapentin
lamotrigine
magnesium sulfate
paraldehyde
paramethadione
phenacemide
phenobarbital
primidone
tiagabine
topiramate
valproate/valproic acid, divalproex sodium
zonisamide

ANTIDEPRESSANTS

Action: Antidepressants are divided into the tricyclics, MAOIs, and miscellaneous antidepressants (SSRIs). The tricyclics work by blocking reuptake of norepinephrine and serotonin into nerve endings and increasing action of norepinephrine and serotonin in nerve cells. MAOIs act by increasing concentrations of endogenous epinephrine, norepinephrine, serotonin, dopamine in storage sites in CNS by inhibition of MAO; increased concentration reduces depression.

Uses: Antidepressants are used for depression and, in some cases, enuresis in children.

Side effects: The most serious adverse reactions are paralytic ileus, acute renal failure, hypertension, and hypertensive crisis, depending on the specific product. Common side effects are dizziness, drowsiness, diarrhea, dry mouth, urinary retention, and orthostatic hypotension.

Contraindications: The contraindications to antidepressants are convulsive disorders, prostatic hypertrophy and severe renal, hepatic, cardiac disease depending on the type of medication.

Precautions: Antidepressants should be used cautiously in suicidal patients, severe depression, schizophrenia, hyperactivity, diabetes mellitus, pregnancy, and the geriatric.

Pharmacokinetics: Onset, peak, and duration vary widely among products. Most products are metabolized in the liver and excreted in urine.

Interactions: Please check individual monographs since interactions vary widely among products.

Possible nursing diagnoses:
• Coping, ineffective *[uses]*
• Injury, risk for *[uses/adverse reactions]*
• Knowledge, deficient *[teaching]*

Nursing Considerations

Assess:
• B/P (lying, standing), pulse q4h; if systolic B/P drops 20 mm Hg, hold drug, notify prescriber; take vital signs q4h in patients with cardiovascular disease
• Blood studies: CBC, leukocytes, differential, cardiac enzymes if patient is receiving long-term therapy
• Hepatic studies: AST, ALT, bilirubin, creatinine

• Weight qwk; appetite may increase with drug
• EPS, primarily in geriatric: rigidity, dystonia, akathisia
• Mental status: mood, sensorium, affect, suicidal tendencies, increase in psychiatric symptoms: depression, panic
• Urinary retention, constipation; constipation is more likely to occur in children, geriatric
• Withdrawal symptoms: headache, nausea, vomiting, muscle pain, weakness; do not usually occur unless drug was discontinued abruptly
• Alcohol consumption; if alcohol is consumed, hold dose until morning

Administer:
• Increased fluids if urinary retention occurs, bulk in diet, if constipation occurs
• With food or milk for GI symptoms

Perform/provide:
• Storage in tight container at room temp; do not freeze
• Assistance with ambulation during beginning therapy, since drowsiness, dizziness occur
• Safety measures including side rails primarily in geriatric
• Checking to see PO medication swallowed
• Gum, hard candy, or frequent sips of water for dry mouth

Evaluate:
• Therapeutic response: decreased depression

Teach patient/family:
• That therapeutic effects may take 2-3 wk
• To use caution in driving, other activities requiring alertness because of drowsiness, dizziness, blurred vision
• To avoid alcohol ingestion, other CNS depressants

• Not to discontinue medication quickly after long-term use; may cause nausea, headache, malaise

• To wear sunscreen or wide-brimmed hat, since photosensitivity may occur

Selected Generic Names

Tetracyclics
mirtazapine
Tricyclics
amitriptyline
amoxapine
clomiPRAMINE
desipramine
doxepin
imipramine
nortriptyline
trimipramine
Miscellaneous
buPROPion
duloxetine
trazodone
venlafaxine
MAOIs
phenelzine
tranylcypromine
SSRIs
citalopram
escitalopram
fluoxetine
fluvoxamine
paroxetine
sertraline

ANTIDIABETICS

Action: Antidiabetics are divided into the insulins that decrease blood glucose, phosphate, and potassium and increase blood pyruvate and lactate; and oral antidiabetics that cause functioning β-cells in the pancreas to release insulin, improve the effect of endogenous and exogenous insulin.

Uses: Insulins are used for ketoacidosis and diabetes mellitus types 1 and 2; oral antidiabetics are used for stable adult-onset diabetes mellitus type 2.

Side effects: The most common side effect of insulin and oral antidiabetics is hypoglycemia. Other adverse reactions to oral antidiabetics include blood dyscrasias, hepatotoxicity, and rarely, cholestatic jaundice. Adverse reactions to insulin products include allergic responses and, more rarely, anaphylaxis.

Contraindications: Hypersensitive reactions may occur, and allergies should be identified before these products are given. Oral antidiabetics should not be used in juvenile or brittle diabetes, diabetic ketoacidosis, severe renal disease, or severe hepatic disease.

Precautions: Oral antidiabetics should be used with caution in the geriatric, in cardiac disease, pregnancy, lactation, and in the presence of alcohol.

Pharmacokinetics: Onset, peak, and duration vary widely among products. Oral antidiabetics are metabolized in the liver, with metabolites excreted in urine, bile, and feces.

Interactions: Interactions vary widely among products. Check individual monographs for specific information.

Possible nursing diagnoses:
• Imbalanced nutrition: more than body requirements *[uses]*

Nursing Considerations

Assess:
• Blood, urine glucose levels during

treatment to determine diabetes control (oral products)
• Fasting blood glucose, 2 hr PP (60-100 mg/dl normal fasting level) (70-130 mg/dl normal 2-hr level)
• Hypoglycemic reaction that can occur during peak time

Administer:
• Insulin after warming to room temp by rotating in palms to prevent lipodystrophy from injecting cold insulin
• Human insulin to those allergic to beef or pork
• Oral antidiabetic 30 min before meals

Perform/provide:
• Rotation of injection sites when giving insulin; use abdomen, upper back, thighs, upper arm, buttocks; rotate sites within one of these regions; keep a record of sites

Evaluate:
• Therapeutic response, including decrease in polyuria, polydipsia, polyphagia, clear sensorium, absence of dizziness, stable gait

Teach patient/family:
• To avoid alcohol and salicylates except on advice of prescriber
• Symptoms of ketoacidosis: nausea, thirst, polyuria, dry mouth, decreased B/P; dry, flushed skin; acetone breath, drowsiness, Kussmaul respiration
• Symptoms of hypoglycemia: headache, tremors, fatigue, weakness; and that candy or sugar should be carried to treat hypoglycemia
• To test urine for glucose/ketones tid if this drug is replacing insulin
• To continue weight control, dietary restrictions, exercise, hygiene
• Obtain yearly eye exams

Selected Generic Names

chlorproPAMIDE
glipiZIDE
glyBURIDE
insulin aspart
insulin detemir
insulin glargine
insulin glulisine
insulin, inhaled
insulin lispro
insulin, regular
insulin, regular concentrated
insulin, zinc suspension (Lente)
insulin, zinc suspension extended (Ultralente)
metformin
miglitol
pioglitazone
repaglinide
rosiglitazone
sitagliptin

ANTIDIARRHEALS

Action: Antidiarrheals work by various actions, including direct action on intestinal muscles to decrease GI peristalsis; by inhibiting prostaglandin synthesis responsible for GI hypermotility; by acting on mucosal receptors responsible for peristalsis; or by decreasing water content of stools.

Uses: Antidiarrheals are used for diarrhea of undetermined causes.

Side effects: The most serious adverse reactions of some products are paralytic ileus, toxic megacolon, and angioneurotic edema. The most common side effects are constipation, nausea, dry mouth, and abdominal pain.

Contraindications: Persons with severe ulcerative colitis, pseudomembranous colitis with some products.

Precautions: Antidiarrheals should be used with caution in the geriatric, pregnancy, lactation, children, dehydration.

Pharmacokinetics: Onset, peak, and duration vary widely among products. Most products are metabolized in the liver and excreted in urine.

Interactions: Please check individual monographs since interactions vary widely among products.

Possible nursing diagnoses:
- Diarrhea *[uses]*
- Constipation *[adverse reactions]*
- Fluid volume, deficient *[adverse reactions]*
- Knowledge, deficient *[teaching]*

Nursing Considerations

Assess:
- Electrolytes (K, Na, Cl) if on long-term therapy
- Bowel pattern before; for rebound constipation after termination of medication
- Response after 48 hr; if no response, drug should be discontinued
- Dehydration in children

Administer:
- For 48 hr only

Evaluate:
- Therapeutic response: decreased diarrhea

Teach patient/family:
- To avoid OTC products
- Not to exceed recommended dose

Selected Generic Names

bismuth subsalicylate
kaolin/pectin
loperamide

ANTIDYSRHYTHMICS

Action: Antidysrhythmics are divided into four classes and miscellaneous antidysrhythmics:
- Class I increases the duration of action potential and effective refractory period and reduces disparity in the refractory period between a normal and infarcted myocardium; further subclasses include Ia, Ib, Ic
- Class II decreases the rate of SA node discharge, increases recovery time, slows conduction through the AV node, and decreases heart rate, which decreases O_2 consumption in the myocardium
- Class III increases the duration of action potential and the effective refractory period
- Class IV inhibits calcium ion influx across the cell membrane during cardiac depolarization; decreases SA node discharge, decreases conduction velocity through the AV node
- Miscellaneous antidysrhythmics include those such as adenosine, which slows conduction through the AV node, and digoxin, which decreases conduction velocity and prolongs the effective refractory period in the AV node

Uses: These products are used for PVCs, tachycardia, hypertension, atrial fibrillation, angina pectoris.

Side effects: Side effects and adverse reactions vary widely among products.

Contraindications: Contraindications vary widely among products.

Precautions: Precautions vary widely among products.

Pharmacokinetics: Onset, peak, and duration vary widely among products.

Interactions: Interactions vary

widely among products; check individual monographs for specific information.

Possible nursing diagnoses:
- Cardiac output, decreased *[uses]*
- Tissue perfusion, ineffective *[uses]*
- Diarrhea *[adverse reactions]*
- Gas exchange, impaired *[adverse reactions]*

Nursing Considerations

Assess:
- ECG continuously to determine drug effectiveness, PVCs, or other dysrhythmias
- IV infusion rate to avoid causing nausea, vomiting
- For dehydration or hypovolemia
- B/P continuously for hypotension, hypertension
- I&O ratio
- Serum potassium
- Edema in feet and legs daily

Evaluate:
- Therapeutic response, including decrease in B/P in hypertension; decreased B/P, edema, moist crackles in CHF

Teach patient/family:
- To comply with dosage schedule, even if patient is feeling better
- To report bradycardia, dizziness, confusion, depression, fever

Selected Generic Names

Class I
moricizine
Class Ia
disopyramide
procainamide
quinidine
Class Ib
lidocaine
mexiletine
phenytoin
tocainide
Class Ic
flecainide
propafenone
Class II
acebutolol
esmolol
propranolol
sotalol
Class III
amiodarone
ibutilide
Class IV
verapamil
Miscellaneous
adenosine
atropine
digoxin

ANTIFUNGALS (SYSTEMIC)

Action: Antifungals act by increasing cell membrane permeability in susceptible organisms by binding sterols and decreasing potassium, sodium, and nutrients in the cell.

Uses: Antifungals are used for infections of histoplasmosis, blastomycosis, coccidioidomycosis, cryptococcosis, aspergillosis, phycomycosis, candidiasis, sporotrichosis causing severe meningitis, septicemia, and skin infections.

Side effects: The most serious adverse reactions include renal tubular acidosis, permanent renal impairment, anuria, oliguria, hemorrhagic gastroenteritis, acute hepatic failure, and blood dyscrasias. Some common side effects include hypokalemia, nausea, vomiting, anorexia, headache, fever, and chills.

Contraindications: Persons with severe bone depression or hypersensitivity should not use these products.

Precautions: Antifungals should be used with caution in renal disease, pregnancy, and hepatic disease.

Pharmacokinetics: Onset, peak, and duration vary widely among products. Most products are metabolized in the liver and excreted in urine.

Interactions: Please check individual monographs since interactions vary widely among products.

Possible nursing diagnoses:
• Infection, risk for *[uses]*
• Injury, risk for *[adverse reactions]*
• Knowledge, deficient *[teaching]*

Nursing Considerations

Assess:
• VS q15-30min during first infusion; note changes in pulse, B/P
• I&O ratio; watch for decreasing urinary output, change in specific gravity; discontinue drug to prevent permanent damage to renal tubules
• Blood studies: CBC, K, Na, Ca, Mg q2wk
• Weight weekly; if weight increases over 2 lb/wk, edema is present; renal damage should be considered
• For renal toxicity: increasing BUN, if >40 mg/dl or if serum creatinine >3 mg/dl; drug may be discontinued or dosage reduced
• For hepatotoxicity: increasing AST, ALT, alk phos, bilirubin
• For allergic reaction: dermatitis, rash; drug should be discontinued, antihistamines (mild reaction) or epINEPHrine (severe reaction) administered
• For hypokalemia: anorexia, drowsiness, weakness, decreased reflexes, dizziness, increased urinary output, increased thirst, paresthesias
• For ototoxicity: tinnitus (ringing, roaring in ears), vertigo, loss of hearing (rare)

Administer:
• IV using in-line filter (mean pore diameter >1 µm) using distal veins; check for extravasation, necrosis q8h
• Drug only after C&S confirms organism, drug needed to treat condition; make sure drug is used in life-threatening infections

Perform/provide:
• Protection from light during infusion, cover with foil
• Symptomatic treatment as ordered for adverse reactions: aspirin, antihistamines, antiemetics, antispasmodics
• Storage protected from moisture and light; diluted sol is stable for 24 hr

Evaluate:
• Therapeutic response: decreased fever, malaise, rash, negative C&S for infecting organism

Teach patient/family:
• That long-term therapy may be needed to clear infection (2 wk-3 mo depending on type of infection)

Selected Generic Names

amphotericin B
anidulafungin
caspofungin
fluconazole
griseofulvin
itraconazole
ketoconazole
micafungin
nystatin
posaconazole
voriconazole

ANTIHISTAMINES

Action: Antihistamines compete with histamines for H_1-receptor sites. They antagonize in varying degrees most of the pharmacologic effects of histamines.

Uses: Products are used to control the symptoms of allergies, rhinitis, and pruritus.

Side effects: Most products cause drowsiness; however, fexofenadine and loratadine produce little, if any, drowsiness. Other common side effects are headache and thickening of bronchial secretions. Serious blood dyscrasias may occur, but are rare. Urinary retention, GI effects occur with many of these products.

Contraindications: Hypersensitivity to H_1-receptor antagonists occurs rarely. Patients with acute asthma and lower respiratory tract disease should not use these products since thick secretions may result. Other contraindications include narrow-angle glaucoma, bladder neck obstruction, stenosing peptic ulcer, symptomatic prostatic hypertrophy, newborn, lactation.

Precautions: These products must be used cautiously in conjunction with intraocular pressure since they increase intraocular pressure. Caution should also be used in patients with renal and cardiac disease, hypertension, seizure disorders, pregnancy, lactation, and in the geriatric.

Pharmacokinetics: Onset varies from 20-60 min, with duration lasting 4-24 hr. In general, pharmacokinetics vary widely among products.

Interactions: Barbiturates, opioids, hypnotics, tricyclic antidepressants, or alcohol can increase CNS depression when taken with antihistamines.

Possible nursing diagnoses:
• Airway clearance, ineffective *[uses]*

Nursing Considerations

Assess:
• I&O ratio; be alert for urinary retention, frequency, dysuria; drug should be discontinued if these occur
• CBC during long-term therapy, since hemolytic anemia, although rare, may occur
• Blood dyscrasias: thrombocytopenia, agranulocytosis (rare)
• Respiratory status, including rate, rhythm, increase in bronchial secretions, wheezing, chest tightness
• Cardiac status, including palpitations, increased pulse, hypotension

Administer:
• With food or milk to decrease GI symptoms; absorption may be decreased slightly
• Whole (sustained-release tabs)

Perform/provide:
• Hard candy, gum, frequent rinsing of mouth for dryness

Evaluate:
• Therapeutic response, including absence of allergy symptoms, itching

Teach patient/family:
• To notify prescriber if confusion, sedation, hypotension occur
• To avoid driving, other hazardous activity if drowsiness occurs
• To avoid concurrent use of alcohol, other CNS depressants
• To discontinue a few days before skin testing

Selected Generic Names

brompheniramine
budesonide

cetirizine
chlorpheniramine
cyproheptadine
desloratadine
diphenhydrAMINE
fexofenadine
loratadine
promethazine

ANTIHYPERTENSIVES

Action: Antihypertensives are divided into angiotensin-converting enzyme (ACE) inhibitors, β-adrenergic blockers, calcium channel blockers, centrally acting adrenergics, diuretics, peripherally acting antiadrenergics, and vasodilators. β-Blockers, calcium channel blockers, and diuretics are discussed in separate sections. Angiotensin-converting enzyme inhibitors act by selectively suppressing renin-angiotensin I to angiotensin II; dilation of arterial and venous vessels occurs. Centrally acting adrenergics act by inhibiting the sympathetic vasomotor center in the CNS that reduces impulses in the sympathetic nervous system; blood pressure, pulse rate, and cardiac output decrease. Peripherally acting antiadrenergics inhibit sympathetic vasoconstriction by inhibiting release of norepinephrine and/or depleting norepinephrine stores in adrenergic nerve endings. Vasodilators act on arteriolar smooth muscle by producing direct relaxation or vasodilation; a reduction in blood pressure, with concomitant increases in heart rate and cardiac output, occurs.

Uses: Used for hypertension, and some products are used for heart failure not responsive to conventional therapy. Some products are used in hypertensive crisis, angina, and for some cardiac dysrhythmias.

Side effects: The most common side effects are hypotension, bradycardia, tachycardia, headache, nausea, and vomiting. Side effects and adverse reactions may vary widely between classes and specific products.

Contraindications: Hypersensitive reactions may occur, and allergies should be identified before these products are given. Antihypertensives should not be used in patients with heart block or in children.

Precautions: Antihypertensives should be used with caution in the geriatric, in dialysis patients, and in the presence of hypovolemia, leukemia, and electrolyte imbalances.

Pharmacokinetics: Onset, peak, and duration vary widely among products. Most products are metabolized in the liver, with metabolites excreted in urine, bile, and feces.

Interactions: Interactions vary widely among products; check individual monographs for specific information.

Possible nursing diagnoses:
• Tissue perfusion, ineffective *[uses]*
• Cardiac output, decreased *[uses]*
• Diarrhea *[adverse reactions]*
• Gas exchange, impaired *[adverse reactions]*

Nursing Considerations

Assess:
• Blood studies: neutrophil; decreased platelets occur with many of the products
• Renal studies: protein, BUN, creatinine; watch for increased levels that may indicate nephrotic syndrome; obtain baselines in renal and hepatic

function studies before beginning treatment
- Edema in feet and legs daily
- Allergic reaction, including rash, fever, pruritus, urticaria: drug should be discontinued if antihistamines fail to help
- Symptoms of CHF: edema, dyspnea, wet crackles, B/P
- Renal symptoms: polyuria, oliguria, frequency

Perform/provide:
- Supine or Trendelenburg position for severe hypotension

Evaluate:
- Therapeutic response, including decrease in B/P in hypotension; decreased B/P, edema, moist crackles in CHF

Teach patient/family:
- To comply with dosage schedule, even if feeling better
- To rise slowly to sitting or standing position to minimize orthostatic hypotension

Selected Generic Names

Aldosterone receptor antagonist
eplerenone

Angiotensin-converting enzyme inhibitors
benazepril
enalapril
fosinopril
lisinipril
quinapril
ramipril
trandolapril

Angiotensin II receptor blockers
candesartan
eprosartan
irbesartan
losartan
olmesartan
telmisartan
valsartan

Centrally acting adrenergics
clonidine
guanfacine
methyldopa

Peripherally acting antiadrenergics
doxazosin
prazosin
reserpine
terazosin

Vasodilators
diazoxide
fenoldopam
hydrALAZINE
minoxidil
nitroprusside

Antiadrenergic combined α-/β-blocker
labetalol

ANTIINFECTIVES

Action: Antiinfectives are divided into several groups, which include but are not limited to penicillins, cephalosporins, aminoglycosides, sulfonamides, tetracyclines, monobactam, erythromycins, and quinolones. These drugs act by inhibiting the growth and replication of susceptible bacterial organisms.

Uses: Used for infections of susceptible organisms. These products are effective against bacterial, rickettsial, and spirochetal infections.

Side effects: The most common side effects are nausea, vomiting, and diarrhea. Adverse reactions include bone marrow depression and anaphylaxis.

Contraindications: Hypersensitivity reactions may occur, and allergies should be identified before these products are given. Cross-sensitivity can occur between products of different classes (penicillins and cephalosporins). Many persons allergic to penicillins are also allergic to cephalosporins.

Precautions: Antiinfectives should be used with caution in persons with renal and hepatic disease.

Pharmacokinetics: Onset, peak, and duration vary widely among products. Most products are metabolized in the liver, and metabolites are excreted in urine, bile, and feces.

Interactions: Interactions vary widely among products; check individual monographs for specific information.

Possible nursing diagnoses:
• Infection, risk for *[uses]*
• Diarrhea *[adverse reactions]*

Nursing Considerations

Assess:
• Nephrotoxicity, including increased BUN, creatinine
• Blood studies: AST, ALT, CBC, Hct, bilirubin; test monthly if patient is on long-term therapy
• Bowel pattern daily; if severe diarrhea occurs, drug should be discontinued
• Urine output; if decreasing, notify prescriber; may indicate nephrotoxicity
• Allergic reaction, including rash, fever, pruritus, urticaria; drug should be discontinued
• Bleeding: ecchymosis, bleeding gums, hematuria, stool guaiac daily
• Overgrowth of infection: perineal itching, fever, malaise, redness, pain, swelling, drainage, rash, diarrhea, change in cough, sputum

Administer:
• For 10-14 days to ensure organism death, prevention of superinfection
• Drug after C&S completed; drug may be taken as soon as C&S is drawn

Evaluate:
• Therapeutic response, including absence of fever, fatigue, malaise, draining wounds

Teach patient/family:
• To comply with dosage schedule, even if feeling better
• To report sore throat, bruising, bleeding, joint pain; may indicate blood dyscrasias (rare)

Selected Generic Names

Aminoglycosides
amikacin
azithromycin
clarithromycin
gentamicin
kanamycin
neomycin
streptomycin
tobramycin

Cephalosporins
cefaclor
cefadroxil
cefazolin
cefdinir
cefditoren
cefepime
cefixime
cefonicid
cefoperazone
cefotaxime
cefprozil
ceftibuten
cefuroxime
cephalexin

cephapirin
cephradine
Fluoroquinolones
alatrofloxacin/trovafloxacin
ciprofloxacin
enoxacin
gemifloxacin
levofloxacin
lomefloxacin
norfloxacin
ofloxacin
sparfloxacin
Ketolides
telithromycin
Miscellaneous
adefovir dipivoxil
daptomycin
ertapenem
meropenem
peginterferon alfa-2a
Penicillins
amoxicillin/clavulanate
ampicillin/sulbactam
cloxacillin
dicloxacillin
imipenem/cilastatin
mezlocillin
nafcillin
oxacillin
penicillin G benzathine
penicillin G
penicillin G procaine
penicillin V
piperacillin
ticarcillin
ticarcillin/clavulanate
Sulfonamides
sulfasalazine
sulfiSOXAZOLE
Tetracyclines
demeclocycline
doxycycline
minocycline
tetracycline

ANTILIPIDEMICS

Action: Antilipidemics are divided into three categories or subclassifications; HMG-CoA reductase inhibitors (statins), bile acid sequestrants, and miscellaneous products. The HMG-CoA reductase inhibitors work by reduction of an enzyme that is responsible for the beginning step in cholesterol production, and bile acid sequestrants work by binding cholesterol in the GI system. The miscellaneous products work by various actions.

Uses: Primary hypercholesterolemia in individuals as an adjunct with other lifestyle changes.

Side effects: The most common side effects are headache, dizziness, fatigue, insomnia, peripheral edema, dysrhythmias, sinusitis, pharyngitis, abdominal pain, diarrhea, constipation, flatulence, and back pain.

Contraindications: Persons with hypersensitivity to any product or severe hepatic disease, or those breastfeeding (some products), should not take these products. Antilipidemics are identified as pregnancy category X on some products.

Precautions: Some products are identified as pregnancy category C.

Pharmacokinetics: All pharmacokinetics and pharmacodynamics vary with each product.

Interactions: Check individual monographs because drug interactions vary widely with each product.

Possible nursing diagnoses:
Constipation *[adverse reactions]*
Diarrhea *[adverse reactions]*
Knowledge, deficit *[teaching]*
Noncompliance *[teaching]*

Nursing Considerations

Assess:
• Obtain a diet and lifestyle history, including exercise, smoking, alcohol, and stress-related activities

Administer:
• As directed by health care provider; times will vary with medication used

Perform/provide:
• Protection from sunlight and heat

Evaluate:
• Therapeutic outcome: decrease in triglycerides and LDL cholesterol levels

Teach patient/family:
• Of all aspects of medication use
• To combine medication with lifestyle changes, including low-cholesterol diet, decreasing LDL in diet; avoid smoking, alcohol, and sedentary daily routine

Selected Generic Names

HMG-CoA reductase inhibitors
atorvastatin
fluvastatin
lovastatin
pravastatin
rosovastatin
simvastatin
Bile acid sequestrants
cholestyramine
colesevelam
colestipol
Miscellaneous
ezetimibe
fenofibrate
gemfibrozil
niacin
niacinamide

ANTINEOPLASTICS

Action: Antineoplastics are divided into alkylating agents, antimetabolites, antibiotic agents, hormonal agents, and miscellaneous agents. Alkylating agents act by cross-linking strands of DNA. Antimetabolites act by inhibiting DNA synthesis. Antibiotic agents act by inhibiting RNA synthesis and by delaying or inhibiting mitosis. Hormones alter the effects of androgens, luteinizing hormone, follicle-stimulating hormone, and estrogen by changing the hormonal environment.

Uses: Uses vary widely among products and classes of drugs. They are used to treat leukemia, Hodgkin's disease, lymphomas, and other tumors throughout the body.

Side effects: Most products cause thrombocytopenia, leukopenia, and anemia, and if these reactions occur, the drug may have to be stopped until the problem is corrected. Other side effects include nausea, vomiting, glossitis, and hair loss. Some products also cause hepatotoxicity, nephrotoxicity, and cardiotoxicity.

Contraindications: Hypersensitive reactions may occur, and allergies should be identified before these products are given. Also, persons with severe hepatic and renal disease should not use these products unless the benefits outweigh the risks.

Precautions: Persons with bleeding, severe bone marrow depression, or renal or hepatic disease should be watched closely.

Pharmacokinetics: Onset, peak, and duration vary widely among products. Most products cross the placenta and are excreted in breast milk and in urine.

Interactions: Toxicity may occur when used with other antineoplastics or radiation.

Possible nursing diagnoses:
• Infection, risk for *[adverse reactions]*
• Nutrition: less than body requirements, imbalanced *[adverse reactions]*
• Oral mucous membrane, impaired *[adverse reactions]*

Nursing Considerations

Assess:
• CBC, differential, platelet count weekly; withhold drug if WBC is <4000/mm³ or platelet count is <75,000/mm³; notify prescriber of results
• Renal function studies, including BUN, creatinine, serum uric acid, and urine CCr before and during therapy
• I&O ratio; report fall in urine output of 30 ml/hr
• Monitor temp q4h (may indicate beginning infection)
• Liver function tests before and during therapy (bilirubin, AST, ALT, LDH) as needed or monthly
• Bleeding, including hematuria, guaiac, bruising or petechiae, mucosa, or orifices q8h; obtain prescription for viscous Xylocaine (lidocaine)
• Yellowing of skin, sclera, dark urine, clay-colored stools, itchy skin, abdominal pain, fever, diarrhea
• Edema in feet, joint pain, stomach pain, shaking
• Inflammation of mucosa, breaks in skin

Administer:
• Checking IV site for irritation; phlebitis
• EpINEPHrine for hypersensitivity reaction
• Antibiotics for prophylaxis of infection

Perform/provide:
• Strict asepsis, protective isolation if WBC levels are low
• Comprehensive oral hygiene, using careful technique and soft-bristle brush

Evaluate:
• Therapeutic response, including decreased tumor size

Teach patient/family:
• To report signs of infection, including increased temp, sore throat, malaise
• To report signs of anemia, including fatigue, headache, faintness, shortness of breath, irritability
• To report bleeding and avoid use of razors or commercial mouthwash

Selected Generic Names

Alkylating agents
busulfan
carboplatin
carmustine
chlorambucil
cisplatin
cyclophosphamide
dacarbazine
lomustine
mechlorethamine
melphalan
oxaliplatin
thiotepa

Antimetabolites
capecitabine
cytarabine
decitabine
etoposide
fludarabine
fluorouracil
mercaptopurine
pemetrexed
thioguanine (6-TG)

Antibiotic agents
bleomycin
dactinomycin

DAUNOrubicin
DOXOrubicin
epirubicin
methotrexate
mitomycin
mitoxantrone
plicamycin
Hormonal agents
aminoglutethimide
estramustine
flutamide
fulvestrant
goserelin
irinotecan
leuprolide
megestrol
mitotane
nilutamide
tamoxifen
testolactone
topotecan
Miscellaneous
alemtuzumab
altretamine
anastrozole
arsenic trioxide
asparaginase
azacitidine
bortezomib
cetuximab
cladribine
dasatinib
erlotinib
gefitinib
gemcitabine
ibritumomab
imatinib
interferon alfa-2a
interferon alfa-2b
irinotecan
panitumumab
pentostatin
porfimer
procarbazine
ranibizumab
rituximab

sunitinib
vinBLAStine
vinCRIStine
vinorelbine

ANTIPARKINSON AGENTS

Action: Antiparkinson agents are divided into cholinergics and dopamine agonists. Cholinergics work by blocking or competing at central acetylcholine receptors; dopamine agonists work by decarboxylation to dopamine or by activation of dopamine receptors; monoamine oxidase type B inhibitors work by increasing dopamine activity by inhibiting MAO type B activity.

Uses: Antiparkinson agents are used alone or in combination for patients with Parkinson's disease.

Side effects: Side effects and adverse reactions vary widely among products. The most common side effects include involuntary movements, headache, numbness, insomnia, nightmares, nausea, vomiting, dry mouth, and orthostatic hypotension.

Contraindications: Persons with hypersensitivity, narrow-angle glaucoma, and undiagnosed skin lesions should not use these products.

Precautions: Antiparkinson agents should be used with caution in pregnancy, lactation, children, renal, cardiac, and hepatic disease, and affective disorder.

Pharmacokinetics: Onset, peak, and duration vary widely among products. Most products are metabolized in the liver and excreted in urine.

Interactions: Please check individual monographs since interactions vary widely among products.

Possible nursing diagnoses:
- Injury, risk for *[uses]*
- Mobility, physical, impaired *[uses]*
- Knowledge, deficient *[teaching]*

Nursing Considerations

Assess:
- B/P, respiration
- Mental status: affect, mood, behavioral changes, depression, complete suicide assessment

Administer:
- Drug up until NPO before surgery
- Adjust dosage depending on patient response
- With meals; limit protein taken with drug
- Only after MAOIs have been discontinued for 2 wk

Perform/provide:
- Assistance with ambulation, during beginning therapy
- Testing for diabetes mellitus, acromegaly if on long-term therapy

Evaluate:
- Therapeutic response: decrease in akathisia, increased mood

Teach patient/family:
- To change positions slowly to prevent orthostatic hypotension
- To report side effects: twitching, eye spasm; indicate overdose
- To use drug exactly as prescribed; if drug is discontinued abruptly, parkinsonian crisis may occur

Selected Generic Names

amantadine
apomorphine
benztropine
biperiden
bromocriptine
cabergoline
carbidopa-levodopa
levodopa
pramipexole
rasagiline
selegiline
tolcapone
trihexyphenidyl

ANTIPSYCHOTICS

Action: Antipsychotics/neuroleptics are divided into several subgroups: phenothiazines, thioxanthenes, butyrophenones, dibenzoxazepines, dibenzodiazepines, and indolones and other heterocyclic compounds. Although chemically different, these subgroups share many pharmacologic and clinical properties. All antipsychotics work to block postsynaptic dopamine receptors in the brain that are responsible for psychotic behavior, including hallucinations, delusions, and paranoia.

Uses: Antipsychotic behavior is decreased in conditions such as schizophrenia, paranoia, and mania. These agents are also effective for severe anxiety, intractable hiccups, nausea, vomiting, behavioral problems in children, and for relaxation before surgery.

Side effects: The most common side effects include EPS such as pseudoparkinsonism, akathisia, dystonia, and tardive dyskinesia, which may be controlled by use of antiparkinson agents. Serious adverse reactions such as hypotension, agranulocytosis, cardiac arrest, and laryngospasm have occurred. Other common side effects include dry mouth and photosensitivity.

Contraindications: Persons with hepatic damage, severe hypertension or coronary disease, cerebral arteriosclerosis, blood dyscrasias, bone marrow depression, parkinsonism, severe depression, narrow-angle glaucoma, children <12 yr, or persons withdrawing from alcohol or barbiturates should not use antipsychotics until these conditions are corrected.

Precautions: Caution must be used when antipsychotics are given to the geriatric since metabolism is slowed and adverse reactions can occur rapidly. Hepatic and renal disease may cause poor metabolism and excretion of the drug. Seizure threshold is decreased with these products; increases in the dose of anticonvulsants may be required. Persons with diabetes mellitus, prostatic hypertrophy, chronic respiratory disease, and peptic ulcer disease should be monitored closely.

Pharmacokinetics: Onset, peak, and duration vary widely with different products and routes. Products are metabolized by the liver, are excreted in urine as metabolites, are highly bound to plasma proteins, cross the placenta, and enter breast milk. Half-life can be extended over 3 days.

Interactions: Because other CNS depressants can cause oversedation, these combinations should be used carefully. Anticholinergics may decrease the therapeutic actions of phenothiazines and also cause increased anticholinergic effects.

Possible nursing diagnoses:
• Thought processes, disturbed [uses]
• Sensory perception, disturbed [uses]

Nursing Considerations

Assess:
• Bilirubin, CBC, hepatic studies qmo, since these drugs are metabolized in the liver and excreted in urine
• I&O ratio: palpate bladder if low urinary output occurs, since urinary retention occurs with many of these products
• Affect, orientation, LOC, reflexes, gait, coordination, sleep pattern disturbances
• Dizziness, faintness, palpitations, tachycardia on rising
• B/P lying and standing; wide fluctuations between lying and standing B/P may require dosage or product change, since orthostatic hypotension is occurring
• EPS, including akathisia, tardive dyskinesia, pseudoparkinsonism

Administer:
• Antiparkinson agent if EPS occur
• Liquid concentrates mixed in glass of juice or cola, since taste is unpleasant; avoid contact with skin when preparing liquid concentrate or parenteral medications
• Patient should remain lying down for at least 30 min after IM injections

Perform/provide:
• Supervised ambulation until stabilized on medication; do not involve in strenuous exercise program because fainting is possible; patient should not stand still for long periods
• Increased fluids to prevent constipation
• Sips of water, candy, gum for dry mouth

Evaluate:
• Therapeutic response: decrease in excitement, hallucinations, delusions, paranoia, reorganization of thought patterns, speech

Teach patient/family:
• To rise from sitting or lying position gradually, since fainting may occur
• To avoid hot tubs, hot showers, or tub baths, since hypotension may occur
• To wear a sunscreen or protective clothing to prevent burns
• To take extra precautions during hot weather to stay cool; heat stroke can occur
• To avoid driving, other activities requiring alertness until response to medication is known
• That drowsiness or impaired mental/motor activity is evident the first 2 wk, but tends to decrease over time

Selected Generic Names

Phenothiazines
chlorproMAZINE
fluphenazine
perphenazine
prochlorperazine
thioridazine
thiothixene
trifluoperazine
Butyrophenone
haloperidol
Miscellaneous
aripiprazole
loxapine
olanzapine
quetiapine
risperidone
ziprasidone

ANTITUBERCULARS

Action: Antituberculars act by inhibiting RNA or DNA, or interfering with lipid and protein synthesis, thereby decreasing tubercle bacilli replication.

Uses: Antituberculars are used for pulmonary tuberculosis.

Side effects: They vary widely among products. Most products can cause nausea, vomiting, anorexia, and rash. Serious adverse reactions include renal failure, nephrotoxicity, ototoxicity, and hepatic necrosis.

Contraindications: Persons with severe renal disease or hypersensitivity should not use these products.

Precautions: Antituberculars should be used with caution with pregnancy, lactation, and hepatic disease.

Pharmacokinetics: Onset, peak, and duration vary widely among products. Most products are metabolized in the liver and excreted in urine.

Interactions: Please check individual monographs since interactions vary widely among products.

Possible nursing diagnoses:
• Infection, risk for [uses]
• Injury, risk for [adverse reactions]
• Knowledge, deficient [teaching]
• Noncompliance [teaching]

Nursing Considerations

Assess:
• Signs of anemia: Hct, Hgb, fatigue
• Hepatic studies qwk: ALT, AST, bilirubin
• Renal status before, qmo: BUN, creatinine, output, specific gravity, urinalysis
• Hepatic status: decreased appetite, jaundice, dark urine, fatigue
Administer:
• For some of these agents on empty stomach, 1 hr before meals (only for

isoniazid and rifampin) or 2 hr after meals
• Antiemetic if vomiting occurs
• After C&S is completed; qmo to detect resistance

Evaluate:
• Therapeutic response: decreased symptoms of TB, culture negative

Teach patient/family:
• That compliance with dosage schedule, duration is necessary
• That scheduled appointments must be kept; relapse may occur
• To avoid alcohol while taking drug
• To report flulike symptoms: excessive fatigue, anorexia, vomiting, sore throat; unusual bleeding, yellowish discoloration of skin/eyes

Selected Generic Names

ethambutol
isoniazid
pyrazinamide
rifabutin
rifampin
streptomycin

ANTITUSSIVES/EXPECTORANTS

Action: Antitussives act by suppressing the cough reflex by direct action on the cough center in the medulla. Expectorants act by liquefying and reducing the viscosity of thick, tenacious secretions.

Uses: Antitussives/expectorants are used to treat cough occurring in pneumonia, bronchitis, TB, cystic fibrosis, and emphysema; as an adjunct in atelectasis (expectorants); and nonproductive cough (antitussives).

Side effects: The most common side effects are drowsiness, dizziness, and nausea.

Contraindications: Some products are contraindicated in hypothyroidism, pregnancy, and lactation.

Precautions: Some products should be used cautiously in asthmatic, geriatric, and debilitated patients.

Pharmacokinetics: Onset, peak, and duration vary widely among products. Some products are metabolized in the liver and excreted in urine.

Interactions: Please check individual monographs since interactions vary widely among products.

Possible nursing diagnoses:
• Breathing pattern, ineffective *[uses]*
• Airway clearance, ineffective *[uses]*
• Knowledge, deficient *[teaching]*

Nursing Considerations

Assess:
• Cough: type, frequency, character (including sputum)

Administer:
• Decreased dose to geriatric patients; their metabolism may be slowed

Perform/provide:
• Increased fluids to liquefy secretions
• Humidification of patient's room

Evaluate:
• Therapeutic response: absence of cough

Teach patient/family:
• To avoid driving, other hazardous activities until patient is stabilized on this medication
• To avoid smoking, smoke-filled rooms, perfumes, dust, environmen-

tal pollutants, cleaners that increase cough

Selected Generic Names

acetylcysteine
ammonium chloride
benzonatate
codeine
dextromethorphan
diphenhydrAMINE
guaifenesin
hydrocodone

ANTIVIRALS/ANTIRETROVIRALS

Action: Antivirals act by interfering with DNA synthesis that is needed for viral replication.

Uses: Antivirals are used for mucocutaneous herpes simplex virus, herpes genitalis (HSV_1, HSV_2), advanced HIV infections, herpes simplex virus encephalitis, varicella-zoster encephalomyelitis.

Side effects: Serious adverse reactions are fatal metabolic encephalopathy, blood dyscrasias, and acute renal failure. Common side effects are nausea, vomiting, anorexia, diarrhea, headache, vaginitis, and moniliasis.

Contraindications: Persons with hypersensitivity, or immunosuppressed individuals with herpes zoster should not use these products.

Precautions: Antivirals should be used with caution in renal disease, hepatic disease, lactation, pregnancy, and dehydration.

Pharmacokinetics: Onset, peak, and duration vary widely among products. Most products are metabolized in the liver and excreted in urine.

Interactions: Please check individual monographs since interactions vary widely among products.

Possible nursing diagnoses:
• Infection, risk for *[uses]*
• Injury, risk for *[adverse reactions]*
• Knowledge, deficient *[teaching]*

Nursing Considerations

Assess:
• Signs of infection, anemia
• I&O ratio; report hematuria, oliguria, fatigue, weakness; may indicate nephrotoxicity; check for protein in urine during treatment
• Any patient with compromised renal system, since drug is excreted slowly in poor renal system function; toxicity may occur rapidly
• Hepatic studies: AST, ALT
• Blood studies: WBC, RBC, Hct, Hgb, bleeding time; blood dyscrasias may occur; drug should be discontinued
• Renal studies: urinalysis, protein, BUN, creatinine, CCr
• C&S before drug therapy; drug may be taken as soon as culture is taken; repeat C&S after treatment
• Bowel pattern before, during treatment; if severe abdominal pain with bleeding occurs, drug should be discontinued
• Skin eruptions: rash, urticaria, itching
• Allergies before treatment, reaction of each medication; record allergies on chart in bright red letters

Administer:
• Increased fluids to 3 L/day to decrease crystalluria when given IV

Perform/provide:
• Storage at room temp for up to 12 hr after reconstitution

• Adequate intake of fluids (2 L) to prevent deposit in kidneys

Evaluate:

• Therapeutic response: absence or control of infection

Teach patient/family:

• That drug does not cure infection, just controls symptoms

• To report sore throat, fever, fatigue; could indicate superinfection

• That drug must be taken in equal intervals around the clock to maintain blood levels for duration of therapy

• To notify prescriber of side effects of bruising, bleeding, fatigue, malaise; may indicate blood dyscrasias

Selected Generic Names

abacavir
acyclovir
amantadine
atazanavir
cidofovir
darunavir
delavirdine
didanosine
emtricitabine
enfuvirtide
famciclovir
fosamprenavir
foscarnet
ganciclovir
indinavir
nelfinavir
nevirapine
rimantadine
ritonavir
saquinavir
stavudine
telbivudine
tenofovir
valganciclovir
zalcitabine
zidovudine

BARBITURATES

Action: Barbiturates act by decreasing impulse transmission to the cerebral cortex.

Uses: All forms of epilepsy can be controlled, since the seizure threshold is increased. Uses also include febrile seizures in children, sedation, insomnia, hyperbilirubinemia, chronic cholestasis with some of these products. Ultra–short-acting barbiturates are used as anesthetics.

Side effects: The most common side effects are drowsiness and nausea. Serious adverse reactions such as Stevens-Johnson syndrome and blood dyscrasias may occur with high doses and long-term treatment.

Contraindications: Hypersensitivity may occur, and allergies should be identified before administering. Barbiturates are identified as pregnancy category D and should not be used in pregnancy. Other contraindications include porphyria and marked impairment of hepatic function.

Precautions: Caution must be used when these products are given to the elderly or debilitated; usually smaller doses are needed since metabolism is slowed. Persons with renal and hepatic disease may show delayed excretion. Barbiturates may produce excitability in children.

Pharmacokinetics: Onset of action can be slow, up to 1 hr, with a peak of 8 hr and a duration of 3-10 hr. These drugs are metabolized by the liver, excreted by the kidneys, cross the placenta, and enter breast milk.

Interactions: Increased CNS depressant effect may occur with alcohol, MAOIs, sedatives, or opioids. These products should be used together cautiously. Oral anticoagulants, corticosteroids, griseofulvin, quinidine, oral contraceptives, and theophylline may show a decreased effect when used with barbiturates.

Possible nursing diagnoses:
• Sleep pattern, disturbed *[uses]*
• Injury, risk for *[adverse reactions]*

Nursing Considerations

Assess:
• Hepatic and renal studies: AST, ALT, bilirubin, creatinine, LDH, alk phos, BUN if patient is on long-term therapy, since these products are metabolized and excreted by the liver and kidneys
• Blood studies: CBC, hematocrit, hemoglobin, and prothrombin time if patient is on long-term therapy, since these products increase the possibility of bleeding and blood dyscrasias
• Barbiturate toxicity: hypotension, pulmonary constriction; cold, clammy skin; cyanosis of lips, insomnia, nausea, vomiting, hallucinations, delirium, weakness

Evaluate:
• Therapeutic response, including appropriate sedation or seizure control

Teach patient/family:
• That physical dependency may result when used for extended periods (45-90 days, depending on dose)
• To avoid driving, activities that require alertness since drowsiness and dizziness may occur
• To abstain from alcohol or other psychotropic medications unless directed by prescriber
• Not to discontinue medication abruptly after long-term use; withdrawal symptoms will occur

Selected Generic Names
pentobarbital
phenobarbital
secobarbital
thiopental

BENZODIAZEPINES

Action: Benzodiazepines potentiate the effects of γ-aminobutyric acid (GABA), including any other inhibitory transmitters in the CNS, resulting in decreased anxiety.

Uses: Anxiety is relieved in conditions such as phobic disorders. Benzodiazepines are also used for acute alcohol withdrawal to relieve the possibility of delirium tremens, and some products are used for relaxation before surgery.

Side effects: The most common side effects are dizziness, drowsiness, blurred vision, and orthostatic hypotension. Most adverse effects are mediated through the CNS. There is a risk of physical dependence and abuse.

Contraindications: Hypersensitivity, acute narrow-angle glaucoma, children <6 mo, hepatic disease (clonazepam), lactation (diazepam).

Precautions: Caution must be used when these products are given to the geriatric or debilitated; usually smaller doses are needed, since metabolism is slowed. Persons with renal and hepatic disease may show delayed excretion. Clonazepam may increase incidence of seizures.

Pharmacokinetics: Onset of action is ½-1 hr, with a peak of 1-2 hr and a duration of 4-6 hr. These drugs are metabolized by the liver, excreted by the kidneys, cross the placenta, and enter breast milk.

Interactions: Increased CNS depressant effect may occur with other CNS depressants. These products should be used together cautiously. Alcohol should not be used; fatal reactions can occur. The serum concentration and toxicity of digoxin may be increased.

Possible nursing diagnoses:
• Anxiety *[uses]*
• Injury, risk for *[adverse reactions]*

Nursing Considerations

Assess:
• B/P (lying, standing), pulse; if systolic B/P drops 20 mm Hg, hold drug, notify prescriber; orthostatic hypotension is severe
• Hepatic and renal studies: AST, ALT, bilirubin, creatinine, LDH, alk phos
• Physical dependency, withdrawal symptoms, including headache, nausea, vomiting, muscle pain, weakness after long-term use

Administer:
• With food or milk for GI symptoms; may give crushed if patient is unable to swallow medication whole

Evaluate:
• Therapeutic response, including relaxation or decreased anxiety

Teach patient/family:
• That drug should not be used for everyday stress or long-term; not to take more than prescribed amount since drug is habit-forming
• To avoid driving and activities that require alertness since drowsiness and dizziness occur

• To abstain from alcohol, other psychotropic medications unless directed by prescriber
• Not to discontinue medication abruptly after long-term use; withdrawal symptoms will occur

Selected Generic Names

alprazolam
chlordiazepoxide
clonazepam
diazepam
flurazepam
lorazepam
midazolam
oxazepam
temazepam
triazolam

BETA-ADRENERGIC BLOCKERS

Action: β-Blockers are divided into selective and nonselective blockers. Nonselective blockers produce a fall in blood pressure without reflex tachycardia or reduction in heart rate through a mixture of β-blocking effects; elevated plasma renins are reduced. Selective β-blockers competitively block stimulation of $β_1$-receptors in cardiac smooth muscle; these drugs produce chronotropic and inotropic effects.

Uses: β-Blockers are used for hypertension, ventricular dysrhythmias, and prophylaxis of angina pectoris.

Side effects: The most common side effects are orthostatic hypotension, bradycardia, diarrhea, nausea, vomiting. Serious adverse reactions include blood dyscrasias, bronchospasm, and CHF.

Contraindications: Hypersensitive reactions may occur, and allergies should be identified before these products are given. β-Adrenergic blockers should not be used in heart block, CHF, or cardiogenic shock.

Precautions: β-Blockers should be used with caution in the elderly or in renal and thyroid disease, COPD, CAD, diabetes mellitus, pregnancy, or asthma.

Pharmacokinetics: Onset, peak, and duration vary widely among products. Most products are metabolized in the liver, with metabolites excreted in urine, bile, and feces.

Interactions: Interactions vary widely among products; check individual monographs for specific information.

Possible nursing diagnoses:
• Tissue perfusion, ineffective *[uses]*
• Cardiac output, decreased *[uses]*
• Diarrhea *[adverse reactions]*
• Gas exchange, impaired *[adverse reactions]*

Nursing Considerations

Assess:
• Renal studies, including protein, BUN, creatinine; watch for increased levels that may indicate nephrotic syndrome; obtain baselines in renal and hepatic function studies before beginning treatment
• I&O, weight daily
• B/P during beginning treatment and periodically thereafter; pulse q4h, note rate, rhythm, quality
• Apical/radial pulse before administration; notify prescriber of significant changes
• Edema in feet and legs daily

Administer:
• PO ac, bedtime; tablets may be crushed or swallowed whole
• Reduced dosage in renal dysfunction

Evaluate:
• Therapeutic response, including decrease in B/P in hypertension, decreased B/P, edema, moist crackles in CHF

Teach patient/family:
• To comply with dosage schedule, even if feeling better
• To rise slowly to sitting or standing position to minimize orthostatic hypotension
• To report bradycardia, dizziness, confusion, depression, fever
• To take pulse at home; advise when to notify prescriber
• To comply with weight control, dietary adjustment, modified exercise program
• To wear support hose to minimize effects of orthostatic hypotension
• Not to discontinue drug abruptly; taper over 2 wk; may precipitate angina

Selected Generic Names

Selective β₁-receptor blockers
acebutolol
atenolol
esmolol
metoprolol

Combined α₁-, β₁-, and β₂-receptor blocker
labetalol

Nonselective β₁- and β₂-blockers
carteolol
nadolol
pindolol
propranolol
timolol

BRONCHODILATORS

Action: Bronchodilators are divided into anticholinergics, α/β-adrenergic agonists, β-adrenergic agonists, and phosphodiesterase inhibitors. Anticholinergics act by inhibiting interaction of acetylcholine at receptor sites on bronchial smooth muscle; α/β-adrenergic agonists by relaxing bronchial smooth muscle and increasing diameter of nasal passages; β-adrenergic agonists by action on β_2-receptors, which relaxes bronchial smooth muscle; phosphodiesterase inhibitors by blocking phosphodiesterase and increasing cAMP, which mediates smooth muscle relaxation in the respiratory system.

Uses: Bronchodilators are used for bronchial asthma, bronchospasm associated with bronchitis, emphysema, or other obstructive pulmonary diseases, Cheyne-Stokes respirations, prevention of exercise-induced asthma.

Side effects: The most common side effects are tremors, anxiety, nausea, vomiting, and irritation in throat. The most serious adverse reactions include bronchospasm and dyspnea.

Contraindications: Persons with hypersensitivity, narrow-angle glaucoma, tachydysrhythmias, and severe cardiac disease should not use some of these products.

Precautions: Bronchodilators should be used with caution in lactation, pregnancy, hyperthyroidism, hypertension, prostatic hypertrophy, and seizure disorders.

Pharmacokinetics: Onset, peak, and duration vary widely among products. Most products are metabolized in the liver and excreted in urine.

Interactions: Please check individual monographs since interactions vary widely among products.

Possible nursing diagnoses:
• Airway clearance, ineffective *[uses]*
• Activity intolerance *[uses]*
• Injury, risk for *[adverse reactions]*
• Knowledge, deficient *[teaching]*

Nursing Considerations

Assess:
• Respiratory function: vital capacity, forced expiratory volume, ABGs, lung sounds, heart rate and rhythm

Administer:
• After shaking, exhale, place mouthpiece in mouth, inhale slowly, hold breath, remove, exhale slowly
• PO with meals to decrease gastric irritation

Perform/provide:
• Storage in light-resistant container, do not expose to temps over 86° F (30° C)
• Gum, sips of water for dry mouth

Evaluate:
• Therapeutic response: absence of dyspnea, wheezing

Teach patient/family:
• Not to use OTC medications; extra stimulation may occur
• Use of inhaler; review package insert with patient
• To avoid getting aerosol in eyes
• To wash inhaler in warm water daily and dry
• To avoid smoking, smoke-filled rooms, persons with respiratory infections

Selected Generic Names

albuterol
aminophylline

arformoterol
atropine
bitolterol
dyphylline
epHEDrine
epINEPHrine
formoterol
ipratropium
isoproterenol
levalbuterol
metaproterenol
pirbuterol
terbutaline
theophylline
tiotropium

CALCIUM CHANNEL BLOCKERS

Action: These products act by inhibiting calcium ion influx across the cell membrane in cardiac and vascular smooth muscle. This action produces relaxation of coronary vascular smooth muscle, dilates coronary arteries, slows SA/AV node conduction, and dilates peripheral arteries.

Uses: These products are used for chronic stable angina pectoris, vasospastic angina, dysrhythmias, hypertension, and unstable angina.

Side effects: The most common side effects are dysrhythmias and edema. Also common are headache, fatigue, drowsiness, and flushing.

Contraindications: Persons with 2nd- or 3rd-degree heart block, sick sinus syndrome, hypotension of <90 mm Hg systolic, Wolff-Parkinson-White syndrome, or cardiogenic shock should not use these products since worsening of those conditions may occur.

Precautions: CHF may worsen since edema may be increased. Hypotension may worsen since B/P is decreased. Patients with renal and hepatic disease should use these products cautiously since they are metabolized in the liver and excreted by the kidneys.

Pharmacokinetics: Onset, peak, and duration vary widely with route of administration. Drugs are metabolized by the liver and excreted in the urine primarily as metabolites.

Interactions: Increased levels of digoxin and theophylline may occur when used with these products. Increased effects of β-blockers and antihypertensives may occur with calcium channel blockers.

Possible nursing diagnoses:
• Tissue perfusion, ineffective *[uses]*
• Cardiac output, decreased *[adverse reactions]*

Nursing Considerations

Assess:
• Cardiac system, including B/P, pulse, respirations, ECG intervals (PR, QRS, QT)

Administer:
• PO before meals and at bedtime

Evaluate:
• Therapeutic response, including decreased anginal pain, decreased B/P, dysrhythmias

Teach patient/family:
• How to take pulse before taking drug; patient should record or graph pulses to identify changes
• To avoid hazardous activities until stabilized on this drug, since dizziness commonly occurs
• Need for compliance in all areas of medical regimen, including diet, exercise, stress reduction, drug therapy

Selected Generic Names

amlodipine
diltiazem
felodipine
isradipine
niCARdipine
NIFEdipine
verapamil

CARDIAC GLYCOSIDES

Action: Products act by inhibiting sodium and potassium ATPase and then making more calcium available to activate contracted proteins. Cardiac contractility and cardiac output are increased.

Uses: These products are used for CHF, atrial fibrillation, atrial flutter, atrial tachycardia, and rapid digitalization in these disorders.

Side effects: The most common side effects are cardiac disturbances, headache, hypotension, GI symptoms. Also common are blurred vision and yellow-green halos.

Contraindications: Hypersensitive reactions may occur, and allergies should be identified before these products are given. Also, persons with ventricular tachycardia, ventricular fibrillation, and carotid sinus syndrome should not use these products.

Precautions: Persons with acute MI and those who have or may develop serum potassium, calcium, or magnesium imbalances should use these products cautiously. Also, persons with AV block, severe respiratory disease, hypothyroidism, or renal and hepatic disease and the geriatric should exercise caution when these drugs are prescribed.

Pharmacokinetics: Onset, peak, and duration vary widely with the route of administration. Digitoxin is inactivated by the liver, and inactive metabolites are excreted in urine. Digoxin is excreted in urine mainly as the parent drug and metabolites.

Interactions: Toxicity may occur when used with diuretics, succinylcholine, quinidine, and thioamines. Increased blood levels may occur with propantheline bromide, spironolactone, quinidine, verapamil, aminoglycosides (PO), amiodarone, anticholinergics, and quinine. Diuretics may increase toxicity.

Possible nursing diagnoses:
• Tissue perfusion, ineffective *[uses]*
• Cardiac output, decreased *[adverse reactions]*

Nursing Considerations

Assess:
• Cardiac system, including B/P, pulse, respirations, and increased urine output
• Apical pulse for 1 min before giving drug; if pulse <60 bpm, take again in 1 hr; if still <60 bpm, notify prescriber
• Electrolytes, including K, Na, Cl, Mg; renal function studies, including BUN and creatinine; and blood studies, including AST, ALT, bilirubin
• I&O ratio, daily weights
• Monitor therapeutic drug levels

Administer:
• K supplements if ordered for K levels <3 mg/dl

Evaluate:
• Therapeutic response, including decreased weight, edema, pulse, respiration, and increased urine output

Teach patient/family:
- How to take pulse before taking drug; patient should record or graph pulse to identify changes
- To avoid hazardous activities until stabilized on this drug, since dizziness commonly occurs
- Need for compliance in all areas of medical regimen, including diet, exercise, stress reduction, drug therapy

Selected Generic Name

digoxin

CHOLINERGICS

Action: Cholinergics act by preventing destruction of acetylcholine, which increases concentration at sites where acetylcholine is released; this exaggerates the effects of acetylcholine and facilitates transmission of impulses across the myoneural junction. Cholinergics may also act by stimulating receptors for acetylcholine.

Uses: Cholinergics are used for myasthenia gravis, as antagonists of nondepolarizing neuromuscular blockade, postoperative bladder distention and urinary distention, and postoperative ileus.

Side effects: The most serious adverse reactions are respiratory depression, bronchospasm, constriction, laryngospasm, respiratory arrest, seizures, and paralysis. The most common side effects are nausea, diarrhea, and vomiting.

Contraindications: Persons with obstruction of the intestine or renal system should not use these products.

Precautions: Caution should be used in patients with bradycardia, hypotension, seizure disorders, bronchial asthma, coronary occlusion, hyperthyroidism, lactation, and in children.

Pharmacokinetics: Onset, peak, and duration vary widely among products. Most products are metabolized in the liver and excreted in urine.

Interactions: Please check individual monographs since interactions vary widely among products.

Possible nursing diagnoses:
- Urinary elimination, impaired *[uses]*
- Breathing pattern, ineffective *[uses]*
- Knowledge, deficient *[teaching]*
- Noncompliance *[teaching]*

Nursing Considerations

Assess:
- VS, respiration q8h
- I&O ratio; check for urinary retention or incontinence
- Bradycardia, hypotension, bronchospasm, headache, dizziness, seizures, respiratory depression; drug should be discontinued if toxicity occurs

Administer:
- Only with atropine sulfate available for cholinergic crisis
- Only after all other cholinergics have been discontinued
- Increased doses if tolerance occurs
- Larger doses after exercise or fatigue
- On empty stomach for better absorption

Perform/provide:
- Storage at room temp

Evaluate:

• Therapeutic response: increased muscle strength, hand grasp, improved muscle gait, absence of labored breathing (if severe)

Teach patient/family:

• That drug is not a cure; it only relieves symptoms (myasthenia gravis)

• To carry emergency ID specifying myasthenia gravis, drugs taken

Selected Generic Names

bethanechol
edrophonium
neostigmine
physostigmine
pyridostigmine

CHOLINERGIC BLOCKERS

Action: Cholinergic blockers inhibit or block acetylcholine at receptor sites in the autonomic nervous system.

Uses: Many products are used to decrease secretions before surgery, to reverse neuromuscular blockade, and to decrease motility of GI, biliary, urinary tracts. Other products are used for parkinsonian symptoms, including dystonia associated with neuroleptic drugs.

Side effects: The most common side effects are dryness of the mouth and constipation, which can be prevented by frequent rinsing of the mouth and by increasing water and bulk in the diet.

Contraindications: Hypersensitivity can occur, and allergies should be identified before administering these products. Persons with GI and GU obstruction should not use these products since constipation and urinary retention may occur. They are also contraindicated in angle-closure glaucoma and myasthenia gravis.

Precautions: Caution must be used when these products are given to the geriatric, since metabolism is slowed. Also, persons with tachycardia or prostatic hypertrophy should use these products with caution.

Pharmacokinetics: Onset, peak, and duration vary with route.

Interactions: Increase in anticholinergic effect occurs when used with opioids, barbiturates, antihistamines, MAOIs, phenothiazines, and amantadine.

Possible nursing diagnoses:

• Mobility, physical, impaired *[uses]*

• Chronic pain *[uses]*

Nursing Considerations

Assess:

• I&O ratio; be alert for urinary retention, frequency, dysuria; drug should be discontinued if these occur

• Urinary hesitancy, retention; palpate bladder if retention occurs

• Constipation; increase fluids, bulk, exercise

• For tolerance over long-term therapy, dose may have to be increased or changed

• Mental status: affect, mood, CNS depression, worsening of mental symptoms during early therapy

Administer:

• With food or milk to decrease GI symptoms

• Parenteral dose with patient recumbent to prevent postural hypotension; give parenteral dose slowly, monitoring vital signs

Perform/provide:

• Hard candy, gum, frequent rinsing of mouth for dryness

Evaluate:
- Therapeutic response, including absence of cramps and EPS

Teach patient/family:
- To avoid driving, other hazardous activity if drowsiness occurs
- To avoid concurrent use of cough, cold preparations with alcohol, antihistamines unless directed by prescriber
- To use with caution in hot weather since medication may increase susceptibility to heat stroke

Selected Generic Names

atropine
benztropine
biperiden
glycopyrrolate
scopolamine
trihexyphenidyl

CORTICOSTEROIDS

Action: Corticosteroids are divided into glucocorticoids and mineralocorticoids. Glucocorticoids decrease inflammation by the suppression of migration of polymorphonuclear leukocytes, fibroblasts, increased capillary permeability, and lysosomal stabilization. They also have varied metabolic effects and modify the body's immune responses to many stimuli. Mineralocorticoids act by increasing resorption of sodium by increasing hydrogen and potassium excretion in the distal tubule.

Uses: Glucocorticoids are used to decrease inflammation and for immunosuppression. In addition, some products may be given for allergy, adrenal insufficiency, or cerebral edema. Mineralocorticoids are given for adrenal insufficiency or adrenogenital syndrome.

Side effects: The most common side effects include change in behavior, including insomnia and euphoria; GI irritation, including peptic ulcer; metabolic reactions, including hypokalemia, hyperglycemia, and carbohydrate intolerance; and sodium and fluid retention. Most adverse reactions are dose dependent.

Contraindications: Hypersensitivity may occur and should be identified before administering. Since these products mask infection, they should not be used in systemic fungal infections or amebiasis. Mothers taking pharmacologic doses of corticosteroids should not nurse.

Precautions: Caution must be used when these products are prescribed for diabetic patients since hyperglycemia may occur. Also, patients with glaucoma, seizure disorders, peptic ulcer, impaired renal function, CHF, hypertension, ulcerative colitis, or myasthenia gravis should be monitored closely if corticosteroids are given. Use with caution in children and the geriatric and during pregnancy.

Pharmacokinetics: For oral preparations, the onset of action occurs between 1 and 2 hr, and duration can be up to 2 days, with a half-life of 2-4 days. Pharmacokinetics vary widely among products. These products cross the placenta and appear in breast milk.

Interactions: Decreased corticosteroid effect may occur with barbiturates, rifampin, phenytoin; corticosteroid dose may have to be increased. There is a possibility of GI bleeding when used with salicylates, indomethacin. Steroids may reduce salicylate levels. When using with digitalis glycosides, potassium-depleting diuretics, and amphotericin, serum potassium levels should be monitored.

Possible nursing diagnoses:

• Infection, risk for *[adverse reactions]*

• Body image, disturbed *[adverse reactions]*

• Suicide, risk for *[adverse reactions]*

Nursing Considerations

Assess:

• Potassium, blood glucose, urine glucose while on long-term therapy; hypokalemia and hyperglycemia are common

• Weight daily; notify prescriber of weekly gain >5 lb, since these products alter fluid and electrolyte balance

• I&O ratio; be alert for decreasing urinary output and increasing edema

• Plasma cortisol levels during long-term therapy (normal level is 138-635 nmol/L SI units when drawn at 8 AM)

• Infection, including increased temp, WBC, even after withdrawal of medication; drug masks symptoms of infection

• Adrenal insufficiency: nausea, anorexia, fatigue, dizziness, dyspnea, weakness, joint pain

• Potassium depletion, including paresthesias, fatigue, nausea, vomiting, depression, polyuria, dysrhythmias, weakness

• Mental status, including affect, mood, behavioral changes, aggression; if severe personality changes occur, including depression, drug may have to be tapered and then discontinued

Administer:

• With food or milk to decrease GI symptoms

• Take single daily or alternate-day doses in the morning before 9 AM (for replacement therapy)

Evaluate:

• Therapeutic response, including decreased inflammation

Teach patient/family:

• That emergency ID as steroid user should be carried

• Not to discontinue this medication abruptly, or adrenal crisis can result

• Teach patient all aspects of drug use, including cushingoid symptoms

• To take with meals or a snack

• If taking immunosuppressives, avoid exposure to chickenpox or measles

Selected Generic Names

Glucocorticoids
beclomethasone
betamethasone
cortisone
dexamethasone
hydrocortisone
hydrocortisone sodium phosphate
methylPREDNISolone
prednisoLONE
predniSONE
triamcinolone
Mineralocorticoid
fludrocortisone

DIURETICS

Action: Diuretics are divided into subgroups: thiazides and thiazide-like diuretics, loop diuretics, carbonic anhydrase inhibitors, osmotic diuretics, and potassium-sparing diuretics. Each one of these subgroups has its own mechanism of action. Thiazides and thiazide-like diuretics increase excretion of water and sodium by inhibiting resorption in the early distal tubule. Loop diuretics inhibit resorption of sodium and chloride in the thick ascending limb of the loop of Henle. Carbonic anhydrase inhibitors increase sodium excretion by decreasing sodium-hydrogen ion exchange throughout the renal tubule. Carbonic anhydrase inhibitors also decrease secretion of aqueous humor in the eye and thus decrease intraocular pressure. Osmotic diuretics increase the osmotic pressure of glomerular filtrate, thus decreasing net absorption of sodium. The potassium-sparing diuretics interfere with sodium resorption at the distal tubule, thus decreasing potassium excretion.

Uses: B/P is reduced in hypertension; edema is reduced in CHF; intraocular pressure is decreased in glaucoma.

Side effects: Hypokalemia, hyperuricemia, and hyperglycemia occur most frequently with thiazide diuretics. Aplastic anemia, blood dyscrasias, volume depletion, and dehydration may occur when thiazide-like diuretics, loop diuretics, or carbonic anhydrase inhibitors are given. Side effects and adverse reactions vary widely for the miscellaneous products.

Contraindications: Persons with electrolyte imbalances (Na, Cl, K), dehydration, or anuria should not be given these products until the problem is corrected.

Precautions: Caution must be used when diuretics are given to the geriatric, since electrolyte disturbances and dehydration can occur rapidly. Hepatic and renal disease may cause poor metabolism and excretion of the drug.

Pharmacokinetics: Onset, peak, and duration vary widely among the different subgroups of these drugs.

Interactions: Cholestyramine and colestipol will decrease the absorption of thiazide diuretics. Concurrent use of thiazides with diazoxide may increase hyperuricemia, hyperglycemia, and antihypertensive effects of thiazides. Ototoxicity may occur when loop diuretics are used with aminoglycosides. Thiazide and loop diuretics may increase therapeutic and toxic effects of lithium.

Possible nursing diagnoses:
• Fluid volume, excess *[uses]*
• Cardiac output, decreased *[adverse reactions]*

Nursing Considerations

Assess:
• Weight, I&O daily to determine fluid loss; check skin turgor for dehydration
• Electrolytes: K, Na, Cl; include BUN, blood glucose, CBC, serum creatinine, blood pH, ABGs, uric acid, Ca; electrolyte imbalances may occur quickly
• B/P lying, standing; postural hypotension may occur since fluid loss occurs first from intravascular spaces
• Signs of metabolic alkalosis, including drowsiness and restlessness
• Signs of hypokalemia with some products, including postural hypotension, malaise, fatigue, tachycardia, leg cramps, weakness

Administer:
- In AM to avoid interference with sleep if using drug as a diuretic
- K replacement if K is less than 3 mg/dl

Evaluate:
- Therapeutic response: improvement in edema of feet, legs, sacral area daily if medication is being used in CHF; improvement in B/P if medication is being used as a diuretic; improvement in intraocular pressure if medication is being used to decrease aqueous humor in the eye

Teach patient/family:
- To take drug early in the day (diuretic) to prevent nocturia

Selected Generic Names

Thiazides
chlorothiazide
hydrochlorothiazide
Thiazide-like
chlorthalidone
indapamide
metolazone
Loop
bumetanide
furosemide
torsemide
Carbonic anhydrase inhibitor
acetaZOLAMIDE
Potassium-sparing
amiloride
spironolactone
triamterene
Osmotics
mannitol
urea

HISTAMINE H₂ ANTAGONISTS

Action: Histamine H₂ antagonists act by inhibiting histamine at the H₂-receptor site in parietal cells, which inhibits gastric acid secretion.

Uses: Histamine H₂ antagonists are used for short-term treatment of duodenal and gastric ulcers and maintenance therapy for duodenal ulcer; gastroesophageal reflux disease.

Side effects: The most serious adverse reactions are agranulocytosis, thrombocytopenia, neutropenia, aplastic anemia, exfoliative dermatitis. The most common side effects are confusion (not with ranitidine), headache, and diarrhea.

Contraindications: Persons with hypersensitivity should not use these products.

Precautions: Caution should be used in pregnancy, lactation, child <16 yr, organic brain syndrome, hepatic disease, renal disease.

Pharmacokinetics: Onset, peak, and duration vary widely among products. Most products are metabolized in the liver and excreted in urine.

Interactions: Antacids interfere with absorption of histamine H₂ antagonists. Check individual monographs for other interactions.

Possible nursing diagnoses:
- Chronic pain [uses]
- Injury, risk for [bleeding]
- Knowledge, deficient [teaching]

Nursing Considerations

Assess:
- Gastric pH (>5 should be maintained)
- I&O ratio, BUN, creatinine

Administer:
- With meals for prolonged drug effect
- Antacids 1 hr before or 1 hr after cimetidine

• IV slowly; bradycardia may occur; give over 30 min

Perform/provide:

• Storage of diluted sol at room temp for up to 48 hr

Evaluate:

• Therapeutic response: decreased pain in abdomen

Teach patient/family:

• That gynecomastia, impotence may occur, but are reversible

• To avoid driving, other hazardous activities until patient is stabilized on this medication

• To avoid black pepper, caffeine, alcohol, harsh spices, extremes in temp of food

• To avoid OTC preparations: aspirin, cough, cold preparations

• That drug must be continued for prescribed time to be effective

• To report bruising, fatigue, malaise; blood dyscrasias may occur

Selected Generic Names

cimetidine
famotidine
ranitidine

IMMUNOSUPPRESSANTS

Action: Immunosuppressants act by inhibiting lymphocytes (T).

Uses: Most products are used for organ transplants to prevent rejection.

Side effects: The most serious adverse reactions are albuminuria, hematuria, proteinuria, renal failure, and hepatotoxicity. The most common side effects are overgrowth of oral *Candida,* gum hyperplasia, tremors, and headache. The most serious adverse reactions for azathioprine are hematologic (leukopenia and thrombocytopenia) and GI (nausea and vomiting). There is a risk of secondary infection.

Contraindications: Products are contraindicated in hypersensitivity.

Precautions: Caution should be used in severe renal disease, severe hepatic disease, and pregnancy.

Pharmacokinetics: Onset, peak, and duration vary widely among products. Most products are metabolized in the liver and excreted in urine.

Interactions: Please check individual monographs since interactions vary widely among products.

Possible nursing diagnoses:

• Infection, risk for *[adverse reactions]*

• Injury, risk for *[uses]*

• Knowledge, deficient *[teaching]*

Nursing Considerations

Assess:

• Renal studies: BUN, creatinine at least qmo during treatment, 3 mo after treatment

• Hepatic studies: alk phos, AST (SGOT), ALT (SGPT), bilirubin

• Drug blood levels during treatment

• Hepatotoxicity: dark urine, jaundice, itching, light-colored stools; drug should be discontinued

Administer:

• For several days before transplant surgery

• With meals for GI upset or drug mixed with chocolate milk

• With oral antifungal for *Candida* infections

Evaluate:

• Therapeutic response: absence of rejection

Teach patient/family:
• To report fever, chills, sore throat, fatigue, since serious infections may occur
• To use contraceptive measures during treatment, for 12 wk after ending therapy

Selected Generic Names

azathioprine
basiliximab
cycloSPORINE
muromonab-CD3
sirolimus
tacrolimus

LAXATIVES

Action: Laxatives are divided into bulk products, lubricants, osmotics, saline laxative stimulants, and stool softeners. Bulk laxatives work by absorbing water and expanding to increase moisture content and bulk in the stool. Lubricants increase water retention in the stool, causing reabsorption of water in the bowel. Stimulants act by increasing peristalsis by direct effect on the intestine. Saline draws water into the intestinal lumen. Osmotics increase distention and promote peristalsis. Stool softeners reduce surface tension of liquids of the bowel.

Uses: Laxatives are used as a preparation for bowel and rectal exam, constipation, and stool softener.

Side effects: The most common side effects are nausea, abdominal cramps, and diarrhea.

Contraindications: Persons with GI obstruction, perforation, gastric retention, toxic colitis, megacolon, abdominal pain, nausea, vomiting, or fecal impaction should not use these products.

Precautions: Caution should be used in rectal bleeding, large hemorrhoids, and anal excoriation.

Pharmacokinetics: Onset, peak, and duration vary among products.

Interactions: Please check individual monographs since interactions vary widely among products.

Possible nursing diagnoses:
• Constipation *[uses]*
• Diarrhea *[adverse reactions]*
• Knowledge, deficient *[teaching]*

Nursing Considerations

Assess:
• Blood, urine electrolytes if drug is used often by patient
• I&O ratio: to identify fluid loss
• Cause of constipation; identify whether fluids, bulk, or exercise missing from lifestyle
• Cramping, rectal bleeding, nausea, vomiting; if these symptoms occur, drug should be discontinued

Administer:
• Swallow tabs whole; do not break, crush, or chew
• Alone only with water for better absorption; do not take within 1 hr of antacids, milk, or cimetidine

Evaluate:
• Therapeutic response: decrease in constipation

Teach patient/family:
• Not to use laxatives for long-term therapy; bowel tone will be lost
• That normal bowel movements do not always occur daily
• Not to use in presence of abdominal pain, nausea, vomiting
• To notify prescriber of abdominal pain, nausea, vomiting
• To notify prescriber if constipation is unrelieved or if symptoms of elec-

trolyte imbalance: muscle cramps, pain, weakness, dizziness

Selected Generic Names

Bulk laxatives
calcium polycarbophil
methylcellulose
psyllium
Osmotic agents
glycerin
lactulose
Saline laxatives
magnesium salts
sodium biphosphate/phosphate
Stimulants
bisacodyl
cascara sagrada
senna
Stool softener
docusate

NEUROMUSCULAR BLOCKING AGENTS

Action: Neuromuscular blocking agents are divided into depolarizing and nondepolarizing blockers. They act by inhibiting transmission of nerve impulses by binding with cholinergic receptor sites.

Uses: Neuromuscular blocking agents are used to facilitate endotracheal intubation and skeletal muscle relaxation during mechanical ventilation, surgery, or general anesthesia.

Side effects: The most serious adverse reactions are prolonged apnea, bronchospasm, cyanosis, respiratory depression, and malignant hyperthermia. The most common side effects are bradycardia and decreased motility.

Contraindications: Persons who are hypersensitive should not be given this product.

Precautions: Caution should be used in pregnancy, thyroid disease, collagen disease, cardiac disease, lactation, children <2 yr, electrolyte imbalances, dehydration, neuromuscular disease (myasthenia gravis), and respiratory disease.

Pharmacokinetics: Onset, peak, and duration vary widely among products. Most products are metabolized in the liver and excreted in urine.

Interactions: Aminoglycosides potentiate neuromuscular blockade. See individual monographs.

Possible nursing diagnoses:
• Breathing pattern, ineffective *[uses]*
• Injury, risk for *[adverse reactions]*
• Knowledge, deficient *[teaching]*

Nursing Considerations

Assess:
• For electrolyte imbalances (K, Mg); may lead to increased action of this drug
• VS (B/P, pulse, respirations, airway) q15min until fully recovered; rate, depth, pattern of respirations, strength of hand grip
• I&O ratio; check for urinary retention, frequency, hesitancy
• Recovery: decreased paralysis of face, diaphragm, leg, arm, rest of body
• Allergic reactions: rash, fever, respiratory distress, pruritus; drug should be discontinued

Administer:
• Using nerve stimulator by anesthesia provider to determine neuromuscular blockade

• Anticholinesterase to reverse neuromuscular blockade
• IV undiluted over 1-2 min (only by qualified person, usually an anesthesiologist)

Perform/provide:
• Storage in light-resistant container, cool area
• Reassurance if communication is difficult during recovery from neuromuscular blockade

Evaluate:
• Therapeutic response: paralysis of jaw, eyelid, head, neck, rest of body

Selected Generic Names

atracurium
doxacurium
gallamine
mivacurium
pancuronium
pipecuronium
rocuronium
succinylcholine
tubocurarine
vecuronium

NONSTEROIDAL ANTIINFLAMMATORIES

Action: Nonsteroidals decrease prostaglandin synthesis by inhibiting an enzyme needed for biosynthesis.
Uses: Nonsteroidal antiinflammatories are used to treat mild to moderate pain, osteoarthritis, rheumatoid arthritis, and dysmenorrhea.
Side effects: The most serious adverse reactions are nephrotoxicity (dysuria, hematuria, oliguria, azotemia), blood dyscrasias, and cholestatic hepatitis. The most common side effects are nausea, abdominal pain, anorexia, dizziness, and drowsiness.
Contraindications: Persons with hypersensitivity, asthma, severe renal disease, and severe hepatic disease should not use these products.
Precautions: Caution should be used in pregnancy, lactation, children, bleeding disorders, GI disorders, cardiac disorders, hypersensitivity to other antiinflammatory agents, and the geriatric.
Pharmacokinetics: Onset, peak, and duration vary widely among products. Most products are metabolized in the liver and excreted in urine.
Interactions: Please check individual monographs since interactions vary widely among products.
Possible nursing diagnoses:
• Pain, chronic [uses]
• Mobility, physical, impaired [uses]
• Knowledge, deficient [teaching]
• Noncompliance [teaching]

Nursing Considerations

Assess:
• Renal, hepatic, blood studies: BUN, creatinine, AST, ALT, Hgb, before treatment, periodically thereafter
• Audiometric, ophthalmic examination before, during, and after treatment
• For eye, ear problems: blurred vision, tinnitus; may indicate toxicity

Administer:
• With food to decrease GI symptoms; however, best to take on empty stomach to facilitate absorption

Perform/provide:
• Storage at room temp

Evaluate:
• Therapeutic response: decreased pain, stiffness in joints, decreased

swelling in joints, ability to move more easily

Teach patient/family:
• To report blurred vision, ringing, roaring in ears; may indicate toxicity
• To avoid driving, other hazardous activities if dizziness, drowsiness occur, especially geriatric
• To report change in urine pattern, increased weight, edema, increased pain in joints, fever, blood in urine; indicate nephrotoxicity
• That therapeutic effects may take up to 1 mo

Selected Generic Names

celecoxib
diclofenac
etodolac
fenoprofen
ibuprofen
indomethacin
ketoprofen
ketorolac
nabumetone
naproxen
piroxicam
sulindac

OPIOID ANALGESICS

Action: Opioid analgesics act by depressing pain impulse transmission at the spinal cord level by interacting with opioid receptors. Products are divided into opiates and nonopiates.

Uses: Most products are used to control moderate to severe pain and are used before and after surgery.

Side effects: GI symptoms, including nausea, vomiting, anorexia, constipation, and cramps, are the most common side effects. Other common side effects include light-headedness, dizziness, sedation. Serious adverse reactions such as respiratory depression, respiratory arrest, circulatory depression, and increased intracranial pressure may result but are less common and usually dose dependent.

Contraindications: Hypersensitive reactions occur frequently. Check for sensitivity before administering. These drugs should be used cautiously if opiate addiction is suspected.

Precautions: Caution must be used when these products are given to a person with an addictive personality since the possibility of addiction is so great. Also, they may worsen intracranial pressure. Persons with severe heart disease, hepatic or renal disease, respiratory conditions, or seizure disorders should be monitored closely for worsening condition.

Pharmacokinetics: Onset of action is immediate by IV route and rapid by IM and PO routes. Peak occurs from 1-2 hr, depending on route, with a duration of 2-8 hr. These agents cross the placenta and appear in breast milk.

Interactions: Barbiturates, other opioids, hypnotics, antipsychotics, or alcohol can increase CNS depression when taken with opioids.

Possible nursing diagnoses:
• Acute pain [uses]
• Gas exchange, impaired [adverse reactions]

Nursing Considerations

Assess:
• I&O ratio; be alert for urinary retention, frequency, dysuria; drug

should be discontinued if these occur

• Respiratory dysfunction, including respiratory depression, rate, rhythm, character; notify prescriber if respirations are <12/min

• CNS changes: dizziness, drowsiness, hallucinations, euphoria, LOC, pupil reaction

• Allergic reactions: rash, urticaria

• Need for pain medication; use pain scoring

Administer:

• With antiemetic if nausea or vomiting occurs

• When pain is beginning to return; determine dosage interval by response

Perform/provide:

• Assistance with ambulation; patient should not be ambulating during drug peak

Evaluate:

• Therapeutic response, including decrease in pain

Teach patient/family:

• To report any symptoms of CNS changes, allergic reactions, or shortness of breath

• That physical dependency may result when used for extended periods

• That withdrawal symptoms may occur, including nausea, vomiting, cramps, fever, faintness, anorexia

• To avoid alcohol and other CNS depressants

Selected Generic Names

alfentanil
buprenorphine
butorphanol
codeine
fentanyl
fentanyl transdermal
hydromorphone
meperidine
methadone
morphine
nalbuphine
oxycodone
oxymorphone
pentazocine
propoxyphene
remifentanil

SALICYLATES

Action: Salicylates have analgesic, antipyretic, and antiinflammatory effects. The antiinflammatory and analgesic activities may be mediated through the inhibition of prostaglandin synthesis. Antipyretic action results from inhibition of the hypothalamic heat-regulating center.

Uses: The primary uses of salicylates are relief of mild to moderate pain and fever and in inflammatory conditions such as arthritis, thromboembolic disorders, and rheumatic fever.

Side effects: The most common side effects are GI symptoms and rash. Serious blood dyscrasias and hepatotoxicity may result when used for long periods at high doses. Tinnitus or impaired hearing may indicate that blood salicylate levels are reaching or exceeding the upper limit of the therapeutic range.

Contraindications: Hypersensitivity to salicylates is common. Check for sensitivity before administering. Persons with bleeding disorders, GI bleeding, and vit K deficiency should not use these products since salicylates increase prothrombin time. Children should not use these products since salicylates have been associated with Reye's syndrome.

Precautions: Caution is needed when salicylates are given to patients with anemia, hepatic or renal disease, or Hodgkin's disease. Caution should also be exercised in pregnancy and lactation.

Pharmacokinetics: Onset of action occurs in 15-30 min, with a peak of 1-2 hr and a duration up to 6 hr. These drugs are metabolized by the liver and excreted by the kidneys.

Interactions: Increased effects of anticoagulants, insulin, methotrexate, heparin, valproic acid, and oral sulfonylureas may occur when used with salicylates. Aspirin may decrease serum concentrations of nonsteroidal antiinflammatory agents.

Possible nursing diagnoses:
• Acute, chronic pain *[uses]*
• Mobility, physical, impaired *[uses]*
• Activity intolerance *[uses]*
• Sensory/perceptual alterations: auditory *[adverse reactions]*
• Thermoregulation, ineffective *[uses]*

Nursing Considerations

Assess:
• Hepatic and renal studies: AST, ALT, bilirubin, creatinine, LDH, alk phos, BUN if patient is on long-term therapy, since these products are metabolized and excreted by the liver and kidney
• Blood studies: CBC, hematocrit, hemoglobin, and prothrombin time if patient is on long-term therapy, since these products increase the possibility of bleeding and blood dyscrasias
• Hepatotoxicity: dark urine, clay-colored stools; yellowing of skin,

sclera; itching, abdominal pain, fever, diarrhea, which may occur with long-term use
• Ototoxicity: tinnitus; ringing, roaring in ears; audiometric testing is needed before and after long-term therapy

Administer:
• With food or milk to decrease gastric irritation; give 30 min before or 1 hr after meals with a full glass of water

Evaluate:
• Therapeutic response, including decreased pain, fever

Teach patient/family:
• That blood glucose levels should be monitored closely if patient is diabetic
• Not to exceed recommended dosage; acute poisoning may result
• That therapeutic response takes 2 wk in arthritis
• To avoid use of alcohol, since GI bleeding may result
• To notify prescriber of ringing in the ears or persistent GI pain
• To take with full glass of water to reduce risk of lodging in esophagus

Selected Generic Names

aspirin
choline salicylate
magnesium salicylate
salsalate

THROMBOLYTICS

Action: Thrombolytics act by activating conversion of plasminogen to plasmin (fibrinolysin): plasmin is able to break down clots (fibrin).

Uses: Thrombolytics are used to treat deep vein thrombosis, pulmonary embolism, arterial thrombosis, arterial embolism, arteriovenous cannula occlusion, lysis of coronary artery thrombi after MI, and acute, evolving transmural MI.

Side effects: Serious adverse reactions include GI, GU, intracranial retroperitoneal bleeding, and anaphylaxis. The most common side effects are decreased Hct, urticaria, headache, and nausea.

Contraindications: Persons with hypersensitivity, active bleeding, intraspinal surgery, neoplasms of the CNS, ulcerative colitis/enteritis, severe hypertension, renal disease, hepatic disease, hypocoagulation, COPD, subacute bacterial endocarditis, rheumatic valvular disease, cerebral embolism/thrombosis/hemorrhage, recent intraarterial diagnostic procedure or surgery (10 days), and recent major surgery should not use these products.

Precautions: Caution should be used in arterial emboli from left side of heart and pregnancy.

Pharmacokinetics: Onset, peak, and duration vary widely among products. Most products are metabolized in the liver and excreted in urine.

Interactions: Please check individual monographs since interactions vary widely among products.

Possible nursing diagnoses:
• Injury, risk for *[uses]*

Nursing Considerations

Assess:
• VS, B/P, pulse, resp, neurologic signs, temp at least q4h; temp >104° F (40° C) indicator of internal bleeding; cardiac rhythm following intracoronary administration; systolic pressure increase of >25 mm Hg should be reported to prescriber
• For neurologic changes that may indicate intracranial bleeding
• Retroperitoneal bleeding: back pain, leg weakness, diminished pulses
• Allergy: fever, rash, itching, chill; mild reaction may be treated with antihistamines
• For bleeding during 1st hr of treatment: hematuria, hematemesis, bleeding from mucous membranes, epistaxis, ecchymosis
• Blood studies (Hct, platelets, PTT, PT, TT, aPTT) before starting therapy; PT or APTT must be less than 2× control before starting therapy; or PT q3-4h during treatment

Administer:
• As soon as thrombi identified; not useful for thrombi over 1 wk old
• Cryoprecipitate or fresh, frozen plasma if bleeding occurs
• Loading dose at beginning of therapy; may require increased loading doses
• Heparin after fibrinogen level is over 100 mg/dl; heparin infusion to increase PTT to 1.5-2 × baseline for 3-7 days
• About 10% of patients have high streptococcal antibody titers requiring increased loading doses
• IV therapy using 0.8 µm filter

Perform/provide:
• Storage of reconstituted drug in refrigerator; discard after 24 hr
• Bed rest during entire course of treatment
• Avoidance of venous or arterial puncture, inj, rectal temp
• Treatment of fever with acetaminophen or aspirin

- Pressure for 30 sec to minor bleeding sites; inform prescriber if this does not attain hemostasis; apply pressure dressing

Evaluate:
- Therapeutic response: resolution of thrombosis, embolism

Selected Generic Names

alteplase
anistreplase
drotrecogin alfa
streptokinase
tenecteplase
urokinase

THYROID HORMONES

Action: Acts by increasing metabolic rates, resulting in increased cardiac output, O_2 consumption, body temp, blood volume, growth, development at cellular level, respiratory rate, enzyme system activity.

Uses: Products are used for thyroid replacement.

Side effects: The most common side effects include insomnia, tremors, tachycardia, palpitations, angina, dysrhythmias, weight loss, and changes in appetite. Serious adverse reactions include thyroid storm.

Contraindications: Persons with adrenal insufficiency, myocardial infarction, or thyrotoxicosis should not use these products.

Precautions: The elderly and patients with angina pectoris, hypertension, ischemia, cardiac disease, or diabetes mellitus or insipidus should be watched closely when using these products. Caution should be used in pregnancy (A) and lactation.

Pharmacokinetics: Pharmacokinetics vary widely among products; check specific monographs.

Interactions:
- Impaired absorption of thyroid products may occur when administered with cholestyramine, iron products (separate by 4-5 hr)
- Increased effects of anticoagulants, sympathomimetics, tricyclic antidepressants, catecholamines may occur
- Decreased effects of digitalis, glycosides, insulin, hypoglycemics may occur
- Decreased effects of thyroid products may occur with estrogens

Possible nursing diagnoses:
- Knowledge, deficient *[teaching]*
- Noncompliance *[teaching]*
- Body image, disturbed *[adverse reactions]*

Nursing Considerations

Assess:
- B/P, pulse before each dose
- I&O ratio
- Weight daily in same clothing, using same scale, at same time of day
- PT should be closely monitored and dosage of anticoagulant therapy may need adjustment
- Height, growth rate if given to a child
- T_3, T_4, which are decreased; radioimmunoassay of TSH, which is increased; ratio uptake, which is decreased if patient is on too low a dosage of medication
- Increased nervousness, excitability, irritability; may indicate overdosage, usually after 1-3 wk of treatment

• Cardiac status: angina, palpitation, chest pain, change in VS

Administer:

• At same time each day to maintain drug level

• Only for hormone imbalances, not to be used for obesity, male infertility, menstrual conditions, lethargy

Perform/provide:

• Removal of medication 4 wk before RAIU test

Evaluate:

• Therapeutic response: absence of depression; increased weight loss; diuresis; pulse; appetite; absence of constipation; peripheral edema; cold intolerance; pale, cool, dry skin; brittle nails; alopecia; coarse hair; menorrhagia; night blindness; paresthesias; syncope; stupor; coma; rosy cheeks

Teach patient/family:

• That hair loss will occur in child and is temporary

• To report excitability, irritability, anxiety, chest pain, palpitations, increased pulse, excessive sweating, heat intolerance; indicates overdose

• Not to switch brands unless directed by prescriber

• That hypothyroid child will show almost immediate behavior/personality change

• That treatment drug is not to be taken to reduce weight

• To avoid OTC preparations with iodine; read labels

• To avoid iodine in food, iodinized salt, soybeans, tofu, turnips, some seafood, some bread

Selected Generic Names

levothyroxine (T_4)

liothyronine (T_3)

liotrix

thyroid USP

VASODILATORS

Action: Vasodilators have various modes of action. Please check individual monographs for specific action.

Uses: Vasodilators are used to treat intermittent claudication, arteriosclerosis obliterans, vasospasm and muscular ischemia, ischemic cerebral vascular disease, hypertension, and angina.

Side effects: The most common side effects are headache, nausea, hypotension or hypertension, and ECG changes.

Contraindications: Some drugs are contraindicated in acute MI, paroxysmal tachycardia, and thyrotoxicosis.

Precautions: Caution should be used in uncompensated heart disease or peptic ulcer disease.

Pharmacokinetics: Onset, peak, and duration vary widely among products. Most products are metabolized in the liver and excreted in urine.

Interactions: Please check individual monographs since interactions vary widely among products.

Possible nursing diagnoses:

• Cardiac output, decreased *[uses]*

- Tissue perfusion, ineffective *[uses]*
- Knowledge, deficient *[teaching]*

Nursing Considerations

Assess:
- Bleeding time in individuals with bleeding disorders
- Cardiac status: B/P, pulse, rate, rhythm, character; watch for increasing pulse

Administer:
- With meals to reduce GI symptoms

Perform/provide:
- Storage in tight container at room temp

Evaluate:
- Therapeutic response: ability to walk without pain, increased temp in extremities, increased pulse volume

Teach patient/family:
- That medication is not cure; may need to be taken continuously
- That it is necessary to quit smoking to prevent excessive vasoconstriction
- That improvement may be sudden, but usually occurs gradually over several wk
- To report headache, weakness, increased pulse, as drug may have to be decreased or discontinued
- To avoid hazardous activities until stabilized on medication; dizziness may occur

Selected Generic Names

amyl nitrite
bosentan
dipyridamole
hydrALAZINE
isoxsuprine
midodrine
minoxidil
nesiritide
papaverine

VITAMINS

Action: Action varies widely among products and classes; check specific monographs.

Uses: Vitamins are used to correct and prevent vitamin deficiencies.

Side effects: There are no side effects or adverse reactions with the water-soluble vitamins (C, B). However, fat-soluble vitamins (A, D, E, K) may accumulate in the body and cause adverse reactions (see specific monographs).

Contraindications: Hypersensitive reactions may occur, and allergies should be identified before these products are given.

Pharmacokinetics: Onset, peak, and duration vary widely among products; check individual monographs for specific information.

Possible nursing diagnoses:
- Nutrition: less than body requirements, imbalanced *[uses]*

Nursing Considerations

Administer:
- PO with food for better absorption

Perform/provide:
- Storage in tight, light-resistant container

Evaluate:
- Therapeutic response: no vitamin deficiency

Teach patient/family:
- Not to take more than prescribed amount

Selected Generic Names

Fat-soluble
phytonadione (vitamin K_1)
vitamin A
vitamin D
vitamin E

Water-soluble
ascorbic acid (C)
cyanocobalamin (B_{12})
pyridoxine (B_6)
riboflavin (B_2)
thiamine (B_1)

Miscellaneous
multivitamins

MECHANISMS AND SITES OF ACTION

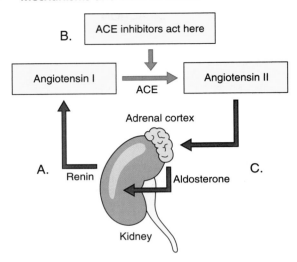

Plate 1:   Sites of Action – ACE Inhibitors

The renin-angiotensin-aldosterone system plays a major role in regulating BP. Any condition that decreases renal blood flow, reduces BP, or stimulates beta$_1$-adrenergic receptors prompts the kidneys to release renin (A). Renin acts on angiotensinogen, which is converted to angiotensin I, a weak vasoconstrictor. Angiotensin-converting enzyme (ACE) converts angiotensin I to angiotensin II, which causes systemic and renal blood vessels to constrict (B). Systemic vasoconstriction increases peripheral vascular resistance, raising the BP. Renal vasoconstriction decreases glomerular filtration, resulting in sodium and water retention and increasing blood volume and BP. In addition, angiotensin II also acts on the adrenal cortex causing it to release aldosterone (C). This makes the kidneys retain additional sodium and water, which further increases the BP.

ACE inhibitors, such as captopril, enalapril, and lisinopril, block the action of ACE. As a result, angiotensin II can't form, which prevents systemic and renal vasoconstriction and the release of aldosterone. (From Prosser S, Worster B, Dewar K: *Applied Pharmacology for Nurses and Other Health Care Professionals*, St. Louis, 2000, Mosby.)

Plate 2:   Mechanisms of Action – Adrenocortical Steroids
Adrenocortical steroids (also called corticosteroids) are available in many forms,
such as predniSONE, and produce a wide range of effects, such as
immunosupression and antiinflammation. Here's how these drugs work at the
cellular level.

Corticosteroids are hormones that are naturally produced by the body
(endogenous hormones). Synthetic corticosteroids work much the same as the
endogenous hormones. When a corticosteroid enters a cell, it binds to corticosteroid
receptors (CRs) in the cell's cytoplasm, forming a complex. The complex moves to
the nucleus, where it causes the transcription of corticosteroid responsive genes
(CRGs) to messenger ribonucleic acid (mRNA), eventually translating to a protein
that produces a steroid response in target tissues. (From Taylor: *Mosby's Crash
Course Pharmacology*, St. Louis, 1998, Mosby.)

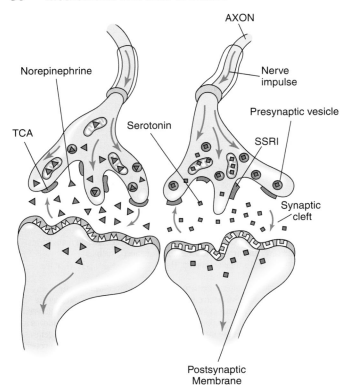

Plate 3:   Mechanisms of Action – Antidepressants
Depression is thought to occur when levels of neurotransmitters, such as
norepinephrine and serotonin, are reduced at postsynaptic receptor sites. These
neurotransmitters affect a wide array of functions, including mood, obsessions,
appetite, and anxiety. Antidepressants work by increasing the availability of these
neurotransmitters at postsynaptic membranes and by enhancing and prolonging
their effects. As a result, these agents improve mood, reduce anxiety, and minimize
obsessions.

Antidepressants typically are classified as tricyclic antidepressants (TCAs),
monoamine oxidase inhibitors (not shown), selective serotonin reuptake inhibitors
(SSRIs), and atypical antidepressants (not shown). TCAs, such as amitriptyline and
desipramine, primarily block norepinephrine reuptake at presynaptic membranes,
thereby increasing the norepinephrine concentration at synapses and making more
available at postsynaptic receptors.

SSRIs, such as fluoxetine and paroxetine, selectively inhibit serotonin uptake at
presynaptic membranes. This action leads to increased serotonin availability at
postsynaptic receptors. (From Gutierrez K: *Pharmacotherapeutics: Clinical
Decision Making in Nursing*, Philadelphia, 1999, Saunders.)

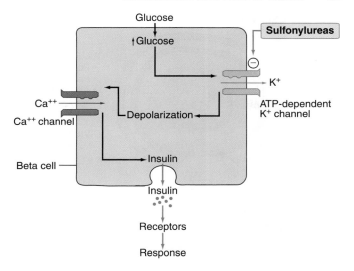

Plate 4:   Mechanisms of Action – Antidiabetic Agents

Diabetes mellitus takes two forms: type 1 diabetes, characterized by a complete lack of insulin, and type 2 diabetes, which is marked by insufficient insulin secretion, insulin resistance in peripheral tissues, or both. Normally, the beta cells in the pancreatic islets of Langerhans are responsible for secreting insulin. When glucose levels rise in the beta cell, it triggers adenosine triphosphate (ATP)–dependent potassium (K^+) channels in the membranes of beta cells to close. Then the beta cells depolarize and calcium (Ca^{++}) enters the cell through Ca^{++} channel, and insulin is released from the cell. When circulating insulin engages with insulin receptors on cell membranes, it facilitates the movement of glucose into the cell, among other actions.

Type 1 diabetes is treated with the use of exogenous insulin, which mimics natural insulin in the body. Insulin takes many forms with varying degrees of onset, peak, and duration, including rapid, regular, intermediate, and long-acting.

Type 2 diabetes is usually treated with oral agents. Sulfonylureas, such as glyburide, block ATP-dependent K^+ channels in the cell membranes of beta cells, ultimately resulting in the release of insulin. (From Taylor: *Mosby's Crash Course Pharmacology*, St. Louis, 1998, Mosby.)

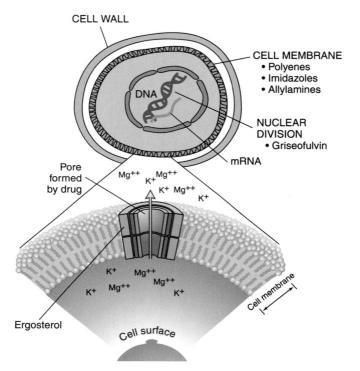

CELL WALL

CELL MEMBRANE
• Polyenes
• Imidazoles
• Allylamines

DNA

NUCLEAR
DIVISION
• Griseofulvin

mRNA

Pore
formed
by drug

Mg^{++} Mg^{++}
K^+ K^+ Mg^{++}
K^+

K^+ Mg^{++} Mg^{++}
K^+ Mg^{++} K^+

Ergosterol

Cell membrane

Cell surface

Plate 5:   Sites and Mechanisms of Action – Antifungal Agents
Antifungal agents primarily affect fungi at one of two sites: the cell membrane or the
cell nucleus. Most of these agents, such as polyene, imidazole, and allylamine
antifungals, act on the fungal cell membrane. Polyene antifungals, such as
amphotericin B, bind to ergosterol and increase cell membrane permeability.
Imidazole antifungals, such as fluconazole and ketoconazole, interfere with
ergosterol synthesis by inhibiting the cytochrome P450 enzyme system, altering the
cell membrane, and inhibiting fungal growth. Allylamine antifungals, such as
terbinafine, inhibit the enzyme squaline epoxidase, which disrupts ergosterol
production—and cell membrane integrity. When cell membrane permeability
increases, cellular components, including potassium (K^+) and magnesium (Mg^{++}),
leak out. Loss of these cellular components leads to cell death.
    Another antifungal agent, griseofulvin, directly affects the fungal nucleus,
interfering with mitosis. By binding to structures in the mitotic spindle, it prevents
cells from dividing, which eventually leads to their death. (From Gutierrez K:
Pharmacotherapeutics: Clinical Decision Making in Nursing, Philadelphia, 1999,
Saunders.)

Cell wall synthesis
- Penicillins
- Cephalosporins
- Carbapenems
- Monobactams
- Tricyclic glycopeptides

Folic acid metabolism
- Trimethoprim

Cell membrane permeability
- Polyene antifungals

DNA synthesis
- Antitubercular agent
- Nitroimidazoles
- Antiviral agents
- Antiretroviral agents
- Quinolones

RNA synthesis

Protein synthesis
- Aminoglycosides
- Macrolides
- Tetracyclines
- Lincosamides
- Chloramphenicol

DNA, mRNA, Folinic acid, Folic acid, Ribosomes, 50 30

Plate 6:   Sites and Mechanisms of Action – Antiinfective Agents

The goal of antiinfective therapy is to kill or inhibit the growth of microorganisms, such as bacteria, viruses, and fungi. To achieve this goal, antiinfective agents must reach their targets, which usually occurs through absorption and distribution by the circulatory system. When the target is reached, a drug can kill or suppress microorganisms by:

- Inhibiting cell wall synthesis or activating enzymes that disrupt the cell wall, which leads to cellular weakening, lysis, and death. Penicillins (ampicillin), cephalosporins (cefazolin), carbapenems (imipenem), monobactams (aztreonam), and tricyclic glycopeptides (vancomycin) act in this way.
- Altering cell membrane permeability through direct action on the cell wall, which allows intracellular substances to leak out and destabilizes the cell. Polyene antifungals (amphotericin) work by this mechanism.
- Altering protein synthesis by binding to bacterial ribosomes (50/30) or affecting ribosomal function, which leads to cell death or slowed growth, respectively. Aminoglycosides (gentamicin), macrolides (erythromycin), tetracyclines (doxycycline), lincosamides (clindamycin), and the miscellaneous antiinfective chloramphenicol act in this way.
- Inhibiting DNA or RNA, including messenger RNA (mRNA), by synthesis by binding to nucleic acids or interacting with enzymes required for their synthesis. Antitubercular agents (rifampin), nitroimidazoles (metronidazole), antiviral agents (acyclovir), antiretroviral agents (stavudine), and quinolones (ciprofloxacin) act like this.
- Inhibiting the metabolism of folic acid and folinic acid or other cellular components that are essential for bacterial cell growth. The miscellaneous anti-infective trimethoprim employs this mechanism of action. (From Page C, et al: *Integrated Pharmacology*, ed 2, St. Louis, 2002, Mosby.)

Platelet Activation

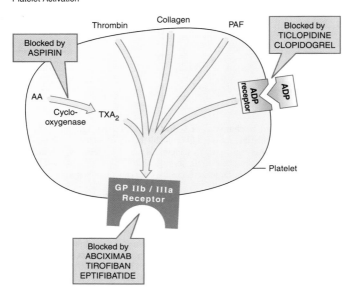

Plate 7:   Sites and Mechanisms of Action – Antiplatelet Agents

Antiplatelet drugs are prescribed to prevent arterial thrombosis because they prevent platelet aggregation. These drugs include aspirin, adenosine diphosphate (ADP) receptor antagonists, or glycoprotein (GP) receptor IIb/IIIa antagonists. The degree of antiplatelet activity exerted by each drug or drug class depends on where the drug acts in the platelet activation pathway.

Aspirin suppresses platelet aggregation and vasoconstriction by inhibiting cylooxygenase, an enzyme that's needed to create thromboxane A_2 (TXA_2) from arachidonic acid (AA). TXA_2 is responsible for platelet activation and vasoconstriction.

ADP receptor antagonists, such as ticlopidine and clopidogrel, block ADP receptors on the surface of platelets, preventing platelet aggregation.

GP receptor IIb/IIIa inhibitors, such as abciximab, tirofiban, and eptifibatide, are powerful antiplatelet agents because they prevent platelet aggregation in the common pathway, whether aggregation is triggered by thromboxane, ADP, or another factor. These drugs block GP IIb/IIIa receptors from the effects of fibrinogen, thrombin, platelet activating factor (PAF), collagen, and other adhesive molecules. (From Lehne RA: *Pharmacology for Nursing Care*, ed 5, St. Louis, 2004, Saunders.)

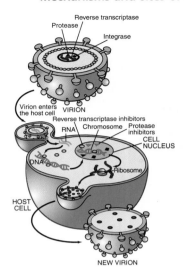

Plate 8: Mechanisms and Sites of Action – Antiretroviral Agents

To understand how antiretroviral agents work, you need to know how viruses reproduce. First, the infectious viral particle or virion enters the host cell. The virion attaches to the cell's surface and then inserts itself into the host cell. Once inside, the virion uncoats, and the enzyme reverse transcriptase makes two copies of the viral RNA: one copy is identical; the other is a mirror image. These two copies merge to form double-stranded viral DNA. This newly formed viral DNA enters the host cell's nucleus, where it inserts itself into the host cell's DNA with the help of the enzyme integrase. Then viral DNA reprograms the host cell to produce additional viral RNA, which begins the process of forming new viruses. Specifically, messenger RNA (mRNA) instructs ribosomal RNA (rRNA) to produce a new chain of proteins and enzymes that are used to form new viruses. Protease, another enzyme, cuts the chains of proteins, creating individual proteins. These individual proteins combine with new RNA to create new virions, which bud and are then released from the host cell.

Antiretroviral agents target specific enzymes during viral reproduction. Many of them work to inhibit reverse transcriptase. Nucleoside reverse transcriptase inhibitors, such as stavudine, interfere with the action of reverse transcriptase by mimicking naturally occurring nucleosides. Nucleotide reverse transcriptase inhibitors, such as tenofovir, block reverse transcriptase by competing with the natural substrate deoxyadenosine triphosphate and by causing DNA chain termination. Nonnucleoside reverse transcriptase inhibitors, such as delavirdine, work by directly binding to reverse transcriptase. All of these actions block the conversion of single-stranded viral RNA into double-stranded DNA. As a result, no viral DNA is available to insert itself into the host cell's DNA. Protease inhibitors, such as indinavir, bind to and interefere with the action of protease. By blocking protease, the new chain of proteins formed by rRNA can't be cut into individual proteins to make new viruses. (From Gutierrez K: *Pharmacotherapeutics: Clinical Decision Making in Nursing*, Philadelphia, 1999, Saunders.)

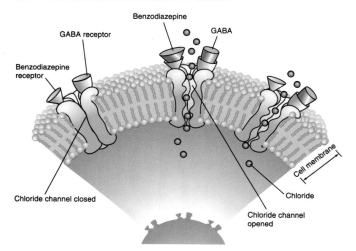

Plate 9: Mechanisms of Action – Benzodiazepines
Benzodiazepines reduce anxiety by stimulating the action of the inhibitory
neurotransmitter, gamma-aminobutyric acid (GABA), in the limbic system. The
limbic system plays an important role in the regulation of human behavior.
Dysfunction of GABA neurotransmission in the limbic system may be linked to the
development of certain anxiety disorders.

The limbic system contains a highly dense area of benzodiazepine receptors that
may be linked to the antianxiety effects of benzodiazepines. These benzodiazepine
receptors are located on the surface of neuronal cell membranes and are adjacent to
GABA receptors. The binding of a benzodiazepine to its receptor enhances the affinity
of a GABA receptor for GABA. In the absence of a benzodiazepine, the binding of
GABA to its receptor causes the chloride channel in the cell membrane to open,
which increases the influx of chloride into the cell. This influx of chloride results in
hyperpolarization of the neuronal cell membrane and reduces the neuron's ability to
fire, which is why GABA is considered an inhibitory neurotransmitter.

A benzodiazepine acts only in the presence of GABA. When it binds to a
benzodiazepine receptor, it prolongs the time that the chloride channel remains
open. This results in greater depression of neuronal function and a reduction in
anxiety. (From Gutierrez K: *Pharmacotherapeutics: Clinical Decision Making in
Nursing*, Philadelphia, 1999, Saunders.)

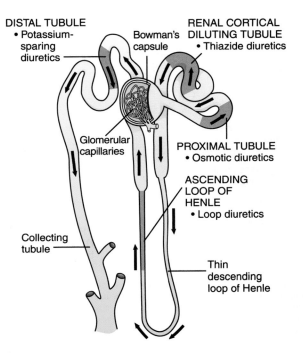

DISTAL TUBULE
• Potassium-sparing diuretics

RENAL CORTICAL DILUTING TUBULE
• Thiazide diuretics

Bowman's capsule

Glomerular capillaries

PROXIMAL TUBULE
• Osmotic diuretics

ASCENDING LOOP OF HENLE
• Loop diuretics

Collecting tubule

Thin descending loop of Henle

Plate 10: Sites of Action – Diuretics

Diuretics act primarily to increase water and sodium excretion by the kidneys, thereby increasing urine output. In the process, chloride, potassium, and other electrolytes may also be excreted. Most diuretics act by blocking sodium, water, and chloride reabsorption by peritubular capillaries in the nephrons. Water and electrolytes remain in the convoluted tubules to be excreted as urine. The increased water and electrolyte excretion reduces blood volume—and ultimately blood pressure.

Diuretics belong to four major subclasses:

1. Thiazide diuretics, such as hydrochlorothiazide, act in the cortical diluting segment. These drugs block sodium, chloride, and water reabsorption and promote their excretion along with potassium.

2. Loop diuretics, such as furosemide, act primarily in the thick ascending limb of the loop of Henle, blocking sodium, water, and chloride reabsorption. Then these substances are excreted along with potassium.

3. Potassium-sparing diuretics, such as spironolactone, act in the late portion of the distal convoluted tubule and collecting tubule. Here, they inhibit the action of aldosterone, leading to sodium excretion and potassium retention. Although triamterene and amiloride act at the same site, they do not affect aldosterone. Instead, these drugs directly block the exchange of sodium and potassium, leading to decreased sodium reabsorption and decreased potassium excretion.

4. Osmotic diuretics, such as mannitol, work in the proximal convoluted tubule. As their name implies, these diuretics increase the osmotic pressure of the glomerular filtrate, inhibiting the passive reabsorption of water, sodium, and chloride. (From Gutierrez K: *Pharmacotherapeutics: Clinical Decision Making in Nursing*, Philadelphia, 1999, Saunders.)

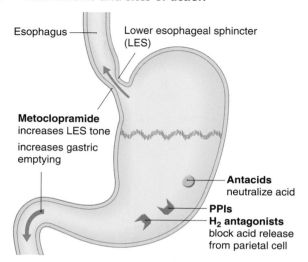

Esophagus — / Lower esophageal sphincter (LES)

Metoclopramide increases LES tone

increases gastric emptying

Antacids neutralize acid

PPIs
H₂ antagonists block acid release from parietal cell

Plate 11: Sites of Action – Drugs Used to Treat GERD
Gastroesophageal reflux disease (GERD) occurs when acidic stomach contents regurgitate into the esophagus, causing heartburn. The disorder may result from a weakness or incompetence of the lower esophageal sphincter (LES). Because the malfunctioning LES makes the reflux leave the esophagus and reenter the stomach slowly, the esophageal mucosa is exposed to the acid for a long time. Because the enzymatic action of parietal cells in the stomach makes the reflux highly acidic, GERD causes irritation and possible erosion of the esophageal mucosa.

Treatment of GERD can employ drugs from several classes: histamine (H_2) antagonists, proton pump inhibitors (PPIs), the miscellaneous GI agent metoclopramide, and antacids. H_2 antagonists, such as cimetidine, act in parietal cells of the stomach. Normally, H_2-receptor stimulation results in gastric acid secretion. By blocking these receptors, H_2 antagonists decrease the amount and acidity of gastric secretion, including secretion that occurs with fasting, food consumption at night, and stomach distension.

PPIs, such as esomeprazole, also suppress gastric acid secretion. However, they do it by inhibiting the hydrogen-potassium-adenosine triphosphatase enzyme system, which is located on the surface of parietal cells and controls their gastric acid secretion. PPIs block acid secretion that results from fasting or abdominal distension caused by food ingestion.

Metoclopramide increases the tone and motility of the upper GI tract. It works by stimulating the release of acetylcholine from GI nerve endings, which improves LES tone and leads to decreased reflux. The drug also stimulates gastric emptying, which reduces gastric contents.

Antacids, such as aluminum hydroxide, act primarily in the stomach by chemically combining with the hydrogen ions (H^+) in gastric acid and raising the pH of gastric contents. They don't prevent reflux. However, they make the reflux less acidic, so it causes less damage to the esophageal mucosa. (From Page C, et al: *Integrated Pharmacology*, ed 2, St. Louis, 2002, Mosby.)

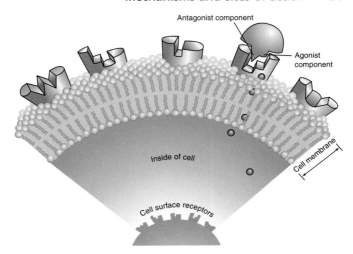

Plate 12:   Mechanisms of Action – Narcotic Agonist-Antagonist Analgesics
Cell membranes have different types of opioid receptors, such as mu, kappa, and
delta receptors. Opioid agonist-antagonists work by stimulating one type of receptor,
while simultaneously blocking another type. As agonists, they work primarily by
activating kappa receptors to produce analgesia and such other effects as CNS and
respiratory depression, decreased GI motility, and euphoria. As antagonists, they
compete with opioids at mu receptors, helping to reverse or block some of the other
effects of agonists. (From Gutierrez K: *Pharmacotherapeutics: Clinical Decision
Making in Nursing*, Philadelphia, 1999, Saunders.)

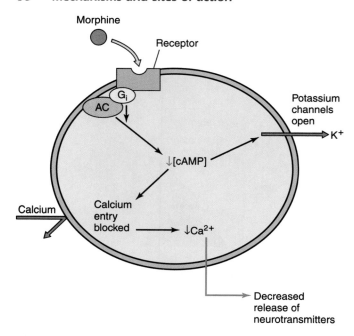

Plate 13:   Mechanisms of Action – Narcotic Analgesics

Narcotic analgesics bind to three types of opioid receptors: mu, kappa, and delta receptors. They produce analgesia primarily by activating mu receptors. However, they also engage with and activate kappa and delta receptors, producing other effects, such as sedation and vasomotor stimulation.

When morphine or another narcotic analgesic binds to opioid receptors, activation occurs. The receptors send signals to the enzyme adenyl cyclase (AC) to slow activity by way of G proteins (G_i). Decreased adenyl cyclase activity causes less cyclic adenosine monophosphate (cAMP) to be produced. A secondary messenger substance, cAMP is important for regulating cell membrane channels. A reduced cAMP level allows fewer potassium ions to leave the cell and blocks calcium ions from entering the cell. This ion imbalance—especially the reduced intracellular calcium level—ultimately decreases the release of neurotransmitters from the cell, thereby blocking or reducing pain impulse transmission. (From Brody TM, Larner J, Minneman KP: *Human Pharmacology: Molecular to Clinical*, ed 3, St. Louis, 1998, Mosby.)

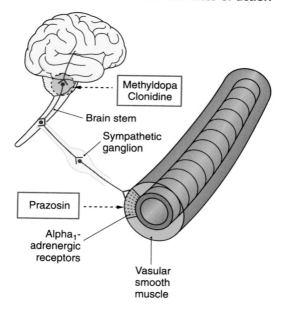

Plate 14:   Sites of Action – Sympatholytics

Sympatholytics inhibit sympathetic nervous system (SNS) activity, which plays a major role in regulating BP. Normally when the SNS is stimulated, nerve impulses travel from the cardiovascular center of the CNS to the sympathetic ganglia. From there, the impulses travel along postganglionic fibers to specific effector organs, such as the heart and blood vessels. SNS stimulation also triggers the release of norepinephrine, which acts primarily at alpha-adrenergic receptors.

Sympatholytics fall into two subclasses: central-acting alpha$_2$ agonists and peripheral-acting alpha$_1$-adrenergic antagonists. Central-acting alpha$_2$ agonists, such as methyldopa and clonidine, stimulate alpha$_2$-adrenergic receptors in the cardiovascular center of the CNS and reduce activity in the vasomotor center of the brain, interfering with sympathetic stimulation of the heart and blood vessels. This causes blood vessel dilation and decreased cardiac output, which leads to reduced BP.

Peripheral-acting alpha$_1$-adrenergic antagonists, such as prazosin, inhibit the stimulation of alpha$_1$-adrenergic receptors by norepinephrine in vascular smooth muscle, interfering with SNS-induced vasoconstriction. As a result, the blood vessels dilate, reducing peripheral vascular resistance and venous return to the heart. These effects, in turn, lead to decreased BP. (From Prosser S, Worster B, Dewar K: *Applied Pharmacology for Nurses and Other Health Care Professionals*, St. Louis, 2000, Mosby.)

abacavir (Ŗ)
(ah-bak'ah-veer)
Ziagen
Func. class.: Antiretroviral
Chem. class.: Nucleoside reverse transcriptase inhibitor (NRTI)

Action: A synthetic nucleoside analog with inhibitory action against HIV-1; inhibits replication of the virus by incorporating into cellular DNA by viral reverse transcriptase, thereby terminating the cellular DNA chain

Uses: In combination with other antiretroviral agents for HIV-1 infection (not to be used with lamivudine or tenofovir)

DOSAGE AND ROUTES
• *Adult:* **PO** 300 mg bid or 600 mg daily with other antiretrovirals
• *Adolescents and child ≥3 mo:* **PO** 8 mg/kg bid, max 300 mg bid with other antiretrovirals
Hepatic dose
• *Adult:* **PO** (oral sol) (Child-Pugh 5-6) 200 mg bid
Available forms: Tabs 300 mg; oral sol 20 mg/ml

SIDE EFFECTS
CNS: Fever, headache, malaise, insomnia, paresthesia
GI: Nausea, vomiting, diarrhea, anorexia, cramps, abdominal pain, increased AST, ALT, **hepatotoxicity**
HEMA: **Granulocytopenia, anemia, lymphopenia**
INTEG: Rash, urticaria, hypersensitivity reactions
META: **Lactic acidosis**
OTHER: Increased CPK, **fatal hypersensitivity reactions**
RESP: Dyspnea
Contraindications: Hypersensitivity, lactic acidosis
Precautions: Pregnancy (C), granulocyte count <1000/mm^3 or Hgb <9.5 g/dl, lactation, children, severe renal disease, impaired hepatic function, child < 3 mo

PHARMACOKINETICS
50% plasma protein binding; extensively metabolized to inactive metabolites, half-life 1½ hr; excreted in urine, feces (unchanged)

INTERACTIONS
Increase: possible lactic acidosis—ribavirin
Increase: abacavir levels—alcohol
Decrease: levels of methadose

NURSING CONSIDERATIONS
Assess:
• For symptoms of HIV and for possible infections
⚠ For lactic acidosis (elevated lactate levels, increased LFTs) severe hepatomegaly with steatosis, discontinue treatment and do not restart; may have large liver, elevated AST, ALT, lactate levels
⚠ For fatal hypersensitivity reactions: fever, rash, nausea, vomiting, fatigue, cough, dyspnea, diarrhea, abdominal discomfort; treatment should be discontinued and not restarted
• For blood dyscrasias (anemia, granulocytopenia): bruising, fatigue, bleeding, poor healing
• For increased temp, may indicate beginning infection
• Renal studies: BUN, serum uric acid, CCr before, during therapy; these may be elevated throughout treatment
• Hepatic studies before and during therapy: bilirubin, AST, ALT, amylase, alk phos, creatine phosphokinase, creatinine, q mo
• Blood counts q2wk; monitor viral load and CD4 counts during treatment; watch for decreasing granulocytes, Hgb; if low, therapy may have to be discontinued and restarted after hematologic recovery; blood transfusions may be required
Administer:
• Give in combination with other antiretrovirals with or without food
• Reduce dose in hepatic disease, use oral sol

Side effects: *italics* = common; **bold** = life-threatening

Perform/provide:
• Storage in cool environment; protect from light; oral sol stored at room temp; do not freeze

Evaluate:
• Therapeutic response: increased CD4 count, decrease viral load

Teach patient/family:
• That drug is not a cure for AIDS but will control symptoms
• To notify prescriber of sore throat, swollen lymph nodes, malaise, fever; other infections may occur; to stop drug if skin rash, fever, cough, shortness of breath, GI symptoms, notify prescriber immediately; advise all health care providers that allergic reaction has occurred with abacavir
• That patient is still infective, may pass AIDS virus on to others
• That follow-up visits must be continued since serious toxicity may occur; blood counts must be done
• To use contraception during treatment
• Give patient Medication Guide and Warning Card, discuss points on guide
• That other drugs may be necessary to prevent other infections
• Do not drink alcohol while taking this drug

---

abarelix (℞)
(a-ba-rel′iks)
Plenaxis
Func. class.: Gonadotropin-releasing hormone antagonist
Chem. class.: Synthetic decapeptide

Action: Inhibitor of pituitary gonadotropin secretion; inhibits LH, FSH, thereby reducing testosterone
Uses: Palliative treatment of prostate cancer

DOSAGE AND ROUTES
• *Adult:* **IM** 100 mg in buttock on day 1, 15, 29 (wk 4), and every 4 wk thereafter
Available forms: Powder for inj 113 mg

SIDE EFFECTS
CNS: Headache, dizziness, fatigue, sleep disturbance
ENDO: Breast enlargement, nipple tenderness
GI: Nausea, constipation, diarrhea
GU: Dysuria, frequency, retention, UTI
INTEG: Pain on inj; local site reactions
MISC: Pain including back pain, hot flashes
SYST: **Anaphylaxis, systemic allergic reaction,** decreased bone density (long-term treatment)
Contraindications: Pregnancy (X), hypersensitivity, latex allergy, lactation, children

PHARMACOKINETICS
Excreted in urine, half-life depends on dosage, protein binding 96%-99%

NURSING CONSIDERATIONS
Assess:
• Anaphylaxis: swelling of face, throat, eyes, tongue, chest tightness, difficulty breathing; hypotension, fainting, shock; if these occur, usually occur within ½ hr of administration
• For ALT, AST, GGT, alk phos

Administer:
• Reconstitute 1 vial with provided diluent (50 mg/ml)
• Before reconstituting gently shake vial; hold at 45-degree angle and tap lightly to break caking; withdraw 2.2 ml of 0.9% NaCl inj using 18-gauge, 1½-inch needle and 3-ml syringe enclosed; discard remaining unused diluent
• Keeping vial upright, insert needle all the way in the vial and inject diluent quickly; withdraw needle, removing 2.2 ml of air; shake for several seconds; allow vial to stand for 2 min; tap to remove foam, swirl

Perform/provide:
• Storage at 59°-80° F; use within 1 hr of reconstitution

Evaluate:
• Therapeutic response: reduction in growth of tumor

Teach patient/family:
• To notify prescriber if family members have QTc interval prolongation
• To notify prescriber immediately of chest, throat tightness, flushing, lightheadedness, shortness of breath
⚠ Chances of serious or life-threatening allergic reaction may increase with each inj

abatacept (℞)
(ab-a-ta'sept)
Orencia
Func. class.: Antirheumatic agent (disease modifying); biologic response modifier

Action: A selective costimulation modulator, inhibits T-lymphocytes, inhibits tumor necrosis factor (TNF-α), interferon-γ, interleukin-2, which are involved in immune and inflammatory reactions
Uses: Acute, chronic rheumatoid arthritis that has not responded to other disease-modifying agents, may use in combination with DMARDs; do not use with TNF antagonists (adalimumab, etanercept, infliximab); anakinra

DOSAGE AND ROUTES
• *Adult >100 kg:* IV INF 1 g
• *Adult 60-100 kg:* IV INF 750 mg
• *Adult <60 kg:* IV INF 500 mg over 30 min; give 2-4 wk after 1st **INF,** then q4wk
Available forms: Lyophilized powder, single use vials 250 mg

SIDE EFFECTS
CNS: Headache, asthenia, dizziness
CV: Hypertension, hypotension
GI: Abdominal pain, dyspepsia, nausea
INTEG: Rash, *inj site reaction,* flushing, urticaria, pruritus
RESP: Pharyngitis, cough, URI, non-URI, *rhinitis,* wheezing
SYST: **Anaphylaxis, malignancies, angioedema**
Contraindications: Hypersensitivity, TB

Precautions: Pregnancy (C), lactation, children, geriatric, recurrent infections, COPD

PHARMACOKINETICS
Terminal half-life 13-16 days, steady state 60 days

INTERACTIONS
• Do not give concurrently with vaccines; immunizations should be brought up to date before treatment
• Do not use with TNF antagonists: (adalimumab, etanercept, infliximab); anakinra
• Do not use with corticosteroids, immunosuppressives

NURSING CONSIDERATIONS
Assess:
• For latent/active TB before beginning treatment
• Pain, stiffness, ROM, swelling of joints during treatment
• For inj site pain, swelling
• Patient's overall health on each visit; product should not be given with active infections
Administer:
• To reconstitute, remove plastic flip top from vial and wipe the top with alcohol wipe; insert syringe needle into vial and direct stream of sterile water for inj on the wall of vial; rotate vial until mixed; vent with needle to rid foam after reconstitution 25 mg/ml; further dilute in 100 ml from a 100-ml infusion bag/bottle; withdraw the needed volume (2 vials remove 20 mg; 3 vials remove 30 ml, 4 vials remove 40 ml); slowly add the reconstituted Orencia sol from each vial into the infusion bag/bottle using the same disposable syringe supplied; mix gently, discard unused portions of vials; do not use if particulate is present or discolored; give over 30 min; use non–protein binding filter (0.2-1.2 mcg)
• Do not admix with other sol or medications

Perform/provide:
• Storage in refrigerator; do not use expired vials
Evaluate:
• Therapeutic response: decreased inflammation, pain in joints
Teach patient/family:
• That drug must be continued for prescribed time to be effective
• To use caution when driving; dizziness may occur
• Not to have vaccinations while taking this product
• Regarding patient information included in packaging

Rarely Used⚠ High Alert

abciximab (℞)
(ab-six'i-mab)
ReoPro
Func. class.: Platelet aggregation inhibitor

Uses: Used with heparin and aspirin to prevent acute cardiac ischemia following percutaneous transluminal coronary angioplasty (PTCA) in patients at high risk for reclosure of affected arteries

DOSAGE AND ROUTES
Percutaneous coronary intervention (PCI)
• *Adult:* **IV BOL** 250 mcg (0.25 mg)/kg 10-60 min prior to PCI, followed by 125 mcg/kg/min **CONT INF** for 12 hr
MI
• *Adult:* **IV BOL** 0.25 mg over 5 min, then 0.125 mcg/kg/min, max 10 mcg/min; **IV INF** for 12 hr unless complications
Contraindications: Hypersensitivity to this drug or murine protein; GI, GU bleeding; CVA within 2 yr, bleeding disorders, intracranial neoplasm, intracranial arteriovenous malformations, intracranial aneurysm, platelet count <100,000/mm^3, recent surgery, aneurysm, uncontrolled severe hypertension, vasculitis, coagulopathy

Rarely Used

acamprosate (℞)
(a-kam-proe'sate)
Campral
Func. class.: Antialcoholic agent

Uses: For maintenance of abstinence from alcohol in alcohol dependence

DOSAGE AND ROUTES
• *Adult:* **PO** 666 mg tid
Renal dose
• *Adult:* **PO** 333 mg tid
Contraindications: Hypersensitivity, severe renal disease, CCr <30 ml/min

acarbose (℞)
(ay-car'bose)
Precose
Func. class.: Oral antidiabetic
Chem. class.: α-Glucosidase inhibitor

Do not confuse:
Precose/preCare
Action: Delays digestion of ingested carbohydrates by inhibiting α glucosidase, results in smaller rise in postprandial blood glucose after meals; does not increase insulin production
Uses: Type 1 diabetes mellitus, alone or in combination with a sulfonylurea

DOSAGE AND ROUTES
• *Adult:* **PO** 25 mg tid initially, with first bite of meal; maintenance dose may be increased to 50-100 mg tid; dosage adjustment at 4-8 wk intervals
• *Adult <60 kg:* **PO** Not to exceed 50 mg tid
Available forms: Tabs 25, 50, 100 mg

SIDE EFFECTS
GI: Abdominal pain, diarrhea, flatulence, increased serum transaminase level
Contraindications: Hypersensitivity, diabetic ketoacidosis, cirrhosis, inflammatory bowel disease, colonic ulceration,

partial intestinal obstruction, chronic intestinal disease, serum creatinine >2 mg/dl

Precautions: Pregnancy (B), lactation, children, renal/hepatic disease

PHARMACOKINETICS

Peak 1 hr, metabolized in GI tract, excreted as intact drug in urine, half-life 2 hr

INTERACTIONS

Increase: hypoglycemia—sulfonylureas, insulin

Decrease: effect, increase hyperglycemia—digestive enzymes, intestinal absorbents, thiazide diuretics, loop diuretics, corticosteroids, estrogen, progestins, oral contraceptives, sympathomimetics, calcium channel blockers, isoniazid, phenothiazines, digoxin

Drug/Herb

Increase: hypoglycemia—alfalfa, aloe, basil, bay, bilberry, bitter melon, black cohosh, buchu, burdock, chromium, coenzyme Q10, coriander, eyebright (PO), fenugreek, garlic, ginseng *(Panax),* glucomannan, glucosamine, goat's rue, gymnema, horehound, horse chestnut, jambul, myrrh, myrtle, raspberry, Siberian ginseng

Decrease: hypoglycemia—bee pollen, blue cohosh, broom chromium, elecampane, eucalyptus, gotu kola, senega

Drug/Lab Test

Increase: AST, bilirubin

Decrease: Calcium, vit B_6

NURSING CONSIDERATIONS

Assess:

• Hypoglycemia (weakness, hunger, dizziness, tremors, anxiety, tachycardia, sweating), hyperglycemia; even though drug does not cause hypoglycemia, if patient is on sulfonylureas or insulin, hypoglycemia may be additive; if hypoglycemia occurs, treat with dextrose, or if severe, IV glucose or glucagon

• 1 hr postprandial for establishing effectiveness, then A1c q3mo

• Monitor AST, ALT q3mo × 1 yr and periodically thereafter; if elevated, dose may need to be reduced or discontinued; obtain A1c periodically

Administer:

PO route

• Tid with first bite of each meal

Perform/provide:

• Storage in tight container in cool environment

Evaluate:

• Therapeutic response: improved signs/symptoms of diabetes mellitus (decreased polyuria, polydipsia, polyphagia; clear sensorium, absence of dizziness, stable gait)

Teach patient/family:

• The symptoms of hypo/hyperglycemia, what to do about each

• That medication must be taken as prescribed; explain consequences of discontinuing medication abruptly; that insulin may need to be used for stress, including trauma, surgery, fever

• To avoid OTC medications, herbal supplements unless approved by health care provider

• That diabetes is lifelong illness; that this drug is not a cure

• To carry emergency ID for emergency purposes; carry glucagon kit, sugar source

• That diet and exercise regimen must be followed

---

acebutolol (℞)

(a-se-byoo′toe- lole)
Monitan ✦, Sectral
Func. class.: Antihypertensive, antidysrhythmic (II)
Chem. class.: β_1 Blocker

Action: Competitively blocks stimulation of β-adrenergic receptors within vascular smooth muscle; decreases rate of SA node discharge, increases recovery time, slows conduction of AV node resulting in decreased heart rate (negative chronotropic effect), which decreases O_2 consumption in myocardium due to

β_1-receptor antagonism; also decreases renin-aldosterone-angiotensin system at high doses, inhibits β_2-receptors in bronchial system (high doses)

Uses: Mild to moderate hypertension, sinus tachycardia, persistent atrial extrasystoles, tachydysrhythmias, management of PVCs

Unlabeled uses: Prophylaxis of MI, treatment of angina pectoris, tremor, mitral valve prolapse, thyrotoxicosis, idiopathic hypertrophic subaortic stenosis, neurocardiogenic syncope

DOSAGE AND ROUTES

Hypertension
• *Adult:* **PO** 400 mg daily or in 2 divided doses; may be increased to desired response; maintenance 200-1200 mg/daily in 2 divided doses
• *Geriatric:* Not to exceed 800 mg daily

Ventricular dysrhythmia
• *Adult:* **PO** 200 mg bid, may increase gradually; usual range 600-1200 mg daily; should be tapered over 2 wk before discontinuing
• *Geriatric:* Not to exceed 800 mg daily

PVC management
• *Adult:* **PO** 200 mg bid, may increase gradually; usual range 600-1200 mg daily in divided doses
• *Geriatric:* Not to exceed 800 mg daily

Renal dose
• *Adult:* **PO** CCr 25-50 ml/min, reduce dose by 50%; if <25 ml/min reduce dose by 75%

Available forms: Caps 200, 400 mg; tabs 100, 200, 400 mg ✤

SIDE EFFECTS

CNS: Insomnia, fatigue, dizziness, mental changes, memory loss, hallucinations, depression, lethargy, drowsiness, strange dreams, catatonia, headache
CV: **Profound hypotension, bradycardia, CHF,** *cold extremities, postural hypotension,* **2nd-/3rd-degree heart block,** edema
EENT: Sore throat; dry, burning eyes
ENDO: Increased hypoglycemic response to insulin

GI: Nausea, diarrhea, vomiting, **mesenteric arterial thrombosis, ischemic colitis, flatulence**
GU: Impotence, decreased libido, dysuria, nocturia, polyuria
HEMA: **Agranulocytosis, thrombocytopenia, purpura**
INTEG: Rash, flushing, pruritus, sweating, alopecia, dry skin
MISC: Facial swelling, weight gain, decreased exercise tolerance
MS: Joint pain, cramping
RESP: **Bronchospasm,** dyspnea, wheezing, cough

Contraindications: Hypersensitivity to this agent or β-blockers; cardiogenic shock, heart block (2nd, 3rd degree), sinus bradycardia, CHF, cardiac failure
Precautions: Pregnancy (B), major surgery, lactation, peripheral vascular disease, children, diabetes mellitus, thyroid disease, COPD, asthma, well-compensated heart failure, renal/hepatic disease

PHARMACOKINETICS

PO: Onset 1-1½ hr, peak 2-4 hr, duration 10-12 hr, half-life 3-4 hr, metabolized in liver, 30%-40% excreted in urine, protein binding 10%-26%

INTERACTIONS

• Attenuated effects: oral sulfonylureas
• Peripheral ischemia: ergots
Increase: hypotension, bradycardia—reserpine, hydrALAZINE, methyldopa, prazosin, anticholinergics, cardiac glycosides, diltiazem, verapamil, diuretics, other antihypertensives, calcium channel blockers, cimetidine
Increase: hypoglycemic effect—insulin
Decrease: antihypertensive effects—NSAIDs, calcium, cholestyramine, colestipol
Decrease: bronchodilation—theophyllines, β_2-agonists

Drug/Herb
• May increase acebutolol effect—aloe, betel palm, buckthorn bark/berry, butterbur, cascara sagrada bark, cola tree, fig-

---

wort, fumitory, guarana, hawthorn, lily of the valley, motherwort, plantain, rhubarb root, senna leaf/fruits

• Toxicity/death: aconite

Decrease: acebutolol effect—St. John's wort

Decrease: antihypertensive effect—coenzyme Q10, yohimbe

Drug/Lab Test

Increase: Serum lipoprotein levels, BUN, potassium, triglyceride, uric acid, LDH, AST, ALT, blood glucose, alk phos

Positive: ANA titer

NURSING CONSIDERATIONS

Assess:

• B/P during beginning treatment, periodically thereafter; pulse q4h; note rate, rhythm, quality

• Apical/radial pulse before administration; notify prescriber of any significant changes (pulse <50 bpm); signs of CHF (dyspnea, crackles, weight gain, jugular vein distention)

• Baselines in renal, hepatic studies before therapy begins

• Edema in feet, legs daily: monitor I&O

• Skin turgor, dryness of mucous membranes for hydration status, especially geriatric

Administer:

PO route

• Drug before meals, at bedtime, tablet may be crushed or swallowed whole; give with food to prevent GI upset

Perform/provide:

• Storage protected from light, moisture; place in cool environment

Evaluate:

• Therapeutic response: decreased B/P after 1-2 wk; decreased dysrhythmias

Teach patient/family:

⚠ Not to discontinue drug abruptly, severe cardiac reactions may occur, taper over 2 wk; do not double dose; if a dose is missed, take as soon as remembered up to 4 hr before next dose

• Drug may mask signs of hypoglycemia or alter blood glucose levels

• Not to use OTC products containing α-adrenergic stimulants (such as nasal decongestants, OTC cold preparations) unless directed by prescriber

• To report low pulse, dizziness, confusion, depression, fever

• To take pulse, B/P at home, advise when to notify prescriber

• To comply with weight control, dietary adjustments, modified exercise program

• To carry emergency ID to identify drug, allergies

• To avoid hazardous activities if dizziness, drowsiness is present

• To report symptoms of CHF: difficult breathing, especially on exertion or when lying down, night cough, swelling of extremities

• To continue with required lifestyle changes (exercise, diet, weight loss, stress reduction)

Treatment of overdose: Lavage, IV atropine for bradycardia, IV theophylline for bronchospasm, digoxin, O_2, diuretic for cardiac failure, IV glucose for hypoglycemia, IV diazepam (or phenytoin) for seizures

acetaminophen (otc)

(a-seat-a-mee'noe-fen)
Abenol ♣, Acephen, Aceta,
Actimol, Aminofen, Apacet,
APAP, Apo-Acetaminophen ♣,
Arthritis Foundation Pain
Reliever Aspirin-Free, Aspirin-
Free Anacin, Aspirin-Free
Pain Relief, Atasol ♣,
Banesin, Children's Feverall,
Dapa, Dapacin, Datril,
Exdol ♣, FemEtts, Genapap,
Genebs, Halenol, Liquiprin,
Mapap, Maranox, Meda,
Neopap, Oraphen-PD,
Panadol, Redutemp,
Robigesic ♣, Rounax ♣,
Silapap, Tapanol, Tempra,
Tylenol
Func. class.: Nonopioid analgesic,
antipyretic
Chem. class.: Nonsalicylate,
paraaminophenol derivative

Action: May block pain impulses peripherally that occur in response to inhibition of prostaglandin synthesis; does not
possess antiinflammatory properties; antipyretic action results from inhibition of
prostaglandins in the CNS (hypothalamic
heat-regulating center)
Uses: Mild pain or fever

DOSAGE AND ROUTES

• *Adult and child >12 yr:* **PO/RECT**
325-650 mg q4h prn, max 4 g/day
• *Child:* **PO** 10-15 mg/kg q4h
• *Child 6-12 yr:* **RECT** 325 mg q4-6h,
max 2.6 g/day
• *Child 3-6 yr:* **RECT** 125 mg q4-6h,
max 720 mg/day
• *Child 1-3 yr:* **RECT** 80 mg q4h
• *Child 3-11 mo:* **RECT** 80 mg q6h
Available forms: Rect supp 80, 120,
125, 325, 600, 650 mg; soft chew tabs
80, 160 mg; caps 500 mg; elix 120, 160,
325 mg/5 ml; liq 160 mg/5 ml, 500

mg/15 ml; sol 100 mg/1 ml, 120 mg/2.5
ml; granules 80 mg/packet, 80 mg/cap;
tabs 160, 325, 500, 650 mg

SIDE EFFECTS

CNS: Stimulation, drowsiness
GI: Nausea, vomiting, abdominal pain; **hepatotoxicity, hepatic seizure (overdose)**
GU: **Renal failure (high, prolonged
doses)**
HEMA: **Leukopenia, neutropenia, hemolytic anemia (long-term use),
thrombocytopenia, pancytopenia**
INTEG: Rash, urticaria
SYST: Hypersensitivity
TOXICITY: **Cyanosis, anemia, neutropenia, jaundice, pancytopenia, CNS
stimulation, delirium followed by
vascular collapse, convulsions, coma,
death**
Contraindications: Hypersensitivity,
intolerance to tartrazine (yellow dye #5),
alcohol, table sugar, saccharin, depending on product
Precautions: Pregnancy (B), anemia,
renal/hepatic disease, chronic alcoholism, geriatric, lactation

PHARMACOKINETICS

Well absorbed PO, rectal absorption
varies; 85%-90% metabolized by liver,
excreted by kidneys; metabolites may
be toxic if overdose occurs; widely distributed, crosses placenta in low concentrations, excreted in breast milk,
half-life 1-4 hr
PO: Onset 10-30 min, peak ½-2 hr,
duration 3-4 hr
RECT: Onset slow, peak 1-2 hr, duration 3-4 hr

INTERACTIONS

• Hypoprothrombinemia: warfarin, long-
term use, high doses of acetaminophen
• Bone marrow suppression: zidovudine
• Renal adverse reactions: NSAIDs, salicylates

Decrease: effect, increase hepatotoxicity—barbiturates, alcohol, carbamazepine, hydantoins, rifampin, rifabutin, isoniazid, diflunisal, sulfinpyrazone
Decrease: absorption—colestipol, cholestyramine

Drug/Lab Test
Interference: Chemstrip G, Dextrostix, Visidex II, 5-HIAA

NURSING CONSIDERATIONS
Assess:
• Hepatic studies: AST, ALT, bilirubin, creatinine prior to therapy if long-term therapy is anticipated; may cause hepatic toxicity at doses >4 g/day with chronic use
• Renal studies: BUN, urine creatinine, occult blood, albumin, if patient is on long-term therapy; presence of blood or albumin indicates nephritis
• Blood studies: CBC, PT if patient is on long-term therapy
• I&O ratio; decreasing output may indicate renal failure (long-term therapy)
• For fever and pain: type of pain, location, intensity, duration
• For chronic poisoning: rapid, weak pulse; dyspnea; cold, clammy extremities; report immediately to prescriber
• Hepatotoxicity: dark urine; clay-colored stools; yellowing of skin, sclera; itching, abdominal pain; fever; diarrhea if patient is on long-term therapy
• Allergic reactions: rash, urticaria; if these occur, drug may have to be discontinued

Administer:
PO route
• Crushed or whole; chewable tablets may be chewed; give with full glass of water
• With food or milk to decrease gastric symptoms if needed

Perform/provide:
• Storage of suppositories <80° F (27° C)

Evaluate:
• Therapeutic response: absence of pain, fever

Teach patient/family:
⚠ Not to exceed recommended dosage;

acute poisoning with liver damage may result

⚠ That acute toxicity includes symptoms of nausea, vomiting, abdominal pain; prescriber should be notified immediately
• To read label on other OTC drugs; many contain acetaminophen and may cause toxicity if taken concurrently
• To recognize signs of chronic overdose: bleeding, bruising, malaise, fever, sore throat
• To notify prescriber of pain or fever lasting over 3 days

Treatment of overdose: Drug level, gastric lavage, activated charcoal; administer oral acetylcysteine to prevent hepatic damage *(see acetylcysteine monograph),* monitor for bleeding

---

*acetaZOLAMIDE (Ŗ)
(a-set-a-zole′a-mide)
acetaZOLAMIDE,
Apo-Acetazolamide ✤,
Dazamide, Diamox, Diamox
Sequels
Func. class.: Diuretic, carbonic anhydrase inhibitor, antiglaucoma agent, antiepileptic
Chem. class.: Sulfonamide derivative

Do not confuse:
acetaZOLAMIDE/acetoHEXAMIDE
Diamox/Trimox/Dobutrex

Action: Inhibits carbonic anhydrase activity in proximal renal tubules to decrease reabsorption of water, sodium, potassium, bicarbonate resulting in increased urine volume and alkalinization of urine; decreases carbonic anhydrase in CNS, increasing seizure threshold; able to decrease secretion of aqueous humor in eye, which lowers intraocular pressure

Uses: Open-angle glaucoma, narrow-angle glaucoma (preoperatively, if surgery delayed), epilepsy (petit mal, grand mal, mixed), edema in CHF, drug-induced edema, acute mountain sickness

Unlabeled uses: Urine alkalinization, respiratory stimulation in COPD, metabolic alkalosis, decrease CSF production in infants with hydrocephalus

DOSAGE AND ROUTES

Urine alkalinization
• *Adult:* **PO** 5 mg/kg/dose, repeat 2-3× over 24 hr

Respiratory stimulant in COPD
• *Adult:* **PO/IV** 250 mg bid

Closed-angle glaucoma
• *Adult:* **PO/IV** 250 mg q4h or 250 mg bid, to be used for short-term therapy

Open-angle glaucoma
• *Adult:* **PO/IV** 250 mg-1 g/day in divided doses for amounts over 250 mg or 500 mg SR bid

Edema in CHF
• *Adult:* **IV** 250-375 mg/day in ᴀᴍ
• *Child:* **IV** 5 mg/kg/day in ᴀᴍ

Seizures
• *Adult:* **PO/IV** 8-30 mg/kg/day, in 1-4 divided doses, usual range 375-1000 mg/day; **ER** not recommended in seizures
• *Child:* **PO/IV** 8-30 mg/kg/day in divided doses tid or qid, or 300-900 mg/m²/day, not to exceed 1 g/day

Mountain sickness
• *Adult:* **PO** 250 mg q8-12h; **EXT REL** 500 mg q12-24h, start therapy 24-48h prior to ascent and for ≥48 hr after arrival at high altitude

Renal stones
• *Adult:* **PO** 250 mg at bedtime

Infants with hydrocephalus
• *Infant:* **IV** 20-55 mg/kg/24h given in divided doses q8-12h

Renal dose
• *Adult:* **PO/IV** CCr 10-50 ml/min give dose q12h; CCr <10 ml/min, avoid use
• *Geriatric:* **PO** 250 mg bid, use lowest effective dose

Available forms: Tabs 125, 250 mg; ext rel caps 500 mg; inj 500 mg

SIDE EFFECTS

CNS: Anxiety, confusion, **convulsions,** depression, dizziness, *drowsiness,* fatigue, headache, *paresthesia,* stimulation
EENT: Myopia, tinnitus
ENDO: Hyperglycemia
GI: Nausea, vomiting, anorexia, diarrhea, melena, weight loss, **hepatic insufficiency, cholestatic jaundice, fulminant hepatic necrosis,** *taste alterations*
GU: Frequency, polyuria, **uremia,** glucosuria, hematuria, dysuria, crystalluria, renal calculi
HEMA: **Aplastic anemia, hemolytic anemia, leukopenia, thrombocytopenia, purpura, pancytopenia**
INTEG: Rash, pruritus, urticaria, fever, **Stevens-Johnson syndrome,** photosensitivity, flushing
META: Hypokalemia, hyperchloremic acidosis, hyponatremia

Contraindications: Hypersensitivity to sulfonamides, severe renal/hepatic disease, electrolyte imbalances (hyponatremia, hypokalemia), hyperchloremic acidosis, Addison's disease, long-term use in narrow-angle glaucoma, adrenalcortical insufficiency

Precautions: Pregnancy (C), hypercalciuria, lactation, respiratory acidosis, COPD

PHARMACOKINETICS

PO: Onset 1-1½ hr, peak 2-4 hr, duration 8-12 hr
PO-SUS REL: Onset 2 hr, peak 3-6 hr, duration 18-24 hr
IV: Onset 2 min, peak 15 min, duration 4-5 hr, 65% absorbed if fasting (oral), 75% absorbed if given with food; half-life 2½-5½ hr; excreted unchanged by kidneys (80% within 24 hr), crosses placenta

INTERACTIONS

Increase: action of amphetamines, flecainide, memantine, phenytoin, procainamide, quinidine, anticholinergics
Increase: excretion of lithium, primidone
Increase: toxicity—salicylates, cycloSPORINE
Increase: side effects—diflunisal
Decrease: acetaZOLAMIDE effect—methenamine
Decrease: primidone levels

Drug/Lab Test
Decrease: Thyroid iodine uptake
False positive: Urinary protein, 17 hydroxysteroid

NURSING CONSIDERATIONS
Assess:
• Weight daily, I&O daily to determine fluid loss; effect of drug may be decreased if used daily; monitor geriatric for dehydration
• For cross-sensitivity between other sulfonamides and this drug
• B/P lying, standing; postural hypotension may occur
• Electrolytes: K, Na, Cl; also BUN, blood glucose, CBC, serum creatinine, blood pH, ABGs, LFTs; I&O, glucose, patient may need to be on a high-potassium diet
Administer:
• In AM to avoid interference with sleep if using drug as diuretic
• Potassium replacement if potassium level is less than 3 mg/dl
PO route
• Do not break, crush, or chew sus rel caps
• With food if nausea occurs; absorption may be decreased slightly
IV route
• After diluting 500 mg in >5 ml sterile H₂O for injection; direct IV—give at 100-500 mg/min; may be diluted further in LR, D₅W, D₁₀W, 0.45% NaCl, 0.9% NaCl, or Ringer's sol and infused over 4-8 hr; use within 24 hr of dilution
Additive compatibilities: Cimetidine, ranitidine
Perform/provide:
• Storage in dark, cool area; use reconstituted solution within 24 hr
Evaluate:
• Therapeutic response: improvement in edema of feet, legs, sacral area daily if medication is being used in CHF; or decrease in aqueous humor if medication is being used in glaucoma
Teach patient/family:
• To take exactly as prescribed; if dose is missed, take as soon as remembered; do not double dose

• To notify prescriber if sore throat, unusual bleeding, bruising, paresthesias, tremors, flank pain, or skin rash occurs
• To use sunscreen to prevent photosensitivity; to monitor blood glucose and urine for sugar
• To avoid hazardous activities if drowsiness occurs
• Increase fluids to 2-3 L/day if not contraindicated
• Report nausea, vertigo, rapid weight gain, change in stools
Treatment of overdose: Lavage if taken orally; monitor electrolytes; administer dextrose in saline; monitor hydration, CV, renal status

---

acetylcholine ophthalmic
See Appendix C

---

acetylcysteine (℞)
(a-se-teel-sis'tay-een)
Acetadote, Mucomyst ✦, Mucosil, Parvolex ✦
Func. class.: Mucolytic; antidote—acetaminophen
Chem. class.: Amino acid L-cysteine

Action: Decreases viscosity of secretions by breaking disulfide links of mucoproteins; increases hepatic glutathione, which is necessary to inactivate toxic metabolites in acetaminophen overdose
Uses: Acetaminophen toxicity; bronchitis; pneumonia; cystic fibrosis; emphysema; atelectasis; TB; complications of thoracic, cardiovascular surgery; diagnosis in bronchial lab tests
Unlabeled uses: Prevention of contrast medium nephrotoxicity

DOSAGE AND ROUTES
Mucolytic
• *Adult and child:* **INSTILL** 1-2 ml (10%-20% sol) q1-4h prn or 3-5 ml (20% sol) or 6-10 ml (10% sol) tid or qid; nebulization (face mask, mouthpiece,

tracheostomy) 1-10 ml of a 20% sol, or
2-20 ml of a 10% sol, q2-6h; nebulization
(tent, croupette) may require large dose,
up to 300 ml/treatment

Acetaminophen toxicity
• *Adult and child:* **PO** 140 mg/kg, then
70 mg/kg q4h × 17 doses to total of 1330
mg/kg; **IV** loading dose 150 mg/kg over
15 min (dilution 150 mg/kg in 200 ml of
D_5); maintenance dose 1: 50 mg/kg over
4 hr (dilution 50 mg/kg in 500 ml D_5):
maintenance dose 2: 100 mg/kg over 16
hr (dilution 100 mg/kg in 1000 ml D_5)
Available forms: Oral sol 10%, 20%;
inj 20% (200 mg/ml)

SIDE EFFECTS

CNS: Dizziness, drowsiness, headache,
fever, chills
CV: Hypotension
EENT: Rhinorrhea, tooth damage
GI: Nausea, stomatitis, constipation, vomiting, anorexia, **hepatotoxicity**
INTEG: Urticaria, rash, fever, clamminess,
pruritus
RESP: **Bronchospasm,** burning, **hemoptysis,** chest tightness
Contraindications: Hypersensitivity,
increased intracranial pressure, status
asthmaticus
Precautions: Pregnancy (B), hypothyroidism, Addison's disease, CNS depression, brain tumor, asthma, renal/hepatic
disease, COPD, psychosis, alcoholism,
convulsive disorders, lactation

PHARMACOKINETICS

INH/INSTILL: Onset 1 min, duration
5-10 min, metabolized by liver, excreted
in urine, half-life 5.6 hr (adult) 11 hr
(newborn)
IV: Protein binding 83%

INTERACTIONS

• Do not use with iron, copper, rubber
• Do not mix with antibiotics: tetracycline, chlortetracycline, oxytetracycline,
erythromycin lactobionate, amphotericin
B, sodium ampicillin; iodized oil, chymo-
trypsin, trypsin, hydrogen peroxide

NURSING CONSIDERATIONS

Assess:
• Cough: type, frequency, character, including sputum
• Rate, rhythm of respirations, increased
dyspnea; sputum; discontinue if bronchospasm occurs
• VS, cardiac status including checking
for dysrhythmias, increased rate, palpitations
• ABGs for increased CO_2 retention in
asthma patients
• Antidotal use: LFTs, PT, BUN, glucose,
electrolytes, acetaminophen levels; inform
prescriber if dose is vomited or vomiting
is persistent
• Nausea, vomiting, rash; notify prescriber if these occur

Administer:
PO route
• Antidotal use: give within 24 hr; give
with cola or soft drink to disguise taste;
can be given with H_2O through tubes; use
within 1 hr

INSTILL route
• By syringe 2-3 doses of 1-2 ml of 20%
or 2-4 ml of 10% solution
• Decreased dose to geriatric patients;
their metabolisms may be slowed
• Only if suction machine is available
• Before meals ½-1 hr for better absorption, to decrease nausea
• 20% solutions diluted with NS or water
for injection; may give 10% solution undiluted
• Only after patient clears airway by deep
breathing, coughing

IV route
• Dilute with D_5
Incompatibilities: Rubber, metals, sta-
bility with other drugs not known

Perform/provide:
• Storage in refrigerator; use within 96
hr of opening
• Assistance with inhaled dose: bronchodilator if bronchospasm occurs
• Mechanical suction if cough insufficient to remove excess bronchial secretions

• Gum, hard candy, frequent rinsing of mouth for dryness of oral cavity

Evaluate:
• Therapeutic response: absence of purulent secretions when coughing; absence of hepatic damage in acetaminophen toxicity

Teach patient/family:
• About mucolytic use
• That unpleasant odor will decrease after repeated use
• That discoloration of solution after bottle is opened does not impair its effectiveness

---

activated charcoal (OTC)
Actidose-Aqua, CharcoAid, CharcoAid 2000, Liqui-Char
Func. class.: Antiflatulent; antidote

Action: Binds poisons, toxins, irritants; increases adsorption in GI tract; inactivates toxins and binds until excreted
Uses: Poisoning
Unlabeled uses: Diarrhea, flatulence

DOSAGE AND ROUTES
Children should not get more than 1 dose of products with sorbitol
Poisoning
• *Adult and child:* **PO** 30-100 g or 1 g/kg, minimum dose 30 g/250 ml of water, may give 20-40 g q6h for 1-2 days in severe poisoning
Available forms: Powder 15, 25 ✿, 30, 40, 120, 125, 240 g/container; oral susp 12.5 g/60 ml, 15 g/72 ml, 15 g/120 ml, 25 g/120 ml, 30 g/120 ml, 50 g/240 ml; Canada 15 g/120 ml, 25 g/125 ml, 50 g/225 ml, 50 g/250 ml
• Tabs/caps should not be used in poisonings

SIDE EFFECTS
GI: Nausea, black stools, vomiting, constipation, diarrhea
Contraindications: Hypersensitivity to this drug, unconsciousness, semiconsciousness, poisoning of cyanide, mineral acids, alkalis, gag reflex, depression, ethanol intoxication
Precautions: Pregnancy (C)

PHARMACOKINETICS
PO: Excreted in feces

INTERACTIONS
• Inactivation of acetylcysteine

NURSING CONSIDERATIONS
Assess:
• Respiration, pulse, B/P to determine charcoal effectiveness if taken for barbiturate/opiate poisoning, intact gag reflex

Administer:
PO route
• After inducing vomiting unless vomiting contraindicated (i.e., cyanide or alkalis)
• After mixing with water or fruit juice to form thick syrup; do not use dairy products to mix charcoal
• Repeat dose if vomiting occurs soon after dose; give with a laxative to promote elimination
• After spacing at least 1 hr before or after other drugs, or absorption will be decreased
NG route
• Through a nasogastric tube if patient unable to swallow

Perform/provide:
• Container closed tightly to prevent absorption of gases

Evaluate:
• Therapeutic response: LOC alert (poisoning)

Teach patient/family:
• That stools will be black
• How to prevent further poisonings

acyclovir (R)

(ay-sye′kloe-veer)

Avirax ✦, Zovirax

Func. class.: Antiviral

Chem. class.: Acyclic purine nucleoside analog

Action: Interferes with DNA synthesis by conversion to acyclovir triphosphate, causing decreased viral replication, time of lesional healing

Uses: Mucocutaneous herpes simplex virus, herpes genitalis (HSV-1, HSV-2), varicella infections, herpes zoster, herpes simplex encephalitis

DOSAGE AND ROUTES

Renal dose

• *Adult and child:* **PO/IV** CCr >50 ml/min 100% dose q8h, CCr 25-50 ml/min 100% dose q12h, CCr 10-25 ml/min 100% dose q24h, CCr 0-10 ml/min 50% of dose q24h

Herpes simplex

• *Adult and child >12 yr:* **IV INF** 5 mg/kg over 1 hr q8h × 5 days

• *Child <12 yr:* **IV INF** 250 mg/m² or 30 mg/kg/day divided q8h over 1 hr × 5 days

Genital herpes

• *Adult:* **PO** 200 mg q4h (5×/day while awake) for 5 days to 6 mo depending on whether initial, recurrent, or chronic; **IV** 5 mg/kg q8h × 5 days

Herpes simplex encephalitis

• *Adult:* **IV** 10 mg/kg over 1 hr q8h × 10 days

• *Child 3 mo-12 yr:* **IV** 20 mg/kg q8h × 10 days

• *Child birth-3 mo:* **IV** 10 mg/kg q8h × 10 days

Herpes zoster

• *Adult:* **PO** 800 mg q4h while awake × 7-10 days; **IV** 5 mg/kg q8h

Varicella-zoster

• *Adult:* **PO** 1000 mg q6h × 5 days or 600-800 mg q4h (5×/day while awake); **IV** 500 mg/m² q8h or 10 mg/kg q8h × 7 days

• *Child:* **PO** 10-20 mg/kg (max 800 mg) qid × 5 days; **IV** 500 mg/m² q8h or 10 mg/kg q8h × 7 days

Mucosal/cutaneous herpes simplex infections in immunosuppressed patients

• *Adult and child >12 yr:* **IV** 5 mg/kg q8h × 7 days

• *Child <12:* **IV** 10 mg/kg q8h × 7 days

Chickenpox

• *Adult and child >40 kg:* **PO** 800 mg qid × 5 days

• *Child ≥2 yr, <40 kg:* **PO** 20 mg/kg qid × 5 days

Available forms: Caps 200 mg; inj 500 mg, oral susp, tabs 400, 800 mg

SIDE EFFECTS

CNS: Tremors, confusion, lethargy, hallucinations, **seizures,** dizziness, *headache,* encephalopathic changes

EENT: Gingival hyperplasia

GI: Nausea, vomiting, diarrhea, increased ALT, AST, abdominal pain, glossitis, colitis

GU: **Oliguria, proteinuria, hematuria,** vaginitis, moniliasis, **glomerulonephritis, acute renal failure,** changes in menses, polydipsia

HEMA: **Thrombotic thrombocytopenia purpura, hemolytic uremic syndrome** (immunocompromised patients)

INTEG: Rash, urticaria, pruritus, pain or phlebitis at IV site, unusual sweating, alopecia

MS: Joint pain, leg pain, muscle cramps

Contraindications: Hypersensitivity

Precautions: Pregnancy (B), lactation, renal/hepatic disease, electrolyte imbalance, dehydration

PHARMACOKINETICS

Distributed widely; crosses placenta, CSF concentrations are 50% plasma

IV: Onset immediate, peak immediate, duration unknown, half-life 20 min-3 hr (terminal); metabolized by liver, excreted by kidneys as unchanged drug (95%)

PO: Absorbed minimally; onset unknown, peak 1½-2 hr, terminal half-life 3½ hr

INTERACTIONS

- Synergistic effect: interferon
- CNS side effects: zidovudine

Increase: levels, toxicity—probenecid

NURSING CONSIDERATIONS

Assess:

- Signs of infection, anemia

⚠ Any patient with compromised renal system, since drug is excreted slowly in poor renal system function; toxicity may occur rapidly

- Hepatic/renal studies: AST, ALT; BUN, creatinine before and during treatment
- Blood studies: WBC, RBC, Hct, Hgb, bleeding time; blood dyscrasias may occur; drug should be discontinued
- Renal studies: urinalysis, protein, BUN, creatinine, CCr, watch for increasing BUN and serum creatinine or decreased CCr, may indicate nephrotoxicity; I&O ratio; report hematuria, oliguria, fatigue, weakness; may indicate nephrotoxicity; check for protein in urine during treatment
- C&S before drug therapy; drug may be taken as soon as culture is taken; repeat C&S after treatment; determine the presence of other infections
- Bowel pattern before, during treatment; if severe abdominal pain with bleeding occurs, drug should be discontinued
- Skin eruptions: rash, urticaria, itching
- Allergies before treatment, reaction of each medication; place allergies on chart in bright red letters

Administer:

PO route

- Do not break, crush, or chew caps
- May give without regard to meals, with 8 oz of water
- Shake suspension before use
- Lower dose in acute or chronic renal failure

IV route

- Increased fluids to 3 L/day to decrease crystalluria
- After reconstituting with 10 ml compatible sol/500 mg of drug, concentration of 50 mg/ml, shake, further dilute in 50-100 ml compatible sol; use within 12 hr;

give over at least 1 hr (constant rate) by infusion pump to prevent nephrotoxicity; do not reconstitute with sol containing benzyl alcohol in neonates

Additive compatibilities: Fluconazole

Solution compatibilities: D_5W, LR, or NaCl (D_5 0.9% NaCl, 0.9% NaCl) solutions

Y-site compatibilities: Allopurinol, amikacin, ampicillin, amphotericin B, cefazolin, cefonicid, cefoperazone, cefotaxime, cefoxitin, ceftazidime, ceftizoxime, ceftriaxone, cefuroxime, cephapirin, chloramphenicol, cholesteryl sulfate complex, cimetidine, clindamycin, dexamethasone sodium phosphate, dimenhyDRINATE, diphenhydrAMINE, DOXOrubicin, doxycycline, erythromycin, famotidine, filgrastim, fluconazole, gallium, gentamicin, granisetron, heparin, hydrocortisone sodium succinate, hydromorphone, imipenem/cilastatin, lorazepam, magnesium sulfate, melphalan, methylPREDNISolone sodium succinate, metoclopramide, metronidazole, multivitamin, nafcillin, oxacillin, paclitaxel, penicillin G potassium, pentobarbital, perphenazine, piperacillin, potassium chloride, propofol, ranitidine, remifentanil, sodium bicarbonate, tacrolimus, teniposide, theophylline, thiotepa, ticarcillin, tobramycin, trimethoprim-sulfamethoxazole, vancomycin, zidovudine

Perform/provide:

- Storage at room temperature for up to 12 hr after reconstitution; if refrigerated, sol may show a precipitate that clears at room temperature, yellow discoloration does not affect potency
- Adequate intake of fluids (2 L) to prevent deposit in kidneys

Evaluate:

- Therapeutic response: absence of itching, painful lesions; crusting and healed lesions; decreased symptoms of chickenpox

Teach patient/family:

- To take as prescribed; if dose is missed,

Side effects: *italics* = common; **bold** = life-threatening

take as soon as remembered up to 1 hr before next dose; do not double dose; that drug does not cure the condition

• That drug may be taken orally before infection occurs; drug should be taken when itching or pain occurs, usually before eruptions

• That sexual partners need to be told that patient has herpes; they can become infected; condoms must be worn to prevent reinfections

• Not to touch lesions to avoid spreading infection to new sites

• That drug does not cure infection, just controls symptoms and does not prevent infecting others

⚠ To report sore throat, fever, fatigue (may indicate superinfection)

• That drug must be taken in equal intervals around the clock to maintain blood levels for duration of therapy

• To notify prescriber of side effects of bruising, bleeding, fatigue, malaise; may indicate blood dyscrasias

• To seek dental care during treatment to prevent gingival hyperplasia

• That women with genital herpes are more likely to develop cervical cancer; to keep all gynecologic appointments

Treatment of overdose: Discontinue drug, hemodialysis, resuscitate if needed

---

acyclovir topical
See Appendix C

---

adalimumab (℞)
(add-a-lim'yu-mab)
Humira
Func. class.: Antirheumatic agent (disease modifying), immunomodulator
Chem. class.: Recombinant human IgG1 monoclonal antibody, DMARDs

Action: A form of human IgG1 monoclonal antibody specific for human tumor necrosis factor (TNF); elevated levels of TNF

are found in patients with rheumatoid arthritis

Uses: Reduction in signs and symptoms and inhibiting progression of structural damage in patients with moderate to severe active rheumatoid arthritis in patients ≥18 years of age who have not responded to other disease-modifying agents, psoriatic arthritis

Unlabeled uses: Crohn's disease, plaque psoriasis

DOSAGE AND ROUTES
• *Adult:* **SUBCUT** 40 mg every other wk
Available form: Inj 40 mg/0.8 ml

SIDE EFFECTS
CNS: Headache
EENT: Sinusitis
GI: Abdominal pain, nausea
INTEG: Rash, *inj site reaction*
MISC: Flulike symptoms, UTI, hypertension, back pain, lupuslike syndrome, **risk of infection (TB, invasive fungal infections, other opportunistic infections); may be fatal**
RESP: URI

Contraindications: Hypersensitivity, active infections

Precautions: Pregnancy (B), lactation, children, geriatric, CNS demyelinating disease, lymphoma, latent TB

PHARMACOKINETICS
Terminal half-life 2 wk

INTERACTIONS
• Do not give concurrently with vaccines; immunizations should be brought up to date before treatment

NURSING CONSIDERATIONS
Assess:
• Pain, stiffness, ROM, swelling of joints during treatment
• For inj site pain, swelling; usually occur after 2 inj (4-5 days)
⚠ For infections (fever, flulike symptoms, dyspnea, change in urination, redness/swelling around any wounds), stop treatment if present; some serious infections

---

including sepsis may occur, may be fatal; patients with active infections should not be started on this drug

Administer:
SUBCUT route
• Do not admix with other sol or medications; do not use filter; protect from light; give at 45-degree angle using abdomen, thighs; rotate inj sites
• Other DMARDs should be continued during this therapy

Evaluate:
• Therapeutic response: decreased inflammation, pain in joints, decreased joint destruction

Teach patient/family:
• About self-administration if appropriate: inj should be made in thigh, abdomen, upper arm; rotate sites at least 1 inch from old site, do not inject in areas that are bruised, red, hard
• That if medication is not taken when due, inject next dose as soon as remembered and inject next dose as scheduled
• Not to take any live virus vaccines during treatment
• To report signs of infection or allergic reaction

---

adefovir dipivoxil (Ɍ)
(add-ee-foh'veer)
Hepsera
Func. class.: Antiviral
Chem. class.: Adenosine monophosphate analog

Action: Inhibits hepatitis B virus DNA polymerase by competing with natural substrates and by causing DNA termination after its incorporation into viral DNA; causes viral DNA death
Uses: Chronic hepatitis B

DOSAGE AND ROUTES
• *Adult:* PO 10 mg daily, optimal duration unknown
Renal dose
• *Adult:* PO CCr ≥50 ml/min 10 mg q24h; CCr 20-49 ml/min 10 mg q48h; CCr

10-19 ml/min 10 mg q72h; hemodialysis 10 mg q7 days following dialysis
Available forms: Tabs 10 mg

SIDE EFFECTS
CNS: Headache
GI: Dyspepsia, abdominal pain
Contraindications: Hypersensitivity
Precautions: Pregnancy (C), lactation, child, severe renal disease, impaired hepatic disease, geriatric

PHARMACOKINETICS
PO: Rapidly absorbed from GI tract, peak 1¾ hr, excreted by kidneys 45%; terminal half-life 7.48 hr

INTERACTIONS
• Granulocytopenia: acetaminophen, aspirin, indomethacin
Increase: serum concentration and possible toxicity—amphotericin B, dapsone, flucytosine, adriamycin, interferon, vinCRIStine, vinBLAStine, pentamidine, probenecid, experimental nucleoside analogs, benzodiazepines, cimetidine, morphine, sulfonamides, acyclovir, ganciclovir, DOXOrubicin, acetaminophen, indomethacin, fluconazole, phenytoin, trimethoprim

NURSING CONSIDERATIONS
Assess:
• For nephrotoxicity: increasing CCr, BUN
• For HIV before beginning treatment, because HIV resistance may occur in chronic hepatitis B patients
• For lactic acidosis, severe hepatomegaly with stenosis
• Geriatric patients more carefully; may develop renal, cardiac symptoms more rapidly
• For exacerbations of hepatitis after discontinuing treatment, monitor LFTs
Administer:
• By mouth without regard to food
Perform/provide:
• Storage in cool environment; protect from light

Evaluate:
• Therapeutic response: decreased symptoms of chronic hepatitis B, improving LFTs

Teach patient/family:
• That optimal duration of treatment is unknown
• To avoid use with other medications unless approved by prescriber
• To notify prescriber of decreased urinary output

⚠ High Alert

adenosine (℞)
(a-den'oh-seen)
Adenocard, Adenoscan
Func. class.: Antidysrhythmic
Chem. class.: Endogenous nucleoside

Do not confuse:
Adenocard/adenosine phosphate

Action: Slows conduction through AV node, can interrupt reentry pathways through AV node, and can restore normal sinus rhythm in patients with paroxysmal supraventricular tachycardia (PSVT)

Uses: SVT, as a diagnostic aid to assess myocardial perfusion defects in CAD

DOSAGE AND ROUTES

Antidysrhythmic
• *Adult and child >50 kg:* **IV BOL** 6 mg; if conversion to normal sinus rhythm does not occur within 1-2 min, give 12 mg by rapid **IV BOL**; may repeat 12 mg dose again in 1-2 min
• *Infant and child <50 kg:* **IV BOL** 0.05 mg/kg; if not effective, increase dose by 0.05 mg/kg q2min to a max of 0.25 mg/kg or 12 mg

Diagnostic use
• *Adult:* **IV BOL** 140 mcg/kg/min × 6 min

Available forms: Inj 3 mg/ml vial, 6 mg/2 ml vial

SIDE EFFECTS

CNS: Lightheadedness, dizziness, arm tingling, numbness, apprehension, blurred vision, headache

CV: Chest pain, pressure, **atrial tachydysrhythmias**, sweating, palpitations, hypotension, *facial flushing*

GI: Nausea, metallic taste, throat tightness, groin pressure

RESP: Dyspnea, chest pressure, hyperventilation

Contraindications: Hypersensitivity, 2nd- or 3rd-degree heart block, AV block, sick sinus syndrome, atrial flutter, atrial fibrillation

Precautions: Pregnancy (C), lactation, children, asthma, geriatric

PHARMACOKINETICS

Cleared from plasma in <30 sec, half-life 10 sec

INTERACTIONS

• Higher degree of heart block: carbamazepine
• Possible ventricular fibrillation: digoxin
• Smoking: increase tachycardia

Increase: effects of adenosine—dipyridamole

Decrease: activity of adenosine—theophylline or other methylxanthines (caffeine)

Drug/Herb

Increase: toxicity/death—aconite

Increase: adenosine effect—aloe, broom, buckthorn, cascara sagrada, figwort, fumitory, goldenseal, kudzu, licorice, rhubarb, senna

Increase: serotonin effect—horehound

Decrease: adenosine effect—coltsfoot, guarana

NURSING CONSIDERATIONS

Assess:
• I&O ratio, electrolytes (K, Na, Cl)
• Cardiopulmonary status: B/P, pulse, respiration, ECG intervals (PR, QRS, QT); check for transient dysrhythmias (PVCs, PACs, sinus tachycardia, AV block)
• Respiratory status: rate, rhythm, lung fields for crackles, watch for respiratory depression; bilateral crackles may occur

---

in CHF patient; increased respiration, increased pulse, drug should be discontinued
• CNS effects: dizziness, confusion, psychosis, paresthesias, convulsions; drug should be discontinued

Administer:
IV BOLUS route
• Undiluted; give 6 mg or less by rapid inj over 1-2 sec; if using an IV line, use port near insertion site, flush with NS (50 ml)
Intermittent IV INF route
• Give 30 ml vial, undiluted, by peripheral vein
Y-site compatibilities: abciximab
Solution compatibilities: D$_5$LR, D$_5$W, LR, 0.9% NaCl

Perform/provide:
• Storage at room temperature; sol should be clear; discard unused drug

Evaluate:
• Therapeutic response: normal sinus rhythm or diagnosis of perfusion defect

Teach patient/family:
• To report facial flushing, dizziness, sweating, palpitations, chest pain
• To rise from sitting or standing slowly to prevent orthostatic hypotension
Treatment of overdose: Defibrillation, vasopressor for hypotension

---

alatrofloxacin (℞)
(ah-lat-troh-floks'ah-sin)
Trovan IV
trovafloxacin (℞)
(tro-vah-floks'ah-sin)
Trovan (oral)
Func. class.: Antiinfective
Chem. class.: Fluoroquinolone

Do not confuse:
Trovan/Tenormin
Action: Interferes with conversion of intermediate DNA fragments into high-molecular-weight DNA in bacteria; DNA gyrase inhibitor

Uses: Nosocomial pneumonia; *Escherichia coli, Pseudomonas aeruginosa, Haemophilus influenzae, Staphylococcus aureus;* community-acquired pneumonia: *Streptococcus pneumoniae, H. influenzae, S. aureus, Klebsiella pneumoniae, Mycoplasma pneumoniae, Moraxella catarrhalis, Legionella pneumophila, Chlamydia pneumoniae;* chronic bronchitis, acute sinusitis, complicated intraabdominal infections, gynecologic/pelvic infections, skin/skin structure infections, UTIs, chronic bacterial prostatitis, urethral gonorrhea in males, PID, cervicitis caused by susceptible organisms

DOSAGE AND ROUTES
Alatrofloxacin—serious infections
• *Adult:* IV 300 mg q24h
Other infections
• *Adult:* IV 200 mg q24h
Perioperative prophylaxis
• *Adult:* IV 200 mg ½-4 hr prior to surgery
Trovafloxacin—gonorrhea
• *Adult:* PO 100 mg as a single dose
Other infections
• *Adult:* PO 100-200 mg q24h
Perioperative prophylaxis
• *Adult:* PO 200 mg ½-4 hr prior to surgery
Hepatic dose (Child-Pugh Class A/B)
• *Adult:* IV 200 mg q24h or **IV/PO** 100 mg q24h
Available forms: Conc sol for inj 5 mg/ml (200 mg/40 ml, 300 mg/60 ml) (alatrofloxacin); tabs 100, 200 mg (trovafloxacin)

SIDE EFFECTS
CNS: Headache, *dizziness,* insomnia, anxiety, psychosis, **seizures**
GI: Nausea, flatulence, vomiting, diarrhea, abdominal pain, **pseudomembranous colitis, hepatotoxicity, fatal hepatitis**
GU: Vaginitis, crystalluria, increased BUN, creatinine
HEMA: Anemia, **thrombocytopenia, leu-**

kopenia, decreased Hgb, Hct; increased platelets
INTEG: Rash, pruritus, photosensitivity
MS: Arthralgia, myalgia
SYST: **Anaphylaxis, Stevens-Johnson syndrome**
Contraindications: Hypersensitivity to quinolones, seizure disorders, cerebral atherosclerosis, photosensitivity
Precautions: Pregnancy (C), lactation, children, GI disease

PHARMACOKINETICS
Metabolized in liver, excreted in urine unchanged

INTERACTIONS
• May increase warfarin level
Increase: severe hypoglycemia—glyburide
Decrease: absorption of trovafloxacin—IV morphine
Decrease: absorption of trovafloxacin—antacids with aluminum, magnesium, citric acid buffered with sodium citrate, sucralfate, iron products, IV morphine
Drug/Herb
• Do not use acidophilus with antiinfectives; separate by several hours
Increase: antiinfective effect—cola tree

NURSING CONSIDERATIONS
Assess:
• For hepatic toxicity, use only for serious or life-threatening infections
• For previous sensitivity reaction to fluoroquinolones
• For signs and symptoms of infection: characteristics of sputum, WBC >10,000, fever; obtain baseline information before and during treatment
• For CNS disorders, since other quinolones can cause CNS stimulation, seizures
• C&S before beginning drug therapy to identify if correct treatment has been initiated
• For allergic reactions and anaphylaxis: rash, urticaria, pruritus, chills, fever, joint pain; may occur a few days after therapy begins; epINEPHrine and resuscitation

equipment should be available for anaphylactic reaction
• Bowel pattern daily; if severe diarrhea occurs, drug should be discontinued
• For overgrowth of infection, perineal itching, fever, malaise, redness, pain, swelling, drainage, rash, diarrhea, change in cough, sputum
⚠ Hepatic studies: AST; ALT, alk phos, bilirubin; identify hepatotoxicity, fatal hepatitis
• Discontinue if tendon pain occurs; possible tendon rupture
Administer:
• Without regard to meals; separate aluminum, magnesium, iron, or sucralfate by 4 hr; to increase fluid intake to 2 L/day to prevent crystalluria
Intermittent IV INF route
• Dilute with compatible solution to a concentration of 1-2 mg/ml, run over 1 hr
Solution compatibilities: D_5, ½NaCl, D_5 ½NaCl, D_5/0.2% NaCl
Y-site compatibilities: Amikacin, cycloSPORINE, DOPamine, droperidol, fentanyl, gentamicin, ketorolac, lorazepam, midazolam, nitroglycerin, ondansetron, tobramycin, vancomycin
Evaluate:
• Therapeutic response: absence of signs/symptoms of infection (WBC <10,000/mm^3, temp WNL)
Teach patient/family:
• To avoid hazardous activities until response is known
• To contact prescriber if vaginal itching, loose, foul-smelling stools, or furry tongue occurs (may indicate superinfection); to report itching, rash, pruritus, urticaria, tendon pain
• To use frequent rinsing of mouth, sugarless candy or gum for dry mouth
• To avoid other medication unless approved by prescriber
• To contact prescriber if taking theophylline
• To take as prescribed, not to double or miss doses
• To notify prescriber of diarrhea with

---

blood or pus, may indicate pseudomembranous colitis
• To prevent sun exposure or use sunscreen to prevent phototoxicity

---

albumin, normal serum 5%/25% (℞)
(al-byoo'min)
Albuminar 5%, Albuminar 25%, Albutein 5%, Albutein 25%, Buminate 5%, Buminate 25%, Plasbumin 5%, Plasbumin 25%
Func. class.: Blood derivative
Chem. class.: Placental human plasma

Action: Exerts oncotic pressure, which expands volume of circulating blood and maintains cardiac output
Uses: Restores plasma volume in burns, hyperbilirubinemia, shock, hypoproteinemia, prevention of cerebral edema, cardiopulmonary bypass procedures, ARDS, nephrotic syndrome

DOSAGE AND ROUTES
Burns
• *Adult:* IV dose to maintain plasma albumin at 30-50 g/L, use 5% sol initially, then 25% sol after 24 hr
Shock
• *Adult:* IV 500 ml of 5% sol q30 min, as needed
• *Child:* IV 0.5-1 g/kg/dose
Hypoproteinemia
• *Adult:* IV 1000-2000 ml of 5% sol daily, not to exceed 5-10 ml/min or 25-100 g of 25% sol daily, not to exceed 3 ml/min, titrated to patient response
Hyperbilirubinemia/ erythroblastosis fetalis
• *Infant:* IV 1 g of 25% sol/kg before transfusion
Available forms: Inj 50, 250 mg/ml (5%, 25%)

SIDE EFFECTS
CNS: Fever, chills, flushing, headache

CV: Fluid overload, hypotension, erratic pulse, tachycardia
GI: Nausea, vomiting, increased salivation
INTEG: Rash, urticaria
RESP: Altered respirations, **pulmonary edema**
Contraindications: Hypersensitivity, CHF, severe anemia, renal insufficiency
Precautions: Pregnancy (C), decreased salt intake, decreased cardiac reserve, lack of albumin deficiency, renal/hepatic disease

PHARMACOKINETICS
In hyponutrition states, metabolized as protein/energy source

INTERACTIONS
Drug/Lab Test
False increase: Alk phos

NURSING CONSIDERATIONS
Assess:
• Blood studies Hct, Hgb; if serum protein declines, dyspnea, hypoxemia can result
• Decreased B/P, erratic pulse, respiration
• I&O ratio: urinary output may decrease
⚠ CVP, pulmonary wedge pressure will increase if overload occurs
• Allergy: fever, rash, itching, chills, flushing, urticaria, nausea, vomiting, hypotension, requires discontinuation of infusion, use of new lot if therapy reinstituted; premedicate with diphenhydrAMINE
• CVP reading: distended neck veins indicate circulatory overload; shortness of breath, anxiety, insomnia, expiratory crackles, frothy blood-tinged cough, cyanosis indicate pulmonary overload
Administer:
IV route
• Slowly, to prevent fluid overload; dilute with NS for injection or D₅W; 5% may be given undiluted; 25% may be given diluted or undiluted, give over 4 hr, use infusion pump
Solution compatibilities: LR, NaCl, Ringer's, D_5W, $D_{10}W$, $D_{2\frac{1}{2}}W$, dextrose/

---

saline, dextran$_6$ D$_5$, dextran$_6$ NaCl 0.9%, dextrose/Ringer's, dextrose/LR

Y-site compatibilities: Diltiazem

Perform/provide:

• Adequate hydration before, during administration

• Check type of albumin; some stored at room temperature, some need to be refrigerated

Evaluate:

• Therapeutic response: increased B/P, decreased edema, increased serum albumin levels, increased plasma protein

---

albuterol (R)
(al-byoo′ter-ole)
AccuNeb, Airet, albuterol,
Gen-Salbutamol ♣,
Novo-Salmol ♣, Proventil,
Salbutamol, Ventodisk,
Ventolin
Func. class.: Adrenergic β$_2$-agonist, sympathomimetic, bronchodilator

---

Do not confuse:
albuterol/atenolol
Ventolin/Vantin
Volmax/Flomax
Proventil/Prinivil
Salbutamol/salmeterol

Action: Causes bronchodilation by action on β$_2$ (pulmonary) receptors by increasing levels of cAMP, which relaxes smooth muscle; produces bronchodilation, CNS, cardiac stimulation, as well as increased diuresis and gastric acid secretion; longer acting than isoproterenol

Uses: Prevention of exercise-induced asthma, acute bronchospasm, bronchitis, emphysema, bronchiectasis, or other reversible airway obstruction

Unlabeled uses: Hyperkalemia in dialysis patients

DOSAGE AND ROUTES

To prevent exercise-induced bronchospasm

• *Adult:* **INH** (metered dose inhaler) 2 puffs 15 min before exercising

Other respiratory conditions

• *Adult and child ≥12 yr:* **INH** (metered dose inhaler) 2 puffs q4h; **PO** 2-4 mg tid-qid, not to exceed 8 mg; **NEB/IPPB** 2.5 mg tid-qid

• *Geriatric:* **PO** 2 mg tid-qid, may increase gradually to 8 mg tid-qid

• *Child 2-12 yr:* **INH** (metered dose inhaler) 0.1 mg/kg tid (max 2.5 mg tid-qid); **NEB/IPPB** 0.1-0.15 mg/kg/dose tid-qid or 1.25 mg tid-qid for child 10-15 kg or 2.5 mg tid-qid >15 kg

Available forms: Aerosol 90 mcg/actuation; oral sol 2 mg/5 ml; tabs 2, 4 mg; ext rel 4, 8 mg; INH sol 0.5, 0.83, 1, 2, 5 mg/ml; powder for INH (Ventodisk) 200, 400 mcg; INH cap 200 mcg; 100 mcg/spray, 80 INH/canister, 200 INH/canister

SIDE EFFECTS

CNS: Tremors, anxiety, insomnia, headache, dizziness, stimulation, *restlessness,* hallucinations, flushing, irritability

CV: Palpitations, tachycardia, hypertension, angina, hypotension, dysrhythmias

EENT: Dry nose, irritation of nose and throat

GI: Heartburn, nausea, vomiting

MISC: Flushing, sweating, anorexia, bad taste/smell changes, hypokalemia

MS: Muscle cramps

RESP: Cough, wheezing, dyspnea, **bronchospasm,** dry throat

Contraindications: Hypersensitivity to sympathomimetics, tachydysrhythmias, severe cardiac disease, heart block

Precautions: Pregnancy (C), lactation, cardiac disorders, hyperthyroidism, diabetes mellitus, hypertension, prostatic hypertrophy, narrow-angle glaucoma, seizures, exercise-induced bronchospasm (aerosol) in children <12 years, hypoglycemia, seizure disorder

PHARMACOKINETICS

Well absorbed PO, extensively metabolized in the liver and tissues, crosses placenta, breast milk, blood-brain barrier

PO: Onset ½ hr, peak 2-3 hr, duration 4-6 hr, half-life 2.7-6 hr

---

PO-ER: Onset ½ hour; peak 2-3 hr; duration 8-12 hr

INH: Onset 5-15 min, peak 0.5-2 hr, duration 2-6 hr, half-life 4 hr

INTERACTIONS

• ECG changes/hypokalemia: potassium-losing diuretics

Increase: severe hypotension—oxytocics

Increase: toxicity—theophylline

Increase: action of aerosol bronchodilators

Increase: action of albuterol—tricyclics, MAOIs, other adrenergics; do not use together

Increase: CV effects—atomoxetine, selegiline

Decrease: albuterol—other β-blockers

Drug/Herb

Increase: stimulation—caffeine (cola nut, green/black tea, guarana, yerba maté, coffee, chocolate)

NURSING CONSIDERATIONS

Assess:

• Respiratory function: vital capacity, forced expiratory volume, ABGs; lung sounds, heart rate and rhythm, B/P, sputum (baseline and peak)

• That patient has not received theophylline therapy before giving dose

• Patient's ability to self-medicate

• For evidence of allergic reactions

• Paradoxical bronchospasm, hold medication, notify prescriber if bronchospasm occurs

Administer:

PO route

• Do not break, crush, or chew ext rel tabs

• With meals to decrease gastric irritation

• Oral solution to children (no alcohol, sugar)

INH route

• In geriatric patients and children, a spacing device is advised

• After shaking metered dose inhaler, exhale, place mouthpiece in mouth, inhale slowly, while depressing inhaler, hold breath, remove, exhale slowly; give INH at least 1 min apart

• NEB/IPPB diluting 5 mg/ml sol/2.5 ml 0.9% NaCl for INH; other sol do not require dilution; for neb O$_2$ flow or compressed air 6-10 L/min

• Gum, sips of water for dry mouth

Perform/provide:

• Storage in light-resistant container, do not expose to temperatures over 86° F (30° C)

Evaluate:

• Therapeutic response: absence of dyspnea, wheezing after 1 hr, improved airway exchange, improved ABGs

Teach patient/family:

• To use exactly as prescribed; take missed dose when remembered, alter dosing schedule

• Not to use OTC medications; excess stimulation may occur

• Use of inhaler; review package insert with patient; use demonstration, return demonstration

• To avoid getting aerosol in eyes; blurring of vision may result

• To wash inhaler in warm water daily and dry

• To avoid smoking, smoke-filled rooms, persons with respiratory infections

⚠ That paradoxic bronchospasm may occur and to stop drug immediately, call prescriber

• To limit caffeine products such as chocolate, coffee, tea, and colas

Treatment of overdose: Administer a β$_1$-adrenergic blocker

> ### ⚠ High Alert
>
> ### aldesleukin (℞)
> (al-dess-loo'ken)
> Interleukin-2, IL-2, Proleukin
> *Func. class.:* Miscellaneous antineoplastic
> *Chem. class.:* Interleukin-2, human recombinant (cytokine)

Do not confuse:

aldesleukin/oprelvekin

Proleukin/oprelvekin/Prokine

Action: Enhancement of lymphocyte mitogenesis and stimulation of IL-2–dependent cell lines; enhancement of lymphocyte cytotoxicity; induction of killer cell activity; induction of interferon-γ production; results in activation of cellular immunity, production of cytokines, and inhibition of tumor growth

Uses: Metastatic renal cell carcinoma in adults, phase II for HIV in combination with zidovudine; melanoma (metastatic)

Unlabeled uses: Kaposi's sarcoma given with zidovudine, metastatic melanoma given with cyclophosphamide, non-Hodgkin's lymphoma given with lymphokine-activated killer cells, AIDS (phase I) given with zidovudine

DOSAGE AND ROUTES

• *Adult:* **IV INF** 600,000 international units/kg (0.037 mg/kg) over 15 min q8h × 14 doses; off 9 days, repeat schedule for another 14 doses, for a max of 28 doses/course

Available forms: Powder for inj 22 million international units/vial

SIDE EFFECTS

CNS: Mental status changes, dizziness, sensory dysfunction, syncope, motor dysfunction, *fever, chills,* headache, impaired memory, depression, sleep disturbances, hallucinations, rigors, neuropathy

CV: Hypotension, sinus tachycardia, dysrhythmias, bradycardia, PVCs, PACs, myocardial ischemia, **myocardial infarction, cardiac arrest, capillary leak syndrome, CVA**

EENT: Reversible visual changes

GI: Nausea, vomiting, diarrhea, stomatitis, anorexia, GI bleeding, dyspepsia, constipation, **intestinal perforation**/ileus, jaundice, ascites

GU: **Oliguria/anuria, proteinuria, hematuria,** dysuria, **renal failure**

HEMA: Anemia, **thrombocytopenia, leukopenia, coagulation disorders, leukocytosis, eosinophilia**

INTEG: Pruritus, erythema, rash, dry skin, **exfoliative dermatitis,** purpura, petechiae, urticaria

MS: Arthralgia, myalgia

RESP: Pulmonary congestion, *dyspnea,* **pulmonary edema, respiratory failure, apnea,** tachypnea, pleural effusion, wheezing

SYST: Infection

Contraindications: Hypersensitivity, abnormal thallium stress test or pulmonary function tests, organ allografts

Precautions: Pregnancy (C), CNS metastases, bacterial infections, renal/hepatic/cardiac/pulmonary disease, lactation, children, anemia, thrombocytopenia

PHARMACOKINETICS

Renal elimination half-life 85 min; onset 4 wk, duration, variable

INTERACTIONS

• Potentiate hypotension: antihypertensives

• Reduced antitumor effectiveness: glucocorticoids

• Unpredictable reactions: psychotropics

Increase: toxicity—aminoglycosides, indomethacin, cytotoxic chemotherapy, methotrexate, asparaginase, DOXOrubicin

Drug/Lab Test

Increase: Bilirubin, BUN, serum creatinine, transaminase, alk phos; hypomagnesemia, acidosis hypocalcemia, hypophosphatemia, hypokalemia, hyperuricemia, hypoalbuminemia, hypoproteinemia, hyponatremia, hyperkalemia, alkalosis (toxic effect of drug)

NURSING CONSIDERATIONS
Assess:
• CBC, differential, platelet count weekly; withhold drug if WBC is <2000/mm³ or platelet count is <75,000/mm³; notify prescriber of these results

⚠ Capillary leak syndrome including a drop in mean arterial pressure (2-12 hr after initiating therapy); hypotension and hypoperfusion will occur; if B/P <90 mm Hg, use CVP, ECG, VS
• Renal studies: BUN, serum uric acid, urine CCr, electrolytes before, during therapy; I&O ratio; report fall in urine output to <30 ml/hr
• Monitor temp q4h
• Hepatic studies before, during therapy: bilirubin, AST, ALT, alk phos, LDH as needed or monthly
• ECG; ST-T wave changes, low QRS and T, possible dysrhythmias (sinus tachycardia, PVCs)

⚠ Baselines in pulmonary function; document FEV >2 L or ≥75% prior to therapy; check VS q4h, monitor temp q4h, pulse oximetry, dyspnea, crackles, ABGs; watch for respiratory failure, intubate if necessary
• Stress thallium study prior to therapy; document normal ejection fraction, unimpaired wall motion
• Bleeding: hematuria, guaiac, bruising petechiae, mucosa or orifices q8h
• Buccal cavity q8h for dryness, sores, ulceration, white patches, oral pain, bleeding, dysphagia
• Local irritation, pain, burning at inj site
• GI symptoms: frequency of stools, cramping; acidosis, signs of dehydration: rapid respirations, poor skin turgor, decreased urine output, dry skin, restlessness, weakness
Administer:
Intermittent IV INF route
• Hydrocortisone, dexamethasone or sodium bicarbonate (1 mEq/1 ml) for extravasation, apply ice compresses

• Antiemetic 30-60 min before giving drug to prevent vomiting
• IV after diluting 22 million international units (1.3 mg)/1.2 ml sterile H₂O for inj at site of vial and swirl, do not shake; dilute dose with 50 ml D₅W and give over 15 min; use plastic bag; do not use an in-line filter, give through Y-tube or 3-way stopcock
• DOPamine 1-5 kg/min before onset of hypotension; decreased dose preserves kidney output
Y-site compatibilities: Amikacin, amphotericin B, calcium gluconate, diphenhydrAMINE, DOPamine, fluconazole, foscarnet, gentamicin, heparin, IV fat emulsion, magnesium sulfate, metoclopramide, morphine, ondansetron, piperacillin, potassium chloride, ranitidine, ticarcillin, tobramycin, TPN #145, trimethoprim-sulfamethoxazole
Perform/provide:
• Liquid diet: carbonated beverage, gelatin (Jell-O) may be added if patient is not nauseated or vomiting
• Rinsing of mouth tid-qid with water, club soda; brushing of teeth bid-tid with soft brush or cotton-tipped applicators for stomatitis; use unwaxed dental floss
• Increased fluid when able to reduce renal problems
• Storage in refrigerator of diluted drug; protect from light, do not freeze; administer within 48 hr; bring to room temperature before infusing; discard unused portion
Evaluate:
• Therapeutic response: decreased tumor size, spread of malignancy
Teach patient/family:
• To use a nonhormonal contraceptive method during therapy
• To report any complaints, side effects to nurse or prescriber
• To avoid foods with citric acid, hot or rough texture
• To avoid alcohol, NSAIDs, salicylates, vaccinations; GI bleeding may occur

• To report any bleeding, white spots, ulcerations in mouth to prescriber; tell patient to examine mouth daily
• To avoid crowds and persons with infections when granulocyte count is low
• Visual problems may occur, but are reversible

Rarely Used

alefacept (R)
(ah-leh'fa-cept)
Amevive
Func. class.: Immunosuppressive

Uses: Adults with moderate to severe plaque psoriasis

DOSAGE AND ROUTES

• *Adult:* IV BOL 7.5 mg qwk or IM 15 mg qwk, for 12 wk
Contraindications: Hypersensitivity

alemtuzumab (R)
(al-em-tuz'uh-mab)
Campath
Func. class.: Antineoplastic—miscellaneous
Chem. class.: Monoclonal antibody

Action: Composed of recombinant DNA-derived humanized monoclonal antibody (campath-1H), binds to CD52 antigen that is present on surface of B and T lymphocytes, causes lysis of leukemic cells
Uses: B-cell chronic lymphocytic leukemia that has been treated with alkylating agents and that has failed fludarabine therapy
Unlabeled uses: Multiple sclerosis

DOSAGE AND ROUTES

• *Adult:* IV 3 mg over 2 hr daily; when tolerated, increase to 10 mg; when 10 mg tolerated increase to 30 mg daily, maintenance is 30 mg/day 3×/wk on alternate days for 12 wk, titration usually takes 3-7 days, max single dose 30 mg; max weekly dose 90 mg

Available forms: Sol for inj 30 mg/3 ml (single-use ampules)

SIDE EFFECTS

CNS: Dizziness, insomnia, depression, headache, tremor, somnolence, fatigue, drowsiness, weakness
CV: Hypotension, tachycardia, hypertension, edema, chest pain, supraventricular tachycardia
GI: Anorexia, diarrhea, constipation, *nausea, stomatitis, vomiting, abdominal pain, dyspepsia*
HEMA: **Anemia, neutropenia, thrombocytopenia, pancytopenia,** purpura, epistaxis
INTEG: Rash, local reaction, pruritus
MISC: Rigors, fever, *infusion reactions*
MS: Back pain
RESP: Cough, pneumonia, rhinitis, **bronchospasm,** dyspnea, pharyngitis
Contraindications: Hypersensitivity, active systemic infection, immunodeficiency
Precautions: Pregnancy (C), lactation, children

PHARMACOKINETICS

Complete bioavailability, half-life 12 days, steady state 6 wk

INTERACTIONS

Increase: bone marrow depression—radiation, other antineoplastics
Decrease: antibody reaction—live virus vaccines
Drug/Lab Test
Interference: Diagnostic tests using antibodies

NURSING CONSIDERATIONS
Assess:
• CBC, platelets qwk or more often if myelosuppression occurs; CD4+ after therapy until recovery of >200 cells/µl; irradiate blood if transfusions are required to prevent graft vs. host disease
• For symptoms of infection; chills, fever, headache, may be masked by drug

A Safety alert   *"Tall Man" lettering

fever; do not administer drug if infection is present

• CNS reaction: LOC, mental status, dizziness, confusion

• Cardiac status: lung sounds; ECG before and during treatment, especially in those with cardiac disease; monitor B/P hypotensive effect during administration

• Bone marrow depression: bruising, bleeding, blood in stools, urine, sputum, emesis

Administer:

IV route

• Do not give IV push or bolus

• Withdraw amount needed, use 5-micron filter before dilution, check for particulate matter and discoloration; inject into 100 ml sterile 0.9% NaCl or D$_5$W, gently invert to mix; do not add other drugs or infuse in same IV tubing

• Do not shake ampule

• Give diphenhydrAMINE 50 mg and acetaminophen 650 mg ½ hr prior to infusion; give hydrocortisone 200 mg to decrease severe infusion reactions; give trimethoprim-sulfamethoxazole DS bid 3×/wk and famciclovir 250 mg bid; continue for 2 mo or until CD4+ ≥200 cells/mm^3, whichever is later

Perform/provide:

• Storage of reconstituted sol for ≤8 hr at room temperature, do not freeze; protect from light

Evaluate:

• Therapeutic response: decrease in production of malignant lymphocytes

Teach patient/family:

• To take acetaminophen for fever

• To avoid hazardous tasks, because confusion, dizziness may occur

• To report signs of infection: sore throat, fever, diarrhea, vomiting

• To avoid breastfeeding, effects are unknown, do not resume for ≥3 mo after last dose

alendronate (℞)

(al-en-drone′ate)
Fosamax
Func. class.: Bone-resorption inhibitor
Chem. class.: Bisphosphonate

Do not confuse:

Fosamax/Flomax

Action: Absorbs calcium phosphate crystal in bone and may directly block dissolution of hydroxyapatite crystals of bone; inhibits normal and abnormal bone resorption, mineralization

Uses: Treatment and prevention of osteoporosis in postmenopausal women, treatment of osteoporosis in men, Paget's disease, treatment of corticosteroid-induced osteoporosis in postmenopausal women not receiving estrogen and men who are on continuing corticosteroid treatment with low bone mass

DOSAGE AND ROUTES

Osteoporosis in postmenopausal women

• *Adult and geriatric:* **PO** 10 mg daily or 70 mg qwk

Paget's disease

• *Adult and geriatric:* **PO** 40 mg daily × 6 mo, consider retreatment for relapse

Prevention of osteoporosis

• *Adult:* **PO** 5 mg daily or 35 mg qwk

Corticosteroid-induced osteoporosis in postmenopausal women (not receiving estrogen)

• *Adult:* **PO** 10 mg daily

Corticosteroid-induced osteoporosis in men or premenopausal women

• *Adult:* **PO** 5 mg daily

Available forms: Tabs 5, 10, 35, 40, 70 mg; oral sol 70 mg/5 ml

SIDE EFFECTS

CNS: Headache

GI: Abdominal pain, anorexia, constipation, nausea, vomiting, esophageal ulceration, acid reflux, dyspepsia

META: Anemia, hypokalemia, hypomagne-

semia, hypophosphatemia, hypocalcemia
MS: Bone pain

Contraindications: Hypersensitivity to
bisphosphonates, delayed esophageal
emptying, inability to sit or stand for 30
min, hypocalcemia

Precautions: Pregnancy (C), children,
lactation, CCr <35 ml/min, esophageal
disease, ulcers, gastritis

PHARMACOKINETICS

Rapidly cleared from circulation, taken
up mainly by bones, eliminated primarily through kidneys

INTERACTIONS

• Possible GI reactions: NSAIDs, salicy-
lates
Increase: alendronate effect—ranitidine
(IV)
Decrease: absorption—antacids, cal-
cium supplements
Drug/Food
Decrease: absorption when used with
caffeine, orange juice

NURSING CONSIDERATIONS

Assess:
• Hormonal status if a woman, prior to
treatment
• For osteoporosis: bone density test before and during treatment
• For Paget's disease: increased skull
size, bone pain, headache; decreased vision, hearing
• Electrolytes; renal function studies; Ca,
P, Mg, K
• For hypercalcemia: paresthesia, twitching, laryngospasm, Chvostek's, Trousseau's signs
• Alk phos levels, baseline and periodically, 2 × upper limit of normal is indica-
tive of Paget's disease
Administer:
• For 6 months to be effective in Paget's
disease; take with 8 oz of water 30 min
before 1st food, beverage, or medication
of the day

Perform/provide:
• Storage in cool environment, out of direct sunlight
Evaluate:
• Therapeutic response: increased bone
mass, absence of fractures
Teach patient/family:
• To remain upright for 30 min after dose
to prevent esophageal irritation, if dose
is missed, skip dose, do not double doses
or take later in day
• To take in AM before food, other meds,
take with 6-8 oz of water only (no mineral water)
• To take calcium, vit D if instructed by
health care provider
• To use weight-bearing exercise to increase bone density
• To let health care provider know if
pregnant or if pregnancy is planned or if
breastfeeding

Rarely Used

alfentanil (℞)
(al-fen′ta-nil)
Alfenta, Rapifen ✦
Func. class.: Opioid analgesic

Controlled Substance Schedule II
Uses: In combination with other drugs
in general anesthesia, as a primary anesthetic in general surgery, monitored anesthesia care (MAC)

DOSAGE AND ROUTES

Anesthesia <30 min
Combination
• *Adult:* IV 8-50 mcg/kg, may increase
by 3-15 mcg/kg
Anesthetic induction
• *Adult:* IV 3-5 mcg/kg, then 0.5-1.5
mcg/kg/min; total dose is 8-40 mcg/kg
Anesthesia 30-60 min
Induction
• *Adult:* IV 20-50 mcg/kg
Maintenance
• *Adult:* IV 5-15 mcg/kg; may give up to
75 mcg/kg total dose

Continuous anesthesia >45 min
Induction
• *Adult:* IV 50-75 mcg/kg
Maintenance
• *Adult:* IV 0.5-3.0 mcg/kg/min; rate should be decreased by 30%-50% after 1 hr maintenance **INF;** may be increased to 4 mcg/kg/min or **BOL** doses of 7 mcg/kg
Induction of anesthesia >45 min
• *Adult:* IV 130-245 mcg/kg, then 0.5-1.5 mcg/kg/min
MAC
Induction
• *Adult:* IV duration ≤½ hr 3-8 mcg/kg
Maintenance
• *Adult:* IV 3-5 mcg/kg q5-20 min to 1 mcg/kg/min, total dose 3-40 mcg/kg
Contraindications: Child <12 yr, hypersensitivity

---

alfuzosin (℞)
(al-fyoo′zoe-sin)
Uroxatral
Func. class.: Urinary tract, antispasmodic, alpha-$_1$ agonist
Chem. class.: Quinazolone

Action: Binds to α_{1A}-adrenoceptor subtype located mainly in the prostate, relaxing smooth muscles
Uses: Symptoms of benign prostatic hyperplasia

DOSAGE AND ROUTES
• *Adult:* **PO** ext rel 10 mg daily, taken after same meal each day
Available forms: Ext rel tabs 10 mg

SIDE EFFECTS
CNS: Dizziness, headache, fatigue
CV: Postural hypotension (dizziness, lightheadedness, fainting) within a few hours of administration, chest pain, tachycardia
GI: Nausea, abdominal pain, dyspepsia, constipation, diarrhea
INTEG: Rash
GU: Impotence, priapism
MISC: Body pain in general, xerostomia

RESP: Upper respiratory infection, pharyngitis, bronchitis, sinusitis
Contraindications: Hypersensitivity, moderate to severe hepatic impairment, not indicated for use in women or children
Precautions: Pregnancy (B), lactation, coronary artery disease, coronary insufficiency, mild hepatic disease, mild/moderate/severe renal disease, history of QT prolongation or coadministration with meds known to prolong QT interval, prostate cancer

PHARMACOKINETICS
PO: Peak 8 hr, elimination half-life 10 hr; extensively metabolized in liver by CYP3A4 enzyme; excreted via urine (11% unchanged); moderately protein binding (82%-90%)

INTERACTIONS
• Not to be taken with: prazosin, terazosin, doxazosin
Increase: effects of alfuzosin—alcohol
Increase: effects—CYP3A4 inhibitors (ketoconazole, itraconazole, and ritonavir); do not use together
Increase: hypotension—β-blockers, phosphodiesterase 5 inhibitors

NURSING CONSIDERATIONS
Assess:
• Prostatic hyperplasia: change in urinary patterns (hesitancy, dribbling, dysuria, urgency), baseline and throughout treatment
• CBC with diff and LFTs; B/P and heart rate; monitor for orthostatic hypotension; B/P lying and standing
• BUN, uric acid, urodynamic studies (urinary flow rates, residual volume)
• I&O ratios, weight daily, edema, report weight gain or edema
Administer:
PO route
• Do not break, crush, or chew tabs; give with food; take at same time of day

---

Perform/provide:

• Storage in tight container in cool environment

Evaluate:

• Therapeutic response: decreased symptoms of benign prostatic hyperplasia

Teach patient/family:

• To take at same time of day with food; do not double doses

• Not to drive or operate machinery for 4 hr after first dose or after dosage increase, dizziness may occur

• About orthostatic hypotension; to rise slowly from sitting or lying

---

alitretinoin (℞)

(a-li-tret'i-noyn)
Panretin
Func. class.: Retinoid, 2nd generation, topical antineoplastic

---

Action: Controls cellular differentiation and proliferation of neoplastic and healthy cells by binding to retinoid receptors

Uses: Kaposi's sarcoma cutaneous lesions

DOSAGE AND ROUTES

• *Adult:* **TOP** Apply enough gel to cover lesions with a generous coating, allow to dry for 3-5 min, before covering with clothing, do not apply near mucosal areas, apply as long as benefit occurs; do not rub gel into the lesion

Available forms: Gel 0.1%

SIDE EFFECTS

INTEG: Rash, stinging, warmth, redness, erythema, blistering, crusting, peeling, contact dermatitis, *pain*

Contraindications: Pregnancy (D), hypersensitivity to retinoids

Precautions: Lactation, eczema, sunburn, geriatric, cutaneous T-cell lymphoma

PHARMACOKINETICS

TOP: Poor systemic absorption

INTERACTIONS

• Do not use around DEET (an insect repellant agent)

NURSING CONSIDERATIONS

Assess:

• Area of body involved, what helps or aggravates condition; cysts, dryness, itching; lesions may worsen at beginning of treatment

• Dermal toxicity that may start as erythema, then edema, may need to be discontinued and restarted

Administer:

• Bid initially to lesions, can be increased to tid-qid according to tolerance

Perform/provide:

• Storage at room temperature

• Hand washing after application

Evaluate:

• Therapeutic response: decrease in size and number of lesions

Teach patient/family:

• To avoid application on normal skin; getting cream in eyes, nose, other mucous membranes; not to rub into lesion; do not use occlusive dressing; wait 20 min after bath, shower to apply; wait at least 3 hr after using to shower, bathe, swim

• To avoid sunlight, sunlamps, or use protective clothing, sunscreen

• That treatment may cause warmth, stinging, dryness, peeling will occur

• That drug does not cure condition; only relieves symptoms

• That therapeutic results may be seen in 2-3 wk but may not be optimal until after 6 wk

---

⚠ Safety alert   *"Tall Man" lettering

allopurinol (℞)

(al-oh-pure′i-nole)

Aloprim, allopurinol, Apo-Allopurinol ✦, Lopurin, Purimol ✦, Zyloprim

Func. class.: Antigout drug, antihyperuricemic

Chem. class.: Xanthene oxidase inhibitor

Do not confuse:

allopurinol/Apresoline
Lopurin/Lupron

Action: Inhibits the enzyme xanthine oxidase, reducing uric acid synthesis

Uses: Chronic gout, hyperuricemia associated with malignancies, recurrent calcium oxalate calculi, uric acid calculi

DOSAGE AND ROUTES

Increased uric acid levels in malignancies

• *Adult:* **PO** 600-800 mg/day in divided doses, start up to 3 days prior to chemotherapy; **IV INF** 200-400 mg/m²/day, max 600 mg/day

• *Child 6-10 yr:* **PO** 300 mg/day

• *Child <6 yr:* **PO** 150 mg/day

• *Child:* **IV INF** 200 mg/m²/day, initially as a single dose or divided q6-12h

Gout

• *Adult:* **PO** 100 mg/day, increase qwk based on uric acid levels, max 800 mg/day; maintenance dose 100-200 mg bid-tid

Renal dose

• *Adult:* **PO** CCr 60 ml/min 200 mg/day; CCr 40 ml/min 150 mg/day; CCr 20 ml/min 100 mg/day; CCr 10 ml/min 100 mg qod; CCr <10 ml/min 100 mg 3×/wk; **IV** CCr 10-20 ml/min 200 mg/day; CCr 3-10 ml/min 100 mg/day; CCr <3 ml/min 100 mg/day at intervals

Recurrent calculi

• *Adult:* **PO** 200-300 mg daily

Uric acid nephropathy prevention

• *Adult and child >10 yr:* **PO** 600-800 mg daily × 2-3 days

Available forms: Tabs, scored 100, 300 mg; inj 500 mg/vial

SIDE EFFECTS

CNS: Headache, drowsiness, neuritis, paresthesia

EENT: Retinopathy, cataracts, epistaxis

GI: Nausea, vomiting, anorexia, malaise, metallic taste, cramps, peptic ulcer, diarrhea, stomatitis

HEMA: **Agranulocytosis, thrombocytopenia, aplastic anemia, pancytopenia, leukopenia, bone marrow suppression, eosinophilia**

INTEG: Fever, chills, dermatitis, pruritus, purpura, erythema, ecchymosis, alopecia

MISC: Myopathy, arthralgia, hepatomegaly, **cholestatic jaundice, renal failure, exfoliative dermatitis**

Contraindications: Hypersensitivity

Precautions: Pregnancy (C), lactation, renal/hepatic disease, children

PHARMACOKINETICS

PO: Peak 2-4 hr; excreted in feces, urine; half-life 2-3 hr, terminal half-life 18-30 hr

IV: Half-life 1 hr

INTERACTIONS

Increase: kidney stone formation—ammonium chloride, vit C, potassium/sodium phosphate

Increase: rash—ampicillin, amoxicillin

Increase: action of oral anticoagulants, oral antidiabetics, theophylline

Increase: hypersensitivity—ACE inhibitors, thiazides

Increase: bone marrow depression—antineoplastics (mercaptopurine, azathioprine)

NURSING CONSIDERATIONS

Assess:

• Uric acid levels q2wk; uric acid levels should be 6 mg/dl or less

• CBC, AST, BUN, creatinine before starting treatment, periodically

• I&O ratio; increase fluids to 2 L/day to prevent stone formation and toxicity

---

✦ Canada only   Side effects: *italics* = common; **bold** = life-threatening

• For rash, hypersensitivity reactions, discontinue allopurinol
• For gout: joint pain, swelling; may use with NSAIDs for acute gouty attacks

Administer:

PO route

• With meals to prevent GI symptoms; may crush and add to foods or fluids
• A few days before antineoplastic therapy

Intermittent IV INF route

• Reconstitute 30 ml vial with 25 ml of sterile water for inj; dilute to desired conc with 0.9% NaCl for inj or D_5 for inj, begin inf within 10 hr

Solution incompatibilities: Amikacin, amphotericin B, carmustine, cefotaxime, chlorproMAZINE, cimetidine, clindamycin, cytarabine, dacarbazine, DAUNOrubicin, diphenhydrAMINE, DOXOrubicin, doxycycline, droperidol, floxuridine, gentamicin, haloperidol, hydrOXYzine, idarubicin, imipenem, cilastatin, mechlorethamine, meperidine, metoclopramide, methylPREDNISolone, minocycline, nalbuphine, netilmicin, ondansetron, prochlorperazine, promethazine, sodium bicarbonate, streptozocin, tobramycin, vinorelbine

Evaluate:

• Therapeutic response: decreased pain in joints, decreased stone formation in kidneys, decreased uric acid levels

Teach patient/family:

• That tabs may be crushed
• To take as prescribed; if dose is missed, take as soon as remembered; do not double dose
• To increase fluid intake to 2 L/day
• To report skin rash, stomatitis, malaise, fever, aching; drug should be discontinued
• To avoid hazardous activities if drowsiness or dizziness occurs
• To avoid alcohol, caffeine; will increase uric acid levels
• To avoid large doses of vit C; kidney stone formation may occur
• To reduce dairy products, refined sugars, sodium, meat if taking for calcium oxalate stones

---

almotriptan (℞)
(al-moh-trip′tan)
Axert
Func. class.: Antimigraine agent, abortive
Chem. class.: 5-HT$_1$-receptor agonist, triptan

Action: Binds selectively to the vascular 5-HT$_{1B/1D}$-receptors, exerts antimigraine effect

Uses: Acute treatment of migraine with or without aura

DOSAGE AND ROUTES

Adult: **PO** 6.25-12.5 mg; may repeat dose after 2 hr; do not give more than 2 doses/24 hr, 25 mg/day or 4 treatment cycles within any 30-day period

Hepatic/renal dose

• *Adult:* **PO** 6.25 mg initially, max 12.5 mg

Available forms: Tabs 6.25, 12.5 mg

SIDE EFFECTS

CV: Flushing, palpitations, tachycardia, **coronary artery vasospasm, MI, ventricular fibrillation, ventricular tachycardia**
EENT: Throat, mouth, nasal discomfort; vision changes
GI: Nausea, xerostomia
INTEG: Sweating
MS: Weakness, neck stiffness, myalgia
NEURO: Tingling, hot sensation, burning, feeling of pressure, tightness, numbness, dizziness, sedation, headache, anxiety, fatigue, cold sensation
RESP: Chest tightness, pressure

Contraindications: Hypersensitivity, cluster headache, hemiplegia, vascular migraine, ischemic heart disease or risk for, peripheral vascular syndrome, concurrent use of ergotamine-containing preparations, uncontrolled hypertension, basilar or hemiplegic migraine; concurrent MAO inhibitor therapy or within 2 wk

Precautions: Pregnancy (C), postmenopausal women, men >40 yr, risk factors

---

for CAD, MI; hypercholesterolemia, obesity, diabetes, impaired renal/hepatic function, lactation, children <18 yr, geriatric

PHARMACOKINETICS

Onset of pain relief 2 hr; peak 1-3 hr; duration 3-4 hr; metabolized in the liver (metabolite), metabolized by MAO-A, CYP2D6, CYP3A4; excreted in urine (40%), feces (13%); half-life 3-4 hr

INTERACTIONS

Increase: vasospastic effects—ergot, ergot derivatives, other 5-HT₁ agonists; avoid concurrent use

⚠ ***Increase:*** almotriptan effect—MAOIs, CYP2D6 inhibitors; do not use together

Increase: plasma concentration of almotriptan—ketoconazole

Drug/Herb

Increase: almotriptan effect—butterbur, feverfew

NURSING CONSIDERATIONS

Assess:
• Migraine: pain location, aura, duration, intensity, nausea, vomiting
• B/P; signs/symptoms of coronary vasospasms
• Tingling, hot sensation, burning, feeling of pressure, numbness, flushing
• For stress level, activity, recreation, coping mechanisms
• Neurologic status: LOC, blurring vision, nausea, vomiting, tingling in extremities preceding headache
• Ingestion of tyramine foods (pickled products, beer, wine, aged cheese), food additives, preservatives, colorings, artificial sweeteners, chocolate, caffeine, which may precipitate these types of headaches

Administer:
• Avoid using more than 2× per wk, rebound headache may occur
• Swallow tabs whole; do not break, crush, or chew

Perform/provide:
• Quiet, calm environment with decreased stimulation from noise, bright light, excessive talking

Evaluate:
• Therapeutic response: decrease in severity of migraine

Teach patient/family:
• To report chest pain, drowsiness, dizziness, tingling, flushing, pressure
• To use contraception while taking drug, notify prescriber if pregnancy is planned or suspected, avoid breastfeeding
• That if one dose does not relieve migraine to take another after 2 hr
• To provide dark, quiet environment
• That drug does not prevent or reduce number of migraine attacks; use to relieve attack only

---

alprazolam (℞)

(al-pray′zoe-lam)
Apo-Alpraz ✤, Niravam, Novo-Alprazol ✤, Nu-Alpraz ✤, Xanax, Xanax XR
Func. class.: Antianxiety
Chem. class.: Benzodiazepine

Controlled Substance Schedule IV

Do not confuse:
alprazolam/lorazepam
Xanax/Lanoxin/Tylox/Zantac

Action: Depresses subcortical levels of CNS, including limbic system, reticular formation

Uses: Anxiety, panic disorders, anxiety with depressive symptoms

Unlabeled uses: Depression, social phobia, premenstrual dysphoric disorders

DOSAGE AND ROUTES

Anxiety disorder
• *Adult:* **PO** 0.25-0.5 mg tid, not to exceed 4 mg/day in divided doses
• *Geriatric:* **PO** 0.125-0.25 mg bid; increase by 0.125 as needed

Panic disorder
• *Adult:* **PO** 0.5 mg tid may increase, max 10 mg/day; ext rel tabs (Xanax XR) give daily in AM 0.5-1 mg initially, maintenance 1-10 mg daily

Premenstrual dysphoric disorders
• *Adult:* **PO** 0.25 mg bid-qid, starting on day 16-18 of menses, taper over 2-3 days when menses occurs
Social phobia
• *Adult:* **PO** 2-8 mg/day
Hepatic dose
• Reduce dose by 50%
Available forms: Tabs 0.25, 0.5, 1, 2 mg; ext rel tabs (Xanax XR) 0.5, 1, 2, 3 mg; orally disintegrating tabs 0.25, 0.5, 1, 2 mg

SIDE EFFECTS

CNS: Dizziness, drowsiness, confusion, headache, anxiety, tremors, stimulation, fatigue, depression, insomnia, hallucinations
CV: Orthostatic hypotension, **ECG changes, tachycardia,** hypotension
EENT: Blurred vision, tinnitus, mydriasis
GI: Constipation, dry mouth, nausea, vomiting, anorexia, diarrhea
INTEG: Rash, dermatitis, itching
Contraindications: Pregnancy (D), hypersensitivity to benzodiazepines, narrow-angle glaucoma, psychosis, lactation, addiction
Precautions: Geriatric, debilitated, hepatic disease

PHARMACOKINETICS

PO: Well absorbed; widely distributed; onset 30 min; peak 1-2 hr; duration 4-6 hr; therapeutic response 2-3 days; metabolized by liver (CYP3A4), excreted by kidneys; crosses placenta, breast milk; half-life 12-15 hr

INTERACTIONS

Increase: alprazolam action—cimetidine, disulfiram, erythromycin, fluoxetine, isoniazid, ketoconazole, metoprolol, propoxyphene, propanolol, valproic acid
Increase: CNS depression—anticonvulsants, alcohol, antihistamines, sedative/hypnotics, opioids
Decrease: sedation—xanthines
Decrease: alprazolam action—barbiturates, rifampin

Decrease: action of levodopa
Decrease: drug level—cigarette smoking
Drug/Herb
Increase: CNS depression—cat's claw, chamomile, cowslip, echinacea, goldenseal, hops, kava, licorice, Queen Anne's lace, skullcap, St. John's wort, valerian, wild cherry
Drug/Food
Increase: drug level—grapefruit juice
Drug/Lab Test
Increase: AST/ALT, alk phos

NURSING CONSIDERATIONS
Assess:
• Mental status: anxiety, mood, sensorium, affect, sleeping pattern, drowsiness, dizziness, especially in geriatric
• B/P lying, standing; pulse; if systolic B/P drops 20 mm Hg, hold drug, notify prescriber
• Hepatic, blood studies: AST, ALT, bilirubin, creatinine, LDH, alk phos, CBC; may cause neutropenia, decreased Hct, increased LFTs
• For indications of increasing tolerance and abuse
⚠ Physical dependency, withdrawal symptoms: anxiety, panic attacks, agitation, convulsions, headache, nausea, vomiting, muscle pain, weakness; withdrawal seizures may occur after rapid decrease in dose or abrupt discontinuation; since duration of action is short, considered to be the drug of choice in the geriatric
Administer:
PO route
• With food or milk for GI symptoms
• Tabs may be crushed, mixed with food or fluids if patient is unable to swallow medication whole; do not break, crush, or chew ext rel (XR)
• May divide total daily doses into more times/day, if anxiety occurs between doses
• Orally disintegrating tabs on tongue to dissolve
Evaluate:
• Therapeutic response: decreased anxiety, restlessness, sleeplessness

Teach patient/family:

• Not to double doses; take exactly as prescribed; if dose is missed, take within 1 hr as scheduled

• That drug may be taken with food

• Not to use for everyday stress or longer than 4 mo unless directed by prescriber; not to take more than prescribed amount; may be habit forming; memory impairment is a sign of long-term use

• To avoid OTC preparations unless approved by prescriber

• To avoid driving, activities that require alertness, since drowsiness may occur

• To avoid alcohol ingestion or other psychotropic medications unless directed by prescriber

• Not to discontinue medication abruptly after long-term use

• To rise slowly or fainting may occur, especially geriatric

• That drowsiness may worsen at beginning of treatment

Treatment of overdose: Lavage, VS, supportive care, flumazenil

---

Rarely Used

alprostadil (℞)

(al-pros′ta-dil)

Caverject, Edex, Muse, PGEI, prostaglandin E₁, Prostin VR ♣, Prostin VR Pediatric

Func. class.: Hormone

Uses: To maintain patent ductus arteriosus (temporary treatment), erectile dysfunction

DOSAGE AND ROUTES

Patent ductus arteriosus

• *Infant:* **IV INF** 0.1 mcg/kg/min, until desired response, then reduce to lowest effective amount, 0.4 mcg/kg/min not likely to produce greater beneficial effects

Erectile dysfunction of vasculogenic or mixed etiology, psychogenic

• *Men:* **INTRACAVERNOSAL** 2.5 mcg may increase by 2.5 mcg; may then increase by 5-10 mcg until adequate response occurs; **INTRAURETHRAL:** administer as needed to achieve erection

Contraindications: Hypersensitivity, respiratory distress syndrome

---

⚠ High Alert

alteplase (℞)

(al-ti-plaze′)

Activase, Activase rt-PA ♣, Cathflo, Lysatec-rt-PA ♣, tissue plasminogen activator, t-PA

Func. class.: Thrombolytic enzyme

Chem. class.: Tissue plasminogen activator (TPA)

Do not confuse:

alteplase/Altace

Action: Produces fibrin conversion of plasminogen to plasmin; able to bind to fibrin, convert plasminogen in thrombus to plasmin, which leads to local fibrinolysis, limited systemic proteolysis

Uses: Lysis of obstructing thrombi associated with acute MI, ischemic conditions requiring thrombolysis (i.e., PE, DVT, unclotting arteriovenous shunts, acute ischemic CVA)

Unlabeled uses: Unstable angina, occluded central venous catheters

DOSAGE AND ROUTES

MI (standard infusion)

• *Adult >65 kg:* 100 mg total given as: 6-10 mg IV bolus over 1-2 min; 60 mg total over 1st hour; 20 mg over 2nd hr; 30 mg over 3rd hour

• *Adult <65 kg:* 1.25 mg/kg over 3 hr: 60% in 1st hr (10% as a bolus); remaining 40% over next 2 hr

MI (accelerated infusion)

• *Adult >67 kg:* 100 mg total dose: give 15 mg IV bolus, then 50 mg over 30 min, then 35 mg over 60 min

• *Adult <67 kg:* 15 mg IV bolus: 0.75 mg/kg over 30 min; 0.5 mg/kg over 60 min

Venous catheter occlusion

• *Adult <30 kg:* Use 110% of internal

Side effects: *italics* = common; **bold** = life-threatening

lumen volume of catheter; do not exceed 2 mg in 2 ml; may use up to 2 doses (120 min apart)

Pulmonary embolism
• *Adult:* **IV** 100 mg over 2 hr, then heparin

Acute ischemic stroke
• *Adult:* **IV** 0.9 mg/kg, max 90 mg; give as **INF** over 1 hr, give 10% of dose **IV BOL** over 1st min

Available forms: Powder for inj 50 mg (29 million international units/vial), 100 mg (58 million international units/vial); lyophilized powder for inj 2 mg

SIDE EFFECTS

CV: **Sinus bradycardia, ventricular tachycardia, accelerated idioventricular rhythm, bradycardia**
INTEG: Urticaria, rash
SYST: **GI, GU, intracranial, retroperitoneal bleeding,** *surface bleeding,* **anaphylaxis**

Contraindications: Hypersensitivity, active internal bleeding, history of CVA, severe uncontrolled hypertension, intracranial/intraspinal surgery/trauma (within 3 mo), aneurysm, brain tumor, seizures, platelets <100,000 mm^3

Precautions: Pregnancy (C), lactation, children, geriatric, neurologic deficits, mitral stenosis, recent GI, GU bleeding, diabetic retinopathy

PHARMACOKINETICS

Cleared by liver, 80% cleared within 10 min of drug termination, onset immediate, peak 45 min, duration 4 hr, half-life 35 min

INTERACTIONS

Increase: bleeding—anticoagulants, salicylates, dipyridamole, other NSAIDs, abciximab, eptifibatide, tirofiban, clopidogrel, ticlopidine, some cephalosporins, plicamycin, valproic acid

Drug/Herb

Increase: risk of bleeding—agrimony, alfalfa, angelica, anise, basil, bay, bilberry, black haw, bogbean, bromelain, buchu, chondroitin, cinchona bark, dong quai, fenugreek, feverfew, garlic, ginger, ginkgo, ginseng, horse chestnut, Irish moss, kelp, kelpware, khella, lovage, lungwort, meadowsweet, mother wort, mugwort, nettle, papaya, parsley (large amts), pau d'arco, pineapple, poplar, prickly ash, safflower, saw palmetto, tonka bean, tumeric, wintergreen, yarrow

Decrease: anticoagulant effect—chamomile, coenzyme Q10, flax, glucomannan, goldenseal, guar gum

Drug/Lab Test
Increase: PT, APTT, TT

NURSING CONSIDERATIONS

Assess:
• VS, B/P, pulse, respirations, neurologic signs, temperature at least q4h; temp >104° F (40° C) indicates internal bleeding; monitor rhythm closely; ventricular dysrhythmias may occur with hyperfusion; monitor heart, breath sounds, neurologic status, peripheral pulses; assess neurologic status, neurologic change may indicate intracranial bleeding

⚠ For bleeding during first hour of treatment and 24 hr after procedure: hematuria, hematemesis, bleeding from mucous membranes, epistaxis, ecchymosis; guaiac all body fluids, stools. Do not use 150 mg or more total dose; intracranial bleeding may occur

⚠ Hypersensitivity: fever, rash, itching, chills, facial swelling, dyspnea, notify prescriber immediately; stop drug, keep resuscitative equipment nearby; mild reaction may be treated with antihistamines

• Blood studies (Hct, platelets, PTT, PT, TT, APTT) before starting therapy; PT or APTT must be less than 2 × control before starting therapy TT or PT q3-4h during treatment

• ECG continuously, cardiac enzymes, radionuclide myocardial scanning/coronary angiography

Administer:
| **Intermittent IV INF route** |
• After reconstituting with provided diluent, add appropriate amount of sterile water for inj (no preservatives) 20 mg

vial/20 ml or 50 mg vial/50 ml to make 1
mg/ml, mix by slow inversion or dilute
with NaCl, D_5W to a concentration of 0.5
mg/ml; 1.5 to <0.5 mg/ml may result in
precipitation of drug; use 18G needle;
flush line with NaCl after administration,
give over 3 hr for MI, 2 hr for PE
• Heparin therapy after thrombolytic therapy is discontinued, TT, ACT, or APTT less
than 2 × control (about 3-4 hr)
• Reconstituted IV solution within 8 hr
or discard
• Within 6 hr of coronary occlusion for
best results
Additive compatibilities: Lidocaine,
morphine, nitroglycerin
Y-site compatibilities: Lidocaine, metoprolol, propranolol
Perform/provide:
• Avoidance of invasive procedures, injection, rectal temp
• Pressure for 30 sec to minor bleeding
sites; 30 min to sites of atrial puncture,
followed by pressure dressing; inform
prescriber if this does not attain hemostasis; apply pressure dressing
• Storage of powder at room temperature or refrigerate; protect from excessive light
Evaluate:
• Therapeutic response: lysis of thrombi
Teach patient/family:
• The purpose and expected results of
the treatment; to report adverse reactions

Rarely Used

altretamine (℞)
(al-tret'a-meen)
Hexalen, hexamethylmela-
mine, Hexastat ✤
Func. class.: Miscellaneous antineoplastic

Uses: Palliative treatment of recurrent,
persistent ovarian cancer following first-
line treatment with cisplatin or alkylating
agent–based combination
Unlabeled uses: Lymphoma, lung cancer

DOSAGE AND ROUTES
• *Adult:* **PO** 260 mg/m^2/day for 14 or
21 days in a 28-day cycle; give in 4 divided doses after meals and at bedtime
Contraindications: Pregnancy (D),
hypersensitivity, severe bone marrow depression, severe neurologic toxicity

aluminum hydroxide (OTC)
AlternaGEL, Alu-Cap,
Alugel ✤, Aluminet,
aluminum hydroxide, Alu-
Tab, Amphojel, Basal gel,
Dialume
Func. class.: Antacid, hypophospha-
temic, antiulcer
Chem. class.: Aluminum product,
phosphate binder

Action: Neutralizes gastric acidity, binds
phosphates in GI tract; these phosphates
are excreted
Uses: Antacid, hyperphosphatemia in
chronic renal failure; adjunct in gastric,
peptic, duodenal ulcers; hyperacidity, reflux esophagitis, heartburn, stress ulcer
prevention in critically ill, GERD
Unlabeled uses: GI bleeding

DOSAGE AND ROUTES
Antacid
• *Adult:* **SUSP** 5-10 ml 1 hr after meals,
at bedtime; **PO** 600 mg 1 hr after meals,
at bedtime, chewed; max 6 doses per day
Hyperphosphatemia
• *Adult:* **SUSP** 500 mg-2 g bid-qid
GI bleeding
• *Infant:***PO** 2-5 ml/dose q1-2h
• *Child:* **PO** 5-15 ml/dose q1-2h
Available forms: Caps 475, 500 mg;
tabs 300, 500, 600 mg; susp 320 mg/5
ml, 450 mg/5 ml, 600 mg/5 ml, 675 mg/5
ml

SIDE EFFECTS
GI: Constipation, anorexia, **obstruction,**
fecal impaction
META: Hypophosphatemia, hypercalciuria

Contraindications: Hypersensitivity to this drug or aluminum products

Precautions: Pregnancy (C), geriatric, fluid restriction, decreased GI motility, GI obstruction, dehydration, renal disease, sodium-restricted diets, lactation

PHARMACOKINETICS

PO: Onset 20-40 min, duration 1-3 hr, excreted in feces

INTERACTIONS

Decrease: effectiveness of allopurinol, amprenavir, cephalosporins, ciprofloxacin, corticosteroids, delavirdine, diflunisal, digoxin, gabapentin, gatifloxacin, H_2-antagonists, iron salts, isoniazid, ketoconazole, penicillamine, phenothiazines, phenytoin, quinidine, tetracyclines, thyroid hormones, ticlopidine anticholinergics, warfarin; separate by at least 2 hr

Drug/Herb

Decrease: action of buckthorn, cascara sagrada, castor, Chinese rhubarb

NURSING CONSIDERATIONS

Assess:

• Pain: location, intensity, duration, character

• Phosphate levels, since drug is bound in GI system

• Hypophosphatemia: anorexia, weakness, fatigue, bone pain, hyporeflexia

• Constipation; increase bulk in diet if needed

• Urinary pH, Ca^{++}, electrolytes

Administer:

• 2 tsp (10 ml) will neutralize 20 mEq of acid; 2 tabs will neutralize 16 mEq of acid

PO route

• Give with 8 oz water for hyperphosphatemia, unless contraindicated

• Tablets must be chewed well, then give 8 oz water

• Laxatives or stool softeners if constipation occurs, especially geriatric

• After shaking liquid

• With small amount of water or milk

NG route

• By nasogastric tube if patient unable to swallow

Evaluate:

• Therapeutic response: absence of pain, decreased acidity, healed ulcers, decreased phosphate levels

Teach patient/family:

• To increase fluids to 2 L/day unless contraindicated; measures to prevent constipation

• To avoid phosphate foods (most dairy products, eggs, fruits, carbonated beverages) during drug therapy for hyperphosphatemia

• Not to use for prolonged periods in patients with low serum phosphate or if on a low-sodium diet

• To add cheese, corn, pasta, plums, prunes, lentils after drug is discontinued

• That stools may appear white or speckled

• To check with prescriber after 2 wk of self-prescribed antacid use

• To separate other medications by 2 hr

---

amantadine (℞)

(a-man′ta-deen)

amantadine HCl, Symmetrel

Func. class.: Antiviral, antiparkinsonian agent

Chem. class.: Tricyclic amine

Do not confuse:

amantadine/ranitidine/rimantadine

Symmetrel/Synthroid

Action: Prevents uncoating of nucleic acid in viral cell, preventing penetration of virus to host; causes release of DOPamine from neurons

Uses: Prophylaxis or treatment of influenza type A, extrapyramidal reactions, parkinsonism, Parkinson's disease

Unlabeled uses: Neuroleptic malignant syndrome, cocaine dependency, enuresis, MS-associated fatigue

---

⚠ Safety alert　*"Tall Man" lettering

DOSAGE AND ROUTES

Influenza type A
- *Adult and child >12 yr:* **PO** 200 mg/day in single dose or divided bid, max 400 mg/day
- *Geriatric:* **PO** No more than 100 mg daily
- *Child 9-12 yr:* **PO** 100 mg bid
- *Child 1-9 yr:* **PO** 5 mg/kg/day divided bid-tid, not to exceed 150 mg/day

Extrapyramidal reaction/parkinsonism
Adult: **PO** 100 mg bid, up to 400 mg/day in EPS; give for 1 wk, then 100 mg as needed up to 400 mg in parkinsonism

MS-associated fatigue (unlabeled)
- *Adult:* **PO** 200 mg daily or 100 mg bid

Neuroleptic malignant syndrome (unlabeled)
- *Adult:* **PO** 100 mg bid × 3 wk

Renal dose
- *Adult:* **PO** CCr 40-50 ml/min 100 mg/day; CCr 30 ml/min 200 mg 2×/wk; CCr 20 ml/min 100 mg 3×/wk; CCr <10 ml/min 100 mg alternating with 200 mg q7days

Available forms: Caps 100 mg; syr 50 mg/5 ml

SIDE EFFECTS

CNS: Headache, dizziness, drowsiness, fatigue, *anxiety,* psychosis, *depression, hallucinations,* tremors, **convulsions,** confusion, *insomnia*
CV: Orthostatic hypotension, **CHF**
EENT: Blurred vision
GI: Nausea, vomiting, constipation, dry mouth
GU: Frequency, retention
HEMA: **Leukopenia**
INTEG: Photosensitivity, dermatitis, livedo reticularis

Contraindications: Hypersensitivity, lactation, child <1 yr, eczematous rash
Precautions: Pregnancy (C), epilepsy, CHF, orthostatic hypotension, psychiatric disorders, renal/hepatic disease, peripheral edema, geriatric

PHARMACOKINETICS

PO: Onset 48 hr, half-life 24 hr, not metabolized, excreted in urine (90%) unchanged, crosses placenta, excreted in breast milk

INTERACTIONS

Increase: anticholinergic response—atropine, other anticholinergics
Increase: CNS stimulation—CNS stimulants
Decrease: renal excretion of amantadine—triamterene, hydrochlorothiazide
Drug/Herb
Increase: anticholinergic effect—belladonna, henbane
Increase: action/side effects—pheasant's eye, quinine, scopolia root
Decrease: effect—kava

NURSING CONSIDERATIONS

Assess:
- I&O ratio; report frequency, hesitancy
- CHF (weight gain, jugular venous distention, dyspnea, crackles)
- Bowel pattern before, during treatment
- Skin eruptions, photosensitivity after administration of drug
- Respiratory status: rate, character, wheezing, tightness in chest
- Allergies before initiation of treatment, reaction of each medication
- Signs of infection
- Livedo reticularis: mottling of the skin, usually red
- Parkinson's disease: gait, tremors, akinesia, rigidity
- Toxicity: confusion, behavioral changes, hypotension, seizures

Administer:
- Before exposure to influenza; continue for 10 days after contact
- At least 4 hr before bedtime to prevent insomnia
- After meals for better absorption, to decrease GI symptoms
- In divided doses to prevent CNS disturbances: headache, dizziness, fatigue, drowsiness

---

Perform/provide:
• Storage in tight, dry container
Evaluate:
• Therapeutic response: absence of fever, malaise, cough, dyspnea in infection; tremors, shuffling gait in Parkinson's disease
Teach patient/family:
• To change body position slowly to prevent orthostatic hypotension
• About aspects of drug therapy: need to report dyspnea, weight gain, dizziness, poor concentration, dysuria, behavioral changes
• To avoid hazardous activities if dizziness, blurred vision occurs
• To take drug exactly as prescribed; parkinsonian crisis may occur if drug is discontinued abruptly; do not double dose; if a dose is missed, do not take within 4 hr of next dose; caps may be opened and mixed with food
• To avoid alcohol
Treatment of overdose: Withdraw drug, maintain airway, administer epiNEPHrine, aminophylline, O$_2$, IV corticosteroids, physostigmine

---

amifostine (℞)
(a-mi-foss'teen)
Ethyol
Func. class.: Cytoprotective agent for cisplatin

Action: Binds and detoxifies damaging metabolites of cisplatin by converting this drug by alk phos in tissue to an active free thiol compound
Uses: Used to reduce renal toxicity when cisplatin is given repeatedly in ovarian cancer, non–small cell lung cancer; reduces xerostomia (dry mouth) in radiation therapy for head, neck cancer
Unlabeled uses: To prevent or reduce cisplatin-induced neurotoxicity, cyclophosphamide-induced granulocytopenia; prevent or reduce toxicity of radiation therapy; reduce toxicity of paclitaxel

DOSAGE AND ROUTES

Reduction of renal damage with cisplatin
• *Adult:* **IV** 910 mg/m^2 daily, within ½ hr before chemotherapy, give over 15 min; may reduce dose to 740 mg/m^2 if higher dose is poorly tolerated

Xerostomia
• *Adult:* **IV** 200 mg/m^2 daily over 3 min as an infusion 15-30 min before radiation therapy
Available forms: Powder for inj, lyophilized 500 mg/vial

SIDE EFFECTS

CNS: Dizziness, somnolence
CV: Hypotension
EENT: Sneezing
GI: Nausea, vomiting, hiccups
INTEG: Flushing, feeling of warmth
MISC: Hypocalcemia, rash, chills, **anaphylaxis, toxic epidermal necrolysis, Stevens-Johnson syndrome,** *exfoliative dermatitis, erythema multiforme*
Contraindications: Hypersensitivity to mannitol, aminothiol; hypotension, dehydration, lactation
Precautions: Pregnancy (C), geriatric, CV disease, children

PHARMACOKINETICS

Metabolized to free thiol compound, half-life 8 min, onset 5-8 min

INTERACTIONS

Increase: hypotension—antihypertensives

NURSING CONSIDERATIONS
Assess:
• For xerostomia: mouth lesions, dry mouth during therapy
• Fluid status before administration; administer antiemetic prior to administration to prevent severe nausea and vomit-

---

ing; also, dexamethasone 20 mg IV and a serotonin antagonist such as ondansetron, dolasetron, or granisetron

• Calcium levels before and during treatment, may cause hypocalcemia; calcium supplements may be given for hypocalcemia

• B/P prior to and q5min during infusion; antihypertensive should be discontinued 24 hr prior to infusion if severe hypotension occurs, give IV 0.9% NaCl to expand fluid volume, place in modified Trendelenburg position

Administer:

Intermittent IV INF route

• Intermittent inf after reconstituting with 9.5 ml of sterile 0.9% NaCl, further dilute with 0.9% NaCl to a concentration of 5-40 mg/ml, give over 15 min within ½ hr of chemotherapy

• Supine position during infusion

Y-site compatibilities: Amikacin, aminophylline, ampicillin, ampicillin/sulbactam, aztreonam, bleomycin, bumetanide, buprenorphine, butorphanol, calcium gluconate, carboplatin, carmustine, cefazolin, cefonicid, cefotaxime, cefotetan, cefoxitin, ceftazidime, ceftizoxime, ceftriaxone, cefuroxime, cimetidine, ciprofloxacin, clindamycin, cyclophosphamide, cytarabine, dacarbazine, dactinomycin, DAUNOrubicin, dexamethasone, diphenhydrAMINE, DOBUTamine, DOPamine, DOXOrubicin, doxycycline, droperidol, enalaprilat, etoposide, famotidine, floxuridine, fluconazole, fludarabine, fluorouracil, furosemide, gallium, gentamicin, granisetron, haloperidol, heparin, hydrocortisone, hydromorphone, idarubicin, ifosfamide, imipenem-cilastatin, leucovorin, lorazepam, magnesium sulfate, mannitol, mechlorethamine, meperidine, mesna, methotrexate, methylPREDNISolone, metoclopramide, metronidazole, mezlocillin, mitomycin, mitoxantrone, morphine, nalbuphine, netilmicin, ondansetron, piperacillin, plicamycin, potassium chloride, promethazine, ranitidine, sodium bicarbonate, streptozocin, teniposide, thiotepa, ticarcillin, ticarcillin/clavulanate, tobramycin, trimethoprim-sulfamethoxazole, trimetrexate, vancomycin, vinBLAStine, vinCRIStine, zidovudine

Solution compatibility: 0.9% NaCl

Additive incompatibilities: Do not mix with other drugs

Evaluate:

• Therapeutic response: prevention of renal toxicity associated with cisplatin therapy; decreased xerostomia associated with radiation therapy of head, neck cancer

Teach patient/family:

• The reason for the medication and expected results

• That side effects may cause severe nausea, vomiting, decreased B/P, chills, dizziness, somnolence, hiccups, sneezing

• Do not breastfeed

---

amikacin (℞)

(am-i-kay′sin)

amikacin sulfate, Amikin

Func. class.: Antiinfective

Chem. class.: Aminoglycoside

Do not confuse:

Amikin/Amicar

Action: Interferes with protein synthesis in bacterial cell by binding to ribosomal subunit, which causes misreading of genetic code; inaccurate peptide sequence forms in protein chain, causing bacterial death

Uses: Severe systemic infections of CNS, respiratory, GI, urinary tract, bone, skin, soft tissues caused by *Staphylococcus, Pseudomonas aeruginosa, Escherichia coli, Enterobacter, Acinetobacter, Providencia, Citrobacter, Serratia, Proteus, Klebsiella pneumoniae*

Unlabeled uses: *Mycobacterium avium* complex (intrathecal or intraventricular) in combination; aerosolization

DOSAGE AND ROUTES

Severe systemic infections

• *Adult and child:* IV INF 15 mg/kg/day in 2-3 divided doses q8-12h in 100-200 ml D₅W over 30-60 min, not to exceed 1.5 g; use for 7-10 days; decreased doses are needed in poor renal function as de-

termined by blood levels, renal studies;
IM 15 mg/kg/day in divided doses q8-12h; daily or extended interval dosing as an alternative dosing regimen
• *Infant:* **IV/IM** 10 mg/kg initially; then 7.5 mg/kg q12h
• *Neonate:* **IV/IM** 10 mg/kg, initially, 7.5 mg/kg q12h
• *Premature neonate:* 10 mg/kg initially, then 7.5 mg/kg q8-12h
Severe urinary tract infections
• *Adult:* IM 15 mg/kg/day divided q8-12h
Hemodialysis
• *Adult:* IM/IV 7.5 mg/kg followed by 5 mg/kg 3×/week after each dialysis session (for TIW dialysis)
Renal dose
• *Adult:* **IM/IV** 7.5 mg/kg initially, then increased as determined by blood levels, renal function studies
Available forms: Inj 50, 250 mg/ml

SIDE EFFECTS

CNS: Confusion, depression, numbness, tremors, **convulsions,** muscle twitching, **neurotoxicity,** dizziness, vertigo, tinnitus, **neuromuscular blockade with respiratory paralysis**
CV: Hypotension or hypertension, palpitations
EENT: Ototoxicity, deafness, visual disturbances
GI: Nausea, vomiting, anorexia; increased ALT, AST, bilirubin; hepatomegaly, **hepatic necrosis,** splenomegaly
GU: **Oliguria, hematuria, renal damage, azotemia, renal failure, nephrotoxicity**
HEMA: **Agranulocytosis, thrombocytopenia,** leukopenia, eosinophilia, anemia
INTEG: Rash, burning, urticaria, dermatitis, alopecia
Contraindications: Pregnancy (D), mild to moderate infections, hypersensitivity to aminoglycosides, sulfites
Precautions: Neonates, mild renal disease, myasthenia gravis, lactation, hearing deficits, Parkinson's disease, geriatric

PHARMACOKINETICS

IM: Onset rapid, peak 1-2 hr; leads to unpredictable concentrations, IV preferred
IV: Onset immediate, peak 15-30 min; plasma half-life 2-3 hr, prolonged up to 7 hr in infants; not metabolized, excreted unchanged in urine, crosses placental barrier, poor penetration into CSF, removed by hemodialysis

INTERACTIONS

• May increase serum trough and peak: indomethacin
• Inactivation of amikacin: parenteral penicillins, cephalosporins; do not use together
• Mask ototoxicity: dimenhydrinate, ethacrynic acid
• Nephrotoxicity: cephalosporins, acyclovir, vancomycin, amphotericin B, cycloSPORINE
• Do not use with cidofovir
Increase: neuromuscular blockade, respiratory depression—anesthetics, nondepolarizing neuromuscular blockers
Drug/Herb
• Do not use acidophilus with antiinfectives; separate by several hours
• Toxicity: lysine (large amounts)
Drug/Lab Test
Increase: BUN, ALT, AST, bilirubin, LDH, alk phos, creatinine
Decrease: Ca, Na, K, Mg

NURSING CONSIDERATIONS

Assess:
• Weight before treatment; calculation of dosage is usually based on ideal body weight but may be calculated on actual body weight
• I&O ratio; urinalysis daily for proteinuria, cells, casts; report sudden change in urine output
• VS during infusion; watch for hypotension, change in pulse
• IV site for thrombophlebitis including pain, redness, swelling q30 min; change

site if needed; apply warm compresses to discontinued site

• Serum peak, drawn at 30-60 min after IV infusion or 60 min after IM inj, trough level drawn just before next dose; peak 20-30 mcg/ml, trough 4-8 mcg/ml; adjust dosage per levels

• Urine pH if drug is used for UTI; urine should be kept alkaline

• Renal impairment by securing urine for CCr, BUN, serum creatinine; lower dosage should be given in renal impairment (CCr <80 ml/min); nephrotoxicity may be reversible if drug stopped at first sign

⚠ Deafness by audiometric testing, ringing, roaring in ears, vertigo; assess hearing before, during, after treatment

• Dehydration: high specific gravity, decrease in skin turgor, dry mucous membranes, dark urine

• Overgrowth of infection, including increased temp, malaise, redness, pain, swelling, perineal itching, diarrhea, stomatitis, change in cough, sputum

• C&S before starting treatment to identify organism

• Vestibular dysfunction: nausea, vomiting, dizziness, headache; drug should be discontinued if severe

• Inj sites for redness, swelling, abscesses; use warm compresses at site

Administer:
IM route

• Inj in large muscle mass; rotate inj sites

• Bicarbonate to alkalinize urine if ordered for UTI because drug is most active in alkaline environment

Intermittent IV INF route

• Dilute 500 mg of drug/100-200 ml of IV D_5W, D_5RL, D_5NaCl, or 0.9% NaCl and give over ½-1 hr; flush after administration with D_5W or 0.9% NaCl; solution is clear or pale yellow; discard if precipitate or dark color develops

• In evenly spaced doses to maintain blood level

Additive compatibilities: Avoid admixing

Syringe compatibilities: Clindamycin, doxapram

Y-site compatibilities: Acyclovir, ala-

trofloxacin, aldesleukin, amifostine, aminophylline, amiodarone, amsacrine, anidulafungin, aztreonam, cefepime, cisatracurium, cyclophosphamide, dexamethasone, diltiazem, enalaprilat, esmolol, filgrastim, fluconazole, fludarabine, foscarnet, furosemide, granisetron, idarubicin, IL-2, labetalol, lorazepam, magnesium sulfate, melphalan, midazolam, morphine, ondansetron, paclitaxel, perphenazine, remifentanil, sargramostim, teniposide, thiotepa, TPN #54, #61, #91, #203, #204, #212, vinorelbine, warfarin, zidovudine

Perform/provide:

• Adequate fluids of 2-3 L/day, unless contraindicated, to prevent irritation of tubules

• Flush of IV line with NS or D_5W after infusion

• Supervised ambulation, other safety measures with vestibular dysfunction

Evaluate:

• Therapeutic response: absence of fever, draining wounds, negative C&S after treatment

Teach patient/family:

• To report headache, dizziness, symptoms for overgrowth of infection, renal impairment

⚠ To report loss of hearing, ringing, roaring in ears or feeling of fullness in head

• To report hypersensitivity: rash, itching, trouble breathing, facial edema; notify health care provider

Treatment of hypersensitivity: Hemodialysis, exchange transfusion in the newborn, monitor serum levels of drug, may give ticarcillin or carbenicillin

---

amiloride (℞)
(a-mill'oh-ride)
amiloride HCl, Midamor
Func. class.: Potassium-sparing diuretic
Chem. class.: Pyrazine

Do not confuse:
amiloride/amlodipine

Side effects: *italics* = common; **bold** = life-threatening

Action: Inhibits sodium, potassium ATPase in the distal tubule, cortical collecting duct resulting in inhibition of sodium reabsorption and decreasing potassium secretion

Uses: Edema in CHF in combination with other diuretics, for hypertension, adjunct with other diuretics to maintain potassium

DOSAGE AND ROUTES
• *Adult:* PO 5-10 mg daily in 1-2 divided doses; may be increased to 10-20 mg daily if needed
Available forms: Tabs 5 mg

SIDE EFFECTS
CNS: Headache, dizziness, fatigue, weakness, paresthesias, tremor, depression, anxiety
CV: Orthostatic hypotension, dysrhythmias, chest pain
EENT: Blurred vision, increased intraocular pressure
ELECT: **Hyperkalemia**
GI: Nausea, diarrhea, dry mouth, *vomiting, anorexia,* cramps, constipation, abdominal pain, jaundice
GU: Polyuria, dysuria, urinary frequency, impotence
HEMA: **Aplastic anemia, neutropenia**
INTEG: Rash, pruritus, alopecia, urticaria
MS: Cramps
RESP: Cough, dyspnea, shortness of breath
Contraindications: Anuria, hypersensitivity, hyperkalemia, impaired renal function
Precautions: Pregnancy (B), dehydration, diabetes, acidosis, lactation, geriatric

PHARMACOKINETICS
PO: 15%-25% absorbed from GI tract; widely distributed; onset 2 hr, peak 6-10 hr, duration 24 hr; excreted in urine, feces, half-life 6-9 hr

INTERACTIONS
• Hyperkalemia: other potassium-sparing diuretics, potassium products, ACE inhibi-

tors, salt substitutes, cycloSPORINE, tacrolimus
• Lithium toxicity: lithium
Increase: action of antihypertensives
Decrease: effect of amiloride—NSAIDs
Drug/Herb
• Fatal hypokalemia: arginine
• Hypokalemia: bearberry, gossypol, licorice
• Severe photosensitivity: St. John's wort
Increase: effect—cucumber, dandelion, horsetail, licorice, nettle, pumpkin, Queen Anne's lace
Increase: hypotension—khella
Drug/Food
• Possible hyperkalemia: foods high in potassium
Drug/Lab Test
Interference: GTT

NURSING CONSIDERATIONS
Assess:
• Weight, I&O daily to determine fluid loss; effect of drug may be decreased if used daily
• B/P lying, standing; postural hypotension may occur
• Electrolytes: K, Na, Cl; glucose (serum), BUN, CBC, serum creatinine, blood pH, ABGs
Administer:
• In AM to avoid interference with sleep if using drug as a diuretic; if second daily dose is needed, give in late afternoon
• With food; if nausea occurs, absorption may be decreased slightly
Evaluate:
• Therapeutic response: improvement in edema of feet, legs, sacral area daily if medication is being used in CHF
Teach patient/family:
• To take as prescribed; if dose is missed, take when remembered within 1 hr of next dose
• About adverse reactions: muscle cramps, weakness, nausea, dizziness, blurred vision
• To take with food or milk for GI symptoms
• To take early in day to prevent nocturia

• To avoid potassium-rich foods: oranges, bananas; salt substitutes, dried fruits
Treatment of overdose: Lavage if taken orally, monitor electrolytes, administer sodium bicarbonate for potassium >6.5 mEq/L, IV glucose, kacyoxalate is needed, monitor hydration, CV, renal status

---

amino acid injection (℞)
(a-mee'noe)
FreAmine, HepatAmine
Func. class.: Nitrogen product

Action: Needed for anabolism to maintain structure, decrease catabolism, promote healing
Uses: Hepatic encephalopathy, cirrhosis, hepatitis, nutritional support in cancer; to prevent nitrogen loss when adequate nutrition by mouth, gastric, or duodenal tube cannot be used

DOSAGE AND ROUTES

• *Adult:* IV 80-120 g/day; 500 ml of amino acids/500 ml D$_{50}$ given over 24 hr
Available forms: Inj; many strengths, types

SIDE EFFECTS

CNS: Dizziness, headache, confusion, **loss of consciousness**
CV: Hypertension, **CHF, pulmonary edema**
ENDO: Hyperglycemia, rebound hypoglycemia, electrolyte imbalances, hyperosmolar syndrome, hyperosmolar hyperglycemic nonketotic syndrome, alkalosis, acidosis, hypophosphatemia, hyperammonemia, dehydration, hypocalcemia
GI: Nausea, vomiting, liver fat deposits, abdominal pain
GU: Glycosuria, osmotic diuresis
INTEG: Chills, flushing, warm feeling, rash, urticaria, extravasation necrosis, phlebitis at inj site
Contraindications: Hypersensitivity, severe electrolyte imbalances, anuria, severe liver damage, maple syrup urine disease, PKU
Precautions: Pregnancy (C), renal disease, lactation, children, diabetes mellitus, CHF

INTERACTIONS

Decrease: protein sparing effects—tetracycline

NURSING CONSIDERATIONS

Assess:
• Electrolytes (K, Na, Ca, Cl, Mg), blood glucose, ammonia, phosphate, ketones
• Renal, hepatic studies: BUN, creatinine, ALT, AST, bilirubin
• Inj site for extravasation: redness along vein, edema at site, necrosis, pain, hard tender area; site should be changed immediately
• Respiratory function q4h: auscultate lung fields bilaterally for crackles, respirations, quality, rate, rhythm
• Temp q4h for increased fever, indicating infection; if infection suspected, infusion is discontinued, tubing and solution cultured
⚠ For impending hepatic coma: asterixis, confusion, uremic fetor, lethargy
• Hyperammonemia: nausea, vomiting, malaise, tremors, anorexia, convulsions
Administer:
CONT IV route
• Up to 40% protein and dextrose (up to 12.5%) via peripheral vein; stronger solutions require central IV administration
• TPN only mixed with dextrose to promote protein synthesis
• Immediately after mixing under strict aseptic technique; use infusion pump, in-line filter (0.22 μm) unless mixed with fat emulsion and dextrose (3 in 1)
⚠ Using careful monitoring technique; do not speed up infusion; pulmonary edema, glucose overload will result
Additive compatibilities: Amikacin, aminophylline, aztreonam, calcium gluconate, cefazolin, cefepime, cefotaxime, cefoxitin, cefsulodin, ceftazidime, ceftriaxone, cefuroxime, cimetidine, clindamycin, cyanocobalamin, cyclophosphamide,

Side effects: *italics* = common; **bold** = life-threatening

cycloSPORINE, cytarabine, DOPamine, epoetin, erythromycin, famotidine, folic acid, fosphenytoin, furosemide, heparin, insulin (regular), isoproterenol, lidocaine, meperidine, metaraminol, methicillin, methotrexate, methyldopate, methylPREDNISolone, metoclopramide, morphine, nafcillin, netilmicin, nizatidine, norepinephrine, ondansetron, oxacillin, penicillin G potassium, penicillin G sodium, phytonadione, polymyxin B, sodium bicarbonate, tacrolimus, tobramycin, vancomycin

Y-site compatibilities: Amikacin, aminophylline, amoxicillin, ampicillin, ascorbic acid inj, atracurium, azlocillin, aztreonam, bumetanide, buprenorphine, calcium gluconate, carboplatin, cefonicid, cefoperazone, cefotaxime, cefotetan, cefoxitin, ceftazidime, ceftizoxime, ceftriaxone, cefuroxime, cephalothin, cephapirin, chloramphenicol, chlorproMAZINE, cimetidine, clindamycin, clonazepam, dexamethasone, diazepam, digoxin, diphenhydrAMINE, DOBUTamine, DOPamine, doxycycline, droperidol, enalaprilat, epINEPHrine, erythromycin, famotidine, fentanyl, flucloxacillin, fluconazole, folic acid, foscarnet, gentamicin, granisetron, haloperidol, heparin, hydrocortisone, hydromorphone, hydrOXYzine, idarubicin, ifosfamide, IL-2, imipenem/cilastatin, insulin (regular), isoproterenol, kanamycin, leucovorin, levorphanol, lidocaine, lorazepam, magnesium sulfate, mannitol, meperidine, mesna, methicillin, metronidazole, mezlocillin, miconazole, morphine, moxalactam, multivitamins, nafcillin, netilmicin, nitroglycerin, nitroprusside, norepinephrine, octreotide, ofloxacin, ondansetron, oxacillin, paclitaxel, penicillin G, penicillin G potassium, pentobarbital, phenobarbital, piperacillin, potassium chloride, prochlorperazine, ranitidine, salbutamol, sargramostim, tacrolimus, thiotepa, ticarcillin, ticarcillin/clavulanate, tobramycin, trimethoprim-sulfamethoxazole, urokinase, vancomycin, vecuronium, zidovudine

Perform/provide:
• Storage depends on type of solution; consult manufacturer
• Changing dressing and IV tubing to prevent infection q24-48h

Evaluate:
• Therapeutic response: weight gain, decrease in jaundice in liver disorders, increased LOC

Teach patient/family:
• The reason for use of TPN
• If chills, sweating are experienced, report at once
• About infusion pump and blood glucose monitoring

---

amino acid solution (℞)

Aminees, Aminosyn, Branch Amin, FreAmine III, NephrAmine, Novamine, ProcalAmine, Ren Amin, Travasol, Troph Amine

Func. class.: Nitrogen product

Action: Needed for anabolism to maintain structure, decrease catabolism, promote healing

Uses: Nutritional support in cancer, trauma, intestinal obstruction, short bowel syndrome, severe malabsorption

DOSAGE AND ROUTES

• *Adult:* IV 1-1.5 g/kg/day titrated to patient's needs
• *Child:* IV 2-3 g/kg/day titrated to patient's needs

Available forms: Inj, many types, strengths

SIDE EFFECTS

CNS: Dizziness, headache, confusion, **loss of consciousness**
CV: Hypertension, **CHF, pulmonary edema**
ENDO: Hyperglycemia, rebound hypoglycemia, electrolyte imbalances, hyperosmolar syndrome, hyperosmolar hyperglycemic nonketotic syndrome,

alkalosis, acidosis, hypophosphatemia, hyperammonemia, dehydration, hypocalcemia

GI: Nausea, vomiting, liver fat deposits, abdominal pain, jaundice

GU: Glycosuria, osmotic diuresis

INTEG: Chills, flushing, warm feeling, rash, urticaria, extravasation necrosis, phlebitis at inj site

Contraindications: Hypersensitivity, severe electrolyte imbalances, anuria, severe liver damage, maple syrup urine disease, PKU

Precautions: Pregnancy (C), renal disease, lactation, children, diabetes mellitus, CHF

NURSING CONSIDERATIONS

Assess:
• Electrolytes (K, Na, Ca, Cl, Mg), blood glucose, ammonia, phosphate
• Renal, hepatic studies: BUN, creatinine, ALT, AST, bilirubin
• Inj site for extravasation: redness along vein, edema at site, necrosis, pain, hard tender area; site should be changed immediately
• Monitor respiratory function q4h: auscultate lung fields bilaterally for crackles, respirations, quality, rate, rhythm
• Monitor temp q4h for increased fever, indicating infection; if infection suspected, discontinue infusion, culture tubing, bottle
• Urine glucose q6h using Tes-Tape, Clinistix, which are not affected by infusion substances; blood glucose is preferred testing method
• Hyperammonemia: nausea, vomiting, malaise, tremors, anorexia, convulsions

Administer:
CONT IV route
• Up to 40% protein and dextrose (up to 12.5%) via peripheral vein; stronger solutions require central IV administration, use infusion pump
• TPN only mixed with dextrose to promote protein synthesis
• Immediately after mixing in pharmacy under strict aseptic technique using laminar flow hood, use infusion pump, in-

line filter (0.22 µm) unless mixed with fat emulsion and dextrose (3 in 1)

⚠ Using careful monitoring technique; do not speed up infusion; pulmonary edema, glucose overload will result

Y-site compatibilities: Cefazolin, cefoperazone, cefotaxime, cefoxitin, cephalothin, cephapirin, chloramphenicol, clindamycin, digoxin, DOBUTamine, DOPamine, doxycycline, erythromycin lactobionate, fat emulsion, foscarnet, furosemide, gentamicin, isoproterenol, kanamycin, lidocaine, meperidine, methicillin, mezlocillin, miconazole, morphine, nafcillin, netilmicin, norepinephrine, oxacillin, penicillin G potassium, piperacillin, sargramostim, ticarcillin, tobramycin, urokinase, vancomycin

Perform/provide:
• Storage depends on type of solution; consult label
• Dressing and IV tubing change q24-48h to prevent infection

Evaluate:
• Therapeutic response: weight gain, decrease in jaundice in liver disorders, increased serum albumin

Teach patient/family:
• The reason for use of TPN
• That any chills, sweating should be reported at once
• About infusion pump and blood glucose monitoring

Rarely Used

aminocaproic acid (℞)
(a-mee-noe-ka-proe'ik)
Amicar, aminocaproic acid, EACA
Func. class.: Hemostatic

Uses: Hemorrhage from hyperfibrinolysis, adjunctive therapy in hemophilia

DOSAGE AND ROUTES
• *Adult:* **PO/IV** 4-5 g loading dose, then 1-1.25 g q1h

Contraindications: Hypersensitivity, abnormal bleeding, postpartum bleeding, DIC, upper urinary tract bleeding, new burns

---

Rarely Used

aminoglutethimide (℞)
(a-meen-oh-gloo-teth'i-mide)
Cytadren
Func. class.: Antineoplastic, adrenal steroid inhibitor
Chem. class.: Hormone

Uses: Suppression of adrenal function in Cushing's syndrome, adrenal cancer

DOSAGE AND ROUTES
• *Adult:* PO 250 mg qid at 6 hr intervals, may increase by 250 mg/day q1-2wk, not to exceed 2 g/day, concurrent hydrocortisone supplementation is recommended

Contraindications: Pregnancy (D), hypersensitivity, hypothyroidism

---

Rarely Used

aminolevulinic acid (℞)
Levulan Kerastick
Func. class.: Photochemotherapy

Uses: Face/scalp nonhyperkeratotic actinic keratoses

DOSAGE AND ROUTES
• *Adult:* TOP 1 application of solution and 1 dose of illumination/treatment site × 8 wk

Contraindications: Hypersensitivity to porphyrins

---

aminophylline (theophylline ethylenediamine) (℞)
(am-in-off'i-lin)
Phyllocontin, Truphylline
Func. class.: Bronchodilator, spasmolytic
Chem. class.: Methylxanthine

Action: Exact mechanism unknown, relaxes smooth muscle of respiratory system by blocking phosphodiesterase, which increases cAMP; increased cAMP alters intracellular calcium ion movements; produces bronchodilation, increased pulmonary blood flow, relaxation of respiratory tract

Uses: Bronchial asthma, bronchospasm associated with chronic bronchitis, emphysema, bradycardia

Unlabeled uses: Apnea in infancy for respiratory/myocardial stimulation

DOSAGE AND ROUTES
• *Adult:* PO 6 mg/kg, then 3 mg/kg q6h × 2 doses, then 3 mg/kg q8h maintenance, max 900 mg/day or 13 mg/kg; PO in CHF 6 mg/kg, then 2 mg/kg q8h × 2 doses, then 1-2 mg/kg q12h maintenance; IV 4.7 mg/kg, then 0.55 mg/kg/hr × 12 hr, then 0.36/kg/hr maintenance; IV in CHF 4.7 mg/kg, then 0.39 mg/kg/hr × 12 hr, then 0.08-0.16 mg/kg/hr maintenance
• *Geriatric and in cor pulmonale:* PO 6 mg/kg, then 2 mg/kg q6h × 2 doses, then 2 mg/kg q8h maintenance; IV 4.7 mg/kg, then 0.47 mg/kg/hr × 12 hr, then 0.24 mg/kg/hr maintenance
• *Child 9-16 yr:* PO 6 mg/kg, then 3 mg/kg q4h × 3 doses, then 3 mg/kg q6h maintenance, max 18 mg/kg/day 12-16 yr, or 20 mg/kg/day 9-12 yr; IV 4.7 mg/kg, then 0.79 mg/kg/hr × 12 hr, then 0.63 mg/kg/hr maintenance
• *Child 6 mo-9 yr:* PO 4 mg/kg q4h × 3 doses, then 4 mg/kg q6h maintenance, max 24 mg/kg/day; IV 4.7 mg/kg, then

---

A Safety alert   *"Tall Man" lettering

0.95 mg/kg/hr × 12 hr, then 0.79 mg/kg/hr maintenance

• *Infant 6-52 wk:* Dose (0.2 × age in wk) ÷ 5 × kg = 24 hr dose in mg

• *Neonate—up to 40 wk premature postconception age:* **PO/IV** 1 mg/kg q12h

• *Neonate at birth or 40 wk postconception age:* **PO/IV** over 8 wk postnatal 1-3 mg/kg q6h; 4-8 wk postnatal 1-2 mg/kg q8h; up to 4 wk postnatal 1-2 mg/kg q12h

Hepatic disease

• *Adult:* **PO** 6 mg/kg then 2 mg/kg q8h × 2 doses, then 1-2 mg/kg q12h maintenance; **IV** 4.7 mg/kg, then 0.39 mg/kg/hr × 12 hr, then 0.08-0.16 mg/kg/hr maintenance

Available forms: Inj 250 mg/10 ml, 500 mg/20 ml, 100 mg/100 ml in 0.45% NaCl, 200 mg/100 ml in 0.45% NaCl; rect supp 250, 500 mg; oral liq 105 mg/5 ml; tabs 100, 200 mg; con rel tabs 225, 350 mg

SIDE EFFECTS

CNS: Anxiety, restlessness, insomnia, *dizziness,* **seizures,** headache, lightheadedness, muscle twitching, tremors

CV: Palpitations, sinus tachycardia, hypotension, flushing, **dysrhythmias,** edema

GI: Nausea, vomiting, diarrhea, dyspepsia, anal irritation (suppositories), epigastric pain, reflux, anorexia

GU: Urinary frequency, SIADH

INTEG: Flushing, urticaria

MISC: Hyperglycemia

RESP: Tachypnea, increased respiratory rate

Contraindications: Hypersensitivity to xanthines, tachydysrhythmias

Precautions: Pregnancy (C), geriatric, CHF, cor pulmonale, hepatic disease, diabetes mellitus, hyperthyroidism, hypertension, seizure disorder, irritation of the rectum or lower colon, children, lactation, alcoholism, active peptic ulcer disease

PHARMACOKINETICS

Well absorbed PO; ext rel well absorbed slowly, rect supp is erratic, rect sol is absorbed quickly; metabolized by liver (caffeine); excreted in urine; crosses placenta; appears in breast milk; half-life 6.5-10.5 hr; half-life increased in geriatric patients, hepatic disease, CHF, neonates, premature infants, protein binding 40%

PO: Onset ¼ hr, peak 1-2 hr, duration 6-8 hr

PO-ER: Unknown, peak 4-7 hr, duration 8-12 hr

IV: Onset rapid, duration 6-8 hr

REC: Onset erratic, peak 1-2 hr, duration 6-8 hr

INTERACTIONS

• Dose-dependent reversal of neuromuscular blockade

• Dysrhythmias: halothane

• May increase or decrease aminophylline levels: carbamazepine, loop diuretics, isoniazid

Increase: action of aminophylline, toxicity—cimetidine, nonselective β-blockers, erythromycin, clarithromycin, oral contraceptives, corticosteroids, interferons, fluoroquinolones, disulfiram, mexiletine, fluvoxamine, high doses of allopurinol, influenza vaccines, interferon, benzodiazepines

Increase: adverse reactions—tetracyclines

Increase: elimination—smoking

Decrease: effects of lithium

Decrease: effect of aminophylline—nicotine products, adrenergics, barbiturates, phenytoin, ketoconazole, rifampin

Drug/Herb

Increase: effects—cola tree, guarana, yerba maté, tea (black, green), horsetail, ginseng, Siberian ginseng

Decrease: effects—St. John's wort

Drug/Food

Increase: effect—xanthines

Increase: elimination by low-carbohydrate, high-protein diet; charcoal-broiled beef

Decrease: elimination by high-carbohydrate and low-protein diet

Drug/Lab Test
Increase: Plasma-free fatty acids

NURSING CONSIDERATIONS

Assess:
• Theophylline blood levels (therapeutic level is 10-20 mcg/ml); toxicity may occur with small increase above 20 mcg/ml, especially geriatric
• Monitor I&O; diuresis occurs; dehydration may occur in geriatric or children
• Whether theophylline was given recently (24 hr)
• Respiratory rate, rhythm, depth; auscultate lung fields bilaterally; notify prescriber of abnormalities
• Allergic reactions: rash, urticaria; if these occur, drug should be discontinued

Administer:
• Avoid IM inj; pain and tissue damage may occur

PO route
• Do not break, crush, or chew enteric-coated or cont rel tabs
• Avoid giving with food

Rectal route
• If patient is unable to take PO; retain rectal dose for ½ hr
• Remain in bed 15-20 min after rect supp is inserted to avoid removal

IV route
• Only clear sol; flush IV line before dose
• May be diluted for IV INF in 100-200 ml in D_5W, $D_{10}W$, $D_{20}W$, 0.9% NaCl, 0.45% NaCl, LR
• Give loading dose over ½ hr; max rate of inf 25 mg/min, use infusion pump; after loading dose give by cont inf

Additive compatibilities: Amobarbital, bretylium, calcium gluconate, chloramphenicol, cibenzoline, cimetidine, dexamethasone, diphenhydrAMINE, DOPamine, erythromycin lactobionate, esmolol, floxacillin, flumazenil, furosemide, heparin, hydrocortisone, lidocaine, mephentermine, meropenem, methyldopate, metronidazole/sodium bicarbonate, nitroglycerin, pentobarbital, phenobarbital, potassium chloride, ranitidine, secobarbital, sodium bicarbonate, terbutaline

Syringe compatibilities: Heparin, metoclopramide, pentobarbital, thiopental

Y-site compatibilities: Allopurinol, amifostine, amphotericin B, amrinone, aztreonam, ceftazidime, cholesteryl sulfate complex, cimetidine, cladribine, DOXOrubicin liposome, enalaprilat, esmolol, famotidine, filgrastim, fluconazole, fludarabine, foscarnet, gallium, granisetron, heparin sodium with hydrocortisone sodium succinate, labetalol, melphalan, meropenem, netilmicin, paclitaxel, pancuronium, piperacillin/tazobactam, potassium chloride, propofol, ranitidine, remifentanil, sargramostim, tacrolimus, teniposide, thiotepa, tolazoline, vecuronium

Perform/provide:
• Storage of diluted solution for 24 hr if refrigerated

Evaluate:
• Therapeutic response: decreased dyspnea, respiratory stimulation in infancy, clear lung fields bilaterally

Teach patient/family:
• To take doses as prescribed, not to skip dose, not to double dose
• To check OTC medications, current prescription medications for ephedrine; will increase CNS stimulation; not to drink alcohol or caffeine products (tea, coffee, chocolate, colas)
• To avoid hazardous activities; dizziness may occur
• If GI upset occurs, to take drug with 8 oz water; avoid food, since absorption may be decreased
⚠ To notify prescriber of toxicity: insomnia, anxiety, nausea, vomiting, rapid pulse, seizures, flushing, headache, diarrhea; notify prescriber immediately
• To notify prescriber of change in smoking habit; a change in dose may be required
• To increase fluids to 2 L/day to decrease secretion viscosity
• To avoid smoking; decreases blood levels and terminal half-life

⚠ High Alert

amiodarone (℞)

(a-mee-oh′da-rone)

Cordarone, Pacerone

Func. class.: Antidysrhythmic (class III)

Chem. class.: Iodinated benzofuran derivative

Do not confuse:

Amiodarone/Inamrinone

Cordarone/Inocor

Action: Prolongs duration of action potential and effective refractory period, noncompetitive α- and β-adrenergic inhibition; increases PR and QT intervals, decreases sinus rate, decreases peripheral vascular resistance

Uses: Severe ventricular tachycardia, supraventricular tachycardia, atrial fibrillation, ventricular fibrillation not controlled by first-line agents, cardiac arrest

DOSAGE AND ROUTES

Ventricular dysrhythmias

• *Adult:* **PO** loading dose 800-1600 mg/day for 1-3 wk; then 600-800 mg/day × 1 mo; maintenance 400 mg/day; **IV** loading dose (first rapid) 150 mg over the first 10 min then slow 360 mg over the next 6 hr; maintenance 540 mg given over the remaining 18 hr, decrease rate of the slow infusion to 0.5 mg/min

• *Child:* **PO** loading dose 10-15 mg/kg/day in 1-2 divided doses for 4-14 days then 5 mg/kg/day (not recommended in children)

• *Child and infant:* **IV/Intraosseous** 5 mg/kg as a bolus (PALS guidelines)

Perfusion tachycardia

• *Adult:* **IV** 5 mg/kg loading dose given over 20-60 min

Supraventricular tachycardia

• *Adult:* **PO** 600-800 mg/day × 7 days or until desired response, then 400 mg/day × 21 days, then 200-400 mg/day maintenance

• *Child:* **PO** 10 mg/kg/day (800 mg/1.72 m²/day) × 10 days or until desired response, then 5 mg/kg/day (400 mg/1.72 m²/day) × 21-28 days, then 2.5 mg/kg/day (200 mg/1.72 m²/day) (not recommended in children)

Available forms: Tabs 100, 200, 400 mg; inj 50 mg/ml

SIDE EFFECTS

CNS: Headache, dizziness, involuntary movement, tremors, peripheral neuropathy, malaise, fatigue, ataxia, paresthesias, insomnia

CV: Hypotension, bradycardia, **sinus arrest, CHF, dysrhythmias, SA node dysfunction**

EENT: Blurred vision, halos, photophobia, **corneal microdeposits,** dry eyes

ENDO: Hyperthyroidism or hypothyroidism

GI: Nausea, vomiting, diarrhea, abdominal pain, anorexia, constipation, **hepatotoxicity**

INTEG: Rash, photosensitivity, blue-gray skin discoloration, alopecia, spontaneous ecchymosis, **toxic epidermal necrolysis**

MISC: Flushing, abnormal taste or smell, edema, abnormal salivation, coagulation abnormalities

MS: Weakness, pain in extremities

RESP: **Pulmonary fibrosis,** pulmonary inflammation, **ARDS; gasping syndrome if used in neonates**

Contraindications: Pregnancy (D), lactation, 2nd-, 3rd-degree AV block, bradycardia, severe sinus node dysfunction, neonates, infants

Precautions: Goiter, Hashimoto's thyroiditis, electrolyte imbalances, CHF, severe hepatic disease, respiratory disease, children

PHARMACOKINETICS

PO: Onset 1-3 wk; peak 2-7 hr; half-life 15-100 days; metabolized by liver, excreted by kidneys

INTERACTIONS

Increase: bradycardia—β-blockers, calcium channel blockers

Increase: levels of cycloSPORINE, dextromethorphan, digoxin, disopyramide, flecainide, methotrexate, phenytoin, procainamide, quinidine, theophylline
Increase: anticoagulant effects—warfarin

Drug/Herb
Increase: serotonin effect—horehound
Increase: toxicity/death—aconite
Increase: amiodarone effect—aloe, broom, buckthorn, cascara sagrada, Chinese rhubarb, figwort, fumitory, goldenseal, kudzu, licorice, rhubarb, senna
Decrease: amiodarone effect—coltsfoot

Drug/Food
• Toxicity: grapefruit juice

Drug/Lab Test
Increase: T$_4$

NURSING CONSIDERATIONS
Assess:
⚠ Pulmonary toxicity: dyspnea, fatigue, cough, fever, chest pain; drug should be discontinued
• ECG continuously to determine drug effectiveness; measure PR, QRS, QT intervals; check for PVCs, other dysrhythmias, B/P continuously for hypotension, hypertension; report dysrhythmias, slowing heart rate
• I&O ratio; electrolytes (K, Na, Cl); hepatic studies: AST, ALT, bilirubin, alk phos
• Chest x-ray, thyroid function tests
• For dehydration or hypovolemia
• For rebound hypertension after 1-2 hr
• For ARDS, pulmonary fibrosis, crackles, dyspnea, tachypnea
• CNS symptoms: confusion, psychosis, numbness, depression, involuntary movements; if these occur, drug should be discontinued
• Hypothyroidism: lethargy, dizziness, constipation, enlarged thyroid gland, edema of extremities, cool, pale skin
• Hyperthyroidism: restlessness, tachycardia, eyelid puffiness, weight loss, frequent urination, menstrual irregularities, dyspnea; warm, moist skin
• Ophthalmic exams baseline and periodically (PO)

• Cardiac rate, respiration: rate, rhythm, character, chest pain; start with patient hospitalized and monitored up to 1 wk
Administer:
PO route
• Loading dose with food to decrease nausea
IV, direct route
• Give 300 bol; may repeat 150 mg after 3-5 min; used for cardiac arrest
Intermittent IV INF route
• 1000 mg/24 hr during loading/maintenance
• Initial loading: Add 3 ml (150 mg), 100 ml D$_5$W (1.5 mg/ml), give over 10 min
• Loading inf: Add 18 ml (900 mg), 500 ml D$_5$W (1.8 mg/ml), give over next 6 hr
• Maintenance inf: Give remainder of loading inf 540 mg over 18 hr (0.5 mg/min)
CONT INF route
• After 24 hr, give 1-6 mg/ml at 0.5 mg/min, max 30 mg/min
Additive compatibilities: DOBUTamine, lidocaine, potassium chloride, procainamide, verapamil
Y-site compatibilities: Amikacin, bretylium, clindamycin, DOBUTamine, DOPamine, doxycycline, erythromycin, esmolol, gentamicin, insulin, isoproterenol, labetalol, lidocaine, metaraminol, metronidazole, midazolam, morphine, nitroglycerin, norepinephrine, penicillin G potassium, phentolamine, phenylephrine, potassium chloride, procainamide, tobramycin, vancomycin
Solution compatibility: D$_5$W, 0.9% NaCl
Evaluate:
• Therapeutic response: decrease in ventricular tachycardia, supraventricular tachycardia or fibrillation
Teach patient/family:
• To take this drug as directed; avoid missed doses; do not use with grapefruit juice
• To use sunscreen or stay out of sun to prevent burns
• To report side effects immediately
• That skin discoloration is usually reversible

⚠ Safety alert   *"Tall Man" lettering

• That dark glasses may be needed for photophobia

Treatment of overdose: O_2, artificial ventilation, ECG, administer DOPamine for circulatory depression, administer diazepam or thiopental for seizures, isoproterenol

---

amitriptyline (℞)
(a-mee-trip'ti-leen)
amitriptyline HCl,
Apo-Amitriptyline ✤, Endep,
Levate ✤, Novotriptyn ✤
Func. class.: Antidepressant—tricyclic
Chem. class.: Tertiary amine

Do not confuse:

amitriptyline/nortriptyline

Action: Blocks reuptake of norepinephrine, serotonin into nerve endings, increasing action of norepinephrine, serotonin in nerve cells

Uses: Major depression

Unlabeled uses: Chronic pain management, prevention of cluster/migraine headaches, fibromyalgia

DOSAGE AND ROUTES

Depression
• *Adult:* **PO** 75 mg/day in divided doses, may increase to 150 mg daily, not to exceed 300 mg/day; **IM** 20-30 mg qid, or 80-120 mg at bedtime
• *Geriatric and adolescent:* **PO** 30 mg/day in divided doses, may be increased to 100 mg/day
Cluster/migraine headache (unlabeled)
• *Adult:* **PO** 50-150 mg/day
Chronic pain (unlabeled)
• *Adult:* **PO** 75-150 mg/day
Fibromyalgia (unlabeled)
• *Adult:* **PO** 10-50 mg nightly

Available forms: Tabs 10, 25, 50, 75, 100, 150 mg; inj 10 mg/ml; syr 10 mg/5 ml

SIDE EFFECTS

CNS: Dizziness, drowsiness, confusion, headache, anxiety, tremors, stimulation, weakness, insomnia, nightmares, EPS (geriatric), increased psychiatric symptoms, **seizures**

CV: Orthostatic hypotension, **ECG changes, tachycardia, hypertension,** palpitations, **dysrhythmias**

EENT: Blurred vision, tinnitus, mydriasis, ophthalmoplegia

GI: Constipation, dry mouth, weight gain, nausea, vomiting, **paralytic ileus,** increased appetite, cramps, epigastric distress, jaundice, **hepatitis,** stomatitis

GU: Urinary retention

HEMA: **Agranulocytosis, thrombocytopenia, eosinophilia, leukopenia**

INTEG: Rash, urticaria, sweating, pruritus, photosensitivity

Contraindications: Hypersensitivity to tricyclics, recovery phase of myocardial infarction

Precautions: Pregnancy (C), suicidal patients, seizure disorders, prostatic hypertrophy, schizophrenia, psychosis, severe depression, increased intraocular pressure, narrow-angle glaucoma, urinary retention, renal/hepatic/cardiac disease, hyperthyroidism, electroshock therapy, elective surgery, child <12 yr, lactation, geriatric

PHARMACOKINETICS

PO/IM: Onset 45 min, peak 2-12 hr, therapeutic response 4-10 days; metabolized by liver; excreted in urine, feces; crosses placenta, excreted in breast milk, half-life 10-46 hr

INTERACTIONS

⚠ Hyperpyretic crisis, seizures, hypertensive episode: MAOIs

Increase: risk of agranulocytosis—antithyroid agents

Increase: amitriptyline levels, toxicity—cimetidine, fluoxetine, phenothiazines, oral contraceptives, antidepressants, carbamazepine, IC antidysrhythmics

Increase: effects of direct-acting sympathomimetics (epINEPHrine), alcohol, barbiturates, benzodiazepines, CNS depressants, opioids, sedative/hypnotics
Decrease: effects of guanethidine, clonidine, indirect-acting sympathomimetics (epHEDrine)

Drug/Herb
Increase: serotonin syndrome—SAM-e, St. John's wort
Increase: CNS depression—kava, skullcap, hops, chamomile, lavender, valerian
Increase: anticholinergic effect—belladonna leaf/root, henbane leaf, jimsonweed, scopolia
Increase: action of amitriptyline—jimsonweed, scopolia root
Increase: hypertension—yohimbe

Drug/Lab Test
Increase: Serum bilirubin, blood glucose, alk phos

NURSING CONSIDERATIONS
Assess:
• B/P lying, standing; pulse q4h; if systolic B/P drops 20 mm Hg, hold drug, notify prescriber; take vital signs q4h in patients with cardiovascular disease
• Blood studies: CBC, leukocytes, differential, cardiac enzymes if patient is receiving long-term therapy
• Hepatic studies: AST, ALT, bilirubin
• Weight qwk; appetite may increase with drug
• ECG for flattening of T wave, prolongation of QTc interval, bundle branch block, AV block, dysrhythmias in cardiac patients
• EPS primarily in geriatric rigidity, dystonia, akathisia
• Mental status: mood, sensorium, affect, suicidal tendencies; increase in psychiatric symptoms: depression, panic
• Urinary retention, constipation; constipation is most likely to occur in children and geriatric
• Withdrawal symptoms: headache, nausea, vomiting, muscle pain, weakness; do not usually occur unless drug was discontinued abruptly
• Alcohol consumption; if alcohol is consumed, hold dose until morning

Administer:
PO route
• Increased fluids, bulk in diet if constipation, urinary retention occur, especially geriatric
• With food or milk for GI symptoms
• Crushed if patient is unable to swallow medication whole
• Dosage at bedtime if oversedation occurs during day; may take entire dose at bedtime; geriatric may not tolerate once/day dosing

Perform/provide:
• Storage at room temperature; do not freeze
• Assistance with ambulation during beginning therapy, since drowsiness/dizziness occurs
• Gum; hard, sugarless candy; or frequent sips of water for dry mouth

Evaluate:
• Therapeutic response: decrease in depression, absence of suicidal thoughts

Teach patient/family:
• To take medication as directed; do not double dose; that therapeutic effects may take 2-3 wk
• To use caution in driving, other activities requiring alertness because of drowsiness, dizziness, blurred vision; to avoid rising quickly from sitting to standing, especially geriatric
• To avoid alcohol ingestion, other CNS depressants
• Not to discontinue medication quickly after long-term use: may cause nausea, headache, malaise
• To wear sunscreen or large hat, since photosensitivity occurs
• That contraception is recommended during treatment

Treatment of overdose: ECG monitoring, lavage, administer anticonvulsant, sodium bicarbonate

---

amlodipine (℞)

(am-loe'di-peen)
Norvasc
Func. class.: Antianginal, antihypertensive, calcium channel blocker
Chem. class.: Dihydropyridine

Do not confuse:
amlodipine/amiloride
Norvasc/Navane

Action: Inhibits calcium ion influx across cell membrane during cardiac depolarization; produces relaxation of coronary vascular smooth muscle, peripheral vascular smooth muscle; dilates coronary vascular arteries; increases myocardial oxygen delivery in patients with vasospastic angina

Uses: Chronic stable angina pectoris, hypertension, vasospastic angina (Prinzmetal's angina); may coadminister with other antihypertensives, antianginals

DOSAGE AND ROUTES

Angina
• *Adult:* PO 5-10 mg daily
Hypertension
• *Adult:* PO 2.5-5 mg daily initially, max 10 mg/day
Hepatic dose/geriatric
• *Adult:* PO 2.5 mg/day; may increase up to 10 mg/day (antihypertensive); 5 mg/day, may increase up to 10 mg/day (antianginal)
Available forms: Tabs 2.5, 5, 10 mg

SIDE EFFECTS

CNS: Headache, fatigue, dizziness, asthenia, anxiety, depression, insomnia, paresthesia, somnolence
CV: Dysrhythmia, peripheral edema, bradycardia, hypotension, palpitations, syncope, chest pain
GI: Nausea, vomiting, diarrhea, gastric upset, constipation, flatulence, anorexia, gingival hyperplasia, dyspepsia, dysphagia
GU: Nocturia, polyuria, sexual difficulties
INTEG: Rash, pruritus, urticaria, hair loss
OTHER: Flushing, sexual difficulties, muscle cramps, cough, weight gain, tinnitus, epistaxis
Contraindications: Sick sinus syndrome, 2nd- or 3rd-degree heart block, hypersensitivity, severe aortic stenosis, obstructive CAD
Precautions: Pregnancy (C), CHF, hypotension, hepatic injury, lactation, children, geriatric

PHARMACOKINETICS

PO: Onset not determined, peak 6-12 hr, half-life 30-50 hr, increased in geriatric, hepatic disease; metabolized by liver, excreted in urine (90% as metabolites), protein binding >95%

INTERACTIONS

Increase: neurotoxicity—lithium
Increase: hypotension—alcohol, antihypertensives, nitrates
Increase: amlodipine level—diltiazem
Decrease: antihypertensive effect—NSAIDs
Drug/Herb
Increase: effects—barberry, betel palm, burdock, goldenseal, khat, khella, lily of the valley, plantain
Decrease: effect—yohimbe
Drug/Food
Increase: hypotensive effect—grapefruit juice

NURSING CONSIDERATIONS

Assess:
• Cardiac status: B/P, pulse, respiration, ECG; some patients have developed severe angina, acute MI after calcium channel blockers if obstructive CAD is severe
• I&O ratio, weight daily; peripheral edema, dyspnea, jugular vein distention, crackles that are signs of CHF
Administer:
PO route
• Once a day, without regard to meals
Evaluate:
• Therapeutic response: decreased anginal pain, decreased B/P, increased exercise tolerance

---

Side effects: *italics* = common; **bold** = life-threatening

Teach patient/family:
• To take drug as prescribed, do not double or skip dose
• To avoid hazardous activities until stabilized on drug, dizziness is no longer a problem
• To avoid OTC drugs, grapefruit juice unless directed by prescriber
• To comply in all areas of medical regimen: diet, exercise, stress reduction, drug therapy, smoking cessation
• To notify prescriber of irregular heartbeat, shortness of breath, swelling of feet and hands, severe dizziness, constipation, nausea, hypotension
• To use correct technique in monitoring pulse, to contact prescriber if pulse <50 bpm
• To change positions slowly, to prevent orthostatic hypotension
• To continue with good oral hygiene to prevent gingival disease
• To notify all health care providers of this drug use

Treatment of overdose: Defibrillation, β-agonists, IV calcium inotropic agents, diuretics, atropine for AV block, vasopressor for hypotension

---

amoxapine (℞)
(a-mox'a-peen)
amoxapine, Asendin
Func. class.: Antidepressant
Chem. class.: Dibenzoxazepine derivative—secondary amine

Do not confuse:
amoxapine/amoxicillin/Amoxil
Action: Blocks reuptake of norepinephrine, serotonin into nerve endings, increasing action of norepinephrine, serotonin in nerve cells
Uses: Depression

DOSAGE AND ROUTES
• *Adult:* **PO** 50 mg tid, may increase to 100 mg tid on 3rd day of therapy; not to exceed 300 mg/day unless lower doses

have been given for at least 2 wk, may be given daily dose at bedtime, not to exceed 600 mg/day in hospitalized patients
• *Geriatric:* **PO** 25 mg at bedtime, may increase by 25 mg/wk, up to 150 mg/day in divided doses
Available forms: Tabs 25, 50, 100, 150 mg

SIDE EFFECTS
CNS: Dizziness, drowsiness, confusion, headache, anxiety, tremors, stimulation, weakness, insomnia, nightmares, EPS (geriatric), increased psychiatric symptoms, paresthesia, **neuroleptic malignant syndrome,** impairment of sexual functioning
CV: Orthostatic hypotension, ECG changes, tachycardia, hypertension, palpitations
EENT: Blurred vision, tinnitus, mydriasis, ophthalmoplegia
GI: Dry mouth, weight gain, *constipation,* nausea, vomiting, **paralytic ileus,** increased appetite, cramps, epigastric distress, jaundice, **hepatitis,** stomatitis
GU: Urinary retention, **acute renal failure**
HEMA: **Agranulocytosis, thrombocytopenia, eosinophilia, leukopenia**
INTEG: Rash, urticaria, sweating, pruritus, photosensitivity
META: Increased prolactin levels
Contraindications: Hypersensitivity to tricyclics, recovery phase of myocardial infarction, seizure disorders, prostatic hypertrophy, narrow-angle glaucoma
Precautions: Pregnancy (C), suicidal patients, severe depression, increased intraocular pressure, urinary retention, hepatic/cardiac disease, hyperthyroidism, electroshock therapy, elective surgery, geriatric

PHARMACOKINETICS
Steady state 2-7 days; metabolized by liver, excreted by kidneys, crosses placenta, half-life 8 hr

---

⚠ Safety alert   *"Tall Man" lettering

INTERACTIONS

⚠ Hyperpyretic crisis, seizures, hypertensive episode: MAOIs

Increase: CNS depression—CNS depressants

Increase: amoxapine level—cimetidine, fluoxetine, fluvoxamine, paroxetine, sertraline

Increase: hypertensive effect—clonidine, epinephrine, norepinephrine

Decrease: amoxapine effect—barbiturates

Drug/Herb

Increase: CNS depression—chamomile, hops, kava, lavender, skullcap, St. John's wort, valerian

Increase: anticholinergic effects—belladonna, corkwood, henbane, jimsonweed

Increase: action of amoxapine—scopolia root

Drug/Lab Test

Increase: LFTs, blood glucose
Decrease: WBC, blood glucose

NURSING CONSIDERATIONS

Assess:

• B/P lying, standing; pulse q4h; if systolic B/P drops 20 mm Hg, hold drug, notify prescriber; take vital signs q4h in patients with cardiovascular disease

• Blood studies: CBC, leukocytes, differential, cardiac enzymes if patient is receiving long-term therapy

• Blood level: therapeutic 20-100 ng/ml

• Hepatic studies: AST, ALT, bilirubin

• Weight qwk; appetite may increase with drug

• ECG for flattening of T wave, bundle branch block, AV block, dysrhythmias in cardiac patients

• EPS primarily in geriatric: rigidity, dystonia, akathisia

• Mental status: mood, sensorium, affect, suicidal tendencies; increase in psychiatric symptoms: depression, panic; confusion (geriatric)

• Urinary retention, constipation; constipation is more likely to occur in children, geriatric

• Withdrawal symptoms: headache, nausea, vomiting, muscle pain, weakness; do not usually occur unless drug is discontinued abruptly

• Alcohol consumption; if alcohol is consumed, hold dose until morning

Administer:

• Increased fluids, bulk in diet if constipation, urinary retention occur, especially in geriatric

• Crushed if patient is unable to swallow medication whole, with food or milk for GI symptoms

• Dosage at bedtime if oversedation occurs during day; may take entire dose at bedtime; geriatric may not tolerate once/day dosing

Perform/provide:

• Storage at room temperature; do not freeze

• Check to see PO medication swallowed

• Gum, hard candy, or frequent sips of water for dry mouth

Evaluate:

• Therapeutic response: decreased depression, absence of suicidal thoughts

Teach patient/family:

• To take as directed, not to double dose

• That therapeutic effects may take 2-3 wk

• To use caution in driving or other activities requiring alertness because of drowsiness, dizziness, blurred vision

• To avoid alcohol ingestion, other CNS depressants, may potentiate effects

• Not to discontinue medication quickly after long-term use; may cause nausea, headache, malaise

• To wear sunscreen or large hat, since photosensitivity occurs

Treatment of overdose: ECG monitoring, induce emesis, lavage, activated charcoal, administer anticonvulsant

amoxicillin (R)

(a-mox-i-sill'in)
amoxicillin, Amoxil,
Apo-Amoxi ✦ DisperMox,
Novamoxin ✦
Nu-Amoxi ✦ Trimox, Wymox
Func. class.: Antiinfective, antiulcer
Chem. class.: Aminopenicillin

Do not confuse:
amoxicillin/amoxapine/Amoxil
Trimox/Diamox/Tylox
Wymox/Tylox

Action: Interferes with cell wall replication of susceptible organisms; the cell wall, rendered osmotically unstable, swells and bursts from osmotic pressure; bactericidal, lysis mediated by bacterial cell wall autolysins

Uses: Treatment of skin, respiratory, GI, GU infections; otitis media, gonorrhea. For gram-positive cocci *(Staphylococcus aureus, Streptococcus pyogenes, Streptococcus faecalis, Streptococcus pneumoniae)*, gram-negative cocci *(Neisseria gonorrhoeae, Neisseria meningitidis)*, gram-positive bacilli *(Corynebacterium diphtheriae, Listeria monocytogenes)*, gram-negative bacilli *(Haemophilus influenzae, Escherichia coli, Proteus mirabilis, Salmonella)*; prophylaxis of bacterial endocarditis; in combination with other drugs used for treatment of *Helicobacter pylori*

Unlabeled uses: Lyme disease, anthrax treatment, and prophylaxis

DOSAGE AND ROUTES

Systemic infections
• *Adult:* PO 750 mg-1.75 g daily in divided doses q8h
• *Child:* PO 20-50 mg/kg/day in divided doses q8h

Renal disease
• *Adult:* PO CCr 10-30 ml/min 250-500 mg q12h; CCr <10 ml/min 250-500 mg q24h; do not use 875 mg strength if CCr <50 ml/min

Gonorrhea/urinary tract infections
• *Adult:* PO 3 g given with 1 g probenecid as a single dose; followed by tetracycline or erythromycin therapy

Chlamydia trachomatis
• *Adult:* PO 500 mg/tid × 1 wk

Bacterial endocarditis prophylaxis
• *Adult:* PO 2 g 1 hr prior to procedure
• *Child:* PO 50 mg/kg/hr 1 hr prior to procedure; max 2 g

Helicobacter pylori
• *Adult:* PO 1000 mg bid, given with lansoprazole 30 mg bid, clarithromycin 500 mg bid × 2 wk or 1000 mg bid given with omeprazole 20 mg bid, clarithromycin 500 mg bid × 2 wk, or 1000 mg tid given with lansoprazole 30 mg tid × 2 wk

Available forms: Caps 250, 500 mg; chew tabs 125, 200, 250, 400 mg; tabs 500, 875 mg; susp pediatric drops 50 mg/ml; susp 125, 200, 250, 400 mg/5 ml

SIDE EFFECTS

CNS: Headache, **seizures**
GI: Nausea, vomiting, diarrhea, increased AST, ALT, abdominal pain, glossitis, colitis, **pseudomembranous colitis**
HEMA: Anemia, increased bleeding time, **bone marrow depression, granulocytopenia**
INTEG: Urticaria, rash
SYST: **Anaphylaxis, respiratory distress, serum sickness, Stevens-Johnson syndrome**

Contraindications: Hypersensitivity to penicillins

Precautions: Pregnancy (B), lactation, hypersensitivity to cephalosporins, neonates, severe renal disease, acute lymphocytic leukemia

PHARMACOKINETICS

PO: Peak 2 hr, duration 6-8 hr; half-life 1-1⅓ hr, metabolized in liver, excreted in urine, crosses placenta, enters breast milk

---

⚠ Safety alert   *"Tall Man" lettering

INTERACTIONS

Increase: amoxicillin level—probenecid

Increase: anticoagulant action—warfarin

Increase: methotrexate levels—methotrexate

Decrease: effectiveness of oral contraceptives

Drug/Herb

• Do not use acidophilus with antiinfectives; separate by several hours

Decrease: absorption—khat; separate by 2 hr

Drug/Lab Test

False positive: Urine glucose, urine protein, direct Coombs' test

NURSING CONSIDERATIONS

Assess:

• I&O ratio; report hematuria, oliguria, since penicillin in high doses is nephrotoxic

• Any patient with a compromised renal system, since drug is excreted slowly in poor renal system function; toxicity may occur rapidly

• Hepatic studies: AST, ALT

• Blood studies: WBC, RBC, Hgb and Hct, bleeding time

• Renal studies: urinalysis, protein, blood, BUN, creatinine

• C&S before drug therapy; drug may be given as soon as culture is taken

• Bowel pattern before, during treatment; diarrhea, cramping, blood in stools, report to prescriber; pseudomembranous colitis may occur

• Skin eruptions after administration of penicillin to 1 wk after discontinuing drug

• Respiratory status: rate, character, wheezing, tightness in the chest

• Anaphylaxis: rash, itching, dyspnea, facial/laryngeal edema

Administer:

PO route

• Shake suspension well before each dose; may be used alone or mixed in drinks; use immediately; discard unused portion of susp after 14 days

• Give around the clock, caps may be emptied and mixed with liquids if needed

Perform/provide:

• Adrenaline, suction, tracheostomy set, endotracheal intubation equipment on unit

• Adequate intake of fluids (2 L) during diarrhea episodes

• Scratch test to assess allergy after securing order from prescriber; usually done when penicillin is only drug of choice

• Storage in tight container; after reconstituting, oral suspension refrigerated for 14 days

Evaluate:

• Therapeutic response: absence of infection; prevention of endocarditis, resolution of ulcer symptoms

Teach patient/family:

• That caps may be opened and contents taken with fluids; chewable form is available

• To take as prescribed, not to double dose

• All aspects of drug therapy: need to complete entire course of medication to ensure organism death (10-14 days); culture may be taken after completed course of medication

⚠ To report sore throat, fever, fatigue, diarrhea (may indicate superinfection or agranulocytopenia)

• That drug must be taken in equal intervals around the clock to maintain blood levels; take without regard to food

• To wear or carry emergency ID if allergic to penicillins

Treatment of anaphylaxis:

Withdraw drug, maintain airway, administer epINEPHrine, aminophylline, O_2, IV corticosteroids

amoxicillin/clavulanate potassium (℞)

(a-mox-i-sill'in)
Augmentin, Augmentin ES-600, Augmentin XR, Clavulin ✦

Func. class.: Broad-spectrum antiinfective
Chem. class.: Aminopenicillin β-lactamase inhibitor

Action: Bacteriocidal, interferes with cell wall replication of susceptible organisms; the cell wall, rendered osmotically unstable, swells and bursts from osmotic pressure; lysis mediated by bacterial cell wall autolytic enzymes, combination increases spectrum of activity against β-lactamase–resistant organisms

Uses: Sinus infections, pneumonia, otitis media, skin infection, UTI; effective for strains of *Escherichia coli, Proteus mirabilis, Haemophilus influenzae, Streptococcus faecalis, Streptococcus pneumoniae,* and some β-lactamase–producing organisms

DOSAGE AND ROUTES

• *Adult:* **PO** 250-500 mg q8h or 500-875 mg q12h depending on severity of infection
• *Child ≤40 kg:* **PO** 20-40 mg/kg/day in divided doses q8h or 25-45 mg/kg/day in divided doses q12h
Renal disease
• *Adult:* **PO** CCr 10-30 ml/min dose q12h; CCr <10 ml/min dose q24h, do not use 875 mg strength if CCr <30 ml/min; Augmentin XR is contraindicated in renal disease
Available forms: Tabs 250, 500, 875 mg/125 mg clavulanate; chew tabs 125, 200, 250, 400 mg; powder for oral susp 125, 200, 250, 400 mg/5 ml; ext rel tabs (XR) 1000 mg amoxicillin, 62.5 mg clavulanate; powder for oral susp (ES) 600 mg amoxicillin, 42.9 mg clavulanate

SIDE EFFECTS

CNS: Headache, fever, **seizures**
GI: Nausea, diarrhea, vomiting, increased AST, ALT, abdominal pain, glossitis, colitis, black tongue, **pseudomembranous colitis**
GU: Oliguria, proteinuria, hematuria, *vaginitis, moniliasis,* **glomerulonephritis**
HEMA: Anemia, **bone marrow depression, granulocytopenia, leukopenia, eosinophilia,** thrombocytopenic purpura
INTEG: Rash, urticaria, dermatitis, **toxic epidermal necrolysis**
META: Hyperkalemia, hypokalemia, alkalosis, hypernatremia
SYST: **Anaphylaxis, respiratory distress, serum sickness, superinfection, Stevens-Johnson syndrome**
Contraindications: Hypersensitivity to penicillins
Precautions: Pregnancy (B), lactation, hypersensitivity to cephalosporins; neonates, renal/GI disease

PHARMACOKINETICS

PO: Peak 2 hr, duration 6-8 hr; half-life 1-1⅓ hr, metabolized in liver, excreted in urine, crosses placenta, excreted in breast milk, removed by hemodialysis

INTERACTIONS

Increase: amoxicillin levels—probenecid
Increase: anticoagulant effect—warfarin
Increase: skin rash—allopurinol
Decrease: action of oral contraceptives
Drug/Herb
• Delayed/reduced absorption: khat; separate by 2 hr
• Do not use acidophilus with antiinfectives; separate by several hours
Drug/Lab Test
False positive: Urine glucose, urine protein, direct Coombs' test

---

NURSING CONSIDERATIONS
Assess:
• I&O ratio; report hematuria, oliguria since penicillin in high doses is nephrotoxic
• Any patient with a compromised renal system since drug is excreted slowly in poor renal system function; toxicity may occur
• Hepatic studies: AST, ALT
• Blood studies: WBC, RBC, Hgb and Hct, bleeding time
• Renal studies: urinalysis, protein, blood, BUN, creatinine
• C&S before drug therapy; drug may be given as soon as culture is taken
• Bowel pattern before, during treatment; diarrhea, cramping, blood in stools, report to prescriber, pseudomembranous colitis may occur
• Skin eruptions after administration of penicillin to 1 wk after discontinuing drug
• Respiratory status: rate, character, wheezing, tightness in chest
• Anaphylaxis: rash, itching, dyspnea, facial/laryngeal edema

Administer:
PO route
• Do not break, crush, or chew XR (ext rel) product
⚠ Only as directed, 2 (250 mg tab) not equivalent to 1 (500 mg tab) due to strength of clavulanate
• Shake suspension well before each dose, may be used alone or mixed in drinks, use immediately, discard unusual portion of susp after 14 days
• Give around the clock

Perform/provide:
• Adrenaline, suction, tracheostomy set, endotracheal intubation equipment on unit
• Adequate intake of fluids (2 L) during diarrhea episodes
• Scratch test to assess allergy after securing order from prescriber; usually done when penicillin is only drug of choice
• Storage refrigerated for 10 days

Evaluate:
• Therapeutic response: absence of infection
Teach patient/family:
• To take as prescribed, not to double dose
• All aspects of drug therapy: need to complete entire course of medication to ensure organism death (10-14 days); culture may be taken after completed course of medication
⚠ To report sore throat, fever, fatigue (may indicate superinfection or agranulocytosis)
• That drug must be taken in equal intervals around the clock to maintain blood levels
• To wear or carry emergency ID if allergic to penicillins
• To notify prescriber of diarrhea, cramping, blood in stools; pseudomembranous colitis may occur
• To use alternative contraceptive measures, if using oral contraceptives
Treatment of hypersensitivity: Withdraw drug, maintain airway, administer epINEPHrine, aminophylline, O₂, IV corticosteroids for anaphylaxis

amphotericin B desoxycholate
(am-foe-ter′i-sin)
Fungizone
amphotericin B cholesteryl sulfate
Amphotec
amphotericin B lipid based
Abelcet
amphotericin B liposome
AmBisome
Func. class.: Antifungal
Chem. class.: Amphoteric polyene

Action: Increases cell membrane permeability in susceptible fungi by binding sterols; alters cell membrane, causing leakage of cell components and cell death

Uses: Histoplasmosis, blastomycosis, coccidioidomycosis, cryptococcosis, aspergillosis, zygomycosis, candidiasis, sporotrichosis, cryptococcal meningitis; mucomycosis caused by mucormycosis, *Rhizopus, Absidia, Entomorphthora, Basidiobolus*

Unlabeled uses: Candiduria (bladder irrigation)

DOSAGE AND ROUTES

Desoxycholate
• *Adult:* **IV** Give test dose of 1 mg (not required); then 0.25 mg/kg, increase daily slowly to 0.5 mg/kg, may give 1 mg/kg/day or 1.5 mg/kg/day, alternate-day dosing may be used
• *Child:* **IV** 0.25 mg/kg infused initially, increase by 0.25 mg/kg every other day to max of 1 mg/kg/day
• *Adult and child:* **TOP** apply 2-4 × daily
• *Adult and child:* **PO** 1 ml (100 mg) qid
Amphotec
• *Adult and child:* **IV** 3-4 mg/kg/day, max 7.5 mg/kg/day
Abelcet
• *Adult and child:* **IV** 5 mg/kg/day as a 1 mg/ml inf given 2.5 mg/kg/hr
AmBisome
Fungal infections
• *Adult and child:* **IV** 3-5 mg/kg q24h
Visceral leishmaniasis
• *Adult:* **IV** 3-4 mg/kg q24h days 1-5
Available forms: *Amphotericin B desoxycholate:* inj 50 mg vial; oral susp 100 mg/ml; cream, ointment, lotion 3%; *amphotericin B cholesteryl:* powder for inj 50 mg/20 ml, 100 mg/50 ml; *amphotericin B lipid complex:* susp for inj 100 mg/20 ml vial; *amphotericin B liposome:* powder for inj 50 mg vial

SIDE EFFECTS

CNS: Headache, fever, chills, peripheral nerve pain, paresthesias, peripheral neuropathy, **seizures,** dizziness
EENT: Tinnitus, deafness, diplopia, blurred vision
GI: Nausea, vomiting, anorexia, diarrhea, cramps, **hemorrhagic gastroenteritis, acute liver failure**
GU: Hypokalemia, azotemia, hyposthenuria, **renal tubular acidosis,** nephrocalcinosis, **permanent renal impairment, anuria, oliguria**
HEMA: Normochromic, normocytic anemia, **thrombocytopenia, agranulocytosis, leukopenia, eosinophilia,** hypokalemia, hyponatremia, hypomagnesemia
INTEG: Burning, irritation, pain, necrosis at inj site with extravasation, flushing, dermatitis, skin rash (topical route)
MS: **Arthralgia, myalgia,** generalized pain, weakness, weight loss
Contraindications: Hypersensitivity, severe bone marrow depression
Precautions: Pregnancy (B), renal disease, lactation

PHARMACOKINETICS

IV: Peak 1-2 hr, initial half-life 24 hr, metabolized in liver, excreted in urine (metabolites), breast milk, highly bound to plasma proteins; penetrates poorly CSF, bronchial secretions, aqueous humor, muscle, bone

INTERACTIONS

Increase: nephrotoxicity—other nephrotoxic antibiotics (aminoglycosides, cisplatin, vancomycin, cycloSPORINE, polymyxin B)
Increase: hypokalemia—corticosteroids, digoxin, skeletal muscle relaxants, thiazides
Drug/Herb
• Do not use acidophilus with antiinfectives; separate by several hours
Increase: possibility of nephrotoxicity—gossypol

NURSING CONSIDERATIONS

Assess:
• VS q15-30min during first infusion; note changes in pulse, B/P
• I&O ratio; watch for decreasing urinary output, change in specific gravity; discontinue drug to prevent permanent damage to renal tubules

---

⚠ Safety alert   *"Tall Man" lettering

• Blood studies: CBC, K, Na, Ca, Mg q2wk, BUN, creatinine weekly

• Weight weekly; if weight increases over 2 lb/wk, edema is present; renal damage should be considered

⚠ For renal toxicity: increasing BUN, serum creatinine; if BUN is >40 mg/dl or if serum creatinine >3 mg/dl, drug may be discontinued or dosage reduced

⚠ For hepatotoxicity: increasing AST, ALT, alk phos, bilirubin

• For allergic reaction: dermatitis, rash; drug should be discontinued, antihistamines (mild reaction) or epINEPHrine (severe reaction) administered

• For hypokalemia: anorexia, drowsiness, weakness, decreased reflexes, dizziness, increased urinary output, increased thirst, paresthesias

• For ototoxicity: tinnitus (ringing, roaring in ears) vertigo, loss of hearing (rare)

Administer:

• Do not confuse four different types; these are not interchangeable: conventional amphotericin B, amphotericin B cholesteryl, amphotericin B lipid complex, amphotericin B liposome

IV route

• Drug only after C&S confirms organism, drug needed to treat condition; make sure drug is used in life-threatening infections

Desoxycholate

• After diluting 50 mg/10 ml sterile water (no preservatives) (5 mg per 1 ml), shake, dilute with 500 ml of D$_5$W to concentration of 0.1 mg/ml

• Test dose of 1 mg/20 ml D$_5$W; give over 10-30 min

Intermittent IV INF route

• IV using in-line filter (mean pore diameter >1 micron) using distal veins; check for extravasation, necrosis q8h; use an infusion pump; infuse over 2-6 hr; rapid infusion may result in circulation collapse; use central line if possible

Additive compatibilities: Heparin, hydrocortisone, sodium bicarbonate

Syringe compatibilities: Heparin

Y-site compatibilities: Aldesleukin, diltiazem, DOXOrubicin liposome, famoti-

dine, remifentanil, tacrolimus, teniposide, thiotepa, zidovudine

Solution compatibilities: D$_5$W

Cholesteryl

IV route

• Reconstitute 50 mg vial/10 ml, 100 mg vial/20 ml sterile water for inj (5 mg/5 ml); swirl or shake gently until dissolved, further dilute with D$_5$W (0.6 mg/ml); wear gloves when preparing

• Test dose 10 ml of final solution (1.6-8.3 mg) over ½ hr, observe for next ½ hr for reactions

• Give 1 mg/kg/hr using infusion pump, do not give rapidly, may increase infusion, if tolerated

Additive compatibilities: Heparin

Liposomal complex

IV route

• Reconstitute with 12 ml sterile water/50 ml vial (4 mg/ml), shake, use 5-micron filter, dilute in D$_5$W (1-2 mg/ml), give over 2 hr

• Do not admix

Lipid complex

IV route

• Shake vial until dissolved, withdraw dose using 18G needle, replace needle from syringe with drug using 5 micron filter needle (use needle for 4 vials or less), empty contents in IV of D$_5$W (1 mg/ml), give at 2.5 mg/kg/hr, use infusion pump

• Do not admix

Perform/provide:

• Acetaminophen and diphenhydrAMINE 30 min prior to infusion to reduce fever, chills, headache

• Storage protected from moisture and light; diluted solution is stable for 24 hr at room temperature

Evaluate:

• Therapeutic response: decreased fever, malaise, rash, negative C&S for infecting organism

Teach patient/family:

• That long-term therapy may be needed to clear infection (2 wk-3 mo depending on type of infection)

• To notify prescriber of bleeding, bruising, or soft tissue swelling

---

ampicillin (℞)
(am-pi-sill'in)
Ampicin ✦, Apo-Ampi ✦,
Marcillin, NovoAmpicillin ✦,
Nu-Ampi ✦, Omnipen,
Penbriten ✦, Polycillin,
Principen, Totacillin
Func. class.: Broad-spectrum antiinfective
Chem. class.: Aminopenicillin

Do not confuse:
Omnipen/imipenem

Action: Interferes with cell wall replication of susceptible organisms; the cell wall, rendered osmotically unstable, swells, bursts from osmotic pressure, lysis mediated by cell wall autolysins

Uses: Effective for gram-positive cocci *(Staphylococcus aureus, Streptococcus pyogenes, Streptococcus faecalis, Streptococcus pneumoniae)*, gram-negative cocci *(Neisseria gonorrhoeae, Neisseria meningitidis)*, gram-negative bacilli *(Haemophilus influenzae, Proteus mirabilis, Salmonella, Shigella, Listeria monocytogenes)*, gram-positive bacilli

Unlabeled uses: High-risk for infection in patients having C-section

DOSAGE AND ROUTES

Systemic infections
• *Adult and child ≥40 kg:* **PO** 250-500 mg q6h; **IV/IM** 2-8 g daily in divided doses q4-6h
• *Child <40 kg:* **PO** 50-100 mg/kg/day in divided doses q6-8h; **IV/IM** 100-200 mg/kg/day in divided doses q6-8h

Renal disease
• *Adult and child:* CCr 10-30 ml/min dose q8-12h; CCr 30-50 ml/min q6-8hr; <10 ml/min dose q12h

Bacterial meningitis
• *Adult:* **IM/IV** 500 mg-3 g q6h, max 14 g/day
• *Child:* **IM/IV** 200-400 mg/kg/day in divided doses q6h, max 12 g/day

Gonorrhea
• *Adult and child ≥45 kg:* **PO** 3 g given with 1 g probenecid as a single dose; **IM/IV** 500 mg q6h (≥40 kg); **IM/IV** 50 mg/kg/day in divided doses q6-8h (<40 kg)

Prevention of bacterial endocarditis
• *Adult:* **IM/IV** 2 g 30 min before procedure
• *Child:* **IM/IV** 50 mg/kg 30 min prior to procedure, max 2 g

GI/GU infections other than caused by N. gonorrhoeae
• *Adult and child >20 kg:* **PO** 250-500 mg q6h, may use larger dose for more serious infections
• *Child ≤20 kg:* **PO** 50-100 mg/kg/day in divided doses q6h

Available forms: Powder for inj 125, 250, 500 mg, 1, 2, 10 g; IV inj 500 mg, 1, 2 g; caps 250, 500 mg; powder for oral susp 125, 250/5 ml

SIDE EFFECTS

CNS: Lethargy, hallucinations, anxiety, depression, twitching, **coma, seizures**
GI: Nausea, vomiting, diarrhea, **pseudomembranous colitis**
GU: Oliguria, proteinuria, hematuria, *vaginitis, moniliasis,* **glomerulonephritis**
HEMA: Anemia, increased bleeding time, **bone marrow depression, granulocytopenia,** leukopenia, eosinophilia
INTEG: Rash, urticaria, **toxic epidermal necrolysis**
MISC: **Anaphylaxis, serum sickness, Stevens-Johnson syndrome**

Contraindications: Hypersensitivity to penicillins

Precautions: Pregnancy (B), lactation; hypersensitivity to cephalosporins; neonates, renal disease

---

⚠ Safety alert   *"Tall Man" lettering

PHARMACOKINETICS

PO: Peak 2 hr, duration 6-8 hr
IV: Peak 5 min
IM: Peak 1 hr
Half-life 50-110 min; metabolized in liver; excreted in urine, bile, breast milk; crosses placenta, removed by dialysis

INTERACTIONS

Increase: ampicillin concentrations—probenecid
Increase: ampicillin-induced skin rash—allopurinol
Decrease: effectiveness of oral contraceptives
Drug/Herb
• Delayed/reduced absorption—khat; separate by 2 hr
• Do not use acidophilus with antiinfectives; separate by several hours
Drug/Lab Test
Increase: AST, ALT
Decrease: Conjugated estrone in pregnancy, conjugated estriol
False positive: Urine glucose, urine protein, direct Coombs'

NURSING CONSIDERATIONS

Assess:
• I&O ratio; report hematuria, oliguria, since penicillin in high doses is nephrotoxic
⚠ Any patient with compromised renal system, since drug is excreted slowly in poor renal system function; toxicity may occur
• Hepatic studies: AST, ALT
• Blood studies: WBC, RBC, Hgb and Hct, bleeding time
• Renal studies: urinalysis, protein, blood, BUN, creatinine
• C&S before drug therapy; drug may be taken as soon as culture is taken
• Bowel pattern before, during treatment
• Skin eruptions after administration of penicillin to 1 wk after discontinuing drug
• Respiratory status: rate, character, wheezing, tightness in chest
• Anaphylaxis: rash, itching, dyspnea, facial swelling; stop drug, notify prescriber, have emergency equipment available

Administer:
PO route
• On empty stomach, with plenty of water for best absorption (1-2 hr before meals or 2-3 hr after meals)
• Shake suspension well before each dose
IM route
• Reconstitute by adding 0.9-1.2 ml/125 mg vial; 0.9-1.9 ml/250 mg vial; 1.2-1.8 ml/500 mg vial; 2.4-7.4 ml/1 g vial; 6.8 ml/2 g vial
IV route
• After diluting with sterile H_2O 0.9-1.2 ml/125 mg drug, administer over 3-5 min (up to 500 mg), 10-15 min (>500 mg) by direct IV; may be diluted in 50 ml or more of D_5W, D_5 0.45% NaCl to a concentration of 30 mg/ml or less; IV sol is stable for 1 hr; give at prescribed rate
Additive compatibilities: Clindamycin, erythromycin, floxacillin, furosemide
Syringe compatibilities: Chloramphenicol, heparin, procaine
Y-site compatibilities: Acyclovir, allopurinol, amifostine, aztreonam, cyclophosphamide, DOXOrubicin liposome, enalaprilat, esmolol, famotidine, filgrastim, fludarabine, foscarnet, granisetron, heparin, insulin (regular), labetalol, magnesium sulfate, melphalan, meperidine, morphine, multivitamins, ofloxacin, perphenazine, phytonadione, potassium chloride, propofol, remifentanil, tacrolimus, teniposide, theophylline, thiotepa, tolazoline, vit B/C
Perform/provide:
• Adrenaline, suction, tracheostomy set, endotracheal intubation equipment on unit
• Adequate intake of fluids (2 L) during diarrhea episodes
• Scratch test to assess allergy after securing order from prescriber; usually done when penicillin is only drug of choice
• Storage in tight container; after reconstituting, oral suspension refrigerated for 2 wk or stored at room temperature for 1 wk

Evaluate:
• Therapeutic response: absence of temp, draining wounds, other symptoms of infections

Teach patient/family:
• That tabs may be crushed; caps may be opened and mixed with water
• To take oral ampicillin on empty stomach with full glass of water
• All aspects of drug therapy: need to complete entire course of medication to ensure organism death (10-14 days); culture may be taken after completed course of medication
⚠ To report sore throat, fever, fatigue, diarrhea (may indicate superinfection); report rash or other signs of allergy
• That drug must be taken in equal intervals around the clock to maintain blood levels
• To wear or carry emergency ID if allergic to penicillins

Treatment of anaphylaxis: Withdraw drug, maintain airway, administer epINEPHrine, aminophylline, O₂, IV corticosteroids

---

**ampicillin,
sulbactam (℞)**

Unasyn
Func. class.: Broad-spectrum antiinfective
Chem. class.: Aminopenicillin with β-lactamase inhibitor

Action: Interferes with cell wall replication of susceptible organisms; the cell wall, rendered osmotically unstable, swells, bursts from osmotic pressure; lysis due to cell wall autolytic enzymes; combination extends spectrum of activity by β-lactamase inhibition

Uses: Skin infections, intraabdominal infections, pneumonia *(Staphylococcus aureus, Escherichia coli, Klebsiella, Proteus mirabilis, Bacteroides fragilis, Haemophilus influenzae, Enterobacter, Acinetobacter calcoaceticus)*, intraabdominal infections *(Enterobacter, Kleb-siella, Bacteroides, E. coli)*, gynecologic infections *(E. coli, Bacteroides)*, meningitis, septicemia

DOSAGE AND ROUTES

• *Adult and child ≥40 kg:* **IM/IV** 1 g ampicillin, 0.5 g sulbactam to 2 g ampicillin and 1 g sulbactam q6h, not to exceed 4 g/day sulbactam
• *Child ≤40 kg:* **IV** 100-200 mg/kg/day (ampicillin component) divided q6h, max 8 g/day

Renal disease
• *Adult ≥40 kg:* **IM/IV** CCr 15-29 ml/min dose q12h; CCr 5-14 ml/min dose q24h

Available forms: Powder for inj 1.5 g (1 g ampicillin, 0.5 g sulbactam), 3 g (2 g ampicillin, 1 g sulbactam), 10 g (10 g ampicillin, 5 g sulbactam)

SIDE EFFECTS

CNS: Lethargy, hallucinations, anxiety, depression, twitching, **coma, seizures**
GI: Nausea, vomiting, diarrhea, increased AST, ALT, abdominal pain, glossitis, colitis, **pseudomembranous colitis**
GU: Oliguria, proteinuria, hematuria, *vaginitis, moniliasis,* **glomerulonephritis,** dysuria
HEMA: Anemia, increased bleeding time, **bone marrow depression, granulocytopenia, leukopenia, eosinophilia**
MISC: **Anaphylaxis, serum sickness, toxic epidermal necrolysis, Stevens-Johnson syndrome**

Contraindications: Hypersensitivity to penicillins, ampicillin, or sulbactam
Precautions: Pregnancy (B), lactation, hypersensitivity to cephalosporins, neonates, renal disease

PHARMACOKINETICS

IV: Peak 5 min; half-life 50-110 min; little metabolized in liver, 75%-85% of both drugs excreted in urine, diffuses to breast milk, crosses placenta

---

⚠ Safety alert   *"Tall Man" lettering

INTERACTIONS

Increase: ampicillin-induced skin rash—allopurinol

Increase: ampicillin level—probenecid

Increase: methotrexate level—methotrexate

Decrease: oral contraceptive effect

Drug/Herb

• Do not use acidophilus with antiinfectives; separate by several hours

Decrease: absorption—khat; separate by 2 hr

Drug/Lab Test

False positive: Urine glucose, urine protein

NURSING CONSIDERATIONS

Assess:

• Bowel pattern before, during treatment

• Respiratory status: rate, character, wheezing, tightness in chest

• I&O ratio; report hematuria, oliguria, since penicillin in high doses is nephrotoxic

⚠ Any patient with compromised renal system, since drug is excreted slowly in poor renal system function; toxicity may occur rapidly

• Hepatic studies: AST, ALT if on long-term therapy

• Blood studies: WBC, RBC, Hct, Hgb, bleeding time

• Renal studies: urinalysis, protein, blood, BUN, creatinine

• C&S before drug therapy; drug may be given as soon as culture is taken

• Skin eruptions after administration of ampicillin to 1 wk after discontinuing drug

• Allergies before initiation of treatment; reaction of each medication; report allergies

Administer:

IM route

• Reconstitute by adding 3.2 ml sterile water/1.5 g vial; 6.4 ml/3 g vial, give deep in large muscle

IV route

• After diluting 1.5 g/3.2 ml sterile H_2O for inj or 3 g/6.4 ml (250 mg ampicillin/125 mg sulbactam); allow to stand until foaming stops; may give over 15 min as direct IV; dilute further in 50 ml or more of D_5W, NaCl, administer within 1 hr after reconstitution; give as an intermittent inf over 15-30 min

Additive compatibilities: Aztreonam

Y-site compatibilities: Amifostine, aztreonam, cefepime, enalaprilat, famotidine, filgrastim, fluconazole, fludarabine, gallium, granisetron, heparin, insulin (regular), meperidine, morphine, paclitaxel, remifentanil, tacrolimus, teniposide, theophylline, thiotepa

Perform/provide:

• Adrenaline, suction, tracheostomy set, endotracheal intubation equipment on unit for possible anaphylaxis

• Adequate intake of fluids (2 L) during diarrhea episodes

• Scratch test to assess allergy after securing order from prescriber; usually done when penicillin is only drug choice

• Storage in tight container, out of light

Evaluate:

• Therapeutic response: absence of fever, draining wounds, negative C&S

Teach patient/family:

• That oral contraceptives may be reduced and a nonhormonal contraceptive should be taken while on this drug if pregnancy is to be prevented

• To report superinfection: vaginal itching, loose, foul-smelling stools, black furry tongue

⚠ To report immediately pseudomembranous colitis: fever, diarrhea with pus, blood, or mucus; may occur up to 4 wk after treatment

• To wear or carry emergency ID if allergic to penicillin products

Treatment of anaphylaxis: Withdraw drug, maintain airway, administer epiNEPHrine, aminophylline, O_2, IV corticosteroids

---

Side effects: *italics* = common; **bold** = life-threatening

amprenavir (℞)
(am-pren'ah-veer)
Agenerase
Func. class.: Antiretroviral
Chem. class.: Protease inhibitor

Action: Inhibits human immunodeficiency virus (HIV-1) protease, which prevents replication, proliferation of the infectious virus

Uses: HIV-1 in combination with other antiretroviral agents

DOSAGE AND ROUTES

Caps and sol are not interchangeable

• *Adult:* **PO** (cap) 1200 mg bid; **SOL** 1400 mg bid
• *Child ≥50 kg:* **PO** (cap) 1200 mg bid; **SOL** 1400 mg bid
• *Child <50 kg:* **PO** (cap): 20 mg/kg bid or 15 mg/kg tid, max 2400 mg/day; **SOL** 22.5 mg/kg bid or 17 mg/kg tid daily, max 2800 mg/day

Amprenavir/ritonavir regimen
• *Adult:* **PO** 600 mg amprenavir, 100 mg ritonavir bid or 1200 mg amprenavir, 200 mg ritonavir bid

Hepatic dose
• *Adult:* **PO** (Child-Pugh score 5-8) 450 mg bid (caps), 513 mg bid (sol) in combination; (Child-Pugh score 9-12) 300 mg bid (caps), 342 mg bid (sol) in combination

Available forms: Caps 50 mg; oral sol 15 mg/ml

SIDE EFFECTS

CNS: Paresthesia, headache
ENDO: New-onset diabetes, hyperglycemia, exacerbation of preexisting diabetes mellitus, hypertriglyceridemia
GI: Diarrhea, abdominal pain, nausea, **hepatotoxicity**
HEMA: **Acute hemolytic anemia**
INTEG: Rash, **Stevens-Johnson syndrome**

Contraindications: Hypersensitivity; oral sol: renal failure

Precautions: Pregnancy (C), liver/renal disease, lactation, children, hemophilia, sulfonamide sensitivity, geriatric

PHARMACOKINETICS

Rapidly absorbed, peak 1-2 hr, 90% protein bound, metabolized in liver, excreted unchanged in urine/feces (minimal), half-life 7-10½ hr

INTERACTIONS

Toxicity: alprazolam, atorvastatin, bepridil, carbamazepine, clonazepam, clozapine, dapsone, diazepam, diltiazem, ergots, erythromycin, fentanyl, flurazepam, itraconazole, loratadine, lovastatin, midazolam, niCARdipine, NIFEdipine, pimozide, triazolam, verapamil

⚠ Serious life-threatening interactions: amiodarone, lidocaine, quinidine, tricyclics, warfarin

Increase: amprenavir levels—cimetidine, clarithromycin, erythromycin, indinavir, itraconazole, ketoconazole, ritonavir

Decrease: amprenavir levels—antacids, carbamazepine, didanosine, efavirenz, methadone, nevirapine, phenobarbital, phenytoin, rifamycins

Decrease: effects of oral contraceptives, methadone

Drug/Herb
Decrease: amprenavir levels—St. John's wort

Drug/Food
Decrease: bioavailability after high-fat meal

Drug/Lab Test
Increase: Glucose, cholesterol, triglycerides

NURSING CONSIDERATIONS
Assess:

⚠ For renal/hepatic failure, pregnancy, or those receiving disulfiram, metronidazole; oral solution contains propylene glycol in greater quantities
• Signs of infection, anemia

⚠ Safety alert   *"Tall Man" lettering

- Hepatic studies: ALT, AST
- Bowel pattern before, during treatment; if severe abdominal pain with bleeding occurs, drug should be discontinued; monitor hydration
- Viral load, CD4 count throughout treatment
- Skin eruptions, rash, urticaria, itching
- Allergies before treatment, reaction of each medication; place allergies on chart

Administer:
- Do not interchange caps and oral sol; they are not the same on a mg/mg basis.
- With or without food; avoid high-fat meals

Evaluate:
- Therapeutic response: increasing CD4 counts; decreased viral load, resolution of symptoms of HIV

Teach patient/family:
- To take as prescribed with or without food, avoid high-fat foods; if dose is missed, take as soon as remembered up to 1 hr before next dose; do not double dose, do not share with others
- That drug must be taken in equal intervals around the clock to maintain blood levels for duration of therapy
- To use a nonhormonal method of contraception during treatment, use condoms
- To notify prescriber if diarrhea, nausea, vomiting, rash occurs
- That drug does not cure AIDs or prevent transmission to others, only controls symptoms

Rarely Used

amyl nitrite (R)
(am'il nye'trite)
amyl nitrite, Amyl Nitrite Aspirols, Amyl Nitrite Vaporole
Func. class.: Coronary vasodilator

Uses: Acute angina pectoris, cyanide poisoning
Unlabeled uses: Cardiac murmur diagnosis

DOSAGE AND ROUTES
Angina
- *Adult:* **INH** 0.18-0.3 ml as needed, 1-6 inhalations from 1 cap, may repeat in 3-5 min

Cyanide poisoning
- *Adult:* **INH** 0.3 ml ampule inhaled 15 sec until preparation of sodium nitrite infusion is ready

Contraindications: Pregnancy (X), hypersensitivity to nitrites, severe anemia, increased intracranial pressure, hypertension

anagrelide (R)
(a-na'gre-lide)
Agrylin
Func. class.: Antiplatelet
Chem. class.: Imidazo-quinazolinone

Action: Reduces platelet count and prevents early platelet shape changes in response to aggregating agents thus inhibiting platelet aggregation
Uses: Thrombocythemia, secondary to myeloproliferative disorders, to reduce elevated platelet count

DOSAGE AND ROUTES
- *Adult:* **PO** 0.5 mg qid or 1 mg bid, may be adjusted after 1 wk, max 10 mg/day or 2.5 mg single dose; maintenance: titrate to lowest dose to maintain platelets <600,000
Available forms: Caps 0.5, 1 mg

SIDE EFFECTS
CNS: Headache, dizziness, **seizures,** *paresthesia,* **CVA,** *fever*
CV: Postural hypotension, tachycardia, palpitations, **CHF, MI, cardiomyopathy, cardiomegaly, complete heart block, atrial fibrillation,** dysrhythmia, **chest pain**
GI: Diarrhea, abdominal pain, nausea, flatulence, vomiting, anorexia, constipation, pancreatitis
GU: Dysuria

HEMA: **Anemia, thrombocytopenia, ecchymosis, lymphadenoma**
INTEG: Rash, photosensitivity
MISC: Edema, pain,
MS: Asthenia, back pain
RESP: Dyspnea
Contraindications: Hypersensitivity, hypotension
Precautions: Pregnancy (C), lactation, child <16 yr, renal/hepatic/cardiac disease

PHARMACOKINETICS

PO: Peak 1 hr, duration >24 hr: metabolized in liver: excreted in feces/urine

INTERACTIONS

Increase: bleeding risk—abciximab, anticoagulants, aspirin, eptifibatide, NSAIDs, thrombolytics, ticlopidine, tirofiban
Decrease: absorption—sucralfate
Drug/Herb
• Gastric irritation: arginine
Increase: effect—bogbean, dong quai, feverfew, ginger, ginkgo
Increase: bleeding risk; green tea
Decrease: effect—bilberry, saw palmetto
Drug/Food
Decrease: bioavailability, plasma concentrations

NURSING CONSIDERATIONS

Assess:
• Platelet counts q2day × 1 wk, and qwk thereafter, response should begin after 1-2 wk; Hgb, WBC, LFTs, renal function studies
• B/P, pulse during treatment until stable; take B/P lying, standing; orthostatic hypotension is common
• Cardiac status: chest pain, what aggravates or ameliorates condition
Administer:
• May give with food, monitor closely for dosage adjustment, there is better absorption on empty stomach

Perform/provide:
• Storage at room temperature
Evaluate:
• Therapeutic response: decreased platelet count
Teach patient/family:
• That medication is not a cure: may have to be taken continuously in evenly spaced doses only as directed
• That it is necessary to quit smoking to prevent excessive vasoconstriction
• To avoid hazardous activities until stabilized on medication; dizziness may occur
• To rise slowly from sitting or lying to prevent orthostatic hypotension
• Not to use alcohol or OTC medications unless approved by prescriber; to use sunscreen, protective clothing to prevent burns
• To report cardiac reactions, increased bruising, bleeding
• To use contraception (female, childbearing age), fetal harm may occur

anakinra (℞)
(an-ah-kin'rah)
Kineret
Func. class.: Antirheumatic (DMARD), immunomodulator
Chem. class.: Recombinant form of human interleukin-1 receptor antagonist (IL-1Ra)

Action: A form of human interleukin-1 receptor antagonist (IL-1Ra) produced by DNA technology; blocks activity of IL-1, resulting in decreased cartilage degradation and decreased bone resorption
Uses: Reduction in signs and symptoms of moderate to severe active rheumatoid arthritis in patients ≥18 years of age who have not responded to other disease-modifying agents

DOSAGE AND ROUTES
• *Adult:* **SUBCUT** 100 mg daily
Available form: Inj 100 mg/ml prefilled glass syringe

SIDE EFFECTS

CNS: Headache
EENT: Sinusitis
GI: Abdominal pain, nausea, diarrhea
HEMA: **Neutropenia**
INTEG: Rash, *inj site reaction*, allergic reaction
MISC: Flulike symptoms
MS: Worsening of RA, arthralgia
RESP: URI

Contraindications: Hypersensitivity to *Escherichia coli*–derived proteins or this product, sepsis

Precautions: Pregnancy (B), lactation, children, renal impairment, geriatric

PHARMACOKINETICS

Terminal half-life 4-6 hr

INTERACTIONS

• Do not give concurrently with vaccines, immunizations should be brought up to date before treatment
Increase: risk of severe infection—TNF blocking agents (etanercept)
Decrease: antibody reactions

NURSING CONSIDERATIONS
Assess:

• Pain, stiffness, ROM, swelling of joints, baseline periodically during treatment
• For inj site pain, swelling; usually occur after 2 inj (4-5 days)
• For infections (increased WBC, fever, flulike symptoms); stop treatment if present
• Neutrophil counts prior to treatment and monthly × 3 mo and quarterly for up to 1 yr thereafter
• For allergic reactions (rash, dyspnea); discontinue if severe
Administer:

• Do not use if cloudy or discolored or if particulate is present, protect from light
• Do not admix with other sol or medications, do not use filter
Evaluate:

• Therapeutic response: decreased inflammation, pain in joints

Teach patient/family:

• Not to receive vaccines while taking this drug
• About self-administration if appropriate: inj should be made in thigh, abdomen, upper arm; rotate sites at least 1 inch from old site, give at same time of day
• To notify prescriber if pregnancy is planned or suspected, avoid breastfeeding
• To notify prescriber of allergic reaction

anastrozole
(an-a-stroh'zole)
Arimidex
Func. class.: Antineoplastic
Chem. class.: Aromatase inhibitor

Action: Highly selective nonsteroidal aromatase inhibitor that lowers serum estradiol concentrations; many breast cancers have strong estrogen receptors
Uses: Advanced breast carcinoma not responsive to other therapy in estrogen-receptor–positive patients (usually postmenopausal); patients with advanced disease on tamoxifen, adjunct therapy in early breast cancer

DOSAGE AND ROUTES

• *Adult:* **PO** 1 mg daily
Available forms: Tabs 1 mg

SIDE EFFECTS

CNS: Hot flashes, headache, lightheadedness, depression, dizziness, confusion, insomnia, anxiety
CV: Chest pain, hypertension, thrombophlebitis, edema
GI: Nausea, vomiting, altered taste leading to anorexia, diarrhea, constipation, abdominal pain, dry mouth
GU: Vaginal bleeding, vaginal dryness, pelvic pain, pruritus vulvae, UTI
HEMA: **Leukopenia**
INTEG: Rash
MS: Bone pain, myalgia, *asthenia*
RESP: Cough, sinusitis, dyspnea

140   anidulafungin

Contraindications: Pregnancy (D), hypersensitivity
Precautions: Lactation, children, geriatric, hepatic/renal disease

PHARMACOKINETICS

PO: Peak 4-7 hr, half-life 50 hr, excreted in feces, urine

INTERACTIONS

Drug/Lab Test
Increase: GGT, AST, ALT, alk phos, cholesterol, LDL

NURSING CONSIDERATIONS

Assess:
• For side effects during treatment
Administer:
• Give with food
Perform/provide:
• Storage in light-resistant container at room temperature
Evaluate:
• Therapeutic response: decreased tumor size, spread of malignancy
Teach patient/family:
• To report any complaints, side effects to prescriber
• That vaginal bleeding, pruritus, hot flashes are reversible after discontinuing treatment
• To report vaginal bleeding immediately
• If premenopausal, do not breastfeed; use reliable barrier contraception
• That tumor flare—increase in size of tumor, increased bone pain—may occur and will subside rapidly; may take analgesics for pain

---

anidulafungin (℞)
(a-nid-yoo-luh-fun'jin)
Eraxis
Func. class.: Antifungal, systemic
Chem. class.: Echinocandin

Action: Inhibits fungal enzyme synthesis; causes direct damage to fungal cell wall

Uses: *Candida albicans, C. glabrata, C. parapsilosis, C. tropicalis*

DOSAGE AND ROUTES

Candidemia and other candida infections
• *Adult*: IV loading dose 200 mg on day 1, then 100 mg/day until 14 days or more until last positive culture
Esophageal candidiasis
• *Adult*: IV loading dose 100 mg on day 1, then 50 mg/day for at least 14 days and for at least 7 days after symptoms are resolved
Available forms: Powder for inj, lyophilized 50 mg

SIDE EFFECTS

Candidemia/other Candida infections
CNS: **Seizures,** dizziness, *headache*
CV: DVT, **atrial fibrillation, right bundle branch block,** hypotension, **sinus arrhythmia, thrombophlebitis superficial, ventricular extra systoles (rare)**
GI: Nausea, anorexia, vomiting, diarrhea, increased AST, ALT
META: Hypokalemia
Esophageal candidiasis
CNS: Headache
GI: Nausea, anorexia, vomiting, diarrhea, **hepatic necrosis**
HEMA: **Neutropenia, thrombocytopenia, leukopenia, coagulopathy**
INTEG: Rash
META: Hypocalcemia, hyperglycemia, hyperkalemia, hypernatremia, hypomagnesium (rare)
MS: Back pain, rigors
Contraindications: Hypersensitivity to this product, or other echinocandins
Precautions: Pregnancy (C), severe hepatic, lactation, children

PHARMACOKINETICS

Steady state after loading dose, distribution half-life 0.5-1 hr, terminal half-life 40-50 hr, protein binding 84%

⚠ Safety alert   *"Tall Man" lettering

A

INTERACTIONS

Increase: plasma concentrations—cycloSPORINE

Drug/Lab Test

Increase: Amylase, bilirubin, CPK, creatinine, ECG, QT prolongation, lipase
Decrease: Platelets, magnesium, potassium, transferase, urea

NURSING CONSIDERATIONS

Assess:

• For infection, clearing of cultures during treatment; obtain culture baseline and throughout; drug may be started as soon as culture is taken
• CBC (RBC, Hct, Hgb), differential, platelet count periodically; notify prescriber of results
• Renal studies: BUN, serum uric acid, urine CCr, electrolytes before and during therapy
• Hepatic studies before and during treatment: bilirubin, AST, ALT, alk phos, as needed
• Bleeding: hematuria, heme-positive stools, bruising or petechiae, mucosa or orifices; blood dyscrasias can occur
• GI symptoms: frequency of stools, cramping, if severe diarrhea occurs, electrolytes may need to be given

Administer:

IV route

• Reconstitute with provided dilutent 50 mg vial/5 ml (3.33 mg/ml), dilute with D_5 of 0.9% NaCl, only to a concentration of 0.5 mg/ml, run at no more than 1.1 mg/ml
• Do not use if cloudy or precipitated; do not admix

Perform/provide:

• Storage at room temperature, away from light, do not freeze; diluted sol must be used within 24 hr

Evaluate:

• Therapeutic response: decreased symptoms of *Candida* infection, negative culture

Teach patient/family:

• To notify prescriber if pregnancy is suspected or planned; use nonhormonal form of contraception while taking this product
• To avoid breastfeeding while taking this product
• To inform prescriber of renal/hepatic disease
• To report bleeding
• To report signs of infection: increased temp, sore throat, flulike symptoms
• To notify prescriber of nausea, vomiting, diarrhea, jaundice, anorexia, clay-colored stools, dark urine; hepatotoxicity may occur

---

⚠ High Alert

anistreplase (℞)

(ah-nis′tre-place)
anisoylated plasminogen, APSAC, Eminase
Func. class.: Thrombolytic enzyme
Chem. class.: Plasminogen activator

Action: Promotes thrombolysis by promoting conversion of plasminogen to plasmin
Uses: Acute MI for lysis of coronary artery thrombi

DOSAGE AND ROUTES

• *Adult:* **IV** 30 units over 2-5 min as soon as possible after onset of symptoms
Available forms: Powder, lyophilized 30 units/vial

SIDE EFFECTS

CNS: Headache, fever, sweating, agitation, dizziness, paresthesia, tremor, vertigo, **intracranial hemorrhage**
CV: Hypotension, **dysrhythmias,** conduction disorders
GI: Nausea, vomiting
HEMA: Decreased Hct; **GI, GU, intracranial, retroperitoneal,** surface bleeding; **thrombocytopenia**
INTEG: Rash, urticaria, phlebitis at inj site, itching, flushing
MS: Low back pain, arthralgia
RESP: Altered respirations, dyspnea, **bronchospasm, lung edema**
SYST: **Anaphylaxis (rare)**

Contraindications: Hypersensitivity, active internal bleeding, intraspinal or intracranial surgery, neoplasms of CNS, severe, uncontrolled hypertension, cerebral embolism/thrombosis/hemorrhage, hypersensitivity to this drug or streptokinase, recent trauma/history of CVA

Precautions: Pregnancy (C), arterial emboli from left side of heart, ulcerative colitis/enteritis, hepatic/renal disease, hypocoagulation, COPD, subacute bacterial endocarditis, rheumatic valvular disease, intraarterial diagnostic procedure or surgery (10 days), recent major surgery, lactation, geriatric

PHARMACOKINETICS

Inactivated by binding to plasma activators, half-life 70-105 min

INTERACTIONS

Increase: bleeding potential—aspirin, other NSAIDs, heparin, antiplatelets, abciximab, eptifibatide, tirofiban, clopidogrel, ticlopidine, some cephalosporins, plicamycin, valproic acid, anticoagulants, dipyridamole

Decrease: action of anistreplase—aminocaproic acid, aprotinin, trahexamic acid

Drug/Herb

Increase: risk of bleeding—agrimony, alfalfa, angelica, anise, basil, bay, bilberry, black haw, bogbean, bromelain, buchu, chondroitin, cinchona bark, dong quai, fenugreek, feverfew, garlic, ginger, ginkgo, ginseng, horse chestnut, Irish moss, kelp, kelpware, khella, lovage, lungwort, meadowsweet, motherwort, mugwort, nettle, papaya, parsley (large amts), pau d'arco, pineapple, poplar, prickly ash, safflower, saw palmetto, tonka bean, tumeric, wintergreen, yarrow

Decrease: anticoagulant effect—chamomile, coenzyme Q10, flax, glucomannan, goldenseal, guar gum

Drug/Lab Test
Increase: PT, APTT, TT
Decrease: Fibrinogen, plasminogen

NURSING CONSIDERATIONS

Assess:
• VS, B/P, pulse, respirations, neurologic signs, temp at least q4h, temp >104° F (40° C) or indicators of internal bleeding; treat bradycardia, ventricular changes; assess neurologic status, neurologic change may indicate intracranial bleeding; ECG continuously, cardiac enzymes, radionuclide, myocardial scanning/coronary angiography
• Hypersensitivity: fever, rash, itching, chills, facial swelling dyspnea; notify prescriber immediately, stop drug, keep resuscitative equipment nearby; mild reaction may be treated with antihistamines
⚠ Bleeding during first hr of treatment (hematuria, hematemesis, bleeding from mucous membranes, epistaxis, ecchymosis), continue to monitor for 24 hr after treatment
• Blood studies (Hct, platelets, PTT, PT, TT, APTT) before starting therapy; PT or APTT must be less than 2 × control before starting therapy; TT or PT q3-4h during treatment

Administer:
IV, direct route
• Reconstitute single-dose vial/5 ml sterile water for inj (not bacteriostatic water), and roll (not shake) to enhance reconstitution; give over 2-5 min by direct IV, give within ½ hr of reconstitution or discard, do not add other meds to vial or syringe; give within 6 hr of thrombi identification for best results
• Pressure of 30 sec to minor bleeding sites, 30 min to sites of arterial puncture followed by dressing; inform prescriber if hemostasis not attained; apply pressure dressing
• Use powder within 30 min after reconstitution
• Cryoprecipitate or fresh frozen plasma if bleeding occurs

⚠ Safety alert   *"Tall Man" lettering

• Heparin therapy after thrombolytic therapy is discontinued, TT or APTT <2 × control (about 3-4 hr)

• About 10% of patients have high streptococcal antibody titers, requiring increased loading doses

Perform/provide:

• Bed rest during entire course of treatment; handle patient as little as possible during therapy

• Storage of powder in refrigerator

• Avoid invasive procedures: inj, rectal temperature

• Treat fever with acetaminophen

Evaluate:

• Therapeutic response: absence of thrombi formation in MI, improved ventricular function

Teach patient/family:

• Reason for product and expected results

⚠ High Alert

antihemophilic factor VIII (AHF) (℞)

(an-tee-hee-moe-fill'ik)
antihemophilic factor,
Alphanate, Bioclate, Helixate
FS, Hemofil M, Humate-P,
Hyate C, Koate-DVI,
Kogenate, Kogenate FS,
Monoclate-P, Recombinate,
ReFacto

Func. class.: Hemostatic
Chem. class.: Factor VIII

Do not confuse:

Kogenate/Kogenate-2

Action: Necessary for clotting; activates factor X in conjunction with activated factor IX; transforms prothrombin to thrombin

Uses: Hemophilia A, patients with acquired circulating factor VIII inhibitors, factor VIII deficiency

DOSAGE AND ROUTES

Massive hemorrhage

• *Adult and child:* IV 40-50 units/kg, then 20-25 units/kg q8-12h

Overt bleeding

• *Adult and child:* IV 15-25 units/kg, then 8-15 units/kg q8-12h × 4 days

Hemorrhage near vital organs

• *Adult and child:* IV 25 units/kg, then 15 units/kg q8h × 2 days, then 4 units/kg q8h × 2 days

Minor hemorrhage

• *Adult and child:* IV 8-10 units/kg q24h × 2-3 days or 8 units/kg q12h × 2 days, then q24h × 2 days

Joint bleeding

• *Adult and child:* IV 5-15 units/kg q8-12h × 1-2 days

Available forms: Inj 250, 500, 1000, 1500 units/vial (number of units noted on label)

SIDE EFFECTS

CNS: Headache, *lethargy, chills, fever, flushing,* loss of consciousness

CV: Hypotension, tachycardia

GI: Nausea, vomiting, abdominal cramps, constipation, diarrhea, anorexia, jaundice, **viral hepatitis**

HEMA: **Thrombosis, hemolysis, risk of hepatitis B, risk of HIV**

INTEG: Rash, flushing, *urticaria,* stinging at inj site

MISC: **Anaphylaxis,** blurred vision, back pain

RESP: **Bronchospasm,** rhinitis, dyspnea, nosebleeds, wheezing

Contraindications: Hypersensitivity; mouse, hamster, bovine, porcine protein, lactation, HIV, viral infection

Precautions: Pregnancy (C), neonates/infants, hepatic disease; blood types A, B, AB; factor VIII inhibitor

PHARMACOKINETICS

IV: Half-life 4 hr, terminal 15 hr

Side effects: *italics* = common; **bold** = life-threatening

NURSING CONSIDERATIONS
Assess:
• Blood studies (coagulation factors assay by % normal: 5% prevents spontaneous hemorrhage, 30%-50% for surgery, 80%-100% for severe hemorrhage)
• I&O, urine color; notify prescriber if urine becomes orange, red
• Pulse: discontinue infusion if significant increase
• Hct, Coombs' test with blood types A, B, AB
• Test for factor VIII inhibitors before starting treatment, may require concomitant antiinhibitor coagulant complex therapy
• Allergy: fever, rash, itching, jaundice; give diphenhydrAMINE HCl (Benadryl), continue therapy if reaction is mild
• Blood group of patient, donors (if applicable; most factor VIII not from specific blood group donors)
⚠ Bleeding: ankles, knees, elbows, other joints
Administer:
IV route
• To prepare, administer factor VIII concentrates at first sign of danger
• After rotating gently to mix
• Warm to room temperature using plastic syringe to reconstitute and administer; adheres to glass; use another needle as a vent when reconstituting
• After dilution with warm NS, D_5W, LR, give within 3 hr; complete dissolution may take up to 10 min
IV INF route
• Give at ≤2 ml/min if concentration exceeds 34 units/ml or over 3 min if concentration is <34 units/ml
Perform/provide:
• Storage in refrigerator; do not freeze; after reconstitution, do not refrigerate; give within 3 hr
Evaluate:
• Therapeutic response: absence of bleeding
Teach patient/family:
• To report any signs of bleeding: gums, under skin, urine, stools, emesis; review methods to prevent bleeding
• To avoid salicylates, NSAIDs (increase bleeding tendencies)
• To advise health professionals of treatment for hemophilia
• The signs of viral hepatitis, AIDS
• That immunization for hepatitis B may be given first
• To report hives, urticaria, chest tightness, hypotension; may be monoclonal antibody-derived factor VIII
• To be checked q2-3mo for HIV screen
• To carry emergency ID describing disease process

⚠ High Alert

antithrombin III, human (℞)
(an'tee-throm-bin)
ATnativ, Thrombate III
Func. class.: Antithrombin
Chem. class.: Pooled human plasma

Action: Inactivates thrombin and the activated forms of factors IX, X, XI, XII, resulting in inhibition of coagulation
Uses: During surgical or obstetric procedures, or for thromboembolism in patients with known antithrombin III deficiency

DOSAGE AND ROUTES
Dosage is individualized
• Expect a 1.4% rise from baseline for every 1 international unit/kg administered
Units required =
$$\frac{(\text{Desired level} - \text{Baseline}) \times \text{Weight in kg}}{1.4\%}$$

Available forms: 500 international units in 10 ml; 1000 international units in 20 ml

SIDE EFFECTS
CNS: Dizziness, chills, severe lightheadedness
GI: Nausea, cramps, bowel fullness
RESP: Shortness of breath

SYST: **Bleeding,** surface bleeding, **ana-phylaxis,** vasodilatory effects
Precautions: Pregnancy (B), lactation, children

PHARMACOKINETICS
Biologic half-life 2-5 days, peak 15-30 min

INTERACTIONS
• Do not administer with other drugs in syringe or solutions
Increase: anticoagulant effect—anticoagulants

NURSING CONSIDERATIONS
Assess:
• AT-III levels q12h, maintain at >80% of normal activity until stabilized, then daily before dose
• VS, B/P, pulse, respirations, neurologic signs, temp at least q4h, temp 104° F (40° C) or indicators of internal bleeding, cardiac rhythm
⚠ For child born of parents with hereditary AT-III deficiency, obtain AT-III levels immediately after birth
⚠ For neurologic changes that may indicate intracranial bleeding
⚠ Retroperitoneal bleeding: back pain, leg weakness, diminished pulses
Administer:
• Heparin after fibrinogen level is over 100 mg/dl; heparin infusion to increase PTT to 1.5-2 × baseline for 3-7 days
IV route
• After reconstituting 500 international units/10 ml of NS or D₅W; do not shake; rotate to dissolve; allow to warm to room temperature; use within 3 hr of reconstitution; give 50 international units or less/min; do not exceed 100 international units/min using 0.22 or 0.45 microfilter
Evaluate:
• Therapeutic response: absence of thrombi formation
Teach patient/family:
• About drug use and expected results; to report adverse reactions; bleeding, bruising

antithymocyte
See lymphocyte immune globulin

apomorphine (℞)
(a-poe-mor′feen)
Apokyn
Func. class.: Antiparkinson agent
Chem. class.: Dopamine-receptor agonist, nonergot

Action: Selective agonist for D₂ subfamily receptors (presynaptic/postsynaptic sites); binding at D₃ receptor may contribute to antiparkinson effects
Uses: Parkinsonism: for acute, intermittent treatment of hypomobility (off) episodes in advanced Parkinsonism

DOSAGE AND ROUTES
• *Adult:* **SUBCUT** 0.2 ml (2 mg) titrate upward, max 0.6 ml (6 mg); administer a test dose of 0.2 ml (2 mg) and closely monitor B/P; to be used concomitantly with antiemetic
Renal dose
• Reduce test dose and starting dose to 0.1 ml (1 mg)
Acute poisoning
• *Child:* **SUBCUT** 0.06-0.1 mg/kg as a single dose, max 60 mg
Available forms: Inj 10 mg/ml

SIDE EFFECTS
CNS: Agitation, psychosis, hallucination, depression, dizziness, headache, confusion, **sleep attacks,** yawning, dyskinesias, drowsiness, somnolence
CV: Orthostatic hypotension, edema, syncope, tachycardia
EENT: Blurred vision, rhinorrhea, sweating
GI: Nausea, vomiting, *anorexia,* constipation, dysphagia, dry mouth
GU: Impotence, urinary frequency
HEMA: **Hemolytic anemia, leukopenia, agranulocytosis**
Contraindications: Hypersensitivity

Precautions: Pregnancy (C), renal/hepatic/cardiac disease, MI with dysrhythmias, affective disorders, psychosis, pre-existing dyskinesias, geriatric, asthma

PHARMACOKINETICS

Minimally metabolized, peak 10-60 min, half-life 30-60 min

INTERACTIONS

⚠ Do not give with 5-HT$_3$ antagonists: ondansetron, granisetron, dolasetron: profound hypotension may occur

Increase: effect of levodopa

Increase: apomorphine levels—levodopa, cimetidine, ranitidine, diltiazem, triamterene, verapamil, quinidine

Decrease: apomorphine levels—DOPamine antagonists, phenothiazines, metoclopramide, butyrophenones

Drug/Herb

Decrease: effect of apomorphine—chaste tree fruit, kava

NURSING CONSIDERATIONS

Assess:

• B/P supine/standing before dose, and 20, 40, 60 min after dose

• Renal/hepatic/cardiac studies baseline

• Involuntary movements in parkinsonism: akinesia, tremors, staggering gait, muscle rigidity, drooling

• Mental status: affect, mood, behavioral changes, depression; complete suicide assessment

• For risk of QT prolongation, this drug may increase QT prolongation and possibility of prodysrhythmias

Administer:

• Adjust dosage to patient response

⚠ Do not give IV; rotate inj sites

• Use a test dose of 0.2 ml (2 mg); those who tolerate this dose but achieve no response, give 0.4 ml (4 mg) at the next "off"

• Give antiemetic, usually trimethobenzamide, 300 mg tid PO 3 days before beginning apomorphine and continue for 2 months

Perform/provide:

• Assistance with ambulation during beginning therapy

• Storage at 77° F, excursion permitted to 59°-86° F

Evaluate:

• Therapeutic response: decrease in end of dose wearing off and unpredictable on/off episodes

Teach patient/family:

• To notify prescriber if pregnancy is planned or suspected

---

apraclonidine ophthalmic

See Appendix C

---

aprepitant (℞)

(ap-re′pi-tant)

Emend

Func. class.: Antiemetic

Chem. class.: Miscellaneous

Action: A selective antagonist of human substance P/neurokinin 1 (NK$_1$) receptors decreasing emetic reflex

Uses: Prevention of nausea, vomiting associated with cancer chemotherapy (highly emetogenic/moderately emetogenic) including high-dose cisplatin, used in combination with other antiemetics

DOSAGE AND ROUTES

Highly emetogenic

• *Adult:* **PO** Day 1 (1 hour prior to chemotherapy) aprepitant 125 mg with 12 mg dexamethasone **PO**, with 32 mg ondansetron IV; day 2 aprepitant 80 mg with 8 mg dexamethasone **PO**; day 3 aprepitant 80 mg with 8 mg dexamethasone **PO**; day 4 only dexamethasone 8 mg **PO**

Moderately emetogenic

• *Adult:* **PO** Day 1 125 mg aprepitant with dexamethasone 12 mg **PO**, with ondansetron 8 mg **PO** ×2; days 2 and 3 80 mg aprepitant only

Available forms: Caps 80, 125 mg

SIDE EFFECTS

CNS: Headache, dizziness, insomnia, anxiety, depression, confusion, peripheral neuropathy

CV: Bradycardia, tachycardia, DVT, hypo/hypertension

GI: Diarrhea, constipation, abdominal pain, anorexia, gastritis, increased AST, ALT, *nausea,* vomiting, heartburn

GU: Increased BUN, serum creatine, proteinuria, dysuria

HEMA: Anemia, **thrombocytopenia, neutropenia**

MISC: Asthenia, fatigue, dehydration, fever, hiccups, tinnitus

Contraindications: Hypersensitivity

Precautions: Pregnancy (B), lactation, children, hepatic disease, geriatric

PHARMACOKINETICS

Absorption 60%-65%, peak 4 hr, metabolized in liver by CYP3A4 enzymes to an active metabolite, half-life 9-12 hr, 95% protein bound, not excreted in kidneys, crosses blood-brain barrier

INTERACTIONS

Increase: aprepitant action—CYP3A4 inhibitors (ketoconazole, itraconazole, nefazodone, troleandomycin, clarithromycin, ritonavir, nelfinavir, diltiazem)

Increase: action of CYP3A4 substrates (pimozide, cisapride, dexamethasone, methylPREDNISolone, midazolam, alprazolam, triazolam, docetaxel, paclitaxel, etoposide, irinotecan, imatinib, ifosfamide, vinorelbine, vinBLAStine, vinCRIStine)

Decrease: aprepitant action—CYP3A4 inducers (rifampin, carbamazepine, phenytoin)

Decrease: action of CYP2C9 substrates (warfarin, tolbutamide, phenytoin), oral contraceptives

Decrease: action of both drugs—paroxetine

Drug/Food

Decrease: effect—grapefruit juice

NURSING CONSIDERATIONS

Assess:

• CV status: hypertension, hypotension, bradycardia, tachycardia, deep vein thrombosis

• For absence of nausea, vomiting during chemotherapy

Administer:

• Do not break, crush, or chew

• PO on 3-day schedule, give with full glass of water 1 hr before chemotherapy

Perform/provide:

• Storage at room temperature; keep in original bottles, blisters

Evaluate:

• Therapeutic response: absence of nausea, vomiting during cancer chemotherapy

Teach patient/family:

• To report diarrhea, constipation

• To take only as prescribed, take 1st dose 1 hr prior to chemotherapy

• To report all medications and herbals to prescriber prior to taking this medication

• Advise to use nonhormonal form of contraception while taking this agent; oral contraceptive effect may be decreased

• Advise those on warfarin to have clotting monitored closely during 2-wk period following administration of aprepitant

• To avoid breastfeeding

---

arformoterol
See Appendix A—Selected New Drugs

⚠ High Alert

argatroban (℞)
(are-ga-troe'ban)
Argatroban
Func. class.: Anticoagulant
Chem. class.: Thrombin inhibitor

Do not confuse:
argatroban/Aggrastat

Action: Direct inhibitor of thrombin, it reversibly binds to the thrombin active site

---

Uses: Anticoagulation prevention/treatment of thrombosis in heparin-induced thrombocytopenia or adjunct to percutaneous coronary intervention (PCI) in those with a history of HIT

DOSAGE AND ROUTES

Heparin-induced thrombocytopenia/thrombosis syndrome (HIT or HITTS)

• *Adult:* **IV:** 2 mcg/kg/min (1 mg/ml), give at 6 ml/hr for 50 kg of weight, at 8 ml/hr for 70 kg of weight, at 11 ml/hr for 90 kg of weight, at 13 ml/hr for 110 kg of weight, at 16 ml/hr for 130 kg of weight

Hepatic dose

• *Adult:* **CONT INF** 0.5 mcg/kg/min, adjust rate based on aPTT
• HIT or HITTS

Percutaneous coronary intervention (PCI) in HIT

• *Adult:* **IV INF** 25 mcg/kg/min and a bolus of 350 mcg/kg given over 3-5 min, check ACT 5-10 min after bolus is completed; proceed if ACT >300 sec if ACT <300 sec, give another 150 mcg/kg **BOL** and increase infusion rate to 30 mcg/kg/min, recheck ACT in 5-10 min; if ACT >450 sec, decrease infusion rate to 15 mcg/kg/min, recheck ACT in 5-10 min; once ACT is therapeutic, continue for duration of procedure

Available forms: Inj 100 mg/ml (2.5 ml) (must dilute 100-fold)

SIDE EFFECTS

CNS: Fever
CV: **Atrial fibrillation, coronary thrombosis, MI, myocardial ischemia, coronary occlusion, ventricular tachycardia, bradycardia,** *chest pain, hypotension*
GI: Nausea, vomiting, abdominal pain, diarrhea, **GI bleeding**
GU: **Hematuria,** abnormal kidney function, UTI
HEMA: **Hemorrhage**
MISC: Back pain, headache, infection
RESP: Pneumonia, dyspnea, coughing, hemoptysis
SYST: **Sepsis**

Contraindications: Hypersensitivity, overt major bleeding

Precautions: Pregnancy (B), intracranial bleeding, renal function impairment, lactation, children, hepatic disease, severe hypertension, after lumbar puncture, spinal anesthesia, major surgery, congenital or acquired bleeding, GI ulcers

PHARMACOKINETICS

Metabolized in the liver by P450 CYP3A 4/5, distributed to extracellular fluid, 54% plasma protein binding, half-life 39-51 min, excreted in feces

INTERACTIONS

Increase: bleeding risk—antiplatelets, NSAIDs, salicylates, dipyridamole, clopidogrel, ticlopidine, heparin, warfarin, glycoprotein IIb/IIIa antagonists (abciximab, tirofiban, eptifibatide), thrombolytics (streptokinase, alteplase, reteplase, urokinase, tenecteplase), other anticoagulants

Drug/Herb

Increase: bleeding risk—agrimony, alfalfa, angelica, anise, bilberry, black currant, black haw, bogbean, buchu, cat's claw, chondroitin, dong quai, fenugreek, feverfew, fish oils, garlic, ginger, ginkgo, ginseng, horse chestnut, Irish moss, kava, kelp, kelpware, khella, licorice, lovage, lungwort, meadowsweet, motherwort, mugwort, nettle, papaya, parsley, pau d'arco, pineapple, poplar, prickly ash, safflower, saw palmetto, senega, skullcap, turmeric, wintergreen

Decrease: argatroban effect—chamomile, coenzyme Q10, flax, glucomannan, goldenseal, guar gum

NURSING CONSIDERATIONS

Assess:

⚠ Obtain baseline in aPTT before treatment; do not start treatment if aPTT ratio ≥2.5, then aPTT 2 hr after initiation of treatment and at least daily thereafter
• aPTT, which should be 1.5-3 × control
⚠ Bleeding gums, petechiae, ecchymosis, black, tarry stools, hematuria/

epistaxis, B/P, vaginal bleeding and possible hemorrhage

⚠ Anaphylaxis: dyspnea, rash during treatment

• Fever, skin rash, urticaria

Administer:

• Avoiding all IM inj that may cause bleeding

IV, direct route

• For PCI: 350 mg/kg bol, then continuous inf of 25 mcg/kg/min

IV INF route

• Dilute in 0.9% NaCl, D_5, LR to a final conc 1 mg/ml; dilute each 2.5-ml vial 100-fold by mixing with 250 ml of diluent, mix by repeated inversion of the diluent bag for 1 min; may be slightly hazy briefly

• Dosage adjustment may be made after review of aPTT, not to exceed 10 mcg/kg/min

Evaluate:

• Therapeutic response: absence or decrease of thrombosis

Teach patient/family:

• To use soft-bristle toothbrush to avoid bleeding gums, avoid contact sports, use electric razor, avoid IM inj

• To report any signs of bleeding: gums, under skin, urine, stools

• To notify prescriber if planning to become pregnant or breastfeeding

---

aripiprazole (℞)

(a-rip-ip-pra′zol)

Abilify

Func. class.: Antipsychotic

Chem. class.: Quinolinone

Action: Exact mechanism unknown; may be mediated through both dopamine type 2 (D_2, D_3) and serotonin type 2 (5-HT$_{1A}$, 5-HT$_{2A}$) antagonism

Uses: Schizophrenia

DOSAGE AND ROUTES

• *Adult:* **PO** 10-15 mg/day; if needed, dosage may be increased to 30 mg daily after 2 wk; maintenance 15 mg/day, periodically reassess

Available forms: Tabs 5, 10, 15, 20, 30 mg

SIDE EFFECTS

CNS: Drowsiness, insomnia, agitation, anxiety, headache, **seizures, neuroleptic malignant syndrome,** *lightheadedness, akathisia, asthenia, tremor*

CV: Orthostatic hypotension, **tachycardia**

EENT: Blurred vision, rhinitis

GI: Constipation, nausea, vomiting, jaundice, *weight gain*

INTEG: Rash

RESP: Cough

Contraindications: Hypersensitivity, lactation, seizure disorders

Precautions: Pregnancy (C), children, renal disease, hepatic disease, geriatric

PHARMACOKINETICS

PO: Absorption 87%, extensively metabolized by liver to a major active metabolite, plasma protein binding >99%, terminal half-life 75-146 hr, excretion urine 25%, feces 55%; clearance decreased in geriatric

INTERACTIONS

Increase: effects of aripiprazole—CYP3A4 inhibitors (ketoconazole, erythromycin), CYP2D6 inhibitors (quinidine, fluoxetine, paroxetine); reduce dose of aripiprazole

Increase: sedation—other CNS depressants, alcohol

Increase: EPS—other antipsychotics, lithium

Increase: dose of aripiprazole—CYP3A4 inducers

Decrease: aripiprazole level—famotidine, valproate

Decrease: effects of aripiprazole—CYP3A4 inducers (carbamazepine)

Drug/Herb

Increase: EPS—betel palm, kava

Increase: neuroleptic effect—cola tree, hops, nettle, nutmeg

Side effects: *italics* = common; **bold** = life-threatening

NURSING CONSIDERATIONS
Assess:
• Mental status before initial administration
• Swallowing of PO medication; check for hoarding or giving of medication to other patients
• I&O ratio; palpate bladder if urinary output is low
• Bilirubin, CBC, LFTs qmo
• Affect, orientation, LOC, reflexes, gait, coordination, sleep pattern disturbances
• B/P standing and lying; also pulse, respirations; take q4h during initial treatment; establish baseline before starting treatment; report drops of 30 mm Hg; watch for ECG changes
• Dizziness, faintness, palpitations, tachycardia on rising
• EPS, including akathisia (inability to sit still, no pattern to movements), tardive dyskinesia (bizarre movements of the jaw, mouth, tongue, extremities), pseudoparkinsonism (rigidity, tremors, pill rolling, shuffling gait)
⚠ For neuroleptic malignant syndrome: hyperthermia, increased CPK, altered mental status, muscle rigidity; notify prescriber immediately
• Constipation, urinary retention daily; if these occur, increase bulk and water in diet; stool softeners, laxatives may be needed

Administer:
• Reduced dose in geriatric

Perform/provide:
• Supervised ambulation until patient is stabilized on medication; do not involve in strenuous exercise program because fainting is possible; patient should not stand still for a long time
• Storage in tight, light-resistant container

Evaluate:
• Therapeutic response: decrease in emotional excitement, hallucinations, delusions, paranoia; reorganization of patterns of thought, speech

Teach patient/family:
• That orthostatic hypotension may occur and to rise from sitting or lying position gradually
• To avoid hot tubs, hot showers, tub baths; hypotension may occur
• To avoid abrupt withdrawal of this drug; EPS may result; drug should be withdrawn slowly
• To avoid OTC preparations (cough, hay fever, cold) unless approved by prescriber, serious drug interactions may occur; avoid use with alcohol, CNS depressants; increased drowsiness may occur
• To avoid hazardous activities if drowsy or dizzy
• Compliance with drug regimen
• To report impaired vision, tremors, muscle twitching, urinary retention
• In hot weather, that heat stroke may occur; take extra precautions to stay cool
• To notify prescriber if pregnant or intend to become pregnant; not to breastfeed

Treatment of overdose:
• Lavage if orally ingested; provide airway; *do not induce vomiting*

⚠ High Alert

arsenic trioxide (℞)
Trisenox
Func. class.: Antineoplastic—miscellaneous

Action: Not understood, causes morphologic changes and DNA fragmentation
Uses: Acute promyelocytic leukemia patients who are refractory to or have relapsed from retinoid and anthracycline chemotherapy

DOSAGE AND ROUTES
Induction
• *Adult:* **IV** 0.15 mg/kg/day until bone marrow remission, max 60 doses
Consolidation treatment
Wait 3-6 wk after completion of induction

⚠ Safety alert   *"Tall Man" lettering

• *Adult:* IV 0.15 mg/kg/day × 25 doses over a period of up to 5 wk

Available forms: Inj 1 mg/ml

SIDE EFFECTS

CNS: Anxiety, confusion, insomnia, headache, paresthesia, depression, dizziness, tremor, seizures, agitation, coma, weakness

CV: Hypotension, hypertension, prolonged QT interval, other ECG changes, chest pain, *tachycardia,* torsades de pointes

GI: Abdominal pain, constipation, diarrhea, dyspepsia, fecal incontinence, GI hemorrhage, dry mouth, *nausea, vomiting, anorexia*

GU: Vaginal hemorrhage, renal failure, incontinence

HEMA: Leukocytosis, anemia, thrombocytopenia, neutropenia, DIC

META: Increased ALT/AST, hyperkalemia, *hypokalemia,* hypomagnesemia, *hyperglycemia*

MISC: Weight gain or loss, fatigue, severe edema, rigors, herpes simplex/zoster

RESP: **Pleural effusion,** *dyspnea, cough,* epistaxis, hypoxia, sinusitis, wheezing, crackles, tachypnea

Contraindications: Pregnancy (D), hypersensitivity

Precautions: Geriatric, lactation, children

PHARMACOKINETICS

Metabolized in the liver, stored in the liver, kidney, heart, lung, hair, nails, excreted in urine

NURSING CONSIDERATIONS

Assess:

⚠ For APL differentiation syndrome: fever, dyspnea, pulmonary infiltrates, pleural or pericardial effusions, weight gain; this condition can be fatal; give high-dose steroids

• For ECG changes: QT interval prolongation, complete AV block; obtain baseline ECG prior to drug therapy; watch drug interactions with other drugs that prolong QT interval

• Electrolytes: K, Ca, Mg, creatine; hematologic, coagulation lab studies twice weekly or more; ECG qwk

Administer:

IV route

• Dilute with 100-250 ml D$_5$ or 0.9% NaCl immediately after withdrawing from ampule, give over 1-2 hr may give over 4 hr if reactions occur

Evaluate:

• Therapeutic response: decrease in malignant cells

Teach patient/family:

• To report planned or suspected pregnancy

• That fertility impairment has not been studied

• Symptoms of APL differentiation syndrome

Treatment of overdose:

• Dimercaprol 3 mg/kg IM q4hr, then 250 mg penicillamine PO, max 4 ×/day (≤1 g/day)

**ascorbic acid
(vit C)** (otc, ℞)
(a-skor'bic)
Apo-C ✦, ascorbic acid,
Ascorbicap, Cebid, Cecon,
Cecore-500, Cemill,
Cenolate, Cetane, Cevalin,
Cevi-Bid, Ce-Vi-Sol, C-Span,
Flavorcee, Mega-C/A Plus,
Ortho/CS, Sunkist
Func. class.: Vitamin C—water-soluble vitamin

Action: Needed for wound healing, collagen synthesis, antioxidant, carbohydrate metabolism

Uses: Vit C deficiency, scurvy, delayed wound and bone healing, chronic disease, urine acidification, before gastrectomy, acidification of urine, dietary supplement

Unlabeled uses: Common cold prevention

Side effects: *italics* = common; **bold** = life-threatening

DOSAGE AND ROUTES
- *Child <6 mo:* **PO** 30 mg/day

Dietary supplementation
- *Adult and child >14 yr:* 50-200 mg daily
- *Child 11-14 yr:* **PO** 50 mg/day
- *Child 4-10 yr:* **PO** 45 mg/day
- *Child 1-3 yr:* **PO** 40 mg/day
- *Child 6 mo-1 yr:* **PO** 35 mg/day

Scurvy
- *Adult:* **PO/SUBCUT/IM/IV** 100 mg-500 mg daily × 2 wk, then 50 mg or more daily
- *Child:* **PO/SUBCUT/IM/IV** 100-300 mg daily × 2 wk, then 35 mg or more daily

Wound healing/chronic disease/fracture (may be given with zinc)
- *Adult:* **SUBCUT/IM/IV/PO** 200-500 mg daily for 1-2 mo
- *Child:* **SUBCUT/IM/IV/PO** 100-200 mg added doses for 1-2 mo

Urine acidification
- *Adult:* 4-12 g daily in divided doses
- *Child:* 500 mg q6-8h

Available forms: Tabs 25, 50, 100, 250, 500, 1000, 1500 mg; effervescent tabs 1000 mg; chewable tabs 100, 250, 500 mg; timed-release tabs 500, 750, 1000, 1500 mg; timed-release caps 500 mg; crys 4 g/tsp; powd 4 g/tsp; liq 35 mg/0.6 ml; sol 100 mg/ml; syr 20 mg/ml, 500 mg/5 ml; inj SUBCUT, IM, IV 100, 250, 500 mg/ml

SIDE EFFECTS
CNS: Headache, insomnia, dizziness, fatigue, flushing
GI: Nausea, vomiting, diarrhea, anorexia, heartburn, cramps
GU: Polyuria, urine acidification, oxalate or urate renal stones, dysuria
HEMA: **Hemolytic anemia in patients with G6PD**
INTEG: Inflammation at inj site

Contraindications: Tartrazine, sulfite sensitivity; G6PD deficiency

Precautions: Pregnancy (C), gout, diabetes, renal calculi (large doses)

PHARMACOKINETICS
PO, INJ: Readily absorbed PO, metabolized in liver, unused amounts excreted in urine (unchanged) and metabolites, crosses placenta, breast milk

INTERACTIONS
None known

Drug/Lab Test
False positive: Negatives in glucose tests
False negative: Occult blood, urine bilirubin, leukocyte determination

NURSING CONSIDERATIONS
Assess:
- I&O ratio
- Ascorbic acid levels throughout treatment if continued deficiency is suspected
- Nutritional status: citrus fruits, vegetables
- Inj sites for inflammation

Administer:
PO route
- Do not crush or chew ext rel tab or caps
- That caps may be opened and contents mixed with jelly

IV, direct route
- Undiluted by direct IV 100 mg over at least 1 min, rapid inf may cause fainting

Intermittent IV INF route
- Diluted with D_5W, D_5NaCl, NS, LR, Ringer's, sodium lactate and given over 15 min

Additive compatibilities: Amikacin, calcium chloride, calcium gluceptate, calcium gluconate, cephalothin, chloramphenicol, chlorproMAZINE, colistimethate, cyanocobalamin, diphenhydrAMINE, heparin, kanamycin, methicillin, methyldopa, penicillin G potassium, polymyxin B, prednisolone, procaine, prochlorperazine, promethazine, verapamil

Syringe compatibilities: Metoclopramide, aminophylline, theophylline

Y-site compatibilities: Warfarin

Evaluate:
• Therapeutic response: absence of anorexia, irritability, pallor, joint pain, hyperkeratosis, petechiae, poor wound healing

Teach patient/family:
• The necessary foods in diet, such as citrus fruits
• That smoking decreases vit C levels, not to exceed prescribed dose; increases will be excreted in urine, except timed release

---

⚠ High Alert

asparaginase (℞)
(a-spare'a-gi-nase)
Elspar, Kidrolase ✦
Func. class.: Antineoplastic
Chem. class.: Escherichia coli enzyme

Action: Indirectly inhibits protein synthesis in tumor cells; without amino acid, DNA, RNA synthesis is halted; asparagine, protein synthesis is halted; G_1 phase of cell cycle specific; a nonvesicant

Uses: Acute lymphocytic leukemia in combination with other antineoplastics

DOSAGE AND ROUTES
In combination
• *Adult and child:* IV 1000 international units/kg/day × 10 days given over 30 min; IM 6000 international units/m²/day
Sole induction
• *Adult and child:* IV 200 international units/kg/day × 28 days
Desensitization
• *Adult and child:* Test dose adult and child ID 2 international units, then double dose q10 min, until total dose is administered or reaction occurs

Available forms: Inj 10,000 international units with mannitol

SIDE EFFECTS
CNS: Neuritis, dizziness, headache, **coma,** depression, fatigue, confusion, hallucinations, lethargy, drowsiness, agitation, Parkinson-like syndrome, **seizures,** chills, fever

CV: Chest pain
ENDO: Hyperglycemia
GI: Nausea, vomiting, anorexia, diarrhea, weight loss, cramps, stomatitis, **hepatotoxicity, pancreatitis**
GU: Urinary retention, **renal failure,** glycosuria, polyuria, azotemia, uric acid neuropathy, proteinuria
HEMA: **Thrombocytopenia, leukopenia, myelosuppression, anemia, decreased clotting factors (V, VII, VIII, IX), decreased fibrinogen**
INTEG: Rash, urticaria, perspiration
RESP: **Fibrosis, pulmonary infiltrate**
SYST: **Anaphylaxis**

Contraindications: Hypersensitivity, infants, lactation, pancreatitis
Precautions: Pregnancy (C), hepatic/renal disease

PHARMACOKINETICS
Half-life 4-9 hr, terminal 1.4-1.8 days

INTERACTIONS
• May decrease response to live virus vaccines
Increase: toxicity—vinCRIStine, predniSONE
Decrease: action of methotrexate, antigout agents
Drug/Lab Test
Increase: Uric acid
Decrease: Thyroid function tests

NURSING CONSIDERATIONS
Assess:
⚠ For signs and symptoms of pancreatitis (nausea, vomiting, severe abdominal pain), anaphylaxis (bronchospasm, dyspnea), cyanosis; more toxic in adults than children
• CBC, differential, platelet count weekly; withhold drug if WBC is <4000 or platelet count is <75,000; notify prescriber of these results
• Pulmonary function tests, chest x-ray studies before, during therapy; chest x-ray

---

Side effects: *italics* = common; **bold** = life-threatening

film should be obtained q2wk during treatment

• Renal studies: BUN, serum uric acid, ammonia urine CCr, electrolytes before, during therapy

• I&O ratio; report fall in urine output of 30 ml/hr

• Monitor temp q4h; elevated temp may indicate beginning infection

• Hepatic studies before, during therapy (bilirubin, AST, ALT, LDH) as needed or monthly

• RBC, Hct, Hgb, since these may be decreased

• Serum, urine glucose levels

• Bleeding: hematuria, guaiac, bruising or petechiae, mucosa or orifices q8h

⚠ Dyspnea, crackles, nonproductive cough, chest pain, tachypnea, fatigue, increased pulse, pallor, lethargy, swelling around eyes or lips; anaphylaxis may occur; risk of hypersensitivity increases with repeated dose

• Jaundice of skin and sclera, dark urine, clay-colored stools, itchy skin, abdominal pain, fever, diarrhea

• Local irritation, pain, burning, discoloration at inj site

• Symptoms indicating severe allergic reaction: rash, pruritus, urticaria, purpuric skin lesions, itching, flushing, dyspnea

• Frequency of stools, characteristics: cramping, acidosis; signs of dehydration: rapid respirations, poor skin turgor, decreased urine output, dry skin, restlessness, weakness

Administer:

• May be mutagenic, teratogenic, carcinogenic to the staff, prepare according to policy using cytoxic handling procedures

• Desensitization may be required before 1st dose, 1 unit may be ordered IV and dose doubled q10min, if no reaction, until amount equals patient's dose for that day; be prepared to treat acute allergic reaction if it occurs

IM route

• Reconstitute with 2 ml NaCl/10,000 units/vial, refrigerate, use within 8 hr; discard sooner if sol becomes cloudy, do not give more than 2 ml **IM** in one inj site

IV, direct route

• After intradermal skin testing and desensitization, give 0.1 ml (2 international units) intradermally after reconstituting with 5 ml sterile H_2O or 0.9% NaCl for inj; then add 0.1 ml of reconstituted drug to 9.9 ml diluent (20 international units/ml); observe for 1 hr, check for wheal

• Allopurinol to reduce uric acid levels, alkalinization of urine

Intermittent IV INF route

• Using 21G, 23G, 25G needle; administer by slow IV infusion via Y-tube or 3-way stopcock of flowing D_5W or NS infusion over 30 min after diluting 10,000 international units/5 ml of sterile H_2O or 0.9% NaCl (no preservatives) (2000 international units/ml); use of filter may be necessary if fibers are present

Y-site compatibilities: Methotrexate, sodium bicarbonate

Perform/provide:

• Deep-breathing exercises with patient 3-4 ×/day; place in semi-Fowler's position

• Increase fluid intake to 2-3 L/day to prevent urate deposits, calculi formation

• Brushing of teeth 2-3 ×/day with soft brush or cotton-tipped applicators for stomatitis; use unwaxed dental floss

• Warm compresses at inj site for inflammation

Evaluate:

• Therapeutic response: decreased exacerbations in ALL

Teach patient/family:

• To report any changes in breathing or coughing

• Not to obtain vaccination while taking this drug

• To use reliable contraception, since drug is teratogenic; not to breastfeed

Treatment of anaphylaxis:

• Administer epINEPHrine, diphenhydrAMINE, IV corticosteroids, O_2

⚠ Safety alert   *"Tall Man" lettering

aspirin (otc)

(as'pir-in)

acetylsalicylic acid, Acuprin, Apo-ASA ✤, Apo-Asen ✤, Arthrinol ✤, Arthrisin ✤, Artria S.R., A.S.A., Aspergum, Aspirin ✤, Aspir-Low, Aspirtab, Astrin ✤, Bayer Aspirin, Coryphen ✤, Easprin, Ecotrin, 8-Hour Bayer Timed Release, Empirin, Entrophen ✤, Halfprin, Norwich Extra-Strength, Novasen ✤, PMS-ASA ✤, Sloprin, St. Joseph Children's, Supasa ✤, Therapy Bayer, ZORprin

Func. class.: Nonopioid analgesic, nonsteroidal antiinflammatory, antipyretic, antiplatelet

Chem. class.: Salicylate

Action: Blocks pain impulses in CNS, reduces inflammation by inhibition of prostaglandin synthesis; antipyretic action results from vasodilation of peripheral vessels; decreases platelet aggregation

Uses: Mild to moderate pain or fever including RA, osteoarthritis, thromboembolic disorders; TIAs, rheumatic fever, postmyocardial infarction, prophylaxis of MI, ischemic stroke, angina

Unlabeled uses: Prevention of cataracts (long-term use), prevention of pregnancy loss in women with clotting disorders

DOSAGE AND ROUTES

Arthritis

• *Adult:* **PO** 2.6-5.2 g/day in divided doses q4-6h

• *Child:* **PO** 90-130 mg/kg/day in divided doses q4-6h

Pain/fever

• *Adult:* **PO/RECT** 325-650 mg q4h prn, not to exceed 4 g/day

• *Child:* **PO/RECT** 40-100 mg/kg/day in divided doses q4-6h prn

Kawasaki disease

• *Child:* **PO** 80-120 mg/kg/day in 4 divided doses, maintenance 3-8 mg/kg/day as a single dose × 8 wk

Acute rheumatic fever

• *Adult:* **PO** 5-6 g/day initially

• *Child:* **PO** 100 mg/kg/day × 2 wk, then 75 mg/kg/day × 4-6 wk

Thromboembolic disorders

• *Adult:* **PO** 325-650 mg/day or bid

Transient ischemic attacks

• *Adult:* **PO** 650 mg bid or 350 mg qid

MI, stroke prophylaxis

• *Adult:* **PO** 81-650 mg/day

Available forms: Tabs 81, 162.5, 325, 500, 650, 975 mg; chewable tabs 80, 81 mg; supp 60, 120, 125, 130, 150, 160, 195, 200, 300, 320, 325, 600, 640, 650 mg, 1.2 g; gum 227 mg; dispersible tabs 325, 500 mg, enteric coated 80, 165, 300, 325, 500, 600, 650, 975 mg; ext rel tabs 325, 650, 800 mg; del rel caps 325, 500 mg

SIDE EFFECTS

CNS: Stimulation, drowsiness, dizziness, confusion, **seizures, coma**, headache, flushing, hallucinations, **coma**

CV: Rapid pulse, pulmonary edema

EENT: Tinnitus, hearing loss

ENDO: Hypoglycemia, hyponatremia, hypokalemia

GI: Nausea, vomiting, **GI bleeding**, diarrhea, heartburn, anorexia, **hepatitis**

HEMA: **Thrombocytopenia, agranulocytosis, leukopenia, neutropenia, hemolytic anemia,** increased PT, APTT, bleeding time

INTEG: Rash, urticaria, bruising

RESP: Wheezing, hyperpnea

SYST: **Reye's syndrome (children), anaphylaxis, laryngeal edema**

Contraindications: Pregnancy (D) 3rd trimester, hypersensitivity to salicylates, tartrazine (FDC yellow dye #5), GI bleeding, NSAIDs, bleeding disorders, children <12 yr, children with flulike symptoms, lactation, vit K deficiency, peptic ulcer

Precautions: Anemia, renal/hepatic disease, Hodgkin's disease, pre/postoperatively, gastritis, asthmatic patients with nasal polyps or aspirin sensitivity

Side effects: *italics* = common; **bold** = life-threatening

PHARMACOKINETICS

Well absorbed PO; enteric metabolized by liver, inactive metabolites excreted by kidneys, crosses placenta, excreted in breast milk; half-life 15-20 min, up to 30 hr in large dose; rectal products may be erratic

PO: Onset 15-30 min, peak 1-2 hr, duration 4-6 hr

REC: Onset slow, duration 4-6 hr

INTERACTIONS

• Gastric ulcer: steroids, antiinflammatories, NSAIDs

Increase: bleeding—alcohol, heparin, plicamycin, cefamandole, thrombolytics, ticlopidine, clopidogrel, tirofiban, eptifibatide

Increase: effects of warfarin, insulin, methotrexate, thrombolytic agents, penicillins, phenytoin, valproic acid, oral hypoglycemics, sulfonamides

Increase: salicylate levels—urinary acidifiers, ammonium chloride, nizatidine

Increase: hypotension—nitroglycerin

Decrease: effects of aspirin—antacids (high doses), urinary alkalizers, corticosteroids

Decrease: antihypertensive effect—ACE inhibitors

Decrease: effects of probenecid, spironolactone, sulfinpyrazone, sulfonylamides, NSAIDs, β-blockers, loop diuretics

Drug/Herb

• Gastric irritation: arginine, gossypol

Increase: risk of bleeding—anise, arnica, bilberry, bogbean, chamomile, chondroitin, clove, fenugreek, feverfew, garlic, ginger, ginkgo, ginseng *(Panax)*, horse chestnut, Irish moss, kelpware, licorice, pansy

Drug/Food

• Foods acidifying urine may increase aspirin level

Drug/Lab Test

Increase: Coagulation studies, LFTs, serum uric acid, amylase, CO_2, urinary protein

Decrease: Serum potassium, cholesterol

Interference: Urine catecholamines, pregnancy test, urine glucose tests (Clinistix, Tes-Tape)

NURSING CONSIDERATIONS

Assess:

• Pain: character, location, intensity; ROM before and 1 hr after administration

• Fever: temperature before and 1 hr after administration

• Hepatic studies: AST, ALT, bilirubin, creatinine if patient is on long-term therapy

• Renal studies: BUN, urine creatinine; I&O ratio; decreasing output may indicate renal failure (long-term therapy)

• Blood studies: CBC, Hct, Hgb, PT if patient is on long-term therapy

⚠ Hepatotoxicity: dark urine, clay-colored stools, yellowing of skin, sclera, itching, abdominal pain, fever, diarrhea if patient is on long-term therapy

• Allergic reactions: rash, urticaria; if these occur, drug may have to be discontinued; patients with asthma, nasal polyps, allergies: severe allergic reaction may occur

• Ototoxicity: tinnitus, ringing, roaring in ears; audiometric testing needed before, after long-term therapy

• Salicylate level: therapeutic level 150-300 mcg/ml for chronic inflammation

• Visual changes: blurring, halos; corneal, retinal damage

• Edema in feet, ankles, legs

• Drug history; many drug interactions

Administer:

PO route

• Do not break, crush, or chew enteric product

• Crushed or whole; chewable tablets may be chewed

• ½ hr before planned exercise

• With food or milk to decrease gastric symptoms; separate by 2 hr of enteric product

• With 8 oz H_2O and sit upright for ½ hr after dose to facilitate drug passing into the stomach

---

⚠ Safety alert   *"Tall Man" lettering

Evaluate:
• Therapeutic response: decreased pain, inflammation, fever
Teach patient/family:
• To report any symptoms of hepatotoxicity, renal toxicity, visual changes, ototoxicity, allergic reactions, bleeding (long-term therapy)
• To avoid if allergic to tartrazine
• Not to exceed recommended dosage; acute poisoning may result
• To read label on other OTC drugs; many contain aspirin or salicylates
• That the therapeutic response takes 2 wk (arthritis)
• To report tinnitus, confusion, diarrhea, sweating, hyperventilation
• To avoid alcohol ingestion; GI bleeding may occur
• That patients who have allergies, nasal polyps, asthma may develop allergic reactions
• To discard tabs if vinegar-like smell is detected
• That medication is not to be given to children or teens with flulike symptoms or chickenpox; Reye's syndrome may develop
Treatment of overdose: Lavage, activated charcoal, monitor electrolytes, VS

atazanavir (℞)
(at-a-za-na'veer)
Reyataz
Func. class.: Antiretroviral
Chem. class.: Protease inhibitor

Action: Inhibits human immunodeficiency virus (HIV-1) protease, which prevents maturation of the infectious virus
Uses: HIV-1 infection in combination with other antiretroviral agents

DOSAGE AND ROUTES
Antiretroviral-naive patients
• *Adult:* **PO** 400 mg daily
Antiretroviral-experienced patients
• *Adult:* **PO** 300 mg daily and ritonavir 100 mg daily

Hepatic dose
• *Adult:* **PO** (Child-Pugh B) 300 mg daily; (Child-Pugh C) do not use
Available forms: Caps 100, 150, 200 mg

SIDE EFFECTS
CNS: Headache, depression, dizziness, insomnia, peripheral neurologic symptoms
GI: Vomiting, *diarrhea, abdominal pain, nausea,* **hepatotoxicity**
INTEG: Rash, **Stevens-Johnson syndrome,** *photosensitivity*
MISC: Fatigue, fever, arthralgia, back pain, cough, lipodystrophy, pain, gynecomastia
Contraindications: Hypersensitivity
Precautions: Pregnancy (B), hepatic disease, lactation, children, geriatric

PHARMACOKINETICS
Rapidly absorbed, absorption increased with food, peak 2½ hr, 86% protein bound, extensively metabolized in liver, 27% excreted unchanged in urine/feces (minimal), half-life 7 hr

INTERACTIONS
⚠ *Increase:* levels, increased toxicity of immunosuppressants (cycloSPORINE, sirolimus, tacrolimus, sildenafil), tricylic antidepressants, warfarin, calcium channel blockers, irinotecan, HMG-CoA reductase inhibitors, antidysrhythmics, midazolam, triazolam, ergots, pimozide
Increase: effects of estrogens, oral contraceptives
Increase: hyperbilirubinemia—indinavir
Decrease: atazanavir levels—rifampin, antacids, didanosine, efavirenz, proton pump inhibitors, H₂-receptor antagonists
Drug/Herb
Decrease: atazanavir levels—St. John's wort
Drug/Lab Test
Increase: AST, ALT, total bilirubin, amylase, lipase, CK
Decrease: Hgb, neurophils, platelets

NURSING CONSIDERATIONS

Assess:

⚠ For hepatic failure; hepatic studies: ALT, AST, bilirubin

• Signs of infection, anemia

• Bowel pattern before, during treatment; if severe abdominal pain with bleeding occurs, drug should be discontinued; monitor hydration

• Viral load, CD4 count throughout treatment

• Skin eruptions, rash, urticaria, itching

• Allergies before treatment, reaction of each medication; place allergies on chart

Administer:

• With food

Evaluate:

• Therapeutic response: increasing CD4 counts; decreased viral load, resolution of symptoms of HIV-1 infection

Teach patient/family:

• To take as prescribed with other antiretrovirals as prescribed, if dose is missed, take as soon as remembered up to 1 hr before next dose; do not double dose, do not share with others

• That drug must be taken daily to maintain blood levels for duration of therapy

• May cause photosensitivity, use protective clothing, or stay out of the sun

• To notify prescriber if diarrhea, nausea, vomiting, rash occurs; dizziness, light-headedness, ECG may be altered

• That drug interacts with many drugs and St. John's wort, advise prescriber of all drugs, herbal products used

• That redistribution of body fat may occur, the effect is not known

• That drug does not cure HIV-1 infection or prevent transmission to others, only controls symptoms

• That if taking sildenafil with atazanavir, there may be an increased risk of sildenafil-associated adverse events, including hypotension and prolonged penile erection; notify physician promptly of these symptoms

---

atenolol (℞)

(a-ten'oh-lole)

Apo-Atenol ✦, atenolol ✦, Novo-Atenol ✦, Tenormin

Func. class.: Antihypertensive, antianginal

Chem. class.: β-Blocker, β₁-, β₂-blocker (high doses)

Do not confuse:

atenolol/albuterol

Tenormin/thiamine/Imuran/Trovan

Action: Competitively blocks stimulation of β-adrenergic receptor within vascular smooth muscle; produces negative chronotropic activity, negative inotropic activity (decreases rate of SA node discharge, increases recovery time), slows conduction of AV node, decreases heart rate, decreases O_2 consumption in myocardium; also decreases renin-aldosterone-angiotensin system at high doses, inhibits β_2 receptors in bronchial system at higher doses

Uses: Mild to moderate hypertension, prophylaxis of angina pectoris; suspected or known myocardial infarction (IV use)

Unlabeled uses: Dysrhythmia, mitral valve prolapse, pheochromocytoma, hypertrophic cardiomyopathy, vascular headaches, thyrotoxicosis, tremors, alcohol withdrawal

DOSAGE AND ROUTES

• *Adult:* **PO** 25-50 mg daily, increasing q1-2wk to 100 mg daily; may increase to 200 mg daily for angina or up to 100 mg for hypertension

• *Geriatric:* **PO** 25 mg/day initially

Renal disease

• *Adult:* **PO** CCr 15-35 ml/min, max 50 mg/day; CCr <15 ml/min max dose 25 mg/day; hemodialysis 25-50 mg after dialysis

• *Adult:* **IV** 5 mg, repeat in 10 min if initial dose is well tolerated, then start **PO** dose 10 min after last **IV** dose, (MI)

Available forms: Tabs 25, 50, 100 mg; inj 500 mcg/ml

⚠ Safety alert   ✦ "Tall Man" lettering

SIDE EFFECTS

CNS: Insomnia, fatigue, dizziness, mental changes, memory loss, hallucinations, depression, lethargy, drowsiness, strange dreams, catatonia

CV: **Profound hypotension, bradycardia, CHF,** *cold extremities, postural hypotension, 2nd- or 3rd-degree heart block*

EENT: Sore throat, dry burning eyes, blurred vision, stuffy nose

ENDO: Increased hypoglycemic response to insulin

GI: Nausea, diarrhea, vomiting, **mesenteric arterial thrombosis, ischemic colitis**

GU: Impotence, decreased libido

HEMA: **Agranulocytosis, thrombocytopenia, purpura**

INTEG: Rash, fever, alopecia

RESP: **Bronchospasm,** dyspnea, wheezing, pulmonary edema

Contraindications: Pregnancy (D), hypersensitivity to β-blockers, cardiogenic shock, 2nd- or 3rd-degree heart block, sinus bradycardia, cardiac failure, Raynaud's disease, pulmonary edema

Precautions: Major surgery, lactation, diabetes mellitus, renal disease, thyroid disease, CHF, COPD, asthma, well-compensated heart failure, dialysis, myasthenia gravis

PHARMACOKINETICS

IV: Onset rapid, peak 5 min, duration unknown

PO: Peak 2-4 hr, onset 1 hr, duration 24 hr; half-life 6-9 hr, excreted unchanged in urine, feces, protein binding 5%-15%

INTERACTIONS

• Mutual inhibition: sympathomimetics (cough, cold preparations)

Increase: hypotension, bradycardia—reserpine, hydrALAZINE, methyldopa, prazosin, anticholinergics, digoxin, diltiazem, verapamil, cardiac glycosides, antihypertensives

Increase: atenolol absorption—atropine

Drug/Herb

• Toxicity/death: aconite

Increase: atenolol effect—betel palm, butterbur, cola tree, figwort, fumitory, guarana, hawthorn, jaborandi tree, lily of the valley, motherwort, plantain

Decrease: atenolol effect—coenzyme Q10, yohimbe

Drug/Lab Test

Increase: Blood glucose, BUN, K, triglycerides, uric acid, ANA titer

NURSING CONSIDERATIONS

Assess:

• I&O, weight daily

• B/P, pulse q4h; note rate, rhythm, quality; apical/radial pulse before administration; notify prescriber of any significant changes (<50 bpm)

• Baselines in renal/hepatic studies before therapy begins

Administer:

PO route

• Drug before meals, at bedtime; tablet may be crushed or swallowed whole

• Reduced dosage in renal dysfunction

IV, direct route

• Undiluted over 5 min

IV INF route

• Diluted in 10-50 ml of D_5W, D_5/NaCl, or NS and give as an infusion at prescribed rate

Y-site compatibilities: Meperidine, meropenem, morphine

Perform/provide:

• Storage protected from light, moisture; place in cool environment

Evaluate:

• Therapeutic response: decreased B/P after 1-2 wk

Teach patient/family:

⚠ Not to discontinue drug abruptly, taper over 2 wk (angina), take at same time each day

• Not to use OTC products unless directed by prescriber

• To report bradycardia, dizziness, confusion, depression, fever

• To take pulse at home; advise when to notify prescriber

• To limit alcohol, smoking, sodium intake
• To comply with weight control, dietary adjustments, modified exercise program
• To carry emergency ID to identify drug, allergies, conditions being treated
• To avoid hazardous activities if dizziness is present
• That drug may mask symptoms of hypoglycemia in diabetic patients
• To use contraception while taking this drug, pregnancy category (D)

Treatment of overdose: Lavage, IV atropine for bradycardia, IV theophylline for bronchospasm, dextrose for hypoglycemia, digoxin, O_2, diuretic for cardiac failure, hemodialysis

---

atomoxetine (Ŗ)
(at-o-mox'eh-teen)
Strattera
Func. class.: Psychotherapeutic—miscellaneous
Chem. class.: Selective norepinephrine reuptake inhibitor

Action: A selective norepinephrine reuptake inhibitor; may inhibit the presynaptic norepinephrine transporter.
Uses: Attention deficit hyperactivity disorder

DOSAGE AND ROUTES

• *Child ≤70 kg:* **PO** 0.5 mg/kg, increase after 3 days to a target daily dose of 1.2 mg/kg in AM or evenly divided doses AM, late afternoon; max 1.4 mg/kg/day or 100 mg daily, whichever is less
• *Adult and child >70 kg:* **PO** 40 mg daily, increase after 3 days to a target daily dose of 80 mg in AM or evenly divided doses AM, late afternoon; max 100 mg daily
Hepatic dose
• (Child-Pugh B) reduce dose by 50%
• (Child-Pugh C) reduce dose by 75%
Available forms: Caps 10, 18, 25, 40, 60 mg

SIDE EFFECTS

CNS: Insomnia, dizziness, headache, irritability, crying, mood swings, fatigue
CV: Palpitations, hot flushes
ENDO: Growth retardation
GI: Dyspepsia, nausea, anorexia, dry mouth, weight loss, vomiting, diarrhea, constipation
GU: Urinary hesitancy, retention, dysmenorrhea, erectile disturbance, ejaculation failure, impotence, prostatis, orgasm abnormal
INTEG: **Exfoliative dermatitis,** sweating
MISC: Cough, rhinorrhea, dermatitis, ear infection
Contraindications: Hypersensitivity, narrow-angle glaucoma
Precautions: Pregnancy (C), hypertension, lactation, child <6 yr; hepatic/cardiac/cerebrovascular disease

PHARMACOKINETICS

PO: Peak 1-2 hr, metabolized by liver, excreted by kidneys, 98% protein binding

INTERACTIONS

• Hypertensive crisis: MAOIs or within 14 days of MAOIs, vasopressors
Increase: cardiovascular effects of albuterol, pressor agents
Increase: effects of atomoxetine—CYP 2D6 inhibitors (amiodarone, cimetidine [weak], clomipramine, delavirdine, gefitinib, imatinib, propafenone, quinidine [potent], ritonavir, citalopram, escitalopram, fluoxetine, sertraline, paroxetine, thioridazine, venlafaxine)

NURSING CONSIDERATIONS

Assess:
• VS, B/P; check patients with cardiac disease more often for increased B/P
• Height, growth rate q3mo in children; growth rate may be decreased
• Mental status: mood, sensorium, affect, stimulation, insomnia, aggressiveness
• Appetite, sleep, speech patterns

• For attention span, decreased hyperactivity in ADHD persons

Administer:

• Gum, hard candy, frequent sips of water for dry mouth

Evaluate:

• Therapeutic response: decreased hyperactivity (ADHD)

Teach patient/family:

• To avoid OTC preparations unless approved by prescriber

• To avoid alcohol ingestion

• To avoid hazardous activities until stabilized on medication

• To get needed rest; patients will feel more tired at end of day

---

atorvastatin (℞)

(a-tore′va-stat-in)

Lipitor

Func. class.: Antilipidemic

Chem. class.: HMG-CoA reductase inhibitor

Action: Inhibits HMG-CoA reductase enzyme, which reduces cholesterol synthesis

Uses: As an adjunct in primary hypercholesterolemia (types Ia, Ib), dysbetalipoproteinemia, elevated triglyceride levels, prevention of cardiovascular disease by reduction of heart risk in those with mildly elevated cholesterol

DOSAGE AND ROUTES

• *Adult:* **PO** 10-20 mg daily, usual range 10-80, dosage adjustments may be made in 2-4 wk intervals, max 80 mg/day; patients requiring >45% reduction in LDL may be started at 40 mg daily

Available forms: Tabs 10, 20, 40, 80 mg

SIDE EFFECTS

CNS: Headache, asthenia

EENT: Lens opacities

GI: Abdominal cramps, constipation, diarrhea, flatus, heartburn, dyspepsia, **liver dysfunction,** pancreatitis, nausea, increased serum transaminase

GU: Impotence

INTEG: Rash, pruritus, alopecia

MISC: Hypersensitivity

MS: Arthralgia, myalgia, **rhabdomyolysis**

RESP: Pharyngitis, sinusitis

Contraindications: Pregnancy (X), hypersensitivity, lactation, active hepatic disease

Precautions: Past hepatic disease, alcoholism, severe acute infections, trauma, severe metabolic disorders, electrolyte imbalance

PHARMACOKINETICS

Metabolized in liver, highly protein bound, excreted primarily in urine, half-life 14 hr; protein binding 98%

INTERACTIONS

• Risk of possible rhabdomyolysis: azole antifungals, cycloSPORINE, erythromycin, niacin, gemfibrozil, clofibrate

Increase: serum level of digoxin

Increase: levels of oral contraceptives

Increase: levels of atorvastatin—erythromycin

Increase: effects of warfarin

Decrease: atorvastatin levels—colestipol

Drug/Herb

Increase: effect—glucomannan

Decrease: effect—gotu kola, St. John's wort

Drug/Food

• Possible toxicity when used with grapefruit juice; oat bran may reduce effectiveness

Drug/Lab Test

Increase: Bilirubin, alk phos

Interference: Thyroid function tests

NURSING CONSIDERATIONS

Assess:

• Diet, obtain diet history including fat, cholesterol in diet

• Cholesterol triglyceride levels periodically during treatment; check lipid panel 6 wk after changing dose

• Hepatic studies q1-2mo during the first

Side effects: *italics* = common; **bold** = life-threatening

1½ yr of treatment; AST, ALT, LFTs may be increased
• Renal studies in patients with compromised renal system: BUN, I&O ratio, creatinine

A For muscle pain, tenderness, obtain CPK baseline and if these occur, drug may need to be discontinued

Administer:
• Total daily dose any time of day without regard to meals

Perform/provide:
• Storage in cool environment in tight container protected from light

Evaluate:
• Therapeutic response: decrease in cholesterol to desired level after 6 wk

Teach patient/family:
• That blood work and eye exam will be necessary during treatment
• To report blurred vision, severe GI symptoms, headache, muscle pain, weakness
• That previously prescribed regimen will continue: low-cholesterol diet, exercise program, smoking cessation
• Not to take drug if pregnant
• To stay out of the sun, or use sunscreen, protective clothing to prevent photosensitivity (rare)

---

atovaquone (℞)

(a-toe'va-kwon)
Mepron
Func. class.: Antiprotozoal
Chem. class.: Aromatic diamide derivative, analog of ubiquinone

---

Action: Interferes with DNA/RNA synthesis in protozoa

Uses: *Pneumocystis jiroveci* infections in patients intolerant of trimethoprim-sulfamethoxazole, prophylaxis, *Toxoplasma gondii,* toxoplasmosis

Unlabeled uses: Babesiosis, malaria treatment/prophylaxis, toxoplasmosis prophylaxis, *plasmodium* sp.

DOSAGE AND ROUTES

Acute, mild, moderate Pneumocystis jiroveci *pneumonia*
• *Adult and adolescent 13-16 yr:* **PO** 750 mg with food bid for 21 days

Pneumocystis jiroveci *pneumonia, prophylaxis*
• *Adult and adolescent:* **PO** 1500 mg daily with meal

Available forms: Susp 750 mg/5 ml

SIDE EFFECTS

CNS: Dizziness, headache, anxiety, insomnia
CV: Hypotension
GI: Nausea, vomiting, diarrhea, anorexia, increased AST and ALT, acute pancreatitis, constipation, abdominal pain
HEMA: Anemia, **leukopenia,** neutropenia
INTEG: Pruritus, urticaria, *rash,* oral monilia
META: Hyperkalemia, hypoglycemia, hyponatremia

Contraindications: Hypersensitivity or history of developing life-threatening allergic reactions to any component of the formulation, benzyl alcohol sensitivity
Precautions: Pregnancy (C), blood dyscrasias, hepatic disease, diabetes mellitus, lactation, children, geriatric, GI disease, respiratory insufficiency

PHARMACOKINETICS

Excreted unchanged in feces (94%), highly protein bound (99%)

INTERACTIONS

• Use caution when administering concurrently with other highly plasma protein-bound drugs with narrow therapeutic indices
Decrease: effect of atovaquone—rifampin, rifabutin

NURSING CONSIDERATIONS

Assess:
• Signs of infection, anemia
• Bowel pattern before, during treatment

• Respiratory status: rate, character, wheezing, dyspnea
• Allergies before treatment, reaction of each medication
Administer:
• With high-fat food because of increased absorption of the drug and higher plasma concentrations
Evaluate:
• Therapeutic response: decreased temp, ability to breathe
Teach patient/family:
• To take with food to increase plasma concentrations

Rarely Used

atracurium (℞)
(a-tra-kyoor'ee-um)
Tracrium
Func. class.: Neuromuscular blocker (nondepolarizing)

Uses: Facilitation of endotracheal intubation, skeletal muscle relaxation during mechanical ventilation, surgery, or general anesthesia

DOSAGE AND ROUTES
• *Adult and child >2 yr:* IV BOL 0.3-0.5 mg/kg, then 0.08-0.10 mg/kg 20-45 min after first dose if needed for prolonged procedures
• *Child, 1 mo-2 yr:* IV BOL 0.3-0.4 mg/kg
Contraindications: Hypersensitivity

⚠ High Alert

atropine (℞)
(a'troe-peen)
atropine sulfate, Atro-Pen, Sal-Tropine
Func. class.: Antidysrhythmic, anticholinergic parasympatholytic, antimuscarinic
Chem. class.: Belladonna alkaloid

Do not confuse:
atropine/Akarpine

Action: Blocks acetylcholine at parasympathetic neuroeffector sites; increases cardiac output, heart rate by blocking vagal stimulation in heart; dries secretions by blocking vagus
Uses: Bradycardia <40-50 bpm, bradydysrhythmia, reversal of anticholinesterase agents, insecticide poisoning, blocking cardiac vagal reflexes, decreasing secretions before surgery, antispasmodic with GU, biliary surgery, bronchodilator

DOSAGE AND ROUTES
Bradycardia/bradydysrhythmia
• *Adult:* IV BOL 0.5-1 mg given q3-5min, not to exceed 2 mg
• *Child:* IV BOL 0.01-0.03 mg/kg up to 0.4 mg or 0.3 mg/m^2; may repeat q4-6h; min dose 0.1 mg to avoid paradoxical reaction
Organophosphate poisoning
• *Adult and child:* IM/IV 2 mg qhr until muscarinic symptoms disappear, may need 6 mg qhr
• *Adult and child 90 lb, usually >10 yr:* Atro-pen 2 mg
• *Child 40-90 lb, usually 4-10 yr:* Atro-pen 1 mg
• *Child 15-40 lb, 6 mo-4 yr:* Atro-pen 0.05 mg
Presurgery
• *Adult and child >20 kg:* SUBCUT/IM/IV 0.4-0.6 mg before anesthesia
• *Child <20 kg:* IM/SUBCUT 0.01 mg/kg up to 0.4 mg ½-1 hr preop
Available forms: Inj 0.05, 0.1, 0.3, 0.4, 0.5, 0.8, 1 mg/ml; tabs 0.4 mg; Atropen 0.5, 1, 2 mg inj prefilled auto-injectors

SIDE EFFECTS
CNS: Headache, dizziness, involuntary movement, confusion, psychosis, anxiety, coma, flushing, drowsiness, insomnia, weakness; delirium (geriatric)
CV: Hypotension, paradoxical bradycardia, angina, PVCs, hypertension, **tachycardia,** ectopic ventricular beats
EENT: Blurred vision, photophobia, glaucoma, eye pain, pupil dilation, nasal congestion

GI: Dry mouth, nausea, vomiting, abdominal pain, anorexia, constipation, **paralytic ileus,** abdominal distention, altered taste

GU: Retention, hesitancy, impotence, dysuria

INTEG: Rash, urticaria, contact dermatitis, dry skin, flushing

MISC: Suppression of lactation, decreased sweating

Contraindications: Hypersensitivity to belladonna alkaloids, angle-closure glaucoma, GI obstructions, myasthenia gravis, thyrotoxicosis, ulcerative colitis, prostatic hypertrophy, tachycardia/tachydysrhythmias, asthma, acute hemorrhage, hepatic disease, myocardial ischemia

Precautions: Pregnancy (C), renal/hepatic disease, lactation, CHF, tachydysrhythmia, hyperthyroidism, COPD, child <6 yr, hypertension, geriatric, intraabdominal infection, Down syndrome, spastic paralysis, gastric ulcer

PHARMACOKINETICS

Well absorbed PO, IM, SUBCUT; half-life 13-40 hr, excreted by kidneys unchanged (70%-90% in 24 hr); metabolized in liver, 40%-50% crosses placenta, excreted in breast milk

IV: Peak 2-4 min, duration 4-6 hr

IM/SUBCUT: Onset 15-50 min; peak 30 min, duration 4-6 hr

PO: Onset ½ hr; peak ½-1 hr; duration 4-6 hr

INTERACTIONS

• Mucosal lesions: potassium chloride tab

Increase: anticholinergic effects, tricyclics, amantadine, antiparkinson agents

Decrease: absorption—ketoconazole, levodopa

Decrease: effect of atropine—antacids

Drug/Herb

• Forms insoluble complex: black root

• Serotonin effect: horehound

Increase: atropine effect—aloe, buckthorn, cascara sagrada, figwort, fumitory, goldenseal, jimsonweed, kudzu, licorice, rhubarb, senna, scopolia

Increase: toxicity/death—aconite

Decrease: effect—coltsfoot

NURSING CONSIDERATIONS

Assess:

• I&O ratio; check for urinary retention, daily output

• ECG for ectopic ventricular beats, PVC, tachycardia, in cardiac patients

• For bowel sounds; check for constipation

• Respiratory status: rate, rhythm, cyanosis, wheezing, dyspnea, engorged neck veins

• Increased intraocular pressure: eye pain, nausea, vomiting, blurred vision, increased tearing

• Cardiac rate: rhythm, character, B/P continuously

• Allergic reaction: rash, urticaria

Administer:

PO route

• Increased bulk, water in diet if constipation occurs

• ½ hr before meals

IM route

• Atropine flush may occur in children and is not harmful

Atro-Pen

• Use no more than 3 Atro-Pen inj unless under the supervision of trained medical provider

• Use as soon as symptoms appear (tearing, wheezing, muscles fasciculations, excessive oral secretions)

IV route

• Undiluted or diluted with 10 ml sterile H_2O, give at 0.6 mg/min, give through Y-tube or 3-way stopcock; do not add to IV sol; may cause paradoxical bradycardia lasting 2 min

Additive compatibilities: DOBUTamine, furosemide, meropenem, netilmicin, sodium bicarbonate, verapamil

Syringe compatibilities: Benzquinamide, butorphanol, chlorproMAZINE, cimetidine, dimenhyDRINATE, diphenhydrAMINE, droperidol, fentanyl, glycopyrrolate, heparin, hydromorphone, hydrOXYzine, meperidine, metoclopramide, midazolam, milrinone, morphine, nalbuphine, pentazocine, perphenazine, prochlorperazine, promazine, promethazine, propiomazine, ranitidine, scopolamine, sufentanil

Y-site compatibilities: Amrinone, etomidate, famotidine, heparin, hydrocortisone, meropenem, nafcillin, potassium chloride, sufentanil, vit B/C

Perform/provide:

• Sugarless hard candy, gum, frequent rinsing of mouth for dryness

Evaluate:

• Therapeutic response: decreased dysrhythmias, increased heart rate, secretions; GI, GU spasms; bronchodilation

Teach patient/family:

• To report blurred vision, chest pain, allergic reactions, constipation, urinary retention

• Not to perform strenuous activity in high temperatures; heat stroke may result

• To take as prescribed; not to skip doses

• Not to operate machinery if drowsiness occurs

• Not to take OTC products without approval of prescriber

Treatment of overdose: O$_2$, artificial ventilation, ECG; administer DOPamine for circulatory depression; administer diazepam or thiopental for seizures; assess need for antidysrhythmics

atropine ophthalmic
See Appendix C

Rarely Used

auranofin (℞)
(au-rane'oh-fin)
Ridaura
Func. class.: Antiinflammatory

Do not confuse:
Ridaura/Cardura
Uses: RA; not for first-line therapy

Unlabeled uses: SLE, psoriatic arthritis, pemphigus

DOSAGE AND ROUTES

• *Adult:* PO 6 mg daily or 3 mg bid; may increase to 9 mg/day after 3 mo

Contraindications: Hypersensitivity to gold, necrotizing enterocolitis, bone marrow aplasia, child <6 yr, lactation, pulmonary fibrosis, exfoliative dermatitis, blood dyscrasias, recent radiation therapy, renal/hepatic disease, marked hypertension, uncontrolled CHF

Rarely Used

aurothioglucose (℞)
(aur-oh-thye-oh-gloo'kose)
Solganal
Func. class.: Antiinflammatory

Uses: Rheumatoid arthritis, psoriatic arthritis

DOSAGE AND ROUTES

• *Adult:* IM 10 mg, then 25 mg qwk × 2-3 wk, then 50 mg/wk until total of 1 g is administered, then 25-50 mg q3-4wk if there is improvement without toxicity total of 800 mg-1 g

• *Child 6-12 yr:* IM 0.25 mg/kg/wk 1st wk, increase by 0.25 mg/kg/wk up to 0.75-1 mg/kg/wk, max 25 mg/dose; give for 20 wk

Contraindications: Hypersensitivity to gold, SLE, uncontrolled diabetes mellitus, marked hypertension, recent radiation therapy, CHF, lactation, renal/hepatic disease

⚠ High Alert

azacitidine (℞)
(a-za-sie-ti′deen)
Vidaza
Func. class.: Antineoplastic hormone
Chem. class.: DNA demethylation agent

Action: Cytotoxic by producing damage to double-strand DNA during DNA synthesis

Uses: Myelodysplastic syndrome (MDS)

DOSAGE AND ROUTES

• *Adult:* SUBCUT 75 mg/m^2 daily × 7 days, q4wk, premedicate with antiemetic; dose may be increased to 100 mg/m^2 if no response is seen after 2 treatment cycles, minimum treatment 4 cycles

Available forms: Powdered for inj, lyophilized 100 mg

SIDE EFFECTS

CNS: Anxiety, depression, dizziness, fatigue, headache

CV: Cardiac murmur, hypotension, tachycardia

GI: **Diarrhea,** nausea, vomiting, anorexia, constipation, abdominal pain, distention, tenderness, hemorrhoids, mouth hemorrhage, tongue ulceration, stomatitis, dyspepsia, **hepatotoxicity, hepatic coma**

GU: **Renal failure, renal tubular acidosis,** dysuria, UTI

HEMA: **Leukopenia, anemia, thrombocytopenia, neutropenia,** ecchymosis

INTEG: Irritation at site, rash, sweating, pyrexia

META: Hypokalemia

Contraindications: Pregnancy (D), hypersensitivity to this drug or mannitol, advanced malignant hepatic tumors

Precautions: Lactation, children, geriatric, renal/hepatic disease; a man should not father a child while taking this drug

PHARMACOKINETICS

Rapidly absorbed, peak ½ hr, metabolized in the liver, half-life 35-49 min, excreted in urine

INTERACTIONS

None known

NURSING CONSIDERATIONS

Assess:

• For CNS symptoms: fever, headache, chills, dizziness

• Hematologic response with patients with baseline WBC ≥3 × 10^9/L, absolute neutrophil count (ANC) ≥1.5 × 10^9/L, and platelets ≥75 × 10^9/L, adjust dose; ANC <0.5 × 10^9/L, platelets <25 × 10^9/L, give 50% dose next course; ANC 0.5-1.5 × 10^9/L, platelets 25-50 × 10^9/L, give 67% next course

• Buccal cavity q8h for dryness, sores, or ulceration, white patches, oral pain, bleeding, dysphagia

• Bone marrow depression: bruising, bleeding, blood in stools, urine, sputum, emesis

Administer:

• Antiemetics and dexamethasone 10 mg at least ½ hr before antineoplastics

IV route

• Reconstitute with 4 ml sterile water for inj (25 mg/ml), inject diluent slowly into vial, invert vial 2-3 times and gently rotate; sol will be cloudy, use immediately; divide doses <4 ml into two syringes; resuspend the contents 2-3 times and gently roll syringe between the palms for 30 sec immediately before administration

• Rotate inj site

Perform/provide:

• Increased fluid intake to 2-3 L/day to prevent dehydration, unless contraindicated

• Rinsing of mouth tid-qid with water, club soda; brushing of teeth bid-tid with soft brush or cotton-tipped applicator for stomatitis; use unwaxed dental floss

• Nutritious diet with iron, vitamin supplement, low fiber, few dairy products

---

⚠ Safety alert   *"Tall Man" lettering

Evaluate:

• Therapeutic response: improvement in blood counts in refractory anemia, or refractory anemia with excess blasts

Teach patient/family:

• To avoid crowds, persons with known infections; not to receive immunizations

• To avoid foods with citric acid or hot or rough texture if stomatitis is present; to drink adequate fluids

• To report stomatitis; any bleeding, white spots, ulcerations in mouth; tell patient to examine mouth daily, report symptoms

• To use contraception during therapy; not to breastfeed

• Not to father a child while receiving this drug

---

azathioprine (℞)

(ay-za-thye'oh-preen)

Imuran

Func. class.: Immunosuppressant

Chem. class.: Purine antagonist

Do not confuse:

Imuran/Imferon/Elmiron/IMDUR/Enduron/Tenormin

Action: Produces immunosuppression by inhibiting purine synthesis in cells

Uses: Renal transplants to prevent graft rejection, refractory rheumatoid arthritis, glomerulonephritis, nephrotic syndrome, bone marrow transplant

Unlabeled uses: Myasthenia gravis, chronic ulcerative colitis, Crohn's disease, Behçet's disease

DOSAGE AND ROUTES

Prevention of rejection

• *Adult and child:* **IV** 3-5 mg/kg/day, then maintenance (**PO**) of at least 1-3 mg/kg/day

Refractory rheumatoid arthritis

• *Adult:* **PO** 1 mg/kg/day, may increase dose after 2 mo by 0.5 mg/kg/day, not to exceed 2.5 mg/kg/day

Renal disease

• CCr 10-50 ml/min 75% of dose; CCr <10 ml/min 50% of dose

Available forms: Tabs 50, 75, 100 mg; inj 100 mg

SIDE EFFECTS

GI: Nausea, vomiting, stomatitis, esophagitis, **pancreatitis, hepatotoxicity, jaundice**

HEMA: **Leukopenia, thrombocytopenia, anemia, pancytopenia**

INTEG: Rash, alopecia

MISC: **Serum sickness,** Raynaud's symptoms

MS: Arthralgia, muscle wasting

Contraindications: Pregnancy (D), hypersensitivity, lactation

Precautions: Severe renal/hepatic disease, geriatric

PHARMACOKINETICS

Metabolized in liver, excreted in urine (active metabolite), crosses placenta

INTERACTIONS

• Leukopenia: ACE inhibitors; co-trimoxazole

• Do not admix with other drugs

Increase: myelosuppression—cyclo-SPORINE, antineoplastics

Increase: action of azathioprine—allopurinol

Decrease: immune response—vaccines

Decrease: action of warfarin—warfarin

Drug/Herb

Increase: immunosuppression—astragalus, echinacea, melatonin, safflower

Decrease: immunosuppression—ginseng, maitake, mistletoe, schisandra, St. John's wort, tumeric

Drug/Lab Test

Increase: LFTs

Decrease: Uric acid

Interference: CBC, diff count

NURSING CONSIDERATIONS

Assess:

• For infection: increased temp, WBC; sputum, urine

• For rheumatoid arthritis, pain, mobility, ROM

Side effects: *italics* = common; **bold** = life-threatening

- I&O, weight daily, report decreasing urine output; toxicity may occur
- Blood studies: Hgb, WBC, platelets during treatment monthly; if leukocytes are <3000/mm^3 or platelets <100,000/mm^3, drug should be discontinued
⚠ Hepatotoxicity: dark urine, jaundice, itching, light-colored stools, increased LFTs; drug should be discontinued; hepatic studies: alk phos, AST, ALT, bilirubin
- Arthritis: pain; location, ROM, swelling, before and during treatment

Administer:
- All medications PO if possible, avoiding IM inj, since bleeding may occur

PO route
- With meals to reduce GI upset

IV route
- Prepare in biologic cabinet using gown, gloves, mask
- After diluting 100 mg/10 ml of sterile H$_2$O for inj; rotate to dissolve; may further dilute with 50 ml or more saline or glucose in saline, give over ½-1 hr
- For several days before transplant surgery

Solution compatibilities: D$_5$W, NaCl 0.9%, NaCl 0.45%

Evaluate:
- Therapeutic response: absence of graft rejection, immunosuppression in autoimmune disorders

Teach patient/family:
- To take as prescribed, do not miss doses, if dose is missed on daily regimen, skip dose; if on multiple dosing/day, take as soon as remembered
- That therapeutic response may take 3-4 mo in RA; to continue with prescribed exercise, rest, other medications
- To report fever, rash, severe diarrhea, chills, sore throat, fatigue, since serious infections may occur; report unusual bleeding or bruising
- To use contraceptive measures during treatment, for 16 wk after ending therapy; to avoid vaccinations
- To avoid crowds to reduce risk of infection

- To use soft-bristled toothbrush to prevent bleeding
- That treatment is ongoing to prevent transplant rejection

azelaic acid topical
See Appendix C

azelastine nasal agent
See Appendix C

azelastine ophthalmic
See Appendix C

azithromycin (℞)
(ay-zi-thro-my′sin)
Zithromax
Func. class.: Antiinfective
Chem. class.: Macrolide (azalide)

Do not confuse:
azithromycin/erythromycin
Zithromax/Zinacef

Action: Binds to 50S ribosomal subunits of susceptible bacteria and suppresses protein synthesis; much greater spectrum of activity than erythromycin; more effective against gram-negative organisms

Uses: Mild to moderate infections of the upper respiratory tract, lower respiratory tract, uncomplicated skin and skin structure infections caused by *Moraxella catarrhalis, Streptococcus pneumoniae, Streptococcus pyogenes, Staphylococcus aureus, Streptococcus agalactiae, Mycoplasma pneumoniae, Haemophilus influenzae, Clostridium, Legionella pneumophila;* nongonococcal urethritis or cervicitis due to *Chlamydia trachomatis;* in children: acute otitis media *(H. influenzae, M. catarrhalis, S. pneumoniae)* **PO;** acute pharyngitis/tonsillitis (group A streptococcal) **PO;** acute skin/ soft tissue infections **(PO);** community-

---

⚠ Safety alert   *"Tall Man" lettering

acquired pneumonia *(Chlamydia pneumoniae, H. influenzae, M. pneumoniae, S. pneumoniae)* **PO;** pharyngitis/tonsillitis *(S. pyogenes);* prophylaxis of disseminated *Mycobacterium avium* complex (MAC)

Unlabeled uses: Chlamydial infections, gonococcal infections, prophylaxis after sexual assault, bacterial endocarditis prevention

DOSAGE AND ROUTES

Most infections
• *Adult:* **PO** 500 mg on day 1, then 250 mg daily on days 2-5 for a total dose of 1.5 g
• *Child 2-15 yr:* **PO** 10 mg/kg on day 1, then 5 mg/kg × 4 days

Disseminated MAC infections
• *Adult:* **PO** 600 mg/day in combination with ethambutol

Community-acquired pneumonia
• *Adult:* **PO/IV** 500 mg **IV** q24h × 2 doses, then 500 mg **PO** q24h × 7-10 days

Pelvic inflammatory disease
• *Adult:* **PO/IV** 500 mg **IV** q24h × 2 doses, then 500 mg **PO** q24h × 7-10 days

Cervicitis, chlamydia, chancroid, nongonococcal urethritis
• *Adult:* **PO** 1 g single dose

Gonorrhea
• *Adult:* **PO** 2 g single dose

Endocarditis prophylaxis
• *Adult:* **PO** 500 mg **1** hr prior to procedure
• *Child:* **PO** 15 mg/kg 1 hr prior to procedure

Lower respiratory tract infections, acute skin/soft tissue infections, acute pharyngitis/tonsillitis
• *Child, 3-day regimen:* **PO** 5-10 mg/kg daily × 3 days

Acute otitis media
• *Child:* **PO** 30 mg/kg as a single dose or 10 mg/kg daily × 3 days or 10 mg/kg as a single dose on day 1 (max 500 mg/day), then 5 mg/kg on days 2-5 (max 250 mg/day)

Prevention of acute otitis media
• *Child:* **PO** 10 mg/kg q wk × 6 mo

Available forms: Tabs 250, 500, 600 mg; powder for inj 500 mg; powder for oral susp 1 g/packet; susp 100, 200 mg/5 ml

SIDE EFFECTS

CNS: Dizziness, headache, vertigo, somnolence

CV: Palpitations, chest pain

EENT: Hearing loss, tinnitus

GI: Nausea, vomiting, diarrhea, **hepatotoxicity,** abdominal pain, stomatitis, heartburn, dyspepsia, flatulence, melena, **cholestatic jaundice, pseudomembranous colitis,** tongue discoloration

GU: Vaginitis, moniliasis, nephritis

HEMA: Anemia

INTEG: Rash, urticaria, pruritus, photosensitivity

SYST: **Angioedema**

Contraindications: Hypersensitivity to azithromycin, erythromycin, or any macrolide

Precautions: Pregnancy (B), lactation; renal/hepatic/cardiac disease; geriatric, <6 mo for otitis media, <2 yr for pharyngitis, tonsillitis

PHARMACOKINETICS

PO: Peak 2-4 hr, duration 24 hr; *IV:* peak end of inf, duration 24 hr; half-life 11-57 hr, excreted in bile, feces, urine primarily as unchanged drug

INTERACTIONS

• Toxicity: ergotamine

⚠ Dysrhythmias: pimozide; fatal reaction

Increase: effects of oral anticoagulants—digoxin, theophylline, methylPREDNISolone, cycloSPORINE, bromocriptine, disopyramide, triazolam, carbamazepine, phenytoin

Decrease: clearance of triazolam

Decrease: absorption of azithromycin—aluminum, magnesium antacids

Drug/Herb

• Do not use acidophilus with antiinfectives; separate by several hours

---

Drug/Lab Test

Increase: CPK, ALT, AST, bilirubin, BUN, creatinine, alk phos

NURSING CONSIDERATIONS

Assess:

• I&O ratio; report hematuria, oliguria in renal disease

• Hepatic studies: AST, ALT; CBC with differential

• Renal studies: urinalysis, protein, blood

• C&S before drug therapy; drug may be taken as soon as culture is taken; C&S may be repeated after treatment

• For superinfection: sore throat, mouth, tongue; fever, fatigue, diarrhea, anogenital pruritus

• Bowel pattern before, during treatment

• Respiratory status: rate, character, wheezing, tightness in chest; discontinue drug if these occur

Administer:

PO route

• Susp 1 hr before meals or 2 hr after meals; reconstitute 1 g packet for susp with 60 ml water, mix, rinse glass with more water and have patient drink to consume all medication; packets not for pediatric use

IV route

• Reconstitute 500 mg of drug/4.8 ml sterile water for inj (100 mg/ml); shake, dilute with ≥250 ml 0.9% NaCl, 0.45% NaCl, or LR to 1-2 mg/ml; diluted solution is stable for 24 hr or 7 days if refrigerated

• Give 500 mg or more/hr; never give IM or as a bolus

Perform/provide:

• Storage at room temperature

Evaluate:

• Therapeutic response: C&S negative for infection; decreased signs of infection

Teach patient/family:

⚠ To report sore throat, fever, fatigue, severe diarrhea, anal/genital itching (may indicate superinfection)

• Not to take aluminum/magnesium-containing antacids simultaneously with this drug (PO)

⚠ To notify nurse of diarrhea stools, dark urine, pale stools, yellow discoloration of eyes or skin, severe abdominal pain

• To complete dosage regimen

Treatment of hypersensitivity: Withdraw drug, maintain airway, administer epINEPHrine, aminophylline, O₂, IV corticosteroids

---

Rarely Used

aztreonam (℞)

(az-tree'oh nam)

Azactam

Func. class.: Antibiotic—miscellaneous

Uses: Urinary tract infection; septicemia; skin, muscle, bone infection, lower respiratory tract, intraabdominal infections; and other infections caused by gram-negative organisms

DOSAGE AND ROUTES

Urinary tract infections

• *Adult:* **IV/IM** 500 mg-1 g q8-12h

Systemic infections

• *Adult:* **IV/IM** 1-2 g q8-12h

• *Child:* **IV/IM** 90-120 mg/kg/day divided q6-8h; max 8 g/day **IV**

Severe systemic infections

• *Adult:* **IV/IM** 2 g q6-8h; do not exceed 8 g/day

Continue treatment for 48 hr after negative culture or until patient is asymptomatic

Contraindications: Hypersensitivity to this drug, penicillins, cephalosporins, severe renal disease

---

Rarely Used

bacitracin (℞)
(bass-i-tray'sin)
BACI-IM, Baciguent, Bacitin ✦
Func. class.: Antiinfective—
miscellaneous

Uses: Staphylococcal pneumonia, empyema

DOSAGE AND ROUTES

• *Child:* **IM** 800-1200 units/kg/day in divided doses q8-12h; max 12 days of therapy

• *Infant >2.5 kg:* **IM** 1000 units/kg/day in divided doses q8-12h; max 12 days of therapy

• *Infant ≤2.5 kg:* **IM** 900 units/kg/day in divided doses q8-12h; max 12 days of therapy

Renal dose
• *Adult:* CCr 10-30 ml/min, decrease dose by 50% q6-12h after 0.5-2 g **IV** loading dose; CCr <10 ml/min, decrease dose by 75% q6-12h after 0.5-2 g **IV** loading dose

Contraindications: Hypersensitivity, severe renal disease (IM use)

bacitracin topical
See Appendix C

baclofen (℞)
(bak'loe-fen)
Lioresal, Lioresal Intrathecal
Func. class.: Skeletal muscle relaxant, central acting
Chem. class.: GABA chlorophenyl derivative

Do not confuse:
Lioresal/Lotensin
Action: Inhibits synaptic responses in CNS by stimulating GABAb receptor subtype, which decreases neurotransmitter function; decreases frequency, severity of muscle spasms
Uses: Spasticity in spinal cord injury, multiple sclerosis
Unlabeled uses: Pain in trigeminal neuralgia, hiccups

DOSAGE AND ROUTES

• *Adult:* **PO** 5 mg tid × 3 days, then 10 mg tid × 3 days, then 15 mg tid × 3 days, then 20 mg tid × 3 days, then titrated to response, not to exceed 80 mg/day. **IT:** Use implantable intrathecal **INF** pump; use screening trial of 3 separate **BOL** doses if needed 24 hr apart (50 mcg/ml, 75 mcg/1.5 ml, 100 mcg/2 ml). Patients who do not respond to 100 mcg should not be considered for chronic **IT** therapy. Initial: double screening dose that produced result and give over 24 hr: increase by 10%-30% q24h only. Maintenance: 1200-1500 mcg/day

• *Child >2 yr:* **PO** 10-15 mg/kg/day divided q8h titrate every 3 days by 5-15 mg/day to max 40 mg/day

• *Child ≥8 yr:* as above, max 60 mg/day

• *Child:* **IT** Initial test dose same as adult; for small children, initial dose of 25 mcg/dose may be used; 25-1200 mcg/day infusion, titrated to response in screening phase

Available forms: Tabs 10, 20 mg; intrathecal inj 10 mg/20 ml (500 mcg/ml), 10 mg/5 ml (2000 mcg/ml); pharmacy can prepare extemperaneous liquid preparations

SIDE EFFECTS

CNS: Dizziness, weakness, fatigue, drowsiness, headache, *disorientation,* insomnia, paresthesias, tremors; **seizures, life-threatening CNS depression** (IT)
CV: Hypotension, chest pain, palpitations, edema, **cardiovascular collapse (IT)**
EENT: Nasal congestion, blurred vision, mydriasis, tinnitus
GI: Nausea, constipation, *vomiting,* increased AST, alk phos, abdominal pain, dry mouth, anorexia
GU: Urinary frequency, hematuria

✦ Canada only — Side effects: *italics* = common; **bold** = life-threatening

INTEG: Rash, pruritus
RESP: Dyspnea; respiratory failure (IT)
Contraindications: Hypersensitivity
Precautions: Pregnancy (C), peptic ulcer disease, renal/hepatic disease, stroke, seizure disorder, diabetes mellitus, lactation, geriatric

PHARMACOKINETICS

PO: Onset 3-4 days, peak 2-3 hr, duration >8 hr, half-life 2½-4 hr, partially metabolized in liver, excreted in urine (unchanged)
INTRATHECAL: CSF levels with plasma levels 100 times oral route; peak 4 hr, duration 4-8 hr
BOLUS: Onset ½-1 hr
CONT INF: Onset 6-8 hr, peak 24-48 hr

INTERACTIONS

Increase: CNS depression—alcohol, tricyclics, opiates, barbiturates, sedatives, hypnotics, MAOIs
Drug/Herb
Increase: CNS depression—chamomile, hops, kava, skullcap, valerian
Drug/Lab Test
Increase: AST, alk phos, blood glucose

NURSING CONSIDERATIONS
Assess:
• B/P, weight, blood glucose, and hepatic function periodically
🅐 For increased seizure activity in seizure disorders; this drug decreases seizure threshold
• I&O ratio; check for urinary frequency
• EEG in epileptic patients; poor seizure control has occurred in patients taking this drug
• Allergic reactions: rash, fever, respiratory distress
• Severe weakness, numbness in extremities
• Tolerance: increased need for medication, more frequent requests for medication, increased pain
• For withdrawal symptoms: CNS depression, dizziness, drowsiness, psychiatric symptoms

Administer:
PO route
• With meals for GI symptoms
IT route
• For screening, dilute to a concentration of 50 mcg/ml with NaCl for inj (preservative-free), give test dose over 1 min; watch for decreasing muscle tone or frequency of spasm; if inadequate, use 2 more test doses q24h; maintenance infusion via implantable pump 500-2000 mg/ml
• Dosage, as individual titration is required
• Do not use IT inj IV, IM, SUBCUT, epidural
Additive compatibilities: Morphine
Perform/provide:
• Storage in tight container at room temperature
• Assistance with ambulation if dizziness or drowsiness occurs
Evaluate:
• Therapeutic response: decreased pain, spasticity
Teach patient/family:
• Not to discontinue medication quickly; hallucinations, spasticity, tachycardia will occur; drug should be tapered off over 1-2 wk
• Not to take with alcohol, other CNS depressants
• To avoid hazardous activities if drowsiness or dizziness occurs; rise slowly to prevent orthostatic hypotension
• To avoid using OTC medication: cough preparations, antihistamines, unless directed by prescriber
• To notify prescriber of nausea, headache, tinnitus, insomnia, confusion, constipation, inadequate, painful urination continues
• May require 1-2 months for full response
Treatment of overdose: Induce emesis of conscious patient, lavage, dialysis, physostigmine to reduce life-threatening CNS side effects

---

🅐 Safety alert   *"Tall Man" lettering

balsalazide (℞)
(ball-sal′a-zide)
Colazal
Func. class.: GI antiinflammatory
Chem. class.: Salicylate derivative

Do not confuse:
Colazal/Clozaril
Action: Delivered intact to the colon, bioconverted to 5-ASA
Uses: Active, mild to moderate ulcerative colitis

DOSAGE AND ROUTES
• *Adult:* **PO** 2.25 g tid × 8 wk, may take up to 12 wk
Available forms: Tabs 750 mg

SIDE EFFECTS
CNS: Headache, insomnia, fatigue, fever, dizziness
EENT: Dry eyes, rhinitis, sinusitis, watery eyes, blurred vision
GI: Nausea, vomiting, abdominal pain, diarrhea, rectal bleeding, flatulence, dyspepsia, dry mouth, constipation
MS: Arthralgia, back pain, myalgia
SYST: **Anaphylaxis**
Contraindications: Hypersensitivity to salicylates
Precautions: Pregnancy (B), child <14 yr, lactation; pyloric stenosis

PHARMACOKINETICS
PO: Low and variably absorbed, peak 1½ hr, excreted in urine as metabolites, plasma protein binding 99%

INTERACTIONS
Drug/Lab Test
Increase: AST, ALT, GGT, LDH, bilirubin, alk phos
False positive: Urinary glucose test

NURSING CONSIDERATIONS
Assess:
• Renal studies: BUN, creatinine, urinalysis (long-term therapy)

• Allergic reaction: rash, dermatitis, urticaria, pruritus, dyspnea, bronchospasm
Administer:
• Do not break, crush, or chew tabs
• With food in evenly divided doses
• With resuscitative equipment available; severe allergic reactions may occur
• Total daily dose evenly spaced to minimize GI intolerance
Perform/provide:
• Storage in tight, light-resistant container at room temperature
Evaluate:
• Therapeutic response: absence of fever, mucus in stools, resolution of symptoms of ulcerative colitis
Teach patient/family:
• To notify prescriber if symptoms do not improve, if rash, hives, or respiratory problems occur

⚠ High Alert

basiliximab (℞)
(bas-ih-liks′ih-mab)
Simulect
Func. class.: Immunosuppressant
Chem. class.: Murine/human monoclonal antibody (interleukin-2) receptor antagonist

Action: Binds to and blocks the IL-2 receptor, which is selectively expressed on the surface of activated T lymphocytes; impairs the immune system to antigenic challenges
Uses: Acute allograft rejection in renal transplant patients when used with cycloSPORINE and corticosteroids

DOSAGE AND ROUTES
• *Adult:* **IV** 20 mg × 2 doses; 1st dose within 2 hr before transplant surgery; 2nd dose given 4 days after transplantation
• *Child 2-15 yr:* **IV** 12 mg/m² × 2 doses; 1st dose within 2 hr before transplant surgery; 2nd dose given 4 days after transplantation
Available forms: Powder for inj 20 mg

SIDE EFFECTS

CNS: Pyrexia, chills, tremors, headache, insomnia, weakness
CV: Chest pain, angina, **cardiac failure,** hypotension, *hypertension, edema*
GI: Vomiting, nausea, diarrhea, constipation, abdominal pain, **GI bleeding,** *gingival hyperplasia, stomatitis*
INTEG: Acne, pruritus
META: Acidosis, hypercholesterolemia, hyperuricemia, hyperkalemia, hypocalcemia, hypokalemia, hypophosphatemia
MISC: Infection, moniliasis, **anaphylaxis**
MS: Arthralgia, myalgia
RESP: Dyspnea, wheezing, **pulmonary edema,** *cough*
Contraindications: Hypersensitivity, exposure to viral infections, lactation
Precautions: Pregnancy (B), infections, geriatric, children

PHARMACOKINETICS

Peak ½ hr (adults) terminal half-life 7 days (adult), 9½ days (children)

INTERACTIONS

• Immunosuppression: other immunosuppressants
Drug/Herb
Increase: immunosuppression—astragalus, echinacea, melatonin, safflower
Decrease: immunosuppression—ginseng, maitake, mistletoe, schisandra, St. John's wort, turmeric
Drug/Lab Test
Increase: Cholesterol, BUN, uric acid, creatinine, K, Ca, blood glucose, Hgb, Hct
Decrease: Hgb, Hct, platelets, magnesium, phosphate

NURSING CONSIDERATIONS

Assess:
• For infection: increased temp, WBC, sputum, urine
• Blood studies: Hgb, WBC, platelets during treatment qmo; if leukocytes are <3000/mm³, drug should be discontinued
• Hepatic studies: alk phos, AST, ALT, bilirubin
• Hepatotoxicity: dark urine, jaundice, itching, light-colored stools; drug should be discontinued
⚠ Anaphylaxis, hypersensitivity: dyspnea, wheezing, rash, pruritus, hypotension, tachycardia; if severe hypersensitivity reactions occur, drug should not be used again
Administer:
• All medications PO if possible; avoid IM inj, since infection may occur
IV route
• After adding 5 ml sterile water for inj, shake gently to dissolve, reconstitute to a vol of 50 ml with 0.9% NaCl or D₅, gently invert bag, do not shake, give over ½ hr, do not admix
Evaluate:
• Therapeutic response: absence of graft rejection
Teach patient/family:
• To report fever, chills, sore throat, fatigue, since serious infection may occur
• To avoid crowds, persons with known upper respiratory infections
• To use contraception during treatment

---

beclomethasone (℞)
(be-kloe-meth'a-sone)
Beclodisk ♦, Beclovent, QVAR, Vanceril, Vanceril Double Strength
Func. class.: Corticosteroid, synthetic
Chem. class.: Glucocorticoid

Do not confuse:
Vanceril/Vancenase
Action: Prevents inflammation by suppression of migration of polymorphonuclear leukocytes, fibroblasts, reversal of increased capillary permeability and lysosomal stabilization; does not suppress hypothalamus and pituitary function
Uses: Chronic asthma, rhinitis

⚠ Safety alert   *"Tall Man" lettering

DOSAGE AND ROUTES

• *Adult:* **INH** 2-4 puffs bid-qid, max 20 inhalations/day (42 mcg/actuation); 2 puffs bid, max 10 **INH**/day (84 mcg/actuation)

• *Child 6-12 yr:* **INH** 1-2 puffs tid-qid, max 10 **INH**/day (42 mcg/actuations); 2 puffs bid, max 5 **INH**/day (84 mcg/actuations)

Available forms: Aerosol 40, 80, 250 ✿ mcg/actuation; INH cap 100 ✿, 200 ✿ mcg

SIDE EFFECTS

CNS: Headache

EENT: Hoarseness, candidal infections of oral cavity, sore throat

GI: Dry mouth, dyspepsia

MISC: **Angioedema, adrenal insufficiency,** facial edema, Churg-Strauss syndrome

RESP: **Bronchospasm,** wheezing, cough

Contraindications: Hypersensitivity, status asthmaticus (primary treatment), nonasthmatic bronchial disease; bacterial, fungal, viral infections of mouth, throat, lungs

Precautions: Pregnancy (C), nasal disease/surgery, lactation, children <12 yr

PHARMACOKINETICS

INH: Onset 10 min, excreted in feces, urine (metabolites), half-life 2.8 hr, crosses placenta, metabolized in lungs, liver (by CYP3A)

NURSING CONSIDERATIONS

Assess:

• For fungal infection in mucous membranes

• Adrenal function periodically for HPA axis suppression during prolonged therapy, monitor growth/development

Administer:

• INH with water to decrease possibility of fungal infections

• Titrated dose, use lowest effective dose

Perform/provide:

• Gum, rinsing of mouth for dry mouth

Evaluate:

• Therapeutic response: decreased dyspnea, wheezing, dry crackles

Teach patient/family:

• To carry or wear ID as steroid user

• To gargle/rinse mouth after each use to prevent oral fungal infections

• That in times of stress, systemic corticosteroids may be needed to prevent adrenal insufficiency; do not discontinue oral drug abruptly, taper slowly

• To notify prescriber if therapeutic response decreases; dosage adjustment may be needed

• Proper administration technique

• To wash inhaler with warm water and dry after each use

• All aspects of drug usage, including cushingoid symptoms

• The symptoms of adrenal insufficiency: nausea, anorexia, fatigue, dizziness, dyspnea, weakness, joint pain, depression

---

beclomethasone nasal agent
See Appendix C

---

benazepril (℞)
(ben-aze'uh-pril)
Lotensin
Func. class.: Antihypertensive
Chem. class.: Angiotensin-converting enzyme (ACE) inhibitor

Do not confuse:
Lotensin/Lioresal/Loniten

Action: Selectively suppresses renin-angiotensin-aldosterone system; inhibits ACE, preventing conversion of angiotensin I to angiotensin II

Uses: Hypertension, alone or in combination with thiazide diuretics

Unlabeled uses: CHF

DOSAGE AND ROUTES

• *Adult:* **PO** 10 mg daily initially, then 20-40 mg/day divided bid or daily (with-

---

out a diuretic); 5 mg **PO** daily (with a diuretic); max 80 mg daily
• *Geriatric:* **PO** 5-10 mg/day initially
Renal dose
• *Adult:* **PO** CCr <30 ml/min 5 mg **PO** daily, max 40 mg/day
Available forms: Tabs 5, 10, 20, 40 mg

SIDE EFFECTS

CNS: Anxiety, hypertonia, insomnia, paresthesia, headache, dizziness, fatigue
CV: Hypotension, postural hypotension, syncope, palpitations, angina
GI: Nausea, constipation, vomiting, gastritis, melena, diarrhea
GU: Increased BUN, creatinine, decreased libido, impotence, urinary tract infection
INTEG: Rash, flushing, sweating
META: Hyperkalemia, hyponatremia
MISC: **Angioedema**
MS: Arthralgia, arthritis, myalgia
RESP: Cough, asthma, bronchitis, dyspnea, sinusitis

Contraindications: Pregnancy (D) 2nd/3rd trimester, hypersensitivity to ACE inhibitors, lactation, children
Precautions: Pregnancy (C) 1st trimester, impaired renal/hepatic function, dialysis patients, hypovolemia, blood dyscrasias, CHF, COPD, asthma, geriatric, bilateral renal artery stenosis

PHARMACOKINETICS

PO: Peak 1-2 hr fasting, 2-4 hr after food, protein binding 89%-95%, half-life 10-11 hr, metabolized by liver (metabolites), excreted in urine 33%

INTERACTIONS

Increase: hypotension—phenothiazines, nitrates, acute alcohol ingestion, diuretics, other antihypertensives
Increase: hyperkalemia—potassium-sparing diuretics, potassium supplements
Increase: myelosuppression—azathioprine
Increase: serum levels of lithium, digoxin
Decrease: hypotensive effects—NSAIDs

Drug/Herb
Increase: toxicity/death—aconite
Increase: antihypertensive effect—barberry, betony, black catechu, black cohosh, bloodroot, broom, burdock, cat's claw, dandelion, goldenseal, hawthorn, Irish moss, Jamaican dogwood, kelp, khella, mistletoe, parsley
Increase or decrease: antihypertensive effect—astragalus, cola tree
Decrease: antihypertensive effect—coltsfoot, guarana, khat, licorice, pineapple, yohimbe
Drug/Lab Test
Increase: AST, ALT, alk phos, bilirubin, uric acid, blood glucose
Positive: ANA titer
False positive: ANA titer

NURSING CONSIDERATIONS
Assess:
• Blood studies: neutrophils, decreased platelets; WBC with diff baseline and q3mo, if neutrophils <1000/mm^3 discontinue treatment, recommended in collagen-vascular disease
• B/P at peak/trough level of drug, orthostatic hypotension, syncope when used with diuretic
• Renal studies: protein, BUN, creatinine; increased levels may indicate nephrotic syndrome; monitor urine for protein, increased LFTs, uric acid and glucose may be increased
• Potassium levels, although hyperkalemia rarely occurs
• Allergic reactions: rash, fever, pruritus, urticaria; drug should be discontinued if antihistamines fail to help
• Renal symptoms: polyuria, oliguria, frequency, dysuria
• Edema in feet, legs daily, weight daily in CHF; monitor for cough
Administer:
• Do not discontinue drug abruptly
Perform/provide:
• Storage in tight container at 86° F (30° C) or less
Evaluate:
• Therapeutic response: decrease in B/P

Teach patient/family:

• Not to use OTC products (cough, cold, allergy) unless directed by prescriber; do not use salt substitutes containing potassium without consulting prescriber

• The importance of complying with dosage schedule, even if feeling better

• To notify prescriber of pregnancy, drug will need to be discontinued

• To rise slowly to sitting or standing position to minimize orthostatic hypotension

• To notify prescriber of mouth sores, sore throat, fever, swelling of hands or feet, irregular heartbeat, chest pain

• To report excessive perspiration, dehydration, vomiting, diarrhea; may lead to fall in B/P

• That drug may cause dizziness, fainting, light-headedness; may occur during first few days of therapy

• That drug may cause skin rash or impaired perspiration

• How to take B/P, and normal readings for age group

Treatment of overdose: 0.9% NaCl IV INF, hemodialysis

benzocaine topical
See Appendix C

Rarely Used

benzonatate (℞)
(ben-zoe′na-tate)
Tessalon Perles
Func. class.: Antitussive, nonopioid

Uses: Nonproductive cough

DOSAGE AND ROUTES

• *Adult and child:* **PO** 100 mg tid, not to exceed 600 mg/day
Contraindications: Hypersensitivity

Rarely Used

benzoyl peroxide (OTC)
(ben′zoe-ill per-ox′ide)
Func. class.: Antiacne medication

Uses: Mild to moderate acne

DOSAGE AND ROUTES

• *Adult and child:* **TOP** apply to affected area daily or bid
Contraindications: Hypersensitivity to benzoic acid derivatives

benztropine (℞)
(benz′troe-peen)
Apo-Benztropine ✦,
benztropine mesylate,
Cogentin
Func. class.: Cholinergic blocker, antiparkinson's agent
Chem. class.: Tertiary amine

Action: Blockade of central acetylcholine receptors
Uses: Parkinson's symptoms, EPS associated with neuroleptic drugs, acute dystonic reactions, hypersalivation

DOSAGE AND ROUTES
Drug-induced EPS

• *Adult:* **IM/IV** 1-4 mg daily-bid; give **PO** dose as soon as possible; **PO** 1-2 mg bid/tid, increase by 0.5 mg q5-6 days

• *Child:* **IM/IV** 0.02-0.05 mg/kg/dose 1-2 ×/day

• *Geriatric:* **PO** 0.5 mg daily-bid, increase by 0.5 mg q5-6 days
Parkinson's symptoms

• *Adult:* **PO** 1-2 mg/day in 1-2 divided doses, increase 0.5 mg q5-6 days titrated to patient response, max 6 mg daily
Acute dystonic reactions

• *Adult:* **IM/IV** 1-2 mg, may increase to 1-2 mg bid **(PO)**
Available forms: Tabs 0.5, 1, 2 mg; inj 1 mg/ml

Side effects: *italics* = common; **bold** = life-threatening

SIDE EFFECTS

CNS: Anxiety, restlessness, irritability, delusions, hallucinations, headache, sedation, depression, incoherence, dizziness, memory loss; *confusion,* delirium (geriatric)

CV: Palpitations, tachycardia, hypotension, bradycardia

EENT: Blurred vision, photophobia, dilated pupils, difficulty swallowing, dry eyes, mydriasis, increased intraocular tension, angle-closure glaucoma

GI: Dryness of mouth, constipation, nausea, vomiting, abdominal distress, **paralytic ileus,** epigastric distress

GU: Hesitancy, retention, dysuria

INTEG: Rash, urticaria, dermatoses

MISC: Increased temperature, flushing, decreased sweating, **hyperthermia, heat stroke,** numbness of fingers

MS: Muscular weakness, cramping

Contraindications: Hypersensitivity, narrow-angle glaucoma, myasthenia gravis, GI/GU obstruction, child <3 yr, peptic ulcer, megacolon, prostate hypertrophy

Precautions: Pregnancy (C), lactation, geriatric, tachycardia, renal/hepatic disease, drug abuse history, dysrhythmias, hypotension, hypertension, psychiatric patients, children

PHARMACOKINETICS

IM/IV: Onset 15 min, duration 6-10 hr
PO: Onset 1 hr, duration 6-10 hr

INTERACTIONS

Increase: anticholinergic effect—antihistamines, phenothiazines, tricyclics, disopyramide, quinidine

Decrease: absorption—antidiarrheals

Drug/Herb

Increase: benztropine effect—butterbur, jimsonweed

Increase: constipation—black catechu

Decrease: benztropine effect—jaborandi, kava, pill-bearing spurge

NURSING CONSIDERATIONS

Assess:

• I&O ratio; commonly causes decreased urinary output; urinary hesitancy, retention; palpate bladder if retention occurs

• Parkinsonism, EPS: shuffling gait, muscle rigidity, involuntary movements, loss of balance

• Constipation; increase fluids, bulk, exercise if this occurs

• Mental status: affect, mood, CNS depression, worsening of mental symptoms during early therapy

• Use caution in hot weather; drug may increase susceptibility to stroke by decreasing sweating

• For benztropine "buzz" or "high," patients may imitate EPS

Administer:

PO route

• With or after meals to prevent GI upset; may give with fluids other than water

• At bedtime to avoid daytime drowsiness in patient with parkinsonism

IM route

• Use for dystonic reactions only

IV route

• Undiluted IV (1 mg = 1 ml) give 1 mg/1 min; keep in bed for at least 1 hr after dose

Syringe compatibilities: Metoclopramide

Y-site compatibilities: Fluconazole, tacrolimus

Perform/provide:

• Storage at room temperature

• Hard candy, gum, frequent drinks, to relieve dry mouth

Evaluate:

• Therapeutic response: absence of involuntary movements

Teach patient/family:

• That tabs may be crushed and mixed with food

• Not to discontinue this drug abruptly; to taper off over 1 wk, or withdrawal symptoms may occur (EPS, tremors, insomnia, tachycardia, restlessness)

• To avoid driving, other hazardous activities; drowsiness may occur

A Safety alert   *"Tall Man" lettering

• To avoid OTC medication: cough, cold preparations with alcohol, antihistamines unless directed by prescriber
• To change positions slowly to prevent orthostatic hypotension
• To use good oral hygiene, frequent sips of water, sugarless gum for dry mouth

---

Rarely Used

beractant (R)
(ber-ak'tant)
Survanta
Func. class.: Natural lung surfactant

Uses: Prevention and treatment (rescue) of respiratory distress syndrome in premature infants

DOSAGE AND ROUTES

• **INTRATRACHEAL INSTILL:** 4 doses can be administered in the 1st 48 hr of life; give doses no more frequently than q6h; each dose is 100 mg of phospholipids/kg birth weight (4 ml/kg)

---

betamethasone (R)
(bay-ta-meth'a-sone)
Betnelan ♣, Betnesol ♣,
Celestone, Cel-U-Jec,
Selestoject ♣
Func. class.: Corticosteroid, synthetic, long-acting

Action: Decreases inflammation by suppressing migration of polymorphonuclear leukocytes, fibroblasts, reversal of increased capillary permeability and lysosomal stabilization
Uses: Immunosuppression, severe inflammation, prevention of neonatal respiratory distress syndrome (by administration to mother)

DOSAGE AND ROUTES

• *Adult:* **PO** 0.6-7.2 mg daily; **IM/IV** 0.6-7.2 mg daily in joint or soft tissue (sodium phosphate)
• *Child:* **PO** 17.5 mcg/kg/day in 3 di-

vided doses; **IM** 17.5 mcg/kg/day in 3 divided doses every 3rd day or 5.8-8.75 mcg/kg/day as a single dose (adrenal insufficiency)
• *Child:* **PO** 62.5-250 mcg/kg/day in 3 divided doses; **IM** 20.8-125 mcg/kg/day of the base q12-24h (other uses)
Available forms: Tabs 500, 600 mcg; effervescent tabs 500 mcg ♣, syr 600 mcg/5 ml; ext rel tab 1 mg; sol for inj (phosphate) 3 mg/ml; susp for inj (phosphate/acetate) 6 mg/ml

SIDE EFFECTS

CNS: Depression, flushing, sweating, headache, bruising, mood changes
CV: Hypertension, **circulatory collapse, thrombophlebitis, embolism,** tachycardia, **necrotizing angiitis, CHF**
EENT: Fungal infections, increased intraocular pressure, blurred vision
GI: Diarrhea, nausea, abdominal distention, **GI hemorrhage,** *increased appetite,* **pancreatitis**
HEMA: **Thrombocytopenia**
INTEG: Acne, poor wound healing, ecchymosis, bruising, petechiae
MS: Fractures, osteoporosis, weakness
Contraindications: Psychosis, hypersensitivity, idiopathic thrombocytopenia, acute glomerulonephritis, amebiasis, fungal infections, nonasthmatic bronchial disease, child <2 yr, AIDS, TB
Precautions: Pregnancy (C), lactation, diabetes mellitus, glaucoma, osteoporosis, seizure disorders, ulcerative colitis, CHF, myasthenia gravis, renal disease, esophagitis, peptic ulcer

PHARMACOKINETICS

PO: Onset 1-2 hr, peak 1 hr, duration 3 days
IM/IV: Onset 10 min, peak 4-8 hr, duration 1-1½ days
Metabolized in liver, excreted in urine as steroids, crosses placenta

INTERACTIONS

Increase: GI bleeding—NSAIDs, alcohol, salicylates, indomethacin

---

Side effects: *italics* = common; **bold** = life-threatening

Increase: effects of betamethasone —erythromycin, ketoconazole, itraconazole, ritonavir, saquinavir, indinavir

Increase: hypokalemia—thiazides, loop diuretics, ticarcillin, amphotericin B, piperacillin

Increase: tendon rupture—fluoroquinolones

Decrease: action of betamethasone—barbiturates, rifampin, phenytoin

Decrease: effects of anticoagulants, antidiabetics, insulin, isoniazid, toxoids, vaccines, salicylates, oral contraceptives, somatrem, somatropin

Drug/Herb

Increase: hypokalemia—aloe, buckthorn, cascara sagrada, Chinese rhubarb, rhubarb, senna

Increase: corticosteroid effects—goldenseal, hawthorn, hops, lemon balm, licorice, lily of the valley, mistletoe, perilla, pheasant's eye, squill

Increase: hypokalemia—buckthorn, cascara sagrada, Chinese rhubarb

Drug/Food
• Grapefruit juice should be avoided

Drug/Lab Test

Increase: Cholesterol, sodium, blood glucose, uric acid, calcium, urine glucose

Decrease: Calcium, potassium, T_4, T_3, thyroid ^{131}I uptake test, urine 17-OHCS, 17-KS, PBI

False negative: Skin allergy tests

NURSING CONSIDERATIONS

Assess:
• Potassium, blood glucose, urine glucose while on long-term therapy; hypokalemia and hyperglycemia
• Weight daily; notify prescriber of weekly gain >5 lb
• B/P q4h, pulse; notify prescriber if chest pain occurs
• I&O ratio; be alert for decreasing urinary output and increasing edema
• Plasma cortisol levels during long-term therapy (normal level: 138-635 nmol/L SI units when drawn at 8 AM)

Administer:
PO route
• With food or milk to decrease GI symptoms
IM route
• Inj deeply in large muscle mass, rotate sites, avoid deltoid, use 21G needle
• In one dose in AM to prevent adrenal suppression, avoid SUBCUT administration; may damage tissue
IV route
• Only sodium phosphate product; give >1 min; may be given by IV INF in compatible sol
• After shaking suspension (parenteral)
• Titrated dose; use lowest effective dose
Y-site compatibilities: Heparin, hydrocortisone, potassium chloride, vit B/C

Perform/provide:
• Assistance with ambulation in patient with bone tissue disease to prevent fractures

Evaluate:
• Therapeutic response: ease of respirations, decreased inflammation
• Infection: increased temp, WBC even after withdrawal of medication; drug masks infection symptoms
• Potassium depletion: paresthesias, fatigue, nausea, vomiting, depression, polyuria, dysrhythmias, weakness
• Edema, hypertension, cardiac symptoms
• Mental status: affect, mood, behavioral changes, aggression

Teach patient/family:
• That ID as steroid user should be carried
• To notify prescriber if therapeutic response decreases; dosage adjustment may be needed
⚠ Not to discontinue abruptly; adrenal crisis can result
• To avoid OTC products: salicylates, alcohol in cough products, cold preparations unless directed by prescriber
• All aspects of drug usage including cushingoid symptoms
• The symptoms of adrenal insufficiency: nausea, anorexia, fatigue, dizziness, dyspnea, weakness, joint pain

---

---

betamethasone topical
See Appendix C

betamethasone (augmented) topical
See Appendix C

betaxolol ophthalmic
See Appendix C

bethanechol (R)
(be-than′e-kole)
bethanechol chloride,
Duvoid ✤, Urabeth,
Urecholine
Func. class.: Urinary tract stimulant, cholinergic
Chem. class.: Synthetic choline ester

Action: Stimulates muscarinic ACH receptors directly; mimics effects of parasympathetic nervous system stimulation; stimulates gastric motility, stimulates micturition; increases lower esophageal sphincter pressure

Uses: Urinary retention (postoperative, postpartum), neurogenic atony of bladder with retention

Unlabeled uses: GERD

DOSAGE AND ROUTES

• *Adult:* **PO** 10-50 mg bid-qid; **SUBCUT** 5 mg tid-qid prn
• *Child:* **PO** 0.6 mg/kg/day divided in 3-4 doses/day

Test dose
• *Adult:* **SUBCUT** 2.5 mg repeated 15-30 min intervals × 4 doses to determine effective dose

GERD (Unlabeled)
• *Adult:* **PO** 25 mg qid
Available forms: Tabs 5, 10, 25, 50 mg; inj 5 mg/ml

✤ Canada only

SIDE EFFECTS

CNS: Dizziness, headache, malaise
CV: Hypotension, bradycardia, reflex tachycardia, **cardiac arrest, circulatory collapse**
EENT: Miosis, increased salivation, lacrimation, blurred vision
GI: Nausea, bloody diarrhea, belching, vomiting, cramps, fecal incontinence
GU: Urgency
INTEG: Rash, urticaria, flushing, increased sweating
RESP: **Acute asthma, dyspnea, bronchoconstriction**

Contraindications: Hypersensitivity, severe bradycardia, asthma, severe hypotension, hyperthyroidism, peptic ulcer, parkinsonism, seizure disorders, CAD, COPD, coronary occlusion, mechanical obstruction, peritonitis, recent urinary or GI surgery, GI/GU obstruction
Precautions: Pregnancy (C), hypertension, lactation, child <8 yr

PHARMACOKINETICS

PO: Onset 30-90 min, duration 6 hr
SUBCUT: Onset 5-15 min, duration 2 hr

INTERACTIONS

Increase: severe hypotension—ganglionic blockers
Increase: action or toxicity—cholinergic agonists, anticholinesterase agents
Decrease: action of anticholinergics, procainamide, quinidine
Drug/Herb
Increase: cholinergic effect—jaborandi tree
Decrease: effects—jimsonweed, scopolia
Drug/Lab Test
Increase: AST, lipase/amylase, bilirubin, BSP

NURSING CONSIDERATIONS

Assess:
• B/P, pulse; observe after parenteral dose for 1 hr

Side effects: *italics* = common; **bold** = life-threatening

• I&O ratio; check for urinary retention or urge incontinence
• Bradycardia, hypotension, broncho-spasm, headache, dizziness, seizures, respiratory depression; drug should be discontinued if toxicity occurs

Administer:
• To avoid nausea and vomiting, take on an empty stomach

SUBCUT route
⚠ Parenteral dose by SUBCUT route; use of IM, IV may result in cardiac arrest
⚠ Only with atropine sulfate available for cholinergic crisis
• Only after all other cholinergics have been discontinued
• Increased doses if tolerance occurs

Perform/provide:
• Storage at room temperature
• Bedpan/urinal if given for urinary retention

Evaluate:
• Therapeutic response: absence of urinary retention, abdominal distention

Teach patient/family:
• To take drug exactly as prescribed; 1 hr before meals or 2 hr after meals
• To make position changes slowly; orthostatic hypotension may occur

Treatment of overdose: Administer atropine 0.6-1.2 mg IV or IM (adult)

⚠ High Alert

bevacizumab (℞)
(beh-va-kiz′you-mab)
Avastin
Func. class.: Antineoplastic—miscellaneous
Chem. class.: Monoclonal antibody

Action: DNA-derived monoclonal antibody selectively binds to and inhibits activity of human vascular endothelial growth factor to reduce microvascular growth and inhibition of metastatic disease progression
Uses: Metastatic carcinoma of the colon or rectum in combination with 5-FU IV

Unlabeled uses: Adjunctive in breast, renal cancer

DOSAGE AND ROUTES
• *Adult:* **IV INF** 5 mg/kg q14d given over 90 min; if well tolerated, the next infusion may be given over 60 min; if 60-min infusions are well tolerated, subsequent infusions may be given over 30 min
Available forms: Inj 25 mg/ml

SIDE EFFECTS
CNS: **Asthenia,** dizziness
CV: **Deep vein thrombosis,** hypertension, hypotension, **hypertensive crisis**
GI: Nausea, vomiting, anorexia, diarrhea, constipation, abdominal pain, colitis, stomatitis, **GI hemorrhage**
GU: Proteinuria, urinary frequency/urgency, **nephrotic syndrome**
HEMA: **Leukopenia, neutropenia, thrombocytopenia**
META: Bilirubinemia, hypokalemia
MISC: **Exfoliative dermatitis, hemorrhage**
RESP: Dyspnea, upper respiratory tract infection
Contraindications: Hypersensitivity
Precautions: Pregnancy (C), lactation, children, geriatric, CHF, blood dyscrasias, CV disease, hypertension

PHARMACOKINETICS
Half-life 20 days, steady state 100 days

INTERACTIONS
None known

NURSING CONSIDERATIONS
Assess:
• B/P q3-4wk, more frequently if hypertension develops
• For symptoms of infection; may be masked by drug
• CNS reaction: dizziness, confusion
• For CHF: crackles, jugular vein distention, dyspnea during treatment
⚠ For GI perforation, serious bleeding, nephrotic syndrome, hypertensive crisis, drug should be discontinued permanently;

proteinuria or surgery, drug should be discontinued temporarily

Administer:
• Do not give by IV bolus, or IV push
• Give as IV infusion over 90 min for first dose and 60 min thereafter, if well tolerated

Evaluate:
• Therapeutic response: decrease in size of tumors

Teach patient/family:
• To avoid hazardous tasks, since confusion, dizziness may occur
• To report signs of infection: sore throat, fever, diarrhea, vomiting
• Not to become pregnant while taking this drug or for several months after discontinuing treatment
• Notify prescriber if pregnant or planning a pregnancy
• Report bleeding, changes in urinary patterns, edema
• Avoid immunizations

---

bexarotene (℞)
Targretin
Func. class.: Retinoid, 2nd generation

Action: Selectively binds and activates retinoid X receptors (RXRs) that are partially responsible for cellular proliferation and differentiation. Inhibits some tumor cells

Uses: Cutaneous T-cell lymphoma
Unlabeled uses: Breast cancer, psoriasis (phase II)

DOSAGE AND ROUTES

• *Adult:* **PO** 300 mg/day/m^2, may increase to 400 mg/day with proper monitoring

Available forms: Caps 75 mg

SIDE EFFECTS

CNS: Headache, fatigue, lethargy
GI: Nausea, abdominal pain, diarrhea, **acute pancreatitis**
HEMA: **Leukopenia, neutropenia, anemia**

INTEG: Rash, asthenia, dry skin
SYST: Infection, hypothyroidism

Contraindications: Pregnancy (X), hypersensitivity to retinoids

Precautions: Lactation, sunburn, renal/hepatic disease, children

PHARMACOKINETICS

Unknown

INTERACTIONS

• Limit intake of vit A ≤15,000 international units/day
Increase: action of antidiabetics
Increase: bexarotene levels—azole anti-infectives
Decrease: bexarotene levels—barbiturates, rifampins, phenytoin
Decrease: action of tamoxifen, oral contraceptives

Drug/Food
Increase: bexarotene levels—grapefruit juice

NURSING CONSIDERATIONS

Assess:
• Area of body involved, what helps or aggravates condition; cysts, dryness, itching
• Cholesterol, HDL, triglycerides may be elevated
• CBC for leukopenia, neutropenia, anemia

Administer:
• With food

Perform/provide:
• Storage at room temperature

Evaluate:
• Therapeutic response: decrease in size and number of lesions

Teach patient/family:
• To watch for hypoglycemia in diabetic patients on insulin
• To limit vit A intake to ≤15,000 international units/day to avoid toxicity; not to use grapefruit or grapefruit juice
• To avoid sunlight, sunlamps, or use protective clothing, sunscreen

---

• To avoid pregnancy while taking this drug and ≥1 mo after discontinuing therapy; two forms of birth control recommended; avoid breastfeeding; men need to use contraception also

bicalutamide (℞)
(bye-kal-u′ta-mide)
Casodex
Func. class.: Antineoplastic hormone
Chem. class.: Nonsteroidal anti-androgen

Action: Binds to cytosol androgen in target tissue, which competitively inhibits the action to androgens
Uses: Prostate cancer in combination with luteinizing hormone–releasing hormone (LHRH) analog

DOSAGE AND ROUTES
• *Adult:* **PO** 50 mg daily with LHRH
Available forms: Tabs 50 mg

SIDE EFFECTS
CNS: Dizziness, paresthesia, insomnia, anxiety, neuropathy, headache
CV: **CHF,** edema, *hot flashes,* hypertension, chest pain,
GI: Diarrhea, constipation, nausea, vomiting, increased hepatic enzymes, anorexia, dry mouth, melena, abdominal pain
GU: Nocturia, hematuria, UTI, impotence, gynecomastia, urinary incontinence, frequency, dysuria, retention, urgency, breast tenderness, decreased libido
INTEG: Rash, sweating, dry skin, pruritus, alopecia
MISC: Infection, anemia, dyspnea, bone pain, headache, asthenia, *back pain,* flu-like symptoms
Contraindications: Pregnancy (X), hypersensitivity
Precautions: Renal/hepatic disease, geriatric, lactation

PHARMACOKINETICS
Well absorbed, peak 31½ hr, metabolized by liver, excreted in urine, feces; half-life 5.8 days

INTERACTIONS
Increase: anticoagulation—warfarin
Drug/Lab Test
Increase: AST, ALT, bilirubin, BUN, creatinine
Decrease: Hgb, WBC

NURSING CONSIDERATIONS
Assess:
• For diarrhea, constipation, nausea, vomiting
• For hot flashes, gynecomastia (assure patient that these are common side effects)
• Prostate specific antigen (PSA), LFTs
Administer:
• At same time each day, either AM or PM, with/without food
• With LHRH treatment; start at same time for both drugs
Evaluate:
• Therapeutic response: decreased tumor size, decreased spread of malignancy
Teach patient/family:
• To recognize, report signs of anemia, hepatoxicity, renal toxicity
• That hair may be lost, but this is reversible after therapy is completed
• Not to use other products, unless approved by prescriber
• To report severe diarrhea
• To use contraception while taking this drug

bimatoprost ophthalmic
See Appendix C

biperiden (℞)

(bye-per'i-den)

Akineton

Func. class.: Antiparkinson agent, anticholinergic

Action: Centrally acting competitive anticholinergic

Uses: Parkinson's symptoms, EPS secondary to neuroleptic drug therapy

DOSAGE AND ROUTES

Extrapyramidal symptoms

• *Adult:* **PO** 2 mg daily-tid; **IM/IV** 2 mg q30min, if needed, not to exceed 8 mg/24 hr

• *Child:* **IM** 40 mcg/kg or 1.2 mg/m^2, may repeat q½h

Parkinson's symptoms

• *Adult:* **PO** 2 mg tid-qid; max 16 mg/24 hr

Available forms: Tabs 2 mg; inj 5 mg/ml (lactate)

SIDE EFFECTS

CNS: Confusion, anxiety, restlessness, irritability, delusions, hallucinations, headache, sedation, depression, incoherence, dizziness, euphoria, tremors, memory loss

CV: Palpitations, tachycardia, postural hypotension, bradycardia

EENT: Blurred vision, photophobia, dilated pupils, difficulty swallowing, mydriasis, increased intraocular tension, angle-closure glaucoma

GI: Dryness of mouth, constipation, nausea, vomiting, abdominal distress, **paralytic ileus**

GU: Hesitancy, retention, dysuria

INTEG: Rash, urticaria, dermatoses

MISC: Increased temp, flushing, decreased sweating, hyperthermia, **heat stroke,** numbness of fingers

MS: Weakness, cramping

Contraindications: Hypersensitivity, narrow-angle glaucoma, myasthenia gravis, GI/GU obstruction, megacolon, stenosing peptic ulcers, prostatic hypertrophy

Precautions: Pregnancy (C), geriatric, lactation, tachycardia, dysrhythmias, renal/hepatic disease, drug abuse, hypotension, cognitive impairment, Alzheimer's disease, hypertension, psychiatric patients, children <8 yr

PHARMACOKINETICS

IM/IV: Onset 15 min, duration 6-10 hr

PO: Onset 1 hr, duration 6-10 hr

INTERACTIONS

Increase: schizophrenic symptoms—haloperidol

Increase: anticholinergic effect—antihistamines, phenothiazines, amantadine, tricyclics, quinidine

Increase: sedation—alcohol

Decrease: biperiden absorption—antacids, antidiarrheals

Drug/Herb

Increase: biperiden effect—butterbur, jimsonweed

Increase: constipation—black catechu

Decrease: biperiden effect—jaborandi tree, kava, pill-bearing spurge

NURSING CONSIDERATIONS

Assess:

• I&O ratio; retention commonly causes decreased urinary output

• Parkinsonism, EPS: shuffling gait, muscle rigidity, involuntary movements

• Patient response if anticholinergics are given

• Urinary hesitancy, retention; palpate bladder if retention occurs

• Constipation; increase fluids, bulk, exercise if this occurs, stool softeners, laxatives may be needed

• For tolerance over long-term therapy; dose may have to be increased or changed

• Mental status: affect, mood, CNS depression, confusion, dementia, worsening of mental symptoms during early therapy

Administer:

PO route

• With or after meals to prevent GI upset; may give with fluids other than water

---

• At bedtime to avoid daytime drowsiness in patients with parkinsonism

IM/IV route

• With patient recumbent to prevent postural hypotension, give undiluted 2 mg or less over 1 min or more

Perform/provide:

• Inspection visually for particulate or discoloration

• Storage at room temperature, in light-resistant container

• Hard candy, gum, frequent drinks to relieve dry mouth

Evaluate:

• Therapeutic response: absence of involuntary movements

Teach patient/family:

• To use caution in hot weather; drug may increase susceptibility to heat stroke, decreases sweating

• Not to discontinue this drug abruptly; to taper off over 1 wk

• To avoid driving, other hazardous activities; drowsiness may occur

• To avoid OTC medication: cough, cold preparations with alcohol, antihistamines unless directed by prescriber

---

bisacodyl (Ʀ, otc)

(bis-a-koe′dill)
Bisac-Evac, Bisaco-Lax, Bisacolax ✦, Carter's Little Pills, Dacodyl, Deficol, Dulcagen, Dulcolax, Feen-a-Mint, Fleet Laxative, Laxit ✦, Modane, Reliable Gentle Laxative, Therelax
Func. class.: Laxative, stimulant
Chem. class.: Diphenylmethane

Action: Acts directly on intestine by increasing motor activity; thought to irritate colonic intramural plexus

Uses: Short-term treatment of constipation, bowel or rectal preparation for surgery, examination

DOSAGE AND ROUTES

• *Adult and child ≥12 yr:* **PO** 10-15 mg in PM or AM; may use up to 30 mg for bowel or rectal preparation; **RECT** 10 mg, single dose; 30 ml enema

• *Child 6-11 yr:* **PO** 5 mg as a single dose; **RECT** 5 mg as a single dose

Available forms: Tabs 5 mg; enteric-coated tabs 5 mg; del rel tabs 10 mg; supp 5, 10 mg; enema 10 mg/30 ml

SIDE EFFECTS

CNS: Muscle weakness
GI: Nausea, vomiting, anorexia, cramps, diarrhea, rectal burning (suppositories)
META: Protein-losing enteropathy, alkalosis, hypokalemia, **tetany,** electrolyte, fluid imbalances

Contraindications: Hypersensitivity, rectal fissures, abdominal pain, nausea, vomiting, appendicitis, acute surgical abdomen, ulcerated hemorrhoids, acute hepatitis, fecal impaction, intestinal/biliary tract obstruction

Precautions: Pregnancy (C), lactation

PHARMACOKINETICS

PO: Onset 6-10 hr
RECT: Onset 15-60 min
Small amounts metabolized by liver; excreted in urine, bile, feces, breast milk

INTERACTIONS

Increase: gastric irritation—antacids, milk, H_2-blockers, gastric acid pump inhibitors
Drug/Herb
Increase: action—flax, lily of the valley, pheasant's eye, senna, squill

NURSING CONSIDERATIONS

Assess:

• Blood, urine electrolytes if drug is used often by patient

• I&O ratio to identify fluid loss

• Cause of constipation; identify whether fluids, bulk, or exercise missing from lifestyle, constipating drugs

• Cramping, rectal bleeding, nausea, vomiting; if these symptoms occur, drug should be discontinued

---

Administer:

PO route

• Swallow tabs whole; do not break, crush, or chew tabs

• Alone only with water for better absorption; do not take within 1 hr of other drugs or within 1 hr of antacids, milk, H_2 antagonists, proton pump inhibitors

• In AM or PM

Evaluate:

• Therapeutic response: decrease in constipation

Teach patient/family:

• Not to use laxatives for long-term therapy; bowel tone will be lost

• That normal bowel movements do not always occur daily

• Not to use in presence of abdominal pain, nausea, vomiting

• To notify prescriber if constipation is unrelieved or if symptoms of electrolyte imbalance occur: muscle cramps, pain, weakness, dizziness

---

bismuth subsalicylate (otc)

(bis'muth sub-sal-iss'uh-late)
Bismatrol, Bismatrol Extra Strength, Bismed, Kaopectate, Kao-Tin, Kapectolin, K-pek, Peptic Relief, Pepto-Bismol, Pepto-Bismol Maximum Strength, Pink Bismuth ✿, PMS-Bismuth Subsalicylate
Func. class.: Antidiarrheal
Chem. class.: Salicylate

Action: Inhibits prostaglandin synthesis responsible for GI hypermotility; stimulates absorption of fluid and electrolytes

Uses: Diarrhea (cause undetermined), prevention of diarrhea when traveling; may be included to treat *Helicobacter pylori*

DOSAGE AND ROUTES

Antidiarrheal

• *Adult:* PO 524 mg q½hr or 1048 mg q1hr, max 4.2 mg/24 hr

• *Child 9-12 yr:* PO 262 mg q½-1hr, max 2.1 mg/24 hr

• *Child 6-9 yr:* PO 174.6 mg q½-1hr, max 1.4 mg/24 hr

• *Child 3-6 yr:* PO 88 mg q½-1hr, max 704 mg/24 hr

Available forms: Tabs 262 mg; chewable tabs 262, 300 mg; susp 262 mg/15 ml, 524 mg/15 ml

SIDE EFFECTS

CNS: Confusion, twitching
EENT: Hearing loss, tinnitus, metallic taste, blue gums, black tongue (chew tabs)
GI: Increased fecal impaction (high doses), dark stools
HEMA: Increased bleeding time

Contraindications: Child <3 yr, history of GI bleeding, renal disease, child with chickenpox, flulike symptoms

Precautions: Pregnancy (C), anticoagulant therapy, immobility, geriatric, lactation, gout, diabetes mellitus

PHARMACOKINETICS

PO: Onset 1 hr, peak 2 hr, duration 4 hr

INTERACTIONS

Increase: salicylate toxicity—salicylates
Increase: effects of oral anticoagulants, oral antidiabetics
Decrease: absorption of tetracycline
Drug/Herb
Increase: absorption of bismuth—sarsaparilla
Increase: antidiarrheal effect—nutmeg
Drug/Lab Test
Interference: Radiographic studies of GI system

NURSING CONSIDERATIONS

Assess:

• Electrolytes (K, Na, Cl) if diarrhea is severe or continues long term; assess skin turgor

---

Side effects: *italics* = common; **bold** = life-threatening

- Bowel pattern before drug therapy, after treatment

Administer:
PO route
- Increased fluids to rehydrate the patient
- Shake liquid before using

Evaluate:
- Therapeutic response: decreased diarrhea or absence of diarrhea when traveling

Teach patient/family:
- To chew or dissolve in mouth; do not swallow whole; shake liquid before using
- To avoid other salicylates unless directed by prescriber; not to give to children, possibility of Reye's syndrome
- That stools may turn black; tongue may darken; impaction may occur in debilitated patients
- To stop use if symptoms do not improve within 2 days or become worse, or if diarrhea is accompanied by high fever

---

bisoprolol (℞)
(bis-oh′pro-lole)
Zebeta
Func. class.: Antihypertensive
Chem. class.: β_1-Blocker

Do not confuse:
Zebeta/DiaBeta/Zetia
Action: Preferentially and competitively blocks stimulation of β_1-adrenergic receptors within cardiac muscle (decreases rate of SA node discharge, increases recovery time), slows conduction of AV node, decreases heart rate, which decreases O_2 consumption in myocardium; decreases renin-aldosterone-angiotensin system; inhibits β_2-receptors in bronchial and vascular smooth muscle at high doses
Uses: Mild to moderate hypertension
Unlabeled uses: Stable angina pectoris, stable CHF

DOSAGE AND ROUTES

- *Adult:* **PO** 5 mg daily; may increase if necessary to 20 mg daily; max 40 mg daily

Renal/hepatic dose
- *Adult:* **PO** 2.5 mg, titrate upward
Available forms: Tabs 5, 10 mg

SIDE EFFECTS

CNS: Vertigo, headache, insomnia, fatigue, dizziness, mental changes, memory loss, hallucinations, depression, lethargy, drowsiness, strange dreams, catatonia, peripheral neuropathy
CV: **Ventricular dysrhythmias, profound hypotension, bradycardia, CHF,** cold extremities, postural hypotension, **2nd- or 3rd-degree heart block**
EENT: Sore throat; dry, burning eyes
ENDO: Increased hypoglycemic response to insulin
GI: Nausea, diarrhea, vomiting, **mesenteric arterial thrombosis,** ischemic colitis, flatulence, gastritis, gastric pain
GU: Impotence, decreased libido
HEMA: **Agranulocytosis, thrombocytopenia,** purpura, eosinophilia
INTEG: Rash, flushing, alopecia, pruritus, sweating
MISC: Facial swelling, weight gain, decreased exercise tolerance
MS: Joint pain, arthralgia
RESP: **Bronchospasm,** dyspnea, wheezing, cough, nasal stuffiness

Contraindications: Hypersensitivity to β-blockers, cardiogenic shock, heart block (2nd, 3rd degree), sinus bradycardia, CHF, cardiac failure
Precautions: Pregnancy (C), major surgery, lactation, children, diabetes mellitus, renal/hepatic disease, thyroid disease, COPD, asthma, well-compensated heart failure, aortic or mitral valve disease, peripheral vascular disease, myasthenia gravis

PHARMACOKINETICS

PO: Peak 2-4 hr; half-life 9-12 hr, 50% excreted unchanged in urine, protein binding 30%-36%; metabolized in liver to inactive metabolites

---

⚠ Safety alert   *"Tall Man" lettering

INTERACTIONS

Increase: hypotension—reserpine, guanethidine

Increase: myocardial depression—calcium channel blockers

Increase: antihypertensive effect—ACE inhibitors, α blockers, calcium channel blockers, diuretics

Increase: bradycardia—digoxin, amiodarone

Increase: peripheral ischemia—ergots

Increase: antidiabetic effect—antidiabetics

Decrease: antihypertensive effect—NSAIDs, salicylates

Drug/Herb
• Toxicity/death: aconite

Increase: β-blocking effect—betel palm, butterbur, cola tree, figwort, fumitory, guarana, hawthorn, lily of the valley, motherwort, plantain

Decrease: β-blocking effect—coenzyme Q10, St. John's wort, yohimbe

Drug/Lab Test

Increase: AST, ALT, ANA titer, blood glucose, BUN, uric acid, K, lipoprotein

Interference: Glucose/insulin tolerance tests

NURSING CONSIDERATIONS

Assess:
• B/P during beginning treatment, periodically thereafter; pulse q4h: note rate, rhythm, quality
• Apical/radial pulse before administration; notify prescriber of any significant changes (pulse <50 bpm)
• Baselines in renal, hepatic studies before therapy begins
• I&O, weight daily, watch for CHF: increased weight, jugular vein distention, dyspnea, crackles
• Edema in feet, legs daily
• Skin turgor, dryness of mucous membranes for hydration status, especially geriatric

Administer:
• Drug before meals, bedtime; tablet may be crushed or swallowed whole, may give without regard to meals

• Reduced dosage in renal/hepatic dysfunction

Perform/provide:
• Storage protected from light, moisture; place in cool environment

Evaluate:
• Therapeutic response: decreased B/P after 1-2 wk

Teach patient/family:
• Not to discontinue drug abruptly; may cause precipitate angina, rebound hypertension; evaluate noncompliance
• Not to use OTC products containing α-adrenergic stimulants (such as nasal decongestants, OTC cold preparations) unless directed by prescriber
• To report bradycardia, dizziness, confusion, depression, fever, cold extremities
• To take pulse at home; advise when to notify prescriber
• To avoid alcohol, smoking, sodium intake
• To comply with weight control, dietary adjustments, modified exercise program
• To carry emergency ID to identify drug taking, allergies
• To avoid hazardous activities if dizziness is present
⚠ To report symptoms of CHF: difficulty breathing, especially on exertion or when lying down, night cough, swelling of extremities
• That if diabetic, may mask signs of hypoglycemia, or alter blood glucose levels

Treatment of overdose: Lavage, IV atropine for bradycardia, IV theophylline for bronchospasm; digoxin, O_2, diuretic for cardiac failure; hemodialysis, IV glucose for hypoglycemia; IV diazepam (or phenytoin) for seizures

---

⚠ High Alert

bivalirudin (℞)
(bye-val-i-rue′din)
Angiomax
Func. class.: Anticoagulant
Chem. class.: Thrombin inhibitor

Action: Direct inhibitor of thrombin that is highly specific; able to inhibit free and clot-bound thrombin

Uses: Unstable angina in patients undergoing percutaneous transluminal coronary angioplasty (PTCA), used with aspirin; heparin-induced thrombocytopenia; heparin-induced thrombocytopenia with thrombosis syndrome

DOSAGE AND ROUTES
PCI/PTCA
• *Adult:* **IV BOL** 0.75 mg/kg, then **IV INF** 1.75 mg/kg/hr for 4 hr; another **IV INF** may be used at 0.2 mg/kg/hr for ≤20 hr; this drug is intended to be used with aspirin (325 mg daily) adjusted to body weight
HIT/HITTS
• *Adult:* **IV BOL** 0.75 mg/kg, then **CONT INF** 1.75 mg/kg/hr for duration of procedure
Renal dose
• *Adult:* IV GFR 30-59 ml/min give 1.75 mg/kg/hr; GFR 10-29 ml/min give 1 mg/kg/hr; dialysis-dependent patients (not on dialysis) give 0.25 mg/kg/hr
Available forms: Inj, lyophilized 250 mg/vial

SIDE EFFECTS
CNS: Headache, insomnia, anxiety, nervousness
CV: Hypo/hypertension, bradycardia
GI: Nausea, vomiting, abdominal pain, dyspepsia
HEMA: **Hemorrhage**
MISC: Pain at inj site, pelvic pain, urinary retention, fever
MS: Back pain

Contraindications: Hypersensitivity, active bleeding, cerebral aneurysm, intracranial hemorrhage, recent surgery, CVA
Precautions: Pregnancy (B), renal function impairment, geriatric, lactation, children, hepatic disease, asthma, blood dyscrasias, thrombocytopenia, GI ulcers, hypertension

PHARMACOKINETICS
Excreted in urine, half-life 25 min, duration 1 hr, no protein binding

INTERACTIONS
Increase: bleeding risk—anticoagulants, thrombolytics
Drug/Herb
Increase: bleeding risk—agrimony, alfalfa, angelica, anise, bilberry, black haw, bogbean, buchu, cat's claw, chamomile, chondroitin, devil's claw, dong quai, evening primrose, fenugreek, feverfew, fish oils, garlic, ginger, ginkgo, ginseng, horse chestnut, Irish moss, kava, kelp, kelpware, khella, licorice, lovage, lungwort, meadowsweet, motherwort, mugwort, nettle, papaya, parsley (large amts), pau d'arco, pineapple, poplar, prickly ash, red clover, safflower, saw palmetto, senega, skullcap, tonka bean, turmeric, wintergreen, yarrow
Decrease: anticoagulant effect—coenzyme Q10, flax, glucomannan, goldenseal, guar gum

NURSING CONSIDERATIONS
Assess:
• Baseline and periodic ACT, APTT, PT, INR, TT, platelets, Hgb, Hct
⚠ Bleeding: check arterial and venous sites, IM inj sites, catheters; all punctures should be minimized; fall in B/P or Hct that may indicate hemorrhage
• Fever, skin rash, urticaria
• CV status: BP, watch for hypo/hypertension, bradycardia
• Neuro status: any focal or generalized deficits should be reported immediately

---

⚠ Safety alert   *"Tall Man" lettering

Administer:
- Prior to PTCA, give with aspirin, 325 mg

IV, direct route
- Dilute by adding 5 ml of sterile water for inj/250 mg bivalirudin, swirl until dissolved, further dilute in 50 ml of D₅W or 0.9% NaCl (5 mg/ml), give by bolus inj 0.75 mg/kg, then intermittent infusion

Intermittent INF route
- To each 250 mg vial add 5 ml of sterile water for inj, swirl until dissolved, further dilute in 500 ml D₅W or 0.9% NaCl (0.5 mg/ml); give inf after bolus dose at a rate of 1.75 mg/kg/hr; may give an additional infusion at 0.2 mg/kg/hr

Perform/provide:
- Storage of reconstituted vials in refrigerator up to 24 hr; store diluted concentration at room temperature for 24 hr

Evaluate:
- Therapeutic response: anticoagulation in PTCA; resolution of heparin-induced thrombocytopenia and thrombosis syndrome

Teach patient/family:
- Reason for drug and expected results
- To report black, tarry stools, blood in urine, difficulty breathing

---

⚠ High Alert

bleomycin (℞)
(blee-oh-mye′sin)
Blenoxane
Func. class.: Antineoplastic, antibiotic
Chem. class.: Glycopeptide

Action: Inhibits synthesis of DNA, RNA, protein; derived from *Streptomyces verticillus;* phase specific in the G₂ and M phases; a nonvesicant, sclerosing agent

Uses: Cancer of head, neck, penis, cervix, vulva of squamous cell origin, Hodgkin's/non-Hodgkin's disease, lymphosarcoma, reticulum cell sarcoma, testicular carcinoma, as a sclerosing agent for malignant pleural effusion

DOSAGE AND ROUTES
- *Adult and child:* **SUBCUT/IV/IM** 0.25-0.5 units/kg 1-2 times/wk or 10-20 units/m², then 1 unit/day or 5 units/wk; may also be given by **CONT INF;** do not exceed total dose, 400 units in lifetime

Malignant pleural effusion
- *Adult:* 60 units diluted in 100 ml of 0.9% NaCl intrapleural inj given through a thoracostomy tube following drainage of excess pleural fluid and complete lung expansion, remove after 4 hr

Available forms: Powder for inj, 15, 30 units/vial

SIDE EFFECTS
CNS: Pain at tumor site, headache, confusion

GI: Nausea, vomiting, anorexia, stomatitis, weight loss, ulceration of mouth, lips

IDIOSYNCRATIC REACTION: Hypotension, confusion, fever, chills, wheezing

INTEG: Rash, hyperkeratosis, nail changes, alopecia, pruritus, acne, striae, peeling, hyperpigmentation

RESP: **Fibrosis, pneumonitis,** wheezing, **pulmonary toxicity**

SYST: **Anaphylaxis,** radiation recall, Raynaud's phenomenon

Contraindications: Pregnancy (D), hypersensitivity, prior idiosyncratic reaction, lactation

Precautions: Renal/hepatic, respiratory disease, patients >70 yr old

PHARMACOKINETICS
Half-life 2 hr; when CCr >35 ml/min, half-life is increased in lower clearance; metabolized in liver, 50% excreted in urine (unchanged)

INTERACTIONS
Increase: toxicity—other antineoplastics, radiation therapy, general anesthesia
Decrease: serum phenytoin levels—phenytoin, fosphenytoin

Drug/Lab Test
Increase: Uric acid

NURSING CONSIDERATIONS

Assess:

- IM test dose in lymphoma 1-2 units before 1st 2 doses
- Pulmonary function tests: chest x-ray film before and during therapy; should be obtained q2wk during treatment
- Temp q4h; fever may indicate beginning infection
- Serum creatinine
- Dyspnea, crackles, unproductive cough, chest pain, tachypnea, fatigue, increased pulse, pallor, lethargy
- Effects of alopecia and skin color on body image; discuss feelings about body changes
- Buccal cavity q8h for dryness, sores, ulceration, white patches, oral pain, bleeding, dysphagia
- Local irritation, pain, burning, discoloration at inj site
- **⚠** Symptoms indicating anaphylaxis: rash, pruritus, urticaria, purpuric skin lesions, itching, flushing, wheezing, hypotension; have emergency equipment available

Administer:

- Antiemetic 30-60 min before giving drug to prevent vomiting, continue antiemetics 6-10 hr after treatment
- Topical or systemic analgesics for pain of stomatitis as ordered; antihistamines and antipyretics for fever and chills

IM/SUBCUT route

- After reconstituting 15 units/1-5 ml sterile H₂O, D₅W, 0.9% NaCl, or bacteriostatic water for inj, rotate inj sites; do not use products containing benzyl alcohol when giving to neonates

Intrapleural route

- 60 units/50-100 ml of 0.9% NaCl, administered by MD through thoracotomy tube

IV, direct route

- Using cytotoxic handling procedures
- After reconstituting 15 units or less/5 ml or more of D₅W or 0.9% NaCl; after further diluting with 50-100 ml D₅W or 0.9% NaCl, give 15 units or less/10 min through Y-tube or 3-way stopcock

- In lymphoma, two test doses 2-5 units before initial dose; monitor for anaphylaxis

Additive compatibilities: Amikacin, cephapirin, dexamethasone, diphenhydrAMINE, fluorouracil, gentamicin, heparin, hydrocortisone, phenytoin, streptomycin, tobramycin, vinBLAStine, vinCRIStine

Solution compatibilities: 0.9% NaCl

Syringe compatibilities: Cisplatin, cyclophosphamide, DOXOrubicin, droperidol, fluorouracil, furosemide, heparin, leucovorin, methotrexate, metoclopramide, mitomycin, vinBLAStine, vinCRIStine

Y-site compatibilities: Allopurinol, amifostine, aztreonam, cefepime, cisplatin, cyclophosphamide, DOXOrubicin, DOXOrubicin liposome, droperidol, filgrastim, fludarabine, fluorouracil, granisetron, heparin, leucovorin, melphalan, methotrexate, metoclopramide, mitomycin, ondansetron, paclitaxel, piperacillin/tazobactam, sargramostim, teniposide, thiotepa, vinBLAStine, vinCRIStine, vinorelbine

Perform/provide:

- Storage for 2 wk after reconstituting if refrigerated or 24 hr at room temperature; discard unused portions
- Deep-breathing exercises with patient tid-qid; place in semi-Fowler's position
- Liquid diet: carbonated beverage; gelatin may be added if patient is not nauseated or vomiting
- Rinsing of mouth tid-qid with water, club soda; brushing of teeth with baking soda bid-tid with soft brush or cotton-tipped applicators for stomatitis; use unwaxed dental floss
- HOB raised to facilitate breathing

Evaluate:

- Therapeutic response: decrease in size of tumor

Teach patient/family:

- To report any complaints, side effects to nurse or prescriber
- To report any changes in breathing, coughing, fever

⚠ Safety alert   *"Tall Man" lettering

- That hair may be lost during treatment, and wig or hairpiece may make patient feel better; that new hair may be different in color, texture
- To avoid foods with citric acid, hot or rough texture
- To report any bleeding, white spots, ulcerations in mouth; to examine mouth daily and report symptoms
- To use contraception during treatment, avoid breastfeeding
- Not to receive vaccines during treatment

---

bortezomib (℞)
(bor-tez'oh-mib)
Velcade
Func. class.: Antineoplastic—miscellaneous
Chem. class.: Proteasome inhibitor

Action: A reversible inhibitor of chymotrypsin-like activity in mammalian cells. Causes a delay in tumor growth by disrupting normal homeostatic mechanisms.

Uses: Multiple myeloma when at least two other treatments have failed

Unlabeled uses: Several solid, hematologic tumors

DOSAGE AND ROUTES

- *Adult:* **IV BOL** 1.3 mg/m^2/dose 2×/wk for 2 weeks (days 1, 4, 8, 11) followed by 10-day rest period (days 12 to 21); max 8 cycles

Neuropathic pain

- Grade 1 with pain or grade 2: Reduce to 1 mg/m^2
- Grade 2 with pain or grade 3: Hold drug until toxicity resolves, then start at 0.7 mg/m^2 qwk
- Grade 4 hematologic toxicities, withhold use

Available forms: Lyophilized powder for inj 3.5 mg

SIDE EFFECTS

CNS: Anxiety, insomnia, dizziness, head-

ache, *peripheral neuropathy,* rigors, paresthesia
CV: Hypotension, edema
GI: Abdominal pain, *constipation, diarrhea,* dyspepsia, nausea, *vomiting,* anorexia
HEMA: Anemia, **neutropenia, thrombocytopenia**
MISC: Dehydration, weight loss, herpes zoster, rash, pruritus, blurred vision
MS: Fatigue, malaise, weakness, arthralgia, bone pain, muscle cramps, myalgia, back pain
RESP: Cough, pneumonia, dyspnea, URI
Contraindications: Pregnancy (D), hypersensitivity to this drug, boron, or mannitol; lactation
Precautions: Peripheral neuropathy, geriatric, renal/hepatic disease, hypotension, children

PHARMACOKINETICS

Half-life 9-15 hr, protein binding 83%, metabolized by CYP450 enzymes (3A4, 2D6, 2C19, 2C9, 1A2)

INTERACTIONS

- Oral hypoglycemics: may result in hypo/hyperglycemia

Increase: hypotension—antihypertensives

Increase: peripheral neuropathy—amiodarone, antivirals, isoniazid, nitrofurantoin, statins

Increase: toxicity or decrease efficacy when administered with drugs that induce or inhibit CYP4503A4

NURSING CONSIDERATIONS

Assess:

- Hematologic status: platelets, CBC throughout treatment
- For extravasation at inj site
- B/P, fluid status, peripheral neuropathy symptoms

Administer:

- Reconstitute each vial with 3.5 ml 0.9% NaCl
- Use protective clothing during handling, preparation, avoid contact with skin

---

Evaluate:
• Therapeutic response: improvement of multiple myeloma symptoms
Teach patient/family:
• To use contraception while on this drug, pregnancy (D), avoid breastfeeding
• To monitor blood glucose levels if diabetic
• To contact prescriber of new or worsening peripheral neuropathy, severe vomiting, diarrhea
• To avoid driving, operating machinery until effect is known
• To avoid using other medications unless approved by prescriber

---

bosentan (℞)
(boh'sen-tan)
Tracleer
Func. class.: Vasodilator
Chem. class.: Endothelin receptor antagonist

Action: Peripheral vasodilation occurs via antagonism of the effect of endothelin on endothelium and vascular smooth muscle
Uses: Pulmonary arterial hypertension with WHO class III, IV symptoms
Unlabeled uses: Septic shock to improve microcirculatory blood flow

DOSAGE AND ROUTES
• *Adult >40 kg/>12 yr:* **PO** 62.5 mg bid × 4 wk, then 125 mg bid
• *Adult <40 kg/>12 yr:* **PO** 62.5 mg bid
Available forms: Tabs 62.5, 125 mg

SIDE EFFECTS

CNS: Headache, flushing, fatigue
CV: *Hypotension,* palpitations, edema of lower limbs
GI: Abnormal hepatic function, dyspepsia, **hepatotoxicity**
INTEG: Pruritus
MISC: Anemia
Contraindications: Pregnancy (X), hypersensitivity, CVA, CAD
Precautions: Mitral stenosis, geriatric,

lactation, hepatic function impairment, children

PHARMACOKINETICS

Metabolized by CYP2C9, CYP3A4, and possibly CYP2C19; metabolized by the liver; terminal half-life 5 hr; steady state 3-5 days

INTERACTIONS

• Do not coadminister cycloSPORINE and bosentan; bosentan is increased, cycloSPORINE is decreased
• Do not coadminister glyBURIDE with bosentan; glyBURIDE is decreased significantly, bosentan also is decreased, hepatic enzymes may be increased
Increase: bosentan level—ketoconazole
Decrease: effects of simvastatin, other statins, hormonal contraceptives, warfarin
Drug/Lab Test
Increase: ALT, AST
Decrease: Hgb, Hct

NURSING CONSIDERATIONS
Assess:
• B/P, pulse during treatment until stable
• Hepatic studies: AST, ALT, bilirubin; hepatic enzymes may increase; if ALT/AST >3 and ≤5 × ULN, confirm lab value, decrease dose or interrupt treatment and monitor AST/ALT q2wk; if >8 × ULN, stop treatment
• Blood studies: Hct, Hgb may be decreased
• Hepatic involvement: vomiting, jaundice; drug should be discontinued
Administer:
• Do not stop drug abruptly, taper
Perform/provide:
• Storage at room temperature
Evaluate:
• Therapeutic response: decrease in pulmonary hypertension
Teach patient/family:
• To report jaundice, dark urine, joint pain, fatigue, malaise, bruising, easy bleeding; may indicate blood dyscrasias

---

⚠ Safety alert   *"Tall Man" lettering

• To avoid pregnancy; to use nonhormonal form of contraception
• Lab work will be required periodically

brimonidine ophthalmic
See Appendix C

brinzolamide ophthalmic
See Appendix C

bromfenac ophthalmic
See Appendix C

bromocriptine (Rx)
(broe-moe-krip'teen)
Alti-Bromocriptine ✦,
Apo-Bromocriptine ✦,
Parlodel
Func. class.: Dopamine receptor agonist, antiparkinson agent
Chem. class.: Ergot alkaloid derivative

Do not confuse:
Parlodel/pindolol/Provera

Action: Inhibits prolactin release by activating postsynaptic dopamine receptors; activation of striatal dopamine receptors may be reason for improvement in Parkinson's disease

Uses: Parkinson's disease, amenorrhea/galactorrhea caused by hyperprolactinemia, infertility, acromegaly, pituitary adenomas

Unlabeled uses: Neuroleptic malignant syndrome, alcoholism, premenstrual syndrome, mastalgia, cocaine withdrawal, premenstrual breast symptoms, prevention of lactation after stillbirth or abortion

DOSAGE AND ROUTES
Hyperprolactinemia
• *Adult:* **PO** 1.25-2.5 mg with meals; may increase by 2.5 mg q3-7 days, usual 5-7.5 mg
Acromegaly
• *Adult:* **PO** 1.25-2.5 mg × 3 days at bedtime; may increase by 1.25-2.5 mg q3-7 days; usual range 20-30 mg/day, max 100 mg/day
Parkinson's disease
• *Adult:* **PO** 1.25 mg bid with meals, may increase q2-4wk by 2.5 mg/day, not to exceed 100 mg daily
Pituitary adenoma
• *Adult:* **PO** 1.25 mg bid-tid, may increase over several weeks to 10-20 mg/day
Neuroleptic malignant syndrome (unlabeled)
• *Adult:* **PO** 2.5-5 mg 2-6 times/day
Cocaine withdrawal
• *Adult:* **PO** 0.625 mg qid × 42 days
Alcoholism (unlabeled)
• *Adult:* **PO** 7.5 mg/day
Mastalgia
• *Adult:* **PO** 2.5-7.5 bid, starting 10-14 days prior to menses; discontinue when menses begin

Available forms: Caps 5 mg; tabs 2.5 mg

SIDE EFFECTS

CNS: Headache, depression, restlessness, anxiety, nervousness, confusion, **seizures,** *hallucinations,* dizziness, fatigue, drowsiness, abnormal involuntary movements, psychosis
CV: Orthostatic hypotension, decreased B/P, palpitation, extrasystole, **shock,** dysrhythmias, bradycardia, **MI**
EENT: Blurred vision, diplopia, burning eyes, nasal congestion
GI: Nausea, vomiting, anorexia, cramps, constipation, diarrhea, dry mouth, GI hemorrhage
GU: Frequency, retention, incontinence, diuresis
INTEG: Rash on face, arms, alopecia; coolness, pallor of fingers, toes

---

✦ Canada only   Side effects: *italics* = common; **bold** = life-threatening

Contraindications: Hypersensitivity to ergot, bromocriptine; severe ischemic disease, severe peripheral vascular disease
Precautions: Pregnancy (B), lactation, renal/hepatic disease, children, pituitary tumors, peptic ulcer disease

PHARMACOKINETICS

PO: Peak 1-3 hr, duration 4-8 hr, 90%-96% protein bound, half-life 3 hr, metabolized by liver (inactive metabolites), 85%-98% of dose excreted in feces

INTERACTIONS

• Disulfiram-like reaction: alcohol
Increase: action of antihypertensives, levodopa
Decrease: action of bromocriptine—phenothiazines, oral contraceptives, progestins, estrogens, haloperidol, loxapine, methyldopa, metoclopramide, MAOIs, reserpine
Drug/Herb
Increase: serotonin effect—horehound
Decrease: bromocriptine effect—chaste tree fruit, kava
Drug/Lab Test
Increase: Growth hormone, AST, ALT, CK, BUN, uric acid, alk phos

NURSING CONSIDERATIONS

Assess:
• B/P; establish baseline, compare with other reading; this drug decreases B/P
• Parkinson's symptoms: pill-rolling, shuffling gait, restlessness, tremors, before and during treatment
• For resolution of symptoms of neuroleptic malignant syndrome: decreased temp, seizures, sweating, pulse
• Change in size of soft tissue volume, in acromegaly
Administer:
• With meal to prevent GI symptoms
• At bedtime so dizziness, orthostatic hypotension do not occur
Perform/provide:
• Storage at room temperature in tight, light resistant container
Evaluate:
• Therapeutic response (Parkinson's dis-

ease): decreased dyskinesia, decreased slow movements, decreased drooling
Teach patient/family:
• That tabs may be crushed and mixed with food
• To change position slowly to prevent orthostatic hypotension
• To use contraceptives during treatment with this drug; pregnancy may occur; to use methods other than oral contraceptives
• That therapeutic effect for Parkinson's disease may take 2 mo: galactorrhea, amenorrhea
• To avoid hazardous activity if dizziness occurs
• To report symptoms of MI immediately

brompheniramine (R)
(brome-fen-ir'a-meen)
Bidhist, Bromfenac, brompheniramine, BroveX, BroveX CT, Chlorphed, Dehist, Dimetane, Dimetane Extentabs, Dimetapp Allergy Liqui-Gels, Lo Hist 12 Hour, Lodrane 24, Lodrane XR, Nasahist-B, VaZol
Func. class.: Antihistamine
Chem. class.: Alkylamine, H₁-receptor antagonist

Action: Acts on blood vessels, GI, respiratory system by competing with histamine for H₁-receptor site; decreases allergic response by blocking histamine
Uses: Allergy symptoms, rhinitis

DOSAGE AND ROUTES

• *Adult and child >12 yr:* PO 4-8 mg bid-qid, not to exceed 36 mg/day; **EXT-REL** 6-12 mg bid-tid, not to exceed 36 mg/day
• *Child 6-12 yr:* PO 2 mg bid-qid, not to exceed 12 mg/day; **EXT REL** 6-12 mg daily
• *Child 2-6 yr:* 1 mg bid-qid 6h, max 6 mg/day
• *Child <2 yr:* PO 0.5 mg/kg/day in divided doses (qid)
Available forms: Tabs 4 mg; elix 2 mg/5 ml; caps 4 mg; chew tabs 12 mg;

ext rel tabs 6 mg; ext rel caps 12 mg; liquid 8 mg, 12 mg/5 ml

SIDE EFFECTS

CNS: Dizziness, drowsiness, poor coordination, fatigue, anxiety, euphoria, confusion, paresthesia, neuritis

CV: Hypotension, palpitations, tachycardia

EENT: Blurred vision, dilated pupils, tinnitus, nasal stuffiness, dry nose, throat, mouth

GI: Nausea, vomiting, anorexia, constipation, diarrhea

GU: Retention, dysuria, frequency, impotence

HEMA: **Thrombocytopenia, agranulocytosis, hemolytic anemia (rare)**

INTEG: Photosensitivity

RESP: Increased thick secretions, wheezing, chest tightness

Contraindications: Hypersensitivity to H₁-receptor antagonists, acute asthma attack, lower respiratory tract disease, child <2 yr

Precautions: Pregnancy (C), increased intraocular pressure, renal disease, cardiac disease, hypertension, bronchial asthma, seizure disorder, stenosed peptic ulcers, hyperthyroidism, prostatic hypertrophy, bladder neck obstruction, lactation, angle-closure glaucoma

PHARMACOKINETICS

PO: Peak 2-5 hr, duration to 48 hr; metabolized in liver, excreted by kidneys, excreted in breast milk, half-life 12-34 hr

INTERACTIONS

• Incompatible with aminophylline, insulins, pentobarbital

Increase: CNS depression—barbiturates, opiates, hypnotics, tricyclics, alcohol

Increase: anticholinergic effect—MAOIs

Drug/Herb

Increase: effect—hops, Jamaican dogwood, kava, khat, senega

Increase: anticholinergic effect—corkwood, henbane leaf

Drug/Lab Test

Interference: Skin allergy tests

NURSING CONSIDERATIONS   E

Assess:

• Be alert for urinary retention, frequency, dysuria; drug should be discontinued if these occur

• CBC during long-term therapy

• Blood dyscrasias: thrombocytopenia, agranulocytosis (rare) during long-term therapy

• Respiratory status: rate, rhythm, increase in bronchial secretions, wheezing, chest tightness

Administer:

PO route

• Do not break, crush, or chew ext rel forms

• With meals if GI symptoms occur; absorption may slightly decrease

Perform/provide:

• Hard candy, gum, frequent rinsing of mouth for dryness

• Storage in tight container at room temperature

Evaluate:

• Therapeutic response: absence of running or congested nose or rashes

Teach patient/family:

• All aspects of drug use; to notify prescriber if confusion/sedation/hypotension occurs

• To avoid driving, other hazardous activities if drowsiness occurs

• To avoid use of alcohol, other CNS depressants while taking drug

Treatment of overdose: Administer vasopressors, barbiturates (short-acting)

---

budesonide (℞)
(byoo-des'oh-nide)
Entocort EC, Pulmicort, Rhinocort Aqua
Func. class.: Glucocorticoid
Chem. class.: Nonhalogenated

Action: Prevents inflammation by depression of migration of polymorphonuclear leukocytes, fibroblasts, reversal of increased capillary permeability and lysosomal stabilization; does not suppress hypothalamus and pituitary function

Uses: Rhinitis; prophylaxis for asthma; Crohn's disease

DOSAGE AND ROUTES

Rhinitis (Rhinocort Aqua)
• *Adult and child >6 yr:* **SPRAY/INH** 256 mcg daily (2 sprays in each nostril AM, PM or 4 sprays in each nostril, AM)

Asthma
• *Adult and child ≥6 yr:* **INH** 400-600 mcg/day

Crohn's disease
• *Adult:* **PO** 9 mg daily AM × 8 wk

Available forms: Dry powder for INH 200 mcg/metered dose (Palmicort Turbuhaler); inh susp 0.25 mg/2 ml, 0.5 mg/2 ml; 32 mcg/spray (Rhinocort Aqua); caps 3 mg (Entocort EC)

SIDE EFFECTS

CNS: Headache, insomnia, hypertonia, syncope

EENT: Sinusitis, pharyngitis, rhinitis, oral candidiasis

ENDO: Adrenal insufficiency, growth suppression in children

GI: Dry mouth, dyspepsia, nausea, vomiting, abdominal pain

MISC: Ecchymosis, fever, *hypersensitivity,* flulike symptoms

MS: Back pain, myalgias, fractures

RESP: Nasal irritation, cough, nasal bleeding, *respiratory infections,* **bronchospasm**

Contraindications: Hypersensitivity, status asthmaticus

Precautions: Pregnancy (C), inhaled form (B); lactation, children, TB, fungal, bacterial, systemic viral infections, ocular herpes simplex, nasal septal ulcers; hepatic disease (caps)

PHARMACOKINETICS

Peak: Respules 4-6 wk, Rhinocort Aqua 2 wk, Turbuhaler 1-2 wk, half-life 2-3.6 hr

Onset: Respules 2-8 days; Rhinocort Aqua 10 hr; Turbuhale 24 hr

INTERACTIONS

• Avoid using with drugs metabolized by CYP3A4 inhibition

Decrease: budesonide metabolism—ketoconazole, cimetidine

Drug/Herb

Increase: hypokalemia—aloe, buckthorn, Chinese rhubarb, senna

NURSING CONSIDERATIONS

Assess:

• Respiratory status: rate, rhythm, increase in bronchial secretions, wheezing, chest tightness; provide fluids to 2 L/day to decrease thickness of secretions; check for oral candidiasis

• For bronchospasm, stop treatment and give bronchodilator

• With viral infections, corticosteroid use can mask infections

• For increased intraocular pressure, discontinue use if increase occurs

Administer:

PO route (Crohn's disease)

• Swallow caps whole; do not break, crush, or chew

• May repeat 8-wk course if needed; may taper to 6 mg/day for 2 wk before cessation

INH route (asthma)

• Use scissors to open pouch

• Use Turbuhaler upright to load, prime when using first time, turn grip to the right, then left to click in place; to provide dose turn to right, then to the left, click in place. Place mouthpiece between lips, inhale forcefully, do not exhale through Turbuhaler, rinse after use

Perform/provide:

• Storage at 59°-86° F (15°-30° C); keep away from heat, open flame

Evaluate:

• Therapeutic response: absence of asthma, rhinitis

Teach patient/family:

• To notify prescriber of pharyngitis, nasal bleeding

• Not to exceed recommended dose; adrenal suppression may occur

• To carry emergency ID identifying steroid use
• To read and follow package directions
• To prevent exposure to infections, especially viral
• To avoid taking with grapefruit juice (capsule PO)
• To use good oral hygiene if using nebulizer or inhaler

budesonide nasal agent
See Appendix C

bumetanide (℞)
(byoo-met'a-nide)
Bumex
Func. class.: Loop diuretic, antihypertensive
Chem. class.: Sulfonamide derivative

Do not confuse:
Bumex/Buprenex/Permax
Action: Acts on ascending loop of Henle by inhibiting reabsorption of chloride, sodium
Uses: Edema in CHF, hepatic disease, renal disease

DOSAGE AND ROUTES
• *Adult:* **PO** 0.5-2.0 mg daily; may give 2nd or 3rd dose at 4-5 hr intervals, max 10 mg/day; may be given on alternate days or intermittently; **IV/IM** 0.5-1.0 mg; may give 2nd or 3rd dose at 2-3 hr intervals, not to exceed 10 mg/day
• *Child:* **PO/IM/IV** 0.02-0.1 mg/kg q12h, max 10 mg/day
Available forms: Tabs 0.5, 1, 2 mg; inj 0.25 mg/ml

SIDE EFFECTS
CNS: Headache, fatigue, weakness, dizziness
CV: **Chest pain,** hypotension, **circulatory collapse,** ECG changes, dehydration

EENT: Loss of hearing
ELECT: Hypokalemia, hypochloremic alkalosis, hypomagnesemia, hyperuricemia, hypocalcemia, hyponatremia
ENDO: Hyperglycemia
GI: Nausea, diarrhea, dry mouth, vomiting, anorexia, cramps, upset stomach, abdominal pain, **acute pancreatitis, jaundice**
GU: Polyuria, **renal failure,** glycosuria, premature ejaculation
HEMA: **Thrombocytopenia, leukopenia, granulocytopenia**
INTEG: Rash, pruritus, purpura, **Stevens-Johnson syndrome,** sweating, photosensitivity
MS: Muscular cramps, arthritis, stiffness
Contraindications: Hypersensitivity to sulfonamides, anuria, hepatic coma, severe electrolyte deficiency,
Precautions: Pregnancy (C), dehydration, ascites, severe renal disease, hepatic cirrhosis, lactation, blood dyscrasias, neonates, ototoxicity, hyperuricemia, hypokalemia

PHARMACOKINETICS
PO: Onset ½-1 hr, peak 1-2 hr, duration 3-6 hr
IM: Onset 40 min, peak 1-2 hr, duration 4-6 hr
IV: Onset 5 min, peak 15-30 min, duration 3-6 hr, excreted by kidneys (50% unchanged), feces (20%), crosses placenta, excreted in breast milk, protein binding >91%; half-life 1-1½ hr, 6-15 hr neonates

INTERACTIONS
• Ototoxicity: aminoglycosides
• Hypokalemia: potassium-wasting drugs
Increase: toxicity—lithium, digoxin
Increase: diuresis, electrolyte loss—metolazone
Decrease: diuretic effect—indomethacin, NSAIDs, probenecid
Decrease: antidiabetic effects

Drug/Herb

• Severe photosensitivity: St. John's wort
Increase: effect—aloe, cucumber, dandelion, horsetail, pumpkin, Queen Anne's lace
Increase: hypotension—khella

NURSING CONSIDERATIONS

Assess:

• For tinnitus, obtain audiometric testing for long-term IV treatment
• Weight, I&O daily to determine fluid loss; if urinary output decreases or azotemia occurs, drug should be discontinued; the safest dosage schedule is on alternate days
• B/P lying, standing; postural hypotension may occur
• Electrolytes: K, Na, Cl; include BUN, blood glucose, CBC, serum creatinine, blood pH, ABGs, uric acid, Ca, Mg
• Blood glucose if patient is diabetic; blood uric acid levels in those with gout
• Improvement in edema of feet, legs, sacral area daily if medication is being used in CHF
• Signs of metabolic alkalosis: drowsiness, restlessness
• Signs of hypokalemia: postural hypotension, malaise, fatigue, tachycardia, leg cramps, weakness
• Rashes, temp elevation daily
• Confusion, especially in geriatric; take safety precautions if needed
• For digoxin toxicity in patients taking digoxin products (anorexia, nausea, vomiting, confusion, paresthesia, muscle cramps); lithium toxicity in those taking lithium

Administer:

• In AM to avoid interference with sleep if using drug as a diuretic
• Potassium replacement if potassium is <3.0

PO route

• With food if nausea occurs; absorption may be decreased slightly

IV, direct route

• Direct IV undiluted slowly over at least 2 min through Y-tube or 3-way stopcock or heplock

Intermittent IV route

• Dilute in LR, D_5W, 0.9% NaCl (rarely given by this method), give over 12 hr in renal disease

Additive compatibilities: Floxacillin, furosemide

Syringe compatibilities: Doxapram

Y-site compatibilities: Allopurinol, amifostine, aztreonam, cefepime, cisatracurium, cladribine, clarithromycin, diltiazem, docetaxel, etoposide, filgrastim, granisetron, lorazepam, melphalan, meperidine, morphine, piperacillin/tazobactam, propofol, remifentanil, teniposide, thiotepa, vinorelbine

Evaluate:

• Therapeutic response: decreased edema, B/P

Teach patient/family:

• To increase fluid intake to 2-3 L/day unless contraindicated, to take potassium supplement, to rise slowly from lying or sitting position
• To recognize adverse reactions: muscle cramps, weakness, nausea, dizziness
• To take with food or milk for GI symptoms
• To take early in day to prevent nocturia
• To use sunscreen to prevent photosensitivity

Treatment of overdose: Lavage if taken orally; monitor electrolytes; administer dextrose in saline; monitor hydration, CV, renal status

---

buprenorphine (℞)

(byoo-pre-nor′feen)
Buprenex, Subutex
Func. class.: Opioid analgesic, partial agonist
Chem. class.: Thebaine derivative

Controlled Substance Schedule V
Do not confuse:
Buprenex/Bumex
Action: Depresses pain impulse transmission at the spinal cord level by interacting with opioid receptors
Uses: Moderate to severe pain

⚠ Safety alert   *"Tall Man" lettering

DOSAGE AND ROUTES

• *Adult:* **IM/IV** 0.3 mg q6h prn, reduce dosage in geriatric, may repeat after ½ hr; **EPIDURAL** 60-180 mcg over 48 hr
• *Child 2-12 yr:* **IM/IV** 2-6 mcg/kg q4-6h
• *Geriatric:* **PO** 0.15 mg q6h prn
Available forms: Inj 0.3 mg/ml (1 ml vials)

SIDE EFFECTS

CNS: Drowsiness, dizziness, confusion, headache, sedation, euphoria, **increased intracranial pressure,** amnesia
CV: Palpitations, bradycardia, change in B/P, tachycardia
EENT: Tinnitus, blurred vision, *miosis,* diplopia
GI: Nausea, vomiting, anorexia, constipation, cramps, dry mouth
GU: Increased urinary output, dysuria, urinary retention
INTEG: Rash, urticaria, bruising, flushing, diaphoresis, pruritus
RESP: **Respiratory depression,** dyspnea, hypo/hyperventilation
Contraindications: Hypersensitivity
Precautions: Pregnancy (C), addictive personality, lactation, increased intracranial pressure, MI (acute), severe heart disease, respiratory depression, renal/hepatic disease, hypothyroidism, Addison's disease, addiction (opioid)

PHARMACOKINETICS

IM: Onset 10-30 min, peak ½ hr, duration 3-4 hr
IV: Onset 1 min, peak 5 min, duration 2-5 hr
Metabolized by liver; excreted by kidneys/feces; crosses placenta; excreted in breast milk; half-life 2½-3½ hr; 96% bound to plasma proteins

INTERACTIONS

Increase: effect with other CNS depressants—alcohol, opioids, sedative/hypnotics, antipsychotics, skeletal muscle relaxants, MAOIs

Drug/Herb
Increase: CNS depression—Jamaican dogwood, kava, lavender, mistletoe, nettle, pokeweed, poppy, senega, valerian
Increase: anticholinergic effect—corkwood

NURSING CONSIDERATIONS

Assess:
• I&O ratio; check for decreasing output; may indicate urinary retention
• CNS changes, dizziness, drowsiness, hallucinations, euphoria, LOC, pupil reaction; withdrawal in opioid-dependent persons; if dependence occurs, within 2 wk of discontinuing drug withdrawal symptoms will occur
• Allergic reactions: rash, urticaria
• Respiratory dysfunction: respiratory depression, character, rate, rhythm; notify prescriber if respirations are <12/min
• Need for pain medication, tolerance; location, intensity, severity

Administer:
IM route
• In deep muscle mass
IV, direct route
• Undiluted over 3-5 min (0.3 mg over 2 min), titrate to patient response
• With antiemetic if nausea, vomiting occur
• When pain is beginning to return; determine dosage interval by patient response

Additive compatibilities: Atropine, bupivacaine, diphenhydrAMINE, droperidol, glycopyrrolate, haloperidol, hydrOXYzine, promethazine, scopolamine
Syringe compatibilities: Midazolam
Y-site compatibilities: Allopurinol, amifostine, aztreonam, cefepime, cisatracurium, cladribine, filgrastim, granisetron, melphalan, piperacillin/tazobactam, propofol, remifentanil, teniposide, thiotepa, vinorelbine

Perform/provide:
• Assistance with ambulation if needed
Evaluate:
• Therapeutic response: decrease in pain, absence of grimacing

---

Side effects: *italics* = common; **bold** = life-threatening

Teach patient/family:
• To report any symptoms of CNS changes, allergic reactions
• That tolerance may result when used for extended periods
• To avoid hazardous activities

---

*buPROPion (℞)
(byoo-proe′pee-on)
Budeprion SR, buPROPion, Wellbutrin, Wellbutrin SR, Wellbutrin XL, Zyban
Func. class.: Antidepressant—miscellaneous smoking deterrent
Chem. class.: Aminoketone

Do not confuse:
buPROPion/busPIRone
Zyban/Diovan/Zagam

Action: Inhibits reuptake of dopamine, serotonin, norepinephrine

Uses: Depression (Wellbutrin), smoking cessation (Zyban)

Unlabeled uses: Neuropathic pain, enhancement of weight loss, ADHD (attention deficit hyperactivity disorder)

DOSAGE AND ROUTES

Depression
• *Adult:* PO 100 mg bid initially, then increase after 3 days to 100 mg tid if needed; may increase after 1 mo to 150 mg tid; **SR** 150 mg bid, initially 150 mg AM, increase to 300 mg/day if initial dose is tolerated
• *Geriatric:* PO 50-100 mg/day, may increase by 50-100 mg q3-4 day

Smoking cessation
• *Adult:* PO 150 mg bid, begin with 150 mg daily × 3 days, then 300 mg/day; continue for 7-12 wk; not to exceed 300 mg/day

Available forms: Tabs 75, 100 mg; sus rel tabs (SR) 100, 150, 200 (Zyban); ext rel tab (XL) 150, 300 mg; (SR-12 hr, XL-24 hr)

SIDE EFFECTS

*CNS: Headache, agitation, dizziness, akinesia, bradykinesia, confusion, sei-*zures, delusions, *insomnia, sedation, tremors*

CV: Dysrhythmias, hypertension, palpitations, *tachycardia,* hypotension, **complete AV block**

EENT: Blurred vision, auditory disturbance

GI: Nausea, vomiting, anorexia, diarrhea, *dry mouth,* increased appetite, *constipation*

GU: Impotence, urinary frequency, retention, *menstrual irregularities*

INTEG: Rash, pruritus, *sweating*

MISC: Weight loss or gain

Contraindications: Hypersensitivity, eating disorders, seizure disorders

Precautions: Pregnancy (B), renal/hepatic disease, recent MI, cranial trauma, lactation, children <18 yr, geriatric, seizure disorder

PHARMACOKINETICS

Onset 2-4 wk; half-life 14 hr; extensively metabolized by liver; some conversion to active metabolites; steady state 1½-5 wk

INTERACTIONS

⚠ *Increase:* adverse reactions, seizures—levodopa, MAOIs, phenothiazines, antidepressants, benzodiazepines, alcohol, theophylline, systemic steroids

Increase: buPROPion toxicity—ritonavir
Increase: buPROPion level—cimetidine
Decrease: buPROPion effect—carbamazepine, cimetidine, phenobarbital, phenytoin or other drugs (CYP450)

Drug/Herb
Increase: CNS depression—hops, kava, lavender

Increase: anticholinergic effect—belladonna, corkwood, jimsonweed

NURSING CONSIDERATIONS

Assess:
• Hepatic/renal function in patients with hepatic or kidney impairment
• For increased risk of seizures; if patient has excessively used CNS depres-

---

sants and OTC stimulants, dosage of bu-PROPion should not be exceeded

• For smoking cessation after 7-12 wk; if progress has not been made, drug should be discontinued

• Mental status: mood, sensorium, affect, suicidal tendencies, increase in psychiatric symptoms

Administer:

PO route

• Do not break, crush, or chew sus rel, ext rel tab

• In evenly spaced times to prevent seizures; seizure risk increases with high doses

• Increased fluids, bulk in diet if constipation occurs

• With food or milk for GI symptoms

• Sugarless gum, hard candy, or frequent sips of water for dry mouth

• Avoid giving at night to prevent imsomnia

• Other treatments may be used with this product (nicotine patches)

Perform/provide:

• Assistance with ambulation during beginning therapy, since sedation occurs

• Safety measures, primarily in geriatric

Evaluate:

• Therapeutic response: decreased depression, ability to function in daily activities, ability to sleep throughout the night, smoking cessation

Teach patient/family:

• That therapeutic effects may take 2-4 wk; not to increase dose without prescriber's approval; that treatment for smoking cessation lasts 7-12 wk

• To use caution in driving, other activities requiring alertness; sedation, blurred vision may occur

• To avoid alcohol ingestion, other CNS depressants, alcohol may increase risk of seizures

• Not to use with nicotine patches unless directed by prescriber, may increase B/P

• To notify prescriber immediately if retention occurs

• That risk of seizures is increased when dose is exceeded, or if patient has seizure disorder

• To notify prescriber if pregnancy is suspected or planned

Treatment of overdose: ECG monitoring; induce emesis, lavage, activated charcoal; administer anticonvulsant

---

busPIRone (R̸)
(byoo-spye'rone)
BuSpar
Func. class.: Antianxiety, sedative
Chem. class.: Azaspirodecanedione

Do not confuse:
busPIRone/buPROPion

Action: Acts by inhibiting the action of serotonin (5-HT); has shown little potential for abuse, a good choice in substance abuse

Uses: Management and short-term relief of generalized anxiety disorders

DOSAGE AND ROUTES

• *Adult:* **PO** 5 mg tid; may increase by 5 mg/day q2-3 days, not to exceed 60 mg/day

Available forms: Tabs 5, 10, 15 mg

SIDE EFFECTS

CNS: Dizziness, headache, depression, stimulation, insomnia, nervousness, light-headedness, numbness, paresthesia, incoordination, nightmares, *tremors,* excitement, involuntary movements, confusion, akathisia

CV: Tachycardia, palpitations, hypotension, hypertension, **CVA, CHF, MI**

EENT: Sore throat, tinnitus, blurred vision, nasal congestion; red, itching eyes; change in taste, smell

GI: Nausea, dry mouth, diarrhea, constipation, flatulence, increased appetite, rectal bleeding

GU: Frequency, hesitancy, menstrual irregularity, change in libido

INTEG: Rash, edema, pruritus, alopecia, dry skin

MISC: Sweating, fatigue, weight gain, fever

MS: Pain, weakness, muscle cramps, spasms

Side effects: *italics* = common; **bold** = life-threatening

RESP: Hyperventilation, chest congestion, shortness of breath

Contraindications: Hypersensitivity, child <18 yr

Precautions: Pregnancy (B), lactation, geriatric, impaired hepatic, renal function

PHARMACOKINETICS

Half-life 2-3 hr, rapidly absorbed, metabolized by liver (CYP3A4), excreted in feces

INTERACTIONS

Increase: busPIRone—drug metabolized by CYP450, 3A4 (erythromycin, itraconazole, nefazodone, ketoconazole, ritonavir)

Increase: B/P—MAOIs; do not use together

Increase: CNS depression—psychotropic drugs, alcohol (avoid use)

Decrease: busPIRone effects—rifampin

Decrease: busPIRone action—drugs induced by CYP3A4 (rifampin, phenytoin, phenobarbital, carbamazepine, dexamethasone)

Drug/Herb

Increase: CNS depression—cowslip, kava, Queen Anne's lace, valerian

Drug/Food

Increase: peak concentration of busPIRone—grapefruit juice

NURSING CONSIDERATIONS

Assess:

• B/P (lying, standing), pulse; if systolic B/P drops 20 mm Hg, hold drug, notify prescriber

• CNS reactions, since some reactions may be unpredictable

• Mental status: mood, sensorium, affect, sleeping pattern, drowsiness, dizziness

Administer:

• With food or milk for GI symptoms

• Crushed if patient unable to swallow medication whole

• Sugarless gum, hard candy, frequent sips of water for dry mouth

Perform/provide:

• Assistance with ambulation during beginning therapy; drowsiness, dizziness occur

• Safety measures if drowsiness occurs

• Check to see PO medication swallowed

Evaluate:

• Therapeutic response: decreased anxiety, restlessness, sleeplessness

Teach patient/family:

• That drug may be taken with food

• To avoid OTC preparations unless approved by prescriber

• To avoid activities requiring alertness, since drowsiness may occur

• To avoid alcohol ingestion, other psychotropic medications, unless directed by prescriber

• Not to discontinue medication abruptly after long-term use; if dose is missed, do not double

• To rise slowly because fainting may occur, especially geriatric

• That drowsiness may worsen at beginning of treatment

• That 1-2 wk of therapy may be required before therapeutic effects occur

Treatment of overdose: Gastric lavage, VS, supportive care

⚠ High Alert

busulfan (℞)

(byoo-sul'fan)

Busulfex, Myleran

Func. class.: Antineoplastic alkylating agent

Chem. class.: Nitrosourea

Do not confuse:

Myleran/Leukeran

Action: Changes essential cellular ions to covalent bonding with resultant alkylation; this interferes with normal biologic function of DNA; activity is not phase specific; action is due to myelosuppression

Uses: Chronic myelocytic leukemia

DOSAGE AND ROUTES

Chronic myelocytic (granulocytic) leukemia

• *Adult:* PO 4-8 mg/day initially until WBC levels fall to 15,000/mm³, then drug is stopped until WBC levels raise over 50,000/mm³, then 1-3 mg/day
• *Child:* PO 0.06-0.12 mg/kg or 1.8-4.6 mg/m² day; dose is titrated to maintain WBC levels at 20,000/mm³, but never <10,000/mm³

Allogenic hemopoietic stem cell transplantation in chronic myelogenous leukemia

• *Adult:* IV 0.8 mg/kg q6hr × 4 days (total 16 doses); give cyclophosphamide IV 60 mg/kg over 1 hr daily for 2 days, starting after 16th dose of busulfan
Available forms: Tabs 2 mg; inj 6 mg/ml

SIDE EFFECTS

PO route
CV: Hypotension, thrombosis, chest pain, tachycardia, atrial fibrillation, heart block, pericardial effusion, **cardiac tamponade** (high dose with cyclophosphamide)
GI: Anorexia, constipation, diarrhea, dry mouth, nausea, vomiting
RESP: **Alveolar hemorrhage,** atelectasis, cough, hemoptysis, hypoxia, pleural effusion, pneumonia, sinusitis, **pulmonary fibrosis**

IV route
CNS: **Cerebral hemorrhage, coma, seizures,** *anxiety, depression, dizziness, headache,* encephalopathy, *weakness,* mental changes
EENT: Pharyngitis, epistaxis, cataracts
GI: Nausea, vomiting, *diarrhea, weight loss*
GU: Impotence, sterility, amenorrhea, gynecomastia, **renal toxicity,** hyperuremia, adrenal insufficiency–like syndrome
HEMA: **Thrombocytopenia, leukopenia, pancytopenia, severe bone marrow depression**
INTEG: Dermatitis, hyperpigmentation, alopecia

OTHER: **Chromosomal aberrations**
RESP: **Irreversible pulmonary fibrosis,** pneumonitis
Contraindications: Pregnancy (D) 3rd trimester, radiation, chemotherapy, lactation, blastic phase of chronic myelocytic leukemia, hypersensitivity
Precautions: Childbearing-age women and men, leukopenia, thrombocytopenia, anemia, hepatotoxicity, renal toxicity

PHARMACOKINETICS

Well absorbed orally; excreted in urine; crosses placenta; excreted in breast milk, half-life 2.5 hr

INTERACTIONS

Increase: hepatotoxicity—thioguanine
Increase: cardiac tamponade—cyclophosphamide
Increase: toxicity—other antineoplastics, radiation
Increase: risk of bleeding—anticoagulants, aspirin
Increase: antibody response—live virus vaccines
Decrease: busulfan level—phenytoin
Decrease: busulfan clearance—acetaminophen, itraconazole
Drug/Lab Test
False positive: Breast, bladder, cervix, lung cytology tests

NURSING CONSIDERATIONS

Assess:
• CBC, differential, platelet count weekly; withhold drug if WBC is <15,000/mm³ or platelet count is <150,000/mm³; notify prescriber of results; institute thrombocytopenia precautions
• Bone marrow status prior to chemotherapy; seizure history
• Pulmonary function tests, chest x-ray films before, during therapy; chest film should be obtained q2wk during treatment; pulmonary fibrosis may occur up to 10 yr after treatment with busulfan
• Renal studies: BUN, serum uric acid, urine CCr before, during therapy; moni-

tor ALT, alk phos, bilirubin, uric acid before and during treatment

• I&O ratio; report fall in urine output <30 ml/hr

• Monitor for cold, fever, sore throat (may indicate beginning infection)

• Bleeding: hematuria, guaiac, bruising or petechiae, mucosa or orifices q8h, no rectal temps

• Dyspnea, crackles, nonproductive cough, chest pain, tachypnea

• Inflammation of mucosa, breaks in skin; use viscous xylocaine for oral pain

Administer:

PO route

• Give at same time daily, on empty stomach

IV route

• Prepared in biologic cabinet, using gloves, gown, mask; dilute with 10 times volume of drug with D_5W or 0.9% NaCl, (0.5 mg/ml). When withdrawing drug, use needle with 5-micron filter provided, remove amount needed, remove filter and inject drug into diluent; always add drug to diluent, not vice versa; stable for 8 hr room temperature (using D_5W) or 12 hr refrigerated

• Give antiemetics before IV route, on schedule

• In those with history of seizures give phenytoin prior to IV route, to prevent seizures (using 0.9% NaCl) give by central venous catheter over 2 hr q6h × 4 days, use infusion pump, do not admix

Perform/provide:

• Comprehensive oral hygiene

• Strict medical asepsis, protective isolation if WBC levels are low

• Increase fluid intake to 2-3 L/day to prevent urate deposits, calculi formation

• Store in tight container

Evaluate:

• Therapeutic response: decreased exacerbations of chronic myelocytic leukemia

Teach patient/family:

• About protective isolation precautions

• To avoid use of products containing aspirin or ibuprofen, razors, commercial mouthwash

• Use effective contraception during and at least 3 mo after treatment; avoid breast-feeding

• To report signs of anemia (fatigue, headache, irritability, faintness, shortness of breath); symptoms of infection; jaundice

• To report symptoms of bleeding (hematuria, tarry stools)

• Avoid vaccinations

• Avoid crowds, or persons with known infections

• That impotence or amenorrhea can occur, are reversible after discontinuing treatment

• To report any changes in breathing or coughing even several years after treatment

---

butoconazole vaginal antifungal
See Appendix C

---

butorphanol (℞)
(byoo-tor'fa-nole)
Stadol, Stadol NS
Func. class.: Opioid analgesic
Chem. class.: Opioid antagonist, partial agonist

Controlled Substance Schedule IV
Do not confuse:
Stadol/Haldol/sotalol

Action: Depresses pain impulse transmission at the spinal cord level by interacting with opioid receptors

Uses: Moderate to severe pain

Unlabeled uses: Migraine headache, pain

DOSAGE AND ROUTES

• *Adult:* **IM** 1-4 mg q3-4h prn; **IV** 0.5-2 mg q3-4h prn; **INTRANASAL,** 1 spray in one nostril q3-4h; may give another dose 1-1½ hr later; repeat if needed q3-4h

---

⚠ Safety alert   *"Tall Man" lettering

• *Geriatric:* IV ½ adult dose at 2× the interval; **INTRANASAL,** may repeat q1-2h
Severe pain
• *Adult:* **INTRANASAL,** 1 spray in each nostril q3-4h
Renal disease
• CCr 10-50 ml/min 75% dose; CCr <10 ml/min 50% dose
Available forms: Inj 1, 2 mg/ml; nasal spray 10 mg/ml

SIDE EFFECTS

CNS: Drowsiness, dizziness, confusion, headache, sedation, euphoria, weakness, hallucinations
CV: Palpitations, bradycardia, hypotension
EENT: Tinnitus, blurred vision, miosis, diplopia, nasal congestion
GI: Nausea, vomiting, anorexia, constipation, cramps
GU: Increased urinary output, dysuria, urinary retention
INTEG: Rash, urticaria, bruising, flushing, diaphoresis, pruritus
RESP: **Respiratory depression,** pulmonary hypertension
Contraindications: Hypersensitivity to this drug or preservative, addiction (opioid), CHF, myocardial infarction
Precautions: Pregnancy (C), addictive personality, lactation, increased intracranial pressure, respiratory depression, renal/hepatic disease, child <18 yr

PHARMACOKINETICS

IM: Onset 10-30 min, peak ½ hr, duration 3-4 hr
IV: Onset 1 min, peak 5 min, duration 2-4 hr
INTRANASAL: Onset within 15 min, peak 1-2 hr, duration 4-5 hr
Metabolized by liver; excreted by kidneys; crosses placenta; excreted in breast milk; half-life 2½-3½ hr

INTERACTIONS

⚠ Severe, fatal reactions: MAOIs
Increase: CNS effects—alcohol, opioids, sedative/hypnotics, antipsychotics, skeletal muscle relaxants
Drug/Herb
Increase: anticholinergic effect—corkwood
Increase: CNS depression—chamomile, Jamaican dogwood, kava, lavender, mistletoe, nettle, pokewood, poppy, senega, skullcap, valerian

NURSING CONSIDERATIONS
Assess:
• For decreasing output; may indicate urinary retention
⚠ For withdrawal symptoms in opioid-dependent patients: pulmonary embolus, vascular occlusion, abscesses, ulcerations
• CNS changes: dizziness, drowsiness, hallucinations, euphoria, LOC, pupil reaction
• Allergic reactions: rash, urticaria
• Respiratory dysfunction: respiratory depression, character, rate, rhythm; notify prescriber if respirations are <10/min
• Need for pain medication, physical dependence
Administer:
• With antiemetic if nausea, vomiting occur
• When pain is beginning to return; determine dosage interval by patient response
IM route
• Deeply in large muscle mass
IV route
• Undiluted at a rate of <2 mg/>3-5 min, titrate to patient response
Syringe compatibilities: Atropine, chlorproMAZINE, cimetidine, diphenhydrAMINE, droperidol, fentanyl, hydrOXYzine, meperidine, methotrimeprazine, metoclopramide, midazolam, morphine, pentazocine, perphenazine, prochlorperazine, promethazine, scopolamine, thiethylperazine
Y-site compatibilities: Allopurinol, amifostine, aztreonam, cefepime, cisatra-

curium, cladribine, DOXOrubicin liposome, enalaprilat, esmolol, filgrastim, fludarabine, granisetron, labetalol, melphalan, paclitaxel, piperacillin/tazobactam, propofol, remifentanil, sargramostim, tenoposide, thiotepa, vinorelbine

Perform/provide:
• Storage in light-resistant container at room temperature
• Assistance with ambulation
• Safety measures: night-light, call bell within easy reach, especially geriatric

Evaluate:
• Therapeutic response: decrease in pain

Teach patient/family:
• To report any symptoms of CNS changes, allergic reactions
• That physical dependency may result when used for extended periods
• That withdrawal symptoms may occur: nausea, vomiting, cramps, fever, faintness, anorexia

Treatment of overdose: Naloxone HCl (Narcan) 0.2-0.8 mg IV, O_2, IV fluids, vasopressors

---

calcifediol (℞)

(kal-si-fe-dye′ole)
Calderol
Func. class.: Vit D analog, 25-hydroxyvitamin D_3, fat soluble vitamin
Chem. class.: Sterol

Action: Increases intestinal absorption of calcium, increases renal tubular absorption of phosphate; increases mobilization of calcium from bones, bone resorption

Uses: Metabolic bone disease with chronic renal failure, osteopenia, osteomalacia, hypocalcemia

DOSAGE AND ROUTES

• *Adult:* **PO** 300-350 mcg qwk divided into daily or every other day doses; may increase q4wk or 20-100 mcg/day or 20-200 mcg/day every other day
• *Supplement (geriatric):* **PO** 20 mcg daily

Available forms: Caps 20, 50 mcg

SIDE EFFECTS

CNS: Drowsiness, headache, vertigo, fever, lethargy
CV: Dysrhythmias
EENT: Tinnitus, conjunctivitis, photophobia, rhinorrhea
GI: Nausea, diarrhea, vomiting, jaundice, anorexia, dry mouth, constipation, cramps, metallic taste, thirst
GU: Polyuria, hypercalciuria, hyperphosphatemia, hematuria
MS: Myalgia, arthralgia, decreased bone development, weakness

Contraindications: Hypersensitivity, hyperphosphatemia, hypercalcemia, vit D toxicity

Precautions: Pregnancy (C), renal calculi, lactation, CV disease, geriatric

PHARMACOKINETICS

Absorbed by the small intestine; stored in liver and fat deposits, activated in kidneys, excreted in bile and feces; peak 4 hr, duration 15-20 days; half-life 12-22 days

INTERACTIONS

Increase: hypercalcemia—thiazide diuretics, calcium supplements
Increase: cardiac dysrhythmias—cardiac glycosides
Increase: hypermagnesemia—magnesium antacids
Increase: toxicity—other vit D products
Increase: metabolism of vit D—phenytoin
Decrease: absorption of calcifediol—cholestyramine, colestipol, mineral oil, fat-soluble vitamins
Decrease: effect of this drug—corticosteroids

Drug/Food
• Dairy products, other high-calcium foods may cause hypercalcemia

Drug/Lab Test
False increase: Cholesterol
Interfere: Alk phos, electrolytes

NURSING CONSIDERATIONS

Assess:

• BUN, urinary calcium, AST, ALT, cholesterol, creatinine, uric acid, chloride, magnesium, electrolytes, urine pH, phosphate; may increase; calcium should be kept at 9-10 mg/dl, vit D 50-135 international units/dl, phosphate 70 mg/dl, alk phos may be decreased

• For increased blood level, since toxic reactions may occur rapidly

• For dry mouth, metallic taste, polyuria, bone pain, muscle weakness, headache, fatigue, tinnitus, change in LOC, irregular pulse, dysrhythmias, increased respirations, anorexia, nausea, vomiting, cramps, diarrhea, constipation; may indicate hypercalcemia

• Renal status: decreased urinary output (oliguria, anuria), edema in extremities, weight gain 5 lb, periorbital edema

• Nutritional status, diet for sources of vit D (milk, some seafood), calcium (dairy products, dark green vegetables), phosphates (dairy products)

• For hypocalcemia: muscle twitching paresthesia, dysrhythmias, laryngospasm

Administer:

• Do not break, crush, or chew caps

• May be taken without regard to food

• May be increased q4wk depending on blood level

Perform/provide:

• Storage in tight, light-resistant container at room temperature

• Restriction of sodium, potassium if required; ensure adequate calcium intake

• Restriction of fluids if required for chronic renal failure

Evaluate:

• Therapeutic response: calcium levels 9-10 mg/dl, decreasing symptoms of bone disease

Teach patient/family:

• The symptoms of hypercalcemia (renal stones, nausea, vomiting, anorexia, lethargy, thirst, bone or flank pain)

• About foods rich in calcium

• To advise prescriber of all other medications, supplements taken

---

calcitonin (rDNA) ℞
(kal-sih-toh'nin)
Fortical

calcitonin (salmon) ℞
Calcimar, Miacalcin,
Miacalcin Nasal Spray,
Osteocalcin, Salmonine
Func. class.: Parathyroid agents (calcium regulator)
Chem. class.: Polypeptide hormone

Action: Decreases bone resorption, blood calcium levels; increases deposits of calcium in bones; opposes parathyroid hormone

Uses: Paget's disease, postmenopausal osteoporosis, hypercalcemia

DOSAGE AND ROUTES

rDNA

Paget's disease

• *Adult:* **SUBCUT** 0.5 mg/day initially; may require 0.5 mg bid × 6 mo, then decrease until symptoms reappear

Salmon

Postmenopausal osteoporosis

• *Adult:* **SUBCUT/IM** 100 international units/day; **NASAL** 200 international units (1 spray) daily alternating nostrils daily, activate pump before 1st dose

Paget's disease

• *Adult:* **SUBCUT/IM** 100 international units daily, maintenance 50-100 international units daily or every other day

Hypercalcemia

• *Adult:* **SUBCUT/IM** 4 international units/kg q12h, increase to 8 international units/kg q6h if response is unsatisfactory

Available forms: Inj 200 international units/ml; nasal spray 200 international units/actuation

SIDE EFFECTS

CNS: Headache, tetany, chills, weakness, dizziness, fever
CV: Chest pressure
EENT: Nasal congestion, eye pain
GI: Nausea, diarrhea, vomiting, anorexia, abdominal pain, salty taste, epigastric pain

---

GU: Diuresis, nocturia, urine sediment, frequency
INTEG: Rash, flushing, pruritus of earlobes, edema of feet, reaction at inj site
MS: Swelling, tingling of hands
RESP: Dyspnea
SYST: **Anaphylaxis**

Contraindications: Hypersensitivity
Precautions: Pregnancy (C), renal disease, children, lactation, osteogenic sarcoma, pernicious anemia

PHARMACOKINETICS

IM/SUBCUT: Onset 15 min, peak 4 hr, duration 8-24 hr; metabolized by kidneys, excreted as inactive metabolites via kidneys

NURSING CONSIDERATIONS

Assess:
• GI symptoms, polyuria, flushing, head swelling, tingling, headache; may indicate hypercalcemia
• Nutritional status; diet for sources of vit D (milk, some seafood), calcium (dairy products, dark green vegetables), phosphates
• BUN, creatinine, uric acid, chloride, electrolytes, urine pH, urinary calcium, magnesium, phosphate, urinalysis (calcium should be kept at 9-10 mg/dl, vit D 50-135 international units/dl), alk phos baseline, q3-6mo, monitor urine hydroproline in Paget's disease
• Increased drug level, since toxic reactions occur rapidly; have parenteral calcium on hand if calcium level drops too low; check for tetany (irritability, paresthesia, nervousness, muscle twitching, seizures, tetanic spasms)
• Urine for sediment

Administer:
SUBCUT route (rDNA)
• By SUBCUT route only; rotate inj sites; use within 6 hr of reconstitution; give at bedtime to minimize nausea, vomiting
IM route (Salmon)
• After test dose of 10 international units/ml, 0.1 ml intradermally; watch 15 min; give only with epINEPHrine and emergency meds available
• IM inj slowly in deep muscle mass; rotate sites

Perform/provide:
• Storage at <77° F (25° C); protect from light

Evaluate:
• Therapeutic response: calcium levels 9-10 mg/dl, decreasing symptoms of Paget's disease

Teach patient/family:
• The method of inj if patient will be responsible for self-medication
• To report difficulty swallowing or any change in side effects to prescriber immediately

Nasal
• To use alternating nostrils for nasal spray

---

calcitriol (Ŗ)
(kal-sih-try′ole)
Calcijex, Rocaltrol (1,25-dihydroxycholecalciferol), vitamin D₃
Func. class.: Parathyroid agent (calcium regulator)
Chem. class.: Vit D hormone

Do not confuse:
calcitriol/Calciferol

Action: Increases intestinal absorption of calcium, provides calcium for bones, increases renal tubular resorption of phosphate

Uses: Hypocalcemia in chronic renal disease, hyperparathyroidism pseudohypoparathyroidism

DOSAGE AND ROUTES

Hypocalcemia
• *Adult:* **IV** 0.5 mcg tid, initially; may increase by 0.25-0.5 mcg/dose q2-4wk; 0.5-3 mcg tid maintenance
Predialysis
• *Adult:* **PO** 0.25 mcg/day, max 0.5 mcg/day

- *Child:* **PO** 0.25 mcg/day, max 0.5 mcg/day
- *Child <3 yr:* **PO** 10-15 mcg/kg/day

Hypocalcemia during chronic dialysis
- *Adult:* **PO** 0.5-3 mcg/day
- *Child:* **PO** 0.25-2 mcg/day

Renal osteodystrophy
- *Adult:* **PO** 0.25 mcg every other day-3 mcg/day
- *Child:* **PO** 0.014-0.041 mcg/kg/day

Hypoparathyroidism
- *Adult:* **PO** 0.25-2.7 mcg/day
- *Child:* **PO** 0.04-0.08 mcg/kg/day

Available forms: Caps 0.25, 0.5 mcg; inj 1 mcg, 2 mcg/ml

SIDE EFFECTS

CNS: Drowsiness, headache, vertigo, fever, lethargy
CV: Palpitations
EENT: Blurred vision, photophobia
GI: Nausea, diarrhea, vomiting, jaundice, anorexia, dry mouth, constipation, cramps, metallic taste
GU: Polyuria, hypercalciuria, hyperphosphatemia, hematuria, thirst
MS: Myalgia, arthralgia, decreased bone development, weakness

Contraindications: Hypersensitivity, hyperphosphatemia, hypercalcemia, vit D toxicity

Precautions: Pregnancy (C), renal calculi, lactation, CV disease

PHARMACOKINETICS

PO: Absorbed readily from GI tract, peak 10-12 hr, duration 3-5 days, half-life 3-6 hr; undergoes hepatic recycling, excreted in bile

INTERACTIONS

- Hypercalcemia: thiazide diuretics, calcium supplements
- Cardiac dysrhythmias: cardiac glycosides, verapamil
- Hypermagnesemia: magnesium antacids
- Toxicity: other vit D products
Increase: metabolism of vit D—phenytoin

Decrease: absorption of calcitriol—cholestyramine, mineral oil, fat-soluble vitamins

Drug/Food
- Large amounts of high-calcium foods may cause hypercalcemia

Drug/Lab Test
False increase: Cholesterol
Interfere: Alk phos, electrolytes

NURSING CONSIDERATIONS

Assess:
- BUN, urinary calcium, AST, ALT, cholesterol, creatinine, albumin, uric acid, chloride, magnesium, electrolytes, urine pH, phosphate; may increase calcium, should be kept at 9-10 mg/dl, vit D 50-135 international units/dl, phosphate 70 mg/dl
- Alk phos; may be decreased
- For increased drug level, since toxic reactions may occur rapidly
- For dry mouth, metallic taste, polyuria, bone pain, muscle weakness, headache, fatigue, change in LOC, dysrhythmias, increased respirations, anorexia, nausea, vomiting, cramps, diarrhea, constipation; may indicate hypercalcemia
- Renal status: decreased urinary output (oliguria, anuria), edema in extremities, weight gain 5-7 lb, periorbital edema
- Nutritional status, diet for sources of vit D (milk, some seafood); calcium (dairy products, dark green vegetables), phosphates (dairy products) must be avoided

Administer:
PO route
- Do not break, crush, or chew caps
- Give without regard to meals
IV route
- Give by direct IV over 1 min
Perform/provide:
- Storage protected from light, heat, moisture
- Restriction of sodium, potassium if required
- Restriction of fluids if required for chronic renal failure
Evaluate:
- Therapeutic response: calcium 9-10 mg/dl, decreasing symptoms of hypocalcemia, hypoparathyroidism

Side effects: *italics* = common; **bold** = life-threatening

Teach patient/family:

• The symptoms of hypercalcemia (renal stones, nausea, vomiting, anorexia, lethargy, thirst, bone or flank pain)

• About foods rich in calcium

• To avoid products with sodium: cured meats, dairy products, cold cuts, olives, beets, pickles, soups, meat tenderizers in chronic renal failure

• To avoid products with potassium: oranges, bananas, dried fruit, peas, dark green leafy vegetables, milk, melons, beans in chronic renal failure

• To avoid OTC products containing calcium, potassium, or sodium in chronic renal failure

• To avoid all preparations containing vit D

• To monitor weight weekly

---

calcium carbonate
(PO-OTC, IV-℞)

Alka-Mints, Amitone, Apo-Cal ✦, BioCal, Calcarb, Calci-Chew, Calci-Mix, Calcilac, Calcite ✦, Calglycine ✦, Cal-Plus, Calsan ✦, Caltrate 600, Caltrate Jr., Chooz, Dicarbosil, Equilet, Gencalc, Liquid-Cal, Liquid-Cal-600, Maalox Antacid Caplets, Mallamint, Mylanta Lozenges ✦, Nephro-Calci, Nu-Cal ✦, Os-Cal 500, Oysco 500, Oyster-cal 500, Oyst-Cal 500, Rolaids Calcium Rich, Titralac, Tums, Tums E-X Extra Strength

calcium acetate (OTC)
(kal′see-um ass′e-tate)
Calphron, PhosLo
Func. class.: Antacid, calcium supplement
Chem. class.: Calcium product

Action: Neutralizes gastric acidity
Uses: Antacid, calcium supplement; not suitable for chronic therapy, hyperphosphatemia, hypertension in pregnancy, osteoporosis, prevention, treatment of hypocalcemia, hyperparathyroidism

DOSAGE AND ROUTES

Antacid
• *Adult:* **PO** 0.5-1.5 g or 2 pieces of gum 1 hr after meals and at bedtime
Prevention of hypocalcemia, depletion, osteoporosis
• *Adult:* **PO** 1-2 g daily
Hyperphosphatemia
• *Adult:* **PO** 1 g or more in divided doses
Hypertension in pregnancy
• *Adult:* **PO** 500 mg tid during 3rd trimester

Available forms: *calcium carbonate:* chewable tabs 350, 420, 450, 500, 750, 1000, 1250 mg; tabs 500, 600, 650, 1000, 1250 mg; gum 300, 450, 500 mg; susp 1250 mg/5 ml; lozenges 600 mg; caps 1250 mg; powder 6.5 g/packet; *calcium acetate:* tabs 250 mg (65 mg Ca), 667 mg (169 mg Ca), 668 mg (169 mg Ca), 1 g (250 mg Ca); caps 500 mg (125 mg Ca)

SIDE EFFECTS

GI: Constipation, anorexia, nausea, vomiting, flatulence, diarrhea, rebound hyperacidity, eructation
Contraindications: Hypersensitivity, hypercalcemia, hyperparathyroidism, bone tumors
Precautions: Pregnancy (C), geriatric, fluid restriction, decreased GI motility, GI obstruction, dehydration, renal disease, lactation

PHARMACOKINETICS

⅓ of dose absorbed by small intestine, onset 20 min, duration 20-180 min, excreted in feces and urine, crosses placenta

INTERACTIONS

Increase: plasma levels of quinidine, amphetamines
Decrease: levels of salicylates, calcium channel blockers, ketoconazole, tetracyclines, iron salts, quinolone antibiotics

---

⚠ Safety alert   ✦ "Tall Man" lettering

Drug/Herb

Increase: action/side effects—lily of the valley, pheasant's eye, shark cartilage, squill

Drug/Lab Test

False increase: Chloride
False positive: Benzodiazepines
False decrease: Magnesium, oxylate, lipase

NURSING CONSIDERATIONS

Assess:

• Calcium (serum, urine), calcium should be 8.5-10.5 mg/dl, urine calcium should be 150 mg/day, monitor weekly

⚠ Milk-alkali syndrome: nausea, vomiting, disorientation, headache

• Constipation; increase bulk in the diet if needed

• Hypercalcemia: headache, nausea, vomiting, confusion

Administer:

PO route

• As antacid 1 hr after meals and at bedtime

• As supplement 1½ hr after meals and at bedtime

• Only with regular tablets or capsules; do not give with enteric-coated tablets

• Laxatives or stool softeners if constipation occurs

Evaluate:

• Therapeutic response: absence of pain, decreased acidity

Teach patient/family:

• To increase fluids to 2 L unless contraindicated, to add bulk to diet for constipation, notify prescriber of constipation

• Not to switch antacids unless directed by prescriber, not to use as antacid for >2 wk without approval by prescriber

• That therapeutic dose recommendations are figured as elemental calcium

calcium chloride
calcium gluceptate
calcium gluconate
Kalcinate
calcium lactate (℞)
Cal-Lac

Func. class.: Electrolyte replacement—calcium product

Action: Cation needed for maintenance of nervous, muscular, skeletal function, enzyme reactions, normal cardiac contractility, coagulation of blood; affects secretory activity of endocrine, exocrine glands

Uses: Prevention and treatment of hypocalcemia, hypermagnesemia, hypoparathyroidism, neonatal tetany, cardiac toxicity caused by hyperkalemia, lead colic, hyperphosphatemia, vit D deficiency, osteoporosis prophylaxis, calcium antagonist toxicity (calcium channel blocker toxicity)

DOSAGE AND ROUTES

Calcium gluceptate
• *Adult:* **IV** 5-20 ml; **IM** 2-5 ml
Calcium chloride
• *Adult:* **IV** 500 mg-1 g q1-3d as indicated by serum calcium levels, give at <1 ml/min; **IV** 200-800 mg injected in ventricle of heart
• *Child:* **IV** 25 mg/kg over several min
Calcium gluconate
• *Adult:* **PO** 0.5-2 g bid-qid; **IV** 0.5-2 g at 0.5 ml/min (10% solution); max **IV** dose 3 g
• *Child:* **PO/IV** 500 mg/kg/day in divided doses
Calcium lactate
• *Adult:* **PO** 325 mg-1.3 g tid with meals
• *Child:* **PO** 500 mg/kg/day in divided doses

Available forms: Many; check product listings

SIDE EFFECTS

CV: Shortened QT, heart block, hypotension, bradycardia, **dysrhythmias; cardiac arrest (IV)**

GI: Vomiting, nausea, constipation

HYPERCALCEMIA: Drowsiness, lethargy, muscle weakness, headache, constipation, **coma,** anorexia, nausea, vomiting, polyuria, thirst

INTEG: Pain, burning at IV site, severe venous thrombosis, necrosis, extravasation

Contraindications: Hypercalcemia, digoxin toxicity, ventricular fibrillation, renal calculi

Precautions: Pregnancy (C), lactation, children, renal disease, respiratory disease, cor pulmonale, digitalized patient, respiratory failure

PHARMACOKINETICS

Crosses placenta, enters breast milk, excreted via urine and feces; half-life unknown

PO: Onset, peak, duration unknown; absorption (PO) from GI tract

IV: Onset immediate, duration ½-2 hr

INTERACTIONS

Increase: milk-alkali syndrome—antacids

Increase: dysrhythmias—digitalis glycosides

Increase: toxicity—verapamil

Increase: hypercalcemia—thiazide diuretics

Decrease: absorption of fluoroquinolones, tetracyclines, iron salts, phenytoin, when calcium is taken PO

Decrease: effects of atenolol, verapamil

Drug/Herb

Increase: action/side effects—lily of the valley, pheasant's eye, shark cartilage, squill

Drug/Lab Test

Increase: 11-OHCS

Decrease: 17-OHCS

False decrease: Magnesium

NURSING CONSIDERATIONS

Assess:

• ECG for decreased QT and T wave inversion: hypercalcemia, drug should be reduced or discontinued, consider cardiac monitoring

• Calcium levels during treatment (8.5-11.5 g/dl is normal level)

• Cardiac status: rate, rhythm, CVP (PWP, PAWP if being monitored directly)

• Hypocalcemia: muscle twitching, paresthesia, dysrhythmias, laryngospasm

Administer:

PO route

• With or following meals to enhance absorption

IM route

• IM inj may cause severe burning, necrosis, tissue sloughing; warm sol to body temp before administering (only gluconate/gluceptate)

IV route

• Undiluted or diluted with equal amounts of NS to a 5% sol for inj, give 0.5-1 ml/min

• Through small-bore needle into large vein; if extravasation occurs, necrosis will result (IV)

• Remain recumbent ½ hr after IV dose

Calcium chloride

Additive compatibilities: Amikacin, amphotericin B, ampicillin, ascorbic acid, bretylium, ceftriaxone, cephapirin, chloramphenicol, DOPamine, hydrocortisone, isoproterenol, lidocaine, methicillin, norepinephrine, penicillin G potassium, penicillin G sodium, pentobarbital, phenobarbital, verapamil, vit B/C

Syringe compatibilities: Milrinone

Y-site compatibilities: Amrinone, DOBUTamine, epINEPHrine, esmolol, morphine, paclitaxel

Calcium gluceptate

Additive compatibilities: Ascorbic acid inj, isoproterenol, lidocaine, norepinephrine, phytonadione, sodium bicarbonate

Calcium gluconate

Additive compatibilities: Amikacin, aminophylline, ascorbic acid injection, bretylium, cephapirin, chloramphenicol, cisatracurium, corticotropin, dimenhy-DRINATE, DOXOrubicin liposome, erythromycin, furosemide, heparin, hydrocortisone, lidocaine, magnesium sulfate, methicillin, norepinephrine, penicillin G potassium, penicillin G sodium, phenobarbital, potassium chloride, remifentanil, tobramycin, vancomycin, verapamil, vit B/C

Syringe compatibilities: Aldesleukin, allopurinol, amifostine, aztreonam, cefazolin, cefepime, ciprofloxacin, cladribine, DOBUTamine, enalaprilat, epINEPHrine, famotidine, filgrastim, granisetron, heparin/hydrocortisone, labetalol, melphalan, midazolam, netilmicin, piperacillin/tazobactam, potassium chloride, prochlorperazine, propofol, sargramostim, tacrolimus, teniposide, thiotepa, tolazoline, vinorelbine, vit B/C

Perform/provide:
• Seizure precautions: padded side rails, decreased stimuli (noise, light); place airway suction equipment, padded mouth gag if Ca levels are low
• Store at room temperature

Evaluate:
• Therapeutic response: decreased twitching, paresthesias, muscle spasms, absence of tremors, convulsions, dysrhythmias, dyspnea, laryngospasm, negative Chvostek's sign, negative Trousseau's sign

Teach patient/family:
• To add foods high in vit D
• To add calcium-rich foods to diet: dairy products, shellfish, dark green leafy vegetables; decrease oxalate-rich and zinc-rich foods: nuts, legumes, chocolate, spinach, soy
• To prevent injuries, avoid immobilization

calcium polycarbophil (otc)
(pol-ee-kar'boe-fil)
Equalactin, Fiberall, FiberCon, Fiber-Lax, Mitrolan
Func. class.: Laxative, bulk-forming

Action: Attracts water, expands in intestine to increase peristalsis; also absorbs excess water in stool; decreases diarrhea
Uses: Constipation, irritable bowel syndrome (diarrhea), acute, nonspecific diarrhea

DOSAGE AND ROUTES
• *Adult:* PO 1 g daily-qid prn, max 4 g/24 hr
• *Child 6-11 yr:* PO 500 mg ≤4×/day or prn, max 2 g/day
• *Child 3-5 yr:* PO 500 mg bid prn, not to exceed 1 g/24 hr
Available forms: Chew tabs 500, 1000 mg; tabs 500 mg

SIDE EFFECTS
GI: **Obstruction,** abdominal distention, flatus, laxative dependence
Contraindications: Hypersensitivity, GI obstruction
Precautions: Pregnancy (C), lactation

PHARMACOKINETICS
PO: Onset 12-72 hr, peak 1-3 days

INTERACTIONS
Drug/Herb
Increase: action/side effects—flax, lily of the valley, pheasant's eye, senna, squill

NURSING CONSIDERATIONS
Assess:
• Cause of constipation; identify whether fluids, bulk, or exercise is missing from lifestyle, constipating drugs
• Cramping, rectal bleeding, nausea, vomiting; if these symptoms occur, drug should be discontinued

Administer:
• Alone for better absorption; do not take within 1-2 hr of other drugs
• In morning or evening

Evaluate:
• Therapeutic response: decreased constipation

Teach patient/family:
• Not to use laxatives for long-term therapy; laxative dependence will result
• That normal bowel movements do not always occur daily
• Not to use in presence of abdominal pain, nausea, vomiting
• To notify prescriber if constipation is unrelieved or if symptoms of electrolyte imbalance occur: muscle cramps, pain, weakness, dizziness
• To chew thoroughly (chew tab) and follow with 6-8 oz water

Rarely Used

calfactant (℞)
(cal-fak′tant)
Infasurf
Func. class.: Natural lung surfactant extract

Uses: Prevention and treatment (rescue) of respiratory distress syndrome in premature infants

DOSAGE AND ROUTES
• *Newborn:* **INTRATRACHEAL INSTILL:** 3 ml/kg of birth wt, given as 2 doses of 1.5 ml/kg, repeat doses of 3 ml/kg of birth wt until up to 3 doses 12 hr apart have been given

candesartan (℞)
(can-deh-sar′tan)
Atacand
Func. class.: Antihypertensive
Chem. class.: Angiotensin II receptor (type AT_1)

Action: Blocks the vasoconstrictor and aldosterone-secreting effects of angiotensin II; selectively blocks the binding of angiotensin II to the AT_1 receptor found in tissues

Uses: Hypertension, alone or in combination; CHF NYHA Class II-IV and ejection fraction ≤40%

DOSAGE AND ROUTES
• *Adult:* **PO,** single agent 16 mg daily initially in patients who are not volume depleted, range 8-32 mg/day; with diuretic, or volume depletion 2-32 mg/day as single dose or divided bid
Renal disease
• *Adult:* **PO** give lowest possible dose
Available forms: Tabs 4, 8, 16, 32 mg

SIDE EFFECTS
CNS: Dizziness, fatigue, headache
CV: Chest pain, peripheral edema, hypotension
EENT: Sinusitis, rhinitis, pharyngitis
GI: Diarrhea, nausea, abdominal pain, vomiting
GU: **Renal failure**
MS: Arthralgia, pain
RESP: Cough, upper respiratory infection
SYST: **Angioedema**
Contraindications: Pregnancy (D) 2nd/3rd trimesters, hypersensitivity
Precautions: Pregnancy (C) 1st trimester, hypersensitivity to ACE inhibitors, lactation, children, geriatric, volume-depletion, renal/hepatic impairment

PHARMACOKINETICS
Peak 3-4 hr, protein binding 99%, half-life 9-12 hr, extensively metabolized, excreted in urine (33%) and feces (67%)

INTERACTIONS
Increase: lithium level—lithium
Increase: hypokalemia—potassium, potassium-sparing diuretics
Increase: hypotension—ACE inhibitors, β-blockers, calcium channel blockers, α-blockers
Decrease: effect—salicylates, NSAIDs

▲ Safety alert   *"Tall Man" lettering

Drug/Herb
Increase: effect—barberry, betony, black catechu, black cohosh, bloodroot, broom, burdock, cat's claw, dandelion, goldenseal, Irish moss, Jamaican dogwood, kelp, khella, mistletoe, parsley, Queen Anne's lace, rue
Increase: toxicity/death—aconite
Increase or decrease: effect—astragalus, cola tree
Decrease: effect—coltsfoot, guarana, khat, licorice, yohimbine

NURSING CONSIDERATIONS
Assess:
• For angioedema: facial swelling, difficulty breathing (rare)
• For pregnancy, this drug can cause fetal death when given in pregnancy
• Response and adverse reactions especially in renal disease
• B/P, pulse q4h; note rate, rhythm, quality; electrolytes: K, Na, Cl; baselines in renal, hepatic studies before therapy begins
Administer:
• Without regard to meals
Evaluate:
• Therapeutic response: decreased B/P
Teach patient/family:
• To comply with dosage schedule, even if feeling better
• To notify prescriber of mouth sores, fever, swelling of hands or feet, irregular heartbeat, chest pain
• That excessive perspiration, dehydration, vomiting, diarrhea may lead to fall in blood pressure; to consult prescriber if these occur
• That drug may cause dizziness, fainting; light-headedness may occur
• To rise slowly to sitting or standing position to minimize orthostatic hypotension
• To notify prescriber immediately if pregnant; not to use during lactation
• To avoid all OTC medications, unless approved by prescriber; to inform all health care providers of medication use
• To use proper technique for obtaining B/P and acceptable parameters

capecitabine (℞)
(cap-eh-sit'ah-been)
Xeloda
Func. class.: Antineoplastic, antimetabolite
Chem. class.: Fluoropyrimidine carbamate

Do not confuse:
Xeloda/Xenical

Action: Competes with physiologic substrate of DNA synthesis, thus interfering with cell replication in the S phase of cell cycle (before mitosis), also interferes with RNA and protein synthesis; drug is converted to 5-FU

Uses: Monotherapy for paclitaxel, anthracycline resistant, metastatic breast, colorectal cancer when 5-FU monotherapy is preferred; treatment of colorectal cancer patients who have undergone complete resection of their primary tumor
Unlabeled uses: Pancreatic cancer

DOSAGE AND ROUTES
• *Adult:* **PO** 2500 mg/m²/day in 2 divided doses q12h at end of meal × 2 wk, then 1 wk rest period; given in 3 wk cycles; may be combined with docetaxel, when capecitabine dose is lowered; follow the NCIC (National Cancer Institute of Canada) common toxicity criteria
Renal dose
• *Adult:* **PO** CCr 30-50 ml/min, decrease initial dose to 75% of usual dose
Available forms: Tabs 150, 500 mg

SIDE EFFECTS
CNS: Dizziness, *headache, paresthesia, fatigue,* insomnia
GI: Nausea, vomiting, anorexia, diarrhea, stomatitis, abdominal pain, constipation, dyspepsia, **intestinal obstruction, necrotizing enterocolitis**
HEMA: **Neutropenia, lymphopenia, thrombocytopenia,** anemia
INTEG: Hand and foot syndrome, dermatitis, nail disorder
OTHER: Hyperbilirubinemia, *eye irrita-*

tion, edema, myalgia, limb pain, *pyrexia,* dehydration
RESP: Cough, dyspnea

Contraindications: Pregnancy (D), hypersensitivity to 5-FU, infants, severe renal impairment (CCr <30 ml/min)

Precautions: Renal/hepatic disease, lactation, children, geriatric

PHARMACOKINETICS

Readily absorbed, peak 1½ hr; food decreases absorption; extensively metabolized in the liver; elimination half-life 45 min

INTERACTIONS

Increase: toxicity—leucovorin
Increase: capecitabine levels—antacids (aluminum, magnesium)
⚠ *Increase:* risk of bleeding—warfarin
Increase: phenytoin level—phenytoin
Drug/Food
Increase: absorption, give within 30 min of a meal

NURSING CONSIDERATIONS
Assess:

• CBC (RBC, Hct, Hgb), differential, platelet count weekly; withhold drug if WBC is <4000/mm³, platelet count is <75,000/mm³, or RBC, Hct, Hgb low; notify prescriber of these results; frequently monitor INR in those receiving warfarin concurrently
• Renal studies: BUN, serum uric acid, urine CCr, electrolytes before and during therapy
• Monitor temp q4h; fever may indicate beginning infection; no rectal temps
• Hepatic studies before and during therapy: bilirubin, ALT, AST, alk phos, as needed or monthly
• Bleeding: hematuria, heme-positive stools, bruising or petechiae, mucosa or orifices q8h
• Dyspnea, crackles, unproductive cough, chest pain, tachypnea, fatigue, increased pulse, pallor, lethargy; personality changes, with high doses
• For hand and foot syndrome: paresthe-

sia, tingling, painful/painless swelling, blistering, erythema with severe pain of hands or feet
• For toxicity: severe diarrhea, nausea, vomiting, stomatitis, fever
• Buccal cavity q8h for dryness, sores or ulceration, white patches, oral pain, bleeding, dysphagia
• GI symptoms: frequency of stools, cramping; if severe diarrhea occurs, fluid and electrolytes may need to be given
Administer:
• With water within ½ hour of breakfast and dinner
Perform/provide:
• Rinsing of mouth tid-qid with water, club soda; brushing of teeth bid-tid with soft brush or cotton-tipped applicators for stomatitis; use unwaxed dental floss
Evaluate:
• Therapeutic response: decreased tumor size, spread of malignancy
Teach patient/family:
• To avoid foods with citric acid, hot or rough texture if stomatitis is present; take with water within 30 min of end of meal
• To avoid pregnancy while on this drug; to avoid breastfeeding
• Not to double dose, if dose is missed
⚠ To immediately report severe diarrhea, vomiting, stomatitis, fever over 100° F (37.8° C), hand and foot syndrome, anorexia
• To report signs of infection: increased temp, sore throat, flulike symptoms
• To report signs of anemia: fatigue, headache, faintness, shortness of breath, irritability
• To report bleeding; to avoid use of razors, commercial mouthwash

---

captopril (℞)
(kap′toe-pril)
Capoten, Novo-Captopril ✦
Func. class.: Antihypertensive
Chem. class.: Angiotensin-converting enzyme (ACE) inhibitor

Do not confuse:
captopril/Capitrol/carvedilol

⚠ Safety alert   *"Tall Man" lettering

Action: Selectively suppresses renin-angiotensin-aldosterone system; inhibits ACE; preventing conversion of angiotensin I to angiotensin II

Uses: Hypertension, CHF, left ventricular dysfunction after MI, diabetic nephropathy

DOSAGE AND ROUTES

Malignant hypertension
• *Adult:* PO 25 mg increasing q2h until desired response, not to exceed 450 mg/day

Hypertension
• *Adult:* PO initial dose: 12.5-25 mg bid-tid; may increase to 50 mg bid-tid at 1-2 wk intervals; usual range: 25-150 mg bid-tid; max 450 mg

• *Child:* PO 0.3-0.5 mg/kg/dose, titrate up to 6 mg/kg/day in 2-4 divided doses

• *Neonate:* PO 0.05-0.1 mg/kg bid-tid, may increase as needed

CHF
• *Adult:* PO 25 mg bid-tid; may increase to 50 mg bid-tid; after 14 days, may increase to 150 mg tid if needed

LVD after MI
• *Adult:* PO 50 mg tid, may begin treatment 3 days after MI; give 6.25 mg as a single dose, then 12.5 mg tid, increase to 25 mg tid for several days, then to 50 mg tid

Diabetic nephropathy
• *Adult:* PO 25 mg tid

Renal dose
• *Adult:* PO CCr >50, no change; CCr 10-50, decrease dose by 25%; CCr <10, decrease dose by 50%

Available forms: Tabs 12.5, 25, 50, 100 mg

SIDE EFFECTS

CNS: Fever, chills

CV: Hypotension, postural hypotension, *tachycardia,* angina

GI: Loss of taste, increased LFTs

GU: Impotence, dysuria, nocturia, proteinuria, **nephrotic syndrome, acute reversible renal failure,** polyuria, oliguria, urinary frequency

HEMA: **Neutropenia, agranulocytosis, pancytopenia, thrombocytopenia,** anemia

INTEG: Rash, pruritus

MISC: **Angioedema,** hyperkalemia

RESP: **Bronchospasm,** *dyspnea, cough*

Contraindications: Pregnancy (D) 2nd/3rd trimesters, hypersensitivity, lactation, heart block, children, potassium-sparing diuretics, bilateral renal artery stenosis, angioedema

Precautions: Pregnancy (C) 1st trimester, dialysis patients, hypovolemia, leukemia, scleroderma, SLE, blood dyscrasias, CHF, diabetes mellitus, renal/hepatic/thyroid disease, COPD, asthma

PHARMACOKINETICS

PO: Peak 1 hr; duration 2-6 hr; half-life <2 hr, increased in renal disease; metabolized by liver (metabolites); excreted in urine; crosses placenta; excreted in breast milk, small amounts; protein binding 25%-30%

INTERACTIONS

• Do not use with potassium-sparing diuretics, sympathomimetics, potassium supplements

Increase: possible toxicity—lithium, digoxin

Increase: hypoglycemia—insulin, oral antidiabetics

Increase: hypotension—diuretics, other antihypertensives, phenothiazines, nitrates, acute alcohol ingestion

Decrease: captopril effect—antacids, NSAIDs, salicylates

Drug/Herb

Increase: toxicity/death—aconite

Increase: antihypertensive effect—barberry, betony, black catechu, black cohosh, bloodroot, broom, burdock, cat's claw, dandelion, goldenseal, Irish moss, Jamaican dogwood, kelp, khella, mistletoe, parsley

Increase or decrease: antihypertensive effect—astragalus, cola tree

Decrease: antihypertensive effect—coltsfoot, guarana, khat, licorice, yohimbine

---

Drug/Lab Test
Increase: AST, ALT, alk phos, bilirubin, uric acid, glucose
False positive: Urine acetone, ANA titer

NURSING CONSIDERATIONS
Assess:
• Blood studies: decreased platelets; WBC with diff baseline and periodically q3mo, if neutrophils <1000/mm³, discontinue treatment (recommended with collagen-vascular or renal disease)
• B/P, pulse rates baseline, frequently
• Renal studies: protein, BUN, creatinine; watch for raised levels that may indicate nephrotic syndrome
• Baselines in renal, hepatic studies before therapy begins and periodically, increased LFTs, uric acid and glucose may be increased
• Edema in feet, legs daily, weight daily in CHF
• Allergic reaction: rash, fever, pruritus, urticaria; discontinue drug if antihistamines fail to help
• Symptoms of CHF: edema, dyspnea, wet crackles, B/P
Administer:
• 1 hr before or 2 hr after meals
• May crush tab and dissolve in water; give within ½ hr; make sure tab is completely dissolved
Perform/provide:
• Storage in tight container at 86° F (30° C) or less
Evaluate:
• Therapeutic response: decrease in B/P in hypertension, edema, moist crackles (CHF)
Teach patient/family:
• That tabs may be crushed and mixed with food; to take 1 hr before or 2 hr after meals; not to discontinue drug abruptly; if dose is missed take as soon as remembered, but not if almost time for next dose; do not double doses
• Not to use OTC products (cough, cold, or allergy) unless directed by prescriber; avoid salt substitutes, high-potassium or high-sodium foods

• To avoid sunlight or wear sunscreen if in sunlight; photosensitivity may occur
• To comply with dosage schedule, even if feeling better
• To rise slowly to sitting or standing position to minimize orthostatic hypotension
• To notify prescriber of mouth sores, sore throat, fever, swelling of hands or feet, irregular heartbeat, chest pain, signs of angioedema
• That excessive perspiration, dehydration, vomiting; diarrhea may lead to fall in B/P; consult prescriber if these occur
• That dizziness, fainting, lightheadedness may occur during first few days of therapy
• That skin rash or impaired perspiration may occur
• How to take B/P and when to notify prescriber
• To report if pregnancy is suspected or planned
Treatment of overdose: 0.9% NaCl IV/INF; hemodialysis

carbachol ophthalmic
See Appendix C

carbamazepine (℞)
(kar-ba-maz′e-peen)
Apo-Carbamazepine ✦,
Atretol, Carbatrol, Epitol,
Equetro, Novo-Carbamaz ✦,
Tegretol, Tegretol CR ✦,
Tegretol-XR, Teril
Func. class.: Anticonvulsant
Chem. class.: Iminostilbene derivative

Do not confuse:
Tegretol/Toradol
Action: Exact mechanism unknown; appears to decrease polysynaptic responses and block posttetanic potentiation
Uses: Tonic-clonic, complex-partial, mixed seizures; trigeminal neuralgia, bipolar disorder

⚠ Safety alert   *"Tall Man" lettering

Unlabeled uses: Diabetes insipidus, neurogenic pain, schizophrenia, psychotic behavior with dementia, rectal administration, diabetic neuropathy, restless leg syndrome

DOSAGE AND ROUTES
Seizures
• *Adult and child >12 yr:* **PO** 200 mg bid, may be increased by 200 mg/day in divided doses q6-8h; maintenance 800-1200 mg/day maximum 1600 mg/day (adult); max child 12-15 yr 1000 mg/day; max child >15 yr 1200 mg/day; adjustment is needed to minimum dose to control seizures; **EXT REL** give bid; rectal administration of oral susp 200 mg/10 ml or 6 mg/kg as a single dose
• *Child 6-12 yr:* **PO** tabs 100 mg bid or susp 50 mg qid; may increase by <100 mg qwk; max 1000 mg/day **EXT REL** tabs daily-bid
• *Child <6 yr:* **PO** 10-20 mg/kg/day in 2-3 divided doses, may increase qwk
Trigeminal neuralgia
• *Adult:* **PO** 100 mg bid with meals; may increase 100 mg q12h until pain subsides, not to exceed 1200 mg/day; maintenance is 200-400 mg bid
Bipolar disorder
• *Adult:* **PO** (Equetro only) 200 mg bid, may adjust dose by 200 mg daily to desired response, max 1600 mg/day
Available forms: Chewable tabs 100, 200 mg; tabs 200 mg; ext rel tabs (XR) 100, 200, 400 mg; oral susp 100 mg/5 ml; ext rel caps 100, 200, 300 mg

SIDE EFFECTS
CNS: Drowsiness, dizziness, unsteadiness, confusion, fatigue, **paralysis,** headache, hallucinations, **worsening of seizures,** speech disturbance
CV: **Hypertension, CHF, dysrhythmias, AV block,** hypotension, aggravation of cardiac artery disease
EENT: Tinnitus, dry mouth, blurred vision, diplopia, nystagmus, conjunctivitis
ENDO: SIADH (geriatric)
GI: Nausea, constipation, diarrhea, anorexia, vomiting, abdominal pain, stoma-

titis, glossitis, increased hepatic enzymes, **hepatitis**
GU: Frequency, retention, albuminuria, glycosuria, impotence, increased BUN, **renal failure**
HEMA: **Thrombocytopenia, leukopenia, agranulocytosis, leukocytosis, aplastic anemia, eosinophilia,** increased PT
INTEG: Rash, **Stevens-Johnson syndrome,** urticaria, photosensitivity
RESP: Pulmonary hypersensitivity (fever, dyspnea, pneumonitis)
Contraindications: Pregnancy (D), hypersensitivity to carbamazepine or tricyclics, bone marrow depression, concomitant use of MAOIs
Precautions: Glaucoma, renal/hepatic/cardiac disease, psychosis, lactation, child <6 yr

PHARMACOKINETICS
PO: Onset slow, peak 4-8 hr; metabolized by liver; excreted in urine, feces; crosses placenta, blood-brain barrier; excreted in breast milk; half-life 14-16 hr, protein binding 76%

INTERACTIONS
• CNS toxicity: lithium
⚠ Fatal reaction: MAOIs
Increase: carbamazepine levels—cimetidine, clarithromycin, danazol, diltiazem, erythromycin, fluoxetine, fluvoxamine, isoniazid, propoxyphene, valproic acid, verapamil
Increase: effects of desmopressin, lithium, lypressin, vasopressin
Decrease: effects of benzodiazepines, doxycycline, felbamate, haloperidol, oral contraceptives, phenobarbital, phenytoin, primidone, theophylline, thyroid hormones, warfarin
Decrease: carbamazepine levels—cisplatin, DOXOrubicin, felbamate, rifampin, phenobarbital, phenytoin, primidone, theophylline
Drug/Herb
Decrease: carbamazepine metabolism, increased levels—quinine, ginkgo

Decrease: anticonvulsant effect—ginseng, santonica

Drug/Food

Increase: peak concentration of carbamazepine—grapefruit juice

NURSING CONSIDERATIONS

Assess:

• For seizures: character, location, duration, intensity, frequency, presence of aura

• For trigeminal neuralgia: facial pain including location, duration, intensity, character, activity that stimulates pain

• Renal studies: urinalysis, BUN, urine creatinine q3mo

⚠ Blood studies: RBC, Hct, Hgb, reticulocyte counts qwk for 4 wk then q3-6 months, if on long-term therapy; if myelosuppression occurs, drug should be discontinued

• Hepatic studies: ALT, AST, bilirubin

• Drug levels during initial treatment or when changing dose; should remain at 4-12 mcg/ml; anorexia may indicate increased blood levels

• Mental status: mood, sensorium, affect, behavioral changes; if mental status changes, notify prescriber

• Eye problems: need for ophthalmic examinations before, during, after treatment (slit lamp, funduscopy, tonometry)

• Allergic reaction: purpura, red, raised rash; if these occur, drug should be discontinued

⚠ Blood dyscrasias: fever, sore throat, bruising, rash, jaundice

⚠ Toxicity: bone marrow depression, nausea, vomiting, ataxia, diplopia, cardiovascular collapse, Stevens-Johnson syndrome

Administer:

PO route

• Do not crush or chew ext rel tab; ext rel cap may be opened and the beads sprinkled over food; patient should chew chewable tab, not swallow it whole

• With food, milk to decrease GI symptoms

• Shake oral susp before use

• Mix an equal amount of water, D_5W, 0.9% NaCl when giving by NG tube, flush tube with 100 ml of above sol

Perform/provide:

• Storage at room temperature

• Hard candy, gum, frequent rinsing for dry mouth

Evaluate:

• Therapeutic response: decreased seizure activity, document on patient's chart

Teach patient/family:

• To carry emergency ID stating patient's name, drugs taken, condition, prescriber's name, phone number

• To avoid driving, other activities that require alertness usually the first 3 days of treatment

• Not to discontinue medication quickly after long-term use

• To report immediately chills, rash, light-colored stools, dark urine, yellowing of skin and eyes, abdominal pain, sore throat, mouth ulcers, bruising, blurred vision, dizziness

• That urine may turn pink to brown

Treatment of overdose: Lavage, VS

---

carbidopa-levodopa (℞)

(kar-bi-doe'pa) (lee-voe-doe'pa)
Atamet, carbidopa/levodopa, Parcopa, Sinemet, Sinemet CR
Func. class.: Antiparkinson agent
Chem. class.: Catecholamine

Action: Decarboxylation of levodopa to periphery is inhibited by carbidopa; more levodopa is made available for transport to brain and conversion to dopamine in the brain

Uses: Parkinson's disease, parkinsonism resulting from carbon monoxide, chronic manganese intoxication, cerebral arteriosclerosis

Unlabeled uses: Restless leg syndrome

⚠ Safety alert   *"Tall Man" lettering

DOSAGE AND ROUTES

Beginning therapy for those not taking levodopa

• *Adult:* PO 25 mg carbidopa/100 mg levodopa tid, may increase daily or every other day by 1 tab to desired response (8 tabs/day); **EXT REL** tabs 5 mg carbidopa/200 mg levodopa bid or 10 mg carbidopa/100 mg levodopa 1 tab tid-qid; may increase by 1 tab daily or every other day until 8 tabs reached

For those not taking levodopa ER

• 50 mg carbidopa/200 mg levodopa bid

For those taking levodopa ER

• Begin treatment with 10% more levodopa/day given q4-8h, may increase or decrease dose q3d

For those taking levodopa <1.5 g/day

• *Adult:* PO 25 mg carbidopa/100 mg levodopa tid-qid, may increase daily to desired response

For those taking levodopa >1.5 g/day

• *Adult:* PO 25 mg carbidopa/250 mg levodopa tid-qid, may increase daily to desired response

Restless leg syndrome (RLS) (unlabeled)

• *Adult:* PO 25 mg carbidopa/100 mg levodopa, 1 tab at bedtime, may repeat if awakening within 2 hr or 50 mg carbidopa/200 mg levodopa sus rel tab 1-2 tabs 1 hr before bedtime

Available forms: Tabs 10/100, 25/100, 25 mg carbidopa/250 mg levodopa; ext rel tab 25 mg/100 mg, 50 mg carbidopa/200 mg levodopa (Sinemet CR); oral disintegrating tab (Parcopa) 10 mg carbidopa/100 mg levodopa, 25 mg carbidopa/100 mg levodopa; 25 mg carbidopa/250 mg levodopa

SIDE EFFECTS

CNS: Involuntary choreiform movements, hand tremors, fatigue, headache, anxiety, twitching, numbness, weakness, confusion, agitation, insomnia, nightmares, psychosis, hallucina-

tion, hypomania, severe depression, dizziness

CV: Orthostatic hypotension, tachycardia, hypertension, palpitation

EENT: Blurred vision, diplopia, dilated pupils

GI: Nausea, vomiting, anorexia, abdominal distress, dry mouth, flatulence, dysphagia, bitter taste, diarrhea, constipation

HEMA: **Hemolytic anemia, leukopenia, agranulocytosis**

INTEG: Rash, sweating, alopecia

MISC: Urinary retention, incontinence, weight change, dark urine

Contraindications: Hypersensitivity, narrow-angle glaucoma, malignant melanoma, history of malignant melanoma or undiagnosed skin lesions resembling melanoma

Precautions: Pregnancy (C), diabetes, wide-angle glaucoma, renal/hepatic/cardiac disease, respiratory disease, MI with dysrhythmias, convulsions, peptic ulcer, lactation, depression

PHARMACOKINETICS

PO: Onset 30 min, peak 1-3 hr, excreted in urine (metabolites)

Ext Rel: Onset 4-6 hr

INTERACTIONS

• Hypertensive crisis: MAOIs

Increase: effects of levodopa—antacids, metoclopramide

Decrease: effects of levodopa—anticholinergics, hydantoins, papaverine, pyridoxine, benzodiazepines

Decrease: absorption of levodopa—protein

Drug/Herb

Increase: Parkinson symptoms—kava, octacosanol

Decrease: action, increased EPS—Indian snakeroot

Drug/Food

• Increased pyridoxine will decrease levodopa effect

Drug/Lab Test
Increase: BUN, AST, ALT, bilirubin, alk phos, LDH
Decrease: VMA, BUN, creatinine
False positive: Urine ketones (dipstick), Coombs' test
False negative: Urine glucose
False increase: Uric acid, urine protein

NURSING CONSIDERATIONS
Assess:
• For Parkinson's symptoms: tremors, pill rolling, drooling, akinesia, rigidity before and during treatment
• B/P, respiration; orthostatic B/P
• Mental status: affect, mood, behavioral changes, depression, complete suicide assessment
• Muscle twitching, blepharospasm that may indicate toxicity
• Renal, hepatic, hematopoietic tests, also for diabetes, acromegaly if on long-term therapy
Administer:
• Pyridoxine (B₆) is not effective in reversing Sinemet or Sinemet CR
PO route
• Do not crush or chew ext rel tabs; they may be broken in half
• Oral disintegrating tab by gently removing from bottle, placing on tongue and swallowing with saliva; after it dissolves, liquid is not necessary
• Drug until NPO before surgery
• Adjust dosage to response
• With meals if GI symptoms occur; limit protein taken with drug
• Only after MAOIs have been discontinued for 2 wk; if previously on levodopa, discontinue for at least 12 hr before change to carbidopa-levodopa
Evaluate:
• Therapeutic response: decrease in akathisia, tremor, rigidity, improved mood
Teach patient/family:
• To change positions slowly to prevent orthostatic hypotension
• To report side effects: twitching, eye spasms; indicate overdose
• To use drug exactly as prescribed; if discontinued abruptly, parkinsonian cri-

sis, Neuroleptic Malignant Syndrome (NMS) may occur; gradually taper
• That urine, sweat may darken
• To use physical activities to maintain mobility, lessen spasms
• That improvement may not occur for 2-4 mo

⚠ High Alert

carboplatin (℞)
(kar-boe-pla'-tin)
Paraplatin, Paraplatin-AQ ✦
Func. class.: Antineoplastic alkylating agent
Chem. class.: Platinum coordination compound

Do not confuse:
carboplatin/cisplatin
Paraplatin/Platinol
Action: Produces interstrand DNA cross-links and, to a lesser extent, DNA-protein cross-links; activity is not cell cycle phase specific
Uses: Initial treatment of advanced ovarian cancer in combination with other agents; palliative treatment of ovarian carcinoma recurrent after treatment with other antineoplastic agents
Unlabeled uses: Endometrial, non–small cell lung, head/neck cancer; refractory/relapsed acute leukemia, recurrent benign tumor in children

DOSAGE AND ROUTES
(single agent):
• *Adult:* IV INF initially 300 mg/m² given with cyclophosphamide, q4-6wk; refractory tumors 360 mg/m² single dose, may repeat q4wk, as needed, do not repeat until neutrophils >2000/mm³ and platelets >100,000/mm³
Renal dose
• *Adult:* IV INF CCr 41-59 ml/min 250 mg/m², CCr 16-40 ml/min 200 mg/m², do not use in CCr <15 ml/min
Available forms: Lyophilized powder for inj 50, 150, 450 mg vials; aqueous sol for inj 50 mg/5 ml vial, 150 mg/15 ml

---

⚠ Safety alert   *"Tall Man" lettering

vial, 450 mg/45 ml vial, 600 mg/60 ml vial

SIDE EFFECTS

CNS: **Seizures, central neurotoxicity,** *peripheral neuropathy,* dizziness, confusion

CV: Cardiac abnormalities

EENT: Tinnitus, hearing loss, *vestibular toxicity,* visual changes

GI: *Severe nausea, vomiting,* diarrhea, weight loss, mucositis, anorexia, constipation, taste change

HEMA: **Thrombocytopenia, leukopenia, pancytopenia, neutropenia, anemia,** bleeding

INTEG: *Alopecia,* dermatitis, rash, erythema, pruritus, urticaria

META: Hypomagnesemia, hypocalcemia, hypokalemia, hyponatremia, hyperuremia

SYST: **Anaphylaxis**

Contraindications: Pregnancy (D), lactation, hypersensitivity to this drug, platinum products, mannitol; severe bone marrow depression, significant bleeding, aluminum products used to prepare or administer carboplatin

Precautions: Radiation therapy within 1 mo, other cancer chemotherapy within 1 mo, hepatic disease

PHARMACOKINETICS

Initial half-life 1-2 hr, postdistribution half-life 2½-6 hr, not bound to plasma proteins, excreted by the kidneys

INTERACTIONS

Increase: nephrotoxicity or ototoxicity—aminoglycosides, amphotericin B

Increase: risk of bleeding—aspirin, NSAIDs

Increase: toxicity—radiation, bone marrow suppressants

Increase: myelosuppression—myelosuppressives

Decrease: phenytoin levels

Drug/Lab Test

Increase: AST, BUN, alk phos, bilirubin, creatinine

NURSING CONSIDERATIONS
Assess:

• CBC, differential, platelet count weekly; withhold drug if neutrophil count is <2000/mm^3 or platelet count is <100,000/mm^3; notify prescriber of results

• Renal studies: BUN, creatinine, serum uric acid, urine CCr before and during therapy; I&O ratio; report fall in urine output to <30 ml/hr

• Monitor temp q4h (may indicate beginning of infection)

• Hepatic studies tests before and during therapy (bilirubin, AST, ALT, LDH) as needed or monthly; jaundice of skin, sclera, dark urine, clay-colored stools, itchy skin, abdominal pain, fever, diarrhea

⚠ For anaphylaxis: hypotension, rash, pruritus, wheezing, tachycardia; notify prescriber after discontinuing drug, resuscitation equipment should be available

• Bleeding; hematuria, stool guaiac, bruising or petechiae, mucosa or orifices q8h

• Dyspnea, crackles, unproductive cough, chest pain, tachypnea

• Effects of alopecia on body image; discuss feelings about body changes

Administer:

• Antiemetic 30-60 min before giving drug and prn for vomiting

IV route

• Using cytotoxic handling procedures

• After diluting 10 mg/ml of sterile water for inj, D$_5$W, NS (10 mg/ml); then further dilute with the same sol 1-4 mg/ml; give over 15 min or more (intermittent INF)

• IV INF over 5-6 hr; do not use needles or IV administration sets containing aluminum; may cause precipitate or loss of potency

Additive compatibilities: Cisplatin, etoposide, floxuridine, ifosfamide, ifosfamide/etoposide, paclitaxel

Solution compatibilities: D$_5$/0.2% NaCl, D$_5$/0.45% NaCl, D$_5$/0.9% NaCl, 0.9% NaCl, D$_5$W, sterile water for inj

Y-site compatibilities: Allopurinol, amifostine, aztreonam, cefepime, cladribine, DOXOrubicin liposome, filgrastim, fludarabine, granisetron, melphalan, ondansetron, paclitaxel, piperacillin/tazobactam, propofol, sargramostim, teniposide, thiotepa, vinorelbine

Perform/provide:

• Storage protected from light at room temperature; reconstituted sol stable for 8 hr at room temperature

Evaluate:

• Therapeutic response: decreasing size of tumor, spread of malignancy

Teach patient/family:

• To report ringing/roaring in the ears, numbness, tingling in face, extremities, weight gain

• That impotence or amenorrhea can occur; reversible after treatment is discontinued, to notify prescriber if pregnancy is suspected or planned; contraception should be used if patient is fertile

• Not to breastfeed during treatment

• To avoid OTC drugs with aspirin, NSAIDs, alcohol or receiving vaccinations during treatment

⚠ To notify prescriber immediately of fever, fatigue, sore throat, and bleeding, bruising, chills, back pain, blood in stools, dyspnea

• That hair may be lost during treatment; a wig or hairpiece may make patient feel better; new hair may be different in color, texture

• To avoid crowds, persons with known infections; avoid use of razors, stiff-bristle toothbrush

---

carboprost (℞)

(kar′boe-prost)

Hemabate, Prostin/15M ✦

Func. class.: Oxytocic, abortifacient

Chem. class.: Prostaglandin

Action: Stimulates uterine contractions, causing complete abortion in approximately 16 hr

Uses: Abortion at 13-20 wk gestation, postpartum hemorrhage caused by uterine atony not controlled by other methods

DOSAGE AND ROUTES

To induce abortion

• *Adult:* IM 250 mcg, then 250 mcg q1½-3½hr, may increase to 500 mcg if no response, not to exceed 12 mg total dose

Postpartum hemorrhage

• *Adult:* IM 250 mcg, repeat at 15-90 min intervals; max total dosage 2 mg

Available forms: Inj 250 mcg/ml

SIDE EFFECTS

CNS: Fever, chills, headache

GI: Nausea, vomiting, diarrhea

Contraindications: Hypersensitivity, severe renal/hepatic disease, PID, respiratory disease, cardiac disease

Precautions: Pregnancy (C), asthma, anemia, jaundice, diabetes mellitus, convulsive disorders, past uterine surgery

PHARMACOKINETICS

Onset 15 min, peak 2 hr; metabolized in lungs, liver; excreted in urine (metabolites)

INTERACTIONS

Increase: action—other oxytocics

NURSING CONSIDERATIONS

Assess:

• B/P, pulse; watch for change that may indicate hemorrhage

• Respiratory rate, rhythm, depth; notify prescriber of abnormalities

• For length, duration of contraction; notify prescriber of contractions lasting over 1 min or absence of contractions; watch for signs of uterine rupture

• For incomplete abortion, pregnancy must be terminated by another method; drug is teratogenic

Administer:

• In deep muscle mass; rotate inj sites if additional doses are given

Perform/provide:

• Storage in refrigerator

⚠ Safety alert   ✦"Tall Man" lettering

Evaluate:
• Therapeutic response: expulsion of fetus, control of bleeding
Teach patient/family:
• To report increased blood loss, abdominal cramps, increased temp, foul-smelling lochia

---

carisoprodol (R)
(kar-eye-soe-proe'dole)
carisoprodol, Soma,
Vanadom
Func. class.: Skeletal muscle relaxant, central acting
Chem. class.: Meprobamate congener

Do not confuse:
Soma/Soma Compound
Action: Depresses CNS by blocking interneuronal activity in descending reticular formation, spinal cord, producing sedation
Uses: Relieving pain, stiffness in musculoskeletal disorders

DOSAGE AND ROUTES
• *Adult and child >12 yr:* **PO** 350 mg tid and at bedtime
• *Child 6-12 yr:* **PO** 6.25 mg/kg qid
Available forms: Tabs 350 mg

SIDE EFFECTS

CNS: Dizziness, weakness, drowsiness, headache, tremor, depression, insomnia, ataxia, irritability
CV: Postural hypotension, tachycardia
EENT: Diplopia, temporary loss of vision
GI: Nausea, vomiting, hiccups, epigastric discomfort
HEMA: Eosinophilia
INTEG: Rash, pruritus, fever, facial flushing, **erythema multiforme**
RESP: Asthmatic attacks
SYST: **Angioedema, anaphylaxis**
Contraindications: Hypersensitivity, child <12 yr, intermittent porphyria
Precautions: Pregnancy (C), renal disease, hepatic disease, addictive personality, geriatric, lactation

PHARMACOKINETICS

PO: Onset ½ hr, peak 4 hr, duration 4-6 hr; metabolized by liver; excreted in urine; crosses placenta; excreted in breast milk (large amounts); half-life 8 hr

INTERACTIONS

Increase: CNS depression—alcohol, tricyclics, opioids, barbiturates, sedatives, hypnotics
Drug/Herb
Increase: CNS depression—chamomile, kava, skullcap, valerian
Drug/Lab Test
Increase: AST, alk phos, blood glucose

NURSING CONSIDERATIONS
Assess:
• Pain, stiffness, mobility, activities of daily living baseline and throughout treatment
• ECG in seizure patients; poor seizure control has occurred with patients taking this drug
• Idiosyncratic reaction (weakness, dizziness, blurred vision, confusion, euphoria), anaphylaxis within a few min or hr of 1st to 4th dose
• Allergic reactions: rash, fever, respiratory distress
• CNS depression: dizziness, drowsiness, psychiatric symptoms
Administer:
• With meals for GI symptoms
Perform/provide:
• Storage in tight container at room temperature
• Assistance with ambulation if dizziness, drowsiness occurs, especially geriatric
Evaluate:
• Therapeutic response: decreased pain, spasticity
Teach patient/family:
• Not to take with alcohol, other CNS depressants
• To avoid hazardous activities if drowsiness, dizziness occur
• To avoid using OTC medication: cough

---

preparations, antihistamines, unless directed by prescriber
• To report allergic reaction immediately: rash, swelling of tongue/lips, hives, dyspnea
Treatment of overdose: Induce emesis of conscious patient, dialysis, lavage

---

⚠ High Alert

carmustine (℞)
(kar-mus′teen)
BiCNU, BCNU, Gliadel
Func. class.: Antineoplastic alkylating agent
Chem. class.: Nitrosourea

Action: Alkylates DNA, RNA; is able to inhibit enzymes that allow synthesis of amino acids in proteins; activity is not cell cycle phase specific

Uses: Brain tumors such as glioblastoma, medulloblastoma, brain stem glioma, astrocytoma, ependymoma, metastatic brain tumors; multiple myeloma (with predniSONE), non-Hodgkin's, Hodgkin's disease, other lymphomas; GI, breast, bronchogenic, renal carcinomas, other lymphomas; wafer, as adjunct to surgery/radiation in newly diagnosed high-grade malignant glioma patients; in recurrent glioblastoma multiforme patients as an adjunct to surgery

Unlabeled uses: Primary cutaneous T cell lymphoma, malignant melanoma

DOSAGE AND ROUTES

• *Adult:* IV 75-100 mg/m² over 1-2 hr × 2 days or 150-200 mg/m² × 1 dose q6-8wk or 40 mg/m²/day × 5 days q6wk; if WBC is 3000-3999/mm³ give 50% of dose; if WBC is 2000-2999/mm³ and platelets are 25,000-75,000/mm³ give 25% of dose; withhold dose if WBC is <2000/mm³ and platelets are <25,000/mm³
• *Adult:* **INTRACAVITARY** wafer: 8 inserted into resection cavity
Available forms: Powder for inj 100 mg; wafer 7.7 mg (intracavitary)

SIDE EFFECTS

GI: Nausea, vomiting, anorexia, stomatitis, **hepatotoxicity**
GU: Azotemia, **renal failure**
HEMA: **Thrombocytopenia, leukopenia, myelosuppression, anemia**
INTEG: Pain, burning, hyperpigmentation at inj site
RESP: **Fibrosis, pulmonary infiltrate**
Contraindications: Pregnancy (D), hypersensitivity, leukopenia, thrombocytopenia, lactation

PHARMACOKINETICS

Degraded within 15 min; crosses blood-brain barrier; 70% excreted in urine within 96 hr; 10% excreted as CO_2; fate of 20% is unknown

INTERACTIONS

Increase: risk of bleeding—aspirin, anticoagulants
Increase: myelosuppression—myelosuppressive agents
Increase: toxicity: other antineoplastics, radiation, cimetidine
Increase: adverse reactions, decreased antibody reaction—live vaccines
Decrease: effects of digoxin, phenytoin

NURSING CONSIDERATIONS
Assess:
• CBC, differential, platelet count weekly; withhold drug if WBC is <4000 or platelet count is <100,000; notify prescriber of results
• Hepatic studies: AST, ALT, bilirubin
• Pulmonary function tests, chest x-ray films before, during therapy; chest film should be obtained q2wk during treatment; monitor for dyspnea, cough, pulmonary fibrosis; infiltrate occurs after high doses or several low-dose courses
• Renal studies: BUN, serum uric acid, urine CCr before, during therapy; I&O ratio; report fall in urine output of 30 ml/hr
• Monitor for cold, cough, fever (may indicate beginning infection)
• Bleeding: hematuria, guaiac, bruising, petechiae, mucosa, orifices q8h

---

Administer:

• Blood transfusions or RBC colony-stimulating factors to counter anemia

• Antiemetic 30-60 min before giving drug to prevent vomiting

• All medications PO, if possible, avoid IM inj if platelets are <100,000/mm³

Wafer route

• If wafers are broken in several pieces, they should not be used

• Foil pouches may be kept at room temperature for 6 hr if unopened

IV route

• Prepare in biologic cabinet wearing gown, gloves, mask; avoid contact with skin; can cause burning and staining the skin brown; use cytotoxic handling procedures

• After diluting 100 mg drug/3 ml ethyl alcohol (provided); then further dilute 27 ml sterile H₂O for inj; then dilute with 100-500 ml 0.9% NaCl or D₅W, give over 1 hr or more, reduce rate if discomfort is felt; use only glass containers, protect from light

• Flush IV line after carmustine with 10 ml 0.9% NaCl to prevent irritation at site

Y-site compatibilities: Amifostine, aztreonam, cefepime, filgrastim, fludarabine, granisetron, melphalan, ondansetron, piperacillin/tazobactam, sargramostim, teniposide, thiotepa, vinorelbine

Perform/provide:

• Storage of reconstituted sol in refrigerator for 24 hr, or room temperature for 8 hr, protect from light

• Rinsing of mouth tid-qid with water or club soda; use of sponge brush for stomatitis

• Warm compresses at inj site for inflammation; reduce flow rate if patient complains of burning at infusion site

Evaluate:

• Therapeutic response: decreasing size of tumor, spread of malignancy

Teach patient/family:

• To report any changes in breathing or coughing, avoid smoking

• To avoid foods with citric acid, hot or rough texture if stomatitis is present; to

report any bleeding, white spots, ulceration in mouth to prescriber; tell patient to examine mouth daily

• To avoid use of aspirin, ibuprofen, razors, commercial mouthwash

• To report signs of anemia (fatigue, irritability, shortness of breath, faintness); to report signs of infection (sore throat, fever); pulmonary toxicity can occur up to 15 yr after treatment

• To use contraception during treatment; avoid breastfeeding

• Not to receive vaccinations during treatment

carteolol ophthalmic
See Appendix C

carvedilol (℞)
(kar-ved′i-lole)
Coreg
Func. class.: Antihypertensive, α/β-adrenergic blocker

Do not confuse:
carvedilol/captopril/carteolol

Action: A mixture of nonselective α/β-adrenergic blocking activity; decreases cardiac output, exercise-induced tachycardia, reflex orthostatic tachycardia; causes vasodilation, reduction in peripheral vascular resistance

Uses: Essential hypertension alone or in combination with other antihypertensives, CHF, LV dysfunction following MI

Unlabeled uses: Angina pectoris, idiopathic cardiomyopathy

DOSAGE AND ROUTES
Essential hypertension

• *Adult:* **PO** 6.25 mg bid × 7-14 days; if tolerated well, then increase to 12.5 mg bid × 7-14 days; if tolerated well, may be increased (if needed) to 25 mg bid; not to exceed 50 mg daily

Congestive heart failure

• *Adult:* **PO** 3.125 mg bid × 2 wk; if tolerated well, give 6.25 mg bid × 2 wk,

then double q2wk to max dose, 25 mg bid <85 kg or 50 mg bid >85 kg
Angina pectoris
• *Adult:* PO 25-50 mg bid
Idiopathic cardiomyopathy
• *Adult:* PO 6.25-25 mg bid
Available forms: Tabs 3.125, 6.25, 12.5, 25 mg

SIDE EFFECTS

CNS: Dizziness, fatigue, weakness, somnolence, insomnia, ataxia, hyperesthesia, paresthesia, vertigo, depression, headache

CV: **Bradycardia,** *postural hypotension,* dependent edema, peripheral edema, **AV block,** extrasystoles, hypertension, hypotension, palpitations, peripheral ischemia, **CHF, pulmonary edema**

GI: Diarrhea, abdominal pain, increased alk phos, ALT, AST

GU: Decreased libido, *impotence,* UTI

INTEG: Rash

MISC: Injury, back pain, viral infection, hypertriglyceridemia, **thrombocytopenia,** *hyperglycemia*

RESP: Rhinitis, pharyngitis, dyspnea, **bronchospasm**

Contraindications: Hypersensitivity, bronchial asthma, class IV decompensated cardiac failure, 2nd- or 3rd-degree heart block, cardiogenic shock, severe bradycardia, pulmonary edema

Precautions: Pregnancy (C), cardiac failure, hepatic injury, peripheral vascular disease, anesthesia, major surgery, diabetes mellitus, thyrotoxicosis, geriatric, lactation, children, emphysema, chronic bronchitis, renal disease

PHARMACOKINETICS

Peak 1-2 hr; readily and extensively absorbed PO; >98% protein binding; extensively metabolized by liver; excreted through bile into feces; terminal half-life 7-10 hr with increases in geriatric, hepatic disease

INTERACTIONS

Increase: conduction disturbances —calcium channel blockers

Increase: bradycardia, hypotension —levodopa, MAOIs, reserpine

Increase: hypoglycemia—antidiabetic agents

Increase: concentrations of digoxin

Increase: toxicity of carvedilol—cimetidine, other antihypertensives, nitrates, acute alcohol ingestion

Decrease: heart rate, B/P—clonidine

Decrease: carvedilol levels—rifampin, NSAIDs, thyroid medications

Drug/Herb

Increase: toxicity/death—aconite

Increase: antihypertensive effect—barberry, betony, black catechu, black cohosh, bloodroot, broom, burdock, cat's claw, dandelion, goldenseal, hawthorn, Irish moss, Jamaican dogwood, kelp, khella, mistletoe, parsley

Increase or decrease: antihypertensive effect—astragalus, cola tree

Decrease: antihypertensive effect—coltsfoot, guarana, khat, licorice

Drug/Lab Test

Increase: ANA titer, blood glucose, BUN, potassium, triglycerides, uric acid

NURSING CONSIDERATIONS

Assess:

⚠ Renal studies, including protein, BUN, creatinine; watch for increased levels that may indicate nephrotic syndrome; obtain baselines in renal, hepatic studies before beginning treatment; I&O, weight daily

• Hepatic studies, jaundice; if LFTs are elevated, drug should be discontinued

• B/P during beginning treatment, periodically thereafter; pulse q4h, note rate, rhythm, quality; apical/radial pulse before administration; notify prescriber of significant changes

• Edema in feet, legs daily, fluid overload: dyspnea, weight gain, jugular vein distention, fatigue, crackles

---

⚠ Safety alert   *"Tall Man" lettering

Administer:
• Pulse: if <50 bpm, hold drug, call prescriber
• Drug before meals, bedtime; tablets may be crushed or swallowed whole
• Reduced dosage in renal dysfunction; may give with food
Evaluate:
• Therapeutic response: decreased B/P in hypertension
Teach patient/family:
• To comply with dosage schedule, even if feeling better, that improvement may take several weeks
• To rise slowly to sitting or standing position to minimize orthostatic hypotension
• To report bradycardia, dizziness, confusion, depression, fever, weight gain, SOB, cold extremities, rash, sore throat, bleeding, or bruising
• To take pulse, B/P at home; advise when to notify prescriber
⚠ Not to discontinue drug abruptly, taper over 1-2 wk; life-threatening dysrhythmias may occur
• To avoid hazardous activities until stabilized on medication; dizziness may occur
• To avoid all OTC medications unless approved by prescriber
• To carry emergency ID with drug name, prescriber at all times
• To inform all health care providers of drugs, supplements taken

---

**cascara sagrada/
cascara sagrada
aromatic fluid extract/
cascara sagrada fluid
extract** (otc)
(kas-kar′a)
Func. class.: Laxative, stimulant
Chem. class.: Anthraquinone

Action: Direct chemical irritation in colon; increases propulsion of stool
Uses: Constipation; bowel or rectal preparation for surgery or examination

DOSAGE AND ROUTES
• *Adult and child ≥12 yr:* **PO** tab 325 mg; fluid 2-6 ml as a single dose; aromatic liquid 2.5-5 ml as a single dose
• *Child 2-11 yr:* **PO** ⅕-½ tsp as a single dose
Available forms: Tabs 325 mg; fluid extract 1 g/ml; aromatic fluid extract 1 g/ml

SIDE EFFECTS
GI: Nausea, vomiting, anorexia, cramps, diarrhea, melanosis coli
META: Hypocalcemia, enteropathy, alkalosis, hypokalemia, **tetany**
Contraindications: Hypersensitivity, GI bleeding, obstruction, CHF, lactation, abdominal pain, nausea/vomiting, appendicitis, acute surgical abdomen, alcoholics (aromatic form)
Precautions: Pregnancy (C)

PHARMACOKINETICS
PO: Peak 6-12 hr; metabolized by liver; excreted in urine, feces, breast milk

INTERACTIONS
Decrease: absorption of antibiotics, digoxin, nitrofurantoin, salicylates, tetracyclines, oral anticoagulants
Drug/Herb
Increase: action/side effects—flax, lily of the valley, pheasant's eye, senna, squill

NURSING CONSIDERATIONS
Assess:
• Monitor blood, urine electrolytes if drug is used often by patient; check I&O ratio to identify fluid loss
• Cause of constipation; identify whether fluids, bulk, or exercise missing from lifestyle, constipating drugs
• Cramping, rectal bleeding, nausea, vomiting; if these symptoms occur, drug should be discontinued
Administer:
PO route
• Swallow tabs whole; do not break, crush, or chew

• Alone for better absorption; do not take within 1 hr of other drugs or within 1 hr of antacids, milk
• In morning or evening (oral dose)

Evaluate:
• Therapeutic response: decrease in constipation

Teach patient/family:
• Not to use laxatives for long-term therapy; bowel tone will be lost
• That normal bowel movements do not always occur daily
• Not to use in presence of abdominal pain, nausea, vomiting
• To notify prescriber if constipation unrelieved or of symptoms of electrolyte imbalance: muscle cramps, pain, weakness, dizziness
• Excreted in breast milk, may cause diarrhea in infant

---

caspofungin (℞)

(cas-po-fun′gin)
Cancidas
Func. class.: Antifungal, systemic
Chem. class.: Echinocandin

Action: Inhibits an essential component in fungal cell walls; causes direct damage to fungal cell wall

Uses: Treatment of invasive aspergillosis, and candidemia that has responded to other treatment including peritonitis, intraabdominal abscesses; susceptible species: *A. flavus, A. fumigatus, A. terreus, C. albicans, C. glabrata, C. krusei, C. lusitaniae, C. parapsilosis, C. tropicalis*

Unlabeled uses: *Esophageal candidiasis*

DOSAGE AND ROUTES

• *Adult:* **IV** loading dose 70 mg on day 1; then 50 mg daily maintenance dose

Available forms: Powder for injection 50, 70 mg

SIDE EFFECTS

CNS: Dizziness, *headache*
CV: Sinus tachycardia

GI: Abdominal pain, *nausea, anorexia, vomiting, diarrhea, increased AST, ALT, alk phos*
HEMA: Thrombophlebitis, vasculitis, anemia
INTEG: Rash, pruritus, inj site pain
META: Hypokalemia
MS: Myalgia
RESP: **Acute respiratory distress syndrome (ARDS)**
SYST: **Anaphylaxis**

Contraindications: Hypersensitivity to this product or other echinocandins including mannitol

Precautions: Pregnancy (C), severe hepatic disease, lactation, children, geriatric

PHARMACOKINETICS

Metabolized in liver to inactive metabolites; excretion in feces, urine; phase II terminal half-life 9-11 hr; phase III terminal half-life 40-50 hr; protein binding 97%

INTERACTIONS

Increase: plasma concentrations—cyclo-SPORINE; may need dosage reduction
Decrease: caspofungin levels—carbamazepine, dexamethasone, efavirenz, nelfinavir, nevirapine, phenytoin, rifampin
Decrease: tacrolimus levels

NURSING CONSIDERATIONS

Assess:
• For signs and symptoms of infection; clearing of cultures during treatment; obtain culture baseline and throughout; drug may be started as soon as culture is taken *(esophageal candidiasis);* monitor cultures during HSCT, for prevention of *Candida* infections
• Hepatic studies before and during treatment: bilirubin, AST, ALT, alk phos, as needed; obtain baseline in renal studies
• For hypersensitivity: rash, pruritus, facial swelling; also for phlebitis

---

⚠ Safety alert   *"Tall Man" lettering

• GI symptoms: frequency of stools, cramping; if severe diarrhea occurs, electrolytes may need to be given

Administer:

IV route

• Allow to warm to room temperature
• May administer a loading dose on day 1 of treatment
• Do not admix; do not use with dextrose
• Reconstitute 50 mg vial or 70 mg vial with 10.5 ml 0.9% NaCl, sterile water for inj, or bacteriostatic water for inj (5 mg/ml; or 7 mg/ml); swirl to dissolve, withdraw 10 ml reconstituted solution and further dilute with 250 ml 0.9% NaCl, 0.45% NaCl, 0.225% NaCl, RL; run over 1 hr or more

Perform/provide:

• Storage at room temperature for up to 24 hr, or refrigerated 48 hr; store reconstituted solution at room temperature for 1 hr prior to preparation of solution for administration

Evaluate:

• Therapeutic response: decreased symptoms of *Candida* infections or *Aspergillius* infections

Teach patient/family:

• To notify prescriber if pregnancy is suspected or planned; use nonhormonal form of contraception while taking this product
• To avoid breastfeeding while taking this product
• To inform prescriber of renal/hepatic disease
• To report bleeding, facial swelling, wheezing, difficulty breathing, itching, rash, hives, increasing warmth, flushing; anaphylaxis can occur

cefaclor
See cephalosporins—2nd generation
cefadroxil
cefazolin
See cephalosporins—1st generation
cefdinir
See cephalosporins—3rd generation
cefditoren pivoxil
See cephalosporins—3rd generation
cefepime
cefixime
See cephalosporins—3rd generation
cefotaxime
See cephalosporins—3rd generation
cefotetan
cefoxitin
See cephalosporins—2nd generation
cefpodoxime
See cephalosporins—3rd generation
cefprozil
See cephalosporins—2nd generation
ceftazidime
ceftibuten
ceftizoxime
ceftriaxone
See cephalosporins—3rd generation
cefuroxime
See cephalosporins—2nd generation

▲ High Alert

celecoxib (℞)
(sel-eh-cox'ib)
Celebrex
Func. class.: Nonsteroidal antiinflammatory, antirheumatic
Chem. class.: COX-2 inhibitor

Do not confuse:
Celebrex/Celexa/Cerebra/Cerebyx
Action: Inhibits prostaglandin synthesis by selectively inhibiting cyclooxygenase 2 (COX-2), an enzyme needed for biosynthesis
Uses: Acute, chronic rheumatoid arthritis, osteoarthritis, familial adenomatous

polyposis (FAP), acute pain, primary dysmenorrhea, ankylosing spondylitis
Unlabeled uses: Colorectal polyps

DOSAGE AND ROUTES

Do not exceed recommended dose, deaths have occurred
Acute pain/primary dysmenorrhea
• *Adult:* **PO** 400 mg initially, then 200 mg if needed on first day, then 200 mg bid prn on subsequent days
Osteoarthritis
• *Adult:* **PO** 200 mg/day as a single dose or 100 mg bid
Rheumatoid arthritis
• *Adult:* **PO** 100-200 mg bid
Ankylosing spondylitis
• *Adult:* **PO** 200 mg daily or in divided dose (bid)
Familial adenomatous polyposis (FAP)
• *Adult:* **PO** 400 mg bid
Colorectal polyps
• *Adult:* **PO** 400 mg bid × 6 mo
Hepatic disease (Child-Pugh class II)
• *Adult:* **PO** reduce dose by 50%
Available forms: Caps 100, 200 mg

SIDE EFFECTS

CNS: Fatigue, anxiety, depression, nervousness, paresthesia, dizziness, insomnia
CV: **Stroke, MI, tachycardia, CHF,** angina, palpitations, dysrhythmias, hypertension, fluid retention
EENT: Tinnitus, hearing loss, blurred vision, glaucoma, cataract, conjunctivitis, eye pain
GI: Nausea, anorexia, vomiting, constipation, dry mouth, diverticulitis, gastritis, gastroenteritis, hemorrhoids, hiatal hernia, stomatitis, **GI bleeding**
GU: **Nephrotoxicity:** *dysuria,* **hematuria, oliguria, azotemia,** cystitis, UTI
HEMA: **Blood dyscrasias,** epistaxis, bruising, anemia
INTEG: **Serious, sometimes fatal Stevens-Johnson syndrome, toxic epidermal necrolysis,** purpura, rash, pruritus, sweating, erythema, petechiae, photosensitivity, alopecia
RESP: Pharyngitis, shortness of breath, pneumonia, coughing
Contraindications: Pregnancy (D) 3rd trimester, hypersensitivity to aspirin, iodides, other NSAIDs, sulfonamides, asthma triad, asthma, severe CV disease
Precautions: Pregnancy (C) 1st/2nd trimesters, lactation, bleeding, GI, renal/hepatic/cardiac disorders, hypersensitivity to other antiinflammatory agents, glucocorticoids, anticoagulants, geriatrics, hypertension, severe dehydration, children <18 yr

PHARMACOKINETICS

Well absorbed, crosses placenta, bound to plasma proteins, metabolized in liver, excreted by kidneys, peak 3 hr

INTERACTIONS

Increase: effect of anticoagulants
Increase: adverse reactions—glucocorticoids, NSAIDs, aspirin
Increase: toxicity—lithium, antineoplastics
Increase: celecoxib blood level—fluconazole
Decrease: effect of aspirin, ACE inhibitors, thiazide diuretics, furosemide
Drug/Herb
• Severe photosensitivity: St. John's wort
Increase: celecoxib effect—bearberry, bilberry
Increase: gastric irritation—arginine, gossypol
Increase: bleeding risk—bogbean, saw palmetto, turmeric
Drug/Lab Test
Increase: ALT, AST, BUN

NURSING CONSIDERATIONS

Assess:
• For pain of rheumatoid arthritis, osteoarthritis; check ROM, inflammation of joints, characteristics of pain
• For cardiac disease that may be worse after taking this product

---

- FAP clients for decreasing number of polyps
- Blood counts during therapy; watch for decreasing platelets; if low, therapy may need to be discontinued, restarted after hematologic recovery

⚠ For blood dyscrasias (thrombocytopenia): bruising, fatigue, bleeding, poor healing

- GI toxicity: black, tarry stools; abdominal pain

Administer:
- Do not break, crush, chew, or dissolve caps
- With a full glass of water to enhance absorption
- With food or milk to decrease gastric symptoms, do not increase dose

Evaluate:
- Therapeutic response: decreased pain, inflammation in arthritic conditions; decreased number of polyps

Teach patient/family:
⚠ **Do not exceed recommended dose; notify prescriber immediately of chest pain, skin eruptions; stop drug**
- To check with prescriber to determine when drug should be discontinued prior to surgery
- That drug must be continued for prescribed time to be effective; to avoid other NSAIDs, aspirin, sulfonamides
- To notify prescriber if pregnancy is planned or suspected

⚠ To notify prescriber of GI symptoms: black, tarry stools; cramping or rash; edema of extremities, weight gain

⚠ To report bleeding, bruising, fatigue, malaise since blood dyscrasias do occur

---

cephalexin
See cephalosporins—1st generation

CEPHALOSPORINS—1ST GENERATION

cefadroxil (℞)
(sef-a-drox'ill)
cefadroxil, Duricef

cefazolin (℞)
(sef-a'zoe-lin)
Ancef, cefazolin

cephalexin (℞)
(sef-a-lex'in)
Apo-Cephalex ✦, cephalexin, Keflex, Novo-Lexin ✦, Nu-Cephalex ✦, Panixine

cephradine (℞)
(sef'ra-deen)
cephradine, Velosef

Func. class.: Antiinfective
Chem. class.: Cephalosporin (1st generation)

Do not confuse:
cephalexin/cefaclor

Action: Inhibits bacterial cell wall synthesis, rendering cell wall osmotically unstable, leading to cell death; lysis mediated by cell wall autolytic enzymes

Uses:

cefadroxil: Gram-negative bacilli: *Escherichia coli, Proteus mirabilis, Klebsiella* (UTI only); gram-positive organisms: *Streptococcus pneumoniae, Streptococcus pyogenes, Staphylococcus aureus;* upper, lower respiratory tract, urinary tract, skin infections, otitis media; tonsillitis; and UTIs

cefazolin: Gram-negative bacilli: *Haemophilus influenzae, Escherichia coli, Proteus mirabilis, Klebsiella;* gram-positive organisms: *Staphylococcus aureus;* upper, lower respiratory tract, urinary tract, skin infections, bone, joint, biliary, genital infections, endocarditis, surgical prophylaxis, septicemia

cephalexin: Gram-negative bacilli: *Haemophilus influenzae, Escherichia coli, Proteus mirabilis, Klebsiella;* gram-

---

positive organisms: *Streptococcus pneumoniae, Streptococcus pyogenes, Staphylococcus aureus;* upper, lower respiratory tract, urinary tract, skin, bone infections, otitis media

cephradine: Gram-negative bacilli: *Haemophilus influenzae, Escherichia coli, Proteus mirabilis, Klebsiella;* gram-positive organisms: *Streptococcus pneumoniae, Streptococcus pyogenes, Staphylococcus aureus;* serious respiratory tract, skin infections, UTIs, otitis media

DOSAGE AND ROUTES
cefadroxil
• *Adult:* **PO** 1-2 g daily or q12h in divided doses, give a loading dose of 1 g initially
• *Child:* **PO** 30 mg/kg/day in divided doses bid
Renal dose: CCr 25-50 ml/min 500 mg q12h; CCr 10-24 ml/min 500 mg q24h; CCr <10 ml/min 500 mg q36h
Available forms: Caps 500 mg; tabs 1 g; oral susp 125, 250, 500 mg/5 ml
cefazolin
Life-threatening infections
• *Adult:* **IM/IV** 1-2 g q6h; max 12 g/day
• *Child >1 mo:* **IM/IV** 100 mg/kg in 3-4 divided doses; max 6 g/day
Mild/moderate infections
• *Adult:* **IM/IV** 250 mg-1 g q8h
• *Child >1 mo:* **IM/IV** 25-50 mg/kg in 3-4 equal doses
Renal dose
• *Adult:* **IM/IV** following loading dose CCr 35-54 ml/min, dose q8h; CCr 10-34 ml/min; 50% of dose q12h; CCr <10 ml/min; 50% of dose q18-24h
• *Child:* **IM/IV** CCr >70 ml/min, no dosage adjustment; CCr 40-70 ml/min following loading dose, reduce dose to 7.5-30 mg/kg q12h; CCr 20-39 ml/min, give 3.125-12.5 mg/kg after loading dose q12h; CCr 5-19 ml/min, 2.5-10 mg/kg after loading dose q24h
Available forms: Inj 250, 500 mg, 1, 5, 10, 20 g; infusion 500 mg, 1 g/50 ml vial

cephalexin
Moderate infections
Adult: **PO** 250-500 mg q6h
• *Child:* **PO** 25-50 mg/kg/day in 4 equal doses, max 4/g/day
Moderate skin infections
• *Adult:* **PO** 500 mg q12h
Endocarditis prophylaxis
• 2 g 1 hr before procedure
Severe infections
• *Adult:* **PO** 500 mg-1 g q6h
• *Child:* **PO** 50-100 mg/kg/day in 4 equal doses, max 4 g/day
Renal dose: CCr <40 ml/min give q8-12h; CCr 5-10 ml/min give q12h; CCr <5 ml/min give q24h
Available forms: Caps 250, 500 mg; tabs 250, 500 mg, 1 g; oral susp 125 mg, 250 mg/5ml
cephradine
• *Adult:* **PO** 250 mg-1 g q6-12h
• *Child >1 yr:* **PO** 6-12 mg/kg q6h
Renal dose: CCr >20 ml/min 500 mg q6h; CCr 5-20 ml/min 250 mg q6h
Available forms: Caps 250, 500 mg; oral susp 125 mg, 250 mg/5 ml

SIDE EFFECTS
CNS: Headache, dizziness, weakness, paresthesia, fever, chills, **seizures** (high doses)
GI: Nausea, vomiting, *diarrhea, anorexia,* pain, glossitis, bleeding; increased AST, ALT, bilirubin, LDH, alk phos; abdominal pain, **pseudomembranous colitis**
GU: Proteinuria, vaginitis, pruritus, candidiasis, increased BUN, **nephrotoxicity, renal failure**
HEMA: **Leukopenia, thrombocytopenia, agranulocytosis,** anemia, **neutropenia, lymphocytosis, eosinophilia, pancytopenia, hemolytic anemia**
INTEG: Rash, urticaria, dermatitis
RESP: Dyspnea
SYST: **Anaphylaxis, serum sickness,** superinfection, **Stevens-Johnson syndrome**
Contraindications: Hypersensitivity to cephalosporins, infants <1 mo

---

Precautions: Pregnancy (B), hypersensitivity to penicillins, lactation, renal disease

PHARMACOKINETICS

cefadroxil: Peak 1-1½ hr, duration 12-24 hr, half-life 1-2 hr; 20% bound by plasma proteins; crosses placenta; excreted in breast milk

cefazolin

IM: Peak ½-2 hr, duration 6-12 hr, half-life 1½-2¼ hr

IV: Peak 10 min, duration 6-12 hr; eliminated unchanged in urine; 70%-86% protein bound

cephalexin: Peak 1 hr, duration 6-12 hr, half-life 30-72 min; 5%-15% bound by plasma proteins; 90%-100% eliminated unchanged in urine; crosses placenta; excreted in breast milk

cephradine: Peak 1-2 hr, duration 6-12 hr, half-life 0.75-1.5 hr; 20% bound by plasma proteins; 80%-90% eliminated unchanged in urine; crosses placenta; excreted in breast milk

INTERACTIONS

Increase: toxicity—aminoglycosides, loop diuretics, probenecid

Drug/Herb
• Do not use acidophilus with antiinfectives; separate by several hours

Drug/Lab Test
Increase: AST, ALT, alk phos, LDH, BUN, creatinine, bilirubin
False positive: Urinary protein, direct Coombs' test, urine glucose
Interference: Cross-matching

NURSING CONSIDERATIONS

Assess:
• Sensitivity to penicillin and other cephalosporins
⚠ Nephrotoxicity: increased BUN, creatinine
• I&O daily
• Blood studies: AST, ALT, CBC, Hct, bilirubin, LDH, alk phos, Coombs' test monthly if patient is on long-term therapy

• Electrolytes: K, Na, Cl monthly if patient is on long-term therapy
• Bowel pattern daily; if severe diarrhea occurs, drug should be discontinued; may indicate pseudomembranous colitis
• Urine output: if decreasing, notify prescriber; may indicate nephrotoxicity
⚠ Anaphylaxis: rash, urticaria, pruritus, chills, fever, joint pain; angioedema; may occur few days after therapy begins; discontinue drug, notify prescriber immediately, keep emergency equipment nearby
• Bleeding: ecchymosis, bleeding gums, hematuria, stool guaiac daily
⚠ Overgrowth of infection: perineal itching, fever, malaise, redness, pain, swelling, drainage, rash, diarrhea, change in cough, sputum

Administer:

cefadroxil
• For 10-14 days to ensure organism death, prevent superinfection
• With food if needed for GI symptoms
• Shake susp, refrigerate, discard after 2 wk
• After C&S completed

cefazolin
• IV; check for irritation, extravasation often; dilute in 10 ml sterile H_2O for inj and run over 3-5 min; may be further diluted with 50-100 ml of NS, D_5W sol and run over ½-1 hr by Y-tube or 3-way stopcock
• For 10-14 days to ensure organism death, prevent superinfection
• After C&S completed

Additive compatibilities: Aztreonam, clindamycin, famotidine, fluconazole, metronidazole, verapamil

Syringe compatibilities: Heparin, vit B

Y-site compatibilities: Acyclovir, allopurinol, amifostine, atracurium, aztreonam, calcium gluconate, cyclophosphamide, diltiazem, DOXOrubicin liposome, enalaprilat, esmolol, famotidine, filgrastim, fluconazole, fludarabine, foscarnet, heparin, hydromorphone, insulin (regular), labetalol, lidocaine, magnesium sulfate, melphalan, meperidine, midazolam, morphine, multivitamins, ondansetron, perphenazine, pancuronium, remifentanil, sargramostim, tacrolimus, teniposide, theophylline, thiotepa, vecuronium, vit B/C, warfarin

cephalexin
• Shake susp, refrigerate, discard after 2 wk
• For 10-14 days to ensure organism death, prevent superinfection
• With food if needed for GI symptoms
• After C&S

cephradine
• Shake suspension well before each dose
• For 10-14 days to ensure organism death, prevent superinfection
• With food if needed for GI symptoms
• After C&S

Evaluate:
• Therapeutic response: decreased symptoms of infection, negative C&S

Teach patient/family:
• Not to drink alcohol or use meds with alcohol: reaction may occur
• To use yogurt or buttermilk to maintain intestinal flora, decrease diarrhea
• To take all medication prescribed for length of time ordered

A To report sore throat, bruising, bleeding, joint pain (may indicate blood dyscrasias [rare]); diarrhea with mucus, blood, may indicate pseudomembranous colitis

Treatment of anaphylaxis: EpINEPHrine, antihistamines; resuscitate if needed

---

CEPHALOSPORINS— 2ND GENERATION

cefaclor (℞)
(sef′a-klor)
Ceclor, Raniclor
cefotetan (℞)
(sef′oh-tee-tan)
Cefotan
cefoxitin (℞)
(se-fox′i-tin)
Mefoxin
cefprozil (℞)
(sef-proe′zill)
Cefzil
cefuroxime (℞)
(sef-yoor-ox′eem)
Ceftin, cefuroxime, Zinacef
loracarbef (℞)
(lor-a-kar′beff)
Lorabid
Func. class.: Antiinfective
Chem. class.: Cephalosporin
(2nd generation)

Do not confuse:
cefaclor/cephalexin
Cefotan/Ceftin
cefprozil/cefazolin/cefuroxime
Cefzil/Ceftin

Action: Inhibits bacterial cell wall synthesis, rendering cell wall osmotically unstable, leading to cell death by binding to cell wall membrane

Uses:
cefaclor: Gram-negative bacilli: *Haemophilus influenzae, Escherichia coli, Proteus mirabilis, Klebsiella;* gram-positive organisms: *Streptococcus pneumoniae, Streptococcus pyogenes, Staphylococcus aureus;* respiratory tract, urinary tract, skin, bone, joint infections, otitis media
cefotetan: Gram-negative organisms: *Haemophilus influenzae, Escherichia coli, Enterobacter aerogenes, Proteus mirabilis, Klebsiella, Citrobacter, En-*

terobacter, *Salmonella, Shigella, Acinetobacter, Bacteroides fragilis, Neisseria, Serratia;* gram-positive organisms: *Streptococcus pneumoniae, Streptococcus pyogenes, Staphylococcus aureus;* upper, lower, serious respiratory tract, urinary tract, skin, bone, joint, gynecologic, gonococcal, intraabdominal infections

cefoxitin: Gram-negative bacilli: *Haemophilus influenzae, Escherichia coli, Proteus, Klebsiella, Bacteroides fragilis, Neisseria gonorrhoeae;* gram-positive organisms: *Streptococcus pneumoniae, Streptococcus pyogenes, Staphylococcus aureus;* anaerobes including *Clostridium,* lower respiratory tract, urinary tract, skin, bone, gynecologic, gonococcal infections, septicemia, peritonitis

cefprozil: Pharyngitis/tonsillitis, otitis media, secondary bacterial infection of acute bronchitis, and acute bacterial exacerbation of chronic bronchitis and uncomplicated skin and skin structure infections; acute sinusitis

cefuroxime: Gram-negative bacilli: *Haemophilus influenzae, Escherichia coli, Neisseria, Proteus mirabilis, Klebsiella;* gram-positive organisms: *Streptococcus pneumoniae, Streptococcus pyogenes, Staphylococcus aureus;* serious lower respiratory tract, urinary tract, skin, bone, joint, gonococcal infections, septicemia, meningitis

loracarbef: Gram-negative bacilli: *Haemophilus influenzae, Escherichia coli, Proteus mirabilis, Klebsiella;* gram-positive organisms: *Streptococcus pneumoniae, Streptococcus pyogenes, Staphylococcus aureus;* upper and lower respiratory tract, urinary tract, skin infections, otitis media, pharyngitis, tonsillitis

DOSAGE AND ROUTES
cefaclor
• *Adult:* PO 250-500 mg q8h, not to exceed 4 g/day
• *Child >1 mo:* PO 20-40 mg/kg daily in divided doses q8h, or total daily dose may be divided and given q12h, not to exceed 1 g/day

Available forms: Caps 250, 500 mg; oral susp 125, 187, 250, 375 mg/5 ml; chew tabs (Raniclor) 125, 187, 250, 375 mg
cefotetan
• *Adult:* IV/IM 1-2 g q12h × 5-10 days
Renal dose
• *Adult:* IM/IV CCr 10-30 ml/min, give dose q24h or ½ dose q12h; CCr <10 ml/min, give dose q48h or ½ dose q12h
Perioperative prophylaxis
• *Adult:* IV 1-2 g ½-1 hr before surgery
Available forms: Inj 1, 2, 10 g
cefoxitin
• *Adult:* IM/IV 1-2 g q6-8h
Renal dose: after loading dose CCr 30-50 ml/min 1-2 g q8-12h; CCr 10-29 ml/min 1-2 g q12-24h; CCr <10 ml/min 0.5-1 g q12-24h
Uncomplicated gonorrhea
• 2 g IM as single dose with 1 g PO probenecid at same time
Severe infections
• *Adult:* IM/IV 2 g q4h
• *Child ≥3 mo:* IM/IV 80-160 mg/kg/day divided q4-6h; max 12 g/day
Available forms: Powder for inj 1, 2, 10 g
cefprozil
Renal dose: CCr <30 ml/min 50% of dose
Upper respiratory infections
• *Adult:* PO 500 mg q24h × 10 days
Otitis media
• *Child 6 mo-12 yr:* PO 15 mg/kg q12h × 10 days
Lower respiratory infections
• *Adult:* PO 500 mg q12h × 10 days
Skin/skin structure infections
• *Adult:* PO 250-500 mg q12h × 10 days
Available forms: Tabs 250, 500 mg; susp 125, 250 mg/5 ml
cefuroxime
• *Adult and child:* PO 250 mg q12h; may increase to 500 mg q12h in serious infections
• *Adult:* IM/IV 750 mg-1.5 g q8h for 5-10 days
Urinary tract infections
• *Adult:* PO 125 mg q12h; may increase to 250 mg q12h if needed

Otitis media
- *Child <2 yr:* **PO** 125 mg bid
- *Child >2 yr:* **PO** 250 mg bid

Surgical prophylaxis
- *Adult:* **IV** 1.5 g ½-1 hr preop

Severe infections
- *Adult:* **IM/IV** 1.5 g q6h; may give up to 3 g q8h for bacterial meningitis
- *Child >3 mo:* **IM/IV** 50-100 mg/kg/day; may give up to 200-240 mg/kg/day **IV** in divided doses for bacterial meningitis (not recommended)
- Dosage reduction indicated in severe renal impairment (CCr <20 ml/min)

Uncomplicated gonorrhea
- *Adult:* 1.5 g **IM** as single dose with oral probenecid in 2 separate sites

Available forms: Tabs 125, 250, 500 mg; inj 150, 750 mg, 1.5, 7.5 g; inj 750 mg; 1.5 g powder; susp 125, 250 mg/5 ml

loracarbef
- *Adult and child >13 yr:* **PO** 200-400 mg q12h
- *Child <12 yr:* **PO** 15-30 mg/kg/day in 2 divided doses q12h

Renal dose: CCr 10-49 ml/min 50% of dose; CCr <10 ml/min q3-5 days

Available forms: Caps 200, 400 mg; oral susp 100 mg, 200 mg/5 ml

SIDE EFFECTS

CNS: Dizziness, headache, fatigue, paresthesia, fever, chills, confusion

GI: Diarrhea, nausea, vomiting, anorexia, dysgeusia, glossitis, bleeding; increased AST, ALT, bilirubin, LDH, alk phos; abdominal pain, loose stools, flatulence, heartburn, stomach cramps, colitis, jaundice, **pseudomembranous colitis**

GU: Vaginitis, pruritus, candidiasis, increased BUN, **nephrotoxicity, renal failure,** pyuria, dysuria, reversible interstitial nephritis

HEMA: **Leukopenia, thrombocytopenia, agranulocytosis,** anemia, **neutropenia, lymphocytosis, eosinophilia, pancytopenia, hemolytic anemia, leukocytosis, granulocytopenia**

INTEG: Rash, urticaria, dermatitis, **Stevens-Johnson syndrome**

RESP: Dyspnea

SYST: Anaphylaxis, **serum sickness,** superinfection

Contraindications: Hypersensitivity to cephalosporins or related antibiotics, seizures

Precautions: Pregnancy (B), lactation, children, renal/GI disease

PHARMACOKINETICS

cefaclor
PO: Peak ½-1 hr; half-life 36-54 min; 25% bound by plasma proteins; 60%-85% eliminated unchanged in urine in 8 hr; crosses placenta; excreted in breast milk (low concentrations)

cefotetan
IV/IM: Peak 1½-3 hr; half-life 3-5 hr, 70%-90% bound by plasma proteins, 50%-80% eliminated unchanged in urine, crosses placenta, excreted in breast milk

cefoxitin
IV: Peak 3 min
IM: Peak 15-60 min
Half-life 1 hr, 55%-75% bound by plasma proteins, 90%-100% eliminated unchanged in urine; crosses placenta, blood-brain barrier; eliminated in breast milk, not metabolized

cefprozil
PO: Peak 6-10 hr; plasma protein binding 99%; elimination half-life 25 hr; extensively metabolized to an active metabolite

cefuroxime: 65% excreted unchanged in urine, half-life 1-2 hr in normal renal function

loracarbef
PO: Peak 1 hr, half-life 1 hr; excreted in urine as unchanged drug

INTERACTIONS

- Disulfiram-like reaction: alcohol

Increase: effect/toxicity—aminoglycosides, furosemide, probenecid

Increase: bleeding risk (cefotetan)—anticoagulants, thrombolytics, NSAIDs, antiplatelets, plicamycin, valproic acid

---

⚠ Safety alert   *"Tall Man" lettering

Decrease: absorption of cephalosporin —antacids

Decrease: effect of cephalosporin—H_2-blockers

Drug/Herb
• Do not use acidophilus with antiinfectives; separate by several hours

Increase: bleeding risk (cefotetan)—angelica, anise, arnica, bogbean, boldo, celery, chamomile, clove, fenugreek, feverfew, garlic, ginger, ginkgo, ginseng *(Panax),* horse chestnut, horseradish, licorice, meadowsweet, prickly ash, onion, papain, passion flower, poplar, red clover, turmeric, willow

Drug/Lab Test
False increase: Creatinine (serum urine), urinary 17-KS
False positive: Urinary protein, direct Coombs' test, urine glucose testing (Clinitest)
Interference: Cross-matching

NURSING CONSIDERATIONS
Assess:
⚠ Nephrotoxicity: increased BUN, creatinine
• I&O ratio
• Blood studies: AST, ALT, CBC, Hct, bilirubin, LDH, alk phos, Coombs' test qmo if patient is on long-term therapy
• Electrolytes: K, Na, Cl qmo if patient is on long-term therapy
• Bowel pattern daily; if severe diarrhea occurs, drug should be discontinued; may indicate pseudomembranous colitis
• Urine output; if decreasing, notify prescriber (may indicate nephrotoxicity)
⚠ Anaphylaxis: rash, flushing, urticaria, pruritus, dyspnea, discontinue drug, notify prescriber, have emergency equipment available
• Bleeding: ecchymosis, bleeding gums, hematuria, stool guaiac daily
⚠ Overgrowth of infection: perineal itching, fever, malaise, redness, pain, swelling, drainage, rash, diarrhea, change in cough, sputum
Administer:
• Do not break, crush, or chew ext rel tabs or caps

• On an empty stomach 1 hr before or 2 hr after a meal
cefaclor
• Shake susp, refrigerate, discard after 2 wk
• For 10-14 days to ensure organism death, prevent superinfection
• With food if needed for GI symptoms
• After C&S completed
cefotetan
• IV direct after diluting 1 g/10 ml sterile H_2O for inj and give over 3-5 min; may be diluted further with 50-100 ml of NS or D_5W, shake; run over ½-1 hr by Y-tube or 3-way stopcock; discontinue primary inf during administration
• May be stored 96 hr refrigerated or 24 hr room temperature
Y-site compatibilities: Allopurinol, amifostine, aztreonam, diltiazem, famotidine, filgrastim, fluconazole, fludarabine, heparin, insulin (regular), melphalan, meperidine, morphine, paclitaxel, remifentanil, sargramostim, tacrolimus, teniposide, theophylline, thiotepa
cefoxitin
• IV after diluting 1 g or less/10 ml or more D_5W, NS and give over 3-5 min; may be diluted further with 50-100 ml of normal saline or D_5W; run over ½-1 hr by Y-tube or 3-way stopcock; discontinue primary inf during administration; by cont inf at prescribed rate; may store 96 hr refrigerated or 24 hr room temperature
• For 10-14 days to ensure organism death, prevent superinfection
• After C&S completed
Additive compatibilities: Amikacin, cimetidine, clindamycin, gentamicin, kanamycin, multivitamins, sodium bicarbonate, tobramycin, verapamil, vit B/C
Syringe compatibilities: Heparin, insulin
Y-site compatibilities: Acyclovir, amifostine, amphotericin B cholesteryl sulfate complex, aztreonam, cyclophosphamide, diltiazem, DOXOrubicin liposome, famotidine, fluconazole, foscarnet, hydromorphone, magnesium sulfate, meperidine, morphine, ondansetron, perphenazine, remifentanil, teniposide, thiotepa

Side effects: *italics* = common; **bold** = life-threatening

cefprozil
- For 10-14 days to ensure organism death, prevent superinfection
- After C&S
- Refrigerate/shake susp prior to use

cefuroxime
- For 10-14 days to ensure organism death, prevent superinfection
- With food if needed for GI symptoms
- After C&S

Additive compatibilities: Clindamycin, floxacillin, furosemide, metronidazole, netilmicin

Y-site compatibilities: Acyclovir, allopurinol, amifostine, atracurium, aztreonam, cyclophosphamide, diltiazem, famotidine, fludarabine, foscarnet, hydromorphone, melphalan, meperidine, morphine, ondansetron, pancuronium, perphenazine, remifentanil, sargramostim, tacrolimus, teniposide, thiotepa, vecuronium

loracarbef
- Oral susp should be shaken before giving; store for 2 wk at room temperature, discard after 2 wk
- 1 hr before or 2 hr after a meal
- After C&S is completed
- For 7 days to ensure organism death, prevent superinfection

Evaluate:
- Therapeutic response: negative C&S

Teach patient/family:
- If diabetic, to use blood glucose testing
- Not to drink alcohol or take meds with alcohol or reaction may occur
- To complete full course of drug therapy, to report persistent diarrhea
- To use yogurt or buttermilk to maintain intestinal flora, decrease diarrhea
- To notify prescriber if breastfeeding or of any side effects

⚠ To report sore throat, bruising, bleeding, joint pain (may indicate blood dyscrasias [rare]); diarrhea with mucus, blood, may indicate pseudomembranous colitis

Treatment of anaphylaxis: EpINEPHrine, antihistamines; resuscitate if needed

CEPHALOSPORINS— 3RD GENERATION

cefdinir (℞)
(sef′dih-ner)
Omnicef

cefditoren pivoxil (℞)
(sef-dit′oh-ren pih-vox′il)
Spectracef

cefepime (℞)
(sef′e-peem)
Maxipime

cefixime (℞)
(sef-icks′ime)
Cefixime

cefotaxime (℞)
(sef-oh-taks′eem)
Claforan

cefpodoxime (℞)
(sef-poe-docks′eem)
Vantin

ceftazidime (℞)
(sef′tay-zi-deem)
Ceptaz, Fortaz, Tazicef, Tazidime

ceftibuten (℞)
(sef-ti-byoo′tin)
Cedax

ceftizoxime (℞)
(sef-ti-zox′eem)
Cefizox

ceftriaxone (℞)
(sef-try-ax′one)
Rocephin

Func. class.: Broad-spectrum antibiotic
Chem. class.: Cephalosporin (3rd generation)

Do not confuse:
ceftazidime/ceftizoxime
Vantin/Ventolin

Action: Inhibits bacterial cell wall synthesis, rendering cell wall osmotically unstable, leading to cell death

Uses:

cefdinir: Gram-negative bacilli: *Haemophilus influenzae, Haemophilus parainfluenzae, Moraxella catarrhalis;* gram-positive organisms: *Streptococcus pneumoniae, Streptococcus pyogenes, Staphylococcus aureus,* acute exacerbations of chronic bronchitis

cefditoren pivoxil: Acute bacterial exacerbation of chronic bronchitis caused by *Haemophilus influenzae, Haemophilus parainfluenzae, Streptococcus pneumoniae, Moraxella catarrhalis;* pharyngitis/tonsillitis caused by *Streptococcus pyogenes;* uncomplicated skin and skin structure infections caused by *Staphylococcus aureus, Streptococcus pyogenes*

cefepime: Gram-negative bacilli: *Escherichia coli, Proteus, Klebsiella;* gram-positive organisms: *Streptococcus pneumoniae, Streptococcus pyogenes, Staphylococcus aureus;* lower respiratory tract, urinary tract, skin, bone infections

cefixime: Uncomplicated UTI *(Escherichia coli, Proteus mirabilis),* pharyngitis and tonsillitis *(Streptococcus pyogenes),* otitis media *(Haemophilus influenzae), Moraxella catarrhalis,* acute bronchitis, and acute exacerbations of chronic bronchitis *(Streptococcus pneumoniae, H. influenzae)*

cefotaxime: Gram-negative organisms: *Haemophilus influenzae, Haemophilus parainfluenzae, Escherichia coli, Enterococcus faecalis, Neisseria gonorrhoeae, Neisseria meningitidis, Proteus mirabilis, Klebsiella, Citrobacter, Serratia, Salmonella, Shigella Pseudomonas;* gram-positive organisms: *Streptococcus pneumoniae, Streptococcus pyogenes, Staphylococcus aureus;* serious lower respiratory tract, urinary tract, skin, bone, gonococcal infections; bacteremia, septicemia, meningitis, skin, skin structure infections, CNS infections; perioperative prophylaxis

cefpodoxime: Gram-negative bacilli: *Neisseria gonorrhoeae, Haemophilus influenzae, Escherichia coli, Proteus mirabilis, Klebsiella;* gram-positive organisms: *Streptococcus pneumoniae, Streptococcus pyogenes, Staphylococcus aureus;* upper and lower respiratory tract, urinary tract, skin infections; otitis media, sexually transmitted diseases

ceftazidime: Gram-negative organisms: *Haemophilus influenzae, Escherichia coli, Enterobacter aerogenes, Pseudomonas aeruginosa, Proteus mirabilis, Klebsiella, Citrobacter, Enterobacter, Salmonella, Shigella, Acinetobacter, Bacteroides fragilis, Neisseria, Serratia;* gram-positive organisms: *Streptococcus pneumoniae, Streptococcus pyogenes, Staphylococcus aureus;* serious upper/lower respiratory tract, urinary tract, skin, gynecologic, bone, joint, intraabdominal infections; septicemia, meningitis

ceftibuten: Pharyngitis/tonsillitis, otitis media, secondary bacterial infection of acute bronchitis

ceftizoxime: Gram-negative bacilli: *Haemophilus influenzae, Escherichia coli, Enterobacter aerogenes, Proteus mirabilis, Klebsiella, Enterobacter;* gram-positive organisms: *Streptococcus pneumoniae, Streptococcus pyogenes, Staphylococcus aureus;* serious lower respiratory tract, urinary tract, skin, intraabdominal infections, septicemia, meningitis, bone and joint infections, PID caused by *Neisseria gonorrhoeae*

ceftriaxone: Gram-negative bacilli: *Haemophilus influenzae, Escherichia coli, Enterobacter aerogenes, Proteus mirabilis, Klebsiella, Citrobacter, Enterobacter, Salmonella, Shigella, Acinetobacter, Bacteroides fragilis, Neisseria, Serratia;* gram-positive organisms: *Streptococcus pneumoniae, Streptococcus pyogenes, Staphylococcus aureus;* serious lower respiratory tract, urinary tract, skin, gonococcal, intraabdominal infections; septicemia, meningitis, bone, joint infections

---

DOSAGE AND ROUTES

cefdinir
Uncomplicated skin and skin structure infections/community-acquired pneumonia
- *Adult and child ≥13 yr:* **PO** 300 mg q12h × 10 days
- *Child 6 mo-12 yr:* **PO** 7 mg/kg q12h or 14 mg/kg q24h × 10 days

Acute exacerbations of chronic bronchitis/acute maxillary sinusitis
- *Adult and child ≥13 yr:* **PO** 300 mg q12h or 600 mg q24h × 10 days or 300 mg bid × 5 days in some infections

Pharyngitis/tonsillitis
- *Adult and child ≥13 yr:* **PO** 300 mg q12h or 600 mg q24h × 10 days
- *Child 6 mo-12 yr:* **PO** 7 mg/kg q12h × 5-10 days or 14 mg/kg q24h × 10 days

Renal dose
- CCr <30 ml/min 300 mg daily (adult); 7 mg/kg daily (child)

Available forms: Caps 300 mg; susp 125 mg, 250 mg/5 ml

cefditoren pivoxil
- *Adult:* **PO** 200-400 mg bid

Renal dose
- *Adult:* **PO** CCr 30-50 ml/min, max 200 mg bid; CCr <30 ml/min; max 200 mg daily

Available forms: Tabs 200 mg

cefepime
Urinary tract infections (mild to moderate)
- *Adult:* **IV/IM** 0.5-1 g q12h × 7-10 days

Urinary tract infections (severe)
- *Adult:* **IV** 2 g q12h × 10 days

Pneumonia (moderate to severe)
- *Adult:* **IV** 1-2 g q12h × 10 days
- Dosage reduction indicated in renal impairment (CCr <50 ml/min)

Uncomplicated gonorrhea
- **IM** 2 g as a single dose with 1 g **PO** probenecid at the same time

Available forms: Powder for inj 500 mg, 1, 2 g

cefixime
- *Adult:* **PO** 400 mg daily as a single dose or 200 mg q12h

- *Child >50 kg or >12 yr:* **PO** use adult dosage
- *Child <50 kg or <12 yr:* **PO** 8 mg/kg/day as a single dose or 4 mg/kg q12h

Renal dose
- CCr 21-60 ml/min give 75% of dose; CCr <20 ml/min give 50% of dose

Available forms: Tabs 200, 400 mg; powder for oral susp 100 mg/5 ml

cefotaxime
- *Adult:* **IM/IV** 1-2 g q12h
- *Child 1 mo-12 yr:* **IM/IV** 50-180 mg/kg/day divided q6h

Severe infections
- *Adult:* **IM/IV** 2 g q4h, not to exceed 12 g/day
- *Child 1 mo-12 yr:* **IM/IV** 50-180 mg/kg/day in 4-6 divided doses

Uncomplicated gonorrhea
- *Adult:* **IM** 1 g
- Dosage reduction indicated for severe renal impairment (CCr <30 ml/min)

Available forms: Powder for inj 500 mg, 1, 2, 10 g; inj 1, 2 g premixed frozen

cefpodoxime
- *Adult >13 yr:* Pneumonia: 200 mg q12h for 14 days; *uncomplicated gonorrhea:* 200 mg; single dose; *skin and skin structure:* 400 mg q12h for 7-14 days; *pharyngitis and tonsillitis:* 100 mg q12h for 10 days; *uncomplicated UTI:* 100 mg q12h for 7 days; dosing interval increased in presence of severe renal impairment
- *Child 5 mo-12 yr:* acute otitis media: 5 mg/kg q12h for 10 days; *pharyngitis/tonsillitis:* 5 mg/kg q12h (max 100 mg/dose or 200 mg/day) × 5-10 days

Available forms: Tabs 100, 200 mg; granules for susp 50 mg, 100 mg/5 ml

ceftazidime
- *Adult:* **IV/IM** 1-2 g q8-12h × 5-10 days
- *Child:* **IV** 30-50 mg/kg q8h not to exceed 6 g/day
- *Neonate:* **IV** 30-50 mg/kg q12h

Renal dose: CCr <50 ml/min give q12h; CCr 10-30 ml/min give q24h; CCr <10 ml/min give q48h

Available forms: Inj 250, 500 mg, 1, 2, 6 g

ceftibuten
- *Adult:* **PO** 400 mg daily × 10 days

- *Child 6 mo-12 yr:* **PO** 9 mg/kg daily × 10 days

Renal dose: CCr <50 ml/min give 200 mg q24h; CCr 5-20 ml/min give 100 mg q24h

Available forms: Caps 400 mg; susp 90 mg, 180 mg/5 ml

ceftizoxime

- *Adult:* **IM/IV** 1-2 g q8-12h, may give up to 4 g q8h in life-threatening infections
- *Child >6 mo:* **IM/IV** 50 mg/kg q6-8h

Renal dose: CCr <80 ml/min give 500-1500 mg q8h; CCr 10-49 ml/min give 250-1000 mg q12h

PID

- *Adult:* **IV** 2 g q8h, may increase to 4 g q8h in severe infections

Available forms: Powder for inj 500 mg, 1, 2, 10 g; premixed 1 g, 2 g/50 ml

ceftriaxone

- *Adult:* **IM/IV** 1-2 g daily, max 2 g q12h
- *Child:* **IM/IV** 50-75 mg/kg/day in equal doses q12h

Uncomplicated gonorrhea

- *Adult:* 250 mg **IM** as single dose
- Reduce dosage in severe renal impairment (CCr <10 ml/min)

Meningitis

- *Adult and child:* **IM/IV** 100 mg/kg/day in equal doses q12h, max 4 g/day

Surgical prophylaxis

- *Adult:* **IV** 1 g ½-2 hr preop

Available forms: Inj 250, 500 mg, 1, 2, 10 g

SIDE EFFECTS

CNS: Headache, dizziness, weakness, paresthesia, fever, chills, **seizures**

GI: Nausea, vomiting, diarrhea, anorexia, pain, glossitis, **bleeding;** increased AST, ALT, bilirubin, LDH, alk phos; abdominal pain, **pseudomembranous colitis**

GU: **Proteinuria,** vaginitis, pruritus, candidiasis, increased BUN, **nephrotoxicity, renal failure**

HEMA: **Leukopenia, thrombocytopenia, agranulocytosis,** anemia, **neutropenia,** lymphocytosis, eosinophilia, **pancytopenia, hemolytic anemia**

INTEG: Rash, urticaria, dermatitis

RESP: Dyspnea

SYST: **Anaphylaxis, serum sickness, Stevens-Johnson syndrome**

Contraindications: Hypersensitivity to cephalosporins, infants <1 mo

Precautions: Pregnancy (B), hypersensitivity to penicillins, lactation, renal disease, children, GI disease

PHARMACOKINETICS

cefdinir

Unchanged in urine; crosses placenta, blood-brain barrier; eliminated in breast milk; not metabolized

cefditoren pivoxil

Well absorbed after it is broken down (prodrug); distribution widely; half-life 100 min; onset rapid; peak 0.5-3 hr; duration 12 hr

cefepime

Peak 79 min, half-life 2 hr, 20% bound by plasma proteins, 90% excreted unchanged in urine; crosses placenta, blood-brain barrier; excreted in breast milk; not metabolized

cefixime

PO: Peak 1-2 hr, half-life 3-4 hr, 65% bound by plasma proteins, 50% eliminated unchanged in urine; crosses placenta; excreted in breast milk

cefotaxime

IV: Onset 5 min

IM: Onset 30 min

Half-life 1 hr; 35%-65% is bound by plasma proteins; 40%-65% is eliminated unchanged in urine in 24 hr; 25% metabolized to active metabolites; excreted in breast milk (small amounts)

cefpodoxime

Half-life 2-3 hr; 25% bound by plasma proteins; 30% eliminated unchanged in urine in 8 hr; crosses placenta; excreted in breast milk

ceftazidime

IV/IM: Peak 1 hr, half-life ½-1 hr, 90% bound by plasma proteins, 80% eliminated unchanged in urine, crosses placenta, excreted in breast milk

ceftibuten

PO: Peak 6-10 hr; plasma protein

binding 99%; elimination half-life 25 hr; extensively metabolized to an active metabolite

ceftizoxime
IV: Onset 5 min
IM: Peak 1 hr
Half-life 5-8 hr; 90% bound by plasma proteins; 36%-60% eliminated unchanged in urine; crosses placenta; excreted in breast milk

ceftriaxone
IV: Onset 5 min
IM: Peak 1 hr
Half-life 5-8 hr, 90% bound by plasma proteins; 35%-60% eliminated unchanged in urine; crosses placenta; excreted in breast milk

INTERACTIONS

Increase: bleeding—anticoagulants, thrombolytics, plicamycin, valproic acid, NSAIDs

Increase: toxicity—aminoglycosides, furosemide, probenecid

Decrease: absorption of cefdinir—iron

Drug/Herb
• Do not use acidophilus with antiinfectives; separate by several hours

Increase: bleeding risk (cefoperazone)—angelica, anise, arnica, bogbean, boldo, celery, chamomile, clove, fenugreek, feverfew, garlic, ginger, ginkgo, ginseng *(Panax),* horse chestnut, horseradish, licorice, meadowsweet, prickly ash, onion, papain, passion flower, poplar, red clover, turmeric, willow

Drug/Lab Test
Increase: ALT, AST, alk phos, LDH, bilirubin, BUN, creatinine
False increase: Creatinine (serum urine), urinary 17-KS
False positive: Urinary protein, direct Coombs' test, urine glucose
Interference: Cross-matching

NURSING CONSIDERATIONS

Assess:
• Sensitivity to penicillin, other cephalosporins

⚠ Nephrotoxicity: increased BUN, creatinine; urine output: if decreasing, notify prescriber; may indicate nephrotoxicity
• Blood studies: AST, ALT, CBC, Hct, bilirubin, LDH, alk phos, Coombs' test monthly if patient is on long-term therapy
• Electrolytes: K, Na, Cl monthly if patient is on long-term therapy
• Bowel pattern daily; if severe diarrhea occurs, drug should be discontinued; may indicate pseudomembranous colitis
• IV site for extravasation, phlebitis
⚠ Anaphylaxis: rash, urticaria, pruritus, chills, fever, joint pain, angioedema; may occur few days after therapy begins
• Bleeding: ecchymosis, bleeding gums, hematuria, stool guaiac
⚠ Overgrowth of infection: perineal itching, fever, malaise, redness, pain, swelling, drainage, rash, diarrhea, change in cough, sputum

Administer:
• Change IV site q72 hr

cefdinir
• Oral susp after adding 39 ml water to the 60 ml bottle; 65 ml water to the 120 ml bottle; discard unused portion after 10 days
• After C&S completed

cefditoren pivoxil
• For 10 days to ensure organism death, prevent superinfection
• With food if needed for GI symptoms
• After C&S completed

cefepime
• IV after diluting in 50-100 ml or more D$_5$, NS and give over 30 min
• For 7-10 days to ensure organism death, prevent superinfection

Solution compatibilities: 0.9% NaCl, D$_5$, D$_5$W, 0.5%, 10% lidocaine, bacteriostatic water for inj with parabens/benzyl alcohol

Y-site compatibilities: Doxorubicin liposome

cefixime
• For 10-14 days to ensure organism death, prevent superinfection
• Do not break, crush, or chew

⚠ Safety alert   *"Tall Man" lettering

cefotaxime

- IV after diluting 1 g/10 ml D$_5$W, NS, sterile H$_2$O for inj and give over 3-5 min by Y-tube or 3-way stopcock; may be diluted further with 50-100 ml of normal saline or D$_5$W; run over ½-1 hr; discontinue primary inf during administration; or may be diluted in larger vol of sol and given as a cont inf over 6-24 hr
- For 10-14 days to ensure organism death, prevent superinfection
- Thaw frozen container at room temperature or refrigeration; do not force thaw by immersion or microwave; visually inspect container for leaks

Additive compatibilities: Clindamycin, metronidazole, verapamil

Syringe compatibilities: Heparin, ofloxacin

Y-site compatibilities: Acyclovir, amifostine, aztreonam, cyclophosphamide, diltiazem, famotidine, fludarabine, hydromorphone, lorazepam, magnesium sulfate, melphalan, meperidine, midazolam, morphine, ondansetron, perphenazine, sargramostim, teniposide, thiotepa, tolazoline, vinorelbine

cefpodoxime

- Do not break, crush, or chew tabs
- For 10-14 days to ensure organism death, prevent superinfection
- With food to enhance absorption

Y-site compatibilities: Famotidine, fluconazole, fludarabine, insulin (regular), meperidine, morphine, sargramostim

ceftazidime

- IV after diluting 1 g/10 ml sterile H$_2$O for inj, shake, invert needle, push plunger, insert needle through stopper and keep in sol, expel bubbles and give over 3-5 min; may be diluted further with 50-100 ml of normal saline or D$_5$W; run over ½-1 hr, give through Y-tube or 3-way stopcock, discontinue primary inf during administration; store for 96 hr refrigerated, 24 hr room temperature
- For 5-10 days to ensure organism death, prevent superinfection

Syringe compatibilities: Hydromorphone

Additive compatibilities: Ciprofloxacin, clindamycin, fluconazole, metronidazole, ofloxacin

Y-site compatibilities: Acyclovir, allopurinol, amifostine, aztreonam, ciprofloxacin, diltiazem, enalaprilat, esmolol, famotidine, filgrastim, fludarabine, foscarnet, granisetron, heparin, hydromorphone, labetalol, meperidine, melphalan, morphine, ondansetron, paclitaxel, ranitidine, remifentanil, tacrolimus, teniposide, theophylline, thiotepa, vinorelbine, zidovudine

ceftibuten

- For 10 days to ensure organism death, prevent superinfection

ceftizoxime

- IV after diluting 1 g/10 ml sterile water, shake and give over 3-5 min; may be diluted further with 50-100 ml NS or D$_5$W give through Y-tube or 3-way stopcock; run over ½-1 hr
- For 10-14 days to ensure organism death, prevent superinfection

Additive compatibilities: Clindamycin

Y-site compatibilities: Acyclovir, allopurinol, amphotericin B cholesteryl sulfate complex, aztreonam, DOXOrubicin liposome, enalaprilat, esmolol, famotidine, fludarabine, foscarnet, hydromorphone, labetalol, melphalan, meperidine, morphine, ondansetron, remifentanil, sargramostim, teniposide, vinorelbine

ceftriaxone

- For 10-14 days to ensure organism death, prevent superinfection
- IM inj deeply in large muscle mass
- IV after diluting 250 mg/2.4 ml D$_5$W, H$_2$O for inj, 0.9% NaCl; may be further diluted with 50-100 ml NS, D$_5$W, D$_{10}$W, shake; run over ½-1 hr

Additive compatibilities: Amino acids or sodium bicarbonate, metronidazole

Y-site compatibilities: Acyclovir, allopurinol, aztreonam, cisatracurium, diltiazem, DOXOrubicin liposome, fludarabine, foscarnet, heparin, melphalan, meperidine, methotrexate, morphine, paclitaxel, remifentanil, sargramostim, tac-

Side effects: *italics* = common; **bold** = life-threatening

rolimus, teniposide, theophylline, vinorelbine, warfarin, zidovudine

Evaluate:

• Therapeutic response: decreased symptoms of infection; negative C&S

Teach patient/family:

• If diabetic, to check blood glucose

⚠ To report sore throat, bruising, bleeding, joint pain; may indicate blood dyscrasias (rare); diarrhea with mucus, blood, may indicate pseudomembranous colitis

• To report persistent diarrhea

• Cefditoren can be taken with oral contraceptives

Treatment of anaphylaxis: EpINEPHrine, antihistamines; resuscitate if needed

---

cephradine
See cephalosporins—
1st generation

---

cetirizine (℞)
(se-teer'i-zeen)
Zyrtec
Func. class.: Antihistamine (2nd generation, peripherally selective)
Chem. class.: Piperazine, H_1-histamine antagonist

Do not confuse:

Zyrtec/Xanax/Zantac

Action: Acts on blood vessels, GI, respiratory system by competing with histamine for H_1-receptor site; decreases allergic response by blocking pharmacologic effects of histamine; minimal anticholinergic action

Uses: Rhinitis, allergy symptoms, chronic idiopathic urticaria

DOSAGE AND ROUTES

• *Adult and child ≥6 yr:* **PO** 5-10 mg daily

• *Child 2-5 yr:* **PO** 2.5 mg daily, may increase to 5 mg daily or 2.5 mg bid

• *Child 1-2 yr:* **PO** 2.5 mg daily, may increase to 2.5 mg q12h

• *Child 6-11 mo:* **PO** 2.5 mg daily

• *Geriatric:* **PO** 5 mg daily, may increase to 10 mg/day

Renal dose

• *Adult:* **PO** CCr 11-31 ml/min 5 mg daily

Hemodialysis

• *Adult:* **PO** 5 mg daily

Hepatic dose

• *Adult:* **PO** 5 mg daily

Available forms: Tabs 5, 10 mg; syr 5 mg/5 ml

SIDE EFFECTS

CNS: Headache, stimulation, *drowsiness,* sedation, *fatigue,* confusion, blurred vision, tinnitus, restlessness, tremors, paradoxical excitation in children or geriatric

GI: Dry mouth, increase LFTs

INTEG: Rash, eczema, photosensitivity, urticaria

RESP: Thickening of bronchial secretions, dry nose, throat

Contraindications: Hypersensitivity to this drug or hydrOXYzine, newborn or premature infants, lactation, severe hepatic disease

Precautions: Pregnancy (B), geriatric, children, respiratory disease, narrowangle glaucoma, prostatic hypertrophy, bladder neck obstruction, asthma

PHARMACOKINETICS

Absorption rapid; onset ½ hr; peak 1-2 hr; duration 24 hr; protein binding 93%; half-life decreased in children; increased in renal/hepatic disease

INTERACTIONS

Increase: CNS depression—alcohol, other CNS depressants

Increase: anticholinergic/sedative effect—MAOIs

Drug/Herb

Increase: effect—hops, Jamaican dogwood, kava, senega, valerian

Increase: anticholinergic effect—corkwood

Drug/Food

• Food prolongs absorption by 1.7 hr

Drug/Lab Test
False negative: Skin allergy tests

NURSING CONSIDERATIONS
Assess:
• Allergy symptoms: pruritus, urticaria, watering eyes, baseline and during treatment
• Respiratory status: rate, rhythm, increase in bronchial secretions, wheezing, chest tightness
Administer:
• Without regard to meals
Perform/provide:
• Hard candy, gum, frequent rinsing of mouth for dryness
• Storage in tight, light-resistant container
Evaluate:
• Therapeutic response: absence of running or congested nose or rashes
Teach patient/family:
• All aspects of drug use; to notify prescriber if confusion, sedation, hypotension occur
• To avoid driving, other hazardous activity if drowsiness occurs
• To avoid alcohol, other CNS depressants
• That drug is not recommended during lactation
• To avoid exposure to sunlight; burns may occur
• To use sugarless gum, candy, frequent sips of water to minimize dry mouth
Treatment of overdose: Administer diazepam, vasopressors, barbiturates (short-acting)

---

cetrorelix (℞)
(set-roe-ree′lix)
Cetrotide
Func. class.: Gonadotropin-releasing hormone antagonist
Chem. class.: Synthetic decapeptide

Action: Inhibitor of pituitary gonadotropin secretion; initially increases LH and FSH, induces a rapid suppression of gonadotropin secretion
Uses: For inhibition of premature LH surges in women undergoing controlled ovarian hyperstimulation

DOSAGE AND ROUTES
Single-dose regimen
• *Adult:* **SUBCUT** 3 mg when serum estradiol level is at appropriate stimulation response, usually on stimulation day 7; if hCG has not been given within 4 days after inj of 3 mg cetrorelix, give 0.25 mg daily until day of hCG administration
Multiple-dose regimen
• *Adult:* **SUBCUT** 0.25 mg is given on stimulation day 5 (either morning or evening) or 6 (morning) and continued daily until day hCG is given
Available forms: Inj 0.25, 3 mg

SIDE EFFECTS
CNS: Headache
ENDO: Ovarian hyperstimulation syndrome, abdominal pain (gyn)
GI: Nausea, vomiting, diarrhea
INTEG: Pain on inj; local site reactions
SYST: **Fetal death**
Contraindications: Pregnancy (X), hypersensitivity, latex allergy, lactation

PHARMACOKINETICS
Excreted in feces/urine, half-life depends on dosage, metabolized to metabolites, protein binding 86%

NURSING CONSIDERATIONS
Assess:
• For suspected pregnancy, drug should not be used
• For latex allergy, drug should not be used
• For ALT, AST, GGT, alk phos
Administer:
• SUBCUT using abdomen, around navel or upper thigh, swab inj area with disinfectant, clean a 2-inch circle and allow to dry, pinch up area between thumb and finger, insert needle 45-90 degrees to surface; if positioned correctly, no blood will be drawn back into syringe, reposition needle without removing it

---

Side effects: *italics* = common; **bold** = life-threatening

• Do not administer if patient is pregnant

Perform/provide:
• Protection from light

Evaluate:
• Therapeutic response: pregnancy

Teach patient/family:
• To report abdominal pain, vaginal bleeding, nausea, vomiting, diarrhea, shortness of breath, peripheral edema
• To teach self-administration technique if needed

---

cetuximab (℞)
(se-tux'i-mab)
Erbitux
Func. class.: Antineoplastic—miscellaneous, monoclonal antibody
Chem. class.: Epidermal growth factor receptor inhibitor

Action: Not fully understood; binds to epidermal growth factor receptors (EGFRs); inhibits phosphorylation and activation of receptor-associated kinase, resulting in inhibition of cell growth

Uses: Alone or in combination with irinotecan for EGFRs expressing metastatic colorectal carcinoma

DOSAGE AND ROUTES

• *Adult:* **IV INF** 400 mg/m² loading dose given over 120 min, max infusion rate 5 ml/min; weekly maintenance dose (all other infusions) is 250 mg/m² given over 60 min, max infusion rate 5 ml/min; premedicate with an H_1 antagonist (diphenhydrAMINE 50 mg IV); dosage adjustments are made for infusion reactions or dermatologic toxicity

Available forms: Inj 50 ml, single-use vial with 100 mg of cetuximab (2 mg/ml)

SIDE EFFECTS

CNS: Headache, insomnia, depression
GI: Nausea, diarrhea, vomiting, anorexia, mouth ulceration, dehydration, constipation, abdominal pain
HEMA: **Leukopenia, anemia**

INTEG: Rash, pruritus, acne, dry skin, **toxic epidermal necrolysis, angioedema,** *blepharitis, cheilitis, cellulitis, cysts, alopecia, skin/nail disorder*
MISC: Conjunctivitis, asthma, malaise, fever, **renal failure**
MS: Back pain
RESP: **Interstitial lung disease,** *cough,* **dyspnea, pulmonary embolus,** *peripheral edema*
SYST: **Anaphylaxis, sepsis, infection**

Contraindications: Hypersensitivity to this drug or murine proteins
Precautions: Pregnancy (C), renal/hepatic disease, ocular, pulmonary disorders, lactation, children, geriatric

PHARMACOKINETICS

Half-life 114 hr, steady state by 3rd weekly infusion, peak 168-235 g/ml, trough 41-85 g/ml

INTERACTIONS
None known

NURSING CONSIDERATIONS
Assess:
⚠ Pulmonary changes: lung sounds, cough, dyspnea; interstitial lung disease may occur, may be fatal; discontinue therapy if confirmed
⚠ Toxic epidermal necrosis, angioedema, anaphylaxis
• GI symptoms: frequency of stools, dehydration, abdominal pain, stomatitis
Administer:
IV INF route
• Using cytoxic handling procedures
• By IV infusion only, do not give by IV push or bolus
• Do not shake or dilute
• Infusion pump: draw up volume of a vial using appropriate syringe/needle (a vented spike or other appropriate transfer device); fill Erbitux into sterile evacuated container/bag, repeat until calculated volume has been put into the container; use a new needle for each vial; give through in-line filter (low protein binding 0.22-micrometer); affix infusion

---

line and prime before starting infusion, max rate 5 ml/min; flush line at end of infusion with 0.9% NaCl

• Syringe pump: Draw up volume of a vial using appropriate syringe/needle (a vented spike); place syringe into syringe driver of a syringe pump and set rate; use an in-line filter 0.22-micrometer (low protein binding); connect infusion line and start infusion after priming; repeat until calculated volume has been given

• Use a new needle and filter for each vial, max 5 ml/min rate; use 0.9% NaCl to flush line after infusion

• Do not piggyback to patient infusion line

• Observe patient for adverse reactions for 1 hr after infusion

• Infusion reactions: if mild (grade 1 or 2) reduce all doses by 50%; if severe (grade 3 or 4) permanently discontinue

Perform/provide:

• Storage refrigerated 36°-46° F, discard unused portions

Evaluate:

• Therapeutic response: Decrease growth, spread of EGFR expressing metastatic colorectal carcinoma

Teach patient/family:

• To report adverse reactions immediately: shortness of breath, severe abdominal pain, skin eruptions

• Reason for treatment, expected results

• Use contraception during treatment, pregnancy (C), avoid breastfeeding

• To wear sunscreen and hats to limit sun exposure; sun exposure can exacerbate any skin reactions

• To avoid crowds, persons with known infections

chloral hydrate (℞)

(klor-al hye'drate)
Aquachloral, chloral hydrate, Novo-Chlorhydrate ✦, PMS-chloral hydrate ✦
Func. class.: Sedative/hypnotic
Chem. class.: Chloral derivative

Controlled Substance Schedule IV (USA), Schedule F (Canada)
Action: Reduction product trichloroethanol produces mild cerebral depression, which causes sleep
Uses: Sedation, short-term treatment of insomnia

DOSAGE AND ROUTES

Sedation
• *Adult:* **PO/RECT** 250 mg tid after meals
• *Child:* **PO** 25-50 mg/kg tid, not to exceed 500 mg tid

Insomnia
• *Adult:* **PO/RECT** 500 mg-1 g ½ hr before bedtime
• *Child:* **PO/RECT** 50-75 mg/kg (one dose)

Procedure sedation
• *Child:* **PO/RECT** 25-50 mg/kg, not to exceed 100 mg/kg or 2 g

Renal disease
• *Adult:* **PO/RECT** CCr <50 ml/min avoid use

Available forms: Caps 250, 500, 650 mg; syr 250 mg, 500 mg/5 ml; supp 325, 500 mg

SIDE EFFECTS

CNS: Drowsiness, dizziness, stimulation, nightmares, ataxia, hangover (rare), lightheadedness, headache, paranoia
CV: Hypotension, **dysrhythmias**
GI: Nausea, vomiting, flatulence, diarrhea, unpleasant taste, **gastric necrosis**
HEMA: **Eosinophilia, leukopenia**
INTEG: Rash, urticaria, **angioedema**, fever, purpura, eczema
RESP: **Depression**
Contraindications: Hypersensitivity to this drug or triclofos, severe renal/hepatic

---

Side effects: *italics* = common; **bold** = life-threatening

disease, GI disorders (oral forms), gastritis

Precautions: Pregnancy (C), severe cardiac disease, depression, suicidal individuals, asthma, intermittent porphyria, lactation, geriatric

PHARMACOKINETICS

PO: Onset 30 min-1 hr, duration 4-8 hr

RECT: Onset slow, duration 4-8 hr; metabolized by liver; excreted by kidneys (inactive metabolite) and feces; crosses placenta; excreted in breast milk; metabolite is highly protein bound

INTERACTIONS

Increase: action—oral anticoagulants, furosemide

Increase: action of both drugs—alcohol, CNS depressants

Decrease: effects of phenytoin

Drug/Herb

Increase: sedative effect—catnip, chamomile, clary, cowslip, hops, kava, lavender, mistletoe, nettle, pokeweed, poppy, Queen Anne's lace, senega, skullcap, valerian

Increase: hypotension—black cohosh

Drug/Lab Test

Interference: Urine catecholamines, urinary 17-OHCS

NURSING CONSIDERATIONS

Assess:
• Mental status: mood, sensorium, affect, memory (long and short term)
• Physical dependency: more frequent requests for medication, tremors, anxiety, pinpoint pupils
• Respiratory dysfunction: respiratory depression, character, rate, rhythm; hold drug if respirations <10/min or if pupils dilated (rare)
• History of substance abuse, cardiac disease, gastritis

Administer:
• Do not break, crush, or chew caps
• On empty stomach with full glass of water or juice for best absorption and to decrease corrosion
• After meals to decrease GI symptoms if using for sedation
• ½-1 hr before bedtime for sleeplessness

Perform/provide:
• Assistance with ambulation after receiving dose, especially geriatric
• Safety measure: night-light, call bell within easy reach
• Check to see PO medication swallowed
• Check dose of syrup carefully fatal overdoses have occurred
• Storage in dark container, suppositories in refrigerator

Evaluate:
• Therapeutic response: ability to sleep at night, decreased amount of early morning awakening if taking drug for insomnia

Teach patient/family:
• To avoid driving, other activities requiring alertness
• To avoid alcohol ingestion, CNS depressants; serious CNS depression may result
• Not to discontinue medication quickly after long-term use; drug should be tapered over 1-2 wk, delirium may occur
• That effects may take 2 nights for benefits to be noticed
• Alternative measures to improve sleep (reading, exercise several hours before bedtime, warm bath, warm milk, TV, self-hypnosis, deep breathing)
• Avoid breastfeeding

Treatment of overdose: Lavage, activated charcoal; monitor electrolytes, vital signs

---

chlorambucil (℞)

(klor-am′byoo-sil)
Leukeran
Func. class.: Antineoplastic alkylating agent
Chem. class.: Nitrogen mustard

Do not confuse:
Leukeran/leucovorin/Leukine
Action: Alkylates DNA, RNA; inhibits en-

---

zymes that allow synthesis of amino acids in proteins; activity is not cell cycle phase specific

Uses: Chronic lymphocytic leukemia, non-Hodgkin's/Hodgkin's disease, other lymphomas, nephrotic syndrome, choriocarcinoma

Unlabeled uses: Macroglobulinemia ovarian, testicular carcinoma, non-Hodgkin's lymphoma

DOSAGE AND ROUTES
• *Adult:* **PO** 0.1-0.2 mg/kg/day for 3-6 wk initially, then 4-10 mg/day maintenance
• *Geriatric:* **PO** initially ≤2-4 mg/day
• *Child:* **PO** 0.1-0.2 mg/kg/day (4.5 mg/m²/day) in divided doses or 4.5 mg/m²/day as 1 dose or in divided doses × 3-6 wk

Macroglobulinemia (unlabeled)
• *Adult:* **PO** 2-10 mg daily × 9 days, or 8 mg/m² daily with predniSONE × 10 days, repeat q6-8wk as needed

Nephrotic syndrome
• *Child:* **PO** 0.1-0.2 mg/kg daily with predniSONE × 8-12 wk

Intractable idiopathic uveitis, Behçet's syndrome
• *Adult:* **PO** 6-12 mg or 0.1-0.2 mg/kg × 1 yr or more

Available forms: Tabs 2 mg

SIDE EFFECTS

CNS: **Seizures,** tremors, confusion, agitation, ataxia
GI: Nausea, vomiting, diarrhea, weight loss, **hepatoxicity,** *jaundice*
GU: Hyperuremia
HEMA: **Thrombocytopenia, leukopenia, pancytopenia** (prolonged use), **permanent bone marrow depression**
INTEG: Alopecia (rare), dermatitis, rash, **Stevens-Johnson syndrome**
RESP: **Fibrosis, pneumonitis**

Contraindications: Pregnancy (D), radiation therapy within 1 mo, chemotherapy within 1 mo, thrombocytopenia, recent smallpox vaccination, lactation

Precautions: *Pneumococcus* vaccination, children

PHARMACOKINETICS
Well absorbed orally; metabolized in liver; excreted in urine; half-life 2 hr

INTERACTIONS
Increase: toxicity—other antineoplastics, radiation
Increase: risk of bleeding—anticoagulants, salicylates

NURSING CONSIDERATIONS
Assess:
• Bleeding: hematuria, guaiac, bruising or petechiae, mucosa or orifices q8h
• Jaundice of skin, sclera, dark urine, clay-colored stools, itchy skin, abdominal pain, fever, diarrhea
• Dyspnea, crackles, unproductive cough, chest pain, tachypnea
• Effects of alopecia on body image; discuss feelings about body changes (rare)
• CBC, differential, platelet count weekly; withhold drug if WBC is <2000 or granulocyte count is <1000/mm³; notify prescriber of results
• Pulmonary function tests, chest x-ray films before, during therapy; chest film should be obtained q2wk during treatment
• Renal studies: BUN, serum uric acid, urine CCr before, during therapy; I&O ratio; report urine output of <30 ml/hr
• Monitor temp q4h (may indicate beginning infection)
• Hepatic studies before, during therapy (bilirubin, AST, ALT, LDH) as needed or monthly

Administer:
• All drugs PO if possible, avoid IM inj when platelets <100,000/mm³
• Allopurinol to maintain uric acid levels, alkalinization of urine; increase fluid intake to 2-3 L/day to prevent urate deposits, calculi formation

Perform/provide:
• Storage in tight container, amber glass, store in refrigerator

Evaluate:
• Therapeutic response: decreased size of tumor, spread of malignancy

Teach patient/family:
• To report signs of infection: increased temperature, sore throat, persistent cough, flulike symptoms
• To report signs of anemia: fatigue, headache, faintness, shortness of breath, irritability, seizures, jaundice, bruising
• To report bleeding; avoid use of razors, commercial mouthwash
• To avoid use of aspirin products, ibuprofen
• To avoid vaccinations during treatment
• To use contraception during and several months after completion of therapy; may cause irreversible gonadal suppression; avoid breastfeeding
• To report any changes in breathing or coughing
• To drink 2-3 L of fluid daily unless contraindicated; report drop in urine output

---

chloramphenicol (℞)
(klor-am-fen′i-kole)
chloramphenicol,
Chloromycetin,
Pentamycetin ✦
Func. class.: Antiinfective—
miscellaneous
Chem. class.: Dichloroacetic acid
derivative

Action: Binds to 50S ribosomal subunit, which interferes with or inhibits protein synthesis
Uses: Infections caused by *Haemophilus influenzae, Salmonella typhi, Rickettsia, Neisseria, Staphylococcus, Streptococcus, Escherichia coli* mycoplasma; not to be used if less toxic drugs can be used

DOSAGE AND ROUTES
• *Adult and child:* **IV** 50-75 mg/kg/day in divided doses q6h, 100 mg/kg/day (for meningitis only) max 4 g/day
• *Premature infants and neonates:* **IV** 25 mg/kg/day in divided doses q12-24h
Available forms: Inj 1 g

SIDE EFFECTS
CNS: Headache, *depression,* confusion, peripheral neuritis
CV: **Gray syndrome in newborns: failure to feed, pallor, cyanosis, abdominal distention, irregular respiration, vasomotor collapse**
EENT: Optic neuritis, blindness
GI: Nausea, vomiting, diarrhea, abdominal pain, xerostomia, glossitis, colitis, pruritus ani
HEMA: **Anemia, thrombocytopenia, aplastic anemia, granulocytopenia, leukopenia, acute generalized exanthematous pustulosis (AGEP) (rare)**
INTEG: Itching, urticaria, contact dermatitis, rash
Contraindications: Hypersensitivity, severe renal/hepatic disease, minor infections, labor
Precautions: Pregnancy (C), renal/hepatic disease, infants, children, bone marrow depression (drug-induced), lactation

PHARMACOKINETICS
IV: Peak 1-2 hr; duration 8 hr; half-life 1½-4 hr; conjugated in liver; excreted in urine (up to 15% as free drug, up to 80% in neonates), excreted in breast milk, feces; crosses placenta

INTERACTIONS
Increase: action of barbiturates, anticoagulants, hydantoins, iron products, antidiabetics
Decrease: action of vit B₁₂, folic acid, penicillins, rifampin
Drug/Herb
• Do not use acidophilus with antiinfectives; separate by several hours

NURSING CONSIDERATIONS
Assess:
• Signs of infection, anemia
⚠ Any patient with compromised renal system; drug is excreted slowly in poor renal system function; toxicity may occur rapidly
• Hepatic studies: AST, ALT

⚠ Safety alert   *"Tall Man" lettering

• Blood studies: WBC, RBC, Hct, Hgb, platelets, serum iron, reticulocytes; drug should be discontinued if bone marrow is depressed

• Renal studies: urinalysis, protein, blood, BUN, creatinine

• C&S before drug therapy; may be given as soon as culture is taken

• Drug level in impaired renal, hepatic systems; peak 15-20 mg/ml 3 hr after dose, trough 5-10 mg/ml prior to next dose

• Bowel pattern before, during treatment

• Skin eruptions, itching, dermatitis after administration

• Allergies before treatment, reaction of each medication

⚠ Neonates for beginning Gray syndrome: cyanosis, abdominal distention, irregular respiration, failure to feed; drug should be discontinued immediately

Administer:

• Drug must be taken in equal intervals around clock to maintain blood levels

• IM route not recommended

IV route

• After diluting 1 g/10 ml of sterile H$_2$O for inj or D$_5$W (10% sol); give >1 min; may be further diluted in 50-100 ml of D$_5$W; give through Y-tube, 3-way stopcock, or additive inf set; run over ½-1 hr

Additive compatibilities: Amikacin, aminophylline, ascorbic acid, calcium chloride or gluconate, cephalothin, cephapirin, colistimethate, corticotropin, cyanocobalamin, dimenhyDRINATE, DOPamine, epHEDrine, heparin, hydrocortisone, kanamycin, lidocaine, magnesium sulfate, metaraminol, methicillin, methyldopate, methylPREDNISolone, metronidazole, nafcillin, oxacillin, oxytocin, penicillin G potassium, penicillin G sodium, pentobarbital, phenylephrine, phytonadione, plasma protein fraction, potassium chloride, promazine, ranitidine, sodium bicarbonate, thiopental, verapamil, vit B/C

Syringe compatibilities: Ampicillin, cloxacillin, heparin, methicillin, penicillin G sodium

Y-site compatibilities: Acyclovir, cyclophosphamide, enalaprilat, esmolol, fos-

carnet, hydromorphone, labetalol, magnesium sulfate, meperidine, morphine, perphenazine, tacrolimus

Perform/provide:

• Reconstituted sol at room temperature 30 days

Evaluate:

• Therapeutic response: decreased symptoms of infection

Teach patient/family:

• All aspects of drug therapy: culture may be taken after complete course of medication

• To report sore throat, fever, fatigue, unusual bleeding, bruising; could indicate bone marrow depression (may occur weeks or months after termination of drug)

Treatment of hypersensitivity:

• Withdraw drug, maintain airway, administer epINEPHrine, aminophylline, O$_2$, IV corticosteroids

---

chloramphenicol ophthalmic
See Appendix C

---

chloramphenicol otic
See Appendix C

---

chlordiazepoxide (℞)
(klor-dye-az-e-pox'ide)
Apo-Chlordiazepoxide ✦,
chlordiazepoxide HCl ✦,
Libritabs, Librium,
Novo-Poxide ✦
Func. class.: Antianxiety
Chem. class.: Benzodiazepine

Controlled Substance Schedule IV
Do not confuse:
Librium/Librax
Action: Potentiates the actions of GABA, especially in the limbic system, reticular formation

---

Side effects: *italics* = common; **bold** = life-threatening

Uses: Short-term management of anxiety, acute alcohol withdrawal, preoperatively for relaxation

DOSAGE AND ROUTES
Mild anxiety
• *Adult:* PO 5-10 mg tid-qid
• *Geriatric:* PO 5 mg bid-qid initially, increase as needed
• *Child >6 yr:* PO 5 mg bid-qid, not to exceed 10 mg bid-tid
Severe anxiety
• *Adult:* PO 20-25 mg tid-qid; IM/IV 50-100 mg initially, then 25-50 mg tid or 25-50 mg initially in geriatrics
Preoperatively
• *Adult:* PO 5-10 mg tid-qid on day before surgery; IM 50-100 mg 1 hr before surgery
Alcohol withdrawal
• *Adult:* PO/IM/IV 50-100 mg, not to exceed 300 mg/day
Available forms: Caps 5, 10, 25 mg; inj 100 mg ampule

SIDE EFFECTS

CNS: Dizziness, drowsiness, confusion, headache, anxiety, tremors, stimulation, fatigue, depression, insomnia, hallucinations
CV: Orthostatic hypotension, **ECG changes, tachycardia,** hypotension
EENT: Blurred vision, tinnitus, mydriasis
GI: Constipation, dry mouth, nausea, vomiting, anorexia, diarrhea
INTEG: Rash, dermatitis, itching
Contraindications: Pregnancy (D), hypersensitivity to benzodiazepines, narrow-angle glaucoma, psychosis, lactation, child <6 yr
Precautions: Geriatric, debilitated, renal/hepatic disease

PHARMACOKINETICS

PO: Onset 30 min, peak within 2 hr, duration 4-6 hr; metabolized by liver, excreted by kidneys; crosses placenta, excreted in breast milk; half-life 5-30 hr (increased in geriatric)

INTERACTIONS
Increase: CNS depression—CNS depressants, alcohol
Increase: chlordiazepoxide—cimetidine, disulfiram, fluoxetine, isoniazid, ketoconazole, metoprolol, oral contraceptives, propranolol, valproic acid
Decrease: action of levodopa
Decrease: action of chlordiazepoxide—barbiturates, rifamycins
Drug/Herb
Decrease: effect—cowslip, kava, Queen Anne's lace, valerian
Drug/Lab Test
False increase: 17-OHCS
False positive: Pregnancy test (some methods)

NURSING CONSIDERATIONS
Assess:
• B/P (lying, standing), pulse; if systolic B/P drops 20 mm Hg, hold drug, notify prescriber
• Blood studies: CBC during long-term therapy; blood dyscrasias have occurred rarely
• Hepatic studies: AST, ALT, bilirubin, creatinine, LDH, alk phos during long-term therapy
• I&O; may indicate renal dysfunction
• For ataxia, oversedation in geriatric, debilitated patients
• Mental status: mood, sensorium, affect, sleeping pattern, drowsiness, dizziness
• Physical dependency, withdrawal symptoms: headache, nausea, vomiting, muscle pain, weakness after long-term use
• Suicidal tendencies, paradoxic reactions such as excitement, stimulation, acute rage
• For pregnancy; drug should be avoided during pregnancy
Administer:
PO route
• With food or milk for GI symptoms
• Crushed if patient is unable to swallow medication whole

GI: Nausea, vomiting, anorexia, diarrhea, cramps
HEMA: **Thrombocytopenia, agranulocytosis, hemolytic anemia, leukopenia**
INTEG: Pruritus, pigmentary changes, skin eruptions, lichen planus–like eruptions, eczema, **exfoliative dermatitis**
Contraindications: Hypersensitivity, retinal field changes
Precautions: Pregnancy (C), children, blood dyscrasias, severe GI disease, neurologic disease, alcoholism, hepatic disease, G6PD deficiency, psoriasis, eczema, lactation, seizures, preexisting auditory damage

PHARMACOKINETICS

Metabolized in liver; excreted in urine, feces, breast milk; crosses placenta
PO: Peak 1-3 hr, half-life 3-5 days
IM: Peak 30 min

INTERACTIONS

• Reduced oral clearance and metabolism of chloroquine: cimetidine
Decrease: action of chloroquine—magnesium, aluminum compounds, kaolin

NURSING CONSIDERATIONS
Assess:
• Ophthalmic test if long-term treatment or dosage >150 mg/day
• Hepatic studies qwk: AST, ALT, bilirubin
• Blood studies: CBC, since blood dyscrasias occur
• ECG during therapy; watch for depression of T waves, widening of QRS complex
• Allergic reactions: pruritus, rash, urticaria
• Blood dyscrasias: malaise, fever, bruising, bleeding (rare)
• For ototoxicity (tinnitus, vertigo, change in hearing); audiometric testing should be done before, after treatment

⚠ For toxicity: blurring vision; difficulty focusing; headache; dizziness; decreased knee, ankle reflexes, seizures, CV collapse; drug should be discontinued immediately and IV fluids given
Administer:
• Drug in mg or base; they are different
PO route
• Before or after meals at same time each day to maintain drug level
IM route
• IM after aspirating to avoid inj blood system, which may cause hypotension, asystole, heart block; rotate inj sites
Additive compatibilities: Promethazine
Perform/provide:
• Storage in tight, light-resistant container at room temperature; keep injection in cool environment
Evaluate:
• Therapeutic response: decreased symptoms of infection
Teach patient/family:
• To take with meals or immediately after meals
• To use sunglasses in bright sunlight to decrease photophobia
• That urine may turn rust or brown color
• To report hearing, visual problems, fever, fatigue, bruising, bleeding, which may indicate blood dyscrasias
Treatment of overdose: Induce vomiting, gastric lavage, administer barbiturate (ultrashort-acting), vasopressor; tracheostomy may be necessary

chlorothiazide (℞)
(klor-oh-thye′a-zide)
Diuril
Func. class.: Diuretic
Chem. class.: Thiazide; sulfonamide derivative

Do not confuse:
chlorothiazide/chlorproMAZINE/ chlorthalidone/chlorproPAMIDE
Action: Acts on distal tubule and thick ascending limb of the loop of Henle by

increasing excretion of water, sodium, chloride, potassium, magnesium

Uses: Hypertension, diuresis

DOSAGE AND ROUTES

Hypertension
• *Adult:* **PO/IV** 500 mg-2 g daily may divide bid

Edema
• *Adult:* **IV** 250 mg q6-12h
• *Child >6 mo:* **PO** 10-20 mg/kg/day may divide bid
• *Child <6 mo:* **PO** up to 40 mg/kg/day in 2 doses

Available forms: Tabs 250, 500 mg; powder for inj 500 mg; oral susp 250 mg/5 ml

SIDE EFFECTS

CNS: Paresthesia, headache, *dizziness, fatigue*
CV: Irregular pulse, orthostatic hypotension, volume depletion
EENT: Blurred vision
ELECT: Hypokalemia, hypercalcemia, hyponatremia, hypomagnesemia
GI: Nausea, vomiting, anorexia, constipation, diarrhea, pancreatitis, GI irritation, **hepatitis**
GU: Urinary frequency, polyuria
HEMA: **Aplastic anemia, hemolytic anemia, leukopenia, agranulocytosis, thrombocytopenia, neutropenia**
INTEG: Rash, urticaria, purpura, photosensitivity, fever, alopecia
META: Hyperglycemia, *hyperuricemia,* increased creatinine, BUN

Contraindications: Hypersensitivity to thiazides or sulfonamides, hepatic coma, anuria, renal decompensation, lactation

Precautions: Pregnancy (B), hypokalemia, renal/hepatic disease, gout, COPD, SLE, diabetes mellitus, geriatric, hyperlipidemia

PHARMACOKINETICS

Not well absorbed PO
PO: Onset 2 hr, peak 4 hr, duration 6-12 hr; crosses placenta, excreted in breast milk, excreted unchanged by kidneys; half-life 2 hr

INTERACTIONS

• Hypokalemia: ticarcillin, glucocorticoids, amphotericin, mezlocillin, piperacillin
Increase: toxicity—lithium, nondepolarizing skeletal muscle relaxants, digitalis, allopurinol
Increase: hypotension—other antihypertensives, alcohol, nitrates
Decrease: absorption of thiazides—cholestyramine, colestipol
Decrease: diuretic action—NSAIDs

Drug/Herb
• Hypokalemia: chronic use aloe, buckthorn, cascara sagrada, Chinese rhubarb, gossypol, licorice, nettle, senna
• Severe photosensitivity: St. John's wort
Increase: diuretic effect—aloe, cucumber, dandelion, horsetail, pumpkin, Queen Anne's lace

Drug/Lab Test
Increase: Ca, amylase, parathyroid test, CPK
Decrease: PBI
False negative: Phentolamine and tyramine tests
Interference: Urine steroid tests

NURSING CONSIDERATIONS

Assess:
• Weight, I&O daily to determine fluid loss; effect of drug may be decreased if used daily
• Rate, depth, rhythm of respirations; effect of exertion
• B/P lying, standing; postural hypotension may occur, especially in geriatric
• Electrolytes: K, Na, Cl; include BUN, blood glucose, CBC, serum creatinine, blood pH, ABGs, uric acid, Ca, Mg
• Glucose in urine if patient is diabetic
• Signs of metabolic alkalosis: drowsiness, restlessness
• Rashes, temp elevation daily
• Confusion, especially in geriatric; take safety precautions if needed

Administer:
• In AM to avoid interference with sleep if using drug as a diuretic

• Potassium replacement if potassium < 3 mg/dl

• With food if nausea occurs; absorption may be decreased slightly; dehydration may occur; tablets may be crushed

• After shaking suspension

IV route

• After diluting 0.5 g/18 ml or more of sterile water for inj; may be diluted further with 0.9% NaCl, D_5W, check for extravasation; give over 5 min (0.5 g/5 min)

Additive compatibilities: Cimetidine, lidocaine, nafcillin, ranitidine, sodium bicarbonate

Evaluate:

• Therapeutic response: improvement in edema of feet, legs, sacral area daily if medication is being used for CHF; decreased B/P; increased urinary output

Teach patient/family:

• To rise slowly from lying or sitting position; orthostatic hypotension may occur

• To notify prescriber of muscle weakness, cramps, nausea, dizziness

• That drug may be taken with food or milk; to take at same time each day; not to double dose

• That blood glucose may be increased in diabetics

• To take early in day to avoid nocturia

• To use sunscreen; use protective clothing to prevent photosensitivity

• To weigh weekly and notify prescriber of change of >3 lb

• To eat diet high in potassium if recommended by prescriber; teach high-potassium foods

• Not to take OTC medications without consulting prescriber

Treatment of overdose: Lavage if taken orally; monitor electrolytes; administer dextrose in saline; monitor hydration, CV, renal status

---

chlorpheniramine

(OTC, ℞)

(klor-fen-ir′a-meen)
Aller-Chlor, Allergy, Chlo-Amine, Chlorate, chlorpheniramine maleate, Chlor-Trimeton ♣, Chlor-Tripolon ♣, Novo-Pheniram ♣, PediaCare Allergy Formula, Phenetron, Teldrin, Telachlor

Func. class.: Antihistamine (1st generation, nonselective)
Chem. class.: Alkylamine, H_1-receptor antagonist

Do not confuse:
Teldrin/Tedral

Action: Acts on blood vessels, GI system, respiratory system, by competing with histamine for H_1-receptor site; decreases allergic response by blocking histamine

Uses: Allergy symptoms, rhinitis

DOSAGE AND ROUTES

• *Adult and child ≥12 yr:* **PO** 2-4 mg tid-qid, not to exceed 24 mg/day; **TIME-REL** 8-12 mg bid-tid, not to exceed 24 mg/day; **IM/IV/SUBCUT** 5-40 mg/day, max 40 mg/day

• *Child 6-12 yr:* **PO** 2 mg q4-6h, not to exceed 12 mg/day; **SUS REL** 8 mg bedtime or daily, **SUS REL** not recommended for child <6 yr; **SUBCUT** 87.5 mcg/kg or 2.5 mg/m² q6h

• *Child 2-5 yr:* **PO** 1 mg q4-6h, not to exceed 4 mg/day

Available forms: Chewable tabs 2 mg; tabs 4, 8, 12 mg; ext rel tabs 8, 12 mg; ext rel caps 8, 12 mg; syr 1 mg/5 ml, 2 mg/5 ml, 2.5 mg/5 ml; inj 10, 100 mg/ml

SIDE EFFECTS

CNS: Dizziness, drowsiness, poor coordination, fatigue, anxiety, euphoria, confusion, paresthesia, neuritis
EENT: Blurred vision, dilated pupils, tinni-

---

tus, nasal stuffiness, dry nose, throat, mouth
GI: Nausea, anorexia, diarrhea
GU: Retention, dysuria, urinary frequency
HEMA: **Thrombocytopenia, agranulocytosis, hemolytic anemia**
INTEG: Photosensitivity
RESP: Increased thick secretions, wheezing, chest tightness
Contraindications: Hypersensitivity to H₁-receptor antagonists, acute asthma attack, lower respiratory tract disease, stenosed peptic ulcers, bladder neck obstruction, angle-closure glaucoma, newborns/neonates
Precautions: Pregnancy (B), increased intraocular pressure, renal/cardiac disease, hypertension, bronchial asthma, seizure disorder, hyperthyroidism, prostatic hypertrophy, lactation, geriatric

PHARMACOKINETICS

PO: Onset ½ hr, duration 4-12 hr
PO-ER: Duration 8-24 hr
SUBCUT/IM/IV: duration 4-12 hr; detoxified in liver; excreted by kidneys (metabolites/free drug); half-life 12-15 hr

INTERACTIONS

Increase: CNS depression—barbiturates, opiates, hypnotics, tricyclics, alcohol
Increase: effect of chlorpheniramine—MAOIs
Increase: anticholinergic action—atropine, phenothiazines, quinidine, haloperidol
Drug/Herb
Increase: effect—hops, Jamaican dogwood, kava, khat, senega
Increase: anticholinergic effect—corkwood, henbane leaf
Drug/Lab Test
False negative: Skin allergy tests

NURSING CONSIDERATIONS
Assess:
• Be alert for urinary retention, frequency, dysuria; drug should be discontinued
• Respiratory status: rate, rhythm, in-

crease in bronchial secretions, wheezing, chest tightness
Administer:
• Avoid concurrent use with other CNS depressants
PO route
• Do not break, crush, or chew ext rel forms
• With meals for GI symptoms; absorption may slightly decrease
IV route
• Undiluted at ≥10 mg/1 min
• Use only 10 mg/ml form for IV use
Perform/provide:
• Hard candy, gum, frequent rinsing of mouth for dryness
• Storage in tight container at room temperature
Evaluate:
• Therapeutic response: absence of running, congested nose, rashes
Teach patient/family:
• All aspects of drug use; to notify prescriber of confusion/sedation/hypotension, difficulty voiding
• To avoid driving, other hazardous activity if drowsiness occurs, especially geriatric
• To avoid concurrent use of alcohol
Treatment of overdose: Administer diazepam, vasopressors, barbiturates (short-acting)

---

*chlorproMAZINE (℞)
(klor-proe'ma-zeen)
Chlorpromanyl ✤,
chlorproMAZINE HCl,
Largactil ✤, Novo-
Chlorpromazine ✤,
Thorazine, Thor-Prom
Func. class.: Antipsychotic/antiemetic
Chem. class.: Phenothiazine-aliphatic

Do not confuse:
chlorproMAZINE/chlorproPAMIDE/prochlorperazine
Action: Depresses cerebral cortex, hy-

pothalamus, limbic system, which control activity aggression; blocks neurotransmission produced by dopamine at synapse; exhibits a strong α-adrenergic, anticholinergic blocking action; mechanism for antipsychotic effects is unclear

Uses: Psychotic disorders, mania, schizophrenia, anxiety, intractable hiccups in adults, nausea, vomiting; preoperatively for relaxation; acute intermittent porphyria, behavioral problems in children, nonpsychotic, demented patients, Tourette's syndrome

Unlabeled uses: Vascular headache

DOSAGE AND ROUTES

Psychosis
• *Adult:* **PO** 10-50 mg q1-4h initially, then increase up to 2 g/day if necessary; **IM** 10-50 mg q1-4h, usual dose 300-800 mg/day
• *Geriatric:* 10-25 mg daily-bid, increase by 10-25 mg/day q4-7 days, max 800 mg/day
• *Child >6 mo:* **PO** 0.5 mg/kg q4-6h; **IM** 0.5 mg/kg q6-8h; **RECT** 1 mg/kg q6-8h

Nausea and vomiting
• *Adult:* **PO** 10-25 mg q4-6h prn; **IM** 25-50 mg q3h prn; **RECT** 50-100 mg q6-8h prn, not to exceed 400 mg/day; **IV** 25-50 mg daily-qid
• *Child ≥6 mo:* **PO** 0.55 mg/kg q4-6h; **IM** q6-8h; **RECT** 1.1 mg/kg q6-8h; max **IM** ≤5 yr or ≤22.7 kg, 40 mg; max **IM** 5-10 yr or 22.7-45.5 kg, 75 mg

Intractable hiccups
• *Adult:* **PO** 25-50 mg tid-qid; **IM** 25-50 mg (only if PO dose does not work); **IV** 25-50 mg in 500-1000 ml **NS** (only for severe hiccups)

Available forms: Tabs 10, 25, 50, 100, 200 mg; sus rel caps 30, 75, 150, 200, 300 mg; syr 10, 25, 100 mg/5 ml; conc 30, 40, 100 mg/ml; supp 25, 100 mg; inj 25 mg/ml

SIDE EFFECTS

CNS: EPS: pseudoparkinsonism, akathisia, dystonia, tardive dyskinesia, seizures, *headache,* **neuroleptic malignant syndrome,** dizziness

CV: Orthostatic hypotension, hypertension, **cardiac arrest,** ECG changes, **tachycardia**

EENT: Blurred vision, glaucoma, dry eyes

GI: Dry mouth, nausea, vomiting, anorexia, constipation, diarrhea, jaundice, weight gain

GU: Urinary retention, enuresis, impotence, amenorrhea, gynecomastia, breast engorgement

HEMA: Anemia, **leukopenia, leukocytosis, agranulocytosis**

INTEG: Rash, photosensitivity, dermatitis

RESP: **Laryngospasm,** dyspnea, **respiratory depression**

Contraindications: Hypersensitivity, circulatory collapse, liver damage, cerebral arteriosclerosis, coronary disease, severe hyper/hypotension, blood dyscrasias, coma, child <6 mo, brain damage, bone marrow depression, alcohol/ barbiturate withdrawal, narrow-angle glaucoma

Precautions: Pregnancy (C), lactation, seizure disorders, hypertension, hepatic/cardiac disease, geriatric, prostatic enlargement

PHARMACOKINETICS

PO: Absorption variable, widely distributed; onset erratic 30-60 min, duration 4-6 hr

PO-ER: Onset 30-60 min, peak unknown, duration 10-12 hr

REC: Onset erratic, duration 3 hr

IM: Well absorbed; peak 15-20 min, duration 4-8 hr

IV: Onset 5 min, peak 10 min, duration unknown

Metabolized by liver, excreted in urine (metabolites), crosses placenta, enters breast milk; 95% bound to plasma proteins; elimination half-life 10-30 hr

INTERACTIONS

Increase: other CNS depressants, alcohol, barbiturate anesthetics, antihistamines, sedatives/hypnotics, antidepressants

Increase: toxicity—epINEPHrine

Increase: agranulocystosis—antithyroid agents

Increase: effects of both drugs—β-adrenergic blockers, alcohol

Increase: anticholinergic effects—anticholinergics, antidepressants, antiparkinsonian agents

Increase: valproic acid level

Decrease: lowered seizure threshold—anticonvulsants

Decrease: absorption—aluminum hydroxide, magnesium hydroxide antacids

Decrease: antiparkinson activity—levodopa, bromocriptine

Decrease: serum chlorproMAZINE—lithium, barbiturates

Decrease: anticoagulant effect—warfarin

Drug/Herb

Increase: action—cola tree, hops, nettle, nutmeg

Increase: anticholinergic effect—henbane leaf

Increase: EPS—betel palm, kava

Drug/Lab Test

Increase: Hepatic studies, cardiac enzymes, cholesterol, blood glucose, prolactin, bilirubin, PBI, cholinesterase,^{131}I, alk phos, leukocytes, granulocytes, platelets

Decrease: Hormones (blood and urine)

False positive: Pregnancy tests, PKU

False negative: Urinary steroids, 17-OHCS

NURSING CONSIDERATIONS

Assess:

• Mental status: orientation, mood, behavior, presence and type of hallucinations before initial administration and monthly

• Any potentially reversible causes of behavior problems in the geriatric before and during therapy

• Swallowing of PO medication; check for hoarding or giving of medication to other patients

• I&O ratio; palpate bladder if low urinary output occurs, especially in geriatric

• Bilirubin, CBC, LFTs, ocular exam; agranulocytosis may occur, monthly

• Urinalysis recommended before, during prolonged therapy

• Affect, orientation, LOC, reflexes, gait, coordination, sleep pattern disturbances

• B/P sitting, standing, lying; take pulse and respirations q4h during initial treatment; establish baseline before starting treatment; report drops of 30 mm Hg; obtain baseline ECG, Q-wave and T-wave changes

• Dizziness, faintness, palpitations, tachycardia on rising

A For neuroleptic malignant syndrome: hyperpyrexia, muscle rigidity, increased CPK, altered mental status, for acute dystonia (check chewing, swallowing, eyes, pill rolling)

• EPS including akathisia (inability to sit still, no pattern to movements), tardive dyskinesia (bizarre movements of the jaw, mouth, tongue, extremities), pseudoparkinsonism (rigidity, tremors, pill rolling, shuffling gait)

• Skin turgor daily

• Constipation, urinary retention daily; increase bulk, H_2O in diet

Administer:

• IM, inject in deep muscle mass, do not give SUBCUT

• Rectal after placing in refrigerator for ½ hr if too soft to insert

• Antiparkinsonian agent for EPS if ordered

PO route

• Do not break, crush, or chew ext rel caps

• With full glass of water, milk; or with food to decrease GI upset

• Drug in liquid form mixed in glass of juice or cola if hoarding is suspected

• Periodically attempt dosage reduction in behavioral problems

• Avoid use with CNS depressants

IV route

• After diluting 1 mg/1 ml with NS, give 1 mg or less/2 min or more; may be further diluted in 500-1000 ml of NS

Additive compatibilities: Ascorbic acid, ethacrynate, netilmicin, theophylline, vit B/C

Syringe compatibilities: Atropine, benztropine, butorphanol, diphenhydrAMINE, doxapram, droperidol, fentanyl, glycopyrrolate, hydromorphone, hydrOXYzine, meperidine, metoclopramide, midazolam, morphine, pentazocine, perphenazine, prochlorperazine, promazine, promethazine, scopolamine

Y-site compatibilities: Amsacrine, cisatracurium, cisplatin, cladribine, cyclophosphamide, cytarabine, DOXOrubicin, DOXOrubicin liposome, famotidine, filgrastim, fluconazole, granisetron, heparin, hydrocortisone, ondansetron, potassium chloride, propofol, teniposide, thiotepa, vinorelbine, vit B/C

Perform/provide:
• Supervised ambulation until stabilized on medication; do not involve in strenuous exercise program because fainting is possible; patient should not stand still for long periods
• Increased fluids and roughage to prevent constipation
• Candy, gum, sips of water for dry mouth
• Storage in tight, light-resistant container, oral sol in amber bottle

Evaluate:
• Therapeutic response: decrease in emotional excitement, hallucinations, delusions, paranoia, reorganization of patterns of thought, speech, increase in target behaviors

Teach patient/family:
• To use good oral hygiene; frequent rinsing of mouth, sugarless gum, candy, ice chips for dry mouth
• To avoid hazardous activities until drug response is determined
• That orthostatic hypotension occurs often and to rise gradually from sitting or lying position
• To remain lying down for at least 30 min after IM inj
• To avoid hot tubs, hot showers, tub baths, since hypotension may occur; that in hot weather, heat stroke may occur; take extra precautions to stay cool
• To avoid abrupt withdrawal of this drug or EPS may result; drug should be withdrawn slowly
• To avoid OTC preparations (cough, hay fever, cold) unless approved by prescriber, since serious drug interactions may occur; avoid use with alcohol, increased drowsiness may occur
• To use a sunscreen and sunglasses to prevent burns
• To take antacids 2 hr before or after this drug
• To report sore throat, malaise, fever, bleeding, mouth sores; CBC should be drawn and drug discontinued
• Contraceptive measures
• That urine may turn pink or reddish-brown

Treatment of overdose: Lavage if orally ingested; provide airway; *do not induce vomiting or use epINEPHrine*

Rarely Used

*chlorproPAMIDE (R)
(klor-proe′pa-mide)
Chloronase ✚
ChlorproPAMIDE, Diabinese, Novopropamide ✚
Functional class.: Antidiabetic
Uses: Type 2, non–insulin-dependent diabetes mellitus

Uses: Type 2 diabetes mellitus

DOSAGE AND ROUTES
• *Adult:* **PO** 100-250 mg daily, initially, then 100-500 mg maintenance according to response; not to exceed 750 mg/day

Contraindications: Pregnancy (D), hypersensitivity to sulfonylureas, juvenile or brittle diabetes, lactation, renal failure

chlorthalidone (℞)

(klor-thal'i-done)
Apo-Chlorthalidone ✦,
chlorthalidone, Hygroton,
Thalitone, Uridon ✦
Func. class.: Diuretic
Chem. class.: Thiazide-like phthali-
midine derivative

Do not confuse:
Uridon/Vicodin
Hygroton/Regroton
Action: Acts on distal tubule and by
blocking the reabsorption of sodium and
chloride resulting in increasing excretion
of water, sodium, chloride, potassium,
magnesium, bicarbonate, possible arteriolar dilation
Uses: Edema, hypertension, edema in
CHF

DOSAGE AND ROUTES

Hypertension
• *Adult:* **PO** 25-100 mg/day or 100 mg
3×/wk
Edema
• *Adult:* **PO** 50-100 mg/day or 100 mg
or alternate day, max 200 mg /day
• *Geriatric:* **PO** 12.5-25 mg/day or ev-
ery other day
Available forms: Tabs 25, 50, 100 mg

SIDE EFFECTS

CNS: Paresthesia, headache, *dizziness,*
weakness
CV: Hypertension, orthostatic hypotension,
palpitations, volume depletion
EENT: Blurred vision
ELECT: Hypokalemia, hypomagnesemia,
hypercalcemia, hyponatremia, hypochloremia
GI: Nausea, vomiting, anorexia, constipation, diarrhea, pancreatitis, GI irritation
GU: Urinary frequency, polyuria, **uremia,** glucosuria, impotence
HEMA: **Aplastic anemia, hemolytic anemia, leukopenia, agranulocytosis,
thrombocytopenia, neutropenia**

INTEG: Rash, urticaria, purpura, photosensitivity, fever
META: Hyperglycemia, hyperuremia, increased creatinine, BUN, gout
Contraindications: Hypersensitivity to
thiazides or sulfonamides, anuria, renal
decompensation, lactation
Precautions: Pregnancy (B), hypokalemia, renal/hepatic disease, gout, diabetes
mellitus, geriatric, hyperlipidemia, SLE,
hypotension

PHARMACOKINETICS

PO: Onset 2 hr, peak 6 hr, duration
24-72 hr; excreted unchanged by kidneys; crosses placenta; enters breast
milk; half-life 40 hr

INTERACTIONS

Increase: hyperglycemia, hypotension—
diazoxide
Increase: hypokalemia—glucocorti-
coids, amphotericin B
Increase: toxicity of lithium, nondepolar-
izing skeletal muscle relaxants, allopuri-
nol
Increase: hypotensive effect—alcohol
Decrease: absorption of thiazides—
cholestyramine, colestipol
Drug/Herb
• Potassium deficiency: chronic use of
buckthorn, cascara sagrada, Chinese rhu-
barb, gossypol, licorice, nettle, senna
Increase: severe photosensitivity—St.
John's wort
Increase: hypotension—cucumber, dan-
delion, khella, horsetail, pumpkin, Queen
Anne's lace
Drug/Lab Test
Increase: Amylase, bilirubin, calcium,
cholesterol, creatinine, low-density lipo-
proteins, serum/urine glucose (diabet-
ics), triglycerides, uric acid
Decrease: PBI, parathyroid test, magne-
sium, potassium, sodium, urinary calcium

NURSING CONSIDERATIONS

Assess:

• Weight, I&O daily to determine fluid loss; effect of drug may be decreased if used daily

• Rate, depth, rhythm of respiration, effect of exertion, B/P lying, standing; postural hypotension may occur

• Electrolytes: K, Mg, Na, Cl; include BUN, blood glucose, CBC, serum creatinine, blood pH, ABGs, uric acid, Ca

• Blood glucose levels if patient is diabetic

• Signs of metabolic alkalosis: drowsiness, restlessness

• Signs of hypokalemia: postural hypotension, malaise, fatigue, tachycardia, leg cramps, weakness

• Rashes, temp elevation daily

• Confusion, especially in geriatric; take safety precautions if needed

Administer:

• In AM to avoid interference with sleep if using drug as a diuretic

• Potassium replacement if potassium less than 3 mg/dl

• With food if nausea occurs; absorption may be decreased slightly

Evaluate:

• Therapeutic response: improvement in edema of feet, legs, sacral area daily if medication used in CHF

Teach patient/family:

• To rise slowly from lying or sitting position

• To notify prescriber of muscle weakness, cramps, nausea, dizziness

• That drug may be taken with food or milk

• To maintain adequate potassium intake

• That blood glucose may be increased in diabetics

• To use sunscreen to protect against photosensitivity

• To take early in day to avoid nocturia

Treatment of overdose: Lavage if taken orally, monitor electrolytes, administer dextrose in NS, monitor hydration, CV, renal status

---

chlorzoxazone (℞)

(klor-zox′a-zone)
EZE-DS, chlorzoxazone, Paraflex, Parafon Forte DSC, Relaxazone, Remular, Remular-S, Strifon Forte DSC
Func. class.: Skeletal muscle relaxant, central acting
Chem. class.: Benzoxazole derivative

Do not confuse:

Parafon Forte DSC/Fam-Pren Forte

Action: Inhibits multisynaptic reflex arcs causing skeletal muscle relaxation

Uses: Relieving pain, spasm in musculoskeletal conditions

DOSAGE AND ROUTES

• *Adult:* **PO** 250-750 mg tid-qid

• *Child:* **PO** 20 mg/kg/day in divided doses bid-tid

Available forms: Tabs 250, 500 mg

SIDE EFFECTS

CNS: Dizziness, drowsiness, headache, insomnia, stimulation, malaise

GI: Nausea, vomiting, anorexia, diarrhea, constipation, **GI bleeding, hepatotoxicity**

GU: Urine discoloration

HEMA: **Granulocytopenia, anemia**

INTEG: Rash, pruritus, petechiae, ecchymoses, **angioedema**

SYST: **Anaphylaxis, angioedema**

Contraindications: Hypersensitivity, impaired hepatic function

Precautions: Pregnancy (unknown), lactation, hepatic disease, geriatric

PHARMACOKINETICS

PO: Onset 1 hr, peak 1-2 hr, duration 3-4 hr, half-life 1 hr; metabolized in liver; excreted in urine (metabolites)

INTERACTIONS

Increase: CNS depression—alcohol, tricyclics, opiates, barbiturates, sedatives, hypnotics

---

⚠ Safety alert   *"Tall Man" lettering

Drug/Herb
• May increase CNS depression—kava

NURSING CONSIDERATIONS
Assess:
• Blood studies: CBC, WBC, differential for blood dyscrasias if on long-term therapy
• Allergic reactions: rash, fever, respiratory distress
• CNS depression: dizziness, drowsiness, psychiatric symptoms
• For angioedema, anaphylaxis
Administer:
• With meals for GI symptoms
Perform/provide:
• Storage in tight container at room temperature
Evaluate:
• Therapeutic response: decreased pain, spasticity
Teach patient/family:
• Not to discontinue abruptly; insomnia, nausea, headache, spasticity, tachycardia will occur; drug should be tapered over 1-2 wk
• To notify prescriber if fever, rash, anorexia, RUQ pain, dark urine, or jaundice occur
• Not to take with alcohol, other CNS depressants; take with food
• To avoid hazardous activities if drowsiness, dizziness occurs
• To avoid using OTC medication: cough preparations, antihistamines, unless directed by prescriber
• That urine may be orange or purple
Treatment of overdose: Gastric lavage or induce emesis, then administer activated charcoal; use other supportive treatment as necessary; monitor cardiac function

---

cholestyramine (R)
(koe-less-tir′a-meen)
LoCHOLEST, LoCHOLEST
Light, Prevalite, Questran,
Questran Light
Func. class.: Antilipemic
Chem. class.: Bile acid sequestrant

Action: Absorbs, combines with bile acids to form insoluble complex that is excreted through feces; loss of bile acids lowers cholesterol levels
Uses: Primary hypercholesterolemia, pruritus associated with biliary obstruction
Unlabeled uses: Diarrhea caused by excess bile acid

DOSAGE AND ROUTES
• *Adult:* **PO** 4 g daily or bid, max 24 g/day
• *Child:* **PO** 240 mg/kg/day in 3 divided doses with food or drink, max 8 g/day
Available forms: Powder for susp 4 g cholestyramine/packet or scoop; tab 1 g

SIDE EFFECTS
CNS: Headache, dizziness, drowsiness, vertigo, tinnitus, anxiety
GI: Constipation, abdominal pain, nausea, fecal impaction, hemorrhoids, flatulence, vomiting, steatorrhea, peptic ulcer
HEMA: **Bleeding,** increased PT
INTEG: Rash, irritation of perianal area, tongue, skin
META: Decreased vit A, D, K, red cell folate content; **hyperchloremic acidosis**
MS: Muscle, joint pain
Contraindications: Hypersensitivity; biliary obstruction; hyperlipidemia III, IV, V
Precautions: Pregnancy (C), lactation, children

PHARMACOKINETICS
PO: Excreted in feces, LDL lowered in 4-7 days, serum cholesterol lowered in 1 mo

---

Side effects: *italics* = common; **bold** = life-threatening

INTERACTIONS

Decrease: absorption of warfarin, thiazides, cardiac glycosides, propranolol, corticosteroids, iron, thyroid hormones, fat-soluble vitamins, clindamycin, acetaminophen, amiodarone, penicillin G, tetracyclines, clofibrate, gemfibrozil, glipiZIDE, phenytoin, vit A, D, E, K

Drug/Herb
Increase: effect—glucomannan
Decrease: gotu kola

Drug/Lab Test
Increase: AST, ALT, alk phos
Decrease: Sodium, potassium
Interfere: Cholecystography

NURSING CONSIDERATIONS

Assess:
• Cardiac glycoside level, if both drugs are being administered
• For signs of vit A, D, K deficiency
• Fasting LDL, HDL, total cholesterol, triglyceride levels, electrolytes if on extended therapy
• Bowel pattern daily; increase bulk, H_2O in diet for constipation

Administer:
• Drug daily or bid; give all other medications 1 hr before cholestyramine or 4-6 hr after cholestyramine to avoid poor absorption
• Drug mixed with applesauce or stirred into beverage (2-6 oz); let stand for 2 min; do not take dry, avoid inhaling powder
• Supplemental doses of vit A, D, K, if levels are low

Evaluate:
• Therapeutic response: decreased cholesterol level (hyperlipidemia); diarrhea, pruritus (excess bile acids)

Teach patient/family:
⚠ The symptoms of hypoprothrombinemia: bleeding mucous membranes, dark tarry stools, hematuria, petechiae; report immediately
• The importance of compliance
• That risk factors should be decreased: high-fat diet, smoking, alcohol consumption, absence of exercise

• That GI side effects will resolve with continued use

---

choline salicylate (℞)
(koe′leen sa-liss′ih-late)
Arthropan
choline/magnesium salicylates
CMT, Tricosal, Trilisate
Func. class.: Nonopioid analgesic
Chem. class.: Salicylate

Action: Blocks pain impulses in CNS that occur in response to inhibition of prostaglandin synthesis; antipyretic action results from inhibition of hypothalamic heat-regulating center to produce vasodilation to allow heat dissipation

Uses: Mild to moderate pain or fever including arthritis, juvenile rheumatoid arthritis

DOSAGE AND ROUTES
435 mg of choline salicylate is = 325 mg of aspirin

Choline salicylate
• *Adult and child >12 yr:* **PO** 870-1740 mg qid; max 6×/day

Pain/fever
• *Adult:* **PO** 435-870 mg q3-4h prn

Choline/magnesium salicylates
• *Adult:* **PO** 2-3 g salicylate/day divided bid-tid
• *Child >37 kg:* **PO** 2.2 g of salicylate/day divided bid
• *Child <37 kg:* **PO** 50 mg of salicylate/kg/day divided bid

Available forms: *Choline salicylate:* liq 870 mg/5 ml; *choline/magnesium salicylate:* tabs 500, 750, 1000 mg; liq 500 mg/5 ml

SIDE EFFECTS

CNS: Stimulation, drowsiness, dizziness, confusion, **seizures**, headache, flushing, hallucinations, **coma**
CV: Rapid pulse, pulmonary edema
EENT: Tinnitus, hearing loss

ENDO: Hypoglycemia, hyponatremia, hypokalemia
GI: Nausea, vomiting, GI bleeding, diarrhea, heartburn, anorexia, **hepatitis, hepatotoxicity**
HEMA: **Thrombocytopenia, agranulocytosis, leukopenia, neutropenia, hemolytic anemia,** increased PT
INTEG: Rash, urticaria, bruising, sweating
RESP: Wheezing, hyperpnea, hyperventilation

Contraindications: Hypersensitivity to salicylates, GI bleeding, bleeding disorders, children <3 yr, vit K deficiency, children with flulike symptoms
Precautions: Pregnancy (C), anemia, renal/hepatic disease, Hodgkin's disease, lactation

PHARMACOKINETICS

Absorbed via GI tract, onset 15-30 min; metabolized by liver; crosses placenta; excreted in breast milk, by kidneys, half-life 2-3 hr, large doses 15-30 hr

INTERACTIONS

Increase: gastric ulcer—steroids, antiinflammatories, NSAIDs
Increase: bleeding—alcohol, aspirin, heparin, plicamycin
Increase: effects of warfarin, insulin, methotrexate, thrombolytic agents, penicillins, phenytoin, valproic acid, oral hypoglycemics, sulfonamides
Increase: salicylate levels—urinary acidifiers, ammonium chloride, nizatidine
Decrease: effects of aspirin—antacids (high doses), steroids, urinary alkalizers, corticosteroids
Decrease: effects of probenecid, spironolactone, sulfinpyrazone, sulfonylamides, NSAIDs, β-blockers
Drug/Herb
Increase: bleeding risk—bilberry, bogbean, chondroitin, horse chestnut, Irish moss, kelpware, pansy
Drug/Lab Test
Increase: Coagulation studies, LFTs, serum uric acid, amylase, CO_2, urinary protein

Decrease: Serum K, cholesterol
Interference: VMA, TSH, 5-HIAA

NURSING CONSIDERATIONS
Assess:
• Pain: location, intensity, character baseline and 1-2 hr after dose
• Hepatic studies: AST, ALT, bilirubin, creatinine (long-term therapy)
• Renal studies: BUN, urine creatinine (long-term therapy)
• Blood studies: CBC, Hct, Hgb, PT (long-term therapy)
• I&O ratio; decreasing output may indicate renal failure (long-term therapy)
⚠ Hepatotoxicity: dark urine; clay-colored stools; yellowing of skin, sclera; itching; abdominal pain; fever; diarrhea (long-term therapy)
• Allergic reactions: rash, urticaria; drug may have to be discontinued
• Renal dysfunction: decreased urine output
• Ototoxicity: tinnitus, ringing, roaring in ears; audiometric testing needed before, after long-term therapy
• Visual changes: blurring, halos, corneal, retinal damage
• Edema in feet, ankles, legs
• Drug history; many interactions
Administer:
• Mixed with fruit juice, carbonated beverage, water
Evaluate:
• Therapeutic response: decreased pain, fever, stiffness of joints
Teach patient/family:
• To report any symptoms of hepatotoxicity, renal toxicity, visual changes, ototoxicity, allergic reactions, bleeding (long-term therapy)
• Not to exceed recommended dosage; acute poisoning may result
• To read label on other OTC drugs; many contain aspirin
• That therapeutic response takes 2 wk (arthritis)
• To avoid alcohol ingestion; GI bleeding may occur
• That if anticoagulants are given with this

---

drug, this drug should be decreased 2 wk before surgery

Treatment of overdose: Lavage, activated charcoal, monitor electrolytes, VS

---

cidofovir (℞)
(si-doh-foh'veer)
Vistide
Func. class.: Antiviral
Chem. class.: Nucleotide analog

Action: Suppresses cytomegalovirus (CMV) replication by selective inhibition of viral DNA synthesis

Uses: CMV retinitis in patients with HIV, used with probenecid

DOSAGE AND ROUTES

• *Adult:* IV 5 mg/kg qwk ×2 wk, then 5 mg/kg q2wk, give with probenecid
Renal dose
• *Adult:* IV CCr <50 ml/min reduce dose
Available forms: Inj 75 mg/ml

SIDE EFFECTS

CNS: Fever, chills, **coma,** confusion, abnormal thought, *dizziness,* bizarre dreams, *headache,* psychosis, tremors, somnolence, paresthesia, *amnesia, anxiety, insomnia,* **seizures**
CV: Dysrhythmias, hypertension/hypotension
EENT: Retinal detachment in CMV retinitis
GI: Abnormal LFTs, *nausea, vomiting, anorexia, diarrhea,* abdominal pain, **hemorrhage**
GU: **Hematuria,** increased creatinine, BUN, **nephrotoxicity**
HEMA: **Granulocytopenia, thrombocytopenia, irreversible neutropenia, anemia, eosinophilia**
INTEG: Rash, alopecia, pruritus, acne, urticaria, pain at inj site, phlebitis
RESP: Dyspnea
Contraindications: Hypersensitivity to this drug or probenecid, sulfa drugs
Precautions: Pregnancy (C), preexisting cytopenias, renal function impairment,

lactation, children <6 mo, geriatric, platelet count <25,000/mm^3

PHARMACOKINETICS

Unknown

INTERACTIONS

• Nephrotoxicity: amphotericin B, foscarnet, aminoglycosides, pentamidine IV, NSAIDs, wait 7 days after use to begin cidofovir

NURSING CONSIDERATIONS

Assess:
• Culture before treatment is initiated; cultures of blood, urine, and throat may all be taken; CMV is not confirmed by this method; the diagnosis is made by an ophthalmic exam
• Renal, hepatic, increased hemopoietic studies and BUN; serum creatinine, AST, ALT, creatinine, CCr, A-G ratio, baseline and drip treatment, blood counts should be done q2wk; watch for decreasing granulocytes, Hgb; if low, therapy may have to be discontinued and restarted after hematologic recovery; blood transfusions may be required
• For GI symptoms: severe nausea, vomiting, diarrhea; severe symptoms may necessitate discontinuing drug
• Electrolytes and minerals: calcium, phosphorus, magnesium, sodium, potassium; watch closely for tetany during first administration
• For symptoms of blood dyscrasias (anemia, granulocytopenia); bruising, fatigue, bleeding, poor healing
• Allergic reactions: flushing, rash, urticaria, pruritus
• For leukopenia, neutropenia, thrombocytopenia: WBCs, platelets q2d during 2×/day dosing and qwk thereafter; check for leukopenias, with daily WBC count in patients with prior leukopenia, with other nucleoside analogs, or for whom leuko-

---

⚠ Safety alert   *"Tall Man" lettering

penia counts are <1000 cells/mm³ at start of treatment

• Monitor serum creatinine or CCr at least q2wk; give only to those with creatinine levels ≤1.5 mg/dl, CCr >55 ml/min, urine protein <100 mg/dl

Administer:

IV INF route

• Dilute in 100 ml 0.9% saline sol before administration; probenecid must be given PO 2 g 3 hr prior to the cidofovir infusion and 1 g at 2 and 8 hr after ending the cidofovir infusion; give 1 L of 0.9% saline sol IV with each INF of cidofovir, give saline INF over 1-2 hr period immediately prior to cidofovir; patient should be given a 2nd L if the patient can tolerate the fluid load (2nd L given at time of cidofovir or immediately afterward and should be given over a 1-3 hr period)

• Mix under strict aseptic conditions using gloves, gown, and mask, and using precautions for antineoplastic

• Slowly; do not give by bolus IV, SUBCUT inj

• Use diluted sol within 12 hr, do not refrigerate or freeze; do not use sol with particulate matter or discoloration

• Refrigerate up to 24 hr, allow to warm to room temperature before using

Evaluate:

• Therapeutic response: decreased symptoms of CMV

Teach patient/family:

• To notify prescriber if sore throat, swollen lymph nodes, malaise, fever occur; may indicate other infections

• To report perioral tingling, numbness in extremities, and paresthesias

• That serious drug interactions may occur if OTC products are ingested; check first with prescriber

• That drug is not a cure, but will control symptoms

• That regular ophthalmic exams must be continued

• That major toxicities may necessitate discontinuing drug

• To use contraception during treatment and that infertility may occur; men should use barrier contraception for 90 days after treatment

Treatment of overdose: Discontinue drug; use hemodialysis, and increase hydration

---

cilostazol (℞)

(sih-los′tah-zol)

Pletal

Func. class.: Platelet aggregation inhibitor

Chem. class.: Quinolinone derivative

Do not confuse:

Pletal/Plendil

Action: Reversibly inhibits cellular phosphodiesterase; inhibits platelet aggregation induced by thrombin, ADP, collagen, arachidonic acid, epINEPHrine, stress

Uses: Intermittent claudication

DOSAGE AND ROUTES

• *Adult:* **PO** 100 mg bid taken ≥30 min ac or 2 hr pc breakfast and dinner or 50 mg bid if using drugs that inhibit CYP3A4 and CYP2C19; 12 wk of treatment may be needed for beneficial effect

Available forms: Tabs 50, 100 mg

SIDE EFFECTS

CNS: Dizziness, headache

CV: Palpitations, tachycardia, nodal dysrhythmia, postural hypotension

EENT: Blindness, diplopia, ear pain, tinnitus, retinal hemorrhage

GI: Nausea, vomiting, *diarrhea,* GI discomfort, colitis, cholelithiasis, ulcer, esophagitis, gastritis, anorexia, *flatulence, dyspepsia*

GU: Cystitis, frequency, vaginitis, **vaginal hemorrhage,** hematuria

HEMA: **Bleeding (epistaxis, hematuria, retinal hemorrhage, GI bleeding), thrombocytopenia,** anemia, polycythemia

INTEG: Rash, urticaria, dry skin

MISC: Back pain, headache, infection,

Side effects: *italics* = common; **bold** = life-threatening

myalgia, peripheral edema, chills, fever, malaise, diabetes mellitus

RESP: Cough, pharyngitis, rhinitis, asthma, pneumonia

Contraindications: Hypersensitivity, CHF, acute MI, active bleeding conditions, hemostatic conditions

Precautions: Pregnancy (C), past hepatic disease, renal disease, geriatric, lactation, children, increased bleeding risk, low platelet count, platelet dysfunction, active bleeding

PHARMACOKINETICS

95%-98% protein binding, metabolism-hepatic extensively by CYPP450 enzymes, excreted urine (74%), feces (20%), half-life 11-13 hr

INTERACTIONS

Increase: bleeding tendencies—anticoagulants, NSAIDs, thrombolytics, abciximab, eptifibatide, tirofiban, ticlopidine

Increase: cilostazol levels—diltiazem, erythromycin, verapamil, protease inhibitors, omeprazole; exercise caution when coadministering with fluvoxamine, fluoxetine, ketoconazole, itraconazole, voriconazole, fluconazole and reduce dose to 50 mg bid

Drug/Herb

Increase: bleeding risk—agrimony, alfalfa, angelica, anise, bilberry, black haw, bogbean, buchu, chondroitin, dong quai, fenugreek, feverfew, garlic, ginger, ginkgo, ginseng, green tea, horse chestnut, Irish moss, kelp, kelpware, khella, lovage, lungwort, meadowsweet, motherwort, mugwort, nettle, papaya, parsley (large amt), pau d'arco, pineapple, poplar, prickly ash, safflower, saw palmetto, senega, tonka bean, turmeric, wintergreen, yarrow

Decrease: action—chamomile, coenzyme Q10, flax, glucomannan, goldenseal

Drug/Food

• Do not use with grapefruit juice

NURSING CONSIDERATIONS

Assess:

• For underlying CV disease since CV risk is great; for CV lesions with repeated oral administration; do not administer to patients with CHF of any severity

• Blood studies: CBC q2wk, Hct, Hgb, PT

Administer:

• Give bid 1 hr before or 2 hr after meals; do not give with grapefruit juice

Evaluate:

• Therapeutic response: improved walking distance and duration, decreased pain

Teach patient/family:

• To report any unusual bleeding

• To report side effects such as diarrhea, skin rashes, subcutaneous bleeding

• That effects may take 2-4 wk, treatment of up to 12 wk may be required for necessary effect

• To take 1 hr before or 2 hr after meals

• That reading the patient package insert is necessary

cimetidine (OTC, ℞)
(sye-met'i-deen)
Apo-Cimetidine ✤, cimetidine, Novo-Cimetidine ✤, Peptol ✤ Tagamet, Tagamet HB
Func. class.: H₂-histamine receptor antagonist
Chem. class.: Imidazole derivative

Action: Inhibits histamine at H₂-receptor site in the gastric parietal cells, which inhibits gastric acid secretion

Uses: Short-term treatment of duodenal and gastric ulcers and maintenance; management of GERD (PO) and Zollinger-Ellison syndrome; prevention of upper GI bleeding; prevent, relieve heartburn, acid indigestion

Unlabeled uses: Prevention of aspiration pneumonitis, stress ulcers, upper GI bleeding, herpes infection, hirsutism, cutaneous/nongenital warts, weight loss

⚠ Safety alert   *"Tall Man" lettering

DOSAGE AND ROUTES
Short-term treatment of active ulcers
• *Adult:* PO 300 mg qid with meals, at bedtime × 8 wk or 400 mg bid, 800 mg at bedtime; after 8 wk give bedtime dose only; **IV BOL** 300 mg/20 ml 0.9% NaCl over 1-2 min q6h; **IV INF** 300 mg/50 ml D₅W over 15-20 min; **IM** 300 mg q6h, not to exceed 2400 mg/day
• *Child:* PO 20-40 mg/kg/day; **IM/IV** 5-10 mg/kg q6-8h
Prophylaxis of duodenal ulcer
• *Adult and child >16 yr:* 400 mg at bedtime or 300 mg bid
GERD
• *Adult:* PO 800-1600 mg/day in divided doses
Hypersecretory conditions (Zollinger-Ellison syndrome)
• *Adult:* PO/IM/IV 300-600 mg q6h; may increase to 12 g/day if needed; OTC use up to 200 mg daily or bid, max 2×/wk
Upper GI bleeding prophylaxis
• *Adult:* IV 50 mg/hr; lowered in renal disease
Aspiration pneumonitis prophylaxis
• *Adult:* IM/IV 300 mg IM 1 hr before anesthesia, then 300 mg IV q4h until patient is alert, max 2400 mg/day
Hirsutism
• *Adult:* PO 300 mg qid × 5 days or 1600 mg daily up to 6 mo
Warts
• *Adult:* PO 400-800 mg tid × 12 wk or 30-40 mg/kg/day given tid × 3 mo
Weight loss
• *Adult:* PO 200-400 mg tid × 8-12 wk
Renal disease
• *Adult:* PO/IV CCr 20-40 ml/min 300 mg q8h; CCr <20 ml/min 300 mg q12h
• *Child:* PO 10-15 mg/kg/day
Available forms: Tabs 100, 200, 300, 400, 800 mg; liq 200, 300 mg/5 ml; inj 300 mg/2 ml, 300 mg/50 ml 0.9% NaCl

SIDE EFFECTS
CNS: Confusion, headache, depression, dizziness, anxiety, weakness, psychosis, tremors, **seizures**
CV: Bradycardia, tachycardia, **dysrhythmias**
GI: Diarrhea, abdominal cramps, **paralytic ileus, jaundice**
GU: Gynecomastia, galactorrhea, impotence, increase in BUN, creatinine
HEMA: **Agranulocytosis, thrombocytopenia, neutropenia, aplastic anemia, increase in PT**
INTEG: Urticaria, rash, alopecia, sweating, flushing, **exfoliative dermatitis**
Contraindications: Hypersensitivity
Precautions: Pregnancy (B), lactation, child <16 yr, organic brain syndrome, renal/hepatic disease, geriatric

PHARMACOKINETICS
Well absorbed (PO, IM)
IM/IV: Onset 10 min, peak ½ hr, duration 4-5 hr
PO: Onset 30 min, peak 45-90 min; duration 4-5 hr, half-life 1½-2 hr; 30%-40% metabolized by liver, excreted in urine (unchanged), crosses placenta, enters breast milk

INTERACTIONS
Increase: toxicity due to CYP450 pathway—benzodiazepines, β-blockers, calcium channel blockers, carbamazepine, chloroquine, lidocaine, metronidazole, moricizine, phenytoin, quinidine, quinine, sulfonylureas, theophylline, tricyclics, valproic acid, warfarin
Decrease: absorption of cimetidine—antacids, sucralfate
Decrease: absorption—ketoconazole, itraconazole
Drug/Lab Test
Increase: Alk phos, AST, creatinine, prolactin
False positive: Gastroccult, hemoccult
False negative: TB skin tests

NURSING CONSIDERATIONS
Assess:
• Gastric pH (5 or more should be maintained), also epigastric pain and duration, intensity; aggravating, ameliorating factors

Side effects: *italics* = common; **bold** = life-threatening

• I&O ratio, BUN, creatinine, CBC with differential periodically

Administer:
• With meals for prolonged drug effect; antacids 1 hr before or 1 hr after cimetidine

IV route
• After diluting 300 mg/20 ml of 0.9% NaCl for inj; give ≥5 min; may be diluted 300 mg/50 ml of D₅W; run over 15-20 min; or total daily dose (900 mg) diluted in 100-1000 ml D₅W given over 24 hr

Additive compatibilities: AcetaZOLAMIDE, amikacin, aminophylline, atracurium, cefoperazone, cefoxitin, chlorothiazide, clindamycin, colistimethate, dexamethasone, digoxin, epINEPHrine, erythromycin, ethacrynate, floxacillin, flumazenil, furosemide, gentamicin, insulin (regular), isoproterenol, lidocaine, lincomycin, meropenem, metaraminol, methylPREDNISolone, norepinephrine, nitroprusside, penicillin G potassium, phytonadione, polymyxin B, potassium chloride, protamine, quinidine, tacrolimus, vancomycin, verapamil, vit B/C

Syringe compatibilities: Atropine, butorphanol, cephalothin, diazepam, diphenhydrAMINE, doxapram, droperidol, fentanyl, glycopyrrolate, heparin, hydromorphone, hydrOXYzine, lorazepam, meperidine, midazolam, morphine, nafcillin, nalbuphine, penicillin G sodium, pentazocine, perphenazine, prochlorperazine, promazine, promethazine, scopolamine

Y-site compatibilities: Acyclovir, amifostine, aminophylline, amrinone, atracurium, aztreonam, cisatracurium, cisplatin, cladribine, cyclophosphamide, cytarabine, diltiazem, DOXOrubicin, DOXOrubicin liposome, enalaprilat, esmolol, filgrastim, fluconazole, fludarabine, foscarnet, gallium, granisetron, haloperidol, heparin, hetastarch, idarubicin, labetalol, melphalan, meropenem, methotrexate, midazolam, ondansetron, paclitaxel, pancuronium, piperacillin/tazobactam, propofol, remifentanil, sargramostim, tacrolimus, teniposide, theophylline, thiotepa, tolazoline, vecuronium, vinorelbine, zidovudine

Perform/provide:
• Storage of diluted sol at room temperature up to 48 hr

Evaluate:
• Therapeutic response: decreased pain in abdomen; healing of ulcers, absence of gastroesophageal reflux, gastric pH 5

Teach patient/family:
• That gynecomastia, impotence may occur, are reversible
• To avoid driving, other hazardous activities until patient is stabilized on this medication; drowsiness or dizziness may occur
• To avoid black pepper, caffeine, alcohol, harsh spices, extremes in temperature of food
• To avoid OTC preparations: aspirin, cough, cold preparations; condition may worsen
• That smoking decreases the effectiveness of the drug
• That drug must be taken exactly as prescribed and continued for prescribed time to be effective; doses not to be doubled
• To report bruising, fatigue, malaise; blood dyscrasias may occur
• To report to prescriber diarrhea, black tarry stools, sore throat, rash

cinacalcet (℞)
(sin-a-kal'set)
Sensipar
Func. class.: Calcium receptor agonist
Chem. class.: Polypeptide hormone

Action: Directly lowers PTH levels by increasing sensitivity of calcium sensing receptors to extracellular calcium
Uses: Hypercalcemia in parathyroid carcinoma, secondary hyperparathyroidism in chronic kidney disease on dialysis

DOSAGE AND ROUTES
Parathyroid carcinoma
• *Adult:* **PO** 30 mg bid, titrate q2-4wk, with sequential doses of 30 mg bid, 60 mg bid, 90 mg bid, 90 mg tid-qid to normalize calcium levels

Secondary hyperparathyroidism

• *Adult:* **PO** 30 mg daily, titrate no more frequently than 2-4 wk with sequential doses of 30, 60, 90, 120, 180 mg daily

Available forms: Tabs 30, 60, 90 mg

SIDE EFFECTS

CNS: Dizziness

CV: Hypertension

GI: Nausea, diarrhea, vomiting, anorexia

MISC: Access infection, noncardiac chest pain, asthenia

MS: Myalgia

Contraindications: Hypersensitivity

Precautions: Pregnancy (C), children, lactation, seizure disorders, hepatic disease

PHARMACOKINETICS

93%-97% bound to plasma; proteins metabolized by CYP3A4, 2D6, 1A2; half-life 30-40 hr; renal excretion of metabolites (80% renal, 15% feces)

INTERACTIONS

• Drugs metabolized by CYP3A4 (ketoconazole, erythromycin, itraconazole), CYP2D6 (flecainide, vinBLAStine, thioridazine, tricyclics): adjustments may be necessary

Drug/Food

Increase: action by high-fat meal

NURSING CONSIDERATIONS

Assess:

• Hypocalcemia: cramping, seizures, tetany, myalgia, paresthesia

• Calcium, phosphorous within 1 wk and iPTH 1-4 wk after initiation or dosage adjustment when maintenance is established; measure calcium, phosphorus monthly; iPTH q1-3mo, target range 150-300 pg/ml for iPTH level

• If calcium <8.4 mg/dl, do not start therapy

Administer:

• Swallow tabs whole; do not break, crush, or chew

• Can be used alone or in combination with vit D sterols and/or phosphate binders

Secondary hyperthyroidism

• Titrate q2-4wk to target iPTH consistent with National Kidney Foundation–Kidney Disease Outcomes Quality Initiative (NKF-K/DOQI) for chronic kidney disease patient on dialysis of 150-300 pg/ml; if iPTH drops below 150-300 pg/ml, reduce dose of cinacalcet and/or vit D sterols or discontinue treatment

Perform/provide:

• Storage at <77° F (25° C)

Evaluate:

• Therapeutic response: calcium levels 9-10 mg/dl, decreasing symptoms of hypercalcemia

Teach patient/family:

• Take with food or shortly after a meal

• Report immediately: cramping, seizures, muscle pain, tingling, tetany

---

ciprofloxacin (R)

(sip-ro-floks'a-sin)
Cipro, Cipro IV, Cipro XR
Func. class.: Broad-spectrum antiinfective
Chem. class.: Fluoroquinolone

Do not confuse:

ciprofloxacin/cephalexin

Action: Interferes with conversion of intermediate DNA fragments into high-molecular-weight DNA in bacteria; DNA gyrase inhibitor

Uses: Infection caused by susceptible *Escherichia coli, Enterobacter cloacae, Proteus mirabilis, Klebsiella pneumoniae, Proteus vulgaris, Citrobacter freundii, Serratia marcescens, Pseudomonas aeruginosa, Staphylococcus aureus, Staphylococcus epidermidis, Enterobacter, Campylobacter jejuni, Salmonella;* chronic bacterial prostatitis, acute sinusitis, postexposure inhalation anthrax, infectious diarrhea, typhoid fever, complicated intraabdominal infections, nosocomial pneumonia, urinary tract infections

---

DOSAGE AND ROUTES

Uncomplicated urinary tract infections
• *Adult:* **PO** 100-250 mg q12h × 3 days or 500 mg × q24h × 3 days

Complicated/severe urinary tract infections
• *Adult:* **PO** 500 mg q12h or 1000 mg q24h × 7-14 days; **IV** 400 mg q12h

Pyelonephritis, acute uncomplicated
• *Adult:* **PO** 1000 mg q24h × 7-14 days

Respiratory, bone, skin, joint infections
• *Adult:* **PO** 500-750 mg q12h × 7-14 days; **IV** 400 mg q12h

Nosocomial pneumonia
• *Adult:* **IV** 400 mg q8h × 10-14 days

Intraabdominal infections, complicated
• *Adult:* **PO** 500 mg q12h × 7-14 days; **IV** 400 mg q12h × 7-14 days, usually given with metronidazole

Acute sinusitis, mild/moderate
• *Adult:* **PO** 500 mg q12h × 10 days; **IV** 400 mg q12h × 10 days

Inhalational anthrax (postexposure)
• *Adult:* **PO** 500 mg q12h × 60 days; **IV** 400 mg q12h × 60 days
• *Child:* **PO** 15 mg/kg/dose, max 500 mg/dose; **IV** max 400 mg/dose × 60 days

Infectious diarrhea
• *Adult:* **PO** 500 mg q12h × 5-7 days

Chronic bacterial prostatis
• *Adult:* **PO** 500 mg q12h × 28 days; **IV** 400 mg q12h × 28 days

Renal disease
• CCr 30-50 ml/min **PO** 250-500 mg q12h; CCr 5-29 ml/min **PO** 250-500 mg q18h; **IV** 200-400 mg q18-24h

Available forms: Tabs 100, 250, 500, 750 mg; ext rel tabs (XR) 500, 1000 mg; inj 200 mg/20 ml, 400 mg/40 ml, 200 mg/100 ml D₅, 400 mg/200 ml D₅; oral susp 250 mg, 500 mg/5 ml

SIDE EFFECTS

CNS: Headache, dizziness, fatigue, insomnia, depression, *restlessness,* **seizures,** confusion

GI: Nausea, diarrhea, increased ALT, AST, dry mouth, flatulence, heartburn, *vomiting,* oral candidiasis, dysphagia, **pseudomembranous colitis**

INTEG: Rash, pruritus, urticaria, photosensitivity, flushing, fever, chills, **toxic epidermal necrolysis**

MISC: **Anaphylaxis, Stevens-Johnson syndrome,** visual impairment, QT prolongation

MS: Tremor, arthralgia, tendon rupture

Contraindications: Hypersensitivity to quinolones

Precautions: Pregnancy (C), lactation, children, renal disease, epilepsy, QT prolongation, tendon pain, hypokalemia

PHARMACOKINETICS

PO: Peak 1 hr, half-life 3-4 hr; excreted in urine as active drug, metabolites

INTERACTIONS

Increase: nephrotoxicity—cycloSPORINE
Increase: ciprofloxacin levels—probenecid; monitor for toxicity
Increase: levels of theophylline, warfarin, monitor blood levels
Increase: QT prolongation—astemizole, droperidol, probucol
Decrease: ciproflaxin absorption—antacids containing magnesium, aluminum; zinc, iron, sucralfate, enteral feedings, calcium

Drug/Herb
• Do not use acidophilus with antiinfectives; separate by several hours
• Possible toxicity: yerba maté
Decrease: effect—fennel

Drug/Food
Increase: effect of caffeine
Decrease: absorption—dairy products, food

Drug/Lab Test
Increase: AST, ALT, BUN, creatinine, LDH, bilirubin, alk phos, glucose, proteinuria, albuminuria
Decrease: WBC, glucose

⚠ Safety alert   *"Tall Man" lettering

NURSING CONSIDERATIONS
Assess:
• Infection: WBC, temperature prior to and periodically
• CNS symptoms: headache, dizziness, fatigue, insomnia, depression
• Renal, hepatic studies: BUN, creatinine, AST, ALT
• I&O ratio, urine pH <5.5 is ideal
⚠ Anaphylaxis: fever, flushing, rash, urticaria, pruritus, dyspnea
• For tendon pain, especially in children
Administer:
• Not to use theophylline with this product, will cause toxicity
• Use caution when giving with antidysrhythmics IA & III
PO route
• Do not break, crush, or chew XR (ext rel) product
• 2 hr before or 2 hr after antacids, zinc, iron, calcium
IV route
• Over 1 hr as an INF, comes in pre-mixed plastic INF container or diluted 20- or 40-ml vial to a final conc of 0.5-2 mg/ml of NS or D₅W; give through Y-tube or 3-way stopcock
• After clean-catch urine for C&S
Additive compatibilities: Amikacin, aztreonam, ceftazidime, cycloSPORINE, gentamicin, metronidazole, netilmicin, piperacillin, potassium acetate, potassium chloride, potassium phosphates, predniso-LONE, promethazine, propofol, ranitidine, Ringer's, sodium chloride, tobramycin, vit B/C
Y-site compatibilities: Amifostine, amino acids, aztreonam, calcium gluconate, ceftazidime, cisatracurium, digoxin, diltiazem, diphenhydrAMINE, DOBUTamine, DOPamine, DOXOrubicin liposome, gallium, gentamicin, granisetron, hydrOXYzine, lidocaine, lorazepam, metoclopramide, midazolam, midodrine, piperacillin, potassium acetate, potassium chloride, potassium phosphates, predniso-LONE, promethazine, propofol, ranitidine, remifentanil, Ringer's, sodium chlo-

ride, tacrolimus, teniposide, thiotepa, tobramycin, verapamil
Perform/provide:
• Limited intake of alkaline foods, drugs: milk, dairy products, alkaline antacids, sodium bicarbonate
• Increase in fluids to 3 L/day to avoid crystallization in kidneys
Evaluate:
• Therapeutic response: decreased pain, frequency, urgency, C&S; absence of infection
Teach patient/family:
• Not to take any products containing magnesium or calcium (such as antacids), iron, or aluminum with this drug or within 2 hr of drug
• That photosensitivity may occur; patient should avoid sunlight or use sunscreen to prevent burns
• If dizziness occurs, to ambulate, perform activities with assistance
• To complete full course of drug therapy, not to double or miss doses
• To contact prescriber if adverse reaction occurs or if inflammation or pain in tendon occurs
• To use frequent rinsing of mouth, sugarless candy or gum for dry mouth
• To contact prescriber if taking theophylline

ciprofloxacin ophthalmic
See Appendix C

⚠ High Alert

cisplatin (℞)
(sis'pla-tin)
Platinol ✦, Platinol-AQ
Func. class.: Antineoplastic alkylating agent
Chem. class.: Inorganic heavy metal

Do not confuse:
cisplatin/carboplatin
Platinol/Paraplatin

Action: Alkylates DNA, RNA; inhibits enzymes that allow synthesis of amino acids in proteins; activity is not cell cycle phase specific

Uses: Advanced bladder cancer, adjunctive in metastatic testicular cancer, osteosarcoma, soft tissue sarcomas, adjunctive in metastatic ovarian cancer, head, neck cancer, esophagus, prostate, lung and cervical cancer, lymphoma

DOSAGE AND ROUTES

Dosage protocols may vary

Metastatic testicular cancer
• *Adult:* IV 20 mg/m² daily × 5 days, repeat q3wk for 3 cycles or more, depending on response

Advanced bladder cancer
• *Adult:* IV 50-70 mg/m² q3-4wk

Metastatic ovarian cancer
• *Adult:* IV 100 mg/m² q4wk or 75-100 mg/m² q3wk with cyclophosphamide; mix with 2 L NaCl and 37.5 g mannitol over 6 hr

Available forms: Inj 0.5 ♣, 1 mg/ml; powder for inj 10, 50 mg vials

SIDE EFFECTS

CNS: **Seizures,** peripheral neuropathy
CV: Cardiac abnormalities
EENT: Tinnitus, hearing loss, vestibular toxicity, blurred vision, altered color perception
GI: Severe nausea, vomiting, diarrhea, weight loss
GU: **Renal tubular damage,** renal insufficiency, impotence, sterility, amenorrhea, gynecomastia, hyperuremia
HEMA: **Thrombocytopenia, leukopenia, pancytopenia**
INTEG: Alopecia, dermatitis
META: Hypomagnesemia, hypocalcemia, hypokalemia, hypophosphatemia
RESP: **Fibrosis**
SYST: **Anaphylaxis**
Contraindications: Pregnancy (D), radiation therapy or chemotherapy within 1 mo, thrombocytopenia, recent smallpox vaccination, aluminum products used

to prepare or administer cisplatin, lactation
Precautions: Pneumococcus vaccination

PHARMACOKINETICS

Absorption complete, metabolized in liver, excreted in urine; half-life 30-100 hr, accumulates in body tissues for several months, enters breast milk

INTERACTIONS

Increase: Risk of bleeding—aspirin, NSAIDs, alcohol
Increase: Ototoxicity—bumetanide, ethacrynic acid, furosemide
Increase: myelosuppression—myelosuppressive agents, radiation
Increase: nephrotoxicity—aminoglycosides, loop diuretics
Decrease: effects of phenytoin
Decrease: antibody response—live virus vaccines
Drug/Lab Test
Increase: Uric acid, BUN, creatinine
Decrease: CCr, calcium, phosphate, potassium, magnesium
Positive: Coombs' test

NURSING CONSIDERATIONS
Assess:
For bone marrow depression
• CBC, differential, platelet count weekly; withhold drug if WBC is <4000 or platelet count is <100,000; notify prescriber of results
• Renal studies: BUN, creatinine, serum uric acid, urine CCr before, electrolytes during therapy; dose should not be given if BUN <25 mg/dl; creatinine <1.5 mg/dl; I&O ratio; report fall in urine output of <30 ml/hr
⚠ For anaphylaxis: wheezing, tachycardia, facial swelling, fainting; discontinue drug and report to prescriber; resuscitation equipment should be nearby
• Monitor temp q4h (may indicate beginning infection)

⚠ Safety alert   *"Tall Man" lettering

• Hepatic studies before, during therapy (bilirubin, AST, ALT, LDH) as needed or monthly

⚠ Bleeding: hematuria, guaiac, bruising or petechiae, mucosa or orifices q8h; obtain prescription for viscous lidocaine (Xylocaine)

• Effects of alopecia on body image; discuss feelings about body changes

• Jaundice of skin, sclera; dark urine; clay-colored stools; itchy skin; abdominal pain; fever; diarrhea

• Edema in feet, joint pain, stomach pain, shaking

Administer:

IV route

• Do not use aluminum equipment during any preparation or administration, will form precipitate; do not refrigerate unopened powder or solution, protect from sunlight

• Prepare in biologic cabinet using gown, gloves, mask; do not allow drug to come in contact with skin; use soap and water if contact occurs; use cytoxic handling procedures

• Hydrate patient with 0.9% NaCl over 8-12 hr before treatment

• EpINEPHrine, antihistamines, corticosteroids for hypersensitivity reaction

• Antiemetic 30-60 min before giving drug and prn

• Allopurinol to maintain uric acid levels, alkalinization of urine

• Diuretic (furosemide 40 mg IV) or mannitol after infusion

Intermittent INF route

• Dilute 10 mg/10 ml or 50 mg/50 ml sterile H_2O for inj; withdraw prescribed dose, dilute ½ dose with 1000 ml D_5 0.2 NaCl or D_5 0.45 NaCl with 37.5 g mannitol; IV INF is given over 3-4 hr; use a 0.45-μm filter; total dose 2 L over 6-8 hr; check site for irritation, phlebitis

CONT INF route

• Give over 24 hr × 5 days

Additive compatibilities: Carboplatin, cyclophosphamide with etoposide, etoposide, etoposide with floxuridine, floxuridine, floxuridine with leucovorin, hydrOXYzine, ifosfamide, ifosfamide with etoposide, leucovorin, magnesium sulfate, mannitol, ondansetron

Solution compatibilities: D_5/0.225% NaCl, D_5/0.45% NaCl, D_5/0.9% NaCl, D_5/0.45% NaCl with mannitol 1.875%, D_5/0.33% NaCl with KCl 20 mEq and mannitol 1.875%, 0.9% NaCl, 0.45% NaCl, 0.3% NaCl, 0.225% NaCl

Syringe compatibilities: Bleomycin, cyclophosphamide, doxapram, DOXOrubicin, droperidol, fluorouracil, furosemide, heparin, leucovorin, methotrexate, metoclopramide, mitomycin, vinBLAStine, vinCRIStine

Y-site compatibilities: Allopurinol, aztreonam, bleomycin, chlorproMAZINE, cimetidine, cladribine, cyclophosphamide, dexamethasone, diphenhydrAMINE, DOXOrubicin, DOXOrubicin liposome, droperidol, famotidine, filgrastim, fludarabine, fluorouracil, furosemide, ganciclovir, granisetron, heparin, hydromorphone, leucovorin, lorazepam, melphalan, methotrexate, methylPREDNISolone, metoclopramide, mitomycin, morphine, ondansetron, paclitaxel, prochlorperazine, promethazine, propofol, ranitidine, sargramostim, teniposide, vinBLAStine, vinCRIStine, vinorelbine

Perform/provide:

• Comprehensive oral hygiene

• All medications PO, if possible, avoid IM inj when platelets <100,000/mm³

• Increase fluid intake to 2-3 L/day to prevent urate deposits, calculi formation; promote elimination of drug

Evaluate:

• Therapeutic response: decreased tumor size, spread of malignancy

Teach patient/family:

• To report signs of infection: increased temp, sore throat, flulike symptoms

• To report signs of anemia: fatigue, headache, faintness, shortness of breath, irritability

• To report bleeding, bruising, petechiae; avoid use of razors, commercial mouthwash

• To avoid aspirin, ibuprofen, NSAIDs, alcohol; may cause GI bleeding

---

- To report any complaints or side effects to nurse or prescriber
- That impotence or amenorrhea can occur; reversible after discontinuing treatment
- To report any changes in breathing, coughing
- To maintain adequate fluids; report decreased urine output, flank pain
- That hair may be lost during treatment; a wig or hairpiece may make patient feel better; new hair may be different in color, texture
- To report numbness, tingling in face or extremities, poor hearing or joint pain, swelling
- Not to receive vaccinations during treatment
- To use contraception during treatment and 4 mo after; this drug may cause infertility; avoid breastfeeding

citalopram (Ŗ)
(sigh-tal'oh-pram)
Celexa
Func. class.: Antidepressant
Chem. class.: Selective serotonin reuptake inhibitor (SSRI)

Do not confuse:
Celexa/Celebrex/Cerebyx/Cerebra
Action: Inhibits CNS neuron uptake of serotonin but not of norepinephrine; weak inhibitor of CYP450 enzyme system, making it more appealing than other drugs
Uses: Major depressive disorder
Unlabeled uses: Fibromyalgia, premenstrual disorders, panic disorder, social phobia, impulsive aggression in children, obsessive-compulsive disorder in adolescents, treatment of psychotic symptoms in nondepressed demented patients

DOSAGE AND ROUTES
Depression
- *Adult:* **PO** 20 mg daily AM or PM, may increase if needed to 40 mg/day after 1 wk; maintenance: after 6-8 wk of initial treatment, continue for 24 wk (32 wk total), reevaluate long-term usefulness (max 60 mg/day)
Fibromyalgia
- *Adult:* **PO** 20 mg daily × 4 wk; increase dose to 40 mg daily × 4 wk
Hepatic dose/geriatric
- *Adult:* **PO** 20 mg/day, may increase to 40 mg/day if no response
Panic disorder
- *Adult:* **PO** 20-30 mg/day
Premenstrual dysphoria, social phobia, impulsive aggression in children
- *Adult:* **PO** 20-40 mg/day, used intermittently in premenstrual dysphoria
Available forms: Tabs 10, 20, 40 mg; oral sol 2 mg (as base)/ml

SIDE EFFECTS
CNS: Headache, nervousness, insomnia, drowsiness, anxiety, tremor, dizziness, fatigue, sedation, poor concentration, abnormal dreams, agitation, **convulsions,** *apathy, euphoria, hallucinations, delusions, psychosis,* **suicidal attempts**
CV: Hot flashes, palpitations, angina pectoris, **hemorrhage,** hypertension, tachycardia, 1st-degree AV block, bradycardia, *MI,* thrombophlebitis
EENT: Visual changes, ear/eye pain, photophobia, tinnitus
GI: Nausea, diarrhea, dry mouth, anorexia, dyspepsia, constipation, cramps, vomiting, taste changes, flatulence, decreased appetite
GU: Dysmenorrhea, decreased libido, urinary frequency, UTI, amenorrhea, cystitis, impotence, urine retention
INTEG: Sweating, rash, pruritus, acne, alopecia, urticaria
MS: Pain, arthritis, twitching
RESP: Infection, pharyngitis, nasal congestion, sinus headache, sinusitis, cough, dyspnea, bronchitis, asthma, hyperventilation, pneumonia
SYST: Asthenia, viral infection, fever, allergy, chills
Contraindications: Hypersensitivity
Precautions: Pregnancy (C), lactation, children, geriatric

⚠ Safety alert   *"Tall Man" lettering

PHARMACOKINETICS

PO: Metabolized in liver; excreted in urine; steady state 28-35 days; peak 2-4 hr; half-life 35 hr

INTERACTIONS

⚠ Fatal reactions: do not use with MAOIs
⚠ *Increase:* QT$_c$ interval—pimoside, do not use together
Increase: effect of tricyclics, use cautiously
Increase: risk of bleeding—NSAIDs, salicylates, thrombolytics, anticoagulants
Increase: CNS effects—CNS depressants
Increase: citalopram levels—macrolides, azole antifungals
Increase: plasma levels of β-blockers
Increase: serotonergic effects—lithium
Decrease: citalopram levels—carbamazepine

Drug/Herb
⚠ *Increase:* Serotonin syndrome—St. John's wort, SAM-e; fatal reaction may occur; do not use concurrently
Increase: CNS stimulation—yohimbe

Drug/Lab Test
Increase: Serum bilirubin, blood glucose, alk phos
Decrease: VMA, 5-HIAA
False increase: Urinary catecholamines

NURSING CONSIDERATIONS

Assess:
• Mental status: mood, sensorium, affect, suicidal tendencies, increase in psychiatric symptoms, depression, panic
• B/P (lying/standing), pulse q4h; if systolic B/P drops 20 mm Hg, hold drug, notify prescriber; take vital signs q4h in patients with cardiovascular disease
• Weight qwk; appetite may decrease or increase with drug
• ECG for flattening of T wave, bundle branch, AV block, dysrhythmias in cardiac patients
• Alcohol consumption; if alcohol is consumed, hold dose until AM

Administer:
• With food or milk for GI symptoms

• Crushed if patient is unable to swallow medication whole
• Dosages at bedtime if oversedation occurs during the day; may take entire dose at bedtime

Perform/provide:
• Storage at room temperature; do not freeze
• Assistance with ambulation during therapy, since drowsiness, dizziness occur
• Safety measures primarily in geriatric
• Check to see if PO medication swallowed
• Sugarless gum, hard candy, frequent sips of water for dry mouth

Evaluate:
• Therapeutic response: decreased depression

Teach patient/family:
• That therapeutic effect may take 2-3 wk
• To use caution in driving, other activities requiring alertness because of drowsiness, dizziness, blurred vision
• To avoid alcohol ingestion, other CNS depressants
• To notify prescriber if pregnant or plan to become pregnant or breastfeed

Rarely Used

cladribine (CdA) ($R̶$)
(kla′dri-been)
Leustatin
Func. class.: Antineoplastic antiinfective

Uses: Treatment of active hairy cell leukemia; may be useful in chronic lymphocytic leukemia, non-Hodgkin's lymphomas, acute, chronic myeloid leukemia, autoimmune hemolytic anemia

DOSAGE AND ROUTES

• *Adult:* **IV** 0.09 mg/kg diluted with 0.9% NaCl qs to 100 ml; pass through 0.22 μm microfilter, given for cont inf × 5-7 days
Contraindications: Pregnancy (D), hypersensitivity, lactation

---

clarithromycin (℞)
(klare-ith'row-my-sin)
Biaxin, Biaxin XL
Func. class.: Antiinfective
Chem. class.: Macrolide

Action: Binds to 50S ribosomal subunits of susceptible bacteria and suppresses protein synthesis

Uses: Mild to moderate infections of the upper respiratory tract, lower respiratory tract, uncomplicated skin and skin structure infections caused by *Streptococcus pneumoniae, Mycoplasma pneumoniae, Legionella pneumophila, Moraxella catarrhalis, Neisseria gonorrhoeae, Corynebacterium diphtheriae, Listeria monocytogenes, Haemophilus influenzae, Streptococcus pyogenes, Staphylococcus aureus, Mycobacterium avium (MAC)* complex infection in AIDS patients, *Mycobacterium avium intracellulare, Helicobacter pylori* in combination with omeprazole

DOSAGE AND ROUTES

Acute exacerbation of chronic bronchitis
• *Adult:* **PO** 250-500 mg q12h × 7-14 days or 1000 mg daily × 7 days (XL)

Pharyngitis/tonsillitis
• *Adult:* **PO** 250 mg q12h × 10 days

Community-acquired pneumonia
• *Adult:* **PO** 250 mg q12h × 7-14 days or 1000 mg daily × 7 days (XL)

Endocarditis prophylaxis
• *Adult:* **PO** 500 mg 1 hr before procedure

MAC prophylaxis/treatment
• *Adult:* **PO** 500 mg bid, will require an additional antiinfective for active infection

H. pylori infection
• *Adult:* **PO** 500 mg daily plus omeprazole 2 × 20 mg q ᴀᴍ (days 1-14), then omeprazole 20 mg q ᴀᴍ (days 15-28)

Acute maxillary sinusitis
• *Adult:* **PO** 500 mg q12h × 14 days

Most infections
• *Child:* **PO** 7.5 mg/kg q12h × 10 days, max 500 mg/dose for MAC

Renal dose
• *Adult:* **PO** CCr <30 ml/min 250 mg daily × bid, may use an initial dose of 500 mg
• *Child:* **PO** CCr <30 ml/min reduce dose by 50%

Available forms: Tabs 250, 500 mg; oral susp 125 mg/5 ml, 250 mg/5 ml; ext rel tab (XL) 500 mg

SIDE EFFECTS

CV: **Ventricular dysrhythmias**
GI: Nausea, vomiting, diarrhea, **hepatotoxicity**, *abdominal pain*, stomatitis, heartburn, anorexia, *abnormal taste*, **pseudomembranous colitis**
GU: Vaginitis, moniliasis
HEMA: Leukopenia, thrombocytopenia, increased INR
INTEG: Rash, urticaria, pruritus, **Stevens-Johnson syndrome, toxic epidermal necrolysis**
MISC: Headache, hearing loss

Contraindications: Hypersensitivity to this drug or macrolide antibiotics

Precautions: Pregnancy (C), lactation, renal/hepatic disease, geriatric, QT prolongation

PHARMACOKINETICS

Peak 2 hr, duration 12 hr, half-life 4-6 hr; metabolized by liver; excreted in bile, feces

INTERACTIONS

Increase: dysrhythmias—cisapride, pimozide
Increase: levels, increase toxicity—alprazolam, buspirone, carbamazepine, cycloSPORINE, digoxin, disopyramide, ergots, felodipine, fluconazole, omeprazole, tacrolimus, theophylline
Increase: oral anticoagulants effect—digoxin, theophylline, carbamazepine
Increase: levels of HMG-CoA reductase inhibitors

⚠ Safety alert   *‥"Tall Man" lettering

Increase: action, risk of toxicity—all drugs metabolized by CYP3A enzyme system

Increase: QT prolongation—class IA, III antidysrhythmics

Increase or decrease action: zidovudine

Decrease: levels—rifampin, rifabutin

Drug/Herb

• Do not use acidophilus with antiinfectives; separate by several hours

Drug/Lab Test

Increase: 17-OHCS/17-KS, AST, ALT, BUN, creatinine, LDH, total bilirubin

Decrease: Folate assay, WBC

NURSING CONSIDERATIONS

Assess:

• For infection: wound characteristics, urine, stool, sputum, WBC, temp

• Cardiac function due to QT effects

• For ulcers: abdominal pain, bleeding in stools, emesis

• Renal, hepatic studies; report hematuria, oliguria

• C&S before drug therapy; drug may be given as soon as culture is taken; C&S may be repeated after treatment

• Bowel pattern before, during treatment

• Skin eruptions, itching

• Respiratory status: rate, character, wheezing, tightness in chest; discontinue drug

• Allergies before treatment, reaction of each medication

Administer:

• Do not break, crush, or chew tabs

• Adequate intake of fluids (2 L) during diarrhea episodes

• q12h to maintain serum level

Perform/provide:

• Storage at room temperature

Evaluate:

• Therapeutic response: C&S negative for infection

Teach patient/family:

• To take with full glass H_2O; may give with food to decrease GI symptoms

⚠ To report sore throat, fever, fatigue; may indicate superinfection

⚠ To notify nurse of diarrhea, dark urine, pale stools, yellow discoloration of eyes or skin, severe abdominal pain

• To take at evenly spaced intervals; complete dosage regimen

• To notify prescriber if pregnancy is suspected or planned

Treatment of hypersensitivity: Withdraw drug, maintain airway, administer epINEPHrine, aminophylline, O_2, IV corticosteroids

---

clindamycin HCl (Rx)
(klin-da-my′sin)
Cleocin HCl
clindamycin palmitate (Rx)
Cleocin Pediatric, Dalacin C Palmitate
clindamycin phosphate (Rx)
Cleocin Phosphate, Dalacin C, Dalacin C Phosphate
Func. class.: Antiinfective—miscellaneous
Chem. class.: Lincomycin derivative

Action: Binds to 50S subunit of bacterial ribosomes, suppresses protein synthesis

Uses: Infections caused by staphylococci, streptococci, *Rickettsia, Fusobacterium, Actinomyces, Peptococcus, Bacteroides, Pneumocystis jiroveci*

DOSAGE AND ROUTES

• *Adult:* **PO** 150-450 mg q6h, max 1.8 g/day; **IM/IV** 1.2-1.8 g/day in 2-4 divided doses, max 4800 mg/day

• *Child >1 mo:* **PO** 8-25 mg/kg/day in divided doses q6-8h; **IM/IV** 20-40 mg/kg/day in divided doses q6-8h (3-4 equal doses)

• *Child <1 mo:* **IM/IV** 15-20 mg/kg/day divided q6-8h

PID

• *Adult:* **IV** 600 mg qid plus gentamicin or 900 mg q8h

Bacterial endocarditis prophylaxis

• *Adult:* 600 mg 1 hr prior to procedure

Side effects: *italics* = common; **bold** = life-threatening

P. jiroveci *pneumonia (unlabeled)*
• *Adult:* PO 1200-1800 mg/day in divided doses with 15-30 mg primaquine/day

Available forms: *HCl:* caps 75, 150, 300 mg; *palmitate:* oral sol 75 mg/ml; *phosphate:* inj 150, 300, 600 mg base/4 ml; 900 mg base/ml; inj INF in D_5 300 mg, 600 mg, 900 mg

SIDE EFFECTS

GI: Nausea, vomiting, abdominal pain, diarrhea, **pseudomembranous colitis,** anorexia, weight loss, increased AST, ALT, bilirubin, alk phos; jaundice
GU: **Vaginitis,** urinary frequency
HEMA: **Leukopenia, eosinophilia, agranulocytosis, thrombocytopenia, polyarthritis**
INTEG: Rash, urticaria, pruritus, erythema, pain, abscess at inj site
SYST: **Stevens-Johnson syndrome, exfoliative dermatitis**

Contraindications: Hypersensitivity to this drug or lincomycin, tartrazine dye; ulcerative colitis/enteritis
Precautions: Pregnancy (B), renal/hepatic disease, GI disease, geriatric, lactation, tartrazine sensitivity, asthma, allergy

PHARMACOKINETICS

PO: Peak 45 min, duration 6 hr
IM: Peak 3 hr, duration 8-12 hr; half-life 2½ hr; metabolized in liver; excreted in urine, bile, feces as inactive metabolites; crosses placenta; excreted in breast milk

INTERACTIONS

• May block clindamycin effect: erythromycin, chloramphenicol
Increase: neuromuscular blockade—neuromuscular blockers
Decrease: absorption—kaolin
Drug/Herb
• Do not use acidophilus with antiinfectives; separate by several hours

Drug/Lab Test
Increase: Alk phos, bilirubin, CPK, AST, ALT

NURSING CONSIDERATIONS

Assess:
• Hepatic studies: AST, ALT if on long-term therapy
• Blood studies: WBC, RBC, Hct, Hgb, platelets, serum iron, reticulocytes; drug should be discontinued if bone marrow depression occurs
• C&S before drug therapy; drug may be given as soon as culture is taken
• B/P, pulse in patient receiving drug parenterally
• Bowel pattern before, during treatment; if severe diarrhea occurs, drug should be discontinued; may indicate pseudomembranous colitis
• Skin eruptions, itching, dermatitis after administration
• Respiratory status: rate, character, wheezing, tightness in chest
• Allergies before treatment, reaction of each medication
Administer:
• That drug must be taken in equal intervals around clock to maintain blood levels
PO route
• Do not break, crush, or chew caps
• Orally with at least 8 oz H_2O
IM route
• IM deep inj; rotate sites; do not give >600 mg in single IM inj
IV route
• By infusion only; do not administer bolus dose; dilute 300 mg or less/50 ml or more of D_5W, NS; may be further diluted in greater amounts of D_5W, NS and given as a cont inf in acute PID; give first dose 10 mg/min over ½ hr, then 0.75 mg/min; increased rates may be used to keep serum blood levels higher; run >10 min; no more than 1200 mg in a single 1-hr inf

Additive compatibilities: Amikacin, ampicillin, aztreonam, cefazolin, cefepime, cefonicid, cefotaxime, cefoxitin, ceftazidime, ceftizoxime, cefuroxime,

cephalothin, cimetidine, fluconazole, heparin, hydrocortisone, kanamycin, methylPREDNISolone, metoclopramide, metronidazole, netilmicin, ofloxacin, penicillin G, piperacillin, potassium chloride, sodium bicarbonate, tobramycin, verapamil, vit B/C
Syringe compatibilities: Amikacin, aztreonam, gentamicin, heparin
Y-site compatibilities: Amifostine, amiodarone, amphotericin B cholesteryl, amsacrine, aztreonam, cefpirome, cisatracurium, cyclophosphamide, diltiazem, DOXOrubicin liposome, enalaprilat, esmolol, fludarabine, foscarnet, granisetron, heparin, hydromorphone, labetalol, magnesium sulfate, melphalan, meperidine, midazolam, morphine, multivitamins, ondansetron, perphenazine, piperacillin/tazobactam, propofol, remifentanil, sargramostim, tacrolimus, teniposide, theophylline, thiotepa, vinorelbine, vit B/C, zidovudine
Perform/provide:
• Storage at room temperature (caps) up to 2 wk (reconstituted)
• EpINEPHrine, suction, tracheostomy set, endotracheal intubation equipment on unit
• Adequate intake of fluids (2 L) during diarrhea episodes
Evaluate:
• Therapeutic response: decreased temp, negative C&S
Teach patient/family:
• To take oral drug with full glass H_2O; antiperistaltic drugs may worsen diarrhea
• All aspects of drug therapy: need to complete entire course of medication to ensure organism death (10-14 days); culture may be taken after medication course completed
⚠ To report sore throat, fever, fatigue; may indicate superinfection
• To take with food to reduce GI symptoms
• To notify nurse or prescriber of diarrhea

Treatment of hypersensitivity:
• Withdraw drug; maintain airway; administer epINEPHrine, aminophylline, O_2, IV corticosteroids

clobetasol topical
See Appendix C

Rarely Used

clofazimine (R)
(kloe-fa′zi-meen)
Lamprene
Func. class.: Leprostatic

Uses: Lepromatous leprosy, dapsone-resistant leprosy, lepromatous leprosy complicated by erythema nodosum leprosum

DOSAGE AND ROUTES
Erythema nodosum leprosum
• *Adult:* **PO:** 100-200 mg daily × 3 mo, then taper dosage to 100 mg when disease is controlled; do not exceed 200 mg/day
Dapsone-resistant leprosy
• *Adult:* **PO:** 100 mg/day in combination with at least one other antileprosy drug × 3 yr, then 100 mg daily clofazimine (only)
Contraindications: Hypersensitivity to this drug

Side effects: *italics* = common; **bold** = life-threatening

*clomiPHENE (℞)

(kloe′mi-feen)
Clomid, clomiphene citrate,
Milophene, Serophene
Func. class.: Ovulation stimulant
Chem. class.: Nonsteroidal antiestrogenic

Do not confuse:
clomiPHENE/clomiPRAMINE

Action: Increases LH, FSH release from the pituitary, which increases maturation of ovarian follicle, ovulation, development of corpus luteum

Uses: Female infertility (ovulatory failure)

DOSAGE AND ROUTES

• *Adult:* PO 50-100 mg daily × 5 days or 50-100 mg daily beginning on day 5 of cycle; may be repeated until conception occurs or 3 cycles of therapy have been completed

Available forms: Tabs 50 mg

SIDE EFFECTS

CNS: Headache, depression, restlessness, anxiety, nervousness, fatigue, insomnia, dizziness, flushing

CV: Vasomotor flushing, phlebitis, **deep-vein thrombosis**

EENT: Blurred vision, diplopia, photophobia

GI: Nausea, vomiting, constipation, abdominal pain, bloating

GU: Polyuria, urinary frequency, birth defects, spontaneous abortions, multiple ovulation, breast pain, oliguria, abnormal uterine bleeding

INTEG: Rash, dermatitis, urticaria, alopecia

Contraindications: Pregnancy (X), hypersensitivity, hepatic disease, undiagnosed uterine bleeding, uncontrolled thyroid or adrenal dysfunction, intracranial lesion, ovarian cysts

Precautions: Hypertension, depression, convulsions, diabetes mellitus

PHARMACOKINETICS

Metabolized in liver, excreted in feces

INTERACTIONS

Drug/Lab Test
Increase: FSH/LH, BSP, thyroxine, TBG

NURSING CONSIDERATIONS

Administer:
• After discontinuing estrogen therapy
• At same time daily to maintain drug level

Evaluate:
• Therapeutic response: fertility

Teach patient/family:
• That multiple births are common
• To notify prescriber immediately if low abdominal pain occurs; may indicate ovarian cyst, cyst rupture
• To notify prescriber of photophobia, blurred vision, diplopia, abnormal bleeding, hot flashes, nausea, vomiting, headache
• That if dose is missed, to double it next time; if more than one dose is missed, to call prescriber
• That response usually occurs 4-10 days after last day of treatment
• The method for taking, recording basal body temp to determine whether ovulation has occurred
• If ovulation can be determined (there is a slight decrease in temp, then a sharp increase for ovulation), to attempt coitus 3 days before and every other day until after ovulation
• If pregnancy is suspected, to notify prescriber immediately

*clomiPRAMINE (℞)

(kloe-mip′ra-meen)
Anafranil
Func. class.: Antidepressant, tricyclic
Chem. class.: Tertiary amine

Do not confuse:
clomiPRAMINE/clomiPHENE/
desipramine/Norpramin

Action: Potentiates serotonin and norepinephrine; also increases dopamine metabolism; moderate anticholinergic effect

Uses: Obsessive-compulsive disorder, depression, dysphoria, phobias, anxiety, agoraphobia

Unlabeled uses: Panic disorder, premenstrual symptoms

DOSAGE AND ROUTES

Obsessive-compulsive disorder
• *Adult:* **PO** 25 mg at bedtime and increase gradually over 4 wk to 75-250 mg/day in divided doses
• *Child 10-18 yr:* **PO** 25-50 mg/day gradually increased; or 3 mg/kg/day, whichever is smaller, not to exceed 200 mg/day

Depression
• *Adult:* **PO** 50-150 mg/day in a single or divided dose

Anxiety/agoraphobia
• *Adult:* **PO** 25-75 mg/day

Available forms: Caps 25, 50, 75 mg

SIDE EFFECTS

CNS: Dizziness, tremors, mania, **seizures,** aggressiveness, EPS, drowsiness, headache, **neuroleptic malignant syndrome**

CV: Hypotension, tachycardia, **cardiac arrest**

EENT: Blurred vision

ENDO: Galactorrhea, hyperprolactinemia

GI: Constipation, dry mouth, nausea, dyspepsia, weight gain

GU: Delayed ejaculation, anorgasmia, urinary retention, decreased libido

HEMA: **Agranulocytosis, neutropenia, pancytopenia**

INTEG: Diaphoresis, photosensitivity

META: Hyponatremia

SYST: **Suicide in children/adolescents**

Contraindications: Hypersensitivity, immediate post-MI

Precautions: Pregnancy (C), seizures, suicidal patients, geriatric, lactation, cardiac disease

PHARMACOKINETICS

Onset ≥2 wk (depression) 4-10 wk (OCD); peak 2-6 hr; extensively bound to tissue and plasma proteins; demethylated in liver; active metabolites excreted in urine (50%-60%), feces (24%-32%); half-life 20-30 hr; steady state 1-2 wk

INTERACTIONS

• Hypertensive crisis, seizures, hypertensive episode: MAOIs

Increase: clomiPRAMINE levels—cimetidine, fluoxetine, fluvoxamine, sertraline; do not use together

Increase: hypertensive effect—clonidine, epINEPHrine, norepinephrine

Increase: CNS depression—alcohol, CNS depressants

Decrease: clomiPRAMINE levels—barbiturates, carbamazepine, phenytoin

Drug/Herb
• Serotonin syndrome: SAM-e, St. John's wort; do not use concurrently

Increase: CNS depression—hops, kava, lavender

Increase: anticholinergic effect—belladonna, corkwood, henbane, jimsonweed

Increase: clomiPRAMINE action—scopolia root

Drug/Lab Test
Increase: Prolactin, TBG, AST, ALT

Decrease: Serum thyroid hormone (T_3, T_4)

NURSING CONSIDERATIONS

Assess:
• B/P (lying, standing), pulse q4h; if systolic B/P drops 20 mm Hg, withhold drug, notify prescriber; take vital signs q4h in patients with cardiovascular disease
• For neuroleptic malignant syndrome: hyperpyrexia, rigidity, irregular pulse, diaphoresis
• ECG for flattening of T wave, QTc prolongation, bundle branch block, AV block, dysrhythmias in cardiac patients

---

• Blood studies: CBC, leukocytes, differential, cardiac enzymes if patient is receiving long-term therapy
• Hepatic studies: AST, ALT, bilirubin
• Mental status: mood, sensorium, affect, suicidal tendencies; increase in psychiatric symptoms: depression, panic, frequency of obsessive-compulsive behaviors; watch closely for evidence of suicidal thoughts in children/adolescents, seizure disorders
• Urinary retention, constipation; constipation more likely in children
• Withdrawal symptoms: headache, nausea, vomiting, muscle pain, weakness; not usual unless drug discontinued abruptly
• Alcohol consumption; if alcohol consumed, withhold dose until AM

Administer:
• Do not break, crush, or chew caps
• Increased fluids, bulk in diet for constipation, especially geriatric
• With food or milk for GI symptoms
• After titration, may be given as a single dose at bedtime, to reduce daytime sedation

Perform/provide:
• Storage in tight container at room temperature; do not freeze
• Assistance with ambulation during beginning therapy, since drowsiness/dizziness occurs
• Safety measures, primarily in geriatric
• Checking to see PO medication swallowed
• Gum, hard candy, or frequent sips of water for dry mouth

Evaluate:
• Therapeutic response: decreased anxiety, depression

Teach patient/family:
• That the effects may take 4-6 wk
• About risk of seizures
• To use caution in driving, other activities requiring alertness because of drowsiness, dizziness, blurred vision
• To avoid alcohol ingestion, other CNS depressants
• Not to discontinue medication quickly after long-term use; may cause nausea, headache, malaise

• To wear sunscreen, protective clothing to prevent photosensitivity
• To notify prescriber if pregnancy is planned or suspected
• That men may experience a high incidence of sexual dysfunction
• To watch for suicidal thoughts in children/adolescents

Treatment of overdose: ECG monitoring; induce emesis; lavage, activated charcoal; anticonvulsant

clonazepam (℞)
(kloe-na′zi-pam)
Klonopin, Rivotril ✦,
Syn-Clonazepam ✦
Func. class.: Anticonvulsant
Chem. class.: Benzodiazepine derivative

Controlled Substance Schedule IV
Do not confuse:
clonazepam/lorazepam/clorazepate
Klonopin/clonidine

Action: Inhibits spike, wave formation in absence seizures (petit mal), decreases amplitude, frequency, duration, spread of discharge in minor motor seizures

Uses: Absence, atypical absence, akinetic, myoclonic seizures, Lennox-Gastaut syndrome

Unlabeled uses: Parkinsonian dysarthrosis, acute manic episodes, adjunction schizophrenia, neuralgias, multifocal tic disorders, restless leg syndrome, rectal administration

DOSAGE AND ROUTES
• *Adult:* **PO** not to exceed 1.5 mg/day in 3 divided doses; may be increased 0.5-1 mg q3d until desired response, not to exceed 20 mg/day; rectal 0.02 mg/kg
• *Geriatric:* **PO** 0.25 daily-bid initially, increase by 0.25 daily q7-14d as needed
• *Child <10 yr or <30 kg:* **PO** 0.01-0.03 mg/kg/day in divided doses q8h, not to exceed 0.05 mg/kg/day; may be increased 0.25-0.5 mg q3d until desired response, not to exceed 0.1-0.2 mg/kg/day; rectal 0.05-0.1 mg/kg

⚠ Safety alert   *"Tall Man" lettering

Available forms: Tabs 0.5, 1, 2 mg; orally disintegrating tabs 0.125, 0.25, 0.5, 1, 2 mg

SIDE EFFECTS

CNS: Drowsiness, dizziness, confusion, behavioral changes, tremors, insomnia, headache, **suicidal tendencies,** slurred speech
CV: Palpitations, bradycardia, tachycardia
EENT: Increased salivation, nystagmus, diplopia, abnormal eye movements
GI: Nausea, constipation, polyphagia, anorexia, xerostomia, diarrhea, gastritis, sore gums
GU: Dysuria, enuresis, nocturia, retention, libido changes
HEMA: **Thrombocytopenia, leukocytosis, eosinophilia**
INTEG: Rash, alopecia, hirsutism
RESP: **Respiratory depression,** dyspnea, congestion

Contraindications: Hypersensitivity to benzodiazepines, acute narrow-angle glaucoma, psychosis, severe hepatic disease
Precautions: Pregnancy (C), open-angle glaucoma, chronic respiratory disease, lactation, renal/hepatic disease, geriatric

PHARMACOKINETICS

PO: Peak 1-2 hr; metabolized by liver; excreted in urine; half-life 18-50 hr, duration 6-12 hr

INTERACTIONS

Increase: CNS depression—alcohol, barbiturates, opiates, antidepressants, other anticonvulsants, general anesthetics, hypnotics, sedatives
Decrease: clonazepam effect—carbamazepine, phenobarbital, phenytoin
Drug/Herb
Increase: CNS depression—kava
Increase: clonazepam effect—ginkgo
Decrease: clonazepam effect—ginseng, santonica

Drug/Lab Test
Increase: AST, alk phos

NURSING CONSIDERATIONS
Assess:
• Renal studies: urinalysis, BUN, urine creatinine
• Blood studies: RBC, Hct, Hgb, reticulocyte counts qwk for 4 wk, then qmo
• Hepatic studies: ALT, AST, bilirubin, creatinine
• Drug levels during initial treatment (therapeutic 20-80 ng/ml)
• Signs of physical withdrawal if medication suddenly discontinued
• Mental status: mood, sensorium, affect, oversedation, behavioral changes; if mental status changes, notify prescriber
• Eye problems: need for ophthalmic exam before, during, after treatment (slit lamp, funduscopy, tonometry)
• Allergic reaction: red, raised rash; drug should be discontinued
⚠ Blood dyscrasias: fever, sore throat, bruising, rash, jaundice
• Toxicity: bone marrow depression, nausea, vomiting, ataxia, diplopia, cardiovascular collapse
Administer:
PO route
• With food, milk for GI symptoms
• Avoid use with CNS depressants
Perform/provide:
• Storage at room temperature
• Assistance with ambulation during early part of treatment; dizziness occurs, especially geriatric
Evaluate:
• Therapeutic response: decreased seizure activity, document on patient's chart
Teach patient/family:
• To carry emergency ID bracelet stating name, drugs taken, condition, prescriber's name, phone number
• To avoid driving, other activities that require alertness

• To avoid alcohol ingestion; increased sedation may occur
• Not to discontinue medication quickly after long-term use; taper off over several wk

Treatment of overdose: Lavage, activated charcoal, monitor electrolytes, VS, administer vasopressors

---

clonidine (℞)
(klon'i-deen)
Catapres, Catapres-TTS, clonidine HCl, Dixarit ✦, Duraclon
Func. class.: Antihypertensive
Chem. class.: Central α-adrenergic agonist

Do not confuse:
clonidine/Klonopin/clonazepam
Catapres/Cataflam/Catarase

Action: Inhibits sympathetic vasomotor center in CNS, which reduces impulses in sympathetic nervous system; blood pressure, pulse rate, cardiac output decrease, prevents pain signal transmission in CNS by α-adrenergic receptor stimulation of the spinal cord

Uses: Mild to moderate hypertension, used alone or in combination; severe pain in cancer patients (epidural)

Unlabeled uses: Opioid withdrawal, prevention of vascular headaches, treatment of menopausal symptoms, dysmenorrhea, attention deficit hyperactivity disorder (ADHD), autism, cycloSPORINE nephrotoxicity prophylaxis, diabetic neuropathy, ethanol withdrawal, Tourette's syndrome

DOSAGE AND ROUTES

Hypertension
• *Adult:* **PO/TD** 0.1 mg bid, then increase by 0.1-0.2 mg/day at weekly intervals, until desired response; range 0.2-0.6 mg/day in divided doses
• *Geriatric:* **PO** 0.1 mg at bedtime, may increase gradually
• *Child:* 5-10 mcg/kg/day in divided doses q8-12h, max 0.9 mg/day

Severe pain
• *Adult:* **CONT EPIDURAL INF** 30 mcg/hr
• *Child:* **CONT EPIDURAL INF** 0.5 mcg/kg/hr, then titrate to response

Opioid withdrawal (unlabeled)
• *Adult:* **PO** 0.3-1.2 mg/day; may decrease by 50% × 3 days then decrease by 0.1-0.2 mg/day or discontinue

ADHD (unlabeled)
• *Child:* 5 mcg/kg/day in 3-4 divided doses × 8 wk, max 0.3 mg/day

Menopausal symptoms (unlabeled)
• *Adult:* **TD** 0.1 mg patch q1wk; **PO** 0.05-0.4 mg daily

Available forms: Tabs 0.025 ✦, 0.1, 0.2, 0.3 mg; trans 2.5, 5, 7.5 mg delivering 0.1, 0.2, 0.3 mg/24 hr, respectively; inj 100, 500 mcg/ml

SIDE EFFECTS

CNS: Drowsiness, sedation, headache, fatigue, nightmares, insomnia, mental changes, anxiety, depression, hallucinations, delirium
CV: Orthostatic hypotension, palpitations, **CHF**, ECG abnormalities
EENT: Taste change, parotid pain
ENDO: Hyperglycemia
GI: Nausea, vomiting, malaise, constipation, dry mouth
GU: Impotence, dysuria, nocturia, gynecomastia
INTEG: Rash, alopecia, facial pallor, pruritus, hives, edema, burning papules, excoriation (transdermal patches)
MISC: Withdrawal symptoms
MS: Muscle, joint pain; leg cramps

Contraindications: Hypersensitivity; (epidural) bleeding disorders, anticoagulants

Precautions: Pregnancy (C), MI (recent), diabetes mellitus, chronic renal failure, Raynaud's disease, thyroid disease, depression, COPD, child <12 yr (transdermal), asthma, lactation, geriatric, noncompliant patients

PHARMACOKINETICS

Absorbed well

PO: Onset ½ to 1 hr, peak 2-4 hr, duration 8-12 hr; half-life 6-12 hr

TD: Onset 3 days, duration 1 wk; metabolized by liver (metabolites), excreted in urine (30% unchanged, inactive metabolites), feces; crosses blood-brain barrier, excreted in breast milk

INTERACTIONS

• AV block: verapamil

⚠ Life-threatening elevations of B/P: tricyclics, β-blockers

Increase: CNS depression—opiates, sedatives, hypnotics, anesthetics, alcohol

Increase: hypotensive effects—diuretics, other antihypertensive nitrates

Decrease: hypotensive effects—tricyclics, MAOIs, appetite suppressants, amphetamines, prazosin

Decrease: effect of levodopa

Drug/Herb

• Toxicity/death: aconite

Increase: antihypertensive effect—barberry, betony, black catechu, black cohosh, bloodroot, broom, burdock, cat's claw, dandelion, goldenseal, hawthorn, Irish moss, Jamaican dogwood, kelp, khella, mistletoe, parsley, Queen Anne's lace, rue

Decrease: antihypertensive effect—astragalus, capsicum peppers, cola tree, coltsfoot, guarana, khat, licorice, yohimbine

Drug/Lab Test

Increase: Blood glucose

Decrease: VMA, urinary catecholamines, aldosterone

NURSING CONSIDERATIONS

Assess:

• Blood studies: neutrophils, decreased platelets

• Renal studies: protein, BUN, creatinine; increased levels may indicate nephrotic syndrome

• Baselines in renal, hepatic studies before therapy begins; potassium levels, although hyperkalemia rare

• B/P, pulse if used for hypertension, report significant changes

• For opiate withdrawal including fever, diarrhea, nausea, vomiting, cramps, insomnia, shivering, dilated pupils

• Pain: location, intensity, character; alleviating, aggravating factors, baseline and frequently

• Edema in feet, legs daily; monitor I&O; check for falling output

• Allergic reaction: rash, fever, pruritus, urticaria; drug should be discontinued if antihistamines fail to help

• Allergic reaction from patches: rash, urticaria, angioedema; should not continue to use

• Symptoms of CHF: edema, dyspnea, wet crackles, B/P

• Renal symptoms: polyuria, oliguria, frequency

Administer:

PO route

• Give last dose at bedtime

Transdermal route

• Qwk; apply to site without hair; best absorption over chest or upper arm; rotate sites with each application; clean site before application; apply firmly, especially around edges

Epidural route

• Used for severe cancer pain

• May be used with opiates

• Use only if familiar with epidural infusion devices

Perform/provide:

• Storage of patches in cool environment, tablets in tight container

Evaluate:

• Therapeutic response: decrease in B/P in hypertension, decrease in withdrawal symptoms (opioid), decrease in pain

Teach patient/family:

• To avoid hazardous activities, since drug may cause drowsiness

• To notify all health care providers of medication use

• Not to discontinue drug abruptly or withdrawal symptoms may occur: anxiety, increased B/P, headache, insomnia, increased pulse, tremors, nausea, sweating

---

- Not to use OTC (cough, cold, or allergy) products unless directed by prescriber
- To comply with dosage schedule even if feeling better
- To rise slowly to sitting or standing position to minimize orthostatic hypotension, especially geriatric
- To notify prescriber of mouth sores, sore throat, fever, swelling of hands, feet, irregular heartbeat, chest pain, signs of angioedema
- About excessive perspiration, dehydration, vomiting; diarrhea may lead to fall in blood pressure; consult prescriber if these occur
- That drug may cause dizziness, fainting; lightheadedness may occur during first few days of therapy
- That drug may cause dry mouth; use hard candy, saliva product, or frequent rinsing of mouth
- That compliance is necessary; not to skip or stop drug unless directed by prescriber
- That drug may cause skin rash or impaired perspiration
- To use patch; patch comes in two parts: drug patch and overlay to keep patch in place, do not trim or cut patch
- That response may take 2-3 days if drug is given transdermally; instruct on administration of patch, if switching from tabs to patch, taper tabs to avoid withdrawal

Treatment of overdose: Supportive treatment; administer tolazoline, atropine, DOPamine prn

---

clopidogrel (℞)

(klo-pid′oh-grel)

Plavix

Func. class.: Platelet aggregation inhibitor

Chem. class.: Thienopyridine derivative

Do not confuse:

Plavix/Paxil/Elavil

Action: Inhibits first and second phases of ADP-induced effects in platelet aggregation

Uses: Reducing the risk of stroke, MI, peripheral arterial disease in high-risk patients, acute coronary syndrome, transient ischemic attack (TIA), unstable angina

DOSAGE AND ROUTES

Recent MI, stroke, peripheral arterial disease

- *Adult:* **PO** 75 mg daily with or without food

Acute coronary syndrome

- *Adult:* **PO** loading dose 300 mg then 75 mg daily

Available forms: Tabs 75 mg

SIDE EFFECTS

CNS: Headache, dizziness, depression, syncope, hypesthesia, neuralgia

CV: Edema, hypertension

GI: Nausea, vomiting, diarrhea, GI discomfort, **GI bleeding**

HEMA: Epistaxis, purpura, **bleeding, neutropenia**

INTEG: Rash, pruritus

MISC: UTI, hypercholesterolemia, chest pain, fatigue, **intracranial hemorrhage**

MS: Arthralgia, back pain

RESP: Upper respiratory tract infection, dyspnea, rhinitis, bronchitis, cough

Contraindications: Hypersensitivity, active bleeding

Precautions: Pregnancy (B), past hepatic disease, lactation, children, increased bleeding risk, neutropenia, agranulocytosis, renal disease

PHARMACOKINETICS

Rapidly absorbed; peak 1-3 hr; metabolized by liver (CYP3A); excreted in urine, feces; half-life 8 hr; plasma protein binding 95%; effect on platelets after 3-7 days

INTERACTIONS

Increase: bleeding risk—anticoagulants, aspirin, NSAIDs, abciximab, eptifibatide, tirofiban, thrombolytics, ticlopidine

---

Increase: action of—some NSAIDs, phenytoin, TOLBUTamide, tamoxifen, torsemide, fluvastatin, warfarin

Drug/Herb

Increase: clopidogrel effect—bogbean, dong quai, feverfew, garlic, ginger, ginkgo biloba, green tea, horse chestnut

Increase: gastric irritation—arginine

Decrease: clopidogrel effect—bilberry, saw palmetto

Drug/Lab Test

Increase: AST, ALT, bilirubin, uric acid, total cholesterol, nonprotein nitrogen (NPN)

NURSING CONSIDERATIONS

Assess:

⚠ Thrombotic/thrombocytic purpura: fever, thrombocytopenia, neurolytic anemia

• For symptoms of stroke, MI during treatment

• Hepatic studies: AST, ALT, bilirubin, creatinine (long-term therapy)

• Blood studies: CBC, diff, Hct, Hgb, PT, cholesterol (long-term therapy)

Administer:

• With food to decrease gastric symptoms

Evaluate:

• Therapeutic response: absence of stroke, MI

Teach patient/family:

• That blood work will be necessary during treatment

• To report any unusual bruising, bleeding to prescriber, that it may take longer to stop bleeding

• To take with food or just after eating to minimize GI discomfort

• To report diarrhea, skin rashes, subcutaneous bleeding, chills, fever, sore throat

• To tell all health care providers that clopidogrel is used; may be held 3-7 days before surgery

---

clorazepate (℞)

(klor-az'e-pate)
Apo-Clorazepate ❧, clorazepate, Gen-XENE, Novo-Clopate ❧, Tranxene-SD, Tranxene-SD Half Strength, Tranxene T-tab

Func. class.: Antianxiety, anticonvulsant, sedative/hypnotic

Chem. class.: Benzodiazepine

Controlled Substance Schedule IV

Do not confuse:

clorazepate/clonazepam

Action: Potentiates the actions of GABA, especially in limbic system, reticular formation

Uses: Anxiety, acute alcohol withdrawal, adjunct in seizure disorders

Unlabeled uses: Insomnia

DOSAGE AND ROUTES

Anxiety

• *Adult:* **PO** 15-60 mg/day or 7.5-15 mg 2-4×/day; **EXT REL** 11.25-22.5 mg at bedtime, do not use **EXT REL** to initiate therapy

• *Geriatric:* **PO** 7.5 mg daily-bid

Alcohol withdrawal

• *Adult:* **PO** 30 mg then 30-60 mg in divided doses; day 2, 45-90 mg in divided doses; day 3, 22.5-45 mg in divided doses; day 4, 15-30 mg in divided doses; then gradually reduce daily dose to 7.5-15 mg

Seizure disorders

• *Adult and child >12 yr:* **PO** 7.5 mg tid; may increase by 7.5 mg/wk or less, not to exceed 90 mg/day

• *Child 9-12 yr:* **PO** 3.75-7.5 mg bid; may increase by 3.75 mg/wk or less, not to exceed 60 mg/day

Insomnia (unlabeled)

• *Adult:* **PO** 7.5-15 mg at bedtime

• *Geriatric:* **PO** 3.75-7.5 mg at bedtime; max 15 mg at bedtime

---

Available forms: Tabs 3.75, 7.5, 15 mg; ext rel tab (Tranxene-SD Half Strength) 11.25 mg; (Tranxene-SD) 22.5 mg

SIDE EFFECTS

CNS: Dizziness, drowsiness, confusion, headache, anxiety, tremors, stimulation, fatigue, depression, insomnia, hallucinations, lethargy
CV: Orthostatic hypotension, **ECG changes, tachycardia,** hypotension, chest pain
EENT: Blurred vision, tinnitus, mydriasis
GI: Constipation, dry mouth, nausea, vomiting, anorexia, diarrhea
INTEG: Rash, dermatitis, itching
Contraindications: Pregnancy (D), hypersensitivity to benzodiazepines, narrow-angle glaucoma, psychosis, lactation, child <9 yr
Precautions: Geriatric, debilitated, renal/hepatic disease

PHARMACOKINETICS

PO: Onset 1 hr, peak 1-2 hr, duration up to 24 hr; metabolized by liver, excreted by kidneys; crosses placenta, breast milk; half-life 30-100 hr

INTERACTIONS

Increase: clorazepate effects—CNS depressants, alcohol, valproic acid, antidepressants, MAOIs, cimetidine, oral contraceptives, disulfiram, fluoxetine, isoniazid, ketoconazole, propoxyphene, some β-blockers
Decrease: clorazepate action—rifampin, barbiturates
Drug/Herb
Increase: CNS depression—catnip, chamomile, clary, cowslip, kava, mistletoe, nettle, pokeweed, poppy, Queen Anne's lace, senega, valerian
Increase: hypotension—black cohosh
Drug/Lab Test
Increase: AST, ALT
Decrease: Hct

NURSING CONSIDERATIONS

Assess:
• B/P (lying, standing), pulse; if systolic B/P drops 20 mm Hg, hold drug, notify prescriber
• Blood studies: CBC during long-term therapy; blood dyscrasias have occurred rarely
• Hepatic studies: AST, ALT, bilirubin, creatinine, LDH, alk phos
• I&O; may indicate renal dysfunction
• Mental status: mood, sensorium, affect, sleeping pattern, drowsiness, dizziness; for delirium, tremors, hallucination in alcohol withdrawal
• Physical dependency, withdrawal symptoms: headache, nausea, vomiting, muscle pain, weakness after long-term use
• Suicidal tendencies, anxiety level
• Seizures: location, duration, intensity
Administer:
• Do not break, crush, or chew ext rel product
• With food, milk for GI symptoms
• Crushed if patient cannot swallow whole (tab only)
Perform/provide:
• Assistance with ambulation during beginning therapy because of drowsiness/dizziness, especially geriatric
• Safety measures, including side rails
• Check to see PO medication has been swallowed
• Sugarless gum, hard candy, frequent sips of water for dry mouth
Evaluate:
• Therapeutic response: decreased anxiety, restlessness, insomnia
Teach patient/family:
• That drug may be taken with food
• That drug is not to be used for everyday stress or used longer than 4 mo unless directed by prescriber; not to take more than prescribed amount; may be habit forming
• To avoid OTC preparations unless approved by prescriber
• To avoid driving, activities that require alertness; drowsiness may occur, especially in geriatric

---

⚠ Safety alert   *"Tall Man" lettering

• To avoid alcohol ingestion, other psychotropic medications, unless directed by prescriber
• Not to discontinue medication abruptly after long-term use; restlessness, insomnia, irritability may occur
• To rise slowly because fainting may occur
• That drowsiness may worsen at beginning of treatment
Treatment of overdose: Lavage, VS, supportive care, flumazenil

clotrimazole topical
See Appendix C

clotrimazole vaginal antifungal
See Appendix C

cloxacillin (℞)
(klox-a-sill'in)
Apo-Cloxi ✦, cloxacillin, Cloxapen, Novo-Cloxin ✦, Nu-Clox ✦ Orbenin ✦
Func. class.: Broad-spectrum antiinfective, penicillin
Chem. class.: Penicillinase-resistant penicillin

Action: Interferes with cell wall replication of susceptible organisms; the cell wall, rendered osmotically unstable, swells, bursts from osmotic pressure, lysis mediated by cell wall autolytic enzymes; resists the penicillinase action that inactivates penicillin
Uses: Gram-positive cocci (*Staphylococcus aureus, Streptococcus pyogenes, Streptococcus pneumoniae*), penicillinase-producing staphylococci
Unlabeled uses: Bone/joint infection, endocarditis septicemia

DOSAGE AND ROUTES
• *Adult:* **PO** 1-4 g/day in divided doses q6h, max 6 g/day
• *Child:* **PO** 50-100 mg/kg in divided doses q6h, max 4 g/day
Available forms: Caps 250, 500 mg; oral sol 125 mg/5 ml

SIDE EFFECTS
CNS: Lethargy, hallucinations, anxiety, depression, twitching, **coma, seizures**
GI: Nausea, vomiting, diarrhea, increased AST, ALT, abdominal pain, glossitis, colitis, **pseudomembranous colitis**
GU: **Oliguria, proteinuria,** hematuria, *vaginitis, moniliasis,* **glomerulonephritis**
HEMA: Anemia, increased bleeding time, **bone marrow depression, granulocytopenia**
SYST: **Anaphylaxis, serum sickness**
Contraindications: Hypersensitivity to penicillins; imipenem; neonates, severe renal/hepatic disease
Precautions: Pregnancy (B), lactation, hypersensitivity to cephalosporins

PHARMACOKINETICS
PO: Peak 1 hr, duration 6 hr; half-life 30-60 min; metabolized in liver; excreted in urine, bile, breast milk; crosses placenta, poor penetration in CSF

INTERACTIONS
Increase: cloxacillin concentrations—probenecid
Increase: action of anticoagulants
Decrease: effectiveness of oral contraceptives—cloxacillin
Drug/Herb
• Do not use acidophilus with antiinfectives; separate by several hours
Decrease: absorption—khat
Drug/Food
• Citric juices/food decrease absorption of cloxacillin
Drug/Lab Test
Decrease: Uric acid

False positive: Urine glucose, urine protein

NURSING CONSIDERATIONS
Assess:

⚠ Anaphylaxis: pruritus, rash, dyspnea, laryngeal edema; have emergency equipment available; skin eruptions after administration of penicillin to 1 wk after discontinuing drug
• For infection: temp, draining wounds, WBC, sputum, urine, stool before and during treatment
• I&O ratio; report hematuria, oliguria, since penicillin in high doses is nephrotoxic

⚠ Any patient with compromised renal system, since drug is excreted slowly in poor renal system function; toxicity may occur rapidly
• Hepatic studies: AST, ALT
• Blood studies: WBC, RBC, Hgb, Hct, bleeding time
• Renal studies: urinalysis, protein, blood
• C&S before drug therapy; drug may be taken as soon as culture is taken
• Bowel pattern before, during treatment, report diarrhea

Administer:
• Do not break, crush, or chew caps
• After C&S completed
• Shake suspension well before each dose

Perform/provide:
• Adrenaline, suction, tracheostomy set, endotracheal intubation equipment on unit
• Adequate intake of fluids (2 L) during diarrhea episodes
• Scratch test to assess allergy after securing order from prescriber; usually done when penicillin is only drug of choice
• Storage in tight container; after reconstituting, store in refrigerator for 2 wk, room temperature 3 days

Evaluate:
• Therapeutic response: absence of fever, draining wounds

Teach patient/family:
• All aspects of drug therapy, including need to complete entire course of medi-

cation to ensure organism death (10-14 days); culture may be taken after course of medication completed
• To report sore throat, fever, fatigue (may indicate superinfection)
• To wear or carry emergency ID if allergic to penicillins
• To notify prescriber of diarrhea, fever
• To take on an empty stomach with a full glass of water

Treatment of overdose: Withdraw drug; maintain airway; administer epiNEPHrine, aminophylline, O_2, IV corticosteroids for anaphylaxis

---

clozapine (℞)
(kloz'a-peen)
clozapine, Clozaril, Faza Clo
Func. class.: Antipsychotic
Chem. class.: Tricyclic dibenzodiazepine derivative

Do not confuse:
Clozaril/Clinoril/Colazal

Action: Interferes with dopamine receptor binding with lack of EPS; also acts as an adrenergic, cholinergic, histaminergic, serotonergic antagonist

Uses: Management of psychotic symptoms in schizophrenic patients for whom other antipsychotics have failed, recurrent suicidal behavior; orally disintegrating tabs are not used for recurrent suicidal behavior

Unlabeled uses: Agitation, bipolar disorder, dementia, tremor in Parkinson's disease

DOSAGE AND ROUTES
• *Adult:* **PO** 12.5 mg daily or bid; may increase by 25-50 mg/day; normal range 300-450 mg/day after 2 wk; do not increase dose more than 2 × per wk; max 900 mg/day; use lowest dose to control symptoms

Tremor in Parkinson's disease (unlabeled)
• *Adult:* **PO** 40 mg at bedtime

⚠ Safety alert   *"Tall Man" lettering

*Dementia with multiple behavioral
disturbances (unlabeled)*
• *Geriatric:* **PO** 12.5 mg, may increase
by 12.5 mg every other day, max 50 mg
daily

Available forms: Tabs 12.5, 25, 50,
100, 200 mg; orally disintegrating tabs 25,
100 mg

SIDE EFFECTS

CNS: **Neuroleptic malignant syndrome,**
*sedation, salivation, dizziness, headache,
tremors, sleep problems, akinesia, fever,*
seizures, *sweating, akathisia, confusion, fatigue, insomnia,* depression,
slurred speech, anxiety, *agitation*
*CV: Tachycardia, hypotension, hyperten-
sion,* chest pain, ECG changes, orthostatic hypotension
EENT: Blurred vision
*GI: Drooling or excessive salivation,
constipation, nausea, abdominal discomfort, vomiting, diarrhea,* anorexia,
weight gain, dry mouth, heartburn, *dyspepsia, gastroesophageal reflux*
GU: Urinary abnormalities, incontinence,
ejaculation dysfunction, frequency, urgency, retention, dysuria
HEMA: **Leukopenia, agranulocytosis,
eosinophilia**
MS: Weakness; pain in back, neck, legs;
spasm, *rigidity*
OTHER: Diaphoresis
RESP: Dyspnea, nasal congestion

Contraindications: Hypersensitivity,
myeloproliferative disorders, severe granulocytopenia (WBC <3500 before therapy), severe CNS depression, coma, uncontrolled epilepsy

Precautions: Pregnancy (B); lactation;
children <16; renal/hepatic/cardiac disease; seizures; prostatic enlargement; geriatric, narrow-angle glaucoma

PHARMACOKINETICS

Bioavailability 27%-47%, steady state
2.5 hr; 97% protein bound; completely
metabolized by liver enzymes involved
in metabolism CYP1A2, 2D6, 3A4; excreted in urine (50%) and feces (30%)
(metabolites); half-life 8-12 hr

INTERACTIONS

Increase: CNS depression—CNS depressants, psychoactives, alcohol
Increase: clozapine level—caffeine, citalopram, fluoxetine, sertraline, ritonavir,
risperidone, CYP1A2 inhibitors (fluvoxa-
nine), CYP3A4 inhibitors (ketoconazole,
erythromycin)
Increase: plasma concentration—
warfarin, digoxin, other highly protein-
bound drugs
Increase: hypotension, respiratory, cardiac arrest, collapse—benzodiazepines
Decrease: clozapine level—CYP1A2 inducers (carbamazepine, omeprazole, rifampin); phenobarbital

Drug/Herb
Increase: CNS depression—kava, St.
John's wort
Increase: EPS—betel palm, kava
Increase: clozapine action—cola tree,
hops, nettle, nutmeg

Drug/Lab Test
Increase: LFTs, cardiac enzymes, choles-
terol, blood glucose, bilirubin, PBI,
cholinesterase, [131]I
False positive: Pregnancy tests, PKU
False negative: Urinary steroids, 17-
OHCS

NURSING CONSIDERATIONS

Assess:
• For myocarditis, if suspected, discontinue use; myocarditis usually occurs during first month of treatment
• For seizures, usually occurs with higher
doses
• I&O ratio; obtain baseline before treatment begins; palpate bladder if low urinary output occurs
• Bilirubin, CBC, LFTs monthly; discontinue treatment if WBC <3000/mm^3 or
ANC <1500/mm^3; may resume
when normal; if WBC <2000/mm^3 or ANC
<1000/mm^3 discontinue
• Urinalysis is recommended before, during prolonged therapy
• Affect, orientation, LOC, reflexes, gait,
coordination, sleep pattern disturbances
• B/P standing and lying; take pulse and

respirations q4h during initial treatment; establish baseline before starting treatment; report drops of 30 mm Hg

• Dizziness, faintness, palpitations, tachycardia on rising

• EPS including akathisia (inability to sit still, no pattern to movements), tardive dyskinesia (bizarre movements of the jaw, mouth, tongue, extremities), pseudoparkinsonism (rigidity, tremors, pill rolling, shuffling gait)

A For neuroleptic malignant syndrome: tachycardia, seizures, fever, dyspnea, diaphoresis, increased or decreased B/P, notify prescriber immediately

• Constipation, urinary retention daily; if these occur, increase bulk, water in diet, especially geriatric, stool softeners, laxatives may be needed

• If diabetic, check blood glucose levels

Administer:
• Check for swallowing of PO medication; monitor for hoarding or giving of medication to other patients, if hospitalized; avoid giving patient over 7 days medication if outpatient

• Orally disintegrating tab: do not push through foil, leave in foil blister until ready to take, peel back foil, place tab in mouth, allow to dissolve, swallow; water is not needed

Perform/provide:
• Supervised ambulation until stabilized on medication; do not involve in strenuous exercise program because fainting is possible; patient should not stand still for long periods

• Storage in tight, light-resistant container

Evaluate:
• Therapeutic response: decrease in emotional excitement, hallucinations, delusions, paranoia, reorganization of patterns of thought, speech

Teach patient/family:
• About symptoms of agranulocytosis and need for blood tests qwk for 6 mo, then q2wk; report flulike symptoms

• That orthostatic hypotension often occurs, and to rise gradually from sitting or lying position; to avoid hot tubs, hot showers, tub baths; hypotension may occur

• To avoid abrupt withdrawal of this drug because EPS may result; drug should be withdrawn over 1-2 wk

• To avoid OTC preparations (cough, hay fever, cold) unless approved by prescriber, since serious drug interactions may occur; avoid use with alcohol or CNS depressants, increased drowsiness may occur

• About compliance with drug regimen

• About EPS and necessity for meticulous oral hygiene, since oral candidiasis may occur

• To report sore throat, malaise, fever, bleeding, mouth sores; if these occur, CBC should be drawn and drug discontinued

• That heat stroke may occur in hot weather; take extra precautions to stay cool

• To avoid driving, other hazardous activities; seizures may occur

• To notify prescriber if pregnant or if pregnancy is intended, not to breastfeed

Treatment of overdose: Lavage, activated charcoal; provide an airway; do not induce vomiting

---

A High Alert

coagulation factor VIIa, recombinant (℞)

NovoSeven
Func. class.: Antihemophilic

Action: Promotes hemostasis by activating the intrinsic pathway of coagulation

Uses: Bleeding in hemophilia A or B, with inhibitors to factor VIII or IX

Unlabeled uses: Coumarin toxicity, factor VII deficiency

DOSAGE AND ROUTES

• *Adult:* **IV BOL** 90 mcg/kg q2h until hemostasis occurs, or until therapy is deemed to be inadequate; posthemostatic doses q3-6h may be required

Available forms: Lyophilized powder 1.2 mg/vial (1200 mcg/vial), 4.8 mg/vial (4800 mcg/vial) recombinant human coagulation factor VIIa (rFVIIa)

SIDE EFFECTS

CNS: Fever, headache
INTEG: Pain, redness at inj site, pruritus, purpura, rash
SYST: **Hemorrhage NOS, hemarthrosis, fibrinogen plasma decreased,** hypertension, bradycardia, **DIC, coagulation disorder, thrombosis**
Contraindications: Hypersensitivity to this product or mouse, hamster, or bovine products
Precautions: Pregnancy (C), lactation, children

PHARMACOKINETICS

Half-life 2.3 hr

INTERACTIONS

• Do not use with activated prothrombin complex concentrates or prothrombin complex concentrate

NURSING CONSIDERATIONS
Assess:
• VS, B/P, pulse, respirations, neurologic signs, temp at least q4h, temp 104° F (40° C) or indicators of internal bleeding, cardiac rhythm
• PT, aPTT, plasma FVII clotting
• For thrombosis, dose should be reduced or stopped
Administer:
IV route
• Bring to room temperature; for 1.2 mg vial/2.2 ml sterile water for inj; 4.8 mg vial/8.5 ml sterile water for inj
• Remove caps from stop, cleanse stopper with alcohol, allow to dry, draw back plunger of sterile syringe and allow air into syringe, insert needle of syringe into sterile water for inj, inject the air and withdraw amount required, insert syringe needle with diluent into drug vial, aim to side so liquid runs down vial wall, gently swirl until dissolved, use within 3 hr, give by bol over 3-5 min
• Do not admix, keep refrigerated until ready to use, avoid sunlight
Evaluate:
• Therapeutic response: hemostasis

---

codeine (ꝶ)
(koe'deen)
Paveral ♣
Func. class.: Opiate analgesic, antitussive
Chem. class.: Opiate, phenathrene derivative

Controlled Substance Schedule II, III, IV, V (depends on content)
Do not confuse:
codeine/Lodine/iodine/Cardene
Action: Depresses pain impulse transmission at the spinal cord level by interacting with opioid receptors, decreases cough reflex, GI motility
Uses: Moderate to severe pain, nonproductive cough
Unlabeled uses: Diarrhea

DOSAGE AND ROUTES
Pain
• *Adult:* PO 15-60 mg q4h prn; **IM/SUBCUT** 15-60 mg q4h prn
• *Child:* **PO** 3 mg/kg/day in divided doses q4h prn
Cough
• *Adult:* **PO** 10-20 mg q4-6h, not to exceed 120 mg/day
• *Child:* **PO** 1-1.5 mg/kg/day in 4 divided doses, not to exceed 60 mg/day
Diarrhea (unlabeled)
• *Adult:* **PO** 30 mg; may repeat qid prn
Renal disease
• *Adult:* **PO** CCr 10-50 ml/min 75% of dose; CCr <10 ml/min 50% of dose
Available forms: Inj 30, 60 mg/ml; tabs 15, 30, 60 mg; oral sol 10 mg/5 ml, 15 mg/5 ml

SIDE EFFECTS

CNS: Drowsiness, sedation, dizziness, agitation, dependency, lethargy, restlessness, euphoria, **seizures**
CV: Bradycardia, palpitations, orthostatic hypotension, tachycardia, **circulatory collapse**
GI: Nausea, vomiting, anorexia, constipation

GU: Urinary retention

INTEG: Flushing, rash, urticaria, pruritus

RESP: **Respiratory depression, respiratory paralysis**

SYST: **Anaphylaxis**

Contraindications: Hypersensitivity to opiates, respiratory depression, increased intracranial pressure, seizure disorders, severe respiratory disorders

Precautions: Pregnancy (C), geriatric, cardiac dysrhythmias, lactation, prostatic hypertrophy

PHARMACOKINETICS

Bioavailability 60%-90%, onset 10-30 min, peak ½-1 hr, duration 4-6 hr; metabolized by liver; excreted by kidneys, in breast milk; crosses placenta; half-life 3 hr

INTERACTIONS

Increase: CNS depression—alcohol, opiates, sedative/hypnotics, antipsychotics, skeletal muscle relaxants

⚠ *Increase:* toxicity—MAOIs, use cautiously

Drug/Herb

Increase: CNS depression—Jamaican dogwood, kava, lavender, mistletoe, nettle, pokeweed, poppy, senega, valerian

Increase: anticholinergic effect—corkwood

Drug/Lab Test

Increase: Lipase, amylase

NURSING CONSIDERATIONS

Assess:

• I&O ratio; check for decreasing output; may indicate urinary retention, especially geriatric

• GI function: nausea, vomiting, constipation

• By using pain-scoring method

• For productive cough

• Cough: type, duration, ability to raise secretion

• CNS changes, dizziness, drowsiness, hallucinations, euphoria, LOC, pupil reaction

• Allergic reactions: rash, urticaria

⚠ Respiratory dysfunction: respiratory depression, character, rate, rhythm; notify prescriber if respirations are <10/ min, shallow

• Need for pain medication, tolerance

Administer:

IM/SUBCUT route

• Do not use if precipitate is present

• Usually given IM/SUBCUT

IV route

• Give slowly by direct inj

• With antiemetic for nausea, vomiting

• When pain is beginning to return; determine dosage interval by patient response

Syringe compatibilities: Glycopyrrolate, hydrOXYzine

Perform/provide:

• Storage in light-resistant container at room temperature

• Assistance with ambulation if needed

• Safety measures: top side rails, nightlight, call bell

Evaluate:

• Therapeutic response: decrease in pain, absence of grimacing, decreased cough; decreased diarrhea

Teach patient/family:

• To report any symptoms of CNS changes, allergic reactions

• That physical dependency may result after extended periods

• To change position slowly; orthostatic hypotension may occur

• To avoid hazardous activities if drowsiness, dizziness occurs

• To avoid alcohol, other CNS depressants unless directed by prescriber

---

colchicine (℞)

(kol'chi-seen)

Func. class.: Antigout agent

Chem. class.: Colchicum autumnale alkaloid

Action: Inhibits microtubule formation of lactic acid in leukocytes, which decreases phagocytosis and inflammation in joints

Uses: Gout, gouty arthritis (prevention,

---

treatment); to arrest progression of neurologic disability in multiple sclerosis

Unlabeled uses: Hepatic cirrhosis, Mediterranean fever, pericarditis, amyloidosis, Behçet's syndrome, biliary cirrhosis, dermatitis herpetiformis, idiopathic thrombocytopenic purpura, Paget's disease, pseudogout, pulmonary fibrosis

DOSAGE AND ROUTES

Gout prevention
• *Adult:* **PO** 0.6-1.8 mg daily depending on severity; **IV** 0.5-1 mg 1-2 × day
Gout treatment
• *Adult:* **PO** 0.6-1.2 mg, then 0.5-1.2 mg q1h, until pain decreases or side effects occur; **IV** 2 mg, then 0.5 mg q6h until response, max 4 mg total
Available forms: Tabs 0.5, 0.6, 1 🍁 mg; inj 0.5 mg/ml in 2 ml ampule

SIDE EFFECTS

GI: Nausea, vomiting, anorexia, malaise, metallic taste, cramps, peptic ulcer, diarrhea
GU: Hematuria, **oliguria, renal damage**
HEMA: **Agranulocytosis, thrombocytopenia, aplastic anemia, pancytopenia**
INTEG: Chills, dermatitis, pruritus, purpura, erythema
MISC: Myopathy, alopecia, reversible azoospermia, peripheral neuritis
Contraindications: Pregnancy (D), hypersensitivity; serious GI/renal/hepatic/cardiac disorders
Precautions: Blood dyscrasias, hepatic disease, geriatric, lactation, children

PHARMACOKINETICS

PO: Peak ½-2 hr, half-life 20 min; deacetylates in liver; excreted in feces (metabolites/active drug)

INTERACTIONS

Increase: Toxicity—cycloSPORINE, clarithromycin, erythromycin
Increase: GI effects—NSAIDs, ethanol

Increase: bone marrow depression—radiation, bone marrow depressants, cycloSPORINE
Decrease: action of vit B_{12}, may cause reversible malabsorption
Drug/Lab Test
Increase: Alk phos, AST
False positive: Urine, RBC, Hgb
Interference: Urinary 17-hydroxycorticosteroids

NURSING CONSIDERATIONS

Assess:
• I&O ratio; observe for decrease in urinary output
⚠ CBC, platelets, reticulocytes before, during therapy (q3mo), may cause aplastic anemia, agranulocytosis, decreased platelets
• For toxicity: weakness, abdominal pain, nausea, vomiting, diarrhea; drug should be discontinued
Administer:
PO route
• With food for GI symptoms
IV route
• Do not give IM or SUBCUT
• Do not dilute in D_5W, or change in IV line that contains D_5W
• Give over 2-5 min
• Wait ≥1 wk after giving a full course of IV colchicine before giving subsequent doses
Evaluate:
• Therapeutic response: decreased stone formation on x-ray, decreased pain in kidney region, absence of hematuria, decreased pain in joints
Teach patient/family:
• To avoid alcohol, OTC preparations that contain alcohol
• To report any pain, redness, or hard area, usually in legs; rash, sore throat, fever, bleeding, bruising, weakness, numbness, tingling
• The importance of complying with medical regimen (diet, weight loss, drug therapy); the possibility of bone marrow depression occurring
Treatment of overdose: D/C medication, may need opioids to treat diarrhea

---

🍁 Canada only   Side effects: *italics* = common; **bold** = life-threatening

colesevelam (Ⱥ)

(coal-see-vel'am)
Welchol
Func. class.: Antilipemic
Chem. class.: Bile acid sequestrant

Action: Absorbs, combines with bile acids to form insoluble complex that is excreted through feces; loss of bile acids lowers cholesterol levels

Uses: Elevated LDL cholesterol, alone or in combination with HMG-CoA reductase inhibitor

DOSAGE AND ROUTES

• *Adult:* **PO** Monotherapy: 3 625-mg tabs bid with meals or 6 tabs daily with a meal; may increase to 7 tabs if needed
• *Adult:* **PO** Combination therapy: 3 tabs bid with meals or 6 tabs daily with a meal given with an HMG-CoA reductase inhibitor

Available forms: Tabs 625 mg

SIDE EFFECTS

CNS: Headache, dizziness, drowsiness, vertigo, tinnitus
GI: Constipation, abdominal pain, nausea, fecal impaction, hemorrhoids, flatulence, vomiting, steatorrhea, peptic ulcer
HEMA: Decreased red cell folate content; **bleeding,** increased PT
INTEG: Rash, irritation of perianal area, tongue, skin
META: Decreased vit A, D, K; **hyperchloremic acidosis**
MS: Muscle, joint pain

Contraindications: Hypersensitivity, biliary obstruction, dysphagia, swallowing disorders, bowel disease, primary biliary cirrhosis, triglycerides > 300 mg/dl, fat soluble vitamin deficiency

Precautions: Pregnancy (C), lactation, children

PHARMACOKINETICS

PO: Excreted in feces, peak response 2 wk

INTERACTIONS

Decrease: absorption of diltiazem, gemfibrozil, glipiZIDE, mycophenolate, phenytoin, propranolol, warfarin, thiazides, digitalis, penicillin G, tetracyclines, corticosteroids, iron, thyroid, clindamycin, fat-soluble vitamins

Drug/Herb
Increase: effect—glucomannan
Decrease: antilipidemic effect—gotu kola

Drug/Lab Test
Increase: LFTs

NURSING CONSIDERATIONS

Assess:
• Cardiac glycoside level, if both drugs are being administered
• For signs of vit A, D, K deficiency
• Fasting LDL, HDL, total cholesterol, triglyceride levels, electrolytes if on extended therapy
• Bowel pattern daily; increase bulk, H_2O in diet for constipation

Administer:
• Drug daily or bid with meals; give all other medications 1 hr before colesevelam or 4 hr after colesevelam; to avoid poor absorption take with liquid
• Supplemental doses of vit A, D, K, if levels are low

Evaluate:
• Therapeutic response: decreased total cholesterol level, LDL cholesterol, apolipoproteins (hyperlipidemia); diarrhea, pruritus (excess bile acids)

Teach patient/family:
⚠ The symptoms of hypoprothrombinemia: bleeding mucous membranes, dark tarry stools, hematuria, petechiae; report immediately
• The importance of compliance; toxicity may result if doses missed
• That risk factors should be decreased: high-fat diet, smoking, alcohol consumption, absence of exercise
• Not to discontinue suddenly

⚠ Safety alert   *"Tall Man" lettering

colestipol (℞)

(koe-les'ti-pole)

Colestid

Func. class.: Antilipemic

Chem. class.: Bile acid sequestrant

Action: Absorbs, combines with bile acids to form insoluble complex excreted through feces; loss of bile acids lowers cholesterol levels

Uses: Primary hypercholesterolemia, xanthomas

Unlabeled uses: Digotoxin toxicity/overdose, digoxin overdose, pruritus, diarrhea due to increased bile acids after surgery

DOSAGE AND ROUTES

• *Adult:* **PO** tabs 2 g daily-bid, may increase q1mo, max 16 g/day; powder 5-30 g mixed with liquid daily or in divided doses

Digotoxin toxicity/overdose, digoxin overdose (unlabeled)

• *Adult:* **PO** 10 g, then 5 g q6-8h

Diarrhea/pruritus (unlabeled)

• *Adult:* **PO** granules 5 g daily-bid, may increase by 5 g/day at 1-2 month intervals, max 30 g/day in 1-2 divided doses

Available forms: Powder/packet/scoop 5 g; tabs 1 g

SIDE EFFECTS

GI: Constipation, abdominal pain, nausea, fecal impaction, hemorrhoids, flatulence, vomiting, steatorrhea, peptic ulcer

HEMA: **Bleeding, increased PT**

INTEG: Rash, irritation of perianal area, tongue, skin

META: Decreased vit A, D, K, red folate content; **hyperchloremic acidosis**

Contraindications: Hypersensitivity, biliary obstruction

Precautions: Pregnancy (B), lactation, children, bleeding disorders

PHARMACOKINETICS

PO: Onset 24-48 hr, peak/duration 30 days, excreted in feces

INTERACTIONS

Decrease: action of thiazides, digitalis, warfarin, penicillin G, gemfibrozil, glipiZIDE, propranolol, phenytoin, TOLBUTamide, tetracycline, corticosteroids, iron, thyroid agents, clindamycin, fat-soluble vitamins

Drug/Herb

Increase: lipidemic effect—glucomannan

Decrease: lipidemic effect—gotu kola

Drug/Lab Test

Increase: AST, ALT, alk phos, chloride, PO_4

Decrease: Na, K, Ca

NURSING CONSIDERATIONS

Assess:

• Fat consumption in diet

• Cardiac glycoside levels, if both drugs are being administered

• For signs of vit A, D, K deficiency

• Serum cholesterol, triglyceride levels, electrolytes (extended therapy)

• Bowel pattern daily; increase bulk, water in diet if constipation develops

Administer:

• Swallow tabs whole; do not break, crush, or chew; take tabs one at a time

• Drug daily or bid; give all other medications 1 hr before colestipol or 4 hr after colestipol to avoid poor absorption

• Drug mixed in applesauce or stirred into beverage (2-6 oz); do not take dry; let stand for 2 min

• Supplemental doses of vit A, D, K if levels are low

Evaluate:

• Therapeutic response: decreased LDL cholesterol; decreased pruritus, diarrhea

Teach patient/family:

⚠ The symptoms of hypoprothrombinemia: bleeding mucous membranes; dark, tarry stools; hematuria; petechiae; report immediately

• That compliance is needed; not to miss or double doses

• That risk factors should be decreased: high-fat diet, smoking, alcohol consumption, absence of exercise

Side effects: *italics* = common; **bold** = life-threatening

conivaptan (R)

(kon-ih-vap'-tan)
Vaprisol
Func. class.: Vasopressin receptor antagonist

Action: Dual arginine vasopressin (AVP) antagonist with affinity for V_{1A}, V_2 receptors. Level of circulating AVP in circulating blood is critical for regulation of water, electrolyte balance and is usually elevated in euvolemic/hypervolemic hyponatremia

Uses: Euvolemia hyponatremia in those hospitalized, not indicated for CHF

DOSAGE AND ROUTES

• *Adult:* IV INF Loading dose 20 mg given over 30 min, then **CONT IV** over 24 hr; after 1 day, give for an additional 1-3 days as a **CONT INF** of 20 mg/day total, can be titrated up to 40 mg/day if serum sodium is not rising at the desired rate; max time 4 days

Available forms: 5 mg/ml (20 mg) in single use ampule

SIDE EFFECTS

CNS: Headache, confusion, insomnia
CV: **Atrial fibrillation**, hypo/hypertension, orthostatic hypotension, phlebitis
GI: Nausea, vomiting, constipation, dry mouth
GU: Hematuria, polyuria, UTI, pollaklura
HEMA: Anemia
INTEG: Erythemia, inj site reaction
META: Dehydration, hyperglycemia, hypoglycemia, hypokalemia, hypomagnesia, hyponatremia
MISC: Oral candidiasis, pain, peripheral edema, pneumonia

Contraindications: Hypersensitivity, hypovolemia
Precautions: Pregnancy (C), lactation, orthostatic disease, renal disease

PHARMACOKINETICS

Protein binding 99%, metabolized by CYP3A4, terminal half-life 5 hr

INTERACTIONS

Increase: plasma concentrations of conivaptan—CYP3A4 inhibitors
Decrease: plasma concentration of conivaptan—digoxin

NURSING CONSIDERATIONS

Assess:
• Renal, hepatic function
• Frequent sodium volume status; overly rapid correction of sodium concentration (>12 mEq/L per 24 hr) may result in osmotic demyelination syndrome
• Neurologic status: confusion, headache
• CV status: atrial fibrillation, hyper/hypotension, orthostatic hypotension; monitor B/P, pulse
• Monitor other electrolytes (magnesium and potassium)

Administer:
IV route
• Withdraw 4 ml (20 mg) of conivaptan, add to 100 ml D_5W, gently invert several times to mix, give over 30 min
CONT IV INF route
• Withdraw 4 ml (20 mg) of conivaptan, add to 250 ml D_5W, gently invert several times to mix, give over 24 hr; or 40 mg in 250 ml D_5W, gently invert several times to mix, give over 24 hr

Evaluate:
• Therapeutic response: correction of serum sodium levels

Teach patient/family:
• To avoid pregnancy, breastfeeding while taking this product
• To report neurologic changes: headache, insomnia, confusion
• Administrations procedure and expected result
• To report inj site pain, redness, swelling

⚠ Safety alert   *"Tall Man" lettering

CONTRACEPTIVES, HORMONAL

Monophasic, Oral
ethinyl estradiol/ desogestrel (R)
Apri, Cesia, Desogen, Kariva, Mircette, Ortho-Cept, Reclipsen, Solia, Velivet

ethinyl estradiol/ drospirenone (R)
Yasmin, Yaz 28

ethinyl estradiol/ ethynodiol (R)
Demulen, Demulen 1/35, Kelnor 1/35, Zovia

ethinyl estradiol/ levonorgestrel (R)
Alesse, Aviane-28, Enpresse, Jolessa, Lessina, Levlen, Levlite, Levora, Lutera, Nordette, Portia, Quasense, Seasonique, Svonyx

ethinyl estradiol/ norethindrone (R)
Brevicon, Genora 0.5/35, Genora 1/35, Junel 21 1/20, Junel 21 1.5/20, Loestrin 21 1.5/30, Loestrin 21 1/20, Microgestin, Modicon, N.E.E 1/35, Nelova 0.5/35E, Nelova 1/35E, Norcept-E 1/35, Norethin 1/35E, Norinyl 1+35, Norlestrin 1/50, Norlestrin 2.5/50, Nortrel, Ortho-Novum 1/35, Ovcon 35, Ovcon 50

ethinyl estradiol/ norgestimate (R)
MonoNessa, Ortho-Cyclen, Previfem, Sprintec

ethinyl estradiol/ norgestrel (R)
Cryselle, Lo/Ovral, Low-Ogestrel, Ogestrel, Ovral

mestranol/ norethindrone (R)
Genora 1/50, Nelova 1/50m, Norethin 1/50m, Norinyl 1+50, Ortho-Novum 1/50

Biphasic, Oral
ethinyl estradiol/ norethindrone (R)
Nelova 10/11, Ortho-Novum 10/11

Triphasic, Oral
ethinyl estradiol/ desogestrel (R)
Cyclessa

ethinyl estradiol/ norethindrone (R)
Necor 7/7/7, Nortrel 7/7/7, Ortho-Novum 7/7/7, Tri-Norinyl

ethinyl estradiol/ norgestimate (R)
Ortho Tri-Cyclen, Ortho Tri-Cyclen Lo

ethinyl estradiol/ levonorgestrel (R)
Enpresse, Portia, Tri-Levlen, Triphasil

Extended Cycle, Oral
ethinyl estradiol/ levonorgestrel (R)
Seasonale

Progestin, Oral
norethindrone (R)
Errin, Ortho Micronor, Camila, Jolivette, Nor-Q D

Progressive Estrogen, Oral
ethinyl estradiol/ norethindrone acetate (R)
Estrostep, Estrostep Fe

**Emergency
levonorgestrel/ethinyl
estradiol** (℞)
Preven

levonorgestrel (℞)
Plan B

medroxyprogesterone
(℞)
Depo-Provera

**Intrauterine
levonorgestrel** (℞)
Mirena

**Implant
etonogestrel** (℞)
Implanon

**Vaginal Ring
ethinyl estradiol/
etonogestrel** (℞)
Nuva Ring

**Transdermal
ethinyl estradiol/
norelgestromin** (℞)
Ortho Evra

Action: Prevents ovulation by suppressing FSH, LH; *monophasic:* estrogen/progestin (fixed dose) used during a 21-day cycle; ovulation is inhibited by suppression of FSH and LH; thickness of cervical mucus and endometrial lining prevents pregnancy; *biphasic:* ovulation is inhibited by suppression of FSH and LH; alteration of cervical mucus, endometrial lining prevents pregnancy; *triphasic:* ovulation is inhibited by suppression of FSH and LH; change of cervical mucus, endometrial lining prevents pregnancy; variable doses of estrogen/progestin combinations may be similar to natural hormonal fluctuations; *extended cycle:* estrogen/progestin continuous for 84 days, off for 7 days, result 4 menstrual periods/yr; *progressive estrogen:* con-

stant progestin with 3 progressive doses of estrogen; *progestin-only pill, implant, intrauterine:* change of cervical mucus and endometrial lining prevents pregnancy; ovulation may be suppressed

Uses: To prevent pregnancy, regulation of menstrual cycle, treatment of acne in women over 14 yr that other treatment has failed, emergency contraception; *injection:* inhibits gonadotropin secretion, ovulation, follicular maturation; *emergency:* inhibits ovulation and fertilization, decreases transport of sperm and egg from fallopian tube to uterus; *vaginal ring, trandermal:* inhibits ovulation, prevents sperm entry into uterus; *antiacne:* may decrease sex hormone binding globulin, results in decreased testosterone

DOSAGE AND ROUTES
Monophasic
• *Adult:* **PO** Take first tablet on Sunday after start of menses × 21 days, skip 7 days, then repeat cycle, start on 1st day of menses × 21 days, skip 7 days, then repeat cycle; may contain 7 placebo tabs, where 1 tab is taken daily
Biphasic
• *Adult:* **PO** Take 10 days of small progestin, then large progestin, estrogen is the same during cycle, skip 7 days, repeat cycle; may contain 7 placebo tabs, where 1 tab is taken daily
Triphasic
• *Adult:* **PO** Estrogen dose remains constant, progestin changes throughout 21 day cycle, some may contain 28 tabs per month
Extended cycle
• *Adult:* **PO** Start taking on first day of menses; continue for 84 days of active tab, then 7 days of placebo; repeat cycle
Progestin
• *Adult:* **PO** Start on 1st day of menses, then daily and continuously
Progressive estrogen
• *Adult:* **PO** Progestin dose remains constant, estrogen increases q7 days through-

out 21-day cycle, may include 7 placebo tabs for 28-day cycle

Emergency

• *Adult and adolescent:* Give within 72 hr of intercourse, repeat 12 hr later; **Plan B** 1 tab, then 1 tab 12 hr later; **Preven** 2 tab, then 2 tab 12 hr later; **Ovral (unlabeled)** 2 white tabs; **Lo/Ovral (unlabeled)** 4 white tabs; **Levlen (unlabeled)** 4 white tabs; **Nordette (unlabeled)** 4 orange tabs; **Triphasil (unlabeled), Tri-Levlen (unlabeled)** 4 yellow tabs

Injectable

• *Adult:* **IM (Depo-Provera)** 150 mg within 5 days of start of menses, or within 5 days postpartum (must not be breastfeeding); if breastfeeding, give 6 wk postpartum, repeat q3mo

Intrauterine

• *Adult:* To be inserted using the levonorgestrel releasing intrauterine system (LRIS) by those trained in procedure; inserted into uterine cavity within 7 days of the onset of menstruation; use should not exceed 5 years per implant

Vaginal ring

• *Adult:* **VAG** Insert 1 ring on or prior to day 5 of cycle, leave in place 3 wk; remove for 1 wk, then repeat

Transdermal

• *Adult:* **TD** Apply patch within 7 days of menses, change weekly × 3 wk; no patch wk 4, repeat cycle

Implant

• *Adult:* **Subdermal** In inner side of upper arm on days 1-5 of menses, replace q3yr

Acne

• *Adult:* **PO (Ortho Tri-Cyclen)** Take daily × 21 days, off 7 days

SIDE EFFECTS

CNS: Depression, fatigue, dizziness, nervousness, anxiety, headache
CV: Increased B/P, **cerebral hemorrhage, thrombosis, pulmonary embolism,** fluid retention, edema
EENT: Optic neuritis, retinal thrombosis, cataracts

ENDO: Decreased glucose tolerance, increased TBG, PBI, T_4, T_3
GI: Nausea, vomiting, cramps, diarrhea, bloating, constipation, change in appetite, **cholestatic jaundice**
GU: Breakthrough bleeding, amenorrhea, spotting, dysmenorrhea, galactorrhea, endocervical hyperplasia, vaginitis, cystitis-like syndrome, breast change
HEMA: Increased fibrinogen, clotting factor
INTEG: Chloasma, melasma, acne, rash, urticaria, erythema, pruritus, hirsutism, alopecia, photosensitivity

Contraindications: Pregnancy (X), lactation, reproductive cancer, thrombophlebitis, MI, hepatic tumors, hepatic disease, CAD, women 40 and over, CVA
Precautions: Depression, hypertension, renal disease, seizure disorders, lupus erythematosus, rheumatic disease, migraine headache, amenorrhea, irregular menses, breast cancer (fibrocystic), gallbladder disease, diabetes mellitus, heavy smoking, acute mononucleosis, sickle cell disease

PHARMACOKINETICS

Excreted in breast milk

INTERACTIONS

Decrease: oral contraceptives effectiveness—anticonvulsants, rifampin, analgesics, antibiotics, antihistamines, griseofulvin
Decrease: oral anticoagulants action
Drug/Herb
• Altered action: alfalfa, black cohosh, chaste tree
Decrease: oral contraceptives effect—saw palmetto, St. John's wort
Drug/Food
Increase: peak level—grapefruit juice
Drug/Lab Test
Increase: PT; clotting factors VII, VIII, IX, X; TBG, PBI, T_4, platelet aggregability, BSP, triglycerides, bilirubin, AST, ALT
Decrease: T_3, antithrombin III, folate, metyrapone test, GTT, 17-OHCS

NURSING CONSIDERATIONS
Assess:
- Glucose, thyroid function, LFTs
- Reproductive changes: change in breasts, tumors, positive Pap smear; drug should be discontinued

Administer:
- PO with food for GI symptoms; give at same time each day
- Subdermal implant of 6 caps effective for 5 yr; then should be removed
- IM inj deep in large muscle mass after shaking suspension; ensure patient not pregnant if inj are 2 wk or more apart

Evaluate:
- Therapeutic response: absence of pregnancy, endometriosis, hypermenorrhea

Teach patient/family:
- About detection of clots using Homan's sign
- To use sunscreen or avoid sunlight; photosensitivity can occur
- To take at same time each day to ensure equal drug level
- To report GI symptoms that occur after 4 mo
- To use another birth control method during 1st week of oral contraceptive use
- To take another tablet as soon as possible if one is missed
- That after drug is discontinued, pregnancy may not occur for several months
- To report abdominal pain, change in vision, shortness of breath, change in menstrual flow, spotting, breakthrough bleeding, breast lumps, swelling, headache, severe leg pain
- That continuing medical care is needed: Pap smear and gynecologic examinations q6mo
- To notify health care providers and dentists of oral contraceptive

---

Rarely Used

corticotropin (ACTH) (R)
(kor-ti-koe-troe′pin)
H.P. Acthar Gel
Func. class.: Pituitary hormone

Uses: Testing adrenocortical function, treatment of adrenal insufficiency caused by administration of corticosteroids (long term), multiple sclerosis, infantile spasms

DOSAGE AND ROUTES
Acute exacerbations of multiple sclerosis
- *Adult:* **IM** 80-120 units/day × 14-21 days

Infantile spasms
- *Infant:* **IM GEL** 20 units/day × 2 wks, increase if needed

Contraindications: Hypersensitivity, scleroderma, osteoporosis, CHF, peptic ulcer disease, hypertension, systemic fungal infections, smallpox vaccination, recent surgery, ocular herpes simplex, primary adrenocortical insufficiency/hyperfunction

---

cortisone (R)
(kor′ti-sone)
Cortone ✦, Cortone Acetate
Func. class.: Corticosteroid, synthetic
Chem. class.: Glucocorticoid, short-acting

Action: Decreases inflammation by suppression of migration of polymorphonuclear leukocytes, fibroblasts, reversal of increased capillary permeability and lysosomal stabilization

Uses: Inflammation, severe allergy, adrenal insufficiency, collagen disorders; respiratory, dermatologic, rheumatic disorders

---

⚠ Safety alert   *"Tall Man" lettering

DOSAGE AND ROUTES

• *Adult:* **PO/IM** 25-300 mg daily or q2 days, titrated to response
• *Child:* **PO** 0.7-10 mg/kg/day; **IM** 0.2-5 mg/kg/day

Available forms: Tabs 5, 10, 25 mg; inj 50 mg/ml

SIDE EFFECTS

CNS: Depression, flushing, sweating, headache, mood changes
CV: Hypertension, **circulatory collapse, thrombophlebitis, embolism,** tachycardia, **necrotizing angiitis, CHF,** edema
EENT: Fungal infections, increased intraocular pressure, blurred vision
GI: Diarrhea, nausea, abdominal distention, **GI hemorrhage,** increased appetite, **pancreatitis**
HEMA: **Thrombocytopenia**
INTEG: Acne, poor wound healing, ecchymosis, bruising, petechiae
META: Sodium, fluid retention, potassium loss
MS: Fractures, osteoporosis, weakness, loss of muscle mass

Contraindications: Pregnancy (D), psychosis, hypersensitivity, idiopathic thrombocytopenia, acute glomerulonephritis, amebiasis, fungal infections, nonasthmatic bronchial disease, child <2 yr, AIDS, TB

Precautions: Lactation, diabetes mellitus, glaucoma, osteoporosis, seizure disorders, ulcerative colitis, CHF, myasthenia gravis, renal/hepatic disease, esophagitis, peptic ulcer

PHARMACOKINETICS

Half-life 8-12 hrs
PO: Peak 2 hr, duration 1½ days
IM: Peak 20-48 hr, duration 10 days

INTERACTIONS

Increase: action of cortisone—salicylates, estrogens, indomethacin, oral contraceptives, ketoconazole, macrolide antiinfectives
Increase: side effects—alcohol, salicy-lates, indomethacin, potassium-wasting diuretics
Increase: GI symptoms—salicylates, indomethacin, NSAIDs
Decrease: effects of anticoagulants, antidiabetics, toxoids, vaccines, salicylates
Decrease: cortisone action—barbiturates, rifampin, phenytoin, theophylline, acetylcholinesterases

Drug/Herb

Increase: potassium deficiency—aloe, buckthorn, cascara sagrada, Chinese rhubarb, rhubarb, senna
Increase: steroid effect—aloe, licorice, perilla

Drug/Lab Test

Increase: Cholesterol, Na, blood glucose, uric acid, Ca, urine glucose
Decrease: Ca, K, T_4, T_3, thyroid ^{131}I uptake test, urine 17-OHCS, 17-KS
False negative: Skin allergy tests

NURSING CONSIDERATIONS

Assess:

• Potassium, blood, urine glucose while on long-term therapy; hypokalemia and hyperglycemia
• Weight daily; notify prescriber of weekly gain >5 lb
• B/P q4h, pulse; notify prescriber if chest pain occurs
• I&O ratio; be alert for decreasing urinary output and increasing edema
• Plasma cortisol levels during long-term therapy (normal level: 138-635 nmol/L SI units if drawn at 8 AM)
• Infection: fever, WBC even after withdrawal of medication; drug masks infection
• Potassium depletion: paresthesias, fatigue, nausea, vomiting, depression, polyuria, dysrhythmias, weakness
• Edema, hypertension, cardiac symptoms
• Mental status: affect, mood, behavioral changes, aggression

Administer:

• After shaking suspension (parenteral)
• Titrated dose; use lowest effective dose
• IM inj deeply in large mass; rotate sites; avoid deltoid; use a 21G needle

Side effects: *italics* = common; **bold** = life-threatening

• In one dose in AM to prevent adrenal suppression; avoid SUBCUT administration; tissue may be damaged; never administer by IV route

• With food or milk to decrease GI symptoms

Perform/provide:

• Assistance with ambulation in patient with bone tissue disease to prevent fractures

Evaluate:

• Therapeutic response: ease of respirations, decreased inflammation

Teach patient/family:

• That medical ID as steroid user should be carried at all times

• To notify prescriber if therapeutic response decreases; dosage adjustment may be needed

⚠ Not to discontinue abruptly or adrenal crisis can result

• To avoid OTC products: salicylates, alcohol in cough products, cold preparations unless directed by prescriber

• All aspects of drug usage, including cushingoid symptoms

• The symptoms of adrenal insufficiency: nausea, anorexia, fatigue, dizziness, dyspnea, weakness, joint pain

• Avoid exposure to chickenpox and measles

• To take PO dose in AM with food or fluid (milk)

Rarely Used

cosyntropin (℞)
(koe-sin-troe′pin)
Cortrosyn, Synacthen ✦, Tetracosactrin
Func. class.: Pituitary hormone

Uses: Testing adrenocortical function

DOSAGE AND ROUTES

• *Adult and child >2 yr:* **IM/IV** 0.25-1 mg between blood sampling

• *Child <2 yr:* **IM/IV** 0.125 mg

Contraindications: Hypersensitivity

---

cromolyn (OTC, ℞)
(kroe′moe-lin)
Gastrocrom Intal, Nasalcrom, Rynacrom ✦
Func. class.: Antiasthmatic
Chem. class.: Mast cell stabilizer

Do not confuse:
Nasalcrom/Nasalide

Action: Stabilizes the membrane of the sensitized mast cell, preventing release of chemical mediators after an antigen-IgE interaction

Uses: Severe perennial bronchial asthma, prevention of exercise-induced bronchospasm, acute bronchospasm induced by environmental pollutants, mastocytosis, allergic rhinitis

Unlabeled uses: Food allergy, ulcerative colitis

DOSAGE AND ROUTES

Allergic rhinitis

• *Adult and child >2 yr:* **NASAL SOL** 1 spray in each nostril tid-qid, max 6 doses/day

To prevent exercise-induced bronchospasm

• *Adult and child >5 yr:* **INH** 2 metered sprays inhaled ≤1 hr prior to exercise

Bronchial asthma

• *Adult and child >5 yr:* **INH** 2 metered sprays using inhaler qid; **NEB** 20 mg qid by nebulization

Systemic mastocytosis

• *Adult and child >12 yr:* **PO** 200 mg qid ½ hr before meals and at bedtime

• *Child 2-12 yr:* **PO** 100 mg qid ½ before meals and at bedtime

Ulcerative colitis (unlabeled) gastrocrom

• *Adult:* **PO** 200 mg qid 20 min before meals and at bedtime, may double dose after 2 wks

• *Child 2-14 yr:* **PO** 100 mg qid 20 min before meals and at bedtime, may double dose after 2-3 wk

Available forms: Nasal sol 5.2 mg/ metered spray (40 mg/ml); neb sol 20

---

mg/2 ml; aerosol 800 mcg/actuation; oral conc 100 mg/5 ml

SIDE EFFECTS

CNS: Headache, dizziness, neuritis, confusion, drowsiness
EENT: Throat irritation, cough, nasal congestion, burning eyes, nasal stinging, sneezing
GI: Nausea, vomiting, anorexia, dry mouth, bitter taste
GU: Urinary frequency, dysuria
INTEG: Rash, urticaria, angioedema
MS: Joint pain/swelling

Oral conc
CNS: Dizziness, headache, paresthesia, migraine, seizures, psychosis, anxiety, depression, hallucinations, insomnia
CV: Tachycardia, PVCs, palpitations
GI: Diarrhea, nausea, abdominal pain, constipation, dyspepsia, stomatitis, vomiting
HEMA: Polycythemia, neutropenia, pancytopenia
INTEG: Pruritus, rash, flushing, photosensitivity

Contraindications: Hypersensitivity to this drug or lactose, status asthmaticus, acute asthma
Precautions: Pregnancy (B), lactation, renal/hepatic disease, safety not established; child <5 yr (aerosol); <2 yr (nebulizer); <2 yr (nasal sol); oral <2 yr; cardiac dysrhythmias, coronary artery disease

PHARMACOKINETICS

Excreted unchanged in feces; half-life 80 min; 63%-76% protein binding

NURSING CONSIDERATIONS

Assess:
• Eosinophil count during treatment
• Respiratory status: rate, rhythm, characteristics, cough, wheezing, dyspnea
Administer:
• For oral conc: break open ampule, squeeze contents in glass of water, stir, drink

Perform/provide:
• Gargle, sip of water to decrease irritation in throat (INH/Neb)
Evaluate:
• Therapeutic response: decrease in asthmatic symptoms; congested, runny nose
Teach patient/family:
Nasal sol
• Blow nose, hold pump between fingers, if first use spray in air until fine mist occurs, insert nozzle in nostril, spray and breathe in through nose, repeat in other nostril
Aerosol (not for Acute Asthma)
• Take cover off mouthpiece, shake gently, breathe out slowly, place mouthpiece in mouth, close mouth around it, tilt head back, breathe in as the inhaler is depressed, remove, hold breath, then breathe out slowly
Inhalation
• Do not swallow sol
• Empty ampule into power driven nebulizer as directed; do not combine different meds
Oral
• To take ½ hr before meals and at bedtime

Rarely Used

crotamiton (℞)
(kroe-tam′i-ton)
Eurax
Func. class.: Scabicide

Uses: Scabies, pruritus

DOSAGE AND ROUTES

Scabies
• *Adult and child:* **CREAM** wash area with soap, water; remove visible crusts, apply cream, apply another coat in 24 hr, remove with soap, water in 48 hr
Pruritus
• *Adult and child:* **CREAM** massage into affected area, repeat as necessary
Contraindications: Hypersensitivity, skin inflammation, abrasions, breaks in skin, mucous membranes

cyanocobalamin
(vit B$_{12}$) (OTC, R)
(sye-an-oh-koe-bal'a-min)
Alphamin, Anacobin ✚,
Bedoz ✚, Cobex, Cobolin-M,
Crystamine, Crysti-1000,
Cyanabin ✚, Cyanoject,
Cyomin, Ener-B, Hydrobexan,
Hydro Cobex, Hydro-
Crysti-12

hydroxocobalamin
Hydroxycobal, LA-12,
Nascobal, Neuroforte-R,
Rubesol-1000, Rubramin PC,
Shovite, Vibral LA, Vibral,
Vitamin B$_{12}$
Func. class.: Vit B$_{12}$, water-soluble
vitamin

Action: Needed for adequate nerve functioning, protein and carbohydrate metabolism, normal growth, RBC development,
cell reproduction

Uses: Vit B$_{12}$ deficiency, pernicious anemia, vit B$_{12}$ malabsorption syndrome,
Schilling test, increased requirements with
pregnancy, thyrotoxicosis, hemolytic anemia, hemorrhage, renal and hepatic disease

DOSAGE AND ROUTES
Cyanocobalamin
• *Adult:* **PO** up to 1000 mcg/day
SUBCUT/IM 30-100 mcg/day × 1 wk,
then 100-200 mcg/mo
Schilling test
• *Adult and child:* **IM** 1000 mcg in 1
dose
• *Child:* **PO** up to 1000 mcg/day
SUBCUT/IM 30-50 mcg/day × 2 wk, then
100 mcg/mo; **NASAL** 500 mcg qwk
Hydroxocobalamin
• *Adult:* **SUBCUT/IM** 30-50 mcg/day ×
5-10 days, then 100-200 mcg/mo
• *Child:* **SUBCUT/IM** 30-50 mcg/day ×
5-10 days, then 100 mcg/mo
Available forms: *Cyanocobalamin:*
tabs 25, 50, 100, 250, 500, 1000, 5000
mcg; ext rel tabs 100, 200, 500, 1000
mcg; lozenges 100, 250, 500 mcg; nasal
jel 500 mcg/spray; inj 100, 1000 mcg/
ml; *hydroxocobalamin:* inj 1000 mcg/ml

SIDE EFFECTS
CNS: Flushing, optic nerve atrophy
CV: **CHF**, peripheral vascular thrombosis,
pulmonary edema
GI: Diarrhea
INTEG: Itching, rash, pain at inj site
META: Hypokalemia
SYST: **Anaphylactic shock**
Contraindications: Hypersensitivity,
optic nerve atrophy
Precautions: Pregnancy (A), lactation,
children

PHARMACOKINETICS
Gastric intrinsic factor must be present
for absorption to occur; stored in liver,
kidneys, stomach; 50%-90% excreted
in urine; crosses placenta, excreted in
breast milk

INTERACTIONS
Increase: absorption—predniSONE
Decrease: absorption—aminoglyco-
sides, anticonvulsants, colchicine, chlor-
amphenicol, aminosalicylic acid, potas-
sium preparations, cimetidine
Drug/Herb
Decrease: vit B$_{12}$ absorption—
goldenseal
Drug/Lab Test
False positive: Intrinsic factor

NURSING CONSIDERATIONS
Assess:
• For vit B$_{12}$ deficiency: red, beefy
tongue, psychosis, pallor, neuropathy
• GI function: diarrhea, constipation
• Potassium levels during beginning
treatment in megaloblastic anemia; q6mo
in pernicious anemia; folic acid, plasma
vit B$_{12}$ (after 1 wk), reticulocyte counts
• Nutritional status: egg yolks, fish, or-
gan meats, dairy products, clams, oys-
ters: good sources of vit B$_{12}$
• For pulmonary edema, worsening of
CHF in cardiac patients

Administer:
PO route
• With fruit juice to disguise taste; immediately after mixing
• With meals if possible for better absorption
IM route
• By IM inj for pernicious anemia for life unless contraindicated
Nasal route
• Avoid use within 1 hr of hot fluids/food
IV route
• IV route not recommended but may be admixed in TPN solution
Additive compatibilities: Ascorbic acid, chloramphenicol, metaraminol, vit B/C
Solution compatibilities: Dextrose/Ringer's or lactated Ringer's combinations, dextrose/saline combinations, D_5W, $D_{10}W$, 0.45% NaCl, Ringer's or lactated Ringer's sol
Y-site compatibilities: Heparin, hydrocortisone, potassium chloride, vit B/C
Perform/provide:
• Protection from light and heat
Evaluate:
• Therapeutic response: decreased anorexia, dyspnea on exertion, palpitations, paresthesias, psychosis, visual disturbances
Teach patient/family:
• That treatment must continue for life for pernicious anemia
• To eat well-balanced diet
• To avoid contact with persons with infection; infections common
Treatment of overdose: Discontinue drug

---

cyclobenzaprine (℞)
(sye-kloe-ben′za-preen)
cyclobenzaprine HCl, Flexeril
Func. class.: Skeletal muscle relaxant, central acting
Chem. class.: Tricyclic amine salt

Do not confuse:
cyclobenzaprine/cyproheptadine
Action: Reduction of tonic muscle activity at the brain stem; may be related to antidepressant effects
Uses: Adjunct for relief of muscle spasm and pain in musculoskeletal conditions
Unlabeled uses: Fibromyalgia

DOSAGE AND ROUTES
Muscloskeletal disorders
• *Adult:* **PO** 10 mg tid × 1 wk, not to exceed 60 mg/day × 3 wk
Fibromyalgia (unlabeled)
• *Adult:* **PO** 10 mg at bedtime, titrated up
Available forms: Tabs 10 mg

SIDE EFFECTS
CNS: Dizziness, weakness, drowsiness, headache, tremor, depression, insomnia, confusion, paresthesia
CV: Postural hypotension, tachycardia, **dysrhythmias**
EENT: Diplopia, temporary loss of vision
GI: Nausea, vomiting, hiccups, dry mouth, constipation
GU: Urinary retention, frequency, change in libido
INTEG: Rash, pruritus, fever, facial flushing, sweating
Contraindications: Acute recovery phase of myocardial infarction, dysrhythmias, heart block, CHF, hypersensitivity, child <12 yr, intermittent porphyria, thyroid disease
Precautions: Pregnancy (B), renal/hepatic disease, addictive personality, lactation, geriatric

PHARMACOKINETICS
PO: Onset 1 hr, peak 3-8 hr, duration 12-24 hr, half-life 1-3 days; metabolized by liver; excreted in urine; crosses placenta; excreted in breast milk

INTERACTIONS
• Do not use within 14 days of MAOIs, tramadol
Increase: CNS depression—alcohol, tricyclics, opiates, barbiturates, sedatives, hypnotics

Drug/Herb
Increase: CNS depression—kava

NURSING CONSIDERATIONS

Assess:
• For pain: location, duration, mobility, stiffness, baseline and periodically
• Allergic reactions: rash, fever, respiratory distress
• Severe weakness, numbness in extremities

Administer:
• Without regard to meals

Perform/provide:
• Storage in tight container at room temperature
• Assistance with ambulation if dizziness, drowsiness occur, especially geriatric

Evaluate:
• Therapeutic response: decreased pain, spasticity; muscle spasms of acute, painful musculoskeletal conditions generally short term; long-term therapy seldom warranted

Teach patient/family:
• Not to discontinue medication abruptly; insomnia, nausea, headache, spasticity, tachycardia will occur; drug should be tapered off over 1-2 wk
• Not to take with alcohol, other CNS depressants
• To avoid hazardous activities if drowsiness/dizziness occurs
• To avoid using OTC medication: cough preparations, antihistamines, unless directed by prescriber
• To use gum, frequent sips of water for dry mouth

Treatment of overdose: Empty stomach with emesis, gastric lavage, then administer activated charcoal; use anticonvulsants if indicated; monitor cardiac function

---

cyclopentolate ophthalmic
See Appendix C

⚠ High Alert

cyclophosphamide (Ｒ)
(sye-kloe-foss'fa-mide)
Cytoxan, Neosar, Procytox ✦
Func. class.: Antineoplastic alkylating agent
Chem. class.: Nitrogen mustard

Do not confuse:
cyclophosphamide/cycloSPORINE
Cytoxan/Cytosar/Cytotec/cytarabine
Action: Alkylates DNA is responsible for cross-linking DNA strands; activity is not cell cycle phase specific
Uses: Hodgkin's disease; lymphomas; leukemia; cancer of female reproductive tract, breast; lung, prostate; multiple myeloma; neuroblastoma; retinoblastoma; Ewing's sarcoma

DOSAGE AND ROUTES

• *Adult:* **PO** initially 1-5 mg/kg over 2-5 days, maintenance is 1-5 mg/kg; **IV** initially 40-50 mg/kg in divided doses over 2-5 days, maintenance 10-15 mg/kg q7-10d, or 3-5 mg/kg q3d
• *Child:* **PO/IV** 2-8 mg/kg or 60-250 mg/m² in divided doses for 6 or more days; maintenance 10-15 mg/kg q7-10d or 30 mg/kg q3-4wk; dose should be reduced by half when bone marrow depression occurs
Available forms: Inj 100, 200, 500 mg, 1, 2 g; tabs 25, 50 mg

SIDE EFFECTS

CNS: Headache, dizziness
CV: **Cardiotoxicity (high doses), myocardial fibrosis**
ENDO: Syndrome of inappropriate antidiuretic hormone (SIADH), gonadal suppression
GI: Nausea, vomiting, diarrhea, weight loss, colitis, **hepatotoxicity**
GU: **Hemorrhagic cystitis,** hematuria, neoplasms, amenorrhea, azoospermia, sterility, ovarian fibrosis

---

⚠ Safety alert   *"Tall Man" lettering

HEMA: **Thrombocytopenia, leukope-nia, pancytopenia; myelosuppression**
INTEG: Alopecia, dermatitis
META: Hyperuricemia
MISC: Secondary neoplasms, **anaphylaxis**
RESP: **Pulmonary fibrosis**
Contraindications: Pregnancy (D), lactation, severely depressed bone marrow function, hypersensitivity
Precautions: Radiation therapy

PHARMACOKINETICS

Metabolized by liver; excreted in urine; half-life 4-6½ hr; 50% bound to plasma proteins

INTERACTIONS

Increase: neuromuscular blockade—succinylcholine
Increase: cyclophosphamide toxicity—barbiturates
Increase: action of warfarin
Increase: bone marrow depression—allopurinol, thiazides
Increase: hypoglycemia—insulin
Decrease: digoxin levels—digoxin
Decrease: cyclophosphamide effect—chloramphenicol, corticosteroids
Decrease: antibody response—live virus vaccines
Drug/Lab Test
Increase: Uric acid
Decrease: Pseudocholinesterase
False positive: Pap smear
False negative: PPD, mumps, trichophy-tin, *Candida, Trichophyton,* Pap smear

NURSING CONSIDERATIONS

Assess:
• For hemorrhagic cystitis; renal studies: BUN, serum uric acid, urine CCr before, during therapy; I&O ratio; report fall in urine output <30 ml/hr
• CBC, differential, platelet count baseline, weekly; withhold drug if WBC is <2500 or platelet count is <75,000; notify prescriber of results
• Pulmonary function tests, chest x-ray films before, during therapy; chest film

should be obtained q2wk during treatment
• Monitor temp q4h (elevated temp may indicate beginning infection)
• Hepatic studies before, during therapy (bilirubin, AST, ALT, LDH) as needed or monthly
• Bleeding: hematuria, guaiac, bruising or petechiae, mucosa or orifices q8h
• Dyspnea, crackles, unproductive cough, chest pain, tachypnea
• Effects of alopecia on body image, discuss feelings about body changes
• Jaundice of skin, sclera; dark urine; clay-colored stools; itchy skin; abdominal pain; fever; diarrhea
• Buccal cavity q8h for dryness, sores or ulceration, white patches, oral pain, bleeding, dysphagia; obtain prescription for viscous lidocaine (Xylocaine)
⚠ Symptoms indicating severe allergic reaction: rash, pruritus, urticaria, purpuric skin lesions, itching, flushing
Administer:
• In AM so drug can be eliminated before bedtime
• Fluids IV or PO before chemotherapy to hydrate patient
• Antacid before oral agent, give after evening meal, before bedtime
• Antiemetic 30-60 min before giving drug and prn
• Allopurinol or sodium bicarbonate to maintain uric acid levels, alkalinization of urine
IV route
• Using cytoxic handling procedures
• IV after diluting 100 mg/5 ml of sterile H₂O or bacteriostatic H₂O; shake; let stand until clear; may be further diluted in up to 250 ml D₅ or NS; give 100 mg or less/min through 3-way stopcock of glucose or saline inf
• Using 21, 23, 25G needle; check site for irritation, phlebitis
Additive compatibilities: Cisplatin with etoposide, fluorouracil, hydrOXY-zine, methotrexate, methotrexate/fluorouracil, mitoxantrone, ondansetron

Side effects: *italics* = common; **bold** = life-threatening

Solution compatibilities: Amino acids 4.25%/D₂₅, D₅/0.9% NaCl, D₅W, 0.9% NaCl

Syrinage compatibilities: Bleomycin, cisplatin, doxapram, DOXOrubicin, droperidol, fluorouracil, furosemide, heparin, leucovorin, methotrexate, metoclopramide, mitomycin, vinBLAStine, vinCRIStine

Y-site compatibilities: Allopurinol, amifostine, amikacin, ampicillin, azlocillin, aztreonam, bleomycin, cefamandole, cefazolin, cefepime, cefoperazone, cefotaxime, cefoxitin, cefuroxime, cephalothin, cephapirin, chloramphenicol, chlorproMAZINE, cimetidine, cisplatin, cladribine, clindamycin, dexamethasone, diphenhydrAMINE, DOXOrubicin, DOXOrubicin liposome, doxycycline, droperidol, erythromycin, famotidine, filgrastim, fludarabine, fluorouracil, furosemide, gallium, ganciclovir, gentamicin, granisetron, heparin, hydromorphone, idarubicin, kanamycin, leucovorin, lorazepam, melphalan, methotrexate, methylPREDNISolone, metoclopramide, metronidazole, mezlocillin, minocycline, mitomycin, morphine, moxalactam, nafcillin, ondansetron, oxacillin, paclitaxel, penicillin G potassium, piperacillin, piperacillin/tazobactam, prochlorperazine, promethazine, propofol, ranitidine, sargramostim, sodium bicarbonate, teniposide, thiotepa, ticarcillin, ticarcillin-clavulanate, tobramycin, trimethoprim-sulfamethoxazole, vancomycin, vinBLAStine, vinCRIStine, vinorelbine

Perform/provide:
• Storage in tight container at room temperature
• Strict medical asepsis, protective isolation if WBC levels are low
• Increase fluid intake to 2-3 L/day to prevent urate deposits, calculi formation, reduce incidence of hemorrhagic cystitis
• Diet low in purines: organ meats (kidney, liver), dried beans, peas to maintain alkaline urine
• Rinsing of mouth tid-qid with water, club soda; brushing of teeth bid-tid with soft brush or cotton-tipped applicators for stomatitis; use unwaxed dental floss
• Warm compresses at inj site for inflammation

Evaluate:
• Therapeutic response: decreased tumor size, spread of malignancy

Teach patient/family:
• About protective isolation
• That amenorrhea can occur and may last up to 1 yr after therapy; reversible after stopping treatment
• To report any changes in breathing or coughing
• That hair may be lost during treatment; a wig or hairpiece may make patient feel better; new hair may be different in color, texture
• To avoid foods with citric acid, hot or rough texture
• To report any bleeding, white spots, ulcerations in mouth to prescriber; tell patient to examine mouth daily
• To report signs of infection: increased temperature, sore throat, flulike symptoms
• To report signs of anemia: fatigue, headache, faintness, shortness of breath, irritability
• To report bleeding (bruising, hematuria, petechiae): avoid use of razors, commercial mouthwash
• To use reliable contraception during and for 4 mo after treatment; do not breastfeed
• To avoid use of aspirin products, ibuprofen
• To avoid vaccinations during therapy

cycloSPORINE (℞)
(sye′kloe-spor-een)
Gengraf, Neoral, Sandimmune, Pulminiq
Func. class.: Immunosuppressant
Chem. class.: Fungus-derived peptide

Do not confuse:
cycloSPORINE/cycloSERINE/cyclophosphamide

⚠ Safety alert   *"Tall Man" lettering

Action: Produces immunosuppression by inhibiting lymphocytes (T)

Uses: Organ transplants (liver, kidney, heart) to prevent rejection, rheumatoid arthritis, psoriasis

Unlabeled uses: Recalcitrant ulcerative colitis, aplastic anemia, Crohn's disease, graft vs. host disease (GVHD), thrombocytopenia purpura, lupus nephritis, myasthenia gravis, psoriatic arthritis

DOSAGE AND ROUTES

Prevention of transplant rejection
• *Adult and child:* **PO** 15 mg/kg several hr before surgery, daily for 2 wk, reduce dosage by 2.5 mg/kg/wk to 5-10 mg/kg/day; **IV** 5-6 mg/kg several hr before surgery, daily, switch to PO form as soon as possible

Rheumatoid arthritis (Neoral/Gengraf)
• *Adult:* **PO** 2.5 mg/kg/day divided bid, may increase 0.5-0.75 mg/kg/day after 8-12 wk, max 4 mg/kg/day

Psoriasis (Neoral/Gengraf)
• *Adult:* **PO** 2.5 mg/kg/day divided bid, × 4 wk, then increase by 0.5 mg/kg/day q2wk, max 4 mg/kg/day

Idiopathic thrombocytopenia purpura (unlabeled)
• *Adult:* **PO** 1.25-2.5 mg/kg bid

Severe aplastic anemia (unlabeled)
• *Adult and child:* **PO** 12 mg/kg/day or 15 mg/kg/day (child) with antithymocyte globulin (ATG)

Available forms: Oral sol 100 mg/ml; soft gel cap 25, 50, 100 mg; inj 50 mg/ml; sol for inh 300 mg/4.8 ml

SIDE EFFECTS

CNS: *Tremors, headache,* **seizures, confusion**

GI: Nausea, vomiting, diarrhea, *oral candida, gum hyperplasia,* **hepatotoxicity,** pancreatitis

GU: **Albuminuria, hematuria, proteinuria, renal failure**

INTEG: Rash, acne, *hirsutism*

META: Hyperkalemia, hypomagnesemia, hyperlipidemia, hyperuricemia

MISC: *Infection*

Contraindications: Hypersensitivity to polyxyethylated castor oil (inj only), psoriasis or rheumatoid arthritis in renal disease (Neoral/Gengraf); uncontrolled, malignant hypertension; Gengraf/Neoral used with PUVA/UVB, methotrexate, coal tar, radiation in psoriasis, lactation

Precautions: Pregnancy (C), severe renal/hepatic disease, geriatric

PHARMACOKINETICS

Peak 4 hr, highly protein bound, half-life (biphasic) 1.2 hr, 25 hr; metabolized in liver; excreted in feces; crosses placenta; excreted in breast milk

INTERACTIONS

Increase: action, toxicity of cyclo-SPORINE—allopurinol, amiodarone, amphotericin B, androgens, azole antifungals, β-blockers, bromocriptine, calcium channel blockers, carvedilol, cimetidine, colchicine, corticosteroids, fluoroquinolones, foscarnet, imipenem-cilastatin, macrolides, metoclopramide, oral contraceptives, NSAIDs, melphalan, SSRIs

Increase: effects of digoxin, etoposide, HMG-CoA reductase inhibitors, methotrexate, potassium-sparing diuretics, sirolimus, tacrolimus

Decrease: cycloSPORINE action—anticonvulsants, nafcillin, orlistat, phenobarbital, phenytoin, probucol, rifamycins, sulfamethoxazole-trimethoprim, terbinafine, ticlopidine

Decrease: antibody reaction—live virus vaccines

Drug/Herb
Increase: immunosuppressant effect—safflower

Decrease: immunosuppressant effect—ginseng, maitake, mistletoe, schisandra, St. John's wort, turmeric

Drug/Food
• Slowed metabolism of drug: grapefruit juice, food

NURSING CONSIDERATIONS
Assess:
• Renal studies: BUN, creatinine at least monthly during treatment, 3 mo after treatment
• Drug blood level during treatment
• Hepatic studies: alk phos, AST, ALT, bilirubin; hepatotoxicity: dark urine, jaundice, itching, light-colored stools; drug should be discontinued
• Serum lipids, magnesium, potassium, cycloSPORINE blood concentrations
⚠ For nephrotoxicity: 6 wk postop, acute tubular necrosis, CyA trough level >200 ng/ml, gradual rise in creatinine (0.15 mg/dl/day), creatinine plateau <25% above baseline, intracapsular pressure <40 mm Hg
Administer:
PO route
• Do not break, crush, or chew caps
• Use pipette provided to draw up oral sol; may mix with milk or juice, wipe pipette, do not wash
• For several days before transplant surgery
• With corticosteroids
• With meals for GI upset or in chocolate milk, milk, or orange juice
• With oral antifungal for candida infections
Rheumatoid arthritis
• Give Neoral or Gengraf 2.5 mg/kg/day divided bid, may use with salicylates, NSAIDs, PO corticosteroids
• Always give the daily dose of Neoral/Gengraf in 2 divided doses on consistent schedule
• Give initial sandimmune PO dose 4-12 hr prior to transplantation as a single dose of 15 mg/kg, continue the single daily dose for 1-2 wk, then taper 5%/wk to a maintenance dose 5-10 mg/kg/day
IV route
• After diluting each 50 mg/20-100 ml of 0.9% NaCl or D₅W; run over 2-6 hr, may give as a continuous inf over 24 hr; use an infusion pump, glass inf bottles only

Sandimmune, Parenteral
• For sandimmune parenteral, give ⅓ of PO dose, initial dose 4-12 hr prior to transplantation as a single IV dose 5-6 mg/kg/day, continue the single daily dose until PO can be used
Additive compatibilities: Ciprofloxacin
Solution compatibilities: D₅W, NaCl 0.9%
Y-site compatibilities: Cefmetazole, propofol, sargramostim
Evaluate:
• Therapeutic response: absence of rejection
Teach patient/family:
• To report fever, chills, sore throat, fatigue, since serious infections may occur; tremors, bleeding gums, increased B/P
• To use contraceptive measures during treatment, for 12 wk after ending therapy
• To take at same time of day, every day; do not skip doses or double a missed dose; not to use with grapefruit juice

---

cyproheptadine (℞)
(si-proe-hep′ta-deen)
cyproheptadine HCl,
Periactin,
PMS-Cyproheptadine ✦
Func. class.: Antihistamine, H₁-receptor antagonist
Chem. class.: Piperidine

Do not confuse:
cyproheptadine/cyclobenzaprine
Action: Acts on blood vessels, GI, respiratory system by competing with histamine for H₁-receptor site; decreases allergic response by blocking histamine
Uses: Allergy symptoms, rhinitis, pruritus, cold, urticaria
Unlabeled uses: Appetite stimulant, management of vascular headache, nightmares, posttraumatic stress disorder

DOSAGE AND ROUTES
• *Adult:* **PO** 4 mg tid-qid, not to exceed 0.5 mg/kg/day

⚠ Safety alert   *"Tall Man" lettering

- *Child 6-14 yr:* **PO** 4 mg bid-tid, not to exceed 16 mg/day
- *Child 2-5 yr:* **PO** 2 mg bid-tid, not to exceed 12 mg/day

Nightmares, posttraumatic stress disorder (unlabeled)
- *Adult:* **PO** 4-12 mg nightly, max 32 mg

Available forms: Tabs 4 mg; syr 2 mg/5 ml

SIDE EFFECTS

CNS: Dizziness, drowsiness, poor coordination, fatigue, anxiety, euphoria, confusion, paresthesia, neuritis

CV: Hypotension, palpitations, tachycardia

EENT: Blurred vision, dilated pupils; tinnitus; nasal stuffiness; dry nose, throat, mouth

GI: Constipation, dry mouth, nausea, vomiting, anorexia, diarrhea, weight gain, increased appetite

GU: Retention, dysuria, urinary frequency

HEMA: **Hemolytic anemia, leukopenia, thrombocytosis, agranulocytosis**

INTEG: Rash, urticaria, photosensitivity

RESP: Increased thick secretions, wheezing, chest tightness

SYST: **Anaphylactic shock**

Contraindications: Hypersensitivity to H$_1$-receptor antagonist, acute asthma attack, lower respiratory tract disease

Precautions: Pregnancy (B), increased intraocular pressure, renal/cardiac disease, hypertension, bronchial asthma, seizure disorder, stenosed peptic ulcers, hyperthyroidism, prostatic hypertrophy, bladder neck obstruction, lactation, geriatric

PHARMACOKINETICS

PO: Duration 4-6 hr; metabolized in liver; excreted by kidneys; excreted in breast milk

INTERACTIONS

Increase: CNS depression—barbiturates, opiates, hypnotics, tricyclics, alcohol
Increase: anticholinergic effect—MAOIs

Drug/Herb
Increase: CNS depression—hops, Jamaican dogwood, kava, khat, senega
Increase: anticholinergic effect—corkwood, henbane

Drug/Lab Test
False negative: Skin allergy tests

NURSING CONSIDERATIONS

Assess:
- I&O ratio; be alert for urinary retention, frequency, dysuria; drug should be discontinued
- CBC during long-term therapy
- Respiratory status: rate, rhythm, increase in bronchial secretions, wheezing, chest tightness
- Cardiac status: palpitations, increased pulse, hypotension

Administer:
- With meals for GI symptoms; absorption may slightly decrease

Perform/provide:
- Hard candy, gum, frequent rinsing of mouth for dryness
- Storage in airtight container at room temperature

Evaluate:
- Therapeutic response: absence of running or congested nose, rashes

Teach patient/family:
- All aspects of drug use; to notify prescriber of confusion, sedation, hypotension
- To avoid driving, other hazardous activity if drowsiness occurs, especially geriatric
- To avoid concurrent use of alcohol, other CNS depressants

Treatment of overdose: Ipecac syrup or lavage, diazepam, vasopressors, barbiturates (short-acting)

⚠ High Alert

cytarabine (℞)
(sye-tare′a-been)
Ara-C, Cytosar ✦ Cytosar-U,
cytosine arabinoside,
DepoCyt
Func. class.: Antineoplastic, antimetabolite
Chem. class.: Pyrimidine nucleoside

Do not confuse:
Cytosar/Cytoxan/Cytovene

Action: Competes with physiologic substrate of DNA synthesis, thus interfering with cell replication in the S phase of the cell cycle (before mitosis)

Uses: Acute myelocytic leukemia, acute nonlymphocytic leukemia, chronic myelocytic leukemia, lymphomatous meningitis (IT)

Unlabeled uses: Hodgkin's, non-Hodgkin's lymphoma

DOSAGE AND ROUTES

Acute nonlymphocytic/lymphocytic
• *Adult:* **IV INF** 200 mg/m^2/day × 5 days q2wk as single agent or 2-6 mg/kg/day (100-200 mg/m^2/day) as a single dose or 2-3 divided doses for 5-10 days until remission, used in combination; maintenance 70-200 mg/m^2/day for 2-5 days qmo; **SUBCUT/IM** maintenance 1 mg/kg q1-2×/wk

Refractory acute Hodgkin's/refractory non-Hodgkin's lymphoma (unlabeled)
• *Adult:* **IV** 2 g/m^2/day; on day 5 q21 days, with etoposide, methylPREDNISolone, and cisplatin

Meningeal leukemia
• *Adult and child:* **INTRATHECALLY** 5-75 mg/m^2 variable daily × 4 days to q2-7 days

Available forms: Powder for inj 100, 500 mg, 1, 2 g; sus rel, (DepoCyt) liposomal for intrathecal use 10 mg/ml

SIDE EFFECTS

CNS: Neuritis, dizziness, headache, cerebellar syndrome, personality changes, ataxia, mechanical dysphasia, **coma;** **chemical arachnoiditis** (IT)

CV: Chest pain, **cardiopathy**

CYTARABINE SYNDROME: Fever, myalgia, bone pain, chest pain, *rash,* conjunctivitis, malaise (6-12 hr after administration)

EENT: Sore throat, conjunctivitis

GI: Nausea, vomiting, anorexia, diarrhea, stomatitis, **hepatotoxicity,** abdominal pain, hematemesis, **GI hemorrhage**

GU: Urinary retention, **renal failure, hyperuricemia**

HEMA: Thrombophlebitis, bleeding, **thrombocytopenia, leukopenia, myelosuppression, anemia**

INTEG: Rash, fever, freckling, cellulitis

META: Hyperuricemia

RESP: **Pneumonia,** dyspnea, **pulmonary edema** (high doses)

SYST: **Anaphylaxis**

Contraindications: Pregnancy (D), hypersensitivity, infants

Precautions: Renal/hepatic disease, lactation

PHARMACOKINETICS

INTRATHECAL: Half-life 100-236 hr; metabolized in liver; excreted in urine (primarily inactive metabolite); crosses blood-brain barrier, placenta

IV/SUBCUT: Distribution half-life 10 min, elimination half-life 1-3 hr

INTERACTIONS

Increase: toxicity, bone marrow depression—radiation or other antineoplastics

Decrease: effects of oral digoxin

NURSING CONSIDERATIONS

Assess:
• CBC (RBC, Hct, Hgb), differential, platelet count weekly; withhold drug if WBC is <1000/mm^3, platelet count is <50,000/mm^3, or RBC, Hct, Hgb low; notify prescriber of these results
• Renal studies: BUN, serum uric acid,

⚠ Safety alert   ✦"Tall Man" lettering

urine CCr, electrolytes before and during therapy

• I&O ratio; report fall in urine output to <30 ml/hr

• Monitor temp q4h; fever may indicate beginning infection; no rectal temps

• Hepatic studies before and during therapy: bilirubin, ALT, AST, alk phos, as needed or monthly; check for jaundice of skin, sclera; dark urine; clay-colored stools; pruritus; abdominal pain; fever; diarrhea

• Blood uric acid during therapy

⚠ For anaphylaxis: rash, pruritus, facial swelling, dyspnea; resuscitation equipment should be nearby

⚠ Chemical arachnoiditis (IT): headache, nausea, vomiting, fever; neck rigidity pain, meningism, CSF pleocytosis; may be decreased by dexamethasone

• Cytarabine syndrome 6-12 hr after inf: fever, myalgia, bone pain, chest pain, rash, conjunctivitis, malaise; corticosteroids may be ordered

• Bleeding: hematuria, heme-positive stools, bruising or petechiae, mucosa or orifices q8h

⚠ Dyspnea, crackles, unproductive cough, chest pain, tachypnea, fatigue, increased pulse, pallor, lethargy; personality changes, with high doses; pulmonary edema may be fatal (rare)

• Buccal cavity q8h for dryness, sores or ulceration, white patches, oral pain, bleeding, dysphagia

• Local irritation, pain, burning, discoloration at inj site

• GI symptoms: frequency of stools, cramping, antispasmodic may be used

• Acidosis, signs of dehydration: rapid respirations, poor skin turgor, decreased urine output, dry skin, restlessness, weakness

Administer:

• Antiemetic 30-60 min before giving drug and prn

• Allopurinol to maintain uric acid levels and alkalinization of the urine

• Topical or systemic analgesics for pain

IT route

• Use preservative-free NS, add 5 ml/100 mg vial or 10 ml/500 mg vial; use immediately, discard unused drug

• Use dexamethasone with IT administration

IV route

• After diluting 100 mg/5 ml of sterile H_2O for inj; given by direct IV over 1-3 min through free-flowing tubing (IV); may be further diluted in 50-100 ml NS or D_5W, given over 30 min to 24 hr depending on dose; also may be given by continuous inf

Additive compatibilities: Corticotropin, DAUNOrubicin with etoposide, etoposide, hydrOXYzine, lincomycin, mitoxantrone, ondansetron, potassium chloride, prednisoLONE, sodium bicarbonate, vinCRIStine

Solution compatibilities: Amino acids, D_5/LR, D_5/0.2% NaCl, D_5/0.9% NaCl, D_{10}/0.9% NaCl, D_5W, invert sugar 10% in electrolyte #1, Ringer's LR, 0.9% NaCl, sodium lactate ⅙ mol/L, TPN #57

Syringe compatibilities: Metoclopramide

Y-site compatibilities: Amifostine, amsacrine, aztreonam, cefepime, chlorproMAZINE, cimetidine, cladribine, dexamethasone, diphenhydrAMINE, DOXOrubicin liposome, droperidol, famotidine, filgrastim, fludarabine, gentamicin, granisetron, heparin, hydrocortisone, hydromorphone, idarubicin, lorazepam, melphalan, methotrexate, methylPREDNISolone, metoclopramide, morphine, ondansetron, paclitaxel, piperacillin/tazobactam, prochlorperazine, promethazine, propofol, ranitidine, sargramostim, sodium bicarbonate, teniposide, thiotepa, vinorelbine

Perform/provide:

• Strict medical asepsis and protective isolation if WBC levels are low

• Increase fluid intake to 2-3 L/day to prevent urate deposits and calculi formation, unless contraindicated

• Diet low in purines: absence of organ meats (kidney, liver), dried beans, peas to prevent increased urate deposits

- Rinsing of mouth tid-qid with water, club soda; brushing of teeth bid-tid with soft brush or cotton-tipped applicators for stomatitis; use unwaxed dental floss

Evaluate:

- Therapeutic response: decreased tumor size, spread of malignancy

Teach patient/family:

- To report any coughing, chest pain, changes in breathing; may indicate beginning pneumonia, pulmonary edema
- To avoid foods with citric acid, spicy or rough texture if stomatitis is present, use sponge brush and rinse with water after each meal; to report stomatitis: any bleeding, white spots, ulcerations in mouth; tell patient to examine mouth daily, report any symptoms
- To report signs of infection: increased temp, sore throat, flulike symptoms; avoid crowds, persons with infections
- To report signs of anemia: fatigue, headache, faintness, shortness of breath, irritability
- To report bleeding; avoid use of razors, commercial mouthwash, salicylates, NSAIDs
- To use thrombocytopenia precautions
- To take fluids to 3 L/day to prevent renal damage
- To use reliable contraception during treatment and 4 mo thereafter, do not breastfeed
- To avoid receiving vaccines during treatment,
- That fever, headache, nausea, vomiting are likely to occur

⚠ High Alert

dacarbazine (℞)

(da-kar′ba-zeen)

dacarbazine, DTIC ✦, DTIC-Dome

Func. class.: Antineoplastic alkylating agent

Chem. class.: Cytotoxic triazine

Action: Alkylates DNA, RNA; inhibits DNA, RNA synthesis; also responsible for breakage, cross-linking DNA strands; activity is not cell cycle phase specific

Uses: Hodgkin's disease, sarcomas, neuroblastoma, metastatic malignant melanoma

Unlabeled uses: Malignant pheochromocytoma in combination with cyclophosphamide and vinCRIStine, metastatic soft tissue sarcoma in combination with other agents, carcinoma meningitis, neuroblastoma

DOSAGE AND ROUTES

Metastatic malignant melanoma

- *Adult:* **IV** 2-4.5 mg/kg daily × 10 days or 250 mg/m² daily × 5 days; repeat q3wk depending on response

Hodgkin's disease

- *Adult:* **IV** 150 mg/m² daily × 5 days with other agents, repeat q4wk; or 375 mg/m² on day 1 when given in combination, repeat q15d

Osteogenic sarcoma (unlabeled)

- *Adult and child:* **IV** 250 mg/m² day as a continuous inf × 4 days q28d

Soft tissue sarcoma (unlabeled)

- *Adult and child:* **IV** 250-300 mg/m² day as a continuous inf × 3 days q21-28d

Carcinoma meningitis (unlabeled)

- *Adult:* **INTRATHECAL** 5-30 mg in a fixed dose 2-3 ×/wk until disease controlled

Available forms: Powder for inj 100, 200 mg

SIDE EFFECTS

CNS: Facial paresthesia, flushing, fever, malaise; confusion, headache, **seizures,** blurred vision (high doses)

GI: Nausea, anorexia, vomiting, **hepatotoxicity** (rare)

HEMA: **Thrombocytopenia, leukopenia,** anemia

INTEG: **Alopecia,** dermatitis, pain at inj site, photosensitivity; severe sun reactions (high doses)

MISC: Flulike symptoms, malaise, fever, myalgia

SYST: **Anaphylaxis**

Contraindications: Lactation

⚠ Safety alert   *"Tall Man" lettering

Precautions: Pregnancy (C) 1st trimester, radiation therapy

PHARMACOKINETICS

Metabolized by liver; excreted in urine; half-life 35 min, terminal 5 hr, 5% protein bound

INTERACTIONS

• Toxicity, bone marrow suppression: bone marrow suppressants, radiation, other antineoplastics
• Bleeding: salicylates, anticoagulants
Increase: adverse reaction decrease antibody reaction—live virus vaccines
Increase: nephrotoxicity—aminoglycosides
Increase: ototoxicity—loop diuretics
Decrease: dacarbazine effect—phenytoin, phenobarbital

NURSING CONSIDERATIONS

Assess:

⚠ CBC, differential, platelet count weekly; withhold drug if WBC <4000 or platelet count <75,000; notify prescriber of results
• Monitor temp q4h (may indicate beginning infection)
• Hepatic studies before, during therapy (bilirubin, AST, ALT, LDH) as needed or monthly
• Bleeding: hematuria, guaiac, bruising or petechiae, mucosa or orifices q8h
• Effects of alopecia on body image, discuss feelings about body changes
• Jaundice of skin, sclera; dark urine; clay-colored stools; itchy skin; abdominal pain; fever; diarrhea
• Inflammation of mucosa, breaks in skin
⚠ Hypersensitivity reactions, anaphylaxis, discontinue drug, administer meds for anaphylaxis

Administer:

• Antiemetic 30-60 min before giving drug to prevent vomiting, nausea; vomiting may subside after several doses
• Antibiotics for prophylaxis of infection

IV route

• After diluting 100 mg/9.9 ml of sterile H_2O for inj (10 mg/ml), give by direct IV over 1 min through Y-tube or 3-way stopcock; may be further diluted in 50-250 ml D_5W or NS for inj, given as an inf over ½ hr
• Watch for extravasation; give Na thiosulfate 10% 4 ml plus sterile H_2O 5 ml, 3-5 ml SUBCUT if needed

Additive compatibilities: Bleomycin, carmustine, cyclophosphamide, cytarabine, dactinomycin, DOXOrubicin, fluorouracil, mercaptopurine, methotrexate, ondansetron, vinBLAStine

Additive incompatibilities: Hydrocortisone sodium succinate, cysteine

Y-site compatibilities: Amifostine, aztreonam, filgrastim, fludarabine, granisetron, melphalan, ondansetron, paclitaxel, sargramostim, teniposide, thiotepa, vinorelbine

Perform/provide:

• Storage in light-resistant container, dry area
• Strict medical asepsis, protective isolation if WBC levels are low
• Increase fluid intake to 2-3 L/day to prevent urate deposits, calculi formation
• Warm compresses at infusion site for inflammation

Evaluate:

• Therapeutic response: decreased tumor size, spread of malignancy

Teach patient/family:

• That patient should avoid prolonged exposure to sun, wear sunscreen
• That hair may be lost during treatment; a wig or hairpiece may make the patient feel better; new hair may be different in color, texture
• To report signs of infection: fever, sore throat, flulike symptoms
• To report signs of anemia: fatigue, headache, faintness, shortness of breath, irritability
• To report bleeding; avoid use of razors, commercial mouthwash
• To avoid use of aspirin products or ibuprofen

• To use reliable contraceptives during and for several months after therapy; do not breastfeed

---

⚠ High Alert

daclizumab (℞)
(dah-kliz'uh-mab)
Zenapax
Func. class.: Immunosuppressant
Chem. class.: Humanized IgG1 monoclonal antibody

Action: Binds to the IL-2 (interleukin-2) receptor antagonist
Uses: Acute allograft rejection in renal transplant patients

DOSAGE AND ROUTES

• *Adult:* **IV** 1 mg/kg as part of a regimen that includes cycloSPORINE and corticosteroids, mix calculated vol with 50 ml of 0.9% NaCl and give via peripheral/central vein over 15 min; do not admix
Available forms: Inj 5 mg/ml

SIDE EFFECTS

CNS: Chills, tremors, dizziness, insomnia, headache, prickly sensation
CV: Hypertension, **tachycardia, thrombosis,** bleeding, chest pain
GI: Vomiting, nausea, diarrhea, constipation, abdominal pain, pyrosis
GU: Oliguria, dysuria, **renal tubular necrosis,** renal damage, **hydronephrosis**
INTEG: Acne, impaired wound healing
MISC: Edema, peripheral edema, allergic reaction
RESP: Dyspnea, wheezing, **pulmonary edema,** coughing, atelectasis, congestion, hypoxia
Contraindications: Hypersensitivity
Precautions: Pregnancy (C), child <11 mo, lactation, geriatric

INTERACTIONS

Drug/Herb
Increase: immunosuppressant effect—safflower

Decrease: immunosuppressant effect—ginseng, maitake, mistletoe, schisandra, St. John's wort, turmeric

NURSING CONSIDERATIONS

Assess:
• Blood studies: Hgb, WBC, platelets during treatment qmo; if leukocytes are <3000/mm^3, drug should be discontinued
• Hepatic studies: alk phos, AST, ALT, bilirubin
⚠ Hepatotoxicity: dark urine, jaundice, itching, light-colored stools; drug should be discontinued
⚠ For anaphylaxis, have corticosteroids, epINEPHrine available
• For fluid overload: weight gain; check lung sounds, VS
Administer:
• All other medications PO if possible
• Avoid IM inj, since infection may occur
• Protect undiluted sol from direct light; should be used with drugs for immunosuppression
Solution compatibilities: 0.9% NaCl
Perform/provide:
• Increased fluid intake during treatment
• Storage of unopened vials in refrigerator; do not shake or freeze; protect from light
Evaluate:
• Therapeutic response: absence of graft rejection
Teach patient/family:
• To report fever, chills, sore throat, fatigue, since serious infection may occur; rash, hives, difficulty breathing, since allergic reactions may occur; nausea, constipation, diarrhea, stomach pain, headache, fast heartbeat, swelling, tremors, chest pain, urinary tract bleeding, fever, cough, pain, redness at site
• To use contraception (women) before, during, and for 4 mo after treatment
• To avoid vaccinations during treatment
• To avoid hazardous activities, dizziness, blurred vision may occur
• To avoid crowds, persons with known upper respiratory infections

---

⚠ Safety alert   *"Tall Man" lettering

⚠ High Alert

dactinomycin (℞)
(dak-ti-noe-mye'sin)
Cosmegen
Func. class.: Antineoplastic, antibiotic

Action: Inhibits DNA, RNA, protein synthesis; derived from *Streptomyces parvullus;* replication is decreased by binding to DNA, which causes strand splitting; cell cycle nonspecific; a vesicant

Uses: Sarcomas, trophoblastic tumors in women, testicular cancer, Wilms' tumor, rhabdomyosarcoma

Unlabeled uses: Kaposi's sarcoma, malignant melanoma, osteogenic sarcoma, ovarian cancer, soft tissue sarcoma

DOSAGE AND ROUTES
• *Adult:* **IV** 500 mcg/m^2/day × 5 days; stop drug for 2-4 wk; then repeat cycle
• *Child:* **IV** 15 mcg/kg/day × 5 days, not to exceed 500 mcg/day; stop drug until bone marrow recovery, then repeat cycle
Available forms: Inj 0.5 mg/vial

SIDE EFFECTS
CNS: Malaise, fatigue, lethargy, fever
EENT: Chelitis, dysphagia, esophagitis
GI: Nausea, vomiting, anorexia, stomatitis, **hepatotoxicity,** abdominal pain, diarrhea
HEMA: **Thrombocytopenia, leukopenia, aplastic anemia**
INTEG: Rash, alopecia, pain at inj site, folliculitis, acne, desquamation, **extravasation**
MS: Myalgia
Contraindications: Hypersensitivity, herpes infection, child <6 mo
Precautions: Renal/hepatic disease, pregnancy (C), lactation, bone marrow depression

PHARMACOKINETICS
Half-life 36 hr; IV onset 2-5 min; concentrates in kidneys, liver, spleen; does not cross blood-brain barrier; excreted in feces and urine

INTERACTIONS
Increase: toxicity—other antineoplastics, radiation
Drug/Lab Test
Increase: Uric acid

NURSING CONSIDERATIONS
Assess:
• CBC, differential, platelet count weekly; withhold drug if WBC is <4000/mm^3 or platelet count is <75,000/mm^3; notify prescriber
• Renal studies: BUN, serum uric acid, urine CCr, electrolytes before, during therapy
• I&O ratio; report fall in urine output to <30 ml/hr
• Monitor temp q4h; fever may indicate beginning infection
• Hepatic studies before, during therapy: bilirubin, AST, ALT, alk phos, as needed or monthly; check for jaundice of skin, sclera; dark urine; clay-colored stools; itchy skin; abdominal pain; fever; diarrhea
• Bleeding: hematuria, guaiac stools, bruising, petechiae, mucosa or orifices q8h
• Food preferences; list likes, dislikes
• Effects of alopecia on body image; discuss feelings about body changes
• Inflammation of mucosa, breaks in skin
• Buccal cavity q8h for dryness, sores, ulceration, white patches, oral pain, bleeding, dysphagia
⚠ Symptoms indicating severe allergic reaction: rash, pruritus, urticaria, purpuric skin lesions, itching, flushing
• GI symptoms: frequency of stools, cramping, nausea, vomiting, anorexia
• Acidosis, signs of dehydration: rapid respirations, poor skin turgor, decreased urine output, dry skin, restlessness, weakness, sunken eyeball in children

Administer:
• Antiemetic 30-60 min before giving drug to prevent vomiting
• Increase fluids to 3 L/day

IV route
• After diluting 0.5 mg/1.1 ml of sterile H_2O for inj without preservative; use 2.2 ml (0.25 mg/ml), give by direct IV at 0.5 mg or less/min through Y-tube or 3-way stopcock if inf in progress; may be further diluted if required in 50 ml D_5W or NS for infusion; run over 10-15 min; change needles between reconstitution and direct IV administration
• Hydrocortisone, sodium thiosulfate to infiltration area, and ice compress after stopping infusion

Y-site compatibilities: Allopurinol, amifostine, aztreonam, cefepime, fludarabine, granisetron, melphalan, ondansetron, sargramostim, teniposide, thiotepa, vinorelbine

Perform/provide:
• Strict hand-washing technique, gloves and protective covering
• Liquid diet: carbonated beverages; gelatin may be added if patient is not nauseated or vomiting
• Rinsing of mouth tid-qid with water, club soda; brushing of teeth bid-qid with soft brush or cotton-tipped applicators for stomatitis; use unwaxed dental floss to prevent injury
• Storage in cool, dark environment; do not expose to bright light or freeze
• Fluid increase to 3 L/day

Evaluate:
• Therapeutic response: decreased tumor size, spread of malignancy

Teach patient/family:
• That reliable contraception is needed during treatment and for 4-6 mo after discontinuing therapy; do not breastfeed
• To avoid vaccinations without order by prescriber
• That hair may be lost during treatment after 1-2 wk and that wig or hairpiece may make patient feel better; that new hair may be different in color, texture
• To avoid foods with citric acid, hot or rough texture when stomatitis is present
• To report any bleeding, white spots, ulcerations in mouth to prescriber; tell patient to examine mouth daily
• To avoid crowds, persons with known infection when granulocyte count is low

---

⚠ High Alert

dalteparin (℞)
(dahl'ta-pear-in)
Fragmin
Func. class.: Anticoagulant
Chem. class.: Low molecular weight heparin

Action: Inhibits factor Xa/IIa (thrombin) resulting in anticoagulation

Uses: Unstable angina/non–Q-wave MI; prevention of deep vein thrombosis in abdominal surgery, hip replacement or those with restricted mobility during acute illness

Unlabeled uses: Antiphospholipid antibody, arterial thromboembolism, cerebral thromboembolism, pulmonary embolism

DOSAGE AND ROUTES

Hip replacement surgery/DVT prophylaxis
• *Adult:* **SUBCUT** 2500 international units 2 hr prior to surgery and 2nd dose in the evening the day of surgery (4-8 hr postop), then 5000 international units **SUBCUT** 1st postop day and daily 5-10 days

Unstable angina/non–Q-wave MI
• *Adult:* **SUBCUT** 120 international units/kg × 5-8 days, max 10,000 international units q12h × 5-8 days, with concurrent aspirin, continue until stable

DVT, prophylaxis for abdominal surgery
• *Adult:* **SUBCUT** 2500 international units evening prior to surgery and repeat daily × 5-10 days; in high-risk patients 5000 international units should be used

Available forms: Prefilled syringes, 2500, 5000 international units/0.2 ml;

7500 international units/0.3 ml, 10,000, 25,000 international units/ml

SIDE EFFECTS

CNS: **Intracranial bleeding**
HEMA: **Thrombocytopenia**
INTEG: Pruritus, superficial wound infection
SYST: Hypersensitivity, **hemorrhage, anaphylaxis** possible

Contraindications: Hypersensitivity to this drug, heparin, or pork products, benzyl alcohol; active major bleeding, hemophilia, leukemia with bleeding, thrombocytopenic purpura, cerebrovascular hemorrhage, cerebral aneurysm, those undergoing regional anesthesia for unstable angina, non–Q-wave MI, dalteparin-induced thrombocytopenia

Precautions: Pregnancy (B); lactation; geriatric; hepatic disease; severe renal disease; blood dyscrasias; bacterial endocarditis; acute nephritis; uncontrolled hypertension; recent brain, spine, eye surgery; congenital or acquired disorders; severe cardiac disease; children; recent childbirth; peptic ulcer disease; hemorrhagic stroke; history of HIT; pericarditis; pericardial effusion; recent lumbar puncture; vasculitis; other diseases in which bleeding is possible

PHARMACOKINETICS

87% absorbed, excreted by kidneys, elimination half-life 3-5 hr, peak 4 hr, onset 1-2 hr, duration >12 hr

INTERACTIONS

Increase: risk of bleeding—aspirin, oral anticoagulants, platelet inhibitors, NSAIDs, salicylates, thrombolytics

Drug/Herb
Increase: bleeding risk—agrimony, alfalfa, angelica, anise, bilberry, black haw, bogbean, bromelain, buchu, chondroitin, cinchona bark, dong quai, fenugreek, feverfew, garlic, ginger, ginkgo, ginseng, horse chestnut, Irish moss, kelp, kelpware, khella, lovage, lungwort, meadowsweet, motherwort, mugwort, nettle, papaya, parsley (large amts), pau d'arco, pineapple, poplar, prickly ash, safflower, saw palmetto, senega, tonka bean, turmeric, wintergreen, yarrow

Decrease: anticoagulant action—chamomile, coenzyme, flax, glucomannan, goldenseal, guar gum

NURSING CONSIDERATIONS

Assess:
• For blood studies (Hct, CBC, platelets, occult blood in stools) during treatment since bleeding can occur

⚠ For bleeding gums, petechiae, ecchymosis, black tarry stools, hematuria, epistaxis, decrease in Hct, B/P; may indicate bleeding, possible hemorrhage; notify prescriber immediately, drug should be discontinued

⚠ For neurologic impairment frequently in those when neuraxial anesthesia has been used, spinal/epidural hematomas can occur, with paralysis

• For hypersensitivity: fever, skin rash, urticaria; notify prescriber immediately

• For needed dosage change q1-2wk; dose may need to be decreased if bleeding occurs

Administer:
• Cannot be used interchangeably (unit for unit) with unfractionated heparin or LMWHs

• Do not give IM or IV drug route; approved is SUBCUT only; do not mix with other inj or sol

• Have patient sit or lie down; SUBCUT inj may be 2 in from umbilicus in a U-shape, upper outer side of thigh, around navel, or upper outer quadrangle of the buttocks; rotate inj sites

• Changing needles is not recommended; change inj site daily; use at same time of day

Evaluate:
• Therapeutic response: absence of deep-vein thrombosis

Teach patient/family:
• To avoid OTC preparations that contain aspirin; other anticoagulants, serious drug interaction may occur unless approved by prescriber

---

• To use soft-bristle toothbrush to avoid bleeding gums, avoid contact sports, use electric razor, avoid IM inj
• To report any signs of bleeding: gums, under skin, urine, stools; unusual bruising

Treatment of overdose: Protamine sulfate 1% given IV; 1 mg protamine/100 anti-Xa international units of dalteparin given

---

dantrolene (℞)

(dan'troe-leen)
Dantrium
Func. class.: Skeletal muscle relaxant, direct acting
Chem. class.: Hydantoin

Do not confuse:
Dantrium/danazol

Action: Interferes with intracellular release of calcium from the sarcoplasmic reticulum necessary to initiate contraction; slows catabolism in malignant hyperthermia

Uses: Spasticity in multiple sclerosis, stroke, spinal cord injury, cerebral palsy, malignant hyperthermia

Unlabeled uses: Neuroleptic malignant syndrome

DOSAGE AND ROUTES

Spasticity
• *Adult:* **PO** 25 mg/day; may increase by 25-100 mg bid-qid, not to exceed 400 mg/day × 1 wk
• *Child:* **PO** 1 mg/kg/day given in divided doses bid; dosage may increase gradually, not to exceed 400 mg daily

Prevention of malignant hyperthermia
• *Adult and child:* **PO** 4-8 mg/kg/day in 3-4 divided doses × 1-2 days prior to procedures, give last dose 4 hr preop; **IV** 2.5 mg/kg prior to anesthesia

Malignant hyperthermia
• *Adult and child:* **IV** 1 mg/kg, may repeat to total dose of 10 mg/kg; **PO** 4-8 mg/kg/day in 4 divided doses × 3 days to

prevent further hyperthermia; post-crisis follow-up 4-8 mg/kg/day for 1-3 days

Neuroleptic malignant syndrome (unlabeled)
• *Adult:* **PO** 100-300 mg/day in divided doses; **IV** 1.25-1.5 mg/kg

Available forms: Caps 25, 50, 100 mg; powder for inj 20 mg/vial

SIDE EFFECTS

CNS: Dizziness, weakness, fatigue, drowsiness, headache, disorientation, insomnia, paresthesias, tremors, **seizures**
CV: Hypotension, chest pain, palpitations
EENT: Nasal congestion, blurred vision, mydriasis
GI: **Hepatic injury**, *nausea,* constipation, vomiting, increased AST, alk phos, abdominal pain, dry mouth, anorexia, hepatitis, dyspepsia
GU: Urinary frequency, nocturia, impotence, crystalluria
HEMA: **Eosinophilia**
INTEG: Rash, pruritus, photosensitivity
RESP: Pleural effusion

Contraindications: Hypersensitivity, compromised pulmonary function, active hepatic disease, impaired myocardial function

Precautions: Pregnancy (C), peptic ulcer disease, renal/hepatic disease, stroke, seizure disorder, diabetes mellitus, lactation, geriatric

PHARMACOKINETICS

Oral absorption poor
PO: Peak 5 hr; highly protein bound; half-life 8 hr; metabolized in liver; excreted in urine (metabolites)

INTERACTIONS

• Considered incompatible in sol or syringe; compatibility unknown
Increase: dysrhythmias—verapamil
Increase: hepatotoxicity—estrogens, other hepatotoxics
Increase: CNS depression—alcohol, tricyclics, opiates, barbiturates, sedatives, hypnotics, antihistamines

---

⚠ Safety alert   *"Tall Man" lettering

NURSING CONSIDERATIONS
Assess:
- For increased seizure activity, ECG in epilepsy patient; poor seizure control has occurred
- I&O ratio; check for urinary retention, frequency, hesitancy, especially geriatric
- Hepatic function by frequent determination of AST, ALT, bilirubin, alk phos, GGTP; renal function studies, BUN, creatinine, CBC
- Allergic reactions: rash, fever, respiratory distress
- Severe weakness, numbness in extremities; prescriber should be notified and drug discontinued
- Tolerance: increased need for medication, more frequent requests for medication, increased pain
- CNS depression: dizziness, drowsiness, insomnia, psychiatric symptoms

⚠ Signs of hepatotoxicity: jaundice, yellow sclera, pain in abdomen, nausea, fever; prescriber should be notified, drug should be discontinued

Administer:
- Avoid use with other CNS depressants
PO route
- Do not crush or chew caps
- Caps may be opened, mixed with juice and swallowed
- With meals for GI symptoms
IV route
- IV after diluting 20 mg/60 ml sterile H₂O for inj without bacteriostatic agent (333 mcg/ml); shake until clear; give by rapid IV push through Y-tube or 3-way stopcock; follow by prescribed doses immediately; may also give by intermittent inf over 1 hr prior to anesthesia
Perform/provide:
- Storage in tight container at room temperature; protect diluted sol from light, use reconstituted solution within 6 hr
- Gum, frequent sips of water for dry mouth
- Assistance with ambulation if dizziness/drowsiness occurs

Evaluate:
- Therapeutic response: decreased pain, spasticity
Teach patient/family:
- Not to discontinue medication quickly; hallucinations, spasticity, tachycardia will occur; drug should be tapered off over 1-2 wk; notify prescriber of abdominal pain, jaundiced sclera, clay-colored stools, change in color of urine
- Not to take with alcohol
- That if improvement does not occur within 6 wk, prescriber may discontinue
- To avoid hazardous activities if drowsiness, dizziness occurs
- To avoid using OTC medication: cough preparations, antihistamines, unless directed by prescriber
- To use sunscreen or stay out of the sun to prevent burns
Treatment of overdose: Induce emesis of conscious patient; lavage, dialysis

---

dapiprazole ophthalmic
See Appendix C

---

daptomycin (℞)
(dap′toe-mye-sin)
Cubicin
Func. class.: Antiinfective—miscellaneous
Chem. class.: Lipopeptides

Action: A new class of antiinfective; it binds to the bacterial membrane and results in a rapid depolarization of the membrane potential, thus leading to inhibition of DNA, RNA, and protein synthesis
Uses: Complicated skin, skin structure infections caused by *Staphylococcus aureus* including methicillin-resistant strains, *Streptococcus pyogenes, Streptococcus agalactiae, Streptococcus dysgalactiae, Enterococcus faecalis* (vancomycin-susceptible strains)
Unlabeled uses: Bacteremia endocarditis, UTI, vancomycin-resistant enterococci (VRE)

DOSAGE AND ROUTES

• *Adult:* **IV INF** 4 mg/kg over ½ hr diluted in 0.9% NaCl, give q24h × 7-14 days
Bacteremia, endocarditis, UTI (unlabeled)
• *Adult:* **IV** 6 mg/kg/day
VRE (unlabeled)
• *Adult:* **IV** 4 mg/kg/day
Renal dose
• *Adult:* **IV INF** CCr <30 ml/min, hemodialysis, CAPD 4 mg/kg q48h
Available forms: Lyophilized powder for inj 250, 500 mg

SIDE EFFECTS

CNS: Headache, insomnia, dizziness
CV: Hypotension, hypertension, **heart failure**
GI: Nausea, constipation, diarrhea, vomiting, dyspepsia, **pseudomembranous colitis**
GU: Nephrotoxicity
HEMA: Leukocytosis
INTEG: Rash, pruritus
MISC: Fungal infections, UTI, anemia
MS: Muscle pain or weakness, arthralgia, pain
Contraindications: Hypersensitivity
Precautions: Renal/GI disease, pregnancy (B), children, lactation, geriatric, myopathy

PHARMACOKINETICS

Site of metabolism unknown, protein binding 92%

INTERACTIONS

Increase: myopathy—HMG-CoA reductase inhibitors
Drug/Lab Test
Increase: CPK, AST, ALT, BUN, creatinine, albumin

NURSING CONSIDERATIONS

Assess:
• I&O ratio: report hematuria, oliguria; nephrotoxicity may occur
⚠ Any patient with compromised renal system, toxicity may occur; BUN, creatinine

• Blood studies: CBC
• C&S, drug may be given as soon as culture is taken
• B/P during administration; hypo-, hypertension may occur
• Signs of infection
• Respiratory status: rate, character, wheezing
• Allergies before treatment, reaction of each medication
Administer:
IV route
• After reconstitution with 5 ml 0.9% NaCl (250 mg/5 ml) or 10 ml 0.9% NaCl (500 mg/10 ml), further dilution is needed with 0.9 NaCl, infuse over ½ hr
Solution compatibilities: 0.9% NaCl, LR
Evaluate:
• Therapeutic response: Negative culture
Teach patient/family:
• Allergies before treatment, reaction of each medication
• All aspects of drug therapy
• To report sore throat, fever, fatigue, could indicate superinfection

---

darbepoetin (℞)
(dar'bee-poh'eh-tin)
Aranesp
Func. class.: Hematopoietic agent
Chem. class.: Recombinant human erythropoietin

Action: Stimulates erythropoiesis by the same mechanism as endogenous erythropoietin; in response to hypoxia, erythropoietin is produced in the kidney and released into the bloodstream, where it interacts with progenitor stem cells to increase red cell production
Uses: Anemia associated with chronic renal failure, in patients on and not on dialysis and anemia in nonmyeloid malignancies receiving coadministered chemotherapy

---

DOSAGE AND ROUTES

Correction of anemia in chronic renal failure
• *Adult:* **SUBCUT/IV** 0.45 mcg/kg as a single inj, every week titrate not to exceed a target Hgb of 12 g/dl

Epoetin alfa to darbepoetin conversion
• *Adult:* **SUBCUT/IV** (epoetin alfa <2500 units/wk) 6.25 mcg/wk; (epoetin alfa 2500-4999 units/wk) 12.5 mcg/wk; (epoetin alfa 5000-10,999 units/wk) 25 mcg/wk; (epoetin alfa 11,000-17,999 units/wk) 40 mcg/wk; (epoetin alfa 18,000-33,999 units/wk) 60 mcg/wk; (epoetin alfa 34,000-89,999 units/wk) 100 mcg/wk; (epoetin alfa >90,000 units/wk) 200 mcg/wk

Available forms: Sol for inj 25, 40, 60, 100, 150, 200, 300, 500 mcg/ml

SIDE EFFECTS

CNS: **Seizures,** sweating, headache, dizziness, **stroke,** headache

CV: Hypertension, hypotension, **cardiac arrest,** *angina pectoris,* **thrombosis, CHF, acute MI, dysrhythmias,** chest pain, transient ischemic attacks, edema

GI: Diarrhea, vomiting, nausea, abdominal pain, constipation

MISC: Infection, fatigue, fever, **death,** *fluid overload,* **vascular access hemorrhage,** dehydration, **sepsis**

MS: Bone pain, myalgia, limb pain, back pain

RESP: URI, dyspnea, cough, bronchitis

SYST: Allergic reactions, **anaphylaxis**

Contraindications: Hypersensitivity to mammalian cell–derived products or human albumin, uncontrolled hypertension, red cell aplasia

Precautions: Pregnancy (C), seizure disorder, porphyria, hypertension, lactation, children, sickle cell disease; vit B$_{12}$, folate deficiency, chronic renal failure, dialysis

PHARMACOKINETICS

IV: Onset of increased reticulocyte count 2-6 wk; distributed to vascular space; absorption slow and rate-limiting; terminal half-life 49 hr (SUBCUT), 21 hr (IV); peak concentration at 34 hr; increased Hgb levels not generally observed until 2-6 wk after treatment initiated

INTERACTIONS

⚠ Do not use epoetin alfa with this drug
Increase: darbepoetin alfa effect—androgens
Drug/Lab Test
Increase: WBC, platelets
Decrease: Bleeding time

NURSING CONSIDERATIONS

Assess:
• For symptoms of anemia: fatigue, dyspnea, pallor

⚠ Serious allergic reactions: rash, urticaria; if anaphylaxis occurs, stop drug, administer emergency treatment (rare)

• Renal studies: urinalysis, protein, blood, BUN, creatinine; monitor dialysis shunts; during dialysis, heparin may need to be increased

• Blood studies: ferritin, transferrin qmo; transferrin sat ≥20%, ferritin ≥100 ng/ml; Hgb 2×/wk until stabilized in target range (30%-33%), then at regular intervals; those with endogenous erythropoietin levels of <500 units/L respond to this agent; iron stores should be corrected before beginning therapy

• B/P; check for rising B/P as Hgb rises, antihypertensives may be needed

• CV status: hypertension may occur rapidly leading to hypertensive encephalopathy

• I&O; report drop in output to <50 ml/hr

• For seizures if Hgb is increased within 2 wk by 4 pts institute seizure precautions

• CNS symptoms: sweating, pain in long bones

Side effects: *italics* = common; **bold** = life-threatening

• Dialysis patients: thrill, bruit of shunts, monitor for circulation impairment

Administer:

IV/SUBCUT route

• Without shaking; check for discoloration, particulate matter, do not use if present; do not dilute, do not mix with other drugs or solutions, discard unused portion, do not pool unused portions

• Subcut is typically used with those not requiring dialysis

• IV is given undiluted as direct, or bolus into IV tubing or venous line after completion of dialysis

• Adjust dosage every month or more

Evaluate:

• Therapeutic response: increase in reticulocyte count, Hgb/Hct; increased appetite, enhanced sense of well-being

Teach patient/family:

• To avoid driving or hazardous activity during beginning of treatment

• To monitor B/P, Hgb

• To take iron supplements, vit B_{12}, folic acid as directed

• To report side effects to prescriber, to comply with treatment regimen

• That menses and fertility may return; use contraception if want to

• Home administration procedures, if appropriate

---

darunavir

See Appendix A—Selected New Drugs

---

dasatinib

See Appendix A—Selected New Drugs

⚠ High Alert

***DAUNOrubicin** (℞)

(daw-noe-roo'bi-sin)

Cerubidine

***DAUNOrubicin citrate liposome**

DaunoXome

Func. class.: Antineoplastic, antibiotic

Chem. class.: Anthracycline glycoside

Do not confuse:

DAUNOrubicin/DOXOrubicin

Action: Inhibits DNA synthesis, primarily; derived from *Streptomyces coerulorubidus;* replication is decreased by binding to DNA, which causes strand splitting; cell cycle specific (S phase); a vesicant

Uses: Myelogenous, monocytic leukemia, acute nonlymphocytic leukemia, Ewing's sarcoma, rhabdomyosarcoma; DAUNOrubicin citrate liposome: advanced Kaposi's sarcoma in HIV

DOSAGE AND ROUTES

Use decreased dose for those >60 yr of age

DAUNOrubicin

Single agent

• *Adult:* **IV** 60 mg/m²/day × 3-5 days q4wk

In combination

• *Adult:* **IV** 45 mg/m²/day × 3 days, then 2 days of subsequent courses in combination

• *Child:* **IV** 25-60 mg/m² depending on cycle

DAUNOrubicin citrate liposome

• *Adult:* **IV** 40 mg/m² q2wk

Renal dose

• *Adult:* **IV** serum CCr >3 mg/dl reduce dose by 50%

Hepatic dose

• *Adult:* **IV** serum bilirubin 1.2-3 mg/dl reduce dose by 25%; bilirubin >3 mg/dl reduce dose by 50%

⚠ Safety alert   *"Tall Man" lettering

Available forms: Inj 20 mg powder/vial, sol for inj 5 mg/ml (DaunoXome); *liposome:* dispersion for inj 2 mg/ml

SIDE EFFECTS

DAUNOrubicin
CNS: Fever, chills
CV: **Dysrhythmias, CHF, pericarditis, myocarditis,** peripheral edema
GI: Nausea, vomiting, anorexia, mucositis, **hepatotoxicity**
GU: Impotence, sterility, amenorrhea, gynecomastia, hyperuricemia
HEMA: **Thrombocytopenia, leukopenia, anemia**
INTEG: Rash, **extravasation,** dermatitis, reversible alopecia, cellulitis, thrombophlebitis at inj site
SYST: **Anaphylaxis**

DAUNOrubicin citrate liposome
CNS: Fatigue, headache, depression, insomnia, dizziness, *malaise, neuropathy*
CV: Chest pain, edema
GI: Abdominal pain, stomatitis, *nausea, vomiting, diarrhea,* constipation
INTEG: Alopecia, pruritus, sweating
MISC: Allergic reactions, chest pain, fever, edema, flulike symptoms
MS: Rigors, arthralgia, back pain
RESP: Cough, dyspnea, rhinitis, sinusitis

Contraindications: Pregnancy (D), hypersensitivity, lactation, systemic infections, cardiac disease, bone marrow depression
Precautions: Renal/hepatic disease; gout

PHARMACOKINETICS

Half-life 18½ hr, liposome 55½ hr; metabolized by liver; crosses placenta; excreted in breast milk, urine, bile

INTERACTIONS

Increase: bleeding risk—NSAIDs, salicylates
Increase: toxicity—other antineoplastics, radiation, cyclophosphamide
Decrease: antibody reaction—live virus vaccines

Drug/Lab Test
Increase: Uric acid

NURSING CONSIDERATIONS

Assess:
⚠ CBC, differential, platelet count weekly, leukocyte nadir within 2 wk after administration, recovery within 3 wk; do not administer if absolute granulocyte count is <750/mm^3 (liposome)
• Blood, urine uric acid levels baseline and during therapy
• Renal studies: BUN, urine CCr, electrolytes baseline, before each dose
• I&O ratio; report fall in urine output to <30 ml/hr
• Monitor temp q4h; fever may indicate beginning infection
• Hepatic studies baseline, before each dose: bilirubin, AST, ALT, alk phos; check for jaundice of skin, sclera; dark urine; clay-colored stools; itchy skin; abdominal pain; fever; diarrhea
• Chest x-ray, echocardiography, radionuclide angiography, ECG; watch for ST-T wave changes, low QRS and T, possible dysrhythmias (sinus tachycardia, heart block, PVCs); watch for CHF (jugular vein distention, weight gain, edema, crackles), may occur after 2-6 mo of treatment
• Bleeding: hematuria, guaiac stools, bruising or petechiae, mucosa or orifices q8h
• Effects of alopecia on body image; discuss feelings about body changes
• Buccal cavity q8h for dryness, sores or ulceration, white patches, oral pain, bleeding, dysphagia
• Local irritation, pain, burning at inj site
• GI symptoms: frequency of stools, cramping
• Acidosis, signs of dehydration: rapid respirations, poor skin turgor, decreased urine output, dry skin, restlessness, weakness

Administer:
• Antiemetic 30-60 min before giving drug and 6-10 hr after treatment to prevent vomiting

---

• Allopurinol or sodium bicarbonate to reduce uric acid levels, alkalinization of urine

IV route (Cerubidine)
• After diluting 20 mg/4 ml sterile H_2O for inj (5 mg/ml), rotate, further dilute in 10-15 ml 0.9% NaCl; give over 3-5 min by direct IV through Y-tube or 3-way stopcock of inf of D_5 or 0.9% NaCl; or dilute in 50 ml 0.9% NaCl and give over 10-15 min; or dilute in 100 ml and give over 30 min
• Hydrocortisone for extravasation; apply ice compress after stopping infusion
Additive compatibilities: Cytarabine/etoposide, hydrocortisone; not recommended for admixing
Solution compatibilities: $D_{3.3}$/0.3% NaCl, D_5W, Normosol R, Ringer's, 0.9% NaCl
Y-site compatibilities: Amifostine, filgrastim, granisetron, melphalan, methotrexate, ondansetron, sodium bicarbonate, teniposide, thiotepa, vinorelbine

IV route (DaunoXome)
• Dilute with D_5W to (1 mg/ml) give over 60 min, do not use in-line filter, reconstituted sol may be stored ≤6 hr refrigerated; do not admix
Perform/provide:
• Increased fluid intake to 2-3 L/day to prevent urate and calculi formation
• Rinsing of mouth tid-qid with water, club soda; brushing of teeth bid-qid with soft brush or cotton-tipped applicators for stomatitis; use unwaxed dental floss
Evaluate:
• Therapeutic response: decreased tumor size, spread of malignancy
Teach patient/family:
• To report signs of infection, bleeding, bruising, shortness of breath, swelling, change in heart rate
• That hair may be lost during treatment and wig or hairpiece may make patient feel better; tell patient that new hair may be different in color, texture
• To avoid pregnancy while on this drug, and 4 mo thereafter; do not breastfeed
• To avoid foods with citric acid, hot or rough texture

• To report any bleeding, white spots, ulcerations in mouth; tell patient to examine mouth daily
• That urine and other body fluids may be red-orange for 48 hr
• To avoid vaccines while taking this drug
• To avoid crowds, those with known infections
• To avoid alcohol, aspirin, NSAIDs

---

decitabine (℞)
(de-sit′-a-been)
Dacogen
Func. class.: DNA demethylation agent
Chem. class.: Cytosine analog

Action: Incorporated into DNA and inhibits DNA methylation, halting growth of rapid proliferation of blasts
Uses: Treatment of naïve and experienced myelodysplasic syndrome

DOSAGE AND ROUTES
• *Adult:* **CONT IV** first treatment cycle: 15 mg/m² over 3 hr, q8hr × 3 days; subsequent treatment cycles: repeat above cycle q6wk for at least 4 cycles; a partial or complete response may take more than 4 cycles

Available forms: Powder for injection, lyophilized 50 mg, in single-dose vial

SIDE EFFECTS
CNS: Headache, anxiety, dizziness, hypoesthesia, insomnia, confusion
CV: Edema, murmur, hypotension
GI: Nausea, anorexia, vomiting, diarrhea, constipation, stomatitis, abdominal pain, dyspepsia
HEMA: **Neutropenia, thrombocytopenia, leukopenia, anemia**
INTEG: Alopecia, ecchymosis, erythema, pallor, petechiae, pruritus, rash, swelling face, urticaria, hematoma, cellulitis
META: Decreased potassium, sodium, magnesium, albumin; increased bilirubin, increased/decreased glucose
MS: Myalgia, arthralgia, back pain, chest wall pain, pain in limbs

---

RESP: Cough, crackles, hypoxia, pharyngitis, pneumonia, pulmonary edema
Contraindications: Pregnancy (D), hypersensitivity to this product, severe neurotoxicity, severe blood dyscrasias, lactation, children
Precautions: Severe renal/hepatic disease, men (men should not father a child while receiving treatments or for 2 mo after treatment ends)

PHARMACOKINETICS
Protein binding <1%; may be metabolized by the liver, granulocytes, intestinal epithelium, whole blood; terminal half-life 0.2-0.8 hr; data is limited

INTERACTIONS
• Do not use with live virus vaccines

NURSING CONSIDERATIONS
Assess:
• CBC (RBC, Hct, Hgb), diff, platelet count weekly; withhold drug if WBC <4000/mm^3, platelets <75,000/mm^3, or RBC, Hct, Hgb is low; notify prescriber of results
• Renal studies: BUN, serum uric acid, urine CCr, electrolytes before and during therapy
• Monitor temp q4h; fever may indicate beginning infection; no rectal temps
• Hepatic studies before and during treatment: bilirubin, AST, ALT, alk phos, as needed or monthly
• Bleeding: hematuria, heme-positive stools, bruising or petechiae, mucosa or orifices daily; blood dyscrasias can occur
• Dyspnea, crackles, unproductive cough, chest pain, tachypnea, fatigue, increased pulse, pallor, lethargy, personality changes
• Buccal cavity daily for dryness, ulceration, white patches, oral pain, bleeding, dysphagia
• GI symptoms: frequency of stools, cramping; if severe diarrhea occurs, electrolytes may need to be given

Administer:
• Use procedures for handling and disposal of drugs
Perform/provide:
• Rinsing of mouth tid-qid with water or club soda, brushing teeth tid with soft toothbrush or cotton tipped applicator for stomatitis; use unwaxed dental floss
• Storage at room temperature, away from light
Evaluate:
• Therapeutic response: decreased
Teach patient/family:
• To report bleeding; not to use commercial mouthwashes, razors
• To report signs of infection: increased temp, sore throat, flulike symptoms
• To report signs of anemia: fatigue, headache, faintness, shortness of breath, irritability
• To avoid citric acid, rough textured foods, if stomatitis is present
• To notify prescriber if pregnancy is suspected or planned; use contraception while taking this product
• To avoid breastfeeding while taking this product
• Not to operate machinery or perform other hazardous activities while taking this product
• That men should not father a child while taking this product, pregnancy category (D)
• To inform prescriber of renal/hepatic disease
• Not to receive vaccinations while taking this product

deferasirox
See Appendix A—Selected New Drugs

Rarely Used

deferoxamine (R)
(de-fer-ox′a-meen)
Desferal
Func. class.: Heavy metal chelator

Do not confuse:
deferoxamine/cefuroxime
Uses: Acute, chronic iron intoxication, hemochromatosis, hemosiderosis

DOSAGE AND ROUTES
Acute iron toxicity
• *Adult and child:* **IM/IV** 1 g, then 500 mg q4h × 2 doses, then 500 mg q4-12h × 2 doses, not to exceed 15 mg/kg/hr or 6 g/24 hr
Chronic iron toxicity
• *Adult and child:* **IM** 500 mg-1 g/day plus **IV INF** 2 g given by separate line with each unit of blood, not to exceed 15 mg/kg/hr or 6 g/24 hr; **SUBCUT** 1-2 g over 8-24 hr by SUBCUT inf pump
Iron overload due to transfusion-dependent anemias
• *Adult:* **IM** 1 g/day plus **IV** 2 g per unit of blood, max 1 g/day with no blood, 6 g/day with 3 or more units of blood or packed RBC
Contraindications: Hypersensitivity, anuria, severe renal disease, child <3 yr

delavirdine (R)
(de-la-veer′deen)
Rescriptor
Func. class.: Antiretroviral
Chem. class.: Nonnucleoside reverse transcriptase inhibitor (NNRTI)

Action: Binds directly to reverse transcriptase and blocks RNA, DNA, causing a disruption of the enzyme's site
Uses: HIV-1 in combination with other antiretrovirals

DOSAGE AND ROUTES
• *Adult and child ≥16 yr:* **PO** 400 mg tid, max 1200 mg/day

Available forms: Tabs 100, 200 mg

SIDE EFFECTS
CNS: Headache, fatigue
GI: Diarrhea, abdominal pain, nausea, anorexia, vomiting, dyspepsia, **hepatotoxicity**
GU: **Nephrotoxicity**
HEMA: **Neutropenia, leukopenia, thrombocytopenia, anemia, granulocytopenia**
INTEG: Rash, pruritus
MS: Pain, myalgia
SYST: **Stevens-Johnson syndrome**
Contraindications: Hypersensitivity to this drug or atevirdine
Precautions: Pregnancy (C), lactation, children, renal/hepatic disease, myleosuppression

PHARMOCOKINETICS:
98% protein bound, half-life 5.8 hr, peak 1 hr, duration 8 hr, extensively metabolized, excreted in urine/feces

INTERACTIONS
⚠ Serious life-threatening adverse reaction: amphetamines, ergots, benzodiazepines, calcium channel blockers, sedative/hypnotics, antidysrhythmics, sildenafil, pimozide, cisapride
Increase: levels of alprazolam, clarithromycin, dapsone, ergots, felodipine, midazolam, nifedipine, indinavir, amprenavir, saquinavir, lovastatin, simvastatin, atorvastatin
Increase: delavirdine levels—fluoxetine, ketoconazole
Increase: levels of both drugs—quinidine, warfarin, clarithromycin
Decrease: delavirdine levels—antacids, anticonvulsants, rifamycins, protease inhibitors, didanosine
Decrease: action of oral contraceptives, didanosine

NURSING CONSIDERATIONS
Assess:
• For signs of infection, anemia
• Hepatic studies: ALT, AST; renal studies

• C&S before drug therapy; drug may be taken as soon as culture is taken; repeat C&S after treatment; determine the presence of other sexually transmitted disease
• Bowel pattern before, during treatment; if severe abdominal pain with bleeding occurs, drug should be discontinued; monitor hydration
• For skin eruptions; rash, urticaria, itching
• For allergies before treatment, reaction to each medication; place allergies on chart
• Plasma delavirdine concentrations (trough 10 micromolar)
• CBC, blood chemistry, plasma HIV RNA, absolute CD4+/CD8+/cell counts/%, serum β-2 microglobulin, serum ICD+24 antigen levels
• For signs of delavirdine toxicity: severe nausea/vomiting, maculopapular rash

Administer:
• Dispersion by adding 4 tab/3-4 oz water, let stand, stir, swallow, rinse glass, swallow; use only 100 mg tabs for dispersion
• Do not give within 1 hr of antacids or didanosine

Evaluate:
• Therapeutic response: increased CD4 cell count, decreased viral load, improvement in symptoms of HIV

Teach patient/family:
• To take as prescribed; if dose is missed, take as soon as remembered up to 1 hr before next dose; do not double dose
• That tabs may be dissolved in ½ cup of water, stir, when dissolved, drink right away, rinse cup with water, and drink that to get all medication
• To make sure health care provider knows of all the medications being taken
• That if severe rash, mouth sores, swelling, aching muscles/joints, or eye redness occur, stop taking and notify health care provider
• Not to breastfeed if taking this drug

demecarium ophthalmic
See Appendix C

Rarely Used
demeclocycline (℞)
(dem-e-kloe-sye′kleen)
Declomycin
Func. class.: Antiinfective

Uses: Uncommon gram-positive/gram-negative bacteria, protozoa, *Rickettsia, Mycoplasma, Haemophilus ducreyi, Yersinia pestis, Campylobacter fetus, Chlamydia trachomatis,* psittacosis, granuloma inguinale

DOSAGE AND ROUTES
• *Adult:* PO 150 mg q6h or 300 mg q12h
• *Child >8 yr:* PO 6-12 mg/kg/day in divided doses q6-12h
Gonorrhea
• *Adult:* PO 600 mg, then 300 mg q12h × 4 days, total 3 g
Contraindications: Pregnancy (D), hypersensitivity to tetracyclines, children <8 yr

denileukin diftitox (℞)
(den-ih-loo′kin dif′tih-tox)
Ontak
Func. class.: Antineoplastic— miscellaneous

Action: A recombinant DNA-derived cytotoxic protein that interacts with high-affinity IL-2 receptors on the cell surface and inhibits cellular protein synthesis
Uses: Cutaneous T-cell lymphoma that expresses CD25 component of the IL-2 receptor
Unlabeled uses: Non-Hodgkin's lymphoma, psoriasis

DOSAGE AND ROUTES

• *Adult:* **IV** 9-18 mcg/kg/day given for 5 days q21 days, infused over ≥15 min

Available forms: Sol for inj, frozen 150 mcg/ml

SIDE EFFECTS

CNS: Dizziness, paresthesia, nervousness, confusion, insomnia

CV: Hypotension, vasodilation, tachycardia, thrombosis, hypertension, dysrhythmias

GI: Nausea, anorexia, vomiting, diarrhea, constipation, dyspepsia, dysphagia

GU: Hematuria, albuminuria, pyuria, creatinine increase

HEMA: **Thrombocytopenia, leukopenia,** anemia

INTEG: Rash, pruritus, sweating

META: Hypoalbuminemia, edema, hypocalcemia, weight decrease, dehydration, hypokalemia

MISC: Fever, chills, asthenia, infection, pain, headache, chest pain, flulike symptoms

MS: Myalgia, arthralgia

RESP: Dyspnea, cough, pharyngitis, rhinitis

Contraindications: Hypersensitivity to denileukin, diphtheria toxin, IL-2

Precautions: Pregnancy (C), radiation therapy, lactation, geriatric, children

PHARMACOKINETICS

Concentrates in liver/kidneys; metabolized by proteolytic degradation

INTERACTIONS

Increase: bone marrow depression—radiation, other antineoplastics

Decrease: antibody reaction—live vaccines

NURSING CONSIDERATIONS

Assess:

• CBC, differential, platelet count weekly; withhold drug if WBC <4000/mm³ or platelet count <75,000/mm³; notify prescriber of results

• Monitor temp q4h (may indicate beginning infection)

• Hepatic studies before, during therapy (bilirubin, AST, ALT, LDH) as needed or monthly

• Bleeding: hematuria, guaiac, bruising or petechiae, mucosa or orifices q8h

• Jaundice of skin, sclera; dark urine; clay-colored stools; itchy skin; abdominal pain; fever; diarrhea

• For vascular leak syndrome after 2 wk of treatment (hypotension, edema, hypoalbuminemia); monitor weight, B/P, serum albumin, edema

• Obtain CD25 expression on skin biopsy samples

Administer:

• Antiemetic 30-60 min before giving drug to prevent vomiting

• Antibiotics for prophylaxis of infection

IV route

• Do not shake vigorously

• Prepare and hold sol in plastic syringes or soft plastic IV bags only, no glass containers

• Draw calculated dose from vial, inject into empty IV infusion bag, for each 1 ml of drug removed from vial, no more than 9 ml of sterile saline without preservative should be added to IV bag; infuse over ≥15 min; do not give by bolus; do not admix with other drugs; do not use a filter

• Use within 6 hr, discard unused portions

Perform/provide:

• Storage in light-resistant container, dry area

• Warm compresses at infusion site for inflammation

Evaluate:

• Therapeutic response: decreased tumor size, spread of malignancy

Teach patient/family:

• To report signs of infection: fever, sore throat, flulike symptoms

• To report signs of anemia: fatigue, headache, faintness, shortness of breath, irritability

• To report bleeding; avoid use of razors, commercial mouthwash

---

• To avoid use of aspirin products or ibuprofen
• To use reliable contraception; avoid breastfeeding

---

desipramine (℞)
(dess-ip′ra-meen)
Apo-Desipramine ✦,
desipramine HCl, Norpramin,
Pertofrane ✦
Func. class.: Antidepressant, tricyclic
Chem. class.: Dibenzazepine, secondary amine

Action: Blocks reuptake of norepinephrine, serotonin into nerve endings, increasing action of norepinephrine, serotonin in nerve cells
Uses: Depression
Unlabeled uses: Chronic pain, ADHD, bulimia, diabetic neuropathy, panic disorder, social phobia

DOSAGE AND ROUTES

• *Adult:* **PO** 100-200 mg/day in a single dose or in divided doses; max 300 mg/day
• *Geriatric:* **PO** 25-50 mg/day, may increase to 150 mg/day
• *Child >12 yr:* **PO** 25-50 mg/day in divided doses, max 100 mg/day
• *Child 6-12 yr:* **PO** 10-30 mg/day or 1-5 mg/kg/day in divided doses
Available forms: Tabs 10, 25, 50, 75, 100, 150 mg; caps 25, 50 mg

SIDE EFFECTS

CNS: Dizziness, drowsiness, confusion, headache, anxiety, tremors, stimulation, weakness, insomnia, nightmares, EPS (geriatric), increased psychiatric symptoms, paresthenia
CV: Orthostatic hypotension, ECG changes, tachycardia, hypertension, palpitations
EENT: Blurred vision, tinnitus, mydriasis, ophthalmoplegia
GI: Diarrhea, dry mouth, nausea, vomiting, **paralytic ileus,** increased appetite, cramps, epigastric distress, jaundice, **hepatitis,** stomatitis, constipation
GU: Retention, **acute renal failure**
HEMA: **Agranulocytosis, thrombocytopenia, eosinophilia, leukopenia**
INTEG: Rash, urticaria, sweating, pruritus, photosensitivity
Contraindications: Hypersensitivity to tricyclics, narrow-angle glaucoma
Precautions: Pregnancy (C), suicidal patients, severe depression, increased intraocular pressure, geriatric, lactation, seizure disorder, CV disease, prostatic hypertrophy

PHARMACOKINETICS

Well absorbed, widely distributed, protein binding 92%, extensively metabolized in the liver, excretion is unknown, half-life 12-24 hr

INTERACTIONS

Increase: CNS depression—alcohol, barbiturates, opioids, CNS depressants
Increase: desipramine level—cimetidine, fluvoxamine, fluoxetine, paroxetine, sertraline
Increase: life-threatening B/P elevations, do not use concurrently—clonidine
Increase: hypertension—epINEPHrine, norepinephrine
Increase: hyperpyrexia, seizures, excitation, do not use with 14 days of MAOIs—MAOI inhibitors
Drug/Herb
Increase: serotonin syndrome, avoid concurrent use—St. John's Wort, SAM-e
Increase: CNS depression—chamomile, hops, kava, valerian
Decrease: seizure threshold, do not use concurrently—evening primrose oil
Drug/Lab Test
Increase: Serum bilirubin, blood glucose, alk phos

NURSING CONSIDERATIONS
Assess:
• B/P (lying, standing), pulse q4h; if systolic B/P drops 20 mm Hg, hold drug,

---

notify prescriber; take vital signs q4h in patients with cardiovascular disease
• Blood studies: CBC, leukocytes, differential, cardiac enzymes if patient is receiving long-term therapy
• Hepatic studies: AST, ALT, bilirubin
• Weight qwk; appetite may increase with this drug
• ECG for flattening T wave, bundle branch block, AV block, dysrhythmias in cardiac patients
• EPS primarily in geriatric: rigidity, dystonia, akathisia
• Mental status: mood, sensorium, affect, suicidal tendencies, increase in psychiatric symptoms: depression, panic
• Urinary retention, constipation; constipation most likely in children
• Withdrawal symptoms: headache, nausea, vomiting, muscle pain, weakness; not usual unless drug discontinued abruptly
• Alcohol consumption; if consumed, hold dose until morning

Administer:
• Increased fluids, bulk in diet for constipation, especially in geriatric
• With food or milk for GI symptoms
• Crushed if patient is unable to swallow medication whole
• Dosage at bedtime if oversedation occurs during day; may take entire dose at bedtime; geriatric may not tolerate once a day dosing
• Gum, hard candy, frequent sips of water for dry mouth

Perform/provide:
• Storage at room temperature
• Assistance with ambulation during beginning of therapy for drowsiness/dizziness
• Safety measures, primarily in the geriatric
• Check to see that PO medication is swallowed

Evaluate:
• Therapeutic response: decreased depression

Teach patient/family
• That therapeutic effects may take 2-3 wk

• To use caution in driving, other activities requiring alertness because of drowsiness, dizziness, blurred vision
• To avoid alcohol ingestion, other CNS depressants
• Not to discontinue medication quickly after long-term use; may cause nausea, headache, malaise
• To wear sunscreen or large hat, since photosensitivity occurs

Treatment of overdose: ECG monitoring; induce emesis; lavage, activated charcoal; administer anticonvulsant

---

desirudin (℞)
(des-i-rude'in)
Iprivask
Func. class.: Anticoagulant
Chem. class.: Thrombin inhibitor

Action: Inhibits thrombin resulting in prolongation of clotting time
Uses: Prophylaxis for deep vein thrombosis in those undergoing hip replacement

DOSAGE AND ROUTES

• *Adult:* **SUBCUT** 15 mg, 1st dose 5-15 min before surgery, but after regional block anesthesia, then 15 mg q12h, up to 12 days
Available forms: Lyophilized powder 15 mg

SIDE EFFECTS

MISC: Inj site mass, nausea, deep thrombophelibitis, anemia, hypersensitivity, urinary retention, hypotension, leg edema, fever, abdominal pain, nausea, vomiting, constipation
SYST: **Bleeding, hemorrhage**
Contraindications: Hypersensitivity to natural or synthetic hirudins, active bleeding, irreversible coagulation disorders
Precautions: Pregnancy (C), lactation, children, geriatric, hepatic/renal impairment, patients with increased risks of hemorrhage, severe uncontrolled hypertension, bacterial endocarditis, hemor-

---

rhagic stroke, intracranial/intraoccular bleeding, recent ischemic stroke, GI/pulmonary bleeding

PHARMACOKINETICS

Metabolized and eliminated by the kidney (40%-50% unchanged)

INTERACTIONS

Increase: anticoagulant effect—thrombolytics, anticoagulants, antiplatelets (salicylates, NSAIDS, ketorolac, triclopidine, sulfinpyrazone, clopidogrel, abciximab)

NURSING CONSIDERATIONS

Assess:
• APTT 4 hr after administration in those with increased risk for bleeding
A For neurologic changes that may indicate intracranial bleeding
A Retroperitoneal bleeding: back pain, leg weakness, diminished pulses
• For bleeding: gums, petechiae, ecchymosis, black tarry stool, hematuria; notify prescriber
Administer:
• Alone, do not mix with other drugs or solutions
• For 9-12 days
• Only after screening patient for bleeding disorders
• SUBCUT only, do not give IM
• Give to patient recumbent, rotate inj sites (left/right anterolateral, left/right posterolateral abdominal wall)
• Insert whole length of needle into skin fold held with thumb and forefinger
• Give at same time of day to maintain blood level
• Administer only this drug when ordered, not interchangeable with heparin
Perform/provide:
• Bed rest during entire course of treatment
• Avoidance of venous or arterial puncture, inj, rectal temp
• Treatment of fever with acetaminophen
Evaluate:
• Therapeutic response: absence of deep vein thrombosis

Teach patient/family:
• About drug use and expected results; to report adverse reactions; bleeding, bruising
• To avoid all OTC drugs unless prescribed
• To use soft-bristle toothbrush to avoid bleeding gums, to use electric razor

---

desloratadine (℞)
(des′lor-at′ah-deen)
Clarinex, Clarinex Reditabs
Func. class.: Antihistamine, 2nd generation
Chem. class.: Selective histamine (H$_1$)-receptor antagonist

Action: Binds to peripheral histamine receptors, providing antihistamine action without sedation
Uses: Seasonal allergic rhinitis, chronic idiopathic urticaria

DOSAGE AND ROUTES

• *Adult and child ≥12 yr:* **PO** 5 mg daily
• *Child 6-11 yr:* **PO** 2.5 mg daily
• *Child 1-5 yr:* **PO** 1.25 mg daily
• *Child 6-11 mo:* **PO** 1 mg daily
Hepatic/renal dose
• *Adult:* **PO** 5 mg every other day
Available form: Tabs 5 mg; orally disintegrating tabs 5 mg (Reditabs); syrup 0.5 mg/ml

SIDE EFFECTS

CNS: Sedation (more common with increased doses), headache
Contraindications: Hypersensitivity, acute asthma attacks, lower respiratory tract disease
Precautions: Pregnancy (C), bronchial asthma, renal/hepatic impairment

PHARMACOKINETICS

Onset antihistamine effect 1 hr, relief as early as 1 day, duration up to 24 hr, peak 1½ hr, elimination half-life 8½-28 hr; metabolized in liver to active metabolites, excreted in urine

---

INTERACTIONS

Drug/Food
• Food may prolong time to peak with orally disintegrating tabs

NURSING CONSIDERATIONS

Assess:
• Allergy: hives, rash, rhinitis; monitor respiratory status; test interaction, antigen skin test

Administer:
• Without regard to meals
• Do not remove Redi Tabs from blister until ready to use
• Redi Tabs directly on tongue; may take with or without water

Perform/provide:
• Storage in tight container at room temperature

Evaluate:
• Therapeutic response: absence of running or congested nose, other allergy symptoms

Teach patient/family:
• To avoid driving, other hazardous activities if drowsiness occurs; observe caution until drug's effects on the patient are known
• That drug may cause photosensitivity; use sunscreen or stay out of the sun to prevent burns

---

desmopressin (℞)
(des-moe-press'in)
DDAVP, Octostim, Stimate
Func. class.: Pituitary hormone
Chem. class.: Synthetic antidiuretic hormone

Action: Promotes reabsorption of water by action on renal tubular epithelium; causes smooth muscle constriction, increase in plasma factor VIII levels, which increases platelet aggregation resulting in vasopressor effect, similar to vasopressin
Uses: Hemophilia A, von Willebrand's disease type 1, nonnephrogenic diabetes insipidus, symptoms of polyuria/polydipsia caused by pituitary dysfunction, nocturnal enuresis

DOSAGE AND ROUTES

Primary nocturnal enuresis
• *Adult and child ≥6 yr:* **INTRANASAL** 20 mcg (10 mcg in each nostril) at bedtime, may increase to 40 mcg; **PO** 0.2 mg at bedtime, may be increased to max 0.6 mg at bedtime
Diabetes insipidus
• *Adult:* **INTRANASAL** 0.1-0.4 ml daily in divided doses (1-4 sprays with pump); **IV/SUBCUT** 0.5-1 ml daily in divided doses
• *Child 3 mo to 12 yr:* **INTRANASAL** 0.05-0.3 ml daily in divided doses
Hemophilia/von Willebrand's disease
• *Adult and child >3 mo:* **IV** 0.3 mcg/kg in NaCl over 15-30 min; may repeat if needed
Antihemorrhagic
• *Adult and child >3 mo:* **IV** 0.3 mcg/kg
• *Adult and child <50 kg:* **INTRANASAL** 1 spray in one nostril
• *Adult and child >50 kg:* 1 spray each nostril
Available forms: Inj 4, 15 mcg/ml, Rhihal Tube del 2.5 mg/vial (0.1 mg/ml); tabs 0.1, 0.2 mg; nasal spray pump 10 mcg/spray (0.1 mg/ml); nasal sol 1.5 mg/ml (150 mcg/dose)

SIDE EFFECTS

CNS: Drowsiness, headache, lethargy, flushing
CV: Increased B/P
EENT: Nasal irritation, congestion, rhinitis
GI: Nausea, heartburn, cramps
GU: Vulval pain
SYST: **Anaphylaxis (IV)**
Contraindications: Hypersensitivity, nephrogenic diabetes insipidus
Precautions: Pregnancy (B), coronary artery disease, lactation, hypertension

---

PHARMACOKINETICS

NASAL: Onset 1 hr, peak 1-4 hr, duration 8-20 hr, half-life 8 min, 76 min (terminal)

PO: Onset 1 hr, peak 4-7 hr

IV: Onset 1 min, peak ½ hr, duration more than 3 hr

INTERACTIONS

Increase: antidiuretic action—carbamazepine, chlorpropamide, clofibrate

Decrease: antidiuretic action—lithium, alcohol, demeclocycline, heparin, large doses of epINEPHrine

NURSING CONSIDERATIONS

Assess:

• Pulse, B/P when giving IV or SUBCUT

• I&O ratio, weight daily; check for edema in extremities; if water retention is severe, diuretic may be prescribed

• Water intoxication: lethargy, behavioral changes, disorientation, neuromuscular excitability

• Intranasal use: nausea, congestion, cramps, headache; usually decreased with decreased dose; for nasal mucosa changes: congestion, edema, discharge, scarring (nasal route)

A For severe allergic reaction including anaphylaxis (IV route)

• Urine vol/osmolality and plasma osmolality (diabetes insipidus)

• Factor VIII coagulant activity before using for hemostasis

• Nocturnal enuresis: frequency of enuresis before and during treatment

Administer:

• Undiluted over 1 min in diabetes insipidus

• Diluted, one single dose/50 ml of 0.9% NaCl (adult and child >10 kg), a single dose/10 ml as an IV inf over 15-30 min in von Willebrand's disease or hemophilia A

Perform/provide:

• Storage in refrigerator or cool environment

Evaluate:

• Therapeutic response: absence of severe thirst, decreased urine output, decreased osmolality

Teach patient/family:

• The proper technique for nasal instillation: to insert tube into nostril to instill drug

• To avoid OTC products: cough, hay fever products, since these preparations may contain epINEPHrine, decrease drug response; do not use with alcohol, adverse reactions may occur

• To wear emergency ID specifying therapy

• That if dose is missed, take when remembered up to 1 hr before next dose; do not double dose

• To report to prescriber upper respiratory infection, nasal congestion

desonide
See Appendix A—Selected New Drugs

desoximetasone topical
See Appendix C

desoxyephedrine nasal agent
See Appendix C

dexamethasone (℞)
(dex-ah-meth'a-sone)
Decadron, Deronil ✽
Dexasone ✽, Dexon, Hexadrol, Mymethasone

dexamethasone acetate (℞)
Dalalone DP, Dalalone LA, Decadron-LA, Decaject-LA, Dexacen LA-8, Dexasone-LA, Dexone LA, Solurex-LA

dexamethasone sodium phosphate (℞)
Dalalone, Decadron Phosphate, Decaject, Dexacen-4, Dexone, Hexadrol Phosphate, Solurex

Func. class.: Corticosteroid, synthetic

Chem. class.: Glucocorticoid, long acting

Do not confuse:
Decadron/Percodan

Action: Decreases inflammation by suppression of migration of polymorphonuclear leukocytes, fibroblasts, reversal of increased capillary permeability and lysosomal stabilization

Uses: Inflammation, allergies, neoplasms, cerebral edema, septic shock, collagen disorders

DOSAGE AND ROUTES

Inflammation
• *Adult:* **PO** 0.75-9 mg/day in divided doses q6-12h or phosphate **IM** 0.5-9 mg/day divided q6-12h, or acetate **IM** 4-16 mg q1-3wk
• *Child:* **PO** 0.024-0.34 mg/kg/day in divided doses q6-12h

Shock
• *Adult:* (Phosphate) **IV** single dose 1-6 mg/kg or **IV** 40 mg q2-6h as needed up to 72h

Cerebral edema
• *Adult:* (Phosphate) **IV** 10 mg, then 4-6 mg **IM** q6h × 2-4 days, then taper over 1 wk

• *Child:* Loading dose 1-2 mg/kg (**PO/IM/IV**) then 1-1.5 mg/kg/day, max 16 mg/day divided q4-6hr for 2-4 days, then taper down qwk

Adrenocortical insufficiency
• *Adult:* **PO** 0.5-9 mg/day in divided doses
• *Child:* **PO** 0.03-0.3 mg/kg/day divided in 2-4 doses

Suppression test
• *Adult:* **PO** 1 mg at 11 PM or 0.5 mg q6h × 48 hr

Available forms: *Dexamethasone:* tabs 0.25, 0.5, 0.75, 1, 1.5, 2, 4, 6 mg; elix 0.5 mg/5 ml; oral sol 0.5 mg/5 ml, 1 mg/1 ml; *inj acetate* 8, 16 mg/ml; *inj phosphate* 4, 10, 20, 24 mg/ml

SIDE EFFECTS

CNS: Depression, flushing, sweating, headache, mood changes, euphoria, psychosis, **seizures,** insomnia

CV: Hypertension, **circulatory collapse, thrombophlebitis, embolism,** tachycardia, edema

EENT: Fungal infections, increased intraocular pressure, blurred vision

ENDO: HPA suppression, hyperglycemia, sodium, fluid retention

GI: Diarrhea, nausea, abdominal distention, **GI hemorrhage,** *increased appetite,* **pancreatitis**

HEMA: **Thrombocytopenia**

INTEG: Acne, poor wound healing, ecchymosis, petechiae, hirsutism

META: Hypokalemia

MS: Fractures, osteoporosis, weakness

Contraindications: Psychosis, hypersensitivity, idiopathic thrombocytopenia, acute glomerulonephritis, amebiasis, fungal infections, nonasthmatic bronchial disease, child <2 yr, AIDS, TB

Precautions: Pregnancy (C), lactation, diabetes mellitus, glaucoma, osteoporosis, seizure disorders, ulcerative colitis, CHF, myasthenia gravis, renal disease, peptic ulcer, esophagitis

⚠ Safety alert   *"Tall Man" lettering

PHARMACOKINETICS

PO: Onset 1 hr, peak 1-2 hr, duration 2½ days
IM: (acetate) Peak 8 hr, duration 6 days-3 wk
Half-life 36-54 hr

INTERACTIONS

Increase: side effects—alcohol, salicylates, indomethacin, amphotericin B, digoxin, cycloSPORINE, diuretics
Increase: dexamethasone action—salicylates, estrogens, indomethacin, oral contraceptives, ketoconazole, macrolide antiinfectives
Decrease: dexamethasone action—cholestyramine, colestipol, barbiturates, rifampin, epHEDrine, phenytoin, theophylline, antacids
Decrease: effect of anticoagulant effects, anticonvulsants, antidiabetics, ambenonium, neostigmine, isoniazid, toxoids, vaccines, anticholinesterases, salicylates, somatrem

Drug/Herb
• Potassium deficiency: aloe, buckthorn, cascara sagrada, Chinese rhubarb, senna
Increase: corticosteroid effect—aloe, licorice, perilla

Drug/Lab Test
Increase: Cholesterol, sodium, blood glucose, uric acid, calcium, urine glucose
Decrease: Calcium, K, T_4, T_3, thyroid ^{131}I uptake test, urine 17-OHCS, 17-KS, PBI
False negative: Skin allergy tests

NURSING CONSIDERATIONS

Assess:
• Potassium, blood, urine glucose while on long-term therapy; hypokalemia and hyperglycemia
• Weight daily; notify prescriber of weekly gain >5 lb
• B/P q4h, pulse; notify prescriber of chest pain
• I&O ratio; be alert for decreasing urinary output, increasing edema
• Plasma cortisol levels during long-term therapy (normal: 138-635 nmol/L SI units when drawn at 8 AM)

• Infection: fever, WBC even after withdrawal of medication; drug masks infection
• Potassium depletion: paresthesias, fatigue, nausea, vomiting, depression, polyuria, dysrhythmias, weakness
• Edema, hypertension, cardiac symptoms
• Mental status: affect, mood, behavioral changes, aggression

Administer:
• Titrated dose; use lowest effective dose
• IM inj deeply in large muscle mass; rotate sites; avoid deltoid; use 21G needle
• In one dose in AM to prevent adrenal suppression; avoid SUBCUT administration, may damage tissue
• With food or milk to decrease GI symptoms

IV route
• Undiluted direct over 1 min or less or diluted with 0.9% NaCl or D_5W and give as an IV inf at prescribed rate
• After shaking suspension (parenteral); do not give suspension IV

Dexamethasone sodium phosphate
Additive compatibilities: Aminophylline, bleomycin, cimetidine, floxacillin, furosemide, granisetron, lidocaine, meropenem, mitomycin, nafcillin, netilmicin, ondansetron, prochlorperazine, ranitidine, verapamil
Syringe compatibilities: Granisetron, metoclopramide, ranitidine, sufentanil
Y-site compatibilities: Acyclovir, allopurinol, amifostine, amikacin, amphotericin B cholesteryl, amsacrine, aztreonam, cefepime, cefpirome, cisatracurium, cisplatin, cladribine, cyclophosphamide, cytarabine, DOXOrubicin, DOXOrubicin liposome, famotidine, filgrastim, fluconazole, fludarabine, foscarnet, granisetron, heparin, lorazepam, melphalan, meperidine, meropenem, morphine, ondansetron, paclitaxel, piperacillin/tazobactam, potassium chloride, propofol, remifentanil, sargramostim, sodium bicarbonate, sufentanil, tacrolimus, teniposide, theophylline, thiotepa, vinorelbine, vit B/C, zidovudine

Perform/provide:
• Assistance with ambulation in patient with bone tissue disease to prevent fractures

Evaluate:
• Therapeutic response: ease of respirations, decreased inflammation

Teach patient/family:
• That ID as steroid user should be carried
• To contact prescriber if surgery, trauma, stress occurs; dose may need to be adjusted
• To notify prescriber if therapeutic response decreases; dosage adjustment may be needed
⚠ Not to discontinue abruptly or adrenal crisis can result
• Symptoms of adrenal insufficiency: nausea, anorexia, fatigue, dizziness, dyspnea, weakness, joint pain
• To avoid OTC products: salicylates, alcohol in cough products, cold preparations unless directed by prescriber
• To teach patient all aspects of drug usage, including cushingoid symptoms; to notify health care provider of infection
• Avoid exposure to chickenpox or measles, persons with infection

dexamethasone ophthalmic
See Appendix C

dexamethasone topical
See Appendix C

dexmedetomidine
Precedex
Func. class.: Sedative, α_2 adrenoceptor agonist

Action: Produces α_2 activity seen at low and moderate doses, also α_1 at high doses

Uses: Sedation in mechanically ventilated, intubated patients ICU

DOSAGE AND ROUTES
• *Adult:* **IV** loading dose of 1 mcg/kg over 10 min then 0.2-0.7 mcg/kg/hr, do not use for more than 24 hr
Available forms: Inj 100 mcg/ml

SIDE EFFECTS
CV: Bradycardia, hypotension, hypertension, **atrial fibrillation, infarction**
GI: Nausea, thirst
GU: Oliguria
HEMA: Leukocytosis, anemia
RESP: **Pulmonary edema, pleural effusion, hypoxia**
Contraindications: Hypersensitivity
Precautions: Pregnancy (C), geriatric, respiratory depression, severe respiratory disorders, cardiac dysrhythmias, lactation, children, renal disease

PHARMACOKINETICS
Rapid distribution, excreted in urine, metabolized in liver, protein binding 94%, elimination half-life 2 hr

INTERACTIONS
Increase: CNS depression—alcohol, opioids, sedative/hypnotics, antipsychotics, skeletal muscle relaxants, inhalational anesthetics

NURSING CONSIDERATIONS
Assess:
• Inj site: phlebitis, burning, stinging
• ECG for changes: atrial fibrillation
• CNS changes: movement, jerking, tremors, dizziness, LOC, pupil reaction
• Respiratory dysfunction: respiratory depression, character, rate, rhythm; notify prescriber if respirations are <10/min
Administer:
IV route
• After diluting with D_5W 0.9% NaCl, withdraw 2 ml of drug and add to 48 ml of 0.9% NaCl to a total of 50 ml, shake to mix well

• Only with resuscitative equipment available
• Only by qualified persons trained in ICU sedation

Solution compatibilities: LR, D_5W, 0.9% NaCl, 20% mannitol

Additive compatibilities: Thiopental, etomidate, vecuronium, pancuronium, succinylcholine, atracurium, mivacurium, glycopyrrolate, phenylephrine, atropine, midazolam, morphine, fentanyl

Perform/provide:

• Safety measures: side rails, nightlight, call bell within easy reach

Evaluate:

• Therapeutic response: induction of anesthesia

**dexmethyl-
phenidate** (℞)
(dex′meth-ul-fen′ih-dayt)
Focalin, Focalin XR
Func. class.: Central nervous system (CNS) stimulant, psychostimulant

---

Controlled Substance Schedule II
Action: Increases release of norepinephrine and dopamine into the extraneuronal space, also blocks reuptake of norepinephrine and dopamine into the presynaptic neuron; mode of action in treating attention deficit hyperactivity disorder (ADHD) is unknown
Uses: ADHD

DOSAGE AND ROUTES

• *Child >6 yr:* **PO** 2.5 mg bid with doses at least 4 hr apart, gradually increase to a maximum of 20 mg/day (10 mg bid); for those taking methylphenidate, use ½ of methylphenidate dose initially, then increase as needed to a maximum of 20 mg/day; **EXT REL** 5 mg/day, may adjust to 20 mg/day in 5 mg increments
• *Adult:* **PO EXT REL** 10 mg/day, may adjust to 20 mg/day in 10-mg increments
Available forms: Tabs 2.5, 5, 10 mg; ext rel caps 5, 10, 20 mg (Focalin XR)

SIDE EFFECTS

CNS: Dizziness, headache, drowsiness, nervousness, insomnia, **toxic psychosis, neuroleptic malignant syndrome (rare)**, Gilles de la Tourette's syndrome
CV: Palpitations, B/P changes, angina, **dysrhythmias, tachycardia**
GI: Nausea, anorexia, abnormal hepatic function, **hepatic coma**, *abdominal pain*
HEMA: **Leukopenia, anemia, thrombocytopenic purpura**
INTEG: **Exfoliative dermatitis**, urticaria, rash, erythema multiforme
MISC: Fever, arthralgia, scalp hair loss

Contraindications: Hypersensitivity to methylphenidate, anxiety, history of Gilles de la Tourette's syndrome, lactation, tics, psychosis; children <6 yr, glaucoma, concurrent treatment with MAOIs or within 14 days of discontinuing treatment with MAOIs

Precautions: Pregnancy (C), hypertension, depression, seizures, drug abuse, cardiovascular disorders, alcoholism

PHARMACOKINETICS

PO: Peak 1½ hr, onset ½-1 hr, duration 4 hr
PO-ER: Onset unknown, peak 4 hr, duration 8 hr
Readily absorbed, elimination half-life 2.2 hr, metabolized by liver, excreted by kidneys

INTERACTIONS

⚠ *Increase:* Hypertensive crisis—MAOIs or within 14 days of MAOIs, vasopressors
Increase: sympathomimetic effect—decongestants, vasoconstrictors
Increase: effects of anticonvulsants, tricyclics, SSRIs, coumarin anticoagulants (warfarin)
Decrease: effects of antihypertensives
Drug/Herb
• Synergistic effect: melatonin
Increase: stimulant effect—horsetail, yohimbe

Side effects: *italics* = common; **bold** = life-threatening

NURSING CONSIDERATIONS

Assess:

• VS, B/P; may reverse antihypertensives; check patients with cardiac disease more often for increased B/P

• CBC, differential platelet counts during long-term therapy, urinalysis; in diabetes: blood glucose, urine glucose; insulin changes may have to be made, because eating will decrease

• Height, growth rate q3mo in children; growth rate may be decreased

• Mental status: mood, sensorium, affect, stimulation, insomnia, aggressiveness

⚠ Withdrawal symptoms: headache, nausea, vomiting, muscle pain, weakness

• Appetite, sleep, speech patterns

• For attention span, decreased hyperactivity in persons with ADHD

Administer:

• Twice daily at least 4 hr apart; ext rel once a day

• Without regard to meals

Evaluate:

• Therapeutic response: decreased hyperactivity or ability to stay awake

Teach patient/family:

• To decrease caffeine consumption (coffee, tea, cola, chocolate); may increase irritability, stimulation

• To take early in day to prevent insomnia

• To avoid OTC preparations unless approved by prescriber

• To taper off drug over several weeks to avoid depression, increased sleeping, lethargy

• To avoid alcohol ingestion

• To avoid hazardous activities until stabilized on medication

• To get needed rest; patients will feel more tired at end of day

• Notify all health care workers, including school nurse, of medication and schedule

• Discuss information instructions provided in patient information section

Treatment of overdose: Administer fluids; hemodialysis or peritoneal dialysis; antihypertensive for increased B/P; administer short-acting barbiturate before lavage

---

dextran 40 (℞)

(deks'tran)

Dextran 40, Gentran 40, LMD 10%, Rheomacrodex

Func. class.: Plasma volume expander

Chem. class.: Low-molecular-weight polysaccharide

Action: Similar to human albumin, which expands plasma volume by drawing fluid from interstitial space to intravascular space

Uses: Expand plasma volume, prophylaxis of embolism, thrombosis

DOSAGE AND ROUTES

Shock

• *Adult:* IV INF 500 ml over 15-30 min, total dose in 24 hr not to exceed 20 ml/kg; subsequent doses given slowly; if given >24 hr, not to exceed 10 ml/kg/day; not to exceed therapy >5 days

Thrombosis/embolism

• *Adult:* IV INF 500-1000 ml, then 500 ml/day × 3 days, then 500 ml q2-3 days × 2 wk if needed

Available forms: 10% dextran 40/D_5W, 10% dextran 40/0.9% NaCl

SIDE EFFECTS

CV: Hypotension, **cardiac arrest**

GI: Nausea, vomiting, increased AST, ALT

GU: **Osmotic nephrosis, renal failure, stasis,** hyponatremia

HEMA: Decreased hematocrit, platelet function; **increased bleeding/coagulation times**

INTEG: Rash, urticaria, pruritus, **angioedema,** chills, fever, flushing

RESP: Wheezing, dyspnea, **bronchospasm, pulmonary edema**

SYST: **Anaphylaxis**

Contraindications: Hypersensitivity, renal failure, CHF (severe), extreme dehydration

---

⚠ Safety alert   *"Tall Man" lettering

Precautions: Pregnancy (C), active hemorrhage, sodium restriction

PHARMACOKINETICS

IV: Expands blood vol 1-2 × amount infused; excreted in urine and feces

INTERACTIONS

• Incompatible with chlortetracycline, phytonadione, promethazine

Drug/Lab Test

False increase: Blood glucose, urinary protein, bilirubin, total protein

Interference: Rh test, blood typing/crossmatching

NURSING CONSIDERATIONS

Assess:

• VS q5min × 30 min; Hgb/Hct, if falling by 30%, notify prescriber

• CVP during infusion (5-10 cm H_2O—normal range)

• Urine output q1h; watch for increase in urinary output (common); if output does not increase, decrease or discontinue infusion

• I&O ratio and specific gravity, urine osmolarity; if specific gravity is very low, renal clearance is low, drug should be discontinued

• Allergy: rash, urticaria, pruritus, wheezing, dyspnea, bronchospasm, drug should be discontinued immediately

⚠ Circulatory overload: increased pulse, respirations, SOB, wheezing, chest tightness, chest pain

• Dehydration after infusion: decreased output, decreased specific gravity of urine, increased temp, poor skin turgor, increased specific gravity, dry skin

Administer:

IV route

• After prescribed dilution; may give initial 500 mg at 15-30 min; distribute remainder of daily dose over 8-24 hr

• After crossmatch is drawn, if blood is to be given also

• D_5W sol in heart failure patients as ordered

Additive compatibilities: Cloxacillin

Y-site compatibilities: Enalaprilat, famotidine

Perform/provide:

• Storage at constant temperature (15°-30° C [59°-86° F]); discard unused portions, protect from freezing

Evaluate:

• Therapeutic response: increased plasma volume

---

dextran 70/75 (℞)

(deks'tran)

Dextran 75, Gentran 70, Gentran 75, Macrodex

Func. class.: Plasma volume expander

Chem. class.: High-molecular-weight polysaccharide

Action: Similar to human albumin, which expands plasma volume by drawing fluid from interstitial spaces to intravascular space

Uses: Expand plasma volume in hypovolemic shock or impending shock

DOSAGE AND ROUTES

• *Adult:* **IV INF** 500-1000 ml not to exceed 20-40 ml/min, not to exceed 10 ml/kg/24 hr if therapy >24 hr

Available forms: 70/75 dextran in 0.9% NaCl, D_5%

SIDE EFFECTS

CV: Hypotension, **cardiac arrest**

GI: Nausea, vomiting, increased AST, ALT

GU: **Osmotic nephrosis, renal failure, stasis,** hypernatremia

HEMA: Decreased hematocrit, platelet function; **increased bleeding/coagulation times**

INTEG: Rash, urticaria, pruritus, **angioedema,** chills, fever, flushing

RESP: Wheezing, dyspnea, **bronchospasm, pulmonary edema**

SYST: **Anaphylaxis**

Contraindications: Hypersensitivity, renal failure, CHF (severe), extreme dehydration

---

Side effects: *italics* = common; **bold** = life-threatening

Precautions: Pregnancy (C), active hemorrhage

PHARMACOKINETICS

IV: Onset within mins, duration 12 hr, expands blood vol 1-2 × amount infused; excreted in urine, feces

INTERACTIONS

Drug/Lab Test
False increase: Blood glucose, urinary protein, bilirubin, total protein
Interference: Rh test, blood typing/crossmatching

NURSING CONSIDERATIONS

Assess:
• VS q5min × 30 min; Hgb/Hct, if falling by 30%, notify prescriber
• CVP during infusion (5-10 cm H_2O— normal range)
• Urine output q1h; watch for increase in urinary output (common); if output does not increase, decrease or discontinue infusion
• I&O ratio and specific gravity, urine osmolarity; if specific gravity is very low, renal clearance is low, drug should be discontinued
• Allergy: rash, urticaria, pruritus, wheezing, dyspnea, bronchospasm; drug should be discontinued immediately
⚠ Circulatory overload: increased pulse, respirations, SOB, wheezing, chest tightness, chest pain
• Dehydration after infusion: decreased output, increased temp, poor skin turgor, increased specific gravity, dry skin
Administer:
• After prescribed dilution, may give initial 500 mg at 20-40 ml/min, reduce flow to lowest rate
• After crossmatch is drawn, if blood is to be given also
• D_5W sol in heart failure patients as ordered
Perform/provide:
• Storage at constant temperature (<25° C [77° F]); discard unused portions; do not use unless clear

Evaluate:
• Therapeutic response: increased plasma volume

---

dextroamphetamine (Ⓡ)

(dex-troe-am-fet′a-meen)
Dexedrine, dextroamphetamine, Dexedrine Spansule, DextroStat
Func. class.: Cerebral stimulant
Chem. class.: Amphetamine

Controlled Substance Schedule II
Action: Increases release of norepinephrine, dopamine in cerebral cortex to reticular activating system
Uses: Narcolepsy, attention deficit disorder with hyperactivity (ADHD)
Unlabeled uses: Obesity

DOSAGE AND ROUTES

Narcolepsy
• *Adult:* **PO** 5-60 mg daily in divided doses
• *Child >12 yr:* **PO** 10 mg daily increasing by 10 mg/day at weekly intervals
• *Child 6-12 yr:* **PO** 5 mg daily increasing by 5 mg/wk (max 60 mg/day)
ADHD
• *Adult:* **PO** 5-60 mg/day in divided doses
• *Child >6 yr:* **PO** 5 mg daily-bid increasing by 5 mg/day at weekly intervals
• *Child 3-6 yr:* **PO** 2.5 mg daily increasing by 2.5 mg/day at weekly intervals
Available forms: Tabs 5, 10 mg; sus rel caps (Dexedrine Spansule) 5, 10, 15 mg

SIDE EFFECTS

CNS: Hyperactivity, insomnia, restlessness, talkativeness, dizziness, headache, chills, stimulation, dysphoria, irritability, aggressiveness, tremor, dependence, addiction
CV: Palpitations, tachycardia, hypertension, decrease in heart rate, **dysrhythmias**

⚠ Safety alert   *"Tall Man" lettering

GI: Anorexia, dry mouth, diarrhea, constipation, weight loss, metallic taste
GU: Impotence, change in libido
INTEG: Urticaria

Contraindications: Hypersensitivity to sympathomimetic amines, hyperthyroidism, hypertension, glaucoma, severe arteriosclerosis, drug abuse, cardiovascular disease, anxiety, anorexia nervosa, tartrazine dye hypersensitivity

Precautions: Pregnancy (C), Gilles de la Tourette's disorder, lactation, child <3 yr, depression

PHARMACOKINETICS

PO: Onset 30 min, peak 1-3 hr, duration 4-20 hr; metabolized by liver; urine excretion pH dependent; crosses placenta, breast milk; half-life 10-30 hr

INTERACTIONS

⚠ Hypertensive crisis: MAOIs or within 14 days of MAOIs
Increase: dextroamphetamine effect—acetaZOLAMIDE, antacids, sodium bicarbonate
Increase: CNS effect—haloperidol, tricyclics, phenothiazines
Decrease: absorption of barbiturates, phenytoin
Decrease: dextroamphetamine effect—ascorbic acid, ammonium chloride
Decrease: effect of adrenergic blockers, antidiabetics
Drug/Herb
• Serotonin syndrome: St. John's wort
Increase: stimulant effect—khat
Decrease: stimulant effect—eucalyptus
Drug/Food
Increase: amine effect—caffeine

NURSING CONSIDERATIONS

Assess:
• VS, B/P; this drug may reverse antihypertensives; check patients with cardiac disease often
• CBC, urinalysis; in diabetes: blood glucose, urine glucose; insulin changes may be required, since eating will decrease

• Height, growth rate in children; growth rate may be decreased
• Mental status: mood, sensorium, affect, stimulation, insomnia, irritability
• Tolerance or dependency: an increased amount may be used to get same effect; will develop after long-term use
• Overdose: pain, fever, dehydration, insomnia, hyperactivity

Administer:
• Do not break, crush, or chew sus rel forms; sus rel product should not be used initially
• At least 6 hr before bedtime to avoid sleeplessness

Perform/provide:
• Gum, hard candy, frequent sips of water for dry mouth

Evaluate:
• Therapeutic response: increased CNS stimulation, decreased drowsiness

Teach patient/family:
• To decrease caffeine consumption (coffee, tea, cola, chocolate); may increase irritability, stimulation
• To avoid OTC preparations unless approved by prescriber
• To taper drug over several weeks; depression, increased sleeping, lethargy
• To avoid alcohol ingestion
• To avoid hazardous activities until stabilized on medication
• To get needed rest; patient will feel more tired at end of day

Treatment of overdose: Administer fluids, hemodialysis, or peritoneal dialysis; antihypertensive for increased B/P, ammonium Cl for increased excretion

dextromethorphan
(otc)

(dex-troe-meth-or'fan)
Balminil DM ✦, Benylin DM ✦, Broncho-Grippol-DM ✦, Children's Hold, Creo-Terpin, Delsym, dextromethorphan, Hold DM, Koffex ✦, Neo-DM ✦, Orex DM ✦, Pertussin, Pertussin ES, Robidex ✦, Robitussin Cough Calmers, Robitussin Pediatric, Sedatuss ✦, St. Joseph Cough Suppressant, Scot-Tussin DM, Sucrets Cough Control, Suppress, Vicks Formula 44

Func. class.: Antitussive, nonopioid
Chem. class.: Levorphanol derivative

Action: Depresses cough center in medulla by direct effect
Uses: Nonproductive cough
Unlabeled uses: Neuropathy

DOSAGE AND ROUTES
• *Adult and child ≥12 yr:* **PO** 10-20 mg q4h, or 30 mg q6-8h, not to exceed 120 mg/day; **SUS-REL LIQ** 60 mg q12h, not to exceed 120 mg/day
• *Child 6-12 yr:* **PO** 5-10 mg q4h; **SUS-REL LIQ** 30 mg bid, not to exceed 60 mg/day; **LOZ** 5-10 mg q1-4h, max 60 mg/day
• *Child 2-6 yr:* **PO** 2.5-5 mg q4h, or 7.5 mg q6-8h, not to exceed 30 mg/day
Neuropathy
• *Adult:* **PO** doses vary widely
Available forms: Loz 2.5, 5, 7.5, 15 mg; sol; liq 3.5 mg, 7.5, 15 mg/5 ml, 3.5, 5, 7.5, 10, 15 mg/5 ml; syr 15 mg/15 ml, 10 mg/5 ml; sus action liq equivalent to 30 mg/5 ml; caps 30 mg; ext rel susp 30 mg/5 ml; gel caps 15 mg

SIDE EFFECTS
CNS: Dizziness, sedation
GI: Nausea

Contraindications: Hypersensitivity, asthma/emphysema, productive cough
Precautions: Pregnancy (C), nausea/vomiting, fever, persistent headache

PHARMACOKINETICS
PO: Onset 15-30 min, duration 3-6 hr
SUS: Duration 12 hr

INTERACTIONS
• Do not give with MAOIs or within 2 wk of MAOIs
Increase: CNS depression—alcohol, antidepressants, antihistamines, opioids, sedative/hypnotics
Increase: adverse reactions—amiodarone, fluoxetine, quinidine, sibutramine

NURSING CONSIDERATIONS
Assess:
• Cough: type, frequency, character, including sputum
Administer:
• Decreased dose to geriatric patients; metabolism may be slowed
Perform/provide:
• Increased fluids to liquefy secretions
• Humidification of patient's room
Evaluate:
• Therapeutic response: absence of cough
Teach patient/family:
• To avoid driving, other hazardous activities until patient is stabilized on this medication
• To avoid smoking, smoke-filled rooms, perfumes, dust, environmental pollutants, cleaners that increase cough
• To avoid alcohol, CNS depressants
• To notify prescriber if cough persists over a few days

dextrose
(D-glucose) (Ⓡ)
Glucose, Glutose, Insta-Glucose
Func. class.: Caloric, parenteral solution

Action: Needed for adequate utilization of amino acids; decreases protein, nitrogen loss; prevents ketosis

Uses: Increases intake of calories; increases fluids in patients unable to take adequate fluids, calories orally; acute hypoglycemia

DOSAGE AND ROUTES

• *Adult and child:* **IV** depends on individual requirements

Available forms: Inj 2.5%, 5%, 10%, 20%, 25%, 30%, 38.5%, 40%, 50%, 60%, 70%; oral gel 40%; chew tab 5 g

SIDE EFFECTS

CNS: Confusion, **loss of consciousness,** dizziness

CV: Hypertension, **CHF, pulmonary edema, intracranial hemorrhage**

ENDO: Hyperglycemia, rebound hypoglycemia, hyperosmolar syndrome, hyperglycemic nonketotic syndrome, aluminum toxicity, hypokalemia, hypomagnesium

GI: Nausea

GU: Glycosuria, osmotic diuresis

INTEG: Chills, flushing, warm feeling, rash, urticaria, extravasation necrosis

RESP: Pulmonary edema

Contraindications: Hyperglycemia, delirium tremens, hemorrhage (cranial/spinal), CHF, anuria, allergy to corn products

Precautions: Renal/hepatic/cardiac disease, diabetes mellitus, carbohydrate intolerance

INTERACTIONS

Increase: fluid retention/electrolyte excretion—corticosteroids

NURSING CONSIDERATIONS

Assess:

• Electrolytes (K, Na, Ca, Cl, Mg), blood glucose, ammonia, phosphate

• Inj site for extravasation: redness along vein, edema at site, necrosis; pain; hard, tender area; site should be changed immediately

• Monitor temp q4h for increased fever, indicating infection; if infection suspected, infusion is discontinued, tubing, bottle, catheter tip cultured

• Serum glucose in patients receiving hypotonic glucose 50% and over

• Nutritional status: calorie count by dietitian

Administer:

• Only (4%) protein and dextrose (up to 12.5%) via peripheral vein; stronger sol: central IV administration

• May be given undiluted via prepared sol; give 10% sol, 5 ml/15 sec; 10% sol, 1000 ml/3 hr or more; 20% sol, 500 ml/½-1 hr; 50% sol, 10 ml/min; control rate, rapid infusions may cause fluid shifts

• Oral glucose preparations (gel, chew tabs) are to be used in conscious patients only; check serum blood glucose after first dose

• After changing IV catheter, dressing q24h with aseptic technique

Evaluate:

• Therapeutic response: increased weight

Teach patient/family:

• The reason for dextrose infusion

• To review hypoglycemia/hyperglycemia symptoms

• To review blood glucose monitoring procedure

diazepam (℞)
(dye-az′-e-pam)
Apo-Diazepam ✦,
Diazemuls ✦, diazepam,
Novodiapam ✦,
PMS-Diazepam ✦, Valium,
Vivol ✦
Func. class.: Antianxiety, anticonvulsant, skeletal muscle relaxant, central acting
Chem. class.: Benzodiazepine

Controlled Substance Schedule IV
Do not confuse:
diazepam/Ditropan/lorazepam
Action: Potentiates the actions of GABA, especially in limbic system, reticular formation; enhances presympathetic inhibition, inhibits spinal polysynaptic afferent paths
Uses: Anxiety, acute alcohol withdrawal, adjunct in seizure disorders; preoperatively as a relaxant, skeletal muscle relaxation; rectally for acute repetitive seizures
Unlabeled uses: Panic attacks

DOSAGE AND ROUTES
Anxiety/convulsive disorders
• *Adult:* PO 2-10 mg bid-qid
• *Geriatric:* PO 1-2 mg daily-bid, increase slowly as needed
• *Child >6 mo:* PO 1-2.5 mg tid-qid
Precardioversion
• *Adult:* IV 5-15 mg 5-10 min precardioversion
Preendoscopy
• *Adult:* IV 2.5-20 mg; IM 5-10 mg ½ hr preendoscopy
Muscle relaxation
• *Adult:* PO 2-10 mg tid-qid or **EXT REL** 15-30 mg daily; IV/IM 5-10 mg repeat in 2-4 hr
• *Geriatric:* PO 2-5 mg bid-qid; IV/IM 2-5 mg, may repeat in 2-4 hr
Tetanic muscle spasms
• *Child >5 yr:* IM/IV 5-10 mg q3-4h prn
• *Infant >30 days:* IM/IV 1-2 mg q3-4h prn

Status epilepticus
• *Adult:* IV/IM 5-10 mg, 2 mg/min, may repeat q10-15min, not to exceed 30 mg; may repeat in 2-4 hr if seizures reappear
• *Child >5 yr:* IV/IM 1 mg q2-5min max 10 mg, may repeat in 2-4 hr
• *Child 1 mo-5 yr:* IV/IM 0.2-0.5 mg slowly q2-5min up to 5 mg
• *Adult:* RECT 0.2 mg/kg, may repeat 4-12 hr later
• *Child 6-11 yr:* RECT 0.3 mg/kg, may repeat 4-12 hr later
• *Child 2-5 yr:* RECT 0.5 mg/kg, may repeat 4-12 hr later
Alcohol withdrawal
• *Adult:* PO 10 mg tid-qid in 1st 24 hr, then 5 mg tid-qid; IV/IM 10 mg, then 5-10 mg after 3 hr
Psychoneurotic reactions
• *Adult:* IV/IM 2-10 mg, may repeat in 3-4 hr
Available forms: Tabs 2, 5, 10 mg; inj 5 mg/ml; oral sol 5 mg/5 ml; gel, rectal delivery system 2.5, 5, 10, 15, 20 mg, twin packs

SIDE EFFECTS
CNS: Dizziness, drowsiness, confusion, headache, anxiety, tremors, stimulation, fatigue, depression, insomnia, hallucinations
CV: Orthostatic hypotension, **ECG changes, tachycardia,** hypotension
EENT: Blurred vision, tinnitus, mydriasis, nystagmus
GI: Constipation, dry mouth, nausea, vomiting, anorexia, diarrhea
HEMA: **Neutropenia**
INTEG: Rash, dermatitis, itching
RESP: **Respiratory depression**
Contraindications: Pregnancy (D), hypersensitivity to benzodiazepines, narrow-angle glaucoma, psychosis, lactation, coma, respiratory depression
Precautions: Geriatric, debilitated, renal/hepatic disease, addiction, child <6 mo

---
⚠ Safety alert   *"Tall Man" lettering

PHARMACOKINETICS

PO: Rapidly absorbed, onset ½ hr, duration 2-3 hr

IM: Onset 15-30 min, duration 1-1½ hr, absorption slow and erratic

IV: Onset immediate, duration 15 min–1 hr

Metabolized by liver, excreted by kidneys, crosses placenta, excreted in breast milk, crosses the blood-brain barrier; half-life 20-50 hr, more reliable by mouth

INTERACTIONS

Increase: toxicity—barbiturates, SSRIs, cimetidine, CNS depressants, valproic acid

Increase: CNS depression—CNS depressants, alcohol

Decrease: diazepam metabolism—oral contraceptives, valproic acid, disulfiram, isoniazid, propranolol

Drug/Herb

Increase: diazepam action—cowslip, goldenseal, kava, melatonin, mistletoe, pokeweed, poppy, Queen Anne's lace, valerian

Decrease: diazepam effect—cola tree

Drug/Lab Test

Increase: AST/ALT, serum bilirubin

Decrease: RAIU

False increase: 17-OHCS

NURSING CONSIDERATIONS

Assess:

• B/P (lying, standing), pulse; respiratory rate; if systolic B/P drops 20 mm Hg, hold drug, notify prescriber; respirations q5-15min if given IV

• Blood studies: CBC during long-term therapy; blood dyscrasias (rare)

• Degree of anxiety; what precipitates anxiety and whether drug controls symptoms

• For alcohol withdrawal symptoms, including hallucinations (visual, auditory), delirium, irritability, agitation, fine to coarse tremors

• For seizure control and type, duration, intensity of seizures

• Hepatic studies: AST, ALT, bilirubin, creatinine, LDH, alk phos

• IV site for thrombosis or phlebitis, which may occur rapidly

• Mental status: mood, sensorium, affect, sleeping pattern, drowsiness, dizziness

• Physical dependency, withdrawal symptoms: headache, nausea, vomiting, muscle pain, weakness after long-term use

• Suicidal tendencies

Administer:

• With food or milk for GI symptoms; crushed if patient is unable to swallow medication whole

• Sugarless gum, hard candy, frequent sips of water for dry mouth

• Reduced opioid dose by ⅓ if given concomitantly with diazepam

Rectal route

• Do not use more than 5 ×/mo or for an episode q5d

IV route

• Into large vein; give IV 5 mg or less/1 min or total dose over 3 min or more (children, infants); continuous infusion is not recommended

Additive compatibilities: Netilmicin, verapamil

Syringe compatibilities: Cimetidine

Y-site compatibilities: Cefmetazole, DOBUTamine, nafcillin, quinidine, sufentanil

Perform/provide:

• Assistance with ambulation during beginning therapy, for drowsiness, dizziness, safety measures

• Check to see PO medication has been swallowed

Evaluate:

• Therapeutic response: decreased anxiety, restlessness, insomnia

Teach patient/family:

• That drug may be taken with food

• That drug is not to be used for everyday stress or used longer than 4 mo unless directed by prescriber; no more than prescribed amount; may be habit forming

• To avoid OTC preparations unless approved by prescriber

Side effects: *italics* = common; **bold** = life-threatening

• To avoid driving, activities that require alertness; drowsiness may occur

• To avoid alcohol, other psychotropic medications unless directed by prescriber; that smoking may decrease diazepam effect by increasing diazepam metabolism

• Not to discontinue medication abruptly after long-term use

• To rise slowly or fainting may occur, especially in geriatric

• That drowsiness may worsen at beginning of treatment

• To avoid use during pregnancy

Treatment of overdose: Lavage, VS, supportive care, flumazenil

---

diazoxide (℞)
(dye-az-ox′ide)
diazoxide parenteral,
Hyperstat IV
Func. class.: Antihypertensive
Chem. class.: Vasodilator

Action: Vasodilates arteriolar smooth muscle by direct relaxation; a reduction in blood pressure with concomitant increases in heart rate, cardiac output; reduces release of insulin from the pancreas

Uses: Hypertensive crisis when urgent decrease of diastolic pressure required (IV); increase blood glucose levels in hyperinsulinism

DOSAGE AND ROUTES

Hypoglycemia

• *Adult and child:* **PO** 3-8 mg/kg/day in 2-3 divided doses q8-12h

• *Infants and neonates:* **PO** 8-15 mg/kg/day in 2-3 divided doses 8-12h

Hypertension

• *Adult:* **IV BOL** 1-3 mg/kg rapidly up to a max of 150 mg in a single inj; dose may be repeated at 5-15 min intervals until desired response is achieved; give IV in 30 sec or less

• *Child:* **IV BOL** 1-2 mg/kg rapidly; administration same as adult, not to exceed 150 mg

Available forms: Caps 50 mg; oral susp 50 mg/ml; inj 15 mg/ml, 300 mg/20 ml

SIDE EFFECTS

CNS: *Headache,* sleepiness, euphoria, anxiety, EPS, confusion, tinnitus, blurred vision, dizziness, weakness, **seizures, cerebral ischemia, paralysis**

CV: **Hypotension,** T-wave changes, angina pectoris, palpitations, **supraventricular tachycardia, edema,** rebound hypertension, **shock, MI**

ENDO: Hyperglycemia in diabetics, transient hyperglycemia in nondiabetics, increased uric acid

GI: Nausea, vomiting, dry mouth

GU: Breast tenderness; increased BUN, fluid, electrolyte imbalances; Na, water retention

HEMA: Decreased Hgb, Hct, **thrombocytopenia**

INTEG: Rash

Contraindications: Hypersensitivity to thiazides, sulfonamides, hypertension of aortic coarctation or AV shunt, pheochromocytoma, dissecting aortic aneurysm

Precautions: Pregnancy (C), tachycardia, fluid, electrolyte imbalances, lactation, impaired cerebral or cardiac circulation, children

PHARMACOKINETICS

IV: Onset 1-2 min, peak 5 min, duration 3-12 hr

PO: Onset 1 hr, peak 8-12 hr, duration 4-20 hr, half-life 20-36 hr, excreted slowly in urine, crosses blood-brain barrier, placenta; highly protein bound (>90%)

INTERACTIONS

Increase: hyperglycemia—sulfonylureas

Increase: severe hypotension—antihypertensives

Increase: hyperuricemic, antihypertensive effects of diazoxide—thiazide diuretics

Decrease: anticonvulsant effect—hydantoins

⚠ Safety alert   *"Tall Man" lettering

Decrease: antihypertensive effect—
NSAIDs, salicylates
Drug/Herb
• Toxicity/death: aconite

NURSING CONSIDERATIONS
Assess:
• B/P q5min until stabilized, then q1h × 2 hr, then q4h
• Pulse, jugular venous distention q4h
• Electrolytes, blood studies: K, Na, Cl, CO_2, CBC, serum glucose
• Weight daily, I&O
• Edema in feet, legs daily
• Skin turgor, mucous membranes for hydration status
• Crackles, dyspnea, orthopnea
• IV site for extravasation
• Signs of CHF: dyspnea, edema, wet crackles
• Postural hypotension, take B/P sitting, standing
Administer:
• Undiluted; give over ½ min or less
• To patient in recumbent position; keep in that position for 1 hr after administration
Syringe compatibilities: Heparin
Perform/provide:
• Store protected from light
Evaluate:
• Therapeutic response: decreased B/P, primarily diastolic pressure
Treatment of overdose: DOPamine, or norepinephrine for hypotension, Trendelenburg maneuver

dibucaine topical
See Appendix C

diclofenac ophthalmic
See Appendix C

diclofenac potassium (℞)
(dye-kloe'fen-ak)
Cataflam, Voltaren Rapide ✦
diclofenac sodium
Apo-Dilo ✦, Novo-Difenac ✦, Voltaren, Voltaren-XR
Func. class.: Nonsteroidal antiinflammatory drugs (NSAIDs), nonopioid analgesic
Chem. class.: Phenylacetic acid

Do not confuse:
Cataflam/Catapres
Action: Inhibits prostaglandin synthesis by decreasing enzyme needed for biosynthesis; analgesic, antiinflammatory, antipyretic
Uses: Acute, chronic rheumatoid arthritis, osteoarthritis; ankylosing spondylitis, analgesia, primary dysmenorrhea

DOSAGE AND ROUTES
Osteoarthritis
• *Adult:* **PO** 100-150 mg/day in 2-3 divided doses
Rheumatoid arthritis
• *Adult:* **PO** 100-200 mg/day in 2-4 divided doses (potassium); 50 mg tid-qid, then reduce to lowest dose needed (25 mg tid) (sodium)
Ankylosing spondylitis
• *Adult:* **PO** 100-125 mg/day in 4-5 divided doses, give 25 mg qid and 25 mg at bedtime if needed (potassium)
Analgesia/primary dysmenorrhea
• *Adult:* **PO** 50 mg tid, max 150 mg/day (potassium)
Available forms: *Potassium:* tabs 50 mg; *sodium:* delayed rel tabs (entericcoated) 25, 50, 75 mg; ext rel tabs 100 mg

SIDE EFFECTS
CNS: Dizziness, headache, drowsiness, fatigue, tremors, confusion, insomnia, anxiety, depression, nervousness, paresthesia, muscle weakness
CV: **CHF,** tachycardia, peripheral edema,

palpitations, **dysrhythmias,** hypotension, hypertension, fluid retention

EENT: Tinnitus, hearing loss, blurred vision, **laryngeal edema**

GI: Nausea, anorexia, vomiting, diarrhea, **jaundice, cholestatic hepatitis,** constipation, flatulence, cramps, dry mouth, peptic ulcer, GI bleeding, **hepatotoxicity**

GU: **Nephrotoxicity: dysuria, hematuria, oliguria, azotemia, cystitis, UTI**

HEMA: **Blood dyscrasias,** epistaxis, bruising

INTEG: Purpura, rash, pruritus, sweating, erythema, petechiae, photosensitivity, alopecia

RESP: Dyspnea, hemoptysis, pharyngitis, **bronchospasm,** rhinitis, shortness of breath

SYST: **Anaphylaxis**

Contraindications: Hypersensitivity to aspirin, iodides, other nonsteroidal antiinflammatory agents, asthma, serious CV disease

Precautions: Pregnancy (B) 1st trimester, not recommended in 2nd half of pregnancy, lactation, children, bleeding disorders, GI disorders, cardiac disorders, hypersensitivity to other antiinflammatory agents, CCr <30 ml/min

PHARMACOKINETICS

PO: Peak 2-3 hr, elimination half-life 1-2 hr, 90% bound to plasma proteins, metabolized in liver to metabolite, excreted in urine

INTERACTIONS

• Hyperkalemia: potassium-sparing diuretics

• Need for dosage adjustment: antidiabetics

Increase: anticoagulant effect—anticoagulants

Increase: toxicity—phenytoin, lithium, cycloSPORINE, methotrexate

Increase: GI side effects—aspirin, other NSAIDs

Decrease: antihypertensive effect—β-blockers, diuretics

Drug/Herb

• Severe photosensitivity: St. John's wort

Increase: bleeding risk—bogbean, chondroitin, saw palmetto, turmeric

Increase: gastric irritation—arginine, gossypol

Increase: NSAIDs effect—bearberry, bilberry

NURSING CONSIDERATIONS

Assess:

• For pain: location, character, aggravating, alleviating factors, ROM, before and 1 hr after dose

• Blood counts during therapy; watch for decreasing platelets; if low, therapy may need to be discontinued, restarted after hematologic recovery

• For clients with asthma, aspirin hypersensitivity, nasal polyps; may develop hypersensitivity

• LFTs (may be elevated) and uric acid (may be decreased—serum; increased—urine) periodically; also BUN, creatinine, electrolytes (may be elevated)

⚠ Blood dyscrasias (thrombocytopenia): bruising, fatigue, bleeding, poor healing

Administer:

• Do not break, crush, or chew enteric products

• Take with a full glass of water to enhance absorption, remain upright for ½ hr; if dose is missed, take as soon as remembered within 2 hr if taking 1-2 ×/day; do not double doses

Evaluate:

• Therapeutic response: decreased inflammation in joints, decreased inflammation after cataract surgery

Teach patient/family:

• That drug must be continued for prescribed time to be effective; to contact prescriber prior to surgery as when to discontinue this drug

• To report bleeding, bruising, fatigue, malaise; blood dyscrasias do occur

• To avoid aspirin, alcoholic beverages, NSAIDs, acetaminophen, or other OTC medications unless approved by prescriber

---

⚠ Safety alert   *"Tall Man" lettering

- To take with food, milk, or antacids to avoid GI upset, to swallow whole
- To use caution when driving; drowsiness, dizziness may occur
- To report hepatotoxicity: flulike symptoms, nausea, vomiting, jaundice, pruritus, lethargy
- To use sunscreen to prevent photosensitivity

dicloxacillin (℞)
(dye-klox-a-sill′-in)
dicloxacillin sodium, Dycill, Dynapen, Pathocil
Func. class.: Antiinfective
Chem. class.: Penicillinase-resistant penicillin

Do not confuse:
Pathocil/Bactocill

Action: Interferes with cell wall replication of susceptible organisms; osmotically unstable cell wall swells, bursts from osmotic pressure, lysis is mediated by cell wall autolytic enzymes

Uses: Effective for gram-positive cocci (*Staphylococcus aureus, Streptococcus pyogenes, Streptococcus viridans, Streptococcus faecalis, Streptococcus bovis, Streptococcus pneumoniae*), infections caused by penicillinase-producing *Staphylococcus*

DOSAGE AND ROUTES
- *Adult and child ≥40 kg:* PO 125-250 mg q6h, max 4 g/day
- *Child ≤40 kg:* PO 12.5-25 mg/kg in divided doses q6h, max 4 g/day
Available forms: Caps 250, 500 mg

SIDE EFFECTS

CNS: Lethargy, hallucinations, anxiety, depression, twitching, **coma, seizures**
GI: Nausea, vomiting, diarrhea, increased AST, ALT, abdominal pain, glossitis, **pseudomembranous colitis, GI bleeding**
GU: Oliguria, proteinuria, hematuria, *vaginitis, moniliasis,* **glomerulonephritis**
HEMA: Anemia, increased bleeding time, **bone marrow depression, granulocytopenia, neutropenia**
INTEG: Rash, **toxic epidermal necrolysis**
SYST: **Anaphylaxis, Stevens-Johnson syndrome**

Contraindications: Hypersensitivity to penicillins; neonates
Precautions: Pregnancy (B), hypersensitivity to cephalosporins, lactation, severe renal/hepatic disease, asthma, GI disease

PHARMACOKINETICS
PO: Peak 1 hr, duration 4-6 hr, half-life 30-60 min; metabolized in liver; excreted in urine, bile, breast milk; crosses placenta

INTERACTIONS
Increase: dicloxacillin concentrations—probenecid
Decrease: anticoagulant effect—anticoagulants
Drug/Herb
- Do not use acidophilus with antiinfectives; separate by several hours
Decrease: absorption—khat, separate by 2 hr
Food/Drug
- Citric juices/food decrease absorption of dicloxacillin
Drug/Lab Test
False positive: Urine glucose, urine protein

NURSING CONSIDERATIONS
Assess:
- I&O ratio; report hematuria, oliguria, since penicillin in high doses is nephrotoxic
⚠ Any patient with compromised renal system, since drug is excreted slowly in poor renal system function; toxicity may occur rapidly
- Blood studies: WBC, RBC, Hgb, Hct, bleeding time
- Renal studies: urinalysis, protein, blood

Side effects: *italics* = common; **bold** = life-threatening

- C&S before drug therapy; drug may be given as soon as culture is taken
- WBC and differential, ALT, AST, BUN, creatinine for patients on long-term therapy
- Bowel pattern before, during treatment
- Anaphylaxis: pruritus, rash, dyspnea, laryngeal edema; have emergency equipment available; skin eruptions after administration of penicillin to 1 wk after discontinuing drug
- For infection: temp, draining wounds, WBC, sputum, urine, stool, before, during treatment

Administer:
- Do not break, crush, or chew caps
- Drug after C&S
- On an empty stomach with a full glass of water
- Susp after shaking well before each dose

Perform/provide:
- Adrenalin, suction, tracheostomy set, endotracheal intubation equipment
- Adequate fluid intake (2 L) during diarrhea episodes
- Scratch test to assess allergy after securing order from prescriber; usually done when penicillin is only drug of choice
- Storage in tight container; after reconstituting, store in refrigerator up to 2 wk

Evaluate:
- Therapeutic response: absence of fever, draining wounds

Teach patient/family:
- All aspects of drug therapy, including need to complete course of medication to ensure organism death (10-14 days); culture may be taken after completed course
- To report sore throat, fever, fatigue; may indicate superinfection
- To wear or carry emergency ID if allergic to penicillins
- To notify prescriber of diarrhea, fever

Treatment of anaphylaxis: Withdraw drug; maintain airway; administer epINEPHrine, aminophylline, O_2, IV corticosteroids

---

Rarely Used

dicyclomine (℞)

(dye-sye'kloe-meen)
Antispas, Bentyl, Bentylol ✚, Byclomine, Dibent, dicyclomine HCL, Dilomine, Di-Spaz, Formulex ✚, Lomine ✚, Neoquess, Or-Tyl, Spasmoject
Func. class.: Gastrointestinal anticholinergic

Uses: Treatment of peptic ulcer disease in combination with other drugs; infant colic, urinary incontinence, IBS

DOSAGE AND ROUTES
- *Adult:* **PO** 10-20 mg tid-qid; **IM** 20 mg q4-6h; max 160 mg/day
- *Child >2 yr:* **PO** 10 mg tid-qid
- *Child 6 mo-2 yr:* **PO** 5 mg tid-qid

Contraindications: Hypersensitivity to anticholinergics, narrow-angle glaucoma, GI obstruction, myasthenia gravis, paralytic ileus, GI atony, toxic megacolon

---

didanosine (℞)

(dye-dan'oh-seen)
ddl, dideoxyinosine, Videx, Videx EC
Func. class.: Antiretroviral
Chem. class.: Nucleoside reverse transcriptase inhibitor

Action: Nucleoside analog incorporating into cellular DNA by viral reverse transcriptase, thereby terminating the cellular DNA chain

Uses: HIV-1 infection in combination with other antiretrovirals

DOSAGE AND ROUTES
- *Adult:* **PO** >60 kg, 200 mg bid tabs, or 250 mg bid buffered powder; caps, del rel 400 mg daily; <60 kg, 125 mg bid tabs, or 167 mg bid buffered powder; caps, del rel 250 mg daily
- *Child:* **PO** tabs 90-120 mg/m^2 q12h;

---

buffered powder packets 112.5-150 mg/m^2 q12h; **PO** (child BSA 1.1-1.4 m^2) tab 100 mg q8-12h; recon pedi powder 125 mg q8-12h; **PO** (child BSA 0.8-1 m^2) tabs 75 mg q8-12h; recon pedi powder 94 mg q8-12h; **PO** (child BSA 0.5-0.7 m^2) tabs 50 mg q8-12h; recon pedi powder 62 mg q8-12h; **PO** (child BSA <0.4 m^2) tabs 25 mg q8-12h; recon pedi powder 31 mg q8-12h

Renal dose
• Reduce dosage CCr <60 ml/min

Available forms: Tabs, buffered, chewable/dispersible 25, 50, 100, 150, 200 mg; powder for oral sol 10 mg/ml; del rel caps 125, 200, 250, 400

SIDE EFFECTS

CNS: **Peripheral neuropathy, seizures,** confusion, *anxiety*, hypertonia, abnormal thinking, asthenia, *insomnia,* **CNS depression,** pain, dizziness, chills, fever
CV: Hypertension, vasodilation, dysrhythmia, syncope, **CHF,** palpitation
EENT: Ear pain, otitis, photophobia, visual impairment, retinal depigmentation
GI: **Pancreatitis,** *diarrhea, nausea,* vomiting, *abdominal pain,* constipation, stomatitis, dyspepsia, liver abnormalities, flatulence, taste perversion, dry mouth, oral thrush, melena, increased ALT, AST, alk phos, amylase, **hepatic failure**
GU: Increased bilirubin, uric acid
HEMA: **Leukopenia, granulocytopenia, thrombocytopenia, anemia**
INTEG: *Rash, pruritus,* alopecia, ecchymosis, hemorrhage, petechiae, sweating
MS: Myalgia, arthritis, myopathy, muscular atrophy
RESP: Cough, pneumonia, dyspnea, asthma, epistaxis, hypoventilation, sinusitis
SYST: **Lactic acidosis, anaphylaxis**
Contraindications: Hypersensitivity, lactic acidosis, pancreatitis, phenylketonuria
Precautions: Pregnancy (B), renal/hepatic disease, lactation, children, sodium-restricted diets, elevated amylase, preexisting peripheral neuropathy, hyperuricemia

PHARMACOKINETICS

PO: Peak 0.67 hr; del rel 2 hr; elimination half-life 1.62 hr, extensive metabolism is thought to occur; administration within 5 min of food will decrease absorption, excreted urine/feces

INTERACTIONS

Increase: didanosine level—allopurinol, tenofovir, adjust dose as needed
Increase: side effects from magnesium, aluminum antacids
Decrease: absorption—ketoconazole, dapsone
Decrease: concentrations of fluoroquinolones, other antiretrovirals, itraconazole, tetracyclines
Decrease: didanosine level—methadone
Drug/Food
• Any food decreases rate of absorption
• Do not use with acidic juices

NURSING CONSIDERATIONS
Assess:
• Peripheral neuropathy: tingling or pain in hands and feet, distal numbness; onset usually occurs 2-6 mo after beginning treatment, may persist if drug is not discontinued
⚠ Pancreatitis: abdominal pain, nausea, vomiting, elevated hepatic enzymes; drug should be discontinued, since condition can be fatal
• For anaphylaxis, lactic acidosis
• Children by dilated retinal exam q6mo to rule out retinal depigmentation
• CBC, differential, platelet count qmo; withhold drug if WBC is <4000 or platelet count is <75,000; notify prescriber of results; alk phos, monitor amylase; viral load, CD4 count
• Renal studies: BUN, serum uric acid, urine CCr before, during therapy
• Temp q4h, may indicate beginning infection
• Hepatic studies before, during therapy (bilirubin, AST, ALT) as needed or qmo
Administer:
• Pediatric powder for oral sol after preparation by pharmacist; dilution is re-

quired using purified USP water, then antacid (10 mg/ml), refrigerate, shake before use
• On an empty stomach ≥30 min before or 2 hr after meals
• Adjust dose in renal impairment

Perform/provide:
• Cleanup of powdered products; use wet mop or damp sponge
• Storage of tabs, caps in tightly closed bottle at room temperature; store oral sol after dissolving at room temperature ≤4 hr

Evaluate:
• Therapeutic response: absence of infection; symptoms of HIV

Teach patient/family:
• To avoid use with alcohol
• To report numbness/tingling in extremities
• To take on an empty stomach; not to take dapsone at same time as ddI; do not mix powder with fruit juice; chew tab or crush and dissolve in water; drink powder immediately after mixing
• To report signs of infection: increased temp, sore throat, flulike symptoms
• To report signs of anemia: fatigue, headache, faintness, shortness of breath, irritability
• To report bleeding; avoid use of razors, commercial mouthwash
• That hair may be lost during therapy (rare); a wig or hairpiece may make patient feel better

---

Rarely Used

diflunisal (℞)
(dye-floo′ni-sal)
diflunisal, Dolobid
Func. class.: Nonsteroidal antiinflammatory/analgesic (nonopioid)

Uses: Mild to moderate pain or fever including arthritis; 3-4 times more potent than aspirin

DOSAGE AND ROUTES
• *Adult:* **PO** loading dose 1 g; then 500-1000 mg/day in 2 divided doses, q12h, not to exceed 1500 mg/day
• *Geriatric:* **PO** ½ adult dose
Contraindications: Hypersensitivity to salicylates, GI bleeding, bleeding disorders, children <12 yr, vit K deficiency

---

⚠ High Alert

digoxin (℞)
(di-jox′in)
digoxin, Lanoxicaps, Lanoxin
Func. class.: Cardiac glycoside, inotropic, antidysrhythmic
Chem. class.: Digoxin preparation

Do not confuse:
Lanoxin/Lasix/Lonox/Lomotil/Xanax/Levoxine
Action: Inhibits the sodium-potassium ATPase, which makes more calcium available for contractile proteins, resulting in increased cardiac output (positive inotropic effect); increases force of contraction; decreases heart rate (negative chronotropic effect); decreases AV conduction speed
Uses: Heart failure, atrial fibrillation, atrial flutter, atrial tachycardia, cardiogenic shock, paroxysmal atrial tachycardia, rapid digitalization in these disorders

DOSAGE AND ROUTES
• *Adult:* **IV digitalizing dose** 0.6-1 mg given as 50% of the dose initially, addi-

---

tional fractions given at 4-8 hr intervals; **PO digitalizing dose** 0.75-1.25 mg given as 50% of the dose initially, additional fractions given at 4-8 hr intervals; **maintenance** 0.125-0.5 mg/day (tabs), or 0.350-0.5 mg/day (gelatin cap)

• *Child >10 yr:* **IV digitalizing dose** 8-12 mcg/kg given as 50% of the dose initially, additional fractions given at 4-8 hr intervals; **PO digitalizing dose** 0.01-0.015 mg/kg given as 50% of the dose initially, additional fractions given at 6-8 hr intervals; **maintenance** 25%-35% of the loading dose daily as a single dose

• *Child 5-10 yr:* **IV digitalizing dose** 0.015-0.03 mg/kg given as 50% of the dose initially, additional fractions given at 4-8 hr intervals; **PO digitalizing dose** 0.02-0.035 mg/kg given as 50% of the dose initially, additional fractions given at 6-8 hr intervals; **maintenance** 25%-35% of the loading dose daily in 2 divided doses

• *Child 2-5 yr:* **IV digitalizing dose** 0.025-0.035 mg/kg given as 50% of the dose initially, additional fractions given at 4-8 hr intervals; **PO digitalizing dose** 0.03-0.04 mg/kg given as 50% of the dose initially, additional fractions given at 6-8 hr intervals; **maintenance** 25%-35% of the loading dose daily in 2 divided doses

• *Child 1-2 yr:* **IV digitalizing dose** 0.03-0.05 mg/kg given as 50% of the dose initially, additional fractions given at 4-8 hr intervals; **PO digitalizing dose** 0.035-0.06 mg/kg given as 50% of the dose initially, additional fractions given at 4-8 hr intervals; **maintenance** 25%-35% of the loading dose daily in 2 divided doses

• *Infant:* **IV digitalizing dose** 0.02-0.03 mg/kg given as 50% of the dose initially, additional fractions given at 4-8 hr intervals; **PO digitalizing dose** 0.025-0.035 mg/kg given as 50% of the dose initially, additional fractions given at 6-8 hr intervals; **maintenance** 25%-35% of the loading dose daily in 2 divided doses

• *Infant, premature:* **IV digitalizing dose** 0.015-0.025 mg/kg given as 50% of the dose initially, additional fractions

given at 4-8 hr intervals; **PO digitalizing dose** 0.02-0.03 mg/kg given as 50% of the dose initially, additional fractions given at 6-8 hr intervals; **maintenance** 20%-30% of the loading dose daily in 2 divided doses

Available forms: Caps 0.05, 0.1, 0.2 mg; elix 0.05 mg/ml; tabs 0.125, 0.25, 0.5 mg; inj 0.5 ✚, 0.25 mg/ml; pediatric inj 0.1 mg/ml

SIDE EFFECTS

CNS: Headache, drowsiness, apathy, confusion, disorientation, fatigue, depression, hallucinations
CV: **Dysrhythmias,** *hypotension,* bradycardia, **AV block**
EENT: Blurred vision, yellow-green halos, photophobia, diplopia
GI: Nausea, vomiting, anorexia, abdominal pain, diarrhea
Contraindications: Hypersensitivity to digoxin, ventricular fibrillation, ventricular tachycardia, carotid sinus syndrome, 2nd- or 3rd-degree heart block
Precautions: Pregnancy (C), renal disease, acute MI, AV block, severe respiratory disease, hypothyroidism, geriatric, sinus nodal disease, lactation, hypokalemia

PHARMACOKINETICS

PO: Onset ½-2 hr, peak 6-8 hr, duration 3-4 days
IV: Onset 5-30 min, peak 1-5 hr, duration variable
Half-life 1.5 days, excreted in urine

INTERACTIONS

• Hypercalcemia, hypomagnesemia, digoxin toxicity: thiazides, parenteral calcium
• Hypokalemia, digoxin toxicity: diuretics, amphotericin B, carbenicillin, ticarcillin, corticosteroids
Increase: digoxin levels—propantheline, quinidine, verapamil, amiodarone, anticholinergics, diltiazem, NIFEdipine
Increase: bradycardia—β-adrenergic blockers, antidysrythmics

Increase: cardiac dysrhythmia risk—sympathomimetics
Decrease: digoxin absorption—antacids, kaolin/pectin
Decrease: digoxin level—thyroid agents, cholestyramine, colestipol, metoclopramide

Drug/Herb
• Forms insoluble complex: blackroot
• Bradycardia: Indian snakeroot
• Cardiac toxicity: aconite, hawthorn, horsetail
Increase: digoxin action—aloe, betel palm, broom, buckthorn, cascara sagrada, castor, Chinese rhubarb, figwort, fumitory, hawthorn, khat, kudzu, licorice, lily of the valley, Mayapple, mistletoe, motherwort, night-blooming cereus, oleander, pheasant's eye, purple foxglove, Queen Anne's lace, rhubarb, rue, senna, Siberian ginseng, squill, yellow dock
Increase: hypokalemia—cocoa, coffee, cola, guarana, horsetail, licorice, yerba maté
Decrease: digoxin absorption—psyllium
Decrease: digoxin effect—beth root, goldenseal, St. John's wort

Drug/Lab Test
Increase: CPK

NURSING CONSIDERATIONS
Assess:
• Apical pulse for 1 min before giving drug; if pulse <60 in adult or <90 in an infant, take again in 1 hr; if <60 in adult, call prescriber; note rate, rhythm, character; monitor ECG continuously during parenteral loading dose
• Electrolytes: K, Na, Cl, Mg, Ca; renal function studies: BUN, creatinine; blood studies: ALT, AST, bilirubin, Hct, Hgb before initiating treatment and periodically thereafter
• I&O ratio, daily weights; monitor turgor, lung sounds, edema
• Monitor drug levels (therapeutic level 0.5-2 ng/ml)
• Cardiac status: apical pulse, character, rate, rhythm

Administer:
PO route
• Do not break, crush, or chew caps
• PO with or without food; may crush tabs, only mix with food/fluids
• Potassium supplements if ordered for potassium levels <3, or foods high in potassium: bananas, orange juice
IV route
• Undiluted or 1 ml of drug/4 ml sterile H_2O, D_5, or NS; give >5 min through Y-tube or 3-way stopcock; during digitalization close monitoring is necessary
Additive compatibilities: Bretylium, cimetidine, floxacillin, furosemide, lidocaine, ranitidine, verapamil
Syringe compatibilities: Heparin, milrinone
Y-site compatibilities: Amrinone, cefmetazole, ciprofloxacin, cisatracurium, diltiazem, famotidine, meperidine, meropenem, midazolam, milrinone, morphine, potassium chloride, propofol, remifentanil, tacrolimus, vit B/C
Perform/provide:
• Storage protected from light
Evaluate:
• Therapeutic response: decreased weight, edema, pulse, respiration, crackles; increased urine output; serum digoxin level (0.5-2 ng/ml)
Teach patient/family:
• Not to stop drug abruptly; teach all aspects of drug, to take exactly as ordered; how to monitor heart rate
• To avoid OTC medications, herbal remedies since many adverse drug interactions may occur; do not take antacid at same time
• To notify prescriber of loss of appetite, lower stomach pain, diarrhea, weakness, drowsiness, headache, blurred or yellow vision, rash, depression, toxicity
• The toxic symptoms of this drug and when to notify prescriber
• To maintain a sodium-restricted diet as ordered
• To report shortness of breath, difficulty breathing, weight gain, edema, persistent cough

Treatment of overdose: Discontinue drug; give potassium; monitor ECG; give adrenergic-blocking agent, digoxin immune FAB

digoxin immune FAB (ovine) (℞)
(di-jox'in im-myoon' FAB)
Digibind, DigiFab
Func. class.: Antidote—digoxin specific

Action: Antibody fragments bind to free digoxin or digitoxin to reverse toxicity by not allowing digoxin or digitoxin to bind to sites of action

Uses: Life-threatening digoxin toxicity

DOSAGE AND ROUTES
1 (38 mg) vial binds 0.5 mg digoxin

Digoxin toxicity (known amount) (tabs, oral sol, IM)
• *Adult and child:* **IV** dose (mg) = dose ingested (mg) × 0.8/1000 × 38; if ingested amount is unknown, give 760 mg **IV**

Toxicity (known amount) (cap, IV)
• *Adult and child:* **IV** dose = dose ingested (mg)/0.5 × 38

Toxicity (known amount) by serum digoxin concentrations (SDCs)
• *Adult and child:* **IV** SDC (nanograms/ml) × kg of weight/100 × 38

Digoxin toxicity (unknown amount)
• *Adult and child >20 kg:* **IV** 228 mg (6 vials)
• *Infant and child <20 kg:* **IV** 38 mg (1 vial)

Skin test
• *Adult:* **ID** 9.5 mcg

Available forms: Inj 38 mg/vial (binds 0.5 mg digoxin), 40 mg/vial (binds 0.5 mg digoxin)

SIDE EFFECTS
CV: **CHF,** ventricular rate increase, **atrial fibrillation,** low cardiac output
INTEG: Hypersensitivity, allergic reactions, facial swelling, redness

META: **Hypokalemia**
MISC: **Anaphylaxis** (rare)
RESP: **Impaired respiratory function, rapid respiratory rate**

Contraindications: Mild digoxin toxicity, hypersensitivity to this product or papain

Precautions: Pregnancy (C), children, lactation, geriatric, renal/cardiac disease, allergy to ovine proteins

PHARMACOKINETICS
IV: Peaks after completion of infusion, onset 30 min (variable); not known if crosses placenta, breast milk; half-life biphasic—14-20 hr; prolonged in renal disease; excreted by kidneys

INTERACTIONS
• Considered incompatible with all drugs in syringe or sol
Drug/Lab Test
Interference: Immunoassay digoxin

NURSING CONSIDERATIONS
Assess:
• Hypokalemia: ST depression, flat T waves, presence of U wave, ventricular dysrhythmia; potassium levels may decrease rapidly
• CHF: Dyspnea, crackles, peripheral edema, weight gain >5 lb

Administer:
• Test doses have proven to be ineffective in the general population; only use test dose in those with known allergies or those previously treated with digoxin immune FAB
• For test dose dilute 0.1 ml or reconstituted drug (9.5 mg/ml) in 9.9 ml sterile isotonic saline, inj 0.1 ml (1:100 dilution) ID and observe for wheal with erythema; read in 20 min
• For scratch test place 1 gtt of sol on skin and make a scratch through the drop with a sterile needle; read in 20 min
• After diluting 38 mg/4 ml of sterile H_2O for inj 10 mg/ml mix; may be further diluted with normal saline, sol should be clear, colorless

- By bolus if cardiac arrest is imminent or IV over 30 min using a 0.22-µm filter

Perform/provide:
- Storage of reconstituted sol for up to 4 hr in refrigerator
- Do not freeze DigiFab

Evaluate:
- Therapeutic response: correction of digoxin toxicity; check digoxin levels 0.5-2 ng/ml; digitoxin level 9-25 ng/ml

Teach patient/family:
- The purpose of medication; to report delayed hypersensitivity; fever, chills, itching, swelling, dyspnea

---

dihydrotachysterol (℞)
(dye-hye-droh-tak-iss′ter-ole)
DHT Intensol ✦, Hytakerol
Func. class.: Parathyroid agent (calcium regulator)
Chem. class.: Vit D analog

Action: Increases intestinal absorption of calcium for bones, increases renal tubular absorption of phosphate; regulates calcium levels by regulating calcitonin, parathyroid hormone
Uses: Renal osteodystrophy, hypoparathyroidism, pseudohypoparathyroidism, familial hypophosphatemia, postoperative tetany

DOSAGE AND ROUTES
Hypophosphatemia
- *Adult and child:* **PO** 0.5-2 mg daily, maintenance 0.2-1.5 mg daily
Hypoparathyroidism/pseudohypoparathyroidism
- *Adult:* **PO** 0.8-2.4 mg daily × 4 days, maintenance 0.2-2 mg daily regulated by serum calcium levels
- *Neonate:* **PO** 0.05-0.1 mg/day
- *Infant, young child:* **PO** 0.1-0.5 mg/day
- *Older child:* **PO** 0.5-1 mg/day
Renal osteodystrophy
- *Adult:* **PO** 0.25-0.375 mg/day
- *Child:* **PO** 0.125-0.5 mg/day

Rickets (vit D–resistant)
- *Child:* **PO** 0.25-1 mg/day
Available forms: Tabs 0.125, 0.2, 0.4 mg; caps 0.125 mg; oral sol 0.2, 0.25 mg/5 ml, 0.2 mg/ml ✦ (Intensol)

SIDE EFFECTS
CNS: Drowsiness, headache, vertigo, fever, lethargy, depression
CV: **Dysrhythmias,** hypertension
EENT: Tinnitus
GI: Nausea, diarrhea, vomiting, jaundice, anorexia, dry mouth, constipation, cramps, metallic taste, thirst
GU: Polyuria, hypercalciuria, hyperphosphatemia, hematuria, nocturia, renal calculi
MS: Myalgia, arthralgia, decreased bone development, weakness, ataxia
Contraindications: Hypersensitivity, renal disease, hyperphosphatemia, hypercalcemia
Precautions: Pregnancy (C), renal calculi, lactation, CV disease

PHARMACOKINETICS
PO: Onset 2 wk; readily absorbed from small intestine; metabolized by liver, excreted in feces (active/inactive)

INTERACTIONS
- Hypercalcemia: thiazide diuretics, calcium supplements
- Cardiac dysrhythmias: cardiac glycosides, verapamil
Decrease: dihydrotachysterol absorption —cholestyramine, colestipol mineral oil
Decrease: dihydrotachysterol effect—corticosteroids, phenytoin, barbiturates
Drug/Lab Test
False increase: Cholesterol

NURSING CONSIDERATIONS
Assess:
- BUN, urinary Ca, AST, ALT, cholesterol, creatinine, alk phos, uric acid, chlorine, magnesium, electrolytes, urine pH, phosphate; may increase calcium, should be kept at 9-10 mg/dl, vit D 50-135 international units/dl, phosphate 70 mg/dl

- Alk phos: may be decreased
- For increased blood level, since toxic reactions may occur rapidly
- For dry mouth, metallic taste, polyuria, bone pain, muscle weakness, headache, fatigue, tinnitus, change in LOC, irregular pulse, dysrhythmias, increased respirations, anorexia, nausea, vomiting, cramps, diarrhea, constipation; may indicate hypercalcemia
- Renal status: decreased urinary output (oliguria, anuria), edema in extremities, weight gain >5 lb, periorbital edema
- Nutritional status, diet for sources of vit D (milk, some seafood), calcium (dairy products, dark green vegetables), phosphates (dairy products) must be avoided

Administer:
- Do not break, crush, or chew caps
- PO, may be increased q4wk depending on blood level

Perform/provide:
- Storage in tight, light-resistant containers at room temperature
- Restriction of sodium, potassium if required
- Restriction of fluids if required for chronic renal failure

Evaluate:
- Therapeutic response: prevention of bone deficiencies

Teach patient/family:
- The symptoms of hypercalcemia
- About foods rich in calcium, vit D

⚠ High Alert

diltiazem (℞)

(dil-tye′a-zem)

Apo-Diltiaz ✦, Cardizem, Cardizem LA, Dilacor-XR, Diltia XR, diltiazem, Nu-Diltiaz, Syn-Diltiazem ✦, Tiamate, Tiazac

Func. class.: Calcium channel blocker, antiarrhythmic class IV

Chem. class.: Benzothiazepine

Do not confuse:

Cardizem/Cardene

Action: Inhibits calcium ion influx across cell membrane during cardiac depolarization; produces relaxation of coronary vascular smooth muscle, dilates coronary arteries, slows SA/AV node conduction times, dilates peripheral arteries

Uses: PO: Angina pectoris due to coronary artery spasm, hypertension, **IV:** atrial fibrillation, flutter, paroxysmal supraventricular tachycardia

DOSAGE AND ROUTES

Hypertension
- *Adult:* **PO** 60-120 mg bid (**SUS REL**) (Cardizem SR), max 540 mg/day, or 180-240 mg (**EXT REL**) daily

Prinzmetal's or variant angina, chronic stable angina
- *Adult:* **PO** 30 mg qid, increasing dose gradually to 180-360 mg/day in divided doses or 60-120 mg bid; may increase to 240-360 mg/day or 120 or 180 mg **EXT REL** (LA, CD, XT, XR products) **PO** daily

Atrial fibrillation/flutter, paroxysmal supraventricular tachycardia
- *Adult:* **IV BOL** 0.25 mg/kg over 2 min initially, then 0.35 mg/kg may be given after 15 min; if no response, may give **CONT INF** 5-15 mg/hr for up to 24 hr

Available forms: Tabs 30, 60, 90, 120 mg; ext rel tabs 120, 180, 240, 300, 360, 420 mg; ext rel caps 60, 90, 120, 180, 240, 300, 360, 420 mg; sus rel cap 60,

90, 120 mg; inj 5 mg/ml (5, 10 ml); powder for inj 25 mg

SIDE EFFECTS

CNS: **Headache, fatigue, drowsiness,** dizziness, depression, weakness, insomnia, tremor, paresthesia
CV: **Dysrhythmia, edema, CHF,** bradycardia, hypotension, palpitations, **heart block**
GI: *Nausea,* vomiting, diarrhea, gastric upset, *constipation,* increased LFTs
GU: Nocturia, polyuria, **acute renal failure**
INTEG: *Rash,* flushing, photosensitivity, burning, pruritus at inj site
RESP: Rhinitis, dyspnea, pharyngitis
Contraindications: Sick sinus syndrome, 2nd- or 3rd-degree heart block, hypotension <90 mm Hg systolic, acute MI, pulmonary congestion, intracranial surgery, bleeding aneurysms, severe hypotension (systolic <90 mm Hg or diastolic <60 mm Hg)
Precautions: Pregnancy (C), CHF, hypotension, hepatic injury, lactation, children, renal disease

PHARMACOKINETICS

Onset 30-60 min; peak 2-3 hr immediate rel; 10-14 hr ext rel, 6-11 hr sus rel; half-life 3½-9 hr; metabolized by liver; excreted in urine (96% as metabolites)

INTERACTIONS

Increase: effect, toxicity—theophylline
Increase: effects of β-blockers, digoxin, lithium, carbamazepine, cycloSPORINE, anesthetics, HMG-CoA reductase inhibitors, benzodiazepines, lovastatin
Increase: effects of diltiazem—cimetidine
Drug/Herb
Increase: diltiazem effect—barberry, betel palm, burdock, goldenseal, khat, khella, lily of the valley, plantain
Decrease: diltiazem effect—yohimbe

Drug/Food
Increase: hypotensive effects—grapefruit juice

NURSING CONSIDERATIONS
Assess:
• Cardiac status: B/P, pulse, respiration, ECG and intervals PR, QRS, QT; if systolic B/P <90 mm Hg or HR <60 bpm, hold dose, notify prescriber
Administer:
PO route
• Do not break, crush, or chew sus rel caps or sus rel tabs
• With a full glass of water before meals, bedtime (PO)
• Give ext rel, sus rel products daily; immediate rel qid
• Dilacor-XR on an empty stomach
• May sprinkle on applesauce for administration
IV route
• IV undiluted over 2 min or diluted 125 mg/100 ml, 250 mg/250 ml of D_5W, 0.9% NaCl, D_5/0.45% NaCl, give 10 mg/hr, may increase by 5 mg/hr to 15 mg/hr, continue infusion up to 24 hr
Y-site compatibilities: Albumin, amikacin, amphotericin B, aztreonam, bretylium, bumetanide, cefazolin, cefotaxime, cefotetan, cefoxitin, ceftazidime, ceftriaxone, cefuroxime, cimetidine, ciprofloxacin, clindamycin, digoxin, DOBUTamine, DOPamine, doxycycline, epINEPHrine, erythromycin, esmolol, fentanyl, fluconazole, gentamicin, hetastarch, hydromorphone, imipenem-cilastatin, labetalol, lidocaine, lorazepam, meperidine, metoclopramide, metronidazole, midazolam, milrinone, morphine, multivitamins, niCARdipine, nitroglycerin, norepinephrine, oxacillin, penicillin G potassium, pentamidine, piperacillin, potassium chloride, potassium phosphates, ranitidine, sodium nitroprusside, theophylline, ticarcillin, ticarcillin/clavulanate, tobramycin, trimethoprim-sulfamethoxazole, vancomycin, vecuronium
Perform/provide:
• Storage in tight container at room temperature

Evaluate:
- Therapeutic response: decreased anginal pain, decreased B/P

Teach patient/family:
- How to take pulse before taking drug; record or graph should be kept
- To avoid hazardous activities until stabilized on drug, dizziness is no longer a problem
- To limit caffeine consumption
- To avoid OTC drugs unless directed by prescriber
- The importance of complying with all areas of medical regimen: diet, exercise, stress reduction, drug therapy
⚠ To report dizziness, shortness of breath, palpitations
- Not to discontinue abruptly

Treatment of overdose: Atropine for AV block, vasopressor for hypotension

---

*dimenhyDRINATE
(OTC, ℞)
(dye-men-hye′dri-nate)
Apo-Dimenhydrinate ✹,
Calm-X, Children's
Dramamine,
dimenhyDRINATE, Dimetabs,
Dramamine, Dramanate,
Dymenate, Gravol ✹, Gravol
L/A ✹, Nauseatol ✹,
Novo-Dimenate ✹,
PMS-Dimenhydrinate ✹,
Travamine ✹,
Func. class.: Antiemetic, antihistamine, anticholinergic
Chem. class.: H_1-Receptor antagonist, ethanolamine derivative

Do not confuse:
dimenhyDRINATE/diphenhydrAMINE
Action: Competes with histamine for H_1 receptors in GI tract, blood vessels, respiratory tract; central anticholinergic activity, which results in decreased vestibular stimulation and blockade of chemoreceptor trigger zone
Uses: Motion sickness, nausea, vomiting, vertigo

DOSAGE AND ROUTES
- *Adult:* PO 50-100 mg q4h; **IM/IV** 50 mg q4h as needed (Canada only)
- *Child 6-12 yr:* PO 25-50 mg q6-8 hr prn, max 150 mg/day
- *Child 2-5 yr:* PO 12.5-25 mg q6-8 hr, max 75 mg/day

Available forms: Tabs 50 mg; inj 50 mg/ml ✹; elixir 15 mg/5 ml ✹; chew tabs 50 mg

SIDE EFFECTS
CNS: Drowsiness, restlessness, headache, dizziness, insomnia, confusion, nervousness, tingling, vertigo
CV: Hypertension, *hypotension*, palpitation
EENT: Dry mouth, blurred vision, diplopia, nasal congestion, photosensitivity
GI: Nausea, anorexia, vomiting, *constipation*
INTEG: Rash, urticaria, fever, chills, flushing
MISC: **Anaphylaxis**
Contraindications: Hypersensitivity
Precautions: Pregnancy (B), children, cardiac dysrhythmias, geriatric, asthma, lactation, prostatic hypertrophy, bladder-neck obstruction, narrow-angle glaucoma, stenosing peptic ulcer, pyloro-duodenal obstruction

PHARMACOKINETICS
IM/PO: Onset 15-30 min, duration 4-6 hr

INTERACTIONS
Increase: effect—alcohol, other CNS depressants, anticholinergic, tricyclics, MAOIs
Drug/Herb
Increase: anticholinergic effect—corkwood, henbane, jimsonweed, scopolia
Increase: effect—hops, Jamaican dogwood, khat, senega
Drug/Lab Test
False negative: Allergy skin testing

NURSING CONSIDERATIONS

Assess:
- VS, B/P; check patients with cardiac disease more often
- Signs of toxicity of other drugs or masking of symptoms of disease: brain tumor, intestinal obstruction
- Observe for drowsiness, dizziness

Administer:
- IM inj in large muscle mass; aspirate to avoid IV administration (Canada only)
- Tablets may be swallowed whole, chewed, or allowed to dissolve

IV route (Canada only)
- After diluting 50 mg/10 ml of NaCl inj; give 50 mg or less over 2 min

Additive compatibilities: Amikacin, calcium gluconate, chloramphenicol, corticotropin, erythromycin, heparin, hydrOXYzine, methicillin, norepinephrine, penicillin G potassium, pentobarbital, phenobarbital, potassium chloride, prochlorperazine, vancomycin, vit B/C

Syringe compatibilities: Atropine, diphenhydrAMINE, droperidol, fentanyl, heparin, hydromorphone, meperidine, metoclopramide, morphine, pentazocine, perphenazine, ranitidine, scopolamine

Y-site compatibilities: Acyclovir
- Therapeutic response: absence of nausea, vomiting

Teach patient/family:
- To avoid hazardous activities, activities requiring alertness; dizziness may occur; instruct patient to request assistance with ambulation
- To avoid alcohol, other depressants

Rarely Used

dimercaprol (℞)
(dye-mer-cap′role)
BAL in Oil, British Anti-Lewisite ✦
dimercaptopropanol
Func. class.: Heavy metal chelator

Uses: Arsenic, gold, mercury, lead poisoning

DOSAGE AND ROUTES

Severe gold/arsenic poisoning
- *Adult:* IM 3 mg/kg q4h × 2 days then qid × 1 day, then bid × 10 days or until recovery

Mild gold/arsenic poisoning
- *Adult:* IM 2.5 mg/kg qid × 2 days, then bid × 1 day, then daily × 10 days or until recovery

Acute lead poisoning
- *Adult:* IM 4 mg/kg, then q4h for 2-7 days with edetate calcium disodium 12.5 mg/kg IM, not to exceed 5 mg/kg/dose

Mercury poisoning
- *Adult:* IM 5 mg/kg, then 2.5 mg/kg/day or bid × 10 days

Contraindications: Pregnancy (C), hypersensitivity, anuria, hepatic insufficiency, poisoning of other metals (iron, cadmium, selenium), severe renal disease, child <3 yr

dinoprostone (℞)
(dye-noe-prost′one)
Cervidil Vaginal Insert, Prepidil, Endocervical Gel, Prostin E Vaginal Suppository
Func. class.: Oxytocic, abortifacient
Chem. class.: Prostaglandin E_2

Do not confuse:
Prepidil/bepridil

Action: Stimulates uterine contractions, causing abortion; acts within 30 hr for complete abortion

Uses: Abortion during 2nd trimester, benign hydatidiform mole, expulsion of uterine contents in fetal deaths to 28 wk, missed abortion, to efface and dilate the cervix in pregnancy at term

DOSAGE AND ROUTES

Abortifacient
- *Adult:* VAG SUPP 20 mg, repeat q3-5h until abortion occurs, max dose is 240 mg

Cervical ripening
- *Adult:* GEL warm to room temperature, choose correct length shielded cath-

eter (10 or 20 mm), fill catheter by pushing plunger; patient should remain recumbent for 15-30 min; insert one 10 mg insert

Available forms: Vag supp 20 mg; gel 0.5 mg/3 g (prefilled syringe); vag insert 10 mg

SIDE EFFECTS

CNS: Headache, dizziness, chills, fever
CV: Hypotension, **dysrhythmias**
EENT: Blurred vision
FETAL: Bradycardia (i.e., deceleration)
GI: Nausea, vomiting, diarrhea
GU: Vaginitis, vaginal pain, vulvitis, vaginismus
INTEG: Rash, skin color changes
MS: Leg cramps, joint swelling, weakness
GEL: Uterine contractile abnormality, GI side effects, back pain, fever
INSERT: Uterine hyperstimulation, fever, nausea, vomiting, diarrhea, abdominal pain
SUPPOSITORY: **Uterine rupture, anaphylaxis**

Contraindications: Hypersensitivity, uterine fibrosis, cervical stenosis, pelvic surgery, pelvic inflammatory disease, respiratory disease

Precautions: Pregnancy (C), renal/hepatic/cardiac disease, asthma, anemia, jaundice, diabetes mellitus, convulsive disorders, hypertension, hypotension, glaucoma

INTERACTIONS

Increase: effect—other oxytocics
Decrease: oxytocic effect—alcohol

PHARMACOKINETICS

GEL: Onset 10 min, peak 30-45 min
SUPP: Onset 10 min, duration 2-3 hr
Metabolized in spleen, kidney, lungs; excreted in urine

NURSING CONSIDERATIONS

Assess:
• Cervical ripening: dilation, effacement of cervix and uterine contraction, fetal heart tones, check for contractions over 1 min

• For fever that occurs ½ hr after suppository insertion (abortion)
• Respiratory rate, rhythm, depth; notify prescriber of abnormalities, pulse, B/P, temp
• Vaginal discharge: check for itching, irritation; indicates vaginal infection

Administer:
• By gel: after warming to room temp, remove seal from end of syringe, and remove the protective end cap and insert into plunger stopper assembly; make sure patient is in dorsal position
• Antiemetic/antidiarrheal before administration of this drug

Evaluate:
• Therapeutic response: expulsion of fetus

Teach patient/family:
• To remain supine for 10-15 min after insertion of supp 2 hr after insert, 15-30 min after gel
• To report excessive cramping, bleeding, chills, fever
• Some methods of pain, comfort control
• Avoid intercourse, tub baths, douches, tampon use for at least 2 wk

Side effects: *italics* = common; **bold** = life-threatening

*diphenhydrAMINE
(otc, ℞)

(dye-fen-hye'dra-meen)
Allerdryl ✤, AllerMax ✤,
Allermed, Banophen,
Benadryl, Benadryl 25,
Benadryl Kapseals, Benahist
10, Benahist 50, Ben-
Allergin-50, Benoject-10,
Benoject-50, Benylin Cough,
Bydramine, Compoz,
Diphenadryl, Diphen
Cough, Diphenhist,
diphenhydrAMINE HCl,
Dormin, Genahist,
Hydramine, Hydramyn,
Hydril, Hyrexin-50,
Insomnal ✤, Nidryl,
Nighttime Sleep Aid, Nordryl,
Nordryl Cough, Nytol,
Phendry, Siladryl, Sleep-Eze
3, Sominex 2, Tusstat, Twilite,
Uni-Bent Cough, Wehydryl

Func. class.: Antihistamine (1st
generation, nonselective)

Chem. class.: Ethanolamine derivative, H_1-receptor antagonist

Do not confuse:

diphenhydrAMINE/dicyclomine
diphenhydrAMINE/dimenhyDRINATE

Action: Acts on blood vessels, GI, respiratory system by competing with histamine for H_1-receptor site; decreases allergic response by blocking histamine

Uses: Allergy symptoms, rhinitis, motion
sickness, antiparkinsonism, nighttime sedation, infant colic, nonproductive cough

DOSAGE AND ROUTES

• *Adult and child >12 yr:* **PO** 25-50 mg
q4-6h, not to exceed 400 mg/day; **IM/IV**
10-50 mg, not to exceed 400 mg/day

• *Child <12 yr:* **PO/IM/IV** 5 mg/kg/day
in 4 divided doses, not to exceed 300 mg/
day

Nighttime sleep aid
• *Adult and child ≥12 yr:* **PO** 25-50 mg
at bedtime

Antitussive (syrup only)
• *Adult and child ≥12 yr:* **PO** 25 mg
q4h, max 100 mg/24 hr

• *Child 6-12 yr:* **PO** 12.5 mg q4h, max
75 mg/24 hr

• *Child 2-6 yr:* **PO** 6.25 mg q4h, max
37.5 mg/24 hr

Renal disease
• CCr >50 ml/min give dose q6h; CCr
10-50 ml/min dose q6-12h; CCr <10 ml/
min dose q12-18h

Available forms: Caps 25, 50 mg; tabs
25, 50 mg; chew tabs 12.5 mg; elix 12.5
mg/5 ml; syr 12.5 mg/5 ml; inj 10, 50
mg/ml; orally disintegrating tabs 12.5 mg

SIDE EFFECTS

CNS: Dizziness, drowsiness, poor coordination, fatigue, anxiety, euphoria, confusion, paresthesia, neuritis, **seizures**

EENT: Blurred vision, dilated pupils, tinnitus, nasal stuffiness, dry nose, throat,
mouth

GI: Nausea, anorexia, diarrhea

GU: Retention, dysuria, frequency

HEMA: **Thrombocytopenia, agranulocytosis, hemolytic anemia**

INTEG: Photosensitivity

MISC: **Anaphylaxis**

RESP: Increased thick secretions, wheezing, chest tightness

Contraindications: Hypersensitivity to
H_1-receptor antagonist, acute asthma attack, lower respiratory tract disease

Precautions: Pregnancy (B), increased
intraocular pressure, renal/cardiac disease, hypertension, bronchial asthma, seizure disorder, stenosed peptic ulcers, hyperthyroidism, prostatic hypertrophy,
bladder neck obstruction, lactation

PHARMACOKINETICS

PO: Peak 1-3 hr, duration 4-7 hr
IM: Onset ½ hr, peak 1-4 hr, duration
4-7 hr
IV: Onset immediate, duration 4-7 hr;
metabolized in liver, excreted by

kidneys; crosses placenta, excreted in breast milk; half-life 2-7 hr

INTERACTIONS

Increase: CNS depression—barbiturates, opiates, hypnotics, tricyclics, alcohol
Increase: diphenhydrAMINE effect—MAOIs
Drug/Herb
Increase: anticholinergic effect—corkwood, henbane
Increase: effect—hops, Jamaican dogwood, khat, senega
Drug/Lab Test
False negative: Skin allergy tests

NURSING CONSIDERATIONS

Assess:
• Be alert for urinary retention, frequency, dysuria; drug should be discontinued
• CBC during long-term therapy; blood dyscrasias may occur
• Respiratory status: rate, rhythm, increase in bronchial secretions, wheezing, chest tightness
Administer:
• With meals for GI symptoms; absorption rate may slightly decrease
• Deep IM in large muscle; rotate site
• At bedtime only if using for sleep aid
IV route
• Undiluted; give 25 mg/1 min
Additive compatibilities: Amikacin, aminophylline, ascorbic acid, bleomycin, cephapirin, erythromycin, hydrocortisone, lidocaine, methicillin, methyldopate, nafcillin, netilmicin, penicillin G potassium, penicillin G sodium, polymyxin B, vit B/C
Syringe compatibilities: Atropine, butorphanol, chlorproMAZINE, cimetidine, dimenhyDRINATE, droperidol, fentanyl, fluphenazine, glycopyrrolate, hydromorphone, hydrOXYzine, meperidine, metoclopramide, midazolam, morphine, nalbuphine, pentazocine, perphenazine, prochlorperazine, promazine, promethazine, ranitidine, scopolamine, sufentanil, thiothixene

Y-site compatibilities: Acyclovir, aldesleukin, amifostine, amsacrine, aztreonam, ciprofloxacin, cisatracurium, cisplatin, cladribine, cyclophosphamide, cytarabine, DOXOrubicin, DOXOrubicin liposome, famotidine, filgrastim, fluconazole, fludarabine, gallium, granisetron, heparin, hydrocortisone, idarubicin, melphalan, meperidine, meropenem, methotrexate, ondansetron, paclitaxel, piperacillin/tazobactam, potassium chloride, propofol, remifentanil, sargramostim, sufentanil, tacrolimus teniposide, thiotepa, vinorelbine, vit B/C
Perform/provide:
• Hard candy, gum, frequent rinsing of mouth for dryness
• Storage in tight container at room temperature
Evaluate:
• Therapeutic response: absence of running or congested nose or rashes, improved sleep
Teach patient/family:
• All aspects of drug use; to notify prescriber of confusion, sedation, hypotension
• To avoid driving, other hazardous activity if drowsiness occurs
• That photosensitivity may occur
• To avoid concurrent use of alcohol, other CNS depressants
Treatment of overdose: Administer diazepam, vasopressors, barbiturates (short-acting)

diphenoxylate/ atropine (℞)

(dye-fen-ox′ee-late/a′troe-peen)

Logene, Lomanate, Lomotil, Lonox

difenoxin/atropine (℞)

(dye-fen-ox′in/a′troe-peen)

Motofen

Func. class.: Antidiarrheal
Chem. class.: Phenylpiperidine derivative opiate agonist

Controlled Substance Schedule V
diphenoxylate/atropine

Controlled Substance Schedule IV
difenoxin/atropine (US)

Do not confuse:
Lomotil/Lamictal/Lamisil/Lanoxin/Lasix

Action: Inhibits gastric motility by acting on mucosal receptors responsible for peristalsis

Uses: Acute nonspecific and acute exacerbations of chronic functional diarrhea

DOSAGE AND ROUTES

Diphenoxylate/atropine
• *Adult:* **PO** 5 mg qid titrated to patient response needed, not to exceed 8 tabs/24 hr
• *Child 2-12 yr:* **PO** (liquid only) 0.3-0.4 mg/kg/day in divided dose
Difenoxin/atropine
• *Adult:* **PO** 2 tabs, then 1 tab after each loose stool or q3-4hr prn, max 8 tabs/day

Available forms: *diphenoxylate/atropine:* tabs 2.5 mg with atropine 0.025 mg; liquid 2.5 mg with atropine 0.025 mg/5 ml; *difenoxin/atropine:* tabs 1 mg difenoxin/0.025 atropine

SIDE EFFECTS

CNS: Dizziness, drowsiness, lightheadedness, headache, fatigue, nervousness, insomnia, confusion
EENT: Burning eyes, blurred vision

GI: Nausea, vomiting, dry mouth, epigastric distress, constipation, **paralytic ileus**
MISC: **Anaphylaxis, angioedema**
RESP: **Respiratory depression**

Contraindications: Hypersensitivity, pseudomembranous enterocolitis, jaundice, glaucoma, child <2 yr, severe electrolyte imbalances, diarrhea associated with organisms that penetrate intestinal mucosa

Precautions: Pregnancy (C), renal/hepatic disease, ulcerative colitis, lactation, severe hepatic disease

PHARMACOKINETICS

PO: Onset 40-60 min, peak 2 hr, duration 3-4 hr, terminal half-life 12-14 hr; metabolized in liver to inactive metabolite; excreted in urine, feces

INTERACTIONS

• Do not use with MAOIs; hypertensive crisis may occur
Increase: action of alcohol, opioids, barbiturates, other CNS depressants, anticholinergics
Drug/Herb
Increase: antidiarrheal action—nutmeg

NURSING CONSIDERATIONS

Assess:
• Electrolytes (K, Na, Cl) if on long-term therapy
• Bowel pattern before; for rebound constipation after termination of medication; bowel sounds
• Response after 48 hr; if none, drug should be discontinued
• Abdominal distention, toxic megacolon, which may occur in ulcerative colitis
• Hepatic studies if on long-term therapy
Administer:
• For 48 hr only; if no response, drug should be discontinued
Evaluate:
• Therapeutic response: decreased diarrhea

⚠ Safety alert   *"Tall Man" lettering

Teach patient/family:

- To avoid OTC products unless directed by prescriber (may contain alcohol); do not use alcohol or CNS depressants
- Not to exceed recommended dose
- That drug may be habit forming
- Not to engage in hazardous activities; drowsiness may occur, not to use for longer than 48 hr for acute diarrhea

---

dipivefrin ophthalmic
See Appendix C

---

dipyridamole (R)
(dye-peer-id'a-mole)
Apo-Dipyridamole ✤, Novo-
Dipiradol ✤, Persantine,
Persantine IV
Func. class.: Coronary vasodilator,
antiplatelet agent
Chem. class.: Nonnitrate

Action: Inhibits adenosine uptake, which produces coronary vasodilation; increases oxygen saturation in coronary tissues, coronary blood flow; acts on small resistance vessels with little effect on vascular resistance; may increase development of collateral circulation; decreases platelet aggregation by the inhibition of phosphodiesterase (an enzyme)

Uses: Prevention of transient ischemic attacks, inhibition of platelet adhesion to prevent myocardial reinfarction, thromboembolism, with warfarin in prosthetic heart valves, prevention of coronary bypass graft occlusion with aspirin; IV form used to evaluate coronary artery disease; used as alternative to exercise in thallium myocardial perfusion imaging to evaluate coronary artery disease

DOSAGE AND ROUTES
TIA
- *Adult:* PO 50 mg tid, 1 hr before meals, not to exceed 400 mg daily

Inhibition of platelet adhesion
- *Adult:* PO 50-75 mg qid in combination with aspirin or warfarin
Thallium myocardial perfusion imaging
- *Adult:* IV 570 mcg/kg

Available forms: Tabs 25, 50, 75 mg; inj 10 mg/2 ml

SIDE EFFECTS
CNS: Headache, dizziness, weakness, fainting, syncope; IV: transient cerebral ischemia, weakness
CV: Postural hypotension; IV: **MI**
GI: Nausea, vomiting, anorexia, diarrhea
INTEG: Rash, flushing
RESP: IV: **Bronchospasm**
Contraindications: Hypersensitivity
Precautions: Pregnancy (B), lactation, hypotension

PHARMACOKINETICS
PO: Peak 1.25 hr, duration 6 hr; therapeutic response may take several months; metabolized in liver; excreted in bile; undergoes enterohepatic recirculation

INTERACTIONS
- Prevention of coronary vasodilation: theophylline
Increase: digoxin effect—digoxin
Increase: bleeding risk—NSAIDs, cefamandole, cefotetan, cefoperazone, plicamycin, valproic acid, sulfinpyrazone, anticoagulants, thrombolytics
Drug/Herb
- Gastric irritation: arginine
Increase: antiplatelet effect—bogbean, dong quai, feverfew, garlic, ginger, ginkgo, grapeseed, primrose
Decrease: antiplatelet effect—bilberry, saw palmetto

NURSING CONSIDERATIONS
Assess:
- B/P, pulse during treatment until stable; take B/P lying, standing; orthostatic hypotension is common

• Cardiac status: chest pain, what aggravates or ameliorates condition

Administer:

PO route

• On an empty stomach: 1 hr before meals or 2 hr after; give with 8 oz water for better absorption

IV route

• IV after diluting to at least 1:2 ratio using D_5W, 0.45% NaCl, or 0.9% NaCl to a total vol of 20-50 ml; give over 4 min; do not give undiluted

Perform/provide:

• Storage at room temperature

Evaluate:

• Therapeutic response: decreased platelet adhesion

Teach patient/family:

• That medication is not a cure; may have to be taken continuously in evenly spaced doses only as directed

• To avoid hazardous activities until stabilized on medication; dizziness may occur

• To rise slowly from sitting or lying to prevent orthostatic hypotension

• Not to use alcohol or OTC medications unless approved by prescriber

---

Rarely Used

dirithromycin (℞)

(dye-rith-roe-mye′sin)

Dynabac

Func. class.: Antiinfective

Uses: Infections of the respiratory tract caused by *Moraxella catarrhalis, Streptococcus* sp. (*S. pneumoniae, S. pyogenes, S. agalactiae, S. viridans*), *Legionella pneumophilia, Mycoplasma pneumoniae, Staphylococcus aureus, Bordetella pertussis, Haemophilus influenzae*

DOSAGE AND ROUTES

• *Adult:* **PO** 500 mg daily, given for 7-14 days depending on infections

Contraindications: Hypersensitivity to this drug or any other macrolide, or erythromycin, bacteremias

---

disopyramide (℞)

(dye-soe-peer′a-mide)

disopyramide, Norpace, Norpace CR, Rythmodan ✦, Rythmodan-LA ✦

Func. class.: Antidysrhythmic (Class IA)

Chem. class.: Nonnitrate

Action: Prolongs duration of action potential and effective refractory period; reduces disparity in refractory period between normal and infarcted myocardium; prevents increased myocardial excitability and conduction contractility

Uses: PVCs, ventricular tachycardia, supraventricular tachycardia, atrial flutter, fibrillation

Unlabeled uses: Supraventricular tachycardia (prevention, treatment)

DOSAGE AND ROUTES

• *Adult:* **PO** 100-200 mg q6h, **CONT REL CAPS** 200-400 mg q12h

• *Child 12-18 yr:* **PO** 6-15 mg/kg/day, in divided doses q6h

• *Child 4-12 yr:* **PO** 10-15 mg/kg/day, in divided doses q6h

• *Child 1-4 yr:* **PO** 10-20 mg/kg/day, in divided doses q6h

• *Child <1 yr:* **PO** 10-30 mg/kg/day, in divided doses q6h

Renal dose

• *Adult:* **PO** CCr >40 ml/min 100 mg q6h; CCr 30-40 ml/min dose q8h; CCr 15-30 ml/min dose q12h; CCr <15 ml/min dose q24h

Available forms: Caps 100, 150 mg; ext rel caps (CR) 100, 150 mg; ext rel tabs 150 mg ✦

SIDE EFFECTS

CNS: Headache, dizziness, psychosis, fatigue, depression, paresthesias, insomnia

CV: Hypotension, bradycardia, angina, PVCs, tachycardia, increased QRS, QT seg-

---

ments, **cardiac arrest,** edema, weight gain, AV block, **CHF,** syncope, chest pain
EENT: Blurred vision; dry nose, throat, eyes; narrow-angle glaucoma
GI: Dry mouth, constipation, nausea, anorexia, flatulence, diarrhea, vomiting
GU: Urinary retention, hesitancy, impotence
HEMA: **Thrombocytopenia, agranulocytosis,** anemia (rare), decreased Hgb, Hct
INTEG: Rash, pruritus, urticaria
META: Hypoglycemia, hypokalemia
MS: Weakness, pain in extremities
Contraindications: Hypersensitivity, 2nd- or 3rd-degree block, cardiogenic shock, CHF (uncompensated), sick sinus syndrome, QT prolongation
Precautions: Pregnancy (C), lactation, diabetes mellitus, renal disease, children, hepatic disease, myasthenia gravis, narrow-angle glaucoma, cardiomyopathy, conduction abnormalities, potassium imbalance

PHARMACOKINETICS

PO: Peak 30 min-3 hr, duration 6-12 hr; half-life 4-10 hr; metabolized in liver; excreted in feces, urine, breast milk; crosses placenta

INTERACTIONS

Increase: disopyramide effect—quinidine, procainamide, propranolol, lidocaine, atenolol, other antidysrhythmics, erythromycin
Increase: side effects, urinary retention—anticholinergics
Decrease: disopyramide effect—phenytoin, rifampin, phenobarbital
Drug/Herb
• Toxicity/death: aconite
Increase: action—aloe, broom, buckthorn, cascara sagrada, Chinese rhubarb, figwort, fumitory, goldenseal, kudzu, licorice, senna
Increase: serotonin effect—horehound
Decrease: antiarrhythmic action—coltsfoot

Drug/Lab Test
Increase: Hepatic enzymes, lipids, BUN, creatinine
Decrease: Hgb/Hct, blood glucose

NURSING CONSIDERATIONS
Assess:
• B/P, apical pulse for 1 min; if less than 60, check again in 1 hr; if still less than 60, notify prescriber; for rebound hypertension after 1-2 hr
• ECG; check for increased QT, widening QRS; drug should be discontinued
⚠ CHF: crackles, jugular vein distension, weight gain, peripheral edema, dyspnea
• For dehydration or hypovolemia, I&O ratio, electrolytes (Na, K, Cl)
• Renal, hepatic studies (AST, ALT, bilirubin, BUN, creatinine) during treatment
• Diabetics for signs of hypoglycemia (rare)
• Constipation: increased bulk in diet, water, stool softeners, or laxatives needed
• Cardiac rate, respiration: rate, rhythm, character
• Urinary hesitancy, frequency, or a change in I&O ratio; check for edema daily; check for toxicity
Administer:
• Do not break, crush, or chew sus rel cap; give 1 hr before or 2 hr after meals
• Sugar-free gum, frequent sips of water for dry mouth
Evaluate:
• Therapeutic response: decreased dysrhythmias
Teach patient/family:
• To take drug exactly as prescribed; if dose is missed, take within 3-4 hr of next dose; do not double dose
• To avoid alcohol, or severe hypotension may occur; to avoid OTC drugs, or serious drug interactions may occur
• To make position change slowly during early therapy to prevent orthostatic hypotension
• To avoid hazardous activities if dizziness or blurred vision occurs
• The importance of complying with drug regimen; tell patient that this drug does not cure condition

Treatment of overdose: O_2, artificial ventilation, ECG, DOPamine for circulatory depression, diazepam or thiopental for seizures

---

Rarely Used

disulfiram (Rx)
(dye-sul'fi-ram)
Antabuse, disulfiram
Func. class.: Alcohol deterrent

Uses: Chronic alcoholism (as adjunct)

DOSAGE AND ROUTES
• *Adult:* **PO** 250-500 mg daily × 1-2 wk, then 125-500 mg daily until fully socially recovered
Contraindications: Pregnancy (X), ADD, hypersensitivity, alcohol intoxication, psychoses, CV disease, lactation

---

*DOBUTamine (Rx)
(doe-byoo'ta-meen)
DOBUTamine, Dobutrex
Func. class.: Adrenergic direct-acting β_1-agonist, cardiac stimulant
Chem. class.: Catecholamine

Do not confuse:
DOBUTamine/DOPamine
Dobutrex/Diamox

Action: Causes increased contractility, increased cardiac output without marked increase in heart rate by acting on β_1-receptors in heart; minor α and β_2 effects

Uses: Cardiac decompensation due to organic heart disease or cardiac surgery
Unlabeled uses: Cardiogenic shock in children; congenital heart disease in children undergoing cardiac cath

DOSAGE AND ROUTES
• *Adult and child:* **IV INF** 2.5-10 mcg/kg/min; may increase to 40 mcg/kg/min if needed
Available forms: Inj 12.5 mg/ml

SIDE EFFECTS
CNS: Anxiety, headache, dizziness, fatigue
CV: Palpitations, tachycardia, hypertension, hypotension, PVCs, angina
ENDO: Hypokalemia
GI: Heartburn, nausea, vomiting
MS: Muscle cramps (leg)
RESP: Dyspnea
Contraindications: Hypersensitivity, idiopathic hypertrophic subaortic stenosis
Precautions: Pregnancy (B), lactation, children, hypertension, CAD, MI, hypovolemia, dysrhythmias

PHARMACOKINETICS
IV: Onset 1-2 min, peak 10 min, half-life 2 min; metabolized in liver (inactive metabolites); excreted in urine

INTERACTIONS
Increase: severe hypertension—guanethidine
Increase: dysrhythmias—general anesthetics, bretylium
Increase: pressor effect, dysrhythmias—atomoxetine, COMT inhibitors, tricyclics, MAOIs, oxytocics
Decrease: DOBUTamine action—other β-blockers

NURSING CONSIDERATIONS
Assess:
• Hypovolemia; if present, correct first; administer cardiac glycoside before DOBUTamine
• Oxygenation/perfusion deficit (check B/P, chest pain, dizziness, loss of consciousness)
• Heart failure: S_3 gallop, dyspnea, neck vein distention, bibasilar crackles in patients with CHF, cardiomyopathy, palpate peripheral pulses; report if extremities become cold or mottled or if peripheral pulses decrease
• ECG during administration continuously; if B/P increases, drug is decreased; CVP or PCWP, cardiac output during infusion; report changes
• Serum electrolytes, urine output

A Safety alert   *"Tall Man" lettering

⚠ Sulfite sensitivity, which may be life-threatening

Administer:

IV route

• Diluting each 250 mg/10 ml of sterile H_2O or D_5W for inj; may be further diluted in 50 ml or more given at prescribed rate; should be gradually increased to desired rate; use a CVP catheter or large peripheral vein, use inf pump, titrate to patient response

• Standard concentrations are 250 mcg/ml-1000 mcg/ml, max 5 mg of DOBUTamine/ml

Additive compatibilities: Amiodarone, atracurium, atropine, DOPamine, enalaprilat, epINEPHrine, flumazenil, hydrALAZINE, isoproterenol, lidocaine, meperidine, meropenem, metaraminol, morphine, nitroglycerin, norepinephrine, phentolamine, phenylephrine, procainamide, propranolol, ranitidine

Syringe compatibilities: Heparin, ranitidine

Y-site compatibilities: Amifostine, amiodarone, amrinone, atracurium, aztreonam, bretylium, calcium chloride, calcium gluconate, ciprofloxacin, cisatracurium, cladribine, diazepam, diltiazem, DOPamine, DOXOrubicin liposome, enalaprilat, epINEPHrine, famotidine, fentanyl, fluconazole, granisetron, haloperidol, hydromorphone, insulin (regular), labetalol, lidocaine, lorazepam, magnesium sulfate, meperidine, milrinone, morphine, niCARdipine, nitroglycerin, norepinephrine, pancuronium, potassium chloride, propofol, ranitidine, remifentanil, sodium nitroprusside, streptokinase, tacrolimus, theophylline, thiotepa, tolazoline, vecuronium, verapamil, zidovudine

Perform/provide:

• Storage of reconstituted solution for 24 hr if refrigerated

Evaluate:

• Therapeutic response: increased B/P with stabilization, increased urine output

Teach patient/family:

• The reason for drug administration; to report dyspnea, chest pain, numbness of extremities, headache, IV site discomfort

Treatment of overdose: Administer a β_1-adrenergic blocker; reduce IV or discontinue, ensure oxygenation/ventilation; for severe tachydysrhythmias (ventricular) give lidocaine or propranolol

---

docetaxel (℞)
(doe-se-tax'el)
Taxotere
Func. class.: Antineoplastic—miscellaneous plasic—
Chem. class.: Taxoid

Do not confuse:
Taxotere/Taxol

Action: Inhibits reorganization of microtubule network needed for interphase and mitotic cellular functions; also causes abnormal bundles of microtubules during cell cycle and multiple esters of microtubules during mitosis

Uses: Locally advanced or metastatic breast cancer, non–small-cell lung cancer, androgen independent metastatic prostate cancer, post-surgery operable node-positive breast cancer

DOSAGE AND ROUTES:

Locally advanced or metastatic breast cancer after failure of other chemotherapy

• *Adult:* IV 60-100 mg/m² given over 1 hr q3wk; if neutrophil count is <500 cells/mm³ for >1 wk, reduce dose by 25%

Locally advanced or metastatic non–small-cell lung cancer after failure of cisplatin chemotherapy

• *Adult:* IV 75 mg/m² over 1 hr q3wk; if neutrophil count is <500 cells/mm³ for >1 wk, reduce dose to 55 mg/m²; if patient develops grade 3 peripheral neuropathy, stop drug

Unreactable, locally advanced or metastatic non–small-cell lung cancer previously treated with chemotherapy

• *Adult:* IV 75 mg/m² over 1 hr, then cisplatin 75 mg/m² IV given over 30-60

---

min q3wk; reduce dose to 65 mg/m^2 in those with hematologic or non-hematologic toxicities

Androgen-independent metastatic prostate cancer

• *Adult:* IV 75 mg/m^2 given over 1 hr q3wk, with 5 mg predniSONE **PO** bid continuously; give dexamethasone 8 mg **PO** at 12 hr, 3 hr, and 1 hr prior to docetaxel; if neutrophil count is <500 cells/mm^3 for more than 1 wk or other toxicities occur, reduce dose to 60 mg/m^2

Adjuvant post-surgery treatment of operable node-positive breast cancer

• *Adult:* IV 75 mg/m^2 over 1 hr, given 1 hr after DOXOrubicin 50 mg/m^2, cyclophosphamide 500 mg/m^2 q3wk × 6 cycles

Available forms: Inj 20, 80 mg in single-dose vials

SIDE EFFECTS

CV: Hypotension, fluid retention, peripheral edema, flushing

GI: Nausea, vomiting, diarrhea, **hepatotoxicity**

HEMA: **Neutropenia, leukopenia, thrombocytopenia, anemia,** bleeding, infections, **myelosuppression**

INTEG: Alopecia, nail pain, rash, skin eruptions

MS: Arthralgia, myalgia, back pain

NEURO: Peripheral neuropathy

RESP: Dyspnea, **pulmonary edema**

SYST: Hypersensitivity reactions, **death**

Contraindications: Pregnancy (D), hypersensitivity to this drug or other drugs with polysorbate 80, neutropenia of <1500/mm^3, severe hepatic disease, bilirubin exceeding upper normal limit, or severely elevated ALT, AST, alk phos, lactation

Precautions: Children, cardiovascular disease, pulmonary disorders, bone marrow depression, herpes zoster, pleural effusion

PHARMACOKINETICS

Metabolized in liver, excreted in feces; terminal half-life 11.1 hr

INTERACTIONS

• Altered docetaxel levels: cycloSPORINE, erythromycin, ketoconazole, troleadomycin

Increase: myelosuppression—other antineoplastics, radiation

Decrease: immune response—live virus vaccines

NURSING CONSIDERATIONS

Assess:

• CBC, differential, platelet count prior to and qwk; withhold drug if WBC is <1500/mm^3 or platelet count is <100,000/mm^3, notify prescriber

• Monitor temp q4h (may indicate beginning of infection)

• CV status: B/P, edema, flushing

• Hepatic studies before, during therapy (bilirubin, AST, ALT, LDH) prn or qmo; check for jaundiced skin and sclera, dark urine, clay-colored stools, itchy skin, abdominal pain, fever, diarrhea

• CNS changes: confusion, paresthesias, dysethenia, pain, weakness; if severe, drug should be discontinued

• VS during 1st hr of infusion, check IV site for signs of infiltration

⚠ Hypersensitive reactions, anaphylaxis including hypotension, dyspnea, angioedema, generalized urticaria; discontinue infusion immediately

• Bone marrow depression: bleeding, hematuria, guaiac, bruising or petechiae, mucosa or orifices q8h; obtain prescription for viscous lidocaine (Xylocaine); avoid invasive procedures

• Effects of alopecia on body image; discuss feelings about body changes

Administer:

• Antiemetic 30-60 min before giving drug and prn

IV route

• Using cytotoxic handling procedures

• Allow vials to warm to room temperature; withdraw all diluent and inject in

---

⚠ Safety alert   *"Tall Man" lettering

vial of docetaxel; rotate gently to mix; allow to stand to decrease foaming, then withdraw the required amount (10 mg/ml) and inject in 250 ml of 0.9% wall or D_5W; mix gently; give over 1 hr

Y-site compatibilities: Acyclovir, amikacin, aminophylline, ampicillin/sulbactam, butorphanol, calcium gluconate, cefepime, cefotetan, ceftazidime, ceftriaxone, cimetidine, diphenhydrAMINE, droperidol, famotidine, fluconazole, furosemide, ganciclovir, gentamicin, granisetron, haloperidol, heparin, hydrocortisone, hydromorphone, lorazepam, magnesium sulfate, mannitol, meperidine, mesna, metoclopramide, morphine, ondansetron, potassium chloride, prochlorperazine, ranitidine, sodium bicarbonate, vancomycin, zidovudine

Perform/provide:
• Confirmation that dexamethasone was given 12 hr and 6 hr before infusion begins
• Storage of prepared sol up to 27 hr in refrigerator

Evaluate:
• Therapeutic response: decreased tumor size, spread of malignancy

Teach patient/family:
• To report signs of infection: fever, sore throat, flulike symptoms
• To report signs of anemia: fatigue, headache, faintness, shortness of breath, irritability
• To report bleeding; avoid use of razors, commercial mouthwash
• To avoid use of aspirin, ibuprofen
• To report any complaints or side effects to nurse or prescriber
• That hair may be lost during treatment; a wig or hairpiece may make patient feel better; new hair may be different in color and texture
• That pain in muscles and joints 2-5 days after infusion is common
• To use barrier contraception; avoid breastfeeding
• To avoid receiving vaccinations while on this drug

---

docosanol topical
See Appendix C

---

docusate calcium (OTC)
(dok'yoo-sate cal'see-um)
DC Softgels, Dioctocal, Pro-Cal-Sof, Sulfolax, Surfak

docusate sodium (OTC)
Colace, Correctol Extra Gentle, Diocto, Docu DOK, DOS, DSS, Dulcolax Stool Softener Ex-Lax, Fleet Sof-Lax Modane, Regulex ✦, Silace, Therevac SB

Func. class.: Laxative, emollient; stool softener
Chem. class.: Anionic surfactant

Action: Increases water, fat penetration in intestine; allows for easier passage of stool

Uses: Prevention of dry, hard stools

DOSAGE AND ROUTES
• *Adult:* **PO** 50-300 mg daily (sodium) or 240 mg (calcium or potassium) prn; **ENEMA** 4 ml
• *Child >12 yr:* **ENEMA** 2 ml
• *Child 6-12 yr:* **PO** 40-150 mg daily (sodium) in divided doses
• *Child 3-6 yr:* **PO** 20-60 mg daily (sodium) in divided doses
• *Child <3 yr:* **PO** 10-40 mg daily (sodium) in divided doses

Available forms: *Calcium:* 240 mg; *sodium:* caps 50, 100, 250 mg; tabs 100 mg; syrup 20 mg/5 ml, 50 mg/15 ml, 100 mg/30 ml, 150 mg/15 ml; oral sol 10, 50 mg/ml; enema 283 mg/3.9 cap

SIDE EFFECTS
EENT: Bitter taste, throat irritation
GI: Nausea, anorexia, cramps, diarrhea
INTEG: Rash

Contraindications: Hypersensitivity, obstruction, fecal impaction, nausea/vomiting

Precautions: Pregnancy (C), lactation

Side effects: *italics* = common; **bold** = life-threatening

PHARMACOKINETICS

Onset 12-72 hr

INTERACTIONS

• Toxicity: mineral oil

Drug/Herb

Increase: laxative action—flax, senna

NURSING CONSIDERATIONS

Assess:

• Cause of constipation; identify whether fluids, bulk, or exercise are missing from lifestyle, constipating drugs

• Cramping, rectal bleeding, nausea, vomiting; if these symptoms occur, drug should be discontinued

Administer:

• Swallow tabs whole; do not break, crush, or chew

• Oral sol: diluted in milk, fruit juice to decrease bitter taste

• In morning or evening (oral dose)

Perform/provide:

• Storage in cool environment; do not freeze

Evaluate:

• Therapeutic response: decrease in constipation

Teach patient/family:

• That normal bowel movements do not always occur daily

• Not to use in presence of abdominal pain, nausea, vomiting

• To notify prescriber if constipation unrelieved or if symptoms of electrolyte imbalance occur: muscle cramps, pain, weakness, dizziness, excessive thirst

• Inform patient that drug may take up to 3 days to soften stools

• Take oral prep with a full glass of water unless on fluid restrictions and increase fluid intake

---

dofetilide (R)

Tikosyn

Func. class.: Antidysrhythmic (Class III)

Action: Blocks cardiac ion channel carrying the rapid component of delayed potassium current, no effect on sodium channels

Uses: Atrial fibrillation, flutter, maintenance of normal sinus rhythm

DOSAGE AND ROUTES

• *Adult:* **PO** 125-500 mcg bid depending on CCr, may be adjusted q2-3h to get appropriate increase in QTc

Renal dose

• *Adult:* **PO** CCr >60 ml/min 500 mcg bid; CCr 40-60 ml/min 250 mcg bid; CCr 20-40 ml/min 125 mcg bid; CCr <20 ml/min do not use

Available forms: Caps 125, 250, 500 mcg

SIDE EFFECTS

CNS: Syncope, dizziness, headache

CV: Hypotension, postural hypotension, bradycardia, angina, PVCs, substernal pressure, transient hypertension, precipitation of angina

GI: Nausea, vomiting, severe diarrhea, anorexia

Contraindications: Hypersensitivity, digoxin toxicity, aortic stenosis, pulmonary hypertension, children, QT syndromes, severe renal disease

Precautions: Pregnancy (C), renal disease, lactation

PHARMACOKINETICS

Well absorbed, max plasma conc 2-3 hr, steady state 2-3 days, half-life 10 hr, metabolized by liver, excreted by kidneys

INTERACTIONS

• Do not use with cimetidine, ketoconazole, verapamil, prochlorperazine,

---

A Safety alert   *"Tall Man" lettering

trimethoprim-sulfamethizole, amiloride, metformin, megestrol, triamterene

Increase: hypokalemia—potassium-depleting diuretics

Drug/Herb

Increase: toxicity, death—aconite

Increase: serotonin effect—horehound

Increase: effect—aloe, broom, buckthorn (chronic use), cascara sagrada (chronic use), Chinese rhubarb, figwort, fumitory, goldenseal, kudzu, licorice

Decrease: effect—coltsfoot

NURSING CONSIDERATIONS

Assess:

• ECG continuously to determine drug effectiveness, PVCs, other dysrhythmias; renal function, QTc and baseline q3mo; if QTc >440 msec or 500 msec if ventricular conduction disturbance, discontinue until QTc is at starting level; this drug is only available to facilities that have been educated in this administration, patient must be hospitalized

• AF patients should receive anticoagulation prior to cardioversion

• Cardiac status: rate, rhythm, character, continuously

Administer:

• For 3 days hospitalized

• Give dofetilide after withholding class I or III antidysrhythmic for 3 half-lives of dofetilide

Perform/provide:

• Place patient in supine position unless otherwise ordered; assist with ambulation

Evaluate:

• Therapeutic response: control in atrial fibrillation

Teach patient/family:

• To make position changes slowly; orthostatic hypotension may occur

• Notify prescriber if fast heartbeats with fainting or dizziness occur

• Notify all prescribers of all medications and supplements taken

• That if dose is missed, do not double, take next dose at usual time

• Avoid breastfeeding

dolasetron (℞)

(do-la'se-tron)

Anzemet

Func. class.: Antiemetic

Chem. class.: 5-HT3 receptor antagonist

Action: Prevents nausea, vomiting by blocking serotonin peripherally, centrally, and in the small intestine

Uses: Prevention of nausea, vomiting associated with cancer chemotherapy, radiotherapy, and prevention of postoperative nausea, vomiting

Unlabeled uses: Radiotherapy-induced nausea/vomiting

DOSAGE AND ROUTES

Prevention of nausea/vomiting of cancer chemotherapy

• *Adult and child 2-16 yr:* IV 1.8 mg/kg as a single dose, ½ hr prior to chemotherapy

• *Adult:* PO 100 mg 1 hr prior to chemotherapy

• *Child 2-16 yr:* PO 1.8 mg/kg/hr prior to chemotherapy; max 100 mg

Prevention of postoperative nausea/vomiting

• *Adult:* IV 12.5 mg as a single dose, 15 min before cessation of anesthesia; PO 100 mg 2 hr before surgery (prevention only)

• *Child 2-16 yr:* IV 0.35 mg/kg as a single dose, 15 min before cessation of anesthesia; PO 1.2 mg/kg 2 hr before surgery (prevention only)

Available forms: Tabs 50, 100 mg; inj 20 mg/ml (12.5 mg/0.625 ml)

SIDE EFFECTS

CNS: Headache, dizziness, fatigue, drowsiness

CV: **Dysrhythmias,** ECG changes, hypotension, tachycardia, hypertension, bradycardia

GI: Diarrhea, constipation, increased AST, ALT, abdominal pain, anorexia

GU: Urinary retention, oliguria

MISC: Rash, **bronchospasm**

Side effects: *italics* = common; **bold** = life-threatening

Contraindications: Hypersensitivity
Precautions: Pregnancy (B), lactation, children, geriatric, hypokalemia, electrolyte imbalances; granisetron, ondansetron hypersensitivity

PHARMACOKINETICS

Well absorbed, metabolized to active metabolite, half-life of active metabolite 8 hr

INTERACTIONS

Increase: dysrhythmias—antidysrhythmics
Increase: dolasetron levels—cimetidine
Increase: QT prolongation—thiazide, loop diuretics
Decrease: dolasetron levels—rifampin

NURSING CONSIDERATIONS
Assess:
• For absence of nausea, vomiting during chemotherapy
• For hypersensitivity reaction: rash, bronchospasm
• For cardiac conduction conditions, electrolyte imbalances, or dysrhythmias
Administer:
• By inj 100 mg/½ min or less or diluted in 50 ml compatible sol; give over 15 min
• Not to mix product for oral administration in juice until immediately before administration; apple or apple-grape diluted can be kept for 2 hr at room temp
Perform/provide:
• Storage at room temperature 48 hr after dilution
Evaluate:
• Therapeutic response: absence of nausea, vomiting during cancer chemotherapy
Teach patient/family:
• To report diarrhea, constipation, nausea, vomiting, rash, or changes in respirations
• May cause headache, use analgesic

donepezil (Ŗ)
(don-ep-ee′zill)
Aricept
Func. class.: Reversible cholinesterase inhibitor

Action: Elevates acetylcholine concentrations (cerebral cortex) by slowing degradation of acetylcholine released in cholinergic neurons; does not alter underlying dementia
Uses: Treatment of mild to moderate dementia in Alzheimer's disease
Unlabeled uses: Vascular dementia

DOSAGE AND ROUTES
• *Adult:* **PO** 5 mg daily at bedtime; may increase to 10 mg daily after 4-6 wk
Available forms: Tabs 5, 10 mg

SIDE EFFECTS
CNS: Dizziness, *insomnia,* somnolence, *headache,* fatigue, abnormal dreams, syncope, **seizures**
CV: **Atrial fibrillation,** hypotension or hypertension, **sinus bradycardia**
GI: Nausea, vomiting, anorexia; *diarrhea*
GU: Urinary frequency, UTI, incontinence
INTEG: Rash, flushing
MS: Cramps, arthritis
RESP: Rhinitis, URI, cough, pharyngitis
Contraindications: Hypersensitivity to this drug or piperidine derivatives
Precautions: Pregnancy (C), sick sinus syndrome, history of ulcers, GI bleeding, hepatic disease, bladder obstruction, asthma, lactation, children, seizures, asthma, COPD

PHARMACOKINETICS
Well absorbed PO; metabolized to metabolites by CYP2D6, CYP3A4; elimination half-life 10 hr single dose, 70 hr multiple dosing; protein binding 96%

⚠ Safety alert   *"Tall Man" lettering

INTERACTIONS

Increase: synergistic effect—succinylcholine, cholinesterase inhibitors, cholinergic agonists

Increase: gastric acid secretions—NSAIDs

Decrease: action of anticholinergics

Decrease: donepezil effect—carbamazepine, dexamethasone, phenytoin, phenobarbital, rifampin

NURSING CONSIDERATIONS

Assess:
• B/P: hypotension, hypertension
• Mental status: affect, mood, behavioral changes, depression, complete suicide assessment
• GI status: nausea, vomiting, anorexia, diarrhea
• GU status: urinary frequency, incontinence

Administer:
• Between meals; may be given with meals for GI symptoms
• Dosage adjusted to response no more than q6wk

Perform/provide:
• Assistance with ambulation during beginning therapy; dizziness, ataxia may occur

Evaluate:
• Therapeutic response: decrease in confusion, improved mood

Teach patient/family:
• To report side effects: twitching, nausea, vomiting, sweating; indicates overdose
• To use drug exactly as prescribed; at regular intervals, preferably between meals; may be taken with meals for GI upset
• To notify prescriber of nausea, vomiting, diarrhea (dose increase or beginning treatment), or rash
• Not to increase or abruptly decrease dose; serious consequences may result
• That drug is not a cure, relieves symptoms

Treatment of overdose: Withdraw drug, administer tertiary anticholinergics, provide supportive care

---

⚠ High Alert

***DOPamine** (℞)
(doe′pa-meen)
DOPamine HCl, Intropin, Revimine ✦
Func. class.: Adrenergic
Chem. class.: Catecholamine

D

Do not confuse:
DOPamine/DOBUTamine

Action: Causes increased cardiac output; acts on β_1- and α-receptors, causing vasoconstriction in blood vessels; low dose causes renal and mesenteric vasodilation; β_1 stimulation produces inotropic effects with increased cardiac output

Uses: Shock; increased perfusion; hypotension

Unlabeled uses: COPD, RDS in infants, severe CHF

DOSAGE AND ROUTES

Shock
• *Adult:* **IV INF** 2-10 mcg/kg/min, not to exceed 50 mcg/kg/min, titrate to patient's response
• *Child:* **IV** 5-20 mcg/kg/min adjust depending on response

COPD
• *Adult:* **IV** 4 mcg/kg/min

CHF
• *Adult:* **IV** 3-10 mcg/kg/min

RDS
• *Infant:* **IV** 5 mcg/kg/min

Available forms: Inj 40 mg, 80 mg, 160 mg/ml conc for IV inf; 0.8, 1.6, 3.2 mg/ml in D_5W

SIDE EFFECTS

CNS: Headache, anxiety
CV: Palpitations, tachycardia, hypertension, ectopic beats, angina, wide QRS complex, peripheral vasoconstriction
GI: Nausea, vomiting, diarrhea
INTEG: Necrosis, tissue sloughing with extravasation, **gangrene**
RESP: Dyspnea

Contraindications: Hypersensitivity, ventricular fibrillation, tachydysrhythmias, pheochromocytoma

Precautions: Pregnancy (C), lactation, arterial embolism, peripheral vascular disease

PHARMACOKINETICS

IV: Onset 5 min, duration <10 min; metabolized in liver, kidney, plasma, excreted in urine (metabolites), half-life 2 min

INTERACTIONS

• Do not use within 2 wk of MAOIs; hypertensive crisis may result

Increase: bradycardia, hypotension—phenytoin

Increase: dysrhythmias—general anesthetics

Increase: severe hypertension—ergots

Increase: B/P—oxytocics

Increase: pressor effect—tricyclics, MAOIs

Decrease: DOPamine action—β-blockers, α-blockers

Drug/Lab Test

Increase: Urinary catecholamine, serum glucose

NURSING CONSIDERATIONS

Assess:

• Hypovolemia; if present, correct first

• Oxygenation/perfusion deficit (check B/P, chest pain, dizziness, loss of consciousness)

• Heart failure: S_3 gallop, dyspnea, neck vein distention, bibasilar crackles in patients with CHF, cardiomyopathy, palpate peripheral pulses

• I&O ratio: if urine output decreases, without decrease in B/P, drug may need to be reduced

• ECG during administration continuously; if B/P increases, drug should be decreased; PCWP, CVP during infusion

• B/P and pulse q5min

• Paresthesias and coldness of extremities; peripheral blood flow may decrease

• Injection site: tissue sloughing; if this occurs, administer phentolamine mixed with NS

Administer:

IV route

• IV after diluting 200-400 mg/250-500 ml of D_5W, D_5 0.45% NaCl, D_5 0.9% NaCl, D_5LR, LR; use large vein

• After reconstituting, use infusion pump; give at rate of 0.5-5 mcg/kg/min, increase by 1-4 mcg/kg/min at 10-30 min intervals, until desired response

Y-site compatibilities: Aldesleukin, amifostine, amiodarone, amrinone, atracurium, aztreonam, cefpirome, ciprofloxacin, cisatracurium, cladribine, diltiazem, DOBUTamine, doxorubicin liposome, enalaprilat, epINEPHrine, esmolol, famotidine, fentanyl, fluconazole, foscarnet, granisetron, haloperidol, heparin, hydrocortisone, hydromorphone, labetalol, lidocaine, lorazepam, meperidine, methylPREDNISolone, metronidazole, midazolam, milrinone, morphine, niCARdipine, nitroglycerin, norepinephrine, ondansetron, pancuronium, piperacillin/tazobactam, potassium chloride, propofol, ranitidine, remifentanil, sargramostim, sodium nitroprusside, streptokinase, tacrolimus, theophylline, thiotepa, tolazoline, vecuronium, verapamil, vit B/C, warfarin, zidovudine

Perform/provide:

• Storage of reconstituted sol for up to 24 hr if refrigerated

• Do not use discolored sol; protect from light

Evaluate:

• Therapeutic response: increased B/P with stabilization; increased urine output

Teach patient/family:

• The reason for drug administration

Treatment of overdose: Discontinue IV, may give a short-acting α-adrenergic blocker

Rarely Used

dornase alfa (℞)
(door'nace alfa)
Pulmozyme
Func. class.: Cystic fibrosis agent
(orphan drug)

Uses: Management of cystic fibrosis

DOSAGE AND ROUTES
• *Adult and child >5 yr:* **INH** 2.5 mg
daily by nebulizer

Contraindications: Hypersensitivity to
this drug or Chinese hamster ovary cell
products

dorzolamide
ophthalmic
See Appendix C

Rarely Used ⚠ High Alert

doxacurium (℞)
(dox-a-cure'ee-um)
Nuromax
Func. class.: Neuromuscular
blocker (nondepolarizing)

Uses: Facilitation of endotracheal intubation, skeletal muscle relaxation during
mechanical ventilation, surgery, or general anesthesia

DOSAGE AND ROUTES
• *Adult:* **IV** 0.05 mg/kg; 0.08 mg/kg is
used for prolonged neuromuscular blockade; maintenance 0.005-0.01 mg/kg
• *Child 2-12 yr:* **IV** 0.03-0.05 mg/kg;
may decrease for maintenance dose

Contraindications: Hypersensitivity,
neonates

doxapram (℞)
(dox'a-pram)
Dopram
Func. class.: Analeptic

Action: Respiratory stimulation through
activation of peripheral carotid chemoreceptor; with higher doses, medullary
respiratory centers are stimulated; with
progressive CNS stimulation

Uses: Chronic obstructive pulmonary disease (COPD), postanesthesia respiratory
depression, prevention of acute hypercapnia, drug-induced CNS depression

Unlabeled uses: Neonatal apnea

DOSAGE AND ROUTES
Postanesthesia
• *Adult:* **IV** inj 0.5-1 mg/kg, not to ex-
ceed 1.5 mg/kg total as a single injection;
IV INF 250 mg in 250 ml sol, not to ex-
ceed 4 mg/kg; run at 1-3 mg/min

Drug-induced CNS depression
• *Adult:* **IV** priming dose of 2 mg/kg, repeated in 5 min; repeat q1-2h until patient awakes; **IV INF** priming dose 2
mg/kg at 1-3 mg/min, not to exceed 3
g/day

COPD (hypercapnia)
• *Adult:* **IV INF** 1-2 mg/min, not to exceed 3 mg/min for no longer than 2 hr

Apnea of premature infant
• *Infant:* **IV** 1-1.5 mg/kg/hr loading dose
followed by infusion of 0.5-2.5 mg/kg/hr

Available forms: Inj 20 mg/ml

SIDE EFFECTS
CNS: **Seizures,** (clonus/generalized),
headache, restlessness, dizziness, confusion, paresthesias, flushing, sweating, bilateral Babinski's sign, rigidity, depression

*CV: Chest pain, hypertension, change in
heart rate,* lowered T waves, tachycardia, **dysrhythmias**

EENT: Pupil dilation, sneezing

GI: Nausea, vomiting, diarrhea, desire to
defecate

GU: Retention, incontinence, elevation of
BUN, albuminuria

INTEG: Pruritus, irritation at inj site

RESP: **Laryngospasm, bronchospasm,** rebound hypoventilation, dyspnea, cough, tachypnea, hiccups

Contraindications: Hypersensitivity, seizure disorders, severe hypertension, severe bronchial asthma, severe dyspnea, severe cardiac disorders, flail chest, pneumothorax, pulmonary embolism, severe respiratory disease

Precautions: Pregnancy (B), bronchial asthma, pheochromocytoma, severe tachycardia, dysrhythmias, hypertension, lactation, children, hyperthyroidism

PHARMACOKINETICS

IV: Onset 20-40 sec, peak 1-2 min, duration 5-10 min; metabolized by liver; excreted by kidneys (metabolites); half-life 2.5-4 hr

INTERACTIONS

• Synergistic pressor effect: MAOIs, sympathomimetics
• Cardiac dysrhythmias: halothane, cyclopropane, enflurane; delay use of doxapram for at least 10 min after inhalation anesthetics

NURSING CONSIDERATIONS

Assess:
• BP, heart rate, deep tendon reflexes, ABGs, LOC before administration, q30min
• Po_2, Pco_2, O_2 saturation during treatment
• Hypertension, dysrhythmias, tachycardia, dyspnea, skeletal muscle hyperactivity; may indicate overdosage; discontinue drug
• Respiratory stimulation: increased rate, abnormal rhythm
• Extravasation; change IV site q48h
• Patient closely for ½-1 hr

Administer:

IV route
• Undiluted or diluted with equal parts of sterile H_2O for inj; may be diluted 250 mg/250 ml of D_5W, $D_{10}W$ and run as infusion; rapid infusion may cause hemolysis

• IV undiluted over 5 min; IV inf at 1-3 mg/min; adjust for desired respiratory response, using infusion pump IV; if an inf is used after initial dose, start at 1-3 mg/min depending on patient response; D/C after 2 hr; wait 1-2 hr and repeat
• Only after adequate airway is established
• After O_2, IV barbiturates, resuscitative equipment available

Syringe compatibilities: Amikacin, bumetadine, chlorproMAZINE, cimetidine, cisplatin, cyclophosphamide, DOPamine, doxycycline, epINEPHrine, hydrOXYzine, imipramine, isoniazid, lincomycin, methotrexate, netilmicin, phytonadione, pyridoxine, terbutaline, thiamine, tobramycin, vinCRIStine

Perform/provide:
• Placing patient in Sims' position to prevent aspiration of vomitus
• Discontinue infusion if side effects occur; narrow margin of safety

Evaluate:
• Therapeutic response: increased breathing capacity

Teach patient/family:
• Purpose of medication

---

doxazosin (℞)
(dox-ay'zoe-sin)
Cardura
Func. class.: Peripheral α_1-adrenergic receptor blocker
Chem. class.: Quinazoline

Do not confuse:
Cardura/Coumadin/Cardene/Ridaura

Action: Peripheral blood vessels are dilated, peripheral resistance lowered; reduction in blood pressure results from peripheral α_1-adrenergic receptors being blocked

Uses: Hypertension, urinary outflow obstruction, symptoms of benign prostatic hyperplasia

Unlabeled uses: BPH with finasteride

DOSAGE AND ROUTES
BPH
• *Adult:* **PO** 1 mg daily, increase in stepwise manner to 2, 4, 8 mg daily as needed at 1-2 wk intervals, max 8 mg
Hypertension
• *Adult:* **PO** 1 mg daily, increasing up to 16 mg daily if required; usual range 4-16 mg/day
• *Geriatric:* **PO** 0.5 mg nightly, gradually increase
Available forms: Tabs 1, 2, 4, 8 mg; ext rel tabs 4, 8 mg

SIDE EFFECTS

CNS: Dizziness, headache, drowsiness, anxiety, depression, vertigo, weakness, fatigue, asthenia
CV: Palpitations, *orthostatic hypotension,* tachycardia, edema, **dysrhythmias,** chest pain
EENT: Epistaxis, tinnitus, dry mouth, red sclera, pharyngitis, rhinitis
GI: Nausea, vomiting, diarrhea, constipation, abdominal pain
GU: Incontinence, polyuria, priapism
Contraindications: Hypersensitivity to quinazolines
Precautions: Pregnancy (C), children, lactation, hepatic disease

PHARMACOKINETICS

PO: Onset 2 hr, peak 2-6 hr, duration 6-12 hr; half-life 22 hr; metabolized in liver; excreted via bile/feces (<63%) and in urine (9%); extensively protein bound (98%)

INTERACTIONS

Increase: hypotensive effects—alcohol, other antihypertensives, sildenafil, vardenafil, nitrates
Decrease: antihypertensive effects of clonidine
Drug/Herb
• Toxicity: yohimbe
Increase: doxazosin effect—angelica, hawthorn
Decrease: doxazosin effect—butcher's broom, capsicum peppers

NURSING CONSIDERATIONS
Assess:
• B/P (lying, standing) and pulse 2-6 hr after each dose and with each increase; postural effects may occur, crackles, dyspnea, orthopnea with B/P; pulse; jugular venous distention during beginning treatment
• BUN, uric acid if on long-term therapy
• I&O, weight daily
• Edema in feet, legs daily
• Skin turgor, dryness of mucous membranes for hydration status
Administer:
• Tabs broken, crushed, or chewed; if chewed, will be bitter; XL tabs should not be broken, crushed, or chewed
Perform/provide:
• Storage in tight container in cool environment
Evaluate:
• Therapeutic response: decreased B/P; decreased symptoms of BPH
Teach patient/family:
• That fainting occasionally occurs after first dose; do not drive or operate machinery for 4 hr after first dose or after dosage increase or take first dose at bedtime
• To take 1st dose at bedtime to decrease orthostatic B/P changes, may take 1-2 wk to respond in BPH
Treatment of overdose: Administer volume expanders or vasopressors; discontinue drug; place in supine position

doxepin (℞)
(dox′e-pin)
doxepin HCl, Novo-Doxepin ✦, Sinequan, Triadapin ✦, Zonalon Topical Cream
Func. class.: Antidepressant, tricyclic, antihistamine (topical)
Chem. class.: Dibenzoxepin, tertiary amine

Do not confuse:
Sinequan/Serentil/Sarafem

Side effects: *italics* = common; **bold** = life-threatening

Action: Blocks reuptake of norepinephrine, serotonin into nerve endings, increasing action of norepinephrine, serotonin in nerve cells

Uses: Major depression, anxiety

Unlabeled uses: Chronic pain management, topical pruritus

DOSAGE AND ROUTES

Depression/anxiety
• *Adult:* PO 25-75 mg/day, may increase to 300 mg/day for severely ill
• *Geriatric:* PO 10-25 mg at bedtime, increase qwk by 10-25 mg to desired dose

Pruritus
• *Adult:* PO 10 mg at bedtime, may increase to 25 mg at bedtime; **TOP** apply thin film qid at least 3 hr apart

Available forms: Caps 10, 25, 50, 75, 100, 150 mg; oral conc 10 mg/ml; cream 5%

SIDE EFFECTS

CNS: Dizziness, drowsiness, confusion, headache, anxiety, tremors, stimulation, weakness, insomnia, nightmares, EPS (geriatric), increased psychiatric symptoms, paresthesia

CV: Orthostatic hypotension, ECG changes, tachycardia, **hypertension,** palpitations, **dysrhythmias**

EENT: Blurred vision, tinnitus, mydriasis, ophthalmoplegia, glossitis

GI: Diarrhea, dry mouth, nausea, vomiting, **paralytic ileus,** increased appetite, cramps, epigastric distress, jaundice, **hepatitis,** stomatitis, constipation

GU: Urinary retention, **acute renal failure**

HEMA: **Agranulocytosis, thrombocytopenia, eosinophilia, leukopenia**

INTEG: Rash, urticaria, sweating, pruritus, photosensitivity

Contraindications: Hypersensitivity to tricyclics, urinary retention, narrow-angle glaucoma, prostatic hypertrophy

Precautions: Pregnancy (C), suicidal patients, geriatric, UK-PO lactation, seizures

PHARMACOKINETICS

PO: Steady state 2-8 days; metabolized by liver; excreted by kidneys; crosses placenta; excreted in breast milk; half-life 8-24 hr

INTERACTIONS

Increase: hyperpyretic crisis, seizures, hypertensive episode—MAOIs

Increase: hypertensive action—clonidine, epINEPHrine, norepinephrine

Increase: doxepin effect—cimetidine, fluoxetine, sertraline

Increase: CNS depression—other CNS depressants

Drug/Herb
• Serotonin syndrome: SAM-e, St. John's wort

Increase: anticholinergic effect—belladonna, corkwood, henbane, jimsonweed

Increase: doxepin action—hops, kava, lavender, scopolia

Increase: hypertension—yohimbe

Drug/Lab Test
Increase: Serum bilirubin, blood glucose, alk phos

NURSING CONSIDERATIONS

Assess:
• B/P (lying, standing), pulse q4h; if systolic B/P drops 20 mm Hg, hold drug, notify prescriber; take vital signs q4h in patients with cardiovascular disease
• Blood studies: CBC, leukocytes, differential, cardiac enzymes if patient is receiving long-term therapy
• Hepatic studies: AST, ALT, bilirubin
• Weight qwk; appetite may increase with drug
• ECG for flattening of T wave, bundle branch block, AV block, dysrhythmias in cardiac patients; drug should be discontinued gradually several days before surgery
• EPS primarily in geriatric: rigidity, dystonia, akathisia
• Mental status: mood, sensorium, affect, suicidal tendencies, increase in psychiatric symptoms: depression, panic

---

• Urinary retention, constipation; constipation most likely in children, geriatric
• Withdrawal symptoms: headache, nausea, vomiting, muscle pain, weakness; not usual unless drug is discontinued abruptly
• Alcohol consumption; if alcohol is consumed, hold dose until morning

Administer:
• Oral conc should be diluted with 120 ml of water, milk, orange, grapefruit juice, tomato, prune, pineapple juice; do not mix with grape juice
• Increased fluids, bulk in diet for constipation
• With food, milk for GI symptoms, do not give with carbonated beverages
• Dosage at bedtime for oversedation during day; may take entire dose at bedtime; geriatric may not tolerate daily dosing
• Gum, hard candy, or frequent sips of water for dry mouth
• Topically by applying to affected area, rub slightly

Perform/provide:
• Storage in tight container protected from direct sunlight
• Assistance with ambulation during beginning therapy, since drowsiness/dizziness occurs
• Safety measures primarily for geriatric
• Checking to see PO medication swallowed

Evaluate:
• Therapeutic response: decreased anxiety, depression

Teach patient/family:
• That therapeutic effect (depressions) may take 2-3 wk, antianxiety effects sooner
• To use caution in driving, other activities requiring alertness, because of drowsiness, dizziness, blurred vision
• To avoid alcohol ingestion, other CNS depressants, may potentiate effects
• Not to discontinue medication quickly after long-term use; may cause nausea, headache, malaise
• To wear sunscreen or large hat, since photosensitivity occurs
• To report immediately urinary retention

Treatment of overdose: ECG monitoring; lavage, activated charcoal; administer anticonvulsant, sodium bicarbonate

doxercalciferol (R)

Hectorol
Func. class.: Parathyroid agent (calcium regulator)
Chem. class.: Vit D hormone

Action: Synthetic vit D analog, reduces parathyroid hormone
Uses: To lower high parathyroid hormone levels in patients undergoing chronic kidney dialysis and those in stages 3/4 of chronic renal disease prior to dialysis

DOSAGE AND ROUTES

• *Adult:* **PO** iPTH level >400 pg/ml 10 mcg 3×/wk at dialysis; dose titration iPTH level decreased by <50% and >300 pg/ml increase by 2.5 mcg at 8 wk intervals as necessary; iPTH level 150-300 pg/ml maintain; iPTH levels <100 pg/ml suspend for 1 wk, then resume at a dose that is at least 2.5 mcg lower
• *Adult:* **IV BOL** initial iPTH level >400 pg/ml 4 mcg 3×/wk at the end of dialysis, or approximately every other day; dose titration iPTH level decreased by <50% and >300 pg/ml increase by 1-2 mcg at 8 wk intervals; iPTH level 150-300 pg/ml maintain; iPTH level <100 pg/ml suspend for 1 wk, then resume at a dose that is at least 1 mcg lower

Available forms: Caps 2.5 mcg; inj 2 mcg/ml

SIDE EFFECTS

CNS: Drowsiness, headache, lethargy
GI: Nausea, diarrhea, vomiting, anorexia, dry mouth, constipation, cramps, metallic taste
GU: Polyuria, hypercalciuria, hyperphosphatemia, hematuria

MS: Myalgia, arthralgia, decreased bone development
RESP: SOB

Contraindications: Hypersensitivity, hyperphosphatemia, hypercalcemia, vit D toxicity

Precautions: Pregnancy (C), renal calculi, lactation, CV disease

PHARMACOKINETICS

Metabolism in liver, terminal half-life 96 hr

INTERACTIONS

Decrease: absorption of doxercalciferol—cholestyramine, magnesium antacids, mineral oil, do not use together

NURSING CONSIDERATIONS

Assess:

• BUN, urinary calcium, AST, ALT, cholesterol, creatinine, albumin, uric acid, chloride, magnesium, electrolytes, urine pH, phosphate; may increase calcium, should be kept at 9-10 mg/dl, vit D 50-135 international units/dl, phosphate 70 mg/dl

• Alk phos; may be decreased

• For increased drug level, since toxic reactions may occur rapidly

• For dry mouth, metallic taste, polyuria, bone pain, muscle weakness, headache, fatigue, change in LOC, dysrhythmias, increased respirations, anorexia, nausea, vomiting, cramps, diarrhea, constipation; may indicate hypercalcemia

• Renal status: decreased urinary output (oliguria, anuria), edema in extremities, weight gain 5-7 lb, periorbital edema

• Nutritional status, diet for sources of vit D (milk, some seafood); calcium (dairy products, dark green vegetables), phosphates (dairy products) must be avoided

Administer:

• Do not break, crush, or chew caps

Perform/provide:

• Storage protected from light, heat, moisture

• Restriction of sodium, potassium if required

• Restriction of fluids if required for chronic renal failure

Evaluate:

• Therapeutic response: calcium 9-10 mg/dl, decreasing symptoms of hypocalcemia, hypoparathyroidism

Teach patient/family:

• The symptoms of hypercalcemia

• About foods rich in calcium

• To avoid products with sodium in chronic renal failure: cured meats, dairy products, cold cuts, olives, beets, pickles, soups, meat tenderizers

• To avoid products with potassium in chronic renal failure: oranges, bananas, dried fruit, peas, dark green leafy vegetables, milk, melons, beans

• To avoid OTC products containing calcium, potassium, or sodium in chronic renal failure

• To avoid all preparations containing vit D

• To monitor weight weekly

⚠ High Alert

*DOXOrubicin (℞)
(dox-oh-roo'bi-sin)
Adriamycin PFS, Adriamycin RDF, Rubex
*DOXOrubicin liposome (℞)
Doxil
Func. class.: Antineoplastic, antibiotic
Chem. class.: Anthracycline glycoside

Do not confuse:

DOXOrubicin/Idamycin/DAUNOrubicin
Adriamycin/Aredia/Idamycin

Action: Inhibits DNA synthesis primarily; derived from *Streptomyces peucetius;* replication is decreased by binding to DNA, which causes strand splitting; active throughout entire cell cycle; a vesicant

Uses: Wilms' tumor; bladder, breast, liver, lung, ovarian, stomach, testicular,

---

thyroid cancer; Hodgkin's disease; acute lymphoblastic leukemia; myeloblastic leukemia; neuroblastomas; lymphomas; sarcomas; Doxil: AIDS-related Kaposi's sarcoma, metastatic ovarian carcinoma

DOSAGE AND ROUTES

DOXOrubicin
- *Adult:* IV 60-75 mg/m^2 q3wk, or 30 mg/m^2 on days 1-3 of 4-wk cycle, not to exceed 550 mg/m^2 cumulative dose
- *Child:* IV 30 mg/m^2/day × 3 days, may repeat q4wk

Hepatic dose
- *Adult:* IV bilirubin 1.2-3 mg/dl give 50% of dose; bilirubin 3.1-5 mg/dl give 25% of dose

DOXOrubicin liposome
Kaposi's sarcoma
- *Adult:* IV 20 mg/m^2 q3wk

Ovarian cancer
- *Adult:* IV 50 mg/m^2 (DOXOrubicin equivalent) given 1 mg/min, if no adverse reactions, may increase to finish infusion in 1 hr

Available forms: Inj 10, 20, 50, 100, 150 mg; liposomal dispersion for inj: (Doxil) 20 mg/10 ml, 50 mg/30 ml

SIDE EFFECTS

CV: Increased B/P, **sinus tachycardia, PVCs,** chest pain, **bradycardia, extrasystoles**

GI: Nausea, vomiting, anorexia, *mucositis,* **hepatotoxicity**

GU: Impotence, sterility, amenorrhea, gynecomastia, hyperuricemia

HEMA: **Thrombocytopenia, leukopenia, anemia**

INTEG: Rash, necrosis at inj site, dermatitis, reversible *alopecia,* cellulitis, thrombophlebitis at inj site

Contraindications: Pregnancy (D) 1st trimester, hypersensitivity, lactation, systemic infections, cardiac disorders

Precautions: Renal/hepatic/cardiac disease; gout, bone marrow depression (severe)

PHARMACOKINETICS

Triphasic pattern of elimination; half-life 12 min, 3⅓ hr, 29⅔ hr; metabolized by liver; crosses placenta; excreted in urine, bile, breast milk

INTERACTIONS

Increase: hypersensitivity—mercaptopurine

Increase: toxicity—other antineoplastics or radiation, mercaptopurine

Increase: hemorrhagic cystitis risk, cardiac toxicity—cyclophosphamide

Decrease: antibody response—live virus vaccine

Drug/Lab Test

Increase: Uric acid

NURSING CONSIDERATIONS

Assess:
- CBC, differential, platelet count weekly; withhold drug if WBC is <4000/mm^3 or platelet count is <75,000/mm^3; notify prescriber of these results
- Blood, urine uric acid levels
- Renal studies: BUN, serum uric acid, urine CCr, electrolytes before, during therapy
- I&O ratio; report fall in urine output to <30 ml/hr
- Monitor temp q4h; fever may indicate beginning infection
- Hepatic studies before, during therapy: bilirubin, AST, ALT, alk phos as needed or monthly; check for jaundice of skin and sclera, dark urine, clay-colored stools, itchy skin, abdominal pain, fever, diarrhea
- ECG; watch for ST-T wave changes, low QRS and T, possible dysrhythmias (sinus tachycardia, heart block, PVCs); signs of irreversible cardiomyopathy
- Bleeding: hematuria, guaiac, bruising, or petechiae, mucosa or orifices q8h
- Effects of alopecia on body image; discuss feelings about body changes; almost total alopecia is expected
- Inflammation of mucosa, breaks in skin
- Buccal cavity q8h for dryness, sores,

ulceration, white patches, oral pain, bleeding, dysphagia
• Alkalosis if severe vomiting is present
• Local irritation, pain, burning at inj site
• GI symptoms: frequency of stools, cramping
• Acidosis, signs of dehydration: rapid respirations, poor skin turgor, decreased urine output, dry skin, restlessness, weakness
• Cardiac status: B/P, pulse, character, rhythm, rate, ABGs, ECG
Administer:
• Antiemetic 30-60 min before giving drug to prevent vomiting
• Allopurinol or sodium bicarbonate to maintain uric acid levels, alkalinization of urine
• Topical or systemic analgesics for pain
• Transfusion for anemia
• Antispasmodic for GI symptoms
IV route
• Using cytotoxic handling procedures
⚠ Do not interchange DOXOrubicin with DOXOrubicin liposome
• Hydrocortisone, dexamethasone, or sodium bicarbonate (1 mEq/1 ml) for extravasation; apply ice compresses
• IV after diluting 10 mg/5 ml of NaCl for inj; another 5 ml of diluent/10 mg is recommended; shake; give over 3-5 min; give through Y-tube of free-flowing 5% dextrose INF or NS
• IV liposome inj (Doxil): dilute dose up to 90 mg/250 ml D5W, give over ½ hr; do not admix with other sol or meds
• Dose modifications for toxicity: Grade 1, redose unless patient has experienced previous grade 3 or 4; Grade 2, delay dosing up to 2 wk or until resolved to grades 0 or 1; Grade 3 delay dosing up to 2 wk or until resolved to grades 0 or 1, resume dose at 25% decrease, return to original dosing after interval; Grade 4 delay dosing up to 2 wk or until grade 0 or 1, resume dose at 25% decrease then return to original dose, if after 2 wk there is no resolution, discontinue
Additive compatibilities: Ondansetron
Syringe compatibilities: Bleomycin,

cisplatin, cyclophosphamide, droperidol, leucovorin, methotrexate, metoclopramide, mitomycin, vinCRIStine
Y-site compatibilities: Amifostine, aztreonam, bleomycin, chlorproMAZINE, cimetidine, cisplatin, cladribine, cyclophosphamide, dexamethasone, diphenhydrAMINE, droperidol, famotidine, filgrastim, fludarabine, fluorouracil, granisetron, hydromorphone, leucovorin, lorazepam, melphalan, methotrexate, methylPREDNISolone, metoclopramide, mitomycin, morphine, ondansetron, paclitaxel, prochlorperazine, promethazine, propofol, ranitidine, sargramostim, sodium bicarbonate, teniposide, thiotepa, vinBLAStine, vinCRIStine, vinorelbine
Perform/provide:
• Liquid diet: carbonated beverages, gelatin may be added if patient is not nauseated or vomiting
• Increased fluid intake to 2-3 L/day to prevent urate, calculi formation
• Rinsing of mouth tid-qid with water, club soda; brushing of teeth bid-tid with soft brush or cotton-tipped applicators for stomatitis; use unwaxed dental floss
• Storage at room temperature for 24 hr after reconstituting or 48 hr refrigerated
Evaluate:
• Therapeutic response: decreased tumor size, spread of malignancy
Teach patient/family:
• To add 2-3 L of fluids unless contraindicated prior to and for 24-48 hr after, to decrease possible hemorrhagic cystitis
• To report any complaints, side effects to nurse or prescriber
• That hair may be lost during treatment and wig or hairpiece may make patient feel better; tell patient that new hair may be different in color, texture
• To avoid foods with citric acid, hot or rough texture
• To report any bleeding, white spots, ulcerations in mouth to prescriber; tell patient to examine mouth daily
• That urine and other body fluids may be red-orange for 48 hr
• To avoid crowds and persons with infections when granulocyte count is low

⚠ Safety alert   *"Tall Man" lettering

• That barrier contraceptive measures are recommended during therapy and 4 mo after; avoid breastfeeding
• To avoid vaccinations; reactions may occur; avoid alcohol

---

doxycycline (℞)

(dox-i-sye'kleen)
Adoxa, Apo-Doxy ✦, Doryx, Doxy, Doxycaps, Doxycin ✦, doxycycline, Monodox, Novodoxylin ✦, Periostat, Vibramycin, Vibra-Tabs
Func. class.: Antiinfective
Chem. class.: Tetracycline

Do not confuse:
doxycycline/doxepin

Action: Inhibits protein synthesis, phosphorylation in microorganisms by binding to 30S ribosomal subunits, reversibly binding to 50S ribosomal subunits; bacteriostatic

Uses: Syphilis, *Chlamydia trachomatis,* gonorrhea, *Rickettsia,* lymphogranuloma venereum, uncommon gram-negative/positive organisms, malaria prophylaxis, chronic periodontitis, acne, anthrax, Lyme disease

Unlabeled uses: Traveler's diarrhea, prevention of chronic bronchitis

DOSAGE AND ROUTES

Most infections
• *Adult:* **PO/IV** 100 mg q12h on day 1, then 100 mg/day; **IV** 200 mg in 1-2 inf on day 1, then 100-200 mg/day
• *Child >8 yr:* **PO/IV** 2.2-4.4 mg/kg/day in divided doses q12h

Gonorrhea (uncomplicated) in patients allergic to penicillin
• *Adult:* **PO** 100 mg q12h × 7 days or 300 mg followed 1 hr later by another 300 mg

Malaria prophylaxis
• *Adult:* **PO** 100 mg daily 1-2 days prior to travel, daily during travel, and 4wk after return

C. trachomatis
• *Adult:* **PO** 100 mg bid × 7 days

Syphilis
• *Adult:* **PO** 100 mg bid × 14 days
Anthrax
• *Adult and child >45 kg:* **IV** 100 mg q12h change to **PO** when able × 60 days
• *Child ≤45 kg:* **PO** 2.2 mg/kg bid × 60 days; **IV** 100 mg q12h, change to **PO** when able × 60 days
Lyme disease
• *Adult:* **PO** 100 mg bid
Periodontitis
• *Adult:* 20 mg bid after scaling and root planing for ≤9 mo; give close to meal time AM or PM

Available forms: Tabs 100 mg; caps 50, 100 mg; syr 50 mg/5 ml; inj 100, 200 mg; powder for oral susp 25 mg/5 ml; tabs for mouth products 20 mg; inj 42.5 mg

SIDE EFFECTS

CNS: Fever
CV: Pericarditis
EENT: Dysphagia, glossitis, decreased calcification of deciduous teeth, oral candidiasis, tooth discoloration
GI: Nausea, abdominal pain, vomiting, diarrhea, anorexia, enterocolitis, **hepatotoxicity,** flatulence, abdominal cramps, gastric burning, stomatitis
GU: Increased BUN
HEMA: **Eosinophilia, neutropenia, thrombocytopenia, hemolytic anemia**
INTEG: Rash, urticaria, photosensitivity, increased pigmentation, **exfoliative dermatitis,** pruritus
SYST: **Stevens-Johnson syndrome, angioedema**
Contraindications: Pregnancy (D), hypersensitivity to tetracyclines, children <8 yr, esophageal ulceration
Precautions: Hepatic disease, lactation

PHARMACOKINETICS

PO: Well absorbed, widely distributed peak 1½-4 hr, half-life 14-17 hr; excreted in urine, feces, bile, 90% protein bound, crosses placenta, enters breast milk

Side effects: *italics* = common; **bold** = life-threatening

INTERACTIONS

Increase: effect—warfarin

Decrease: doxycycline effect—antacids, $NaHCO_3$, dairy products, alkali products, iron, kaolin/pectin, barbiturates, carbamazepine, phenytoin, cimetidine sucralfate, cholestyramine, colestipol, rifampin, bismuth

Decrease: effects—penicillins, oral contraceptives, digoxin

Drug/Herb

• Do not use acidophilus with antiinfectives; separate by several hours

Increase: action—bromelain

Drug/Lab Test

Increase: BUN, alk phos, bilirubin, amylase, ALT, AST

False increase: Urinary catecholamines

NURSING CONSIDERATIONS

Assess:

• I&O ratio

• Blood studies: PT, CBC, AST, ALT, BUN, creatinine

• Signs of infection

• Allergic reactions: rash, itching, pruritus, angioedema

• Nausea, vomiting, diarrhea; administer antiemetic, antacids as ordered

• Overgrowth of infection: fever, malaise, redness, pain, swelling, drainage, perineal itching, diarrhea, changes in cough or sputum

• IV site for phlebitis/thrombosis; drug is highly irritating

Administer:

• Do not break, crush, or chew caps

• After C&S

• An empty stomach, or with a full glass of water 2 hr before or after meals; avoid dairy products, antacids, laxatives, iron-containing products; if these must be taken, give 2 hr before or after this agent

IV route

• After diluting 100 mg or less/10 ml of sterile H_2O or NS for inj; further dilute with 100-1000 ml of NaCl, D_5, Ringer's LR D_5LR, Normosol-M, Normosol-R in D_5W; run 100 mg or less over 1-4 hr; do not give IM/SUBCUT; inf must be completed in 6 hr, when diluted in LR sol, or 12 hr in other sol

Additive compatibilities: Ranitidine

Syringe compatibilities: Doxapram

Y-site compatibilities: Acyclovir, amifostine, amiodarone, aztreonam, cisatracurium, cyclophosphamide, diltiazem, filgrastim, fludarabine, granisetron, hydromorphone, magnesium sulfate, melphalan, meperidine, morphine, ondansetron, perphenazine, propofol, remifentanil, sargramostim, tacrolimus, teniposide, theophylline, thiotepa, vinorelbine

Perform/provide:

• Storage in tight, light-resistant container at room temperature; IV stable for 12 hr at room temperature, 72 hr refrigerated; discard if precipitate forms

Evaluate:

• Therapeutic response: decreased temp, absence of lesions, negative C&S

Teach patient/family:

• To avoid sun, since burns may occur; sunscreen does not seem to decrease photosensitivity

• That all prescribed medication must be taken to prevent superinfection

---

⚠ High Alert

droperidol (℞)

(droe-per'i-dole)

droperidol, Inapsine

Func. class.: Sedative/hypnotic

Chem. class.: Butyrophenone

Action: Acts on CNS at subcortical levels, produces tranquilization, sleep; antiemetic; mild α-blockade

Uses: Premedication for surgery; induction, maintenance in general anesthesia; postoperatively for nausea, vomiting

DOSAGE AND ROUTES

Induction, adjunct

• *Adult:* **IV/IM** 1.25-2.5 mg, may give additional 1.25 mg

• *Child 2-12 yr:* **IV** 0.05-0.1 mg/kg, titrate to response

---

Premedication
- *Adult:* **IM** 2.5-10 mg ½-1 hr before surgery, may give 1.25-2.5 mg additionally
- *Child 2-12 yr:* **IM** 0.05-0.1 mg/kg

Available forms: Inj 2.5 mg/ml

SIDE EFFECTS

CNS: EPS (dystonia, akathisia, flexion of arms, fine tremors); dizziness, anxiety, drowsiness, restlessness, hallucination, depression, **seizures,** extrapyramidal symptoms, **neuroleptic malignant syndrome**

CV: Tachycardia, hypotension, prolonged QT

EENT: Upward rotation of eyes, oculogyric crisis

INTEG: Chills, facial sweating, shivering

RESP: **Laryngospasm, bronchospasm**

Contraindications: Hypersensitivity, child <2 yr, lactation

Precautions: Pregnancy (C), geriatric, cardiovascular disease (hypotension, bradydysrhythmias), renal/hepatic disease, Parkinson's disease, pheochromocytoma

PHARMACOKINETICS

IM/IV: Onset 3-10 min, peak ½ hr, duration 3-6 hr; metabolized in liver; excreted in urine as metabolites; crosses placenta, half-life 2-3 hr

INTERACTIONS

Increase: CNS depression—alcohol, opiates, barbiturates, antihistamines, antipsychotics, or other CNS depressants

Increase: hypotension—nitrates, antihypertensives

Increase: side effects of lithium

Drug/Herb

Increase: action—kava

NURSING CONSIDERATIONS

Assess:
- VS q10min during IV administration, q30min after IM dose
- EPS: dystonia, akathisia

⚠ For increasing heart rate or decreasing B/P, notify prescriber at once; do not place patient in Trendelenburg position, or sympathetic blockade may occur, causing respiratory arrest
- ECG prior to and 2-3 hr after administration for serious arrhythmias

Administer:
- Protect solution from light
- Anticholinergics (benztropine, diphenhydrAMINE) for EPS
- Only with crash cart, resuscitative equipment nearby
- IM deep in large muscle mass

IV, direct route
- Undiluted; give through Y-tube at 10 mg or less/min; titrate to patient response

Intermittent INF route
- May be given as an infusion by adding dose to 250 ml LR, D_5W, 0.9% NaCl; give slowly, titrate to patient response

Syringe compatibilities: Atropine, bleomycin, butorphanol, chlorproMAZINE, cimetidine, cisplatin, cyclophosphamide, dimenhyDRINATE, diphenhydrAMINE, DOXOrubicin, fentanyl, glycopyrrolate, hydrOXYzine, meperidine, metoclopramide, midazolam, mitomycin, morphine, nalbuphine, pentazocine, perphenazine, prochlorperazine, promazine, promethazine, scopolamine, vinBLAStine, vinCRIStine

Y-site compatibilities: Amifostine, aztreonam, bleomycin, cisatracurium, cisplatin, cladribine, cyclophosphamide, cytarabine, DOXOrubicin, DOXOrubicin liposome, famotidine, filgrastim, fluconazole, fludarabine, granisetron, hydrocortisone, idarubicin, melphalan, meperidine, metoclopramide, mitomycin, ondansetron, paclitaxel, potassium chloride, propofol, remifentanil, sargramostim, teniposide, thiotepa, vinBLAStine, vinCRIStine, vinorelbine, vit B/C

Evaluate:
- Therapeutic response: decreased anxiety, absence of vomiting during and after surgery

Teach patient/family:
• To rise slowly from sitting or standing to minimize orthostatic hypotension
• To avoid ambulation without assistance

---

drotrecogin alfa (℞)
(droh'treh-koh-jin al'fah)
Xigris
Func. class.: Recombinant human activated protein C

Action: Activated protein C exerts an antithrombotic effect by inhibiting factor Va/VIIIa

Uses: Severe sepsis associated with organ dysfunction

DOSAGE AND ROUTES

• *Adult:* IV INF 24 mcg/kg/hr × 96 hr; based on actual body weight
Available forms: Powder for inj, lyophilized, 5, 20 mg

SIDE EFFECTS

HEMA: Decreased Hct, **bleeding**
SYST: **GI, GU, intracranial, intraabdominal, intrathoracic, retroperitoneal bleeding; surface bleeding**
Contraindications: Hypersensitivity, internal active bleeding, intraspinal surgery, CNS neoplasms, ulcerative colitis, enteritis, hepatic disease, hypocoagulation, hemorrhagic stroke, epidural catheter in place, cerebral embolism/thrombosis/hemorrhage, recent major surgery, trauma
Precautions: Pregnancy (C), recent GI bleeding, PT–INR >3, lactation, children, use >96 hr

PHARMACOKINETICS

Inactivated by endogenous plasma protease inhibitors

INTERACTIONS

• Bleeding potential: aspirin, indomethacin, phenylbutazone, anticoagulants, thrombolytics, glycoprotein IIb/IIIa inhibitors

NURSING CONSIDERATIONS

Assess:

⚠ For bleeding during treatment; hematuria, hematemesis, bleeding from mucous membranes, epistaxis, ecchymosis; may require transfusion (rare), continue to assess for bleeding

• Blood studies (Hct, platelets, PTT, PT, TT, aPTT) before starting therapy; PT or aPTT must be less than 2× control before starting therapy; PTT or PT q3-4h during treatment

• VS, B/P, pulse, respirations, neurologic signs, temp at least q4h; temp >104° F (40° C) indicates internal bleeding; systolic pressure increase >25 mm Hg should be reported to prescriber

⚠ For neurologic changes that may indicate intracranial bleeding

⚠ Retroperitoneal bleeding: back pain, leg weakness, diminished pulses

Administer:
IV route

• Reconstitute 5 mg vial/2.5 ml; 20 mg vial/10 ml sterile water for inj to a concentration of 2 mg/ml; slowly add sterile water for inj, do not shake or invert, gently swirl until dissolved

• Further dilute with 0.9% NaCl, slowly withdraw prescribed amount and add to bag of 0.9% NaCl, direct stream to side of bag, gently invert bag; do not transport infusion bag between locations using mechanical delivery systems

• Use immediately after reconstituting, may be held for only 3 hr at controlled room temperature 59°-86° F; must complete infusion within 12 hr after preparation

• Do not use if discolored or if particulate is present

• If using an infusion pump, usual concentration is 100-200 mcg/ml; if using a syringe pump, usual concentration is 100-1000 mcg/ml

• Use a dedicated IV line, or dedicated lumen of central venous catheter; may use only 0.9% NaCl, LR, dextrose, or dextrose/saline mixtures through same line

---

⚠ Safety alert   *"Tall Man" lettering

• Do not expose to heat or direct sunlight

• Discontinue 2 hr prior to invasive surgery or procedures introducing risk of bleeding; may be reinstated 12 hr after invasive procedures if hemostasis achieved; may restart immediately after less invasive procedures

Perform/provide:

• Refrigerated storage at 2° to 8° C (36° to 46° F); do not freeze

• Protect unreconstituted vials from light; keep in carton until time of use

Evaluate:

• Therapeutic response: Decreasing symptoms of sepsis, lack of mortality

Teach patient/family:

• Reason for therapy and expected results

• That bleeding may occur for up to 1 month after therapy; signs, symptoms of bleeding

---

duloxetine (℞)

(du-lox'uh-teen)

Cymbalta

Func. class.: Antidepressant—miscellaneous

Chem. class.: Serotonin, norepinephrine reuptake inhibitor

Action: Unknown, may potentiate serotonergic, nonadrenergic activity in the CNS; in studies duloxetine is a potent inhibitor of neuronal serotonin and norepinephrine reuptake

Uses: Major depressive disorder (MDD), neuropathic pain associated with diabetic neuropathy

DOSAGE AND ROUTES

Depression

• *Adult:* PO 20 mg bid, may increase to 30 mg bid if needed

Diabetic neuropathy

• *Adult:* PO 60 mg daily

Renal dose

• *Adult:* PO start with 20 mg, gradually increase

Available forms: Caps 20, 30, 60 mg

SIDE EFFECTS

CNS: Insomnia, anxiety, dizziness, tremor, fatigue, decreased appetite, decreased weight

CV: Thrombophlebitis, peripheral edema

EENT: Abnormal vision

GI: Constipation, diarrhea, dysphagia, nausea, vomiting, anorexia, dry mouth, colitis, gastritis

GU: Abnormal ejaculation, urinary hesitation, ejaculation delayed, erectile dysfunction

INTEG: Photosensitivity, bruising, sweating

Contraindications: Hypersensitivity, narrow-angle glaucoma

Precautions: Pregnancy (C), mania, lactation, children, geriatric, hypertension, narrow-angle glaucoma, renal/hepatic/cardiac disease, seizures

PHARMACOKINETICS

Well absorbed, extensively metabolized (CYP2D6, CYP1A2) in the liver to an active metabolite; 70% of drug recovered in urine, 20% in feces; 90% protein binding; half-life 12 hr

INTERACTIONS

• Narrow therapeutic index: CYP2D6 extensively metabolized drugs (flecainide, phenothiazines, propafenone, tricyclics, thioridazine)

⚠ Hyperthermia, rigidity, rapid fluctuations of vital signs, mental status changes, neuroleptic malignant syndrome—MAOIs, coadministration is contraindicated or within 14 days of MAOI use

Increase: CNS depression—opioids, antihistamines, sedative/hypnotics

Increase: action of duloxetine—CYP1A2 inhibitors (fluvoxamine, quinolone antiinfectives); CYP2D6 (fluoxetine, quinidine, paroxetine)

Increase: ALT, bilirubin—alcohol

Drug/Herb

• Serotonin syndrome: SAM-e, St. John's wort

Increase: CNS depression—chamomile, hops, kava, lavender, skullcap, valerian

---

Side effects: *italics* = common; **bold** = life-threatening

Increase: anticholinergic effect—corkwood, jimsonweed
Increase: hypertension—yohimbe

NURSING CONSIDERATIONS
Assess:
• B/P lying, standing; pulse q4h; if systolic B/P drops 20 mm Hg, hold drug, notify prescriber; take VS q4h in patients with CV disease
• Hepatic studies: AST, ALT, bilirubin
• Weight qwk; weight loss or gain; appetite may increase; peripheral edema may occur
• Sugarless gum, hard candy, frequent sips of water for dry mouth
• Mental status: mood, sensorium, affect, suicidal tendencies, increase in psychiatric symptoms; depression, panic
• Withdrawal symptoms: headache, nausea, vomiting, muscle pain, weakness; not usual unless drug is discontinued abruptly
Administer:
• Swallow cap whole; do not break, crush, or chew; do not sprinkle on food or mix with liquid
Perform/provide:
• Storage in tight container at room temperature; do not freeze
• Assistance with ambulation during beginning therapy since drowsiness, dizziness occur
• Checking to see if PO medication swallowed
Evaluate:
• Therapeutic response: decreased depression
Teach patient/family:
• To dispense in small amounts because of suicide potential, especially in the beginning of therapy
• To use with caution when driving or other activities requiring alertness because of drowsiness, dizziness, blurred vision
• To avoid alcohol ingestion, MAOIs, other CNS depressants
• Not to discontinue medication quickly after long-term use; may cause nausea, headache, malaise; taper

• To wear sunscreen or large hat, since photosensitivity may occur
• To notify prescriber if pregnancy is planned or suspected, or if breastfeeding
• Improvement may occur in 1-4 wk

---

dutasteride (℞)
(doo-tass'ter-ide)
Avodart
Func. class.: Sex hormone 5α-reductase inhibitor
Chem. class.: Synthetic 4-azasteroid compound

Action: Inhibits both types 1 and 2 forms of a steroid enzyme that converts testosterone to 5α-dihydrotestosterone (DHT), which is responsible for the initial growth of prostatic tissue
Uses: Treatment of benign prostatic hyperplasia (BPH) in men with an enlarged prostate gland
Unlabeled uses: Alopecia

DOSAGE AND ROUTES
• *Adult:* **PO** 0.5 mg daily
Available form: Caps 0.5 mg

SIDE EFFECTS
GU: Decreased libido, impotence, gynecomastia, ejaculation disorders (rare), mastalgia, teratogenesis
Contraindications: Pregnancy (X), hypersensitivity, lactation, women, children
Precautions: Hepatic disease

PHARMACOKINETICS
Peak 2-3 hr, protein binding 99%; metabolized in liver by CYP3A4, excreted in feces; half-life 5 wk at steady state

INTERACTIONS
Increase: dutasteride concentrations—ritonavir, ketoconazole, verapamil, diltiazem, cimetidine, ciprofloxacin, antiretroviral protease inhibitors, or other drugs metabolized by the CYP3A4 pathway

---

Drug/Lab Test
Increase: TSH
Decrease: PSA

NURSING CONSIDERATIONS
Assess:
• For decreasing symptoms in BPH: decreasing urinary retention, frequency, urgency, nocturia
• PSA levels, digital rectal, urinary obstruction; determine the absence of urinary cancer before starting treatment
• Hepatic studies: ALT, AST, bilirubin
Administer:
• Swallow caps whole; do not break, crush, or chew
• Without regard to meals
Evaluate:
• Therapeutic response: Decreasing symptoms of BPH—decreased urinary frequency, retention, urgency, nocturia
Teach patient/family:
• To read patient information leaflet before starting therapy and reread it upon prescription renewal
• To notify prescriber if therapeutic response decreases; if edema occurs
• Not to discontinue drug abruptly
• About changes in sex characteristics
• That men taking dutasteride should not donate blood for at least 6 mo after last dose, to prevent blood administration to pregnant female
• That caps should not be handled by a pregnant woman because this drug can be absorbed through the skin
• That ejaculate volume may decrease during treatment; that drug rarely interferes with sexual function

D

dyphylline (℞)
(dye′fi-lin)
Dilor, Dyflex-200, Dylline, dyphylline, Lufyllin, Neothylline
Func. class.: Bronchodilator
Chem. class.: Xanthine, theophylline derivative

Action: Relaxes smooth muscle of respiratory system by blocking phosphodiesterase, which increases cyclic AMP; cyclic AMP results in positive inotropic, chronotropic effects, bronchodilation, stimulation of CNS
Uses: Bronchial asthma, bronchospasm in chronic bronchitis and emphysema, COPD

DOSAGE AND ROUTES
• *Adult and child >6 yr:* **PO** 15 mg/kg/dose, max 60 mg/kg/day
Renal dose
• *Adult:* **PO** CCr 50-80 ml/min 75% of original dose; CCr 10-50 ml/min 50% of original dose; CCr <10 ml/min 25% of original dose
Available forms: Tabs 200, 400 mg; elix 33.3 mg, 53.3 mg/5 ml

SIDE EFFECTS
CNS: Anxiety, restlessness, insomnia, dizziness, **seizures,** headache, lightheadedness, muscle twitching
CV: Palpitations, **circulatory failure,** *sinus tachycardia,* hypotension, flushing, **dysrhythmias**
GI: Nausea, diarrhea, *vomiting, anorexia,* dyspepsia, epigastric pain, rectal irritation, bleeding, reflux
INTEG: Flushing, urticaria
OTHER: Fever, dehydration, **albuminuria,** hyperglycemia, increased diuresis
RESP: Tachypnea, **respiratory arrest**
Contraindications: Hypersensitivity to xanthines
Precautions: Pregnancy (C), geriatric, CHF, cor pulmonale, diabetes mellitus, hypertension, children, renal/hepatic dis-

Side effects: *italics* = common; **bold** = life-threatening

ease, lactation, glaucoma, hyperthyroidism, seizure disorder, peptic ulcer

PHARMACOKINETICS

Well absorbed, peak 1 hr, duration 6 hr, half-life 2 hr, excreted in urine (85%) unchanged, and in breast milk

INTERACTIONS

• Cardiotoxicity: β-blockers
Increase: action of dyphylline—cimetidine, propranolol, erythromycin, probenecid
Increase: dyphylline metabolism—barbiturates, phenytoin
Decrease: dyphylline elimination—uricosurics
Decrease: phenytoin levels

NURSING CONSIDERATIONS
Assess:
• Dyphylline blood levels; toxicity may occur with small increase above 20 mcg/ml; assess for drug toxicity: nausea, vomiting, anorexia, cramping, diarrhea, confusion, dysrhythmias, seizures, diuresis, flushing, headache
• Monitor I&O; diuresis occurs; dehydration may be the result in geriatric or children
• Whether theophylline was given recently
• Auscultate lung fields bilaterally; notify prescriber of abnormalities, monitor pulmonary function studies baseline and periodically
• Allergic reactions: rash, urticaria; drug should be discontinued
Administer:
• Give around the clock to maintain blood levels, give daily dose each AM
• PO after meals to decrease GI symptoms; absorption may be affected
Perform/provide:
• Storage protected from light, at room temperature
Evaluate:
• Therapeutic response: decreased dyspnea, respiratory rate, rhythm

Teach patient/family:
• To check OTC medications, current prescription medications for epHEDrine; will increase stimulation; not to drink alcohol, caffeine, or other xanthine products; not to change brands
• To avoid hazardous activities; dizziness, drowsiness, blurred vision may occur
• For GI upset, to take drug with 8 oz water and food
• To avoid smoking, condition may worsen
• To obtain blood levels 6-12 mo

echothiophate ophthalmic
See Appendix C

econazole topical
See Appendix C

Rarely Used

edetate calcium disodium (℞)
(ee'de-tate)
calcium disodium versenate, calcium EDTA, edathamil calcium disodium, sodium calcium edetate
Func. class.: Heavy metal antagonist (antidote)

Uses: Lead poisoning, acute lead encephalopathy

DOSAGE AND ROUTES
Lead mobilization test
• *Adult:* IV 25-30 mg/kg (up to 2 g) in 250-1000 ml D_5W over 1-6 hr
Acute lead encephalopathy (blood levels 20-70 mcg/dl)
• *Adult:* IM 1 g/m^2/day divided q8-12h ×5 days, skip 2-4 days, repeat course

---

⚠ Safety alert   *"Tall Man" lettering

Acute lead poisoning (blood levels 20-70 mcg/dl)
• *Adult:* **IV INF** 1 g/m²/day over 8-12h ×5 days, skip 2-4 days and repeat as needed, max 75 mg/kg/day

Chronic lead poisoning (blood levels 20-70 mcg/dl)
• *Adult:* **IV INF** 1 g/m²/day over 8-12h ×5 days, skip 2-4 days, repeat as needed

Contraindications: Hypersensitivity, anuria, poisoning of other metals, severe renal disease, child <3 yr, hepatitis

---

Rarely Used

edetate disodium (℞)
(ee′de-tate)
Chealamide, Disodium EDTA, Disotate, Endrate
Func. class.: Heavy metal antagonist (chelator)

Uses: Hypercalcemic crisis, control of ventricular dysrhythmias associated with digoxin toxicity

DOSAGE AND ROUTES

Digitalis glucoside toxicity/ ventricular dysrhythmias/ hypercalcemia crisis
• *Adult:* **IV** 50 mg/kg/day given over 3 hr or more, daily ×5 days; skip 2 days; repeat as needed up to 15 doses; max 3 g/day

Contraindications: Hypersensitivity, anuria, hepatic insufficiency, poisoning of other metals, severe renal disease, child <3 yr, seizure disorders, active/inactive TB

---

edrophonium (℞)
(ed-roh-fone′ee-um)
Enlon, Reversol, Tensilon
Func. class.: Cholinergics, anticholinesterase
Chem. class.: Quaternary ammonium compound

Action: Inhibits breakdown of acetylcholine, which increases concentration at sites where acetylcholine is released; this facilitates transmission of impulses across myoneural junction

Uses: To diagnose myasthenia gravis; curare antagonist; differentiation of myasthenic crisis from cholinergic crisis

DOSAGE AND ROUTES

Tensilon test (myasthenia gravis diagnosis)
• *Adult:* **IV** 1-2 mg over 15-30 sec, then 8 mg if no response; **IM** 10 mg; if cholinergic reaction occurs, retest after ½ hr with 2 mg **IM**
• *Child >34 kg:* **IV** 2 mg; if no response in 45 sec, then 1 mg q45sec, not to exceed 10 mg; **IM** 5 mg
• *Child <34 kg:* **IV** 1 mg; if no response in 45 sec, then 1 mg q45sec, not to exceed 5 mg; **IM** 2 mg
• *Infant:* **IV** 0.5 mg

Reversal of nondepolarizing neuromuscular blockers
• *Adult:* **IV** 10 mg over 30-45 sec, may repeat, not to exceed 40 mg

Differentiation of myasthenic crisis from cholinergic crisis
• *Adult:* **IV** 1 mg, if no response in 1 min, may repeat

Available forms: Inj 10 mg/ml

SIDE EFFECTS

CNS: Dizziness, headache, sweating, weakness, **seizures,** incoordination, **paralysis,** drowsiness, **loss of consciousness**
CV: Dysrhythmias, bradycardia, hypotension, **AV block,** ECG changes, **cardiac arrest,** syncope
EENT: Miosis, blurred vision, lacrimation, visual changes
GI: Nausea, diarrhea, vomiting, cramps, increased salivary and gastric secretions, dysphagia, increased peristalsis
GU: Urinary frequency, incontinence, urgency
INTEG: Rash, urticaria
RESP: **Respiratory depression, bronchospasm, constriction, laryngospasm, respiratory arrest,** dyspnea, increased bronchial secretions

---

Side effects: *italics* = common; **bold** = life-threatening

Contraindications: Obstruction of intestine, renal system, hypersensitivity
Precautions: Pregnancy (C), seizure disorders, bronchial asthma, coronary occlusion, hyperthyroidism, dysrhythmias, peptic ulcer, megacolon, poor GI motility, bradycardia, hypotension

PHARMACOKINETICS

IV: Onset 30-60 sec, duration 6-15 min
IM: Onset 2-10 min, duration 12-45 min

INTERACTIONS

• Bradycardia: digoxin
• Prolonged action of depolarizing muscle relaxants
Increase: endrophonium effects—parasympathomimetics; avoid giving concurrently
Decrease: action of edrophonium—procainamide, quinidine, atropine

NURSING CONSIDERATIONS

Assess:
• VS, respiration during test; muscle strength
• Diabetic patient carefully, since this drug lowers blood glucose
Administer:
⚠ Only with atropine sulfate available for cholinergic crisis
• Only after all other cholinergics have been discontinued
IV, direct route
• 2 mg or less over 15-30 sec
Y-site compatibilities: Heparin, hydrocortisone, potassium chloride, vit B/C
Perform/provide:
• Storage at room temperature
Evaluate:
• Therapeutic response: increased muscle strength, hand grasp; improved gait; absence of labored breathing (if severe)
Teach patient/family:
• To wear emergency ID specifying myasthenia gravis, drugs taken
Treatment of overdose: Respiratory support, atropine 1-4 mg (IV)

efalizumab (℞)

(eh-fah-lih'zyoo-mab)
Raptiva
Func. class.: Immunosuppressive

Uses: Adults 18 years of age and older with moderate to severe plaque psoriasis

DOSAGE AND ROUTES

• *Adult:* **SUBCUT** 0.7 mg/kg as a conditioning dose, then **SUBCUT** 1 mg/kg qwk, max single dose 200 mg
Contraindications: Hypersensitivity

efavirenz (℞)

(ef-ah-veer'enz)
Sustiva
Func. class.: Antiretroviral
Chem. class.: Nonnucleoside reverse transcriptase inhibitor (NNRTI)

Action: Binds directly to reverse transcriptase and blocks RNA, DNA causing a disruption of the enzyme's site
Uses: HIV-1 in combination with other antivirals

DOSAGE AND ROUTES

Given in combination with protease inhibitor or nucleoside analog reverse transcriptase inhibitors (NARTIs)
• *Adult and child >40 kg:* **PO** 600 mg daily at bedtime
• *Child 10-15 kg:* **PO** 200 mg daily at bedtime
• *Child 15-20 kg:* **PO** 250 mg daily at bedtime
• *Child 20-25 kg:* **PO** 300 mg daily at bedtime
• *Child 25-32.5 kg:* **PO** 350 mg daily at bedtime
• *Child 32.5-40 kg:* **PO** 400 mg daily at bedtime
Available forms: Caps 50, 100, 200 mg; 600 mg tabs

⚠ Safety alert   *"Tall Man" lettering

SIDE EFFECTS

CNS: Fatigue, impaired concentration, insomnia, abnormal dreams, depression, headache, dizziness, anxiety, drowsiness
GI: Diarrhea, abdominal pain, *nausea,* hyperlipidemia
GU: Hematuria, kidney stones
INTEG: Rash, **erythema multiforme, Stevens-Johnson syndrome, toxic epidermal necrolysis**
Contraindication: Pregnancy (D), hypersensitivity
Precautions: Lactation, children <3 yr, renal/hepatic disease, myelosuppression, depression, seizures

PHARMACOKINETICS

Peak 3–5 hr, well absorbed, metabolized by liver, terminal half-life 52-76 hr, >99% protein binding, excreted in urine/feces

INTERACTIONS

• Do not give together with benzodiazepines, ergots, midazolam, triazolam, cisapride
Increase: CNS depression—alcohol, antidepressants, antihistamines, opioids
Increase: levels of both drugs—ritonavir, estrogens, anticonvulsants
Increase: levels of warfarin, ergots, midazolam, triazolam, statins (except pravastatin, fluvastatin)
Decrease: efavirenz levels—rifamycins
Decrease: levels of indinavir, saquinavir, clarithromycin, methadone
Drug/Herb
Decrease: efavirenz level—St. John's wort, do not use together
Drug/Food
Increase: absorption—high-fat foods
Drug/Lab Test
Increase: ALT
False positive: Cannibinoids

NURSING CONSIDERATIONS
Assess:
• Signs of infection, anemia
• Hepatic studies: ALT, AST; renal studies
• Bowel pattern before, during treatment; if severe abdominal pain with bleeding occurs, drug should be discontinued; monitor hydration
• Skin eruptions; rash, urticaria, itching
• Allergies before treatment, reaction to each medication
• CBC, blood chemistry, plasma HIV RNA, absolute CD4+/CD8+ cell counts/%, serum β_2 microglobulin, serum ICD+24 antigen levels, cholesterol, hepatic enzymes
• Signs of toxicity: severe nausea/vomiting, maculopapular rash
Administer:
• Give on empty stomach; at bedtime to decrease CNS side effects
Evaluate:
• Therapeutic response: increased CD4 cell counts; decreased viral load; slowing progression of HIV
Teach patient/family:
• To take as prescribed; if dose is missed, take as soon as remembered; do not double dose; take with water, juice; taken on empty stomach at bedtime
• To make sure health care provider knows all the medications, supplements, or OTC drugs taken
• That if severe rash occurs, to notify health care provider; that adverse reactions (rash, dizziness, abnormal dreams, insomnia) lessen after a month
• Not to breastfeed or become pregnant if taking this drug, use nonhormonal contraception, serious birth defects have occurred
• To avoid hazardous activities if dizziness/drowsiness occur
• That drug does not cure disease, but controls symptoms, HIV can be transmitted to others even while taking this drug, to continue with safe-sex practices

eletriptan (℞)

(el-ee-trip′tan)

Relpax

Func. class.: Antimigraine agent, abortive

Chem. class.: 5-HT$_1$-1B/1D receptor agonist, triptan

Action: Binds selectively to the vascular 5-HT$_1$-receptor subtype; causes vasoconstriction in cranial arteries

Uses: Acute treatment of migraine with or without aura

DOSAGE AND ROUTES

• *Adult:* **PO** 20 mg, may increase if needed, max 40 mg (single dose); may repeat in 2 hr if headache improves but returns, max 80 mg/24 hr

Available forms: Tabs 20, 40 mg

SIDE EFFECTS

CNS: Dizziness, headache, anxiety, paresthesia, asthenia, somnolence, flushing, fatigue, hot/cold sensation

CV: Chest pain, palpitations, hypertension

GI: Nausea, dry mouth

MS: Weakness

RESP: Chest tightness, pressure

Contraindications: Hypersensitivity, coronary artery vasospasm, peripheral vascular disease, hemiplegic/basilar migraine, concurrent use of ergotamine-containing preparations, uncontrolled hypertension; ischemic bowel, heart disease; severe renal/hepatic disease

Precautions: Pregnancy (C), postmenopausal women, men >40 yr, risk factors of CAD, MI, or other cardiac disease, hypercholesterolemia, obesity, diabetes, impaired renal/hepatic function, lactation, children, geriatric

PHARMACOKINETICS

Onset of pain relief 2 hr; metabolized in the liver; 70% excreted in urine, feces

INTERACTIONS

Increase: plasma concentration of eletriptan—propranolol, CYP3A4 inhibitors (clarithromycin, ketoconazole, erythromycin, itraconazole, ritonavir, nelfinavir)

Drug/Herb

Increase: effect—butterbur

NURSING CONSIDERATIONS

Assess:

• For symptoms of migraine: pain location, character, intensity, nausea, vomiting, aura

• B/P; signs/symptoms of coronary vasospasms

• Tingling, hot sensation, burning, feeling of pressure, numbness, flushing

• For stress level, activity, recreation, coping mechanisms

• Neurologic status: LOC, blurring vision, nausea, vomiting, tingling in extremities preceding headache

• Ingestion of tyramine foods (pickled products, beer, wine, aged cheese), food additives, preservatives, colorings, artificial sweeteners, chocolate, caffeine, which may precipitate these types of headaches

• Urine output; monitor kidney function

Administer:

• Swallow tabs whole; do not break, crush, or chew

• At beginning of headache; if headache returns, repeat dose after 2 hr of first dose; if first dose is ineffective

Perform/provide:

• Quiet, calm environment with decreased stimulation from noise, bright light, excessive talking

Evaluate:

• Therapeutic response: decrease in frequency, severity of migraine

Teach patient/family:

• To report any side effects to prescriber

• To use contraception while taking drug; inform prescriber if pregnant or intend to become pregnant

• To provide dark, quiet environment

• That drug does not prevent or reduce number of migraine attacks

---

⚠ Safety alert   *"Tall Man" lettering

emedastine ophthalmic
See Appendix C

emtricitabine (Ŗ)
(em-tri-sit'uh-bean)
Emtriva
Func. class.: Antiretroviral
Chem. class.: Nucleoside reverse
transcriptase inhibitor (NRTI)

Action: A synthetic nucleoside analog of
cytosine. Inhibits replication of HIV virus
by competing with the natural substrate
and then becoming incorporated into cellular DNA by viral reverse transcriptase,
thereby terminating cellular DNA chain
Uses: HIV-1 infection with other antiretroviral
Unlabeled uses: HBV (hepatitis B virus) infection

DOSAGE AND ROUTES
• *Adult:* **PO** 200 mg daily; oral sol 240
mg (24 ml) daily
• *Child 3 mo-17 yr:* **PO** (caps) 200 mg
daily; oral sol 6 mg/kg daily, max 240 mg
(24 ml)
Renal dose
• *Adult:* **PO** CCr 30-49 ml/min 200 mg
q48h; 15-29 ml/min 200 mg q72h; <15
ml/min 200 mg q96h
Available forms: Cap 200 mg; oral sol
10 mg/ml

SIDE EFFECTS
CNS: Headache, abnormal dreams, *de-
pression,* dizziness, *insomnia,* neuropa-
thy, paresthesia, *asthenia*
*GI: Nausea, vomiting, diarrhea, an-
orexia, abdominal pain, dyspepsia,* **he-
patomegaly with steatosis (may be
fatal)**
INTEG: Rash, skin discolorization
MS: Arthralgia, myalgia
RESP: Cough
SYST: Change in body fat distribution, **lac-
tic acidosis**
Contraindications: Hypersensitivity

Precautions: Pregnancy (B), lactation,
children, geriatric, renal disease, hepatic
insufficiency, chronic hepatitis B virus
(HPV)

PHARMACOKINETICS
Rapidly, extensively absorbed, peak 1-2
hr, protein binding <4%, excreted unchanged in urine (86%), feces (14%);
half-life 10 hr

INTERACTIONS
None known

NURSING CONSIDERATIONS
Assess:
• Renal/hepatic function tests: AST, ALT,
bilirubin, amylase, lipase, triglycerides pe-
riodically during treatment
⚠ For lactic acidosis, severe hepatomeg-
aly with steatosis; if lab reports confirm
these conditions, discontinue treatment;
may be fatal
Administer:
• Give without regard to meals
Perform/provide:
• Storage (caps) at 25° C (77° F); (oral
sol) refrigerated, use within 3 mo
Evaluate:
• Therapeutic response: Decrease in
signs/symptoms of HIV
Teach patient/family:
• That GI complaints resolve after 3-4 wk
of treatment
• Not to breastfeed while taking this drug
• That drug must be taken at same time
of day to maintain blood level
• That drug will control symptoms, but
is not a cure for HIV; patient is still infec-
tious, may pass HIV virus on to others
• That other drugs may be necessary to
prevent other infections
• That changes in body fat distribution
may occur

enalapril/enalaprilat (℞)

(e-nal′a-pril)/(e-nal′a-pril-at)
Vasotec, Vasotec IV
Func. class.: Antihypertensive
Chem. class.: Angiotensin-converting enzyme (ACE) inhibitor

Do not confuse:
enalapril/ramipril/Anafranil/Eldepryl

Action: Selectively suppresses renin-angiotensin-aldosterone system; inhibits ACE; prevents conversion of angiotensin I to angiotensin II, dilation of arterial, venous vessels

Uses: Hypertension, CHF, left ventricular dysfunction

DOSAGE AND ROUTES

Hypertension
• *Adult:* **PO** 2.5-5 mg/day, may increase or decrease to desired response, range 10-40 mg/day; **IV** 0.625-1.25 mg q6h over 5 min
• *Child:* **PO** 0.08 mg/kg/day in 1-2 divided doses, max 0.58 mg/kg/day
• *Child:* **IV** 5-10 mcg/kg/dose q8-24h

Patients on diuretics
• *Adult:* **IV** 0.625 mg over 5 min, may give additional doses of 1.25 mg q6h

Renal impairment
• *Adult:* **PO** 2.5 mg daily (CCr <30 ml/min) increase gradually; **IV** CCr >30 ml/min 1.25 mg q6h; CCr <30 ml/min 0.625 mg as one-time dose, increase as per B/P

CHF
• *Adult:* **PO** 2.5-20 mg/day in 2 divided doses, max 40 mg daily in divided doses

Available forms: enalapril: tabs 2.5, 5, 10, 20 mg; enalaprilat: inj 1.25 mg/ml

SIDE EFFECTS

CNS: Insomnia, dizziness, paresthesias, headache, fatigue, anxiety
CV: Hypotension, chest pain, tachycardia, **dysrhythmias,** syncope, angina, **MI,** orthostatic hypotension
EENT: Tinnitus, visual changes, sore throat, double vision, dry burning eyes

GI: Nausea, vomiting, colitis, cramps, diarrhea, constipation, flatulence, dry mouth, loss of taste
GU: **Proteinuria, renal failure,** increased frequency of polyuria or oliguria
HEMA: **Agranulocytosis, neutropenia**
INTEG: Rash, purpura, alopecia, hyperhidrosis, photosensitivity
META: Hyperkalemia
RESP: Dyspnea, dry cough, crackles, angioedema

Contraindications: Pregnancy (D) 2nd/3rd trimester, hypersensitivity, history of angioedema
Precautions: Renal disease, hyperkalemia, pregnancy (C) 1st trimester, lactation, hepatic failure, dehydration, bilateral renal artery stenosis

PHARMACOKINETICS

Enalapril:
PO: Onset 1 hr, peak 4-6 hr, duration ≥24 hr; half-life 1½ hr; metabolized by liver to active metabolite, excreted in urine
Enalaprilat:
IV: Onset 5-15 min, peak up to 4 hr

INTERACTIONS

Increase: hypersensitivity—allopurinol
Increase: hypotension—diuretics, other antihypertensives, phenothiazines, nitrates, acute alcohol ingestion, general anesthesia
Increase: potassium levels—salt substitutes, potassium-sparing diuretics, potassium supplements, cycloSPORINE, indomethacin
Increase: levels of lithium, digoxin
Decrease: effects of enalapril—antacids, rifampin

Drug/Herb
• Severe photosensitivity: St. John's wort
⚠ Fatal hypokalemia: arginine
Increase: effect—pill-bearing spurge
Decrease: effect—pineapple, yohimbe

Drug/Lab Test
Increase: ALT, AST, bilirubin, alk phos, glucose, uric acid
False positive: ANA titer

⚠ Safety alert   *"Tall Man" lettering

NURSING CONSIDERATIONS

Assess:

- Blood studies: neutrophils, decreased platelets; WBC with diff baseline and q3mo, if neutrophils <1000/mm³, discontinue treatment (recommended in collagen-vascular disease)
- B/P, peak/trough level, orthostatic hypotension, syncope when used with diuretic, pulse q4h; note rate, rhythm, quality
- Electrolytes: K, Na, Cl during 1st 2 wk of therapy
- Baselines in renal, hepatic studies before therapy begins and 1 wk into therapy
- Edema in feet, legs daily
- Skin turgor, dryness of mucous membranes for hydration status
- Symptoms of CHF: edema, dyspnea, wet crackles

Administer:

IV, direct/Intermittent INF route

- Undiluted over 5 min, use diluent provided or 50 ml D₅W, 0.9% NaCl, 0.9% NaCl in D₅W or LR, Isolyte E, give through Y-tube of free-flowing inf of 0.9% NaCl, D₅W, LR, Isolyte E

Additive compatibilities: DOBUTamine, DOPamine, heparin, meropenem, nitroglycerin, nitroprusside, potassium chloride

Y-site compatibilities: Allopurinol, amifostine, amikacin, aminophylline, ampicillin, ampicillin/sulbactam, aztreonam, butorphanol, calcium gluconate, cefazolin, cefoperazone, ceftazidime, ceftizoxime, chloramphenicol, cimetidine, cisatracurium, cladribine, clindamycin, dextran 40, DOBUTamine, DOPamine, DOXOrubicin liposome, erythromycin, esmolol, famotidine, fentanyl, filgrastim, ganciclovir, gentamicin, granisetron, heparin, hetastarch, hydrocortisone, labetalol, lidocaine, magnesium sulfate, melphalan, meropenem, methylPREDNISolone, metronidazole, morphine, nafcillin, niCARdipine, nitroprusside, penicillin G potassium, phenobarbital, piperacillin, piperacillin/tazobactam, potassium chloride, potassium phosphate, propofol, ranitidine, remifentanil, teniposide, thiotepa, tobramycin, trimethoprim-sulfamethoxazole, vancomycin, vinorelbine

Evaluate:

- Therapeutic response: decreased B/P

Teach patient/family:

- Not to use OTC (cough, cold, or allergy) products unless directed by prescriber; to avoid potassium, salt substitutes
- To avoid sunlight or wear sunscreen for photosensitivity
- To comply with dosage schedule, even if feeling better
- To notify prescriber of mouth sores, sore throat, fever, swelling of hands or feet, irregular heartbeat, chest pain, signs of angioedema
- That excessive perspiration, dehydration, vomiting, diarrhea may lead to fall in blood pressure; consult prescriber if these occur
- That drug may cause dizziness, fainting; light-headedness may occur during 1st few days of therapy
- That drug may cause skin rash, impaired perspiration or angioedema; discontinue if angioedema occurs
- Not to discontinue drug abruptly
- That CV adverse reactions may reoccur
- To rise slowly to sitting or standing position to minimize orthostatic hypotension

Treatment of overdose: Lavage, IV atropine for bradycardia, IV theophylline for bronchospasm, digoxin, O₂, diuretic for cardiac failure

---

enfuvirtide (℞)
(en-fyoo'vir-tide)
Fuzeon
Func. class.: Antiretroviral
Chem. class.: Fusion Inhibitor

Action: Inhibitor of the fusion of HIV-1 with CD4+ cells

Uses: Treatment of HIV-1 infection in combination with other antiretrovirals

✤ Canada only

Side effects: *italics* = common; **bold** = life-threatening

DOSAGE AND ROUTES

- *Adult:* **SUBCUT** 90 mg (1 ml) bid
- *Child 6-16 yr:* **SUBCUT** 2 mg/kg bid, max 90 mg bid

Available forms: Powder for inj, lyophilized 108 mg (90 mg/ml when reconstituted)

SIDE EFFECTS

CNS: Anxiety, peripheral neuropathy, taste disturbance, **Guillain-Barré syndrome,** insomnia, depression

GI: Abdominal pain, anorexia, constipation, pancreatitis

GU: **Glomerulonephritis, renal failure**

HEMA: **Thrombocytopenia, neutropenia**

INTEG: Inj site reactions

MISC: Influenza, cough, conjunctivitis, lymphadenopathy, myalgia, hyperglycemia, pneumonia, rhinitis, fatigue

Contraindications: Hypersensitivity, lactation

Precautions: Pregnancy (B), liver disease, children <6 yr, myelosuppression, infections

PHARMACOKINETICS

Peak 8 hr, terminal half-life 3.8 hr, well absorbed, undergoes catabolism, 92% protein binding

INTERACTIONS

None known

NURSING CONSIDERATIONS

Assess:
- Signs of infection, inj site reactions
- Renal studies: BUN, creatinine, renal failure may occur
- Bowel pattern before, during treatment; if severe abdominal pain or constipation occurs, notify prescriber; monitor hydration
- Skin eruptions, rash, urticaria, itching
- Allergies before treatment, reaction to each medication
- CBC, blood chemistry, plasma HIV RNA, absolute CD4+/CD8+ cell counts/%, serum β_2 microglobulin, serum ICD+24 antigen levels, cholesterol

Administer:
- Reconstitute vial with 1.1 ml of sterile water for inj; tap and roll to mix; allow to stand until completely dissolved
- Do not mix with other medications
- SUBCUT, give bid, rotate sites

Evaluate:
- Therapeutic response: increased CD4 cell counts; decreased viral load; slowing progression of HIV-1 infection

Teach patient/family:
- To notify prescriber if pregnancy is suspected, or if breastfeeding
- That pneumonia may occur, to contact prescriber if cough, fever occur
- That hypersensitive reactions may occur, rash, pruritus; stop drug, contact prescriber
- That this drug is not a cure for HIV-1 infection but controls symptoms, HIV-1 can still be transmitted to others
- This drug is to be used in combination only with other antiretrovirals

---

⚠ High Alert

enoxaparin (℞)

(ee-nox′a-par-in)
Lovenox

Func. class.: Anticoagulant, antithrombotic

Chem. class.: Low-molecular-weight heparins (LMWH)

Do not confuse:
enoxaparin/enoxacin
Lovenox/Lotronex

Action: Binds to antithrombin III inactivating factors Xa/IIa resulting in higher ratio of anti–factor Xa to IIa

Uses: Prevention of deep vein thrombosis (inpatient or outpatient), pulmonary emboli (inpatient) in hip and knee replacement, abdominal surgery at risk for thrombosis; unstable angina/non–Q-wave MI

DOSAGE AND ROUTES
DVT prevention before hip/knee surgery
• *Adult:* SUBCUT 30 mg bid given 12-24 hr postop for 7-10 days, until DVT risk is diminished
DVT prevention before hip replacement
• *Adult:* SUBCUT 40 mg daily started 9-15 hr preop or 30 mg bid, started 12-24 hr postop, continued until DVT risk is diminished or is adequately on anticoagulant
DVT prophylaxis before abdominal surgery
• *Adult:* SUBCUT 40 mg daily starting 2 hr prior to surgery × 7-10 days to prevent thromboembolic complications, start 24 hr before surgery
Treatment of DVT/PE
• *Adult:* SUBCUT 1 mg/kg q12h (without PE-outpatient); 1 mg/kg q12h or 1.5 mg/kg daily (with or without PE-inpatient); warfarin should be started within 72 hr and continued until INR is 2-3 (usually 7 days)
Prevention of ischemic complications in unstable angina/non–Q-wave MI
• *Adult:* SUBCUT 1 mg/kg q12h until stable with aspirin 100-325 mg daily × ≥2 days
Available forms: Prefilled syringes/inj 30 mg/0.3 ml, 40 mg/0.4 ml, 60 mg/0.6 ml, 80 mg/0.8 ml, 100 mg/1 ml, 120 mg/0.8 ml, 150 mg/ml; multidose vials 100 mg/ml (3 ml)

SIDE EFFECTS
CNS: Fever, confusion
GI: Nausea
HEMA: **Hemorrhage, hypochromic anemia, thrombocytopenia, bleeding**
INTEG: Ecchymosis, inj site hematoma
SYST: Edema, peripheral edema
Contraindications: Hypersensitivity to this drug, benzyl alcohol, heparin, or pork; active major bleeding hemophilia, leukemia with bleeding, peptic ulcer disease, thrombocytopenic purpura, heparin-induced thrombocytopenia
Precautions: Pregnancy (B), geriatric, severe renal/hepatic disease, blood dyscrasias, severe hypertension, subacute bacterial endocarditis, acute nephritis, lactation, children, recent burn, spinal surgery, indwelling catheters, low weight men (<57 kg), women (<45 kg)

PHARMACOKINETICS
SUBCUT: 90% absorbed, maximum antithrombin activity (3-5 hr), elimination half-life 4½ hr, excreted in urine

INTERACTIONS
Increase: enoxaparin action—anticoagulants, salicylates, NSAIDs, antiplatelets, thrombolytics
Drug/Herb
Increase: risk of bleeding—agrimony, alfalfa, angelica, anise, basil, bay, bilberry, black currant, black haw, bogbean, bromelain, buchu, cat's claw, chondroitin, cinchona bark, dong quai, evening primrose, fenugreek, feverfew, fish oils, garlic, ginger, ginkgo, ginseng, horse chestnut, Irish moss, kava, kelp, kelpware, khella, licorice, lovage, lungwort, meadowsweet, motherwort, mugwort, nettle, papaya, parsley (large amts), pau d'arco, pineapple, poplar, prickly ash, red clover, safflower, saw palmetto, skullcap, tonka bean, turmeric, wintergreen, yarrow
Decrease: anticoagulant effect—chamomile, coenzyme Q10, flax, glucomannan, goldenseal, guar gum
Drug/Lab Test
Increase: AST, ALT
Decrease: Platelet count

NURSING CONSIDERATIONS
Assess:
• Blood studies (Hct, CBC, coagulation studies, platelets, occult blood in stools), anti–factor Xa (should be checked 4 hr after inj); thrombocytopenia may occur
• For bleeding: gums, petechiae, ecchy-

mosis, black tarry stools, hematuria; notify prescriber
• For neurologic symptoms in patients who have received spinal anesthesia

Administer:
• Only after screening patient for bleeding disorders
• SUBCUT only; do not give IM, begin 1 hr prior to surgery, do not aspirate, rotate sites, do not expel bubble from syringe before administration
• To recumbent patient; give SUBCUT; rotate inj sites (left/right anterolateral, left/right posterolateral abdominal wall)
• Insert whole length of needle into skin fold held with thumb and forefinger
• Do not mix with other drugs or infusion fluids
⚠ Only this drug when ordered; not interchangeable with heparin or other LMWHs
• At same time each day to maintain steady blood levels
• Avoid all IM inj that may cause bleeding

Perform/provide:
• Storage at 77° F (25° C); do not freeze

Evaluate:
• Therapeutic response: prevention of deep vein thrombosis

Teach patient/family:
• To use soft-bristle toothbrush to avoid bleeding gums, to use electric razor
• To report any signs of bleeding: gums, under skin, urine, stools
• To avoid OTC drugs containing aspirin unless approved by prescriber

Treatment of overdose: Protamine SO₄ 1% sol; dose should equal dose of enoxaparin

---

entacapone (℞)
(en′ta-kah-pone)
Comtan
Func. class.: Antiparkinson agent
Chem. class.: COMT inhibitor

Action: Inhibits COMT (catechol *O*-methyltransferase) and alters the plasma pharmacokinetics of levodopa. Given with levodopa/carbidopa

Uses: Parkinson's disease in those experiencing end of dose, decreased effect as adjunct to levodopa/carbidopa

DOSAGE AND ROUTES
• *Adult:* **PO** 200 mg given with carbidopa/levodopa, max 1600 mg/day

Available forms: Tabs, film coated 200 mg

SIDE EFFECTS
CNS: Involuntary choreiform movements, hand tremors, fatigue, headache, anxiety, twitching, numbness, dyskinesia, hypokinesia, hyperkinesia, weakness, confusion, agitation, nightmares, psychosis, hallucination, hypomania, severe depression, dizziness, **neuroleptic malignant syndrome**
CV: Orthostatic hypotension
GI: Nausea, vomiting, anorexia, abdominal distress, dry mouth, flatulence, bitter taste, diarrhea, constipation, dyspepsia, gastritis, GI disorder
INTEG: Rash, sweating, alopecia
MISC: Dark urine and other body fluids, back pain, dyspnea, purpura, fatigue, asthenia, bacterial infection, **rhabdomyolysis**

Contraindications: Hypersensitivity
Precautions: Pregnancy (C), renal/hepatic disease, affective disorders, psychosis, lactation, children

PHARMACOKINETICS
Duration up to 8 hr; excreted in urine, feces; well absorbed, protein binding 98%, metabolized in liver extensively, enters breast milk; half-life of levodopa is extended, half-life 0.5 hr initial, 2.5 hr second

INTERACTIONS
• Prevents catecholamine metabolism, do not use together—MAOIs
Increase: B/P, tachycardia, dysrhythmias, avoid use—bitolterol, DOPamine, DO-

---

BUTamine, epINEPHrine, methyldopa, isoetharine, norepinephrine
Decrease: excretion of entacapone—ampicillin, chloramphenicol, probenecid, erythromycin, rifampin
Drug/Herb
Decrease: effect—kava

NURSING CONSIDERATIONS
Assess:
⚠ Neuroleptic malignant syndrome: high temp, increased CPK, rigidity, change in consciousness
• Involuntary movements in Parkinson's disease: akinesia, tremors, staggering gait, muscle rigidity, drooling when given with levodopa/carbidopa
• B/P, respiration during initial treatment
• Mental status: affect, mood, behavioral changes, depression; complete suicide assessment
Administer:
• Only after MAOIs have been discontinued for 2 wk
• Give with a dose of levodopa/carbidopa; this drug has no effect on its own
Perform/provide:
• Assistance with ambulation during beginning therapy
Evaluate:
• Therapeutic response: decrease in akathisia, increased mood when given with levodopa/carbidopa
Teach patient/family:
• That hallucinations, mental changes, nausea, dyskinesia can occur and may mean patient is overmedicated
• To change positions slowly to prevent orthostatic hypotension; not to drive or operate machinery until stabilized on medication and mental performance is not affected
• To use drug exactly as prescribed
• That urine, sweat may darken
• To notify prescriber if pregnancy is suspected; or if lactating, drug is excreted in breast milk

entecavir (℞)
(en-te'ka-veer)
Baraclude
Func. class.: Antiviral
Chem. class.: Guanosine nucleoside analog

Action: Inhibits hepatitis B virus DNA polymerase by competing with natural substrates and by causing DNA termination after its incorporation into viral DNA; causes viral DNA death
Uses: Chronic hepatitis B (HBV), active

DOSAGE AND ROUTES
Chronic hepatitis B (nucleoside treatment–naive)
• *Adult and adolescent ≥16 yr:* **PO** 0.5 mg daily
Chronic hepatitis B while receiving lamivudine or known lamivudine-resistant mutations
• *Adult and adolescent ≥16 yr:* **PO** 1 mg daily
Renal dose
• *Adult:* **PO** CCr ≥50 ml/min 0.5 mg daily; CCr 30-49 ml/min 0.25 mg daily, 0.5 mg daily for lamivudine-refractory patient; CCr 10-29 ml/min 0.15 daily, 0.3 for lamivudine-refractory patient; CCr <10 ml/min 0.05 mg PO daily, 0.1 mg for lamivudine-refractory patient
Available forms: Tabs, film coated 0.5, 1 mg; oral sol 0.05 mg/ml

SIDE EFFECTS
CNS: Headache, fatigue, dizziness, insomnia
GI: Dyspepsia, nausea, vomiting, diarrhea
SYST: **Lactic acidosis, severe hepatomegaly with stenosis**
Contraindications: Hypersensitivity
Precautions: Pregnancy (C), lactation, child, severe renal disease, geriatric

PHARMACOKINETICS

Peak 0.5-1.5 hr, steady state 6-10 days, 100% bioavailability, extensively distributed to tissues, protein binding 13%, terminal half-life 128-149 hr, excreted unchanged (62%-73%) via kidneys

INTERACTIONS

• None known

Drug/Lab Test

Increase: ALT, AST, total bilirubin, amylase, lipase, creatinine, blood glucose, urine glucose

Decrease: Platelets, albumin

NURSING CONSIDERATIONS

Assess:

• For nephrotoxicity: increasing CCr, BUN

• For HIV before beginning treatment, because HIV resistance may occur in chronic hepatitis B patients

⚠ For lactic acidosis, severe hepatomegaly with stenosis

• Geriatric patients more carefully; may develop renal, cardiac symptoms more rapidly

• For exacerbations of hepatitis (jaundice, pruritus, fatigue) after discontinuing treatment, monitor LFTs

Administer:

• By mouth on empty stomach 2 hr before or after food

Perform/provide:

• Storage in cool environment; protect from light

Evaluate:

• Therapeutic response: decreased symptoms of chronic hepatitis B, improving LFTs

Teach patient/family:

• Not to take with food

• To take exactly as prescribed

• Do not stop medication without approval of prescriber

• That optimal duration of treatment is unknown

• To avoid use with other medications unless approved by prescriber

• To notify prescriber of decreased urinary output, blood in urine

• Symptoms of lactic acidosis: muscle pain, severe tiredness, weakness, trouble breathing, stomach pain with nausea/vomiting, coldness in arms/legs, fast/irregular heartbeat, dizziness

• Symptoms of hepatotoxicity: eyes/skin turns yellow, dark urine, light bowel movements, no appetite for days, nausea, stomach pain

• That product does not cure, but lowers the amount of HBV in body

• That product does not stop you from spreading HBV to others by sex, sharing needles, or being exposed to blood

---

⚠ High Alert

epHEDrine (℞)

(e-fed′rin)

epHEDrine sulfate, Pretz-D (OTC)

Func. class.: Bronchodilator, nonselective adrenergic, mixed direct and indirect effects

Chem. class.: Phenylisopropylamine

Do not confuse:

epHEDrine/epINEPHrine

Action: Causes increased contractility and heart rate by acting on β-receptors in the heart; also acts on α-receptors, causing vasoconstriction in blood vessels

Uses: Shock; increased perfusion; hypotension, bronchodilation

DOSAGE AND ROUTES

Hypotension

• *Adult:* **PO** 25 mg daily-qid; **IM/SUBCUT** 25-50 mg; **IV** 10-25 mg, max 150 mg/24 hr

• *Child:* **SUBCUT/IV** 25-100 mg/m²/day in 4-6 divided doses

Bronchodilator

• *Adult and child >12 yr:* **PO** 12.5-50 mg q3-4h prn, max 150 mg/24 hr; **NASAL** 2-3 sprays in each nostril q4h

• *Child 2-12 yr:* **PO** 2-3 mg/kg or 100 mg/m²/day in 4-6 divided doses

Available forms: Inj 25, 30, 50 mg/ml; caps 25, 50 mg

SIDE EFFECTS

CNS: Tremors, anxiety, insomnia, sweating, headache, dizziness, confusion, hallucinations, **seizures, CNS depression, cerebral hemorrhage,** weakness, drowsiness

CV: Palpitations, tachycardia, hypertension, chest pain, **dysrhythmias**

GI: Anorexia, nausea, vomiting

GU: Dysuria, urinary retention

RESP: **Dyspnea**

Contraindications: Hypersensitivity to sympathomimetics, narrow-angle glaucoma, nonanaphylactic shock during general anesthesia, diabetes mellitus, hypertension

Precautions: Pregnancy (C), lactation, cardiac disorders, hyperthyroidism, diabetes mellitus, prostatic hypertrophy, angina

PHARMACOKINETICS

PO: Onset 15-60 min, duration 2-4 hr
IM: Onset 10-20 min, duration 1 hr
IV: Onset 5 min, duration 2 hr
Metabolized in liver; excreted in urine (unchanged), breast milk; crosses blood-brain barrier, placenta; half-life 3-6 hr

INTERACTIONS

• Dysrhythmia: halothane anesthetics, cardiac glycosides, levodopa
Increase: severe hypertension—oxytocics
Increase: hypertensive crisis—ergots, MAOIs
Increase: effect of epHEDrine—urinary alkalizers
Decrease: effect of guanethidine
Decrease: effect of epHEDrine—methyldopa, urinary acidifiers, rauwolfia alkaloids, α-adrenergic blockers, diuretics, tricyclics

NURSING CONSIDERATIONS
Assess:
• I&O ratio
• ECG continuously during administration; if B/P increases, drug is decreased;

B/P and pulse q5min after parenteral route; CVP or PWP during infusion if possible
• For paresthesias and coldness of extremities; peripheral blood flow may decrease; long-term use may produce a pseudoanxiety state requiring sedative; increased lactic acid with severe metabolic acidosis can occur
• Inj site: tissue sloughing; if this occurs, administer phentolamine mixed with 0.9% NaCl
Administer:
IV, direct route
• Through Y-tube or 3-way stopcock; give 10-25 mg slowly; may repeat in 5-10 min, protect from light
Additive compatibilities: Chloramphenicol, lidocaine, metaraminol, nafcillin, penicillin G potassium
Solution compatibilities: D_5W, $D_{10}W$, LR, 0.9% NaCl, 0.45% NaCl, Ringer's
Syringe compatibilities: Pentobarbital
Y-site compatibilities: Etomidate, propofol
Perform/provide:
• Storage of reconstituted sol refrigerated no longer than 24 hr
• Do not use discolored sol
Evaluate:
• Therapeutic response: increased B/P with stabilization
Teach patient/family:
• The reason for drug administration

*epHEDrine nasal agent
See Appendix C

epinastine ophthalmic
See Appendix C

⚠ High Alert

epINEPHrine (℞)
(ep-i-nef'rin)
Adrenalin Ana-Guard, AsthmaHaler Mist, AsthmaNefrin (racepinephrine), Bronitin Mist, Bronkaid Mist, Epinal, epINEPHrine, EpINEPHrine Pediatric, EpiPen, EpiPen Jr., Epitrate, Eppy/N, Medihaler microNefrin, Nephron, Primatene Mist, S-2, Sus-Phrine, Vaponefrin (racepinephrine)

Func. class.: Bronchodilator nonselective adrenergic agonist, vasopressor

Chem. class.: Catecholamine

Do not confuse:
epINEPHrine/epHEDrine

Action: β_1- and β_2-agonist causing increased levels of cAMP producing bronchodilation, cardiac, and CNS stimulation; high doses cause vasoconstriction via α-receptors; low doses can cause vasodilation via β_2-vascular receptors

Uses: Acute asthmatic attacks, hemostasis, bronchospasm, anaphylaxis, allergic reactions, cardiac arrest, adjunct in anesthesia, shock

DOSAGE AND ROUTES

Asthma
• *Adult and child:* **INH** 1-2 puffs of 1:100 or 2.25% racemic q15min
Bronchodilator
• *Adult:* **SUBCUT/IM** 0.3-0.5 mg (1:1000 sol) q10-15min-4h, max 1 mg/dose
Anaphylactic reaction/asthma
• *Adult:* **SUBCUT/IM** 0.3-0.5 mg, repeat q10-15min, max 1 mg/dose; epINEPHrine susp 0.5 mg **SUBCUT,** may repeat 0.5-1.5 mg q6h
• *Child:* **SUBCUT** 0.01 mg/kg, repeat q15min, × 2 doses, then q4h, max 0.5

mg/dose; epINEPHrine susp 0.025 mg/kg **SUBCUT,** may repeat q6h, max 0.75 mg in child ≤30 kg
Cardiac arrest (ACLS)
• *Adult:* **IV** 1 mg q3-5min; **ENDOTRACHEAL** 2-2.5 mg **IC** 0.3-0.5 mg
Symptomatic bradycardia/pulseless arrest (PALS)
• *Child:* **IV** 0.01 mg/kg, may repeat q3-5min up to 0.1-0.2 mg/kg; **ENDOTRACHEAL** give 2-10 × **IV** dose diluted to a volume of 3-5 ml of 0.9% NaCl, followed by positive pressure ventilation
Available forms: Aerosol 0.16 mg/spray, 0.2 mg/spray, 0.25 mg/spray; inj 1:1000 (1 mg/ml), 1:200 (5 mg/ml), 0.01 mg/ml (1:100,000), 0.1 mg/ml (1:10,000), 0.5 mg/ml (1:2000); sol for nebulization 1:100, 1.25%, 2.25% (base)

SIDE EFFECTS

CNS: Tremors, anxiety, insomnia, headache, *dizziness,* confusion, hallucinations, **cerebral hemorrhage**, weakness, drowsiness
CV: Palpitations, tachycardia, hypertension, *dysrhythmias,* increased T wave
GI: Anorexia, nausea, vomiting
MISC: Sweating, dry eyes
RESP: Dyspnea

Contraindications: Hypersensitivity to sympathomimetics, narrow-angle glaucoma, nonanaphylactic shock during general anesthesia

Precautions: Pregnancy (C), lactation, cardiac disorders, hyperthyroidism, diabetes mellitus, prostatic hypertrophy, hypertension, organic brain syndrome, local anesthesia of certain areas, labor, cardiac dilation, coronary insufficiency, cerebral arteriosclerosis, organic heart disease

PHARMACOKINETICS

SUBCUT: Onset 5-15 min, duration 20 min-4 hr
INH: Onset 1-5 min, duration 1-3 hr
Crosses placenta; metabolized in liver

INTERACTIONS
• Do not use with MAOIs or tricyclics; hypertensive crisis may occur
• Toxicity: other sympathomimetics
Decrease: hypertensive effects—α-adrenergic blockers

NURSING CONSIDERATIONS
Assess:
• ECG during administration continuously; if B/P increases, decrease dose; B/P and pulse q5min after parenteral route; CVP, ISVR, PCWP during infusion if possible; inadvertent high arterial B/P can result in angina, aortic rupture, cerebral hemorrhage
• Injection site: tissue sloughing; administer phentolamine with NS
• Sulfite sensitivity, which may be life-threatening
Administer:
• Increased dose of insulin in diabetic patients if glucose is elevated
• Check for correct concentration, route, dosage before administering
IM/SUBCUT route
• Rotate inj sites, massage after inj, shake before using
Endotracheal route
• Give directly via endotracheal tube, use 1:10,000 sol; for small dose further dilute dose prior to administration, follow with quick insufflations
INH route
• Place in nebulizer (10 gtt of a 1% base sol)
• Dilute racepinephrine 2.25% sol
IV route
• Parenteral dose slowly, after reconstituting 1 mg (1:1000 sol)/10 ml or more 0.9% NaCl; to prepare a 1:10,000 sol for maintenance, may be further diluted in 500 ml D5W; give 1 mg or less over 1 min or more through Y-tube or 3-way stopcock; 1 mg = 1 ml of 1:1000 or 10 ml of 1:10,000; protect from light, use large vein
Additive compatibilities: Cimetidine, DOBUTamine, floxacillin, furosemide, metaraminol, ranitidine, verapamil
Syringe compatibilities: Doxapram, heparin, milrinone
Y-site compatibilities: Atracurium, calcium chloride, calcium gluconate, cisatracurium, diltiazem, DOBUTamine, DOPamine, famotidine, fentanyl, furosemide, heparin, hydrocortisone sodium succinate, hydromorphone, labetalol, lorazepam, midazolam, milrinone, morphine, niCARdipine, nitroglycerin, norepinephrine, pancuronium, phytonadione, potassium chloride, propofol, ranitidine, remifentanil, vecuronium, vit B/C, warfarin
Perform/provide:
• Storage of reconstituted sol refrigerated no longer than 24 hr
• Do not use discolored sol
Evaluate:
• Therapeutic response: increased B/P with stabilization or ease of breathing
Teach patient/family:
• The reason for drug administration
• To rinse mouth after use to prevent dryness after inhalation
• Not to take OTC preparations
Treatment of overdose: Administer an α-blocker and a β-blocker

*epINEPHrine/epinephryl borate ophthalmic
See Appendix C

*epINEPHrine nasal agent
See Appendix C

⚠ High Alert

epirubicin (℞)
(ep-ih-roo′bi-sin)
Ellence
Func. class.: Antineoplastic, antibiotic
Chem. class.: Anthracycline

Action: Inhibits DNA synthesis primarily; replication is decreased by binding to DNA, which causes strand splitting; maximum cytotoxic effects at S and for G_2 phases, a vesicant

Uses: Adjuvant therapy for breast cancer with axillary node involvement following resection

Unlabeled uses: Used in combination for treatment of advanced forms of cancer

DOSAGE AND ROUTES

• *Adult:* IV INF 100-120 mg/m² initially, given with other antineoplastics (cyclophosphamide, 5-fluorouracil); given in repeated cycles; 3-4 wk cycles
Epirubicin dosage adjustments
• *Adult:* IV 100 mg/m² on day 1 of each cycle; toxicity nadir platelet counts <50,000 mm³, ANC 250 mm³, neutropenic fever or grade 3 or 4 nonhematologic toxicity; next cycle give 75% of day 1 dose; delay next cycle until platelets are ≥100,000 mm³, ANC ≥1500 mm³, and nonhematologic toxicities have recovered to < grade 1
Hepatic dose
• *Adult:* IV bilirubin 1.2-3 mg/dl or AST 2-4 × normal upper limit 50% of starting dose; bilirubin >3 mg/dl or AST >4 × normal upper limit 25% of starting dose
Available forms: Inj 2 mg/ml

SIDE EFFECTS

CV: Increased B/P, **sinus tachycardia, PVCs,** chest pain, **bradycardia, extrasystoles; CHF confirm for doses >900 mg/m²**
GI: Nausea, vomiting, anorexia, mucositis, diarrhea

GU: Amenorrhea, hot flashes, hyperuricemia
HEMA: **Thrombocytopenia, leukopenia, anemia, neutropenia, secondary AML**
INTEG: Rash, **necrosis, pain at inj site,** *reversible alopecia*
MISC: Infection, febrile neutropenia, lethargy, fever, conjunctivitis

Contraindications: Pregnancy (D), lactation, hypersensitivity to this drug, anthracyclines, anthracenediones, severe hepatic disease, baseline neutrophil count <1500 cell/mm³, severe myocardial insufficiency, recent MI, systemic infections
Precautions: Renal/hepatic/cardiac disease; gout, bone marrow depression (severe), geriatric, children

PHARMACOKINETICS

Triphasic pattern of elimination; half-life 3 min, 2.5 hr, 33 hr; metabolized by liver; crosses placenta; excreted in urine, bile, breast milk

INTERACTIONS

Increase: toxicity—other antineoplastics or radiation, cimetidine
Decrease: antibody response—live virus vaccine

NURSING CONSIDERATIONS

Assess:
• Bone marrow depression, infection: increased temp
• CBC, differential, platelet count weekly; withhold drug if baseline neutrophil ≤1500/mm³; leukocyte nadir occurs 10-14 days after administration, recovery by 21st day; notify prescriber of these results
• Blood, urine uric acid levels; swelling, joint pain primarily in extremities, patient should be well hydrated to prevent urate deposits
• Renal studies: BUN, serum uric acid, urine CCr, electrolytes before, during therapy; I&O ratio; report fall in urine output to <30 ml/hr; dosage adjustment is needed if serum creatinine >5 mg/dl

---

⚠ Safety alert   *"Tall Man" lettering

- Hepatic studies before, during therapy: bilirubin, AST, ALT, alk phos as needed or monthly
- Cardiac status: B/P, pulse, character, rhythm, rate, ABGs, ECG, LVEF, MUGA scan, or ECHO; watch for ST-T wave changes, low QRS and T, possible dysrhythmias (sinus tachycardia, heart block, PVCs)
- Bleeding: hematuria, guaiac, bruising, or petechiae, mucosa or orifices q8h
- Effects of alopecia on body image; discuss feelings about body changes
- Local irritation, pain, burning, necrosis at inj site
- GI symptoms: frequency of stools, cramping

Administer:
- Antiemetic 30-60 min before giving drug to prevent vomiting
- Allopurinol or sodium bicarbonate to maintain uric acid levels, alkalinization of urine

IV route
- Using cytotoxic handling procedures; pregnant women must not handle drug
- Hydrocortisone, dexamethasone, or sodium bicarbonate (1 mEq/1 ml) for extravasation; apply ice compresses
- Given into tubing of free-flowing IV infusion (0.9% NaCl or D₅) give over 3-5 min; do not mix with other drugs in syringe

Perform/provide:
- Strict hand-washing technique, gloves, protective clothing
- Liquid diet: carbonated beverages, gelatin may be added if patient is not nauseated or vomiting
- Increased fluid intake to 2-3 L/day to prevent urate, calculi formation

Evaluate:
- Therapeutic response: decreased tumor size, spread of malignancy

Teach patient/family:
- To report any complaints, side effects to nurse or prescriber
- That hair may be lost during treatment and wig or hairpiece may make patient

feel better; tell patient that new hair may be different in color, texture
- To avoid crowds and persons with infections when granulocyte count is low
- That contraceptive measures are recommended during therapy and 4 mo thereafter for men and women
- To avoid vaccinations, reactions may occur; to avoid cimetidine during therapy
- That urine may appear red for 2 days
- To avoid OTC medications, supplements unless approved by prescriber
- That irreversible myocardial damage, leukopenia, menopause may occur

---

eplerenone (℞)
(ep-ler-ee′known)
Inspra
Func. class.: Antihypertensive
Chem. class.: Selective aldosterone receptor antagonist

Action: Binds to mineralocorticoid receptor and blocks the binding of aldosterone, a component of the renin-angiotensin aldosterone system (RAAS)
Uses: Hypertension, alone or in combination with thiazide diuretics, CHF, post-MI

DOSAGE AND ROUTES
- *Adult:* **PO** 50 mg daily, initially, may increase to 50 mg bid after 4 wk; start dose at 25 mg daily if patient is taking CYP3A4 inhibitors
CHF/Post-MI
- *Adult:* **PO** 25 mg daily initially, may increase to 50 mg max
Available forms: Tabs 25, 50, 100 mg

SIDE EFFECTS
CNS: Headache, dizziness, fatigue
CV: Angina, **MI**
GI: Increased GGT diarrhea, abdominal pain, increased ALT
GU: Increased BUN, creatinine, gynecomastia, mastodynia (males), abnormal vaginal bleeding

META: Hyperkalemia, hyponatremia, hypercholesteremia, hypertriglyceridemia, increased uric acid

RESP: Cough

Contraindications: Hypersensitivity, lactation, children, increased serum creatinine >2 mg/dl (male), >1.8 mg/dl (female), potassium >5.5 mEq/L, type 2 diabetes with microalbuminuria, hepatic disease, CCr <30 ml/min; <50 ml/min in hypertension

Precautions: Pregnancy (B), impaired renal/hepatic function, geriatric, hyperkalemia, lactation

PHARMACOKINETICS

PO: Peak 1½ hr, serum protein binding 50%, half-life 4-6 hr, metabolized by liver (CYP3A4 inhibitor), excreted in urine

INTERACTIONS

Increase: hyperkalemia—ACE inhibitors, angiotensin II antagonists, NSAIDs, potassium supplements, potassium-sparing diuretics

Increase: serum levels of lithium

Increase: levels of eplerenone—CYP3A4 inhibitors (ketoconazole, itraconazole, saquinavir, erythromycin, verapamil, fluconazole), reduce dose of eplerenone

Decrease: antihypertensive effect—NSAIDs

Drug/Herb

Increase: toxicity, death—aconite

Increase: antihypertensive effect—barberry, betony, black catechu, black cohosh, bloodroot, broom, burdock, cat's claw, dandelion, goldenseal, hawthorn, Irish moss, Jamaican dogwood, kelp, khella, mistletoe, parsley

Increase or decrease: antihypertensive effect—astragalus, cola tree

Decrease: antihypertensive effect—coltsfoot, guarana, khat, licorice, yohimbine

Decrease: levels of eplerenone—St. John's wort

Drug/Food

• Grapefruit juice increased drug level by 25%

NURSING CONSIDERATIONS

Assess:

• B/P at peak/trough level of drug, orthostatic hypotension, syncope when used with diuretic; monitor lithium level in those also taking lithium

• Renal studies: protein, BUN, creatinine; increased LFTs, uric acid may be increased

• Potassium levels, hyperkalemia may occur

Perform/provide:

• Storage in tight container at 86° F (30° C) or less

Evaluate:

• Therapeutic response: decreased B/P

Teach patient/family:

• Not to discontinue drug abruptly

• Not to use OTC products (cough, cold, allergy) unless directed by prescriber; do not use salt substitutes containing potassium without consulting prescriber

• Important to comply with dosage schedule, even if feeling better

• That drug may cause dizziness, fainting, light-headedness; may occur during first few days of therapy

• How to take B/P, and normal readings for age-group

---

epoetin (℞)
(ee-poe′e-tin)
EPO, Epogen, Eprex ✦,
Procrit
Func. class.: Antianemic, biologic modifier, hormone
Chem. class.: Amino acid polypeptide

Action: Erythropoietin is one factor controlling rate of red cell production; drug is developed by recombinant DNA technology

Uses: Anemia caused by reduced endogenous erythropoietin production, primarily end-stage renal disease; to correct hemostatic defect in uremia; anemia due to AZT treatment in HIV patients or chemotherapy; reduction of allogenic blood transfusion in surgery patients

Unlabeled uses: Pruritus; anemia in: premature preterm infants, myelodysplastic syndrome, chronic inflammatory disorders

DOSAGE AND ROUTES
Anemia related to chemotherapy
• *Adult:* SUBCUT 150 units/kg 3 ×/wk, may increase after 2 mo up to 300 units/kg 3 ×/wk

Anemia in chronic renal failure
• *Adult:* SUBCUT/IV 50-100 units/kg 3 ×/wk, then adjust to maintain target Hct of 30%-36%
• *Child:* IV/SUBCUT 50 units/kg 3 ×/wk

Anemia secondary to zidovudine treatment
• *Adult:* SUBCUT/IV 100 units/kg 3 ×/wk × 2 mo, may increase by 50-100 units/kg q1-2mo, up to 300 units/kg 3 ×/wk

Surgery
• *Adult:* SUBCUT 300 units/kg/day × 10 days prior to surgery, the day of surgery, and for 4 days postsurgery or 600 units/kg at 3 wk, 2 wk, 1 wk, prior to and on day of surgery

Available forms: Inj 2000, 3000, 4000, 10,000, 20,000, 40,000 units/ml

SIDE EFFECTS
CNS: **Seizures,** coldness, sweating, headache
CV: Hypertension, **hypertensive encephalopathy**
MS: Bone pain

Contraindications: Hypersensitivity to mammalian cell–derived products, or human albumin, uncontrolled hypertension
Precautions: Pregnancy (C), seizure disorder, porphyria, children <1 mo, lactation, multidose preserved formulation contains benzyl alcohol and should not be used in premature infants

PHARMACOKINETICS
IV: Metabolized in body; extent of metabolism unknown; onset of increased reticulocyte count 2-6 wk; peak, immediate

INTERACTIONS
• Need for increased anticoagulant during hemodialysis

E

NURSING CONSIDERATIONS
Assess:
• Renal studies: urinalysis, protein, blood, BUN, creatinine; I&O, report drop in output <50 ml/hr
• Blood studies: ferritin, transferrin monthly; transferrin sat ≥20%, ferritin ≥100 ng/ml; Hct 2 ×/wk until stabilized in target range (30%-36%) then at regular intervals; those with endogenous erythropoietin levels of <500 units/L respond to this agent; monitor Hct 2 ×/wk in chronic renal failure; patients treated with zidovudine or cancer patients should be monitored weekly, then periodically after stabilization
• B/P; check for rising B/P as Hct rises, antihypertensives may be needed; hypertension may occur rapidly leading to hypertensive encephalopathy
• CNS symptoms: coldness, sweating, pain in long bones; for seizures if Hct is increased within 2 wk by 4 pts
• For hypersensitivity reactions: skin rashes, urticaria (rare), antibody development does not occur

⚠ For pure cell aplasia (PRCA) in absence of other causes, evaluate by testing sera for recombinant erythropoetin antibodies; any loss of response to epoetin should be evaluated
• Dialysis patients: thrill, bruit of shunts, monitor for circulation impairment

Administer:
• Do not shake vial

SUBCUT route
• Before injecting preservative free-, single-dose formulation may be admixed using 0.9% NaCl with benzyl alcohol 0.9%

at a 1:1 ratio to reduce injection site discomfort

IV route
• Additional heparin to lower chance of clots
• By direct inj or bolus into IV tubing or venous line at end of dialysis
• Decrease dose by 25 units/kg, if Hct increases by 4% in 2 wk; increase dose if Hct does not increase by 5-6 pts after 8 wk of therapy, suggested target Hct range 30%–36%

Solution compatibilities: Do not dilute or administer with other solutions

Evaluate:
• Therapeutic response: increase in reticulocyte count in 2-6 wk, Hgb/Hct; increased appetite, enhanced sense of well-being

Teach patient/family:
• To avoid driving or hazardous activity during beginning of treatment
• ʹTo monitor B/P
• To take iron supplements, vitamin B_{12}, folic acid as directed

---

eprosartan (℞)
(ep-roh-sarʹtan)
Teveten
Func. class.: Antihypertensive
Chem. class.: Angiotensin II–receptor antagonist (Subtype AT_1)

Action: Blocks the vasoconstrictor and aldosterone-secreting effects of angiotensin II; selectively blocks the binding of angiotensin II to the AT_1 receptor found in tissues

Uses: Hypertension, alone or with other antihypertensives

DOSAGE AND ROUTES
• *Adult:* **PO** 600 mg daily; dose may be divided and given bid with total daily doses from 400-800 mg

Available forms: Tabs 400, 600 mg

SIDE EFFECTS
CNS: Dizziness, depression, fatigue, headache

CV: Chest pain
EENT: Sinusitis
GI: Diarrhea, dyspepsia, abdominal pain
GU: UTI
META: Hypertriglyceridemia
MS: Myalgia, arthralgia
RESP: Cough, upper respiratory infection, rhinitis, pharyngitis, viral infection

Contraindications: Pregnancy (D) 2nd/3rd trimesters, hypersensitivity

Precautions: Pregnancy (C) 1st trimester, hypersensitivity to ACE inhibitors; lactation, children, geriatric, renal/hepatic disease, angioedema

PHARMACOKINETICS
Peak 1-2 hr, food delays absorption, protein binding 98%, moderate renal impairment increases drug levels by 30%, hepatic impairment increases levels by 40%, excreted in urine and feces, half-life 5-9 hr

INTERACTIONS
Decrease: antihypertensive effect—NSAIDs, salicylates

Drug/Herb
Increase: toxicity, death—aconite
Increase: antihypertensive effect—barberry, betony, black catechu, black cohosh, bloodroot, broom, burdock, cat's claw, dandelion, goldenseal, hawthorn, Irish moss, Jamaican dogwood, kelp, khella, mistletoe, parsley
Increase or decrease: antihypertensive effect—astragalus, cola tree
Decrease: antihypertensive effect—coltsfoot, guarana, khat, licorice, yohimbine

Drug/Lab Test
Increase: ALT, AST, alk phos
Decrease: Hgb

NURSING CONSIDERATIONS
Assess:
• B/P with position changes, pulse q4h; note rate, rhythm, quality
• Electrolytes (K, Na, Cl)
• Baselines in renal, hepatic studies before therapy begins

- Edema in feet, legs daily
- Skin turgor, dryness of mucous membranes for hydration status

Administer:
- Without regard to meals

Evaluate:
- Therapeutic response: Decrease B/P

Teach patient/family:
- To comply with dosage schedule, even if feeling better
- To notify prescriber of fever, swelling of hands or feet, chest pain
- That excessive perspiration, dehydration, diarrhea may lead to fall in blood pressure; consult prescriber if these occur
- That drug may cause dizziness, avoid hazardous activities until effect is known
- Not to take this medication if pregnant or breastfeeding, or have had an allergic reaction to this drug
- To take missed dose as soon as possible, unless within 1 hr before next dose

---

⚠ High Alert

eptifibatide (℞)

(ep-tih-fib′ah-tide)

Integrilin

Func. class.: Antiplatelet agent
Chem. class.: Glycoprotein IIb/IIIa inhibitor

Action: Platelet glycoprotein antagonist; this agent reversibly prevents fibrinogen, von Willebrand's factor from binding to the glycoprotein IIb/IIIa receptor, inhibiting platelet aggregation

Uses: Acute coronary syndrome including those undergoing PCI (percutaneous coronary intervention)

DOSAGE AND ROUTES

Acute coronary syndrome
- *Adult:* IV BOL 180 mcg/kg as soon as diagnosed, max 22.6 mg, then **IV CONT** 2 mcg/kg/min until discharge or CABG up to 72 hr, max 15 mg/hr

PCI in patients without acute coronary syndrome
- *Adult:* IV BOL 180 mcg/kg given immediately before PCI; then 2 mcg/kg/min × 18 hr and a second 180-mcg/kg bolus, 10 min after 1st bolus; continue inf for up to 18-24 hr

Renal dose
- *Adult:* IV BOL CCr <50 ml/min: 2-4 mg/dl same loading dose, then ½ usual inf dose

Available forms: Sol for inj 2 mg/ml (10 ml), 0.75 mg/ml (100 ml)

SIDE EFFECTS

CV: **Stroke,** hypotension
GU: Hematuria
HEMA: **Thrombocytopenia**
SYST: **Bleeding, anaphylaxis**

Contraindications: Hypersensitivity, active internal bleeding; history of bleeding, stroke within 1 mo; major surgery with severe trauma, severe hypertension, history of intracranial bleeding, current or planned use of another parenteral GP IIb/IIIa inhibitor, dependence on renal dialysis, coagulopathy

Precautions: Pregnancy (B), bleeding, lactation, children, geriatric, impaired renal function

PHARMACOKINETICS

Half-life 2.5 hr, steady state 4-6 hr, metabolism limited, excretion via kidneys

INTERACTIONS

- Do not give with glycoprotein inhibitors IIb, IIIa

Increase: bleeding—aspirin, heparin, NSAIDs, anticoagulants, ticlopidine, clopidogrel, dipyridamole, thrombolytics, valproate, abciximab

NURSING CONSIDERATIONS

Assess:
⚠ Platelets, Hgb, Hct, creatinine, PT/APTT baseline INR within 6 hr of loading dose and daily therafter, patients undergoing PCI should have ACT monitored; maintain APTT 50-70 sec unless PCI is to be

performed; during PCI, ACT should be 200-300 sec; if platelets drop <100,000/mm³, obtain additional platelet counts; if thrombocytopenia is confirmed, discontinue drug; also, draw Hct, Hgb, serum creatinine

⚠ For bleeding: gums, bruising, ecchymosis, petechiae; from GI, GU tract, cardiac cath sites, IM inj sites

Administer:
• Aspirin and heparin may be given with this drug
• D/C heparin before removing femoral artery sheath, after PCI

IV route
• After withdrawing bolus dose from 10-ml vial, give IV push over 1-2 min; follow bolus dose with continuous inf using pump, give drug undiluted directly from 100-ml vial, spike 100-ml vial with vented infusion set, use caution when centering spike on circle of stopper top

Y-site compatabilities: alteplase, atropine, DOBUTamine, heparin, lidocaine, meperidine, metoprolol, midazolam, morphine, nitroglycerin, verapamil

Solution compatabilities: 0.9% NaCl, D₅/0.9% NaCl

Perform/provide:
• Do not give discolored solutions or those with particulates, discard unused amount
• Discontinue drug prior to CABG
• All medications PO if possible, avoid IM inj and all catheters

Teach patient/family:
• Reason for medication and expected results
• To report bruising, bleeding, chest pain immediately

---

ergonovine (℞)
(er-goe-noe'veen)
ergonovine, Ergotrate
Func. class.: Oxytocic
Chem. class.: Ergot alkaloid

Action: Stimulates uterine contractions and vascular smooth muscle, decreases bleeding

Uses: Postpartum or postabortion hemorrhage

Unlabeled uses: To induce a coronary artery spasm for diagnostic purposes

DOSAGE AND ROUTES

Oxytocic
• *Adult:* **PO/SL** 0.2-0.4 mg q6-12h; **IM** 0.2 mg q2-4h, not to exceed 5 doses; **IV** 0.2 mg given over 1 min

Induced coronary artery spasm
• *Adult:* **IV** 50 mcg q5min up to 400 mcg or when chest pain occurs

Available forms: Inj 0.2, 0.25 ✦ mg/ml; tabs 0.2 mg

SIDE EFFECTS

CNS: Headache, dizziness, fainting
CV: Hypertension, chest pain
EENT: Tinnitus
GI: Nausea, vomiting, diarrhea
GU: Cramping
INTEG: Sweating
RESP: Dyspnea

Contraindications: Hypersensitivity to ergot medication, augmentation of labor, before delivery of placenta, spontaneous abortion (threatened), PID

Precautions: Renal/hepatic/cardiac disease, asthma, anemia, seizure disorders, hypertension, glaucoma, obliterative vascular disease

PHARMACOKINETICS

IM: Onset 2-5 min, duration 3 hr
IV: Onset immediate, duration 45 min
Metabolized in liver, excreted in urine

⚠ Safety alert *"Tall Man" lettering

INTERACTIONS
• Hypertension: sympathomimetics, ergots
Drug/Herb
Increase: serotonin effect—horehound

NURSING CONSIDERATIONS
Assess:
• Ergotism: nausea, vomiting, weakness, muscular pain, insensitivity to cold, paresthesias of extremities; drug should be discontinued
• B/P, pulse; watch for change that may indicate hemorrhage
• Respiratory rate, rhythm, depth; notify prescriber of abnormalities
• Fundal tone, nonphasic contractions; check for relaxation
Administer:
• IM inj deep in large muscle mass; rotate inj sites if additional doses are given
• With emergency equipment available
IV, direct route
• Dilute with 5 ml 0.9% NaCl, give through Y-tube or 3-way stopcock over 1 min
Additive compatibilities: Amikacin, cephapirin, sodium bicarbonate
Evaluate:
• Therapeutic response: decreased blood loss, severe cramping
Teach patient/family:
• To report increased blood loss, increased temp, or foul-smelling lochia; that cramping is normal
• The importance of pad count
• To avoid nicotine products
Treatment of overdose: Stop drug, give vasodilators, heparin, dextran

ergotamine (R)
(er-got′a-meen)
Ergomar ✦, Ergostat, Gynergen ✦
dihydroergotamine
(dye-hye-droe-er-got′a-meen)
DHE45, Dihydroergotamine-Sandoz ✦, Migranal
Func. class.: α-Adrenergic blocker, vascular headache suppressant
Chem. class.: Ergot alkaloid—amino acid

Action: Constricts smooth muscle in peripheral, cranial blood vessels, relaxes uterine muscle; blocks serotonin release
Uses: Vascular headache (migraine, cluster histamine)

DOSAGE AND ROUTES
Ergotamine
• *Adult:* **SL** 1 tab (2 mg), may use q30min, max 3 tabs (6 mg)/24 hr or 10 mg/wk
Dihydroergotamine
• *Adult:* **SUBCUT/IM** 1 mg, may repeat in 1 hr to 3 mg, max 3 mg/day or 6 mg/wk; **IV** 0.5-1 mg, may repeat in 1 hr, max 2 mg/day or 6 mg/wk; **INTRANASAL** 1 spray in each nostril, repeat in 15 min, max 3 mg/24 hr, 4 mg/wk
• *Child ≥6 yr:* **SUBCUT/IM** 0.5 mg, may repeat in 1 hr; **IV:** 0.25 mg, may repeat in 1 hr
Severe acute migraine
• *Child 12-16 yr:* **IV** 0.25-0.5 mg, may repeat q20min for 1-2 doses
Available forms: *Ergotamine:* SL tabs 2 mg; tabs 1 mg; *dihydroergotamine:* inj 1 mg/ml; nasal spray 4 mg/ml

SIDE EFFECTS
CNS: Numbness in fingers, toes, headache, weakness
CV: Transient tachycardia, chest pain, bradycardia, edema, claudication, increase or decrease in B/P, **MI**, peripheral vascular ischemia

GI: Nausea, vomiting, diarrhea, abdominal cramps
MS: Muscle pain

Contraindications: Pregnancy (X), hypersensitivity to ergot preparations, occlusion (peripheral, vascular), coronary artery disease, renal/hepatic disease, peptic ulcer, hypertension, Raynaud's disease, peripheral vascular disease, intermittent claudication, glaucoma, angina, CVA

Precautions: Lactation, children, anemia, geriatric, basilar/hemiplagic migraine

PHARMACOKINETICS

IM/SUBCUT: Peak (IM) 15-30 min, (SUBCUT) 30-60 min; duration (IM) 3-4 hr, (SUBCUT) 8 hr
IV: Peak 3 min, duration 8 hr
PO: Peak 30 min-3 hr; duration up to 48 hr; metabolized in liver; excreted as metabolites in feces; crosses blood-brain barrier; excreted in breast milk; protein binding 90%-93%; half-life 2 hr

INTERACTIONS

Increase: toxicity—CYP4503A4 inhibitors (protease inhibitors, some macrolides, azole antifungals); do not use together
Increase: vasoconstriction—β-blockers, oral contraceptives, nicotine, vasoconstrictors, other migraine agents
Drug/Herb
Increase: serotonin effect—horehound

NURSING CONSIDERATIONS

Assess:
• Migraine characteristics: duration, nausea, vomiting, change in vision, frequency before and at least 1 hr after administration
• Ergotism: nausea, vomiting, weakness, muscular pain, insensitivity to cold, paresthesia of extremities; drug should be discontinued
• Toxicity: dyspnea, hypotension or hypertension, rapid, weak pulse, delirium, nausea, vomiting

Administer:
• At beginning of headache; dose must be titrated to patient response
• Not to pregnant women; harm to fetus may occur
Intranasal route
• Prime nasal sprayer 4 × before dose, use 1 spray in each nostril, wait 15 min, use another spray in each nostril, use nasal applicator for 4 treatments only, discard
IV route
• Give dihydroergotamine undiluted over 1 min
Perform/provide:
• Quiet, calm environment with decreased stimulation for noise, bright light, or excessive talking
Evaluate:
• Therapeutic response: decrease in frequency, severity of headache
Teach patient/family:
• Not to use OTC medications; serious drug interactions may occur
• To maintain dose at approved level; not to increase even if drug does not relieve headache
• To report side effects including increased vasoconstriction starting with cold extremities, then paresthesia, weakness
• That an increase in headaches may occur when this drug is discontinued after long-term use
⚠ To keep drug out of reach of children; death may occur
Treatment of overdose: Induce emesis or gastric lavage if orally ingested; administer saline cathartic; keep warm

---

erlotinib (℞)
(er-loe′tye-nib)
Tarceva
Func. class.: Antineoplastic—miscellaneous
Chem. class.: Epidermal growth factor receptor inhibitor

Action: Not fully understood; inhibits intracellular phosphorylation of cell surface receptors associated with epidermal growth factor receptors

Uses: Non–small cell lung cancer (NSCLC), pancreatic cancer

Unlabeled uses: Squamous cell head and neck cancer

DOSAGE AND ROUTES

Non–small cell lung cancer (NSCLC)
• *Adult:* **PO** 150 mg daily

Pancreatic cancer
• *Adult:* **PO** 100 mg

CYP3A4 inducers concurrently (such as rifampin or phenytoin)
• Dosage increase is advised

CYP3A4 inhibitors (atazanavir, clarithromycin, indinavir, itraconazole, ketoconazole, telithromycin, ritonavir, saquinavir, troleandomycin, nelfinavir)
• Dosage reduction may be needed

Available forms: Tabs 25, 100, 150 mg

SIDE EFFECTS

GI: Nausea, diarrhea, vomiting, anorexia, mouth ulceration
INTEG: Rash
MISC: Conjunctivitis, eye pain, fatigue, infection
RESP: **Interstitial lung disease,** *cough, dyspnea*

Pancreatic cancer
CNS: **CVA,** *anxiety, depression, headache, rigors*
CV: **MI/ischemia**
GI: Nausea, diarrhea, vomiting, anorexia, mouth ulceration
HEMA: **Deep vein thrombosis (DVT)**
INTEG: Rash
MISC: Conjunctivitis, eye pain, fatigue, infection
RESP: **Interstitial lung disease,** *cough, dyspnea*

Contraindications: Pregnancy (D), lactation, hypersensitivity
Precautions: Renal/hepatic/ocular/pulmonary disorders, children, geriatric

PHARMACOKINETICS

Slowly absorbed (60%); peak 3-7 hr; excreted in feces (86%), urine (<4%); metabolized by CYP3A4; terminal half-life 36 hours; protein binding 93%

INTERACTIONS

Increase: erlotinib concentrations—CYP3A4 inhibitors (ketoconazole, itraconazole, erythromycin, clarithromycin, telithromycin)
Increase: plasma concentration of warfarin, metoprolol
Decrease: erlotinib levels—CYP3A4 inducers (phenytoin, rifampin, carbamazepine, phenobarbital)

Drug/Herb
Decrease: erlotinib levels—St. John's wort

NURSING CONSIDERATIONS
Assess:
• For MI/ischemia, CVA in pancreatic cancer patients
⚠ Pulmonary changes: lung sounds, cough, dyspnea; interstitial lung disease may occur, may be fatal; discontinue therapy if confirmed
• Ocular changes: eye irritation, corneal erosion/ulcer, aberrant eyelash growth
• GI symptoms: frequency of stools; if diarrhea is poorly tolerated, therapy may be discontinued for up to 14 days

Administer:
• 1 hr before or 2 hr after food

Evaluate:
• Therapeutic response: decrease non–small cell lung cancer cells, pancreatic cancer cells

Teach patient/family:
⚠ To report adverse reactions immediately: shortness of breath, severe abdominal pain, persistent diarrhea or vomiting, ocular changes, skin eruptions
• Reason for treatment, expected results
• Use reliable contraception during treatment, pregnancy (D), avoid breastfeeding

---

Side effects: *italics* = common; **bold** = life-threatening

ertapenem (R)
(er-tah-pen'em)
Invanz
Func. class.: Antiinfective—
miscellaneous
Chem. class.: Carbapenem

Do not confuse:
Invanz/Avinza

Action: Interferes with cell wall replication of susceptible organisms; osmotically unstable cell wall swells, bursts from osmotic pressure

Uses: Adult patients with moderate to severe infections caused by the following organisms: intraabdominal infections—*Escherichia coli, Clostridium clostridioforme, Eubacterium lentum, Peptostreptococcus* sp., *Bacteroides fragilis, Bacteroides distasonis, Bacteroides ovatus, Bacteroides thetaiotaomicron, Bacteroides uniformis;* complicated skin/skin structure infections—*Staphylococcus aureus* (methicillin-susceptible), *Streptococcus pyogenes, E. coli, Peptostreptococcus* sp.; community-acquired pneumonia—*Streptococcus pneumoniae* (penicillin-susceptible), *Haemophilus influenzae* (β-lactamase–negative), *Moraxella catarrhalis;* complicated UTI—*E. coli, Klebsiella pneumoniae;* acute pelvic infections—*Streptococcus agalactiae, E. coli, B. fragilis, Porphyromonas asaccharolytica, Peptostreptococcus* sp., *Prevotella bivia*

DOSAGE AND ROUTES
Complicated intraabdominal infections
• *Adult:* **IV/IM** 1 g daily × 5-14 days
• *Child 3 mo-12 yr:* **IV/IM** 15 mg/kg bid × 5-14 days
Complicated skin/skin structure infections
• *Adult:* **IV/IM** 1 g daily × 7-14 days
• *Child 3 mo-12 yr:* **IV/IM** 15 mg/kg bid × 7-14 days
Community-acquired pneumonia
• *Adult:* **IV/IM** 1 g daily × 10-14 days
• *Child 3 mo-12 yr:* **IV/IM** 15 mg/kg bid 10-14 days
Complicated UTI
• *Adult:* **IV/IM** 1 g daily × 10-14 days
• *Child 3 mo-12 yr:* **IV/IM** 15 mg/kg bid 10-14 days
Acute pelvic infections
• *Adult:* **IV/IM** 1 g daily × 3-10 days
• *Child 3 mo-12 yr:* **IV/IM** 15 mg/kg bid 3-10 days

Available form: Powder, lyophilized, 1 g

SIDE EFFECTS
CNS: Insomnia, **seizures**, dizziness, *headache*
CV: **Tachycardia**
GI: Diarrhea, nausea, vomiting, **pseudomembranous colitis**
GU: Vaginitis
INTEG: Rash, urticaria, *pruritus,* pain at inj site, *infused vein complication, phlebitis/thrombophlebitis,* erythema at inj site
RESP: Dyspnea, cough, pharyngitis, crackles, respiratory distress
SYST: **Anaphylaxis**

Contraindications: Hypersensitivity to this drug or its components, to amide-type local anesthetics (IM only); anaphylactic reactions to β-lactams
Precautions: Pregnancy (B), lactation, geriatric, children, renal/hepatic/GI disease

PHARMACOKINETICS
IV: Onset immediate, peak dose dependent, half-life 4 hr, metabolized by liver, excreted in urine, feces, breast milk

INTERACTIONS
Increase: ertapenem levels—probenecid; do not coadminister
Drug/Herb
• Do not use acidophilus with antiinfectives; separate by several hours
Drug/Lab Test
Increase: Hepatic enzymes

NURSING CONSIDERATIONS
Assess:
- Sensitivity to carbapenem antibiotics, other β-lactam antibiotics, penicillins
- Renal disease: lower dose may be required
- Bowel pattern daily: if severe diarrhea occurs, drug should be discontinued; may indicate pseudomembranous colitis
- For infection: temp, sputum, characteristics of wound before, during, after treatment
- ⚠ Allergic reactions, anaphylaxis; rash, urticaria, pruritus; may occur a few days after therapy begins
- Overgrowth of infection: perineal itching, fever, malaise, redness, pain, swelling, drainage, rash, diarrhea, change in cough or sputum

Administer:
- By IV or IM
- After C&S is taken

IM route
- Reconstitute 1 g vial of ertapenem with 3.2 ml of 1% lidocaine HCl without epINEPHrine, shake well
- Withdraw contents, administer deep IM in large muscle mass, use within 1 hr

IV route
- Do not confuse or mix with other medications; do not use diluents containing dextrose
- Reconstitute 1 g vial of ertapenem with either 10 ml of water for inj, 0.9% NaCl, or bacteriostatic water for inj
- Shake well to dissolve, transfer contents of reconstituted vial to 50 ml 0.9% NaCl inj
- Complete inf within 6 hr

Evaluate:
- Therapeutic response: negative C&S, absence of signs and symptoms of infection

Teach patient/family:
- To report severe diarrhea; may indicate pseudomembranous colitis
- To report overgrowth of infection: black, furry tongue, vaginal itching, foul-smelling stools
- To avoid breastfeeding; drug is excreted in breast milk

Treatment of overdose: EpINEPHrine, antihistamines; resuscitate if needed (anaphylaxis)

---

erythromycin base (℞)
(eh-rith-roh-my′sin)
Apo-Erythro ✤, E-Mycin, Eramycin, Erybid ✤, Eryc, Ery-Tab, E-Base, Erythromid ✤, Erythromycin Base Filmtab, Erythromycin Delayed-Release, Novo-Rythro Encap ✤, PCE

erythromycin estolate (℞)
Ilosone, Novo-Rythro ✤

erythromycin ethylsuccinate (℞)
Apo-Erythro-Es ✤, E.E.S., Ery Ped, Novo-Rythro ✤

erythromycin gluceptate (℞)

erythromycin lactobionate (℞)
Erythrocin

erythromycin stearate (℞)
Apo-Erythro-S ✤, Novo-Rythro ✤

Func. class.: Antiinfective
Chem. class.: Macrolide

Do not confuse:
erythromycin/azithromycin

Action: Binds to 50S ribosomal subunits of susceptible bacteria and suppresses protein synthesis

Uses: Infections caused by *Neisseria gonorrhoeae;* mild to moderate respiratory tract, skin, soft tissue infections caused by *Bordetella pertussis, Borrelia burgdorferi, Chlamydia trachomatis; Corynebacterium diphtheriae, Haemophilus influenzae* (when used with sulfonamides); *Legionella pneumophila,* Legionnaire's disease, *Listeria monocy-*

Side effects: *italics* = common; **bold** = life-threatening

togenes; *Mycoplasma pneumoniae,
Streptococcus pneumoniae,* syphilis:
Treponema pallidum

DOSAGE AND ROUTES
Soft tissue infections
• *Adult:* **PO** 250-500 mg q6h (base, estolate, stearate); **PO** 400-800 mg q6h
(ethylsuccinate); **IV INF** 15-20 mg/kg/
day (lactobionate) divided q6h
• *Child:* **PO** 30-50 mg/kg/day in divided
doses q6h (salts); **IV** 20-40 mg/kg/day
in divided doses q6h (lactobionate), max
adult dose
Neisseria gonorrhoeae/PID
• *Adult:* **IV** 500 mg q6h × 3 days (gluceptate, lactobionate), then **PO** 250 mg
(base, estolate, stearate) or 400 mg (ethylsuccinate) q6h × 1 wk
Syphilis
• *Adult:* **PO** 500 mg qid × 14 days
Chlamydia
• *Adult:* **PO** 500 mg q6h × 1 wk or 250
mg qid × 2 wk
• *Infant:* **PO** 50 mg/kg/day in 4 divided
doses × 3 wk or more
• *Newborn:* **PO** 50 mg/kg/day in 4 divided doses × 2 wk or more
Intestinal amebiasis
• *Adult:* **PO** 250 mg q6h × 10-14 days
(base, estolate, stearate)
• *Child:* **PO** 30-50 mg/kg/day in divided
doses q6h × 10-14 days (base, estolate,
stearate)
Available forms: *Base:* enteric-coated
tabs 250, 333, 500 mg; film-coated tabs
250, 500 mg; enteric-coated caps 250,
333 mg; *estolate:* tabs 500 mg; caps 125,
250 mg; drops 100 mg/ml; susp 125, 250
mg/5 ml; *stearate:* film-coated tabs 250
mg; *ethylsuccinate:* chewable tabs 200
mg; susp 100 mg/2.5 ml, 200, 400 mg/5
ml; powder for inj 500 mg and 1 g (lactobionate), 1 g (as gluceptate)

SIDE EFFECTS
CV: **Dysrhythmias,** QT prolongation
EENT: Hearing loss, tinnitus
GI: Nausea, vomiting, diarrhea, **hepato-
toxicity,** abdominal pain, stomatitis,

heartburn, anorexia, pruritus ani,
pseudomembranous colitis
GU: Vaginitis, moniliasis
INTEG: Rash, urticaria, pruritus, thrombophlebitis (IV site)
SYST: **Anaphylaxis**
Contraindications: Hypersensitivity,
preexisting hepatic disease (estolate), hepatic disease
Precautions: Pregnancy (B), hepatic
disease, lactation, GI disease, QT prolongation, seizure disorder, geriatric

PHARMACOKINETICS
Peak 4 hr (base), ½–2½ hr (ethylsuccinate); duration 6 hr; half-life 1-2 hr;
metabolized in liver; excreted in bile,
feces; protein binding 75%-90%

INTERACTIONS
⚠ Serious dysrhythmias—diltiazem, itraconazole, ketoconazole, nefazodone, pimozide, protease inhibitors, sparfloxacin,
verapamil
Increase: action, toxicity of alfentanil, al-
prazolam, bromocriptine, busPIRone, car-
bamazepine, cilostazol, clindamycin,
clozapine, cycloSPORINE, diazepam, di-
goxin, disopyramide, ergots, felodipine,
HMG-CoA reductase inhibitors, methyl-
PREDNISolone, midazolam, quinidine,
rifabutin, sildenafil, tacrolimus, tadalafil,
theophylline, triazolam, vardenafil, vin-
BLAStine, warfarin
Drug/Herb
• Do not use acidophilus with antiinfec-
tives; separate by several hours
Drug/Lab Test
Increase: AST/ALT
Decrease: folate assay
False increase: 17-OHCS/17-KS

NURSING CONSIDERATIONS
Assess:
• For infection: temp, characteristics of
wounds, urine, stools, sputum, WBCs,
baseline and periodically
• I&O ratio; report hematuria, oliguria
in renal disease

⚠ Safety alert   *"Tall Man" lettering

- Hepatic studies: AST, ALT, if patient is on long-term therapy
- Renal studies: urinalysis, protein, blood
- C&S before drug therapy; drug may be given as soon as culture is taken; C&S may be repeated after treatment
- Bowel pattern before, during treatment
- Skin eruptions, itching
- Respiratory status: rate, character, wheezing, tightness in chest; discontinue drug if these occur
- Allergies before treatment, reaction of each medication

Administer:
- Do not break, crush, or chew time-rel cap or tab; chew only chewable tabs
- Do not give by IM or IV push
- Enteric-coated tablets may be given with food
- Oral drug with full glass of water; do not give with fruit juice
- Oral drug with food for GI symptoms

IV route
- After diluting 500 mg or less/10 ml sterile H$_2$O without preservatives; dilute further in 80-250 ml of 0.9% NaCl, LR, Normosol-R; may be further diluted to 1 mg/ml and given as cont inf; run 1 g or less/100 ml over ½-1 hr; cont inf over 6 hr, may require buffers to neutralize pH if dilution is <250 ml, use inf pump

Additive compatibilities:
Gluceptate: Calcium gluconate, hydrocortisone, methicillin, penicillin G potassium, potassium chloride, sodium bicarbonate
Lactobionate: Aminophylline, ampicillin, cimetidine, diphenhydrAMINE, hydrocortisone, lidocaine, methicillin, penicillin G potassium or sodium, pentobarbital, polymyxin B, potassium chloride, prednisoLONE, prochlorperazine, promazine, ranitidine, sodium bicarbonate, verapamil

Syringe compatibilities:
Lactobionate: Methicillin
Y-site compatibilities: Acyclovir, amiodarone, cyclophosphamide, diltiazem, enalaprilat, esmolol, famotidine, foscarnet, heparin, hydromorphone, idarubicin, labetalol, lorazepam, magnesium sulfate, meperidine, midazolam, morphine, multivitamins, perphenazine, tacrolimus, theophylline, vit B/C, zidovudine

Perform/provide:
- Storage at room temperature; store susp in refrigerator
- Adequate intake of fluids (2 L) during diarrhea episodes

Evaluate:
- Therapeutic response: decreased symptoms of infection

Teach patient/family:
- To report sore throat, fever, fatigue (could indicate superinfection)
- To notify nurse of diarrhea stools, dark urine, pale stools, jaundice of eyes or skin, and severe abdominal pain
- To take at evenly spaced intervals; complete dosage regimen; take without food unless formulation

Treatment of hypersensitivity: Withdraw drug; maintain airway; administer epINEPHrine, aminophylline, O$_2$, IV corticosteroids

erythromycin ophthalmic
See Appendix C

erythromycin topical
See Appendix C

escitalopram (℞)
(es-sit-tal'oh-pram)
Lexapro
Func. class.: Antidepressant, SSRI (selective serotonin reuptake inhibitor)

Action: Inhibits CNS neuron uptake of serotonin but not of norepinephrine
Uses: General anxiety disorder, major depressive disorder
Unlabeled uses: Panic disorder

DOSAGE AND ROUTES

• *Adult:* **PO** 10 mg daily in AM or PM; after 1 wk if no clinical improvement is noted, dose may be increased to 20 mg daily PM; maintenance 10-20 mg/day, reassess to determine need for treatment
Hepatic dose/geriatric
• *Adult:* **PO** 10 mg/day
Available forms: Tabs 5, 10, 20 mg; oral sol 5 mg (as base)/5 ml

SIDE EFFECTS

CNS: Headache, nervousness, insomnia, drowsiness, anxiety, tremor, dizziness, fatigue, sedation, poor concentration, abnormal dreams, agitation, **seizures,** apathy, euphoria, hallucinations, delusions, psychosis
CV: Hot flashes, palpitations, angina pectoris, **hemorrhage,** hypertension, **tachycardia,** 1st-degree AV block, **bradycardia, MI, thrombophlebitis,** postural hypotension
EENT: Visual changes, ear/eye pain, photophobia, tinnitus
GI: Nausea, diarrhea, dry mouth, anorexia, dyspepsia, constipation, cramps, vomiting, taste changes, flatulence, decreased appetite
GU: Dysmenorrhea, decreased libido, urinary frequency, UTI, amenorrhea, cystitis, impotence, urine retention
INTEG: Sweating, rash, pruritus, acne, alopecia, urticaria, photosensitivity
MS: Pain, arthritis, twitching
RESP: Infection, pharyngitis, nasal congestion, sinus headache, sinusitis, cough, dyspnea, bronchitis, asthma, hyperventilation, pneumonia
SYST: Asthenia, viral infection, fever, allergy, chills
Contraindications: Hypersensitivity
Precautions: Pregnancy (C), lactation, children, geriatric, renal disease, history of seizures

PHARMACOKINETICS

PO: Metabolized in liver; excreted in urine

INTERACTIONS

• Paradoxical worsening of OCD: busPIRone
• Serotonin syndrome: tryptophan, amphetamines, antidepressants, busPIRone, lithium, amantadine, bromocriptine
⚠ Do not use MAOIs with or 14 days before escitalopram
Increase: CNS depression—alcohol, antidepressants, opioids, sedatives
Increase: side effects of escitalopram—highly protein-bound drugs
Increase: effect—haloperidol
Increase: half-life of diazepam
Increase: levels or toxicity of carbamazepine, lithium, warfarin, phenytoin
Increase: levels of tricyclics, phenothiazines
Decrease: escitalopram effect—cyproheptadine
Drug/Herb
• SAM-e, St. John's wort: do not use together
Increase: anticholinergic effect—corkwood, jimsonweed
Increase: CNS effect—hops, kava, lavender
Increase: hypertension—yohimbe
Drug/Lab Test
Increase: Serum bilirubin, blood glucose, alk phos
Decrease: VMA, 5-HIAA
False increase: Urinary catecholamines

NURSING CONSIDERATIONS
Assess:
• Mental status: mood, sensorium, affect, suicidal tendencies, increase in psychiatric symptoms, depression, panic
• Appetite in bulimia nervosa, weight daily, increase nutritious foods in diet, watch for bingeing and vomiting
• Allergic reactions: itching, rash urticaria, drug should be discontinued, may need to give antihistamine
• B/P (lying/standing), pulse q4h; if systolic B/P drops 20 mm Hg, hold drug, notify prescriber; take VS q4h in patients with cardiovascular disease
• Blood studies: CBC, leukocytes, differ-

ential, cardiac enzymes if patient is receiving long-term therapy; check platelets; bleeding can occur

• Hepatic studies: AST, ALT, bilirubin, creatinine

• Weight qwk; appetite may decrease with drug

• ECG for flattening of T wave, bundle branch, AV block, dysrhythmias in cardiac patients

• Alcohol consumption; if alcohol is consumed, hold dose until AM

Administer:

• With food or milk for GI symptoms

• Crushed if patient is unable to swallow medication whole

• Dosage at bedtime if oversedation occurs during the day

• Gum, hard candy, frequent sips of water for dry mouth

Perform/provide:

• Storage at room temperature; do not freeze

• Assistance with ambulation during therapy, since drowsiness, dizziness occur

• Safety measures primarily in geriatric

• Checking to see if PO medication swallowed

Evaluate:

• Therapeutic response: decreased depression

Teach patient/family:

• That therapeutic effect may take 1-4 wk

• To use caution in driving, other activities requiring alertness because of drowsiness, dizziness, blurred vision

• To use sunscreen to prevent photosensitivity

• To avoid alcohol ingestion, other CNS depressants

• To notify prescriber if pregnant or plan to become pregnant or breastfeed

• To change positions slowly, orthostatic hypotension may occur

• To avoid all OTC drugs unless approved by prescriber

• To report immediately signs of urinary retention

---

esmolol (℞)

(ez'moe-lole)
Brevibloc
Func. class.: β-Adrenergic blocker (antidysrhythmic II)

Do not confuse:
esmolol/Osmitrol
Brevibloc/Brevital

Action: Competitively blocks stimulation of β_1-adrenergic receptors in the myocardium; produces negative chronotropic, inotropic activity (decreases rate of SA node discharge, increases recovery time), slows conduction of AV node, decreases heart rate, decreases O_2 consumption in myocardium; also decreases renin-aldosterone-angiotensin system at high doses; inhibits β_2-receptors in bronchial system at higher doses

Uses: Supraventricular tachycardia, noncompensatory sinus tachycardia, hypertensive crisis, intraoperative and postoperative tachycardia and hypertension

DOSAGE AND ROUTES

• *Adult:* **IV** loading dose 500 mcg/kg/min over 1 min; maintenance 50 mcg/kg/min for 4 min; if no response in 5 min, give 2nd loading dose; then increase inf to 100 mcg/kg/min for 4 min; if no response, repeat loading dose, then increase maintenance inf by 50 mcg/kg/min (max of 200 mcg/kg/min), titrate to patient response

• *Child:* **IV** 50 mcg/kg/min, may increase q10min (max 300 mcg/kg/min)

Available forms: Inj 10 mg, 250 mg/ml

SIDE EFFECTS

CNS: Confusion, light-headedness, paresthesia, somnolence, fever, dizziness, fatigue, headache, depression, anxiety, **seizures**

CV: Hypotension, bradycardia, chest pain, peripheral ischemia, shortness of breath, **CHF**, conduction disturbances, 1st-, 2nd-, 3rd-degree heart block

---

Side effects: *italics* = common; **bold** = life-threatening

GI: Nausea, vomiting, anorexia, gastric pain, flatulence, constipation, heartburn, bloating

GU: Urinary retention, impotence, dysuria

INTEG: Induration, inflammation at site, discoloration, edema, erythema, burning pallor, flushing, rash, pruritus, dry skin, alopecia

RESP: **Bronchospasm,** dyspnea, cough, wheeziness, nasal stuffiness

Contraindications: 2nd- or 3rd-degree heart block, cardiogenic shock, CHF, cardiac failure, hypersensitivity

Precautions: Pregnancy (C), hypotension, peripheral vascular disease, diabetes, hypoglycemia, thyrotoxicosis, renal disease, lactation

PHARMACOKINETICS

Onset very rapid, duration short, half-life 9 min; metabolized by hydrolysis of the ester linkage; excreted via kidneys

INTERACTIONS

• Avoid use with MAOIs

Increase: digoxin levels—digoxin

Increase: α-adrenergic stimulation—epHEDrine, epINEPHrine, amphetamine, norepinephrine, phenylephrine, pseudoephedrine

Decrease: action of thyroid hormones

Decrease: action of esmolol—thyroid hormone

Drug/Herb

• Potassium deficiency: aloe, buckthorn, cascara sagrada, senna

Increase: β-blocking effect—betel palm, butterbur, cola tree, figwort, fumitory, guarana, hawthorn, lily of the valley, motherwort, plantain

Increase: CV reactions—jaborandi tree

Decrease: β-blocking effect—coenzyme Q10, yohimbe

Drug/Lab Test

Interference: Glucose/insulin tolerance test

NURSING CONSIDERATIONS
Assess:
• I&O ratio, weight daily, watch for signs of CHF (jugular vein distention, weight gain, crackles, edema)
• B/P, pulse q4h; note rate, rhythm, quality; rapid changes can cause shock; if systolic <100 or diastolic <60, notify prescriber before giving drug
• ECG continuously during inf, hypotension is common
• Baselines in renal, hepatic studies before therapy begins
• Breath sounds and respiratory pattern: wheezing from bronchospasm

Administer:
• Reduced dosage in cool environment, not to discontinue drug suddenly
IV route
• IV diluted 5 g/20 ml of D_5W, D_5R, D_5 0.9% NaCl, 0.45% NaCl, LR, D_5 0.45% NaCl, 0.9% NaCl further dilute in the remaining 480 ml (10 mg/ml) and give as infusion; give loading dose over 1 min, then maintenance over 4 min; may repeat loading dose q5min with increased maintenance dose; maintenance dose should not be >200 mcg/kg/min and be given up to 48 hr; dose should be tapered at 25 mcg/kg/min; use infusion pump

Additive compatibilities: Aminophylline, atracurium, bretylium, heparin

Y-site compatibilities: Amikacin, aminophylline, amiodarone, ampicillin, atracurium, butorphanol, calcium chloride, cefazolin, cefoperazone, ceftazidime, ceftizoxime, chloramphenicol, cimetidine, cisatracurium, clindamycin, diltiazem, DOPamine, enalaprilat, erythromycin, famotidine, fentanyl, gentamicin, heparin, hydrocortisone, insulin (regular), labetalol, magnesium sulfate, methyldopate, metronidazole, midazolam, morphine, nafcillin, nitroglycerin, nitroprusside, norepinephrine, pancuronium, penicillin G potassium, phenytoin, piperacillin, polymyxin B, potassium chloride, potassium phosphate, propofol, ranitidine, remifentanil, streptomycin, tacrolimus, tobramycin, trimethoprim-sulfamethoxazole, vancomycin, vecuronium

Perform/provide:
• Storage protected from light, moisture; in cool environment

Evaluate:
• Therapeutic response: lower B/P immediately, lower heart rate

Teach patient/family:
• To notify prescriber if pain, swelling occurs at IV site

Treatment of overdose: Discontinue drug

---

esomeprazole (Ŗ)
(es'oh-mep'rah-zohl)
Nexium
Func. class.: Antiulcer
Chem. class.: Proton pump inhibitor, benzimidazole

Action: Suppresses gastric secretion by inhibiting hydrogen/potassium ATPase enzyme system in gastric parietal cell; characterized as gastric acid pump inhibitor, because it blocks final step of acid production

Uses: Gastroesophageal reflux disease (GERD), severe erosive esophagitis; treatment of active duodenal ulcers in combination with antiinfectives for *Helicobacter pylori* infection

DOSAGE AND ROUTES

Active duodenal ulcers associated with H. pylori
• *Adult:* **PO** 40 mg daily × 10 days in combination with clarithromycin 500 mg bid × 10 days and amoxicillin 1000 mg bid × 10 days

GERD
• *Adult:* **PO** 20 or 40 mg daily × 4-8 wk; no adjustment needed in renal/liver failure, geriatric; **IV** 20 or 40 mg daily

Hepatic dose
• *Adult:* **PO/IV** max 20 mg daily (severe hepatic disease)

Available forms: Delayed rel caps 20, 40 mg; powder for IV inj 20, 40 mg/vial

SIDE EFFECTS

CNS: Headache, dizziness
GI: Diarrhea, flatulence, abdominal pain, constipation, dry mouth
INTEG: Rash, dry skin
MISC: Dizziness
RESP: Cough

Contraindications: Hypersensitivity
Precautions: Pregnancy (B), lactation, children, geriatric

PHARMACOKINETICS

Well absorbed 90%; protein binding 97%; extensively metabolized liver (CYP2C19); terminal half-life 1-1.5 hr; eliminated in urine as metabolites and in feces; in geriatric, elimination rate decreased, bioavailability increased

INTERACTIONS

Increase: effect, toxicity of diazepam, digoxin, penicillins
Decrease: effect—dapsone, iron, itraconazole, ketoconazole, indinavir, calcium carbonate, vitamin B_{12}

NURSING CONSIDERATIONS

Assess:
• GI system: bowel sounds q8h, abdomen for pain, swelling, anorexia
• Hepatic enzymes: AST, ALT, alk phos during treatment

Administer:
• Swallow caps whole; do not crush or chew; cap may be opened and sprinkled over tbsp of applesauce
• Same time daily, before or with a meal

IV, direct route
• Reconstitute each vial with 5 ml 0.9% NaCl, D_5W, LR; give over 3 min

Intermittent IV INF route
• Dilute reconstituted sol to 50 ml, give over 30 min, do not admix, flush line with D_5W, 0.9% NaCl, LR after infusion

Evaluate:
• Therapeutic response: absence of epigastric pain, swelling, fullness

---

Side effects: *italics* = common; **bold** = life-threatening

Teach patient/family:
• To report severe diarrhea, abdominal pain, black, tarry stools; drug may have to be discontinued
• That diabetic patient should know hypoglycemia may occur
• To avoid hazardous activities; dizziness may occur
• To avoid alcohol, salicylates, NSAIDs; may cause GI irritation

---

estradiol
(es-tra-dye′ole)
Estrace

estradiol cypionate
depGynogen, Depo-Estradiol, Depogen, Dura-Estrin, E-Cypionate, Estragyn LA5, Estro-Cyp, Estrofem, Estroject-LA, Estrol-L.A.

estradiol topical emulsion
Estrasorb

estradiol valerate
Clinigen LA, Delestrogen, Dioval, Duragen, Estra-L, Estro-span, Femogex ✿, Gynogen LA, Menaval, Valergen

estradiol transdermal system
Alora, Climara, Esclim, Estraderm, FemPatch, Vivelle

estradiol vaginal tablet
Vagifem

estradiol vaginal ring
Estring
Func. class.: Estrogen, progestins

Action: Needed for adequate functioning of female reproductive system; affects release of pituitary gonadotropins, inhibits ovulation, adequate calcium use in bone

Uses: Vasomotor symptoms (menopause), inoperable breast cancer (selected cases), prostatic cancer, atrophic vaginitis, kraurosis vulvae, hypogonadism, primary ovarian failure, prevention of osteoporosis

DOSAGE AND ROUTES

Hormone replacement
• *Adult:* TD 0.05-0.1 mg/24 hr, apply 2 ×/wk

Menopause/hypogonadism/castration/ovarian failure
• *Adult:* PO 1-2 mg daily, 3 wk on, 1 wk off or 5 days on, 2 days off; IM 1-5 mg q3-4wk (cypionate); 10-20 mg q4wk (valerate)
• *Adult:* TOP Estraderm 0.05 mg/24 hr applied 2 ×/wk Climara 0.05 mg/hr applied 1 ×/wk in a cyclic regimen; women with hysterectomy may use continuously

Prostatic cancer
• *Adult:* IM 30 mg q1-2wk (valerate); PO 1-2 mg tid (oral estradiol)

Breast cancer
• *Adult:* PO 10 mg tid × 3 mo or longer

Atropic vaginitis/kraurosis vulvae
• *Adult:* VAG CREAM 2-4 g daily × 1-2 wk, then 1 g 1-3 ×/wk cycled; vag tab 1 daily × 2 wk, maintenance 1 tab 2 ×/wk; VAG RING inserted and left in place continuously for 3 mo

Vasomotor symptoms
• *Adult:* TOP After cleaning and drying skin on left thigh, calf, rub in contents of pouch using both hands until completely absorbed; wash hands

Available forms: *Estradiol:* tabs 0.5, 1, 2 mg; *valerate:* inj 10, 20, 40 mg/ml; *transdermal:* 0.025, 0.0375, 0.05, 0.075, 0.1 mg/24 hr release rate; *vag cream:* 100 mcg/g; *vag tab:* 25 mcg; *vag ring:* 2 mg/90 days; *topical emulsion:* 2.5 mg

SIDE EFFECTS

CNS: Dizziness, headache, migraines, depression, **seizures**
CV: Hypotension, thrombophlebitis, edema, **thromboembolism, stroke, pulmonary embolism, myocardial infarction**
EENT: Contact lens intolerance, increased myopia, astigmatism

---

⚠ Safety alert   *"Tall Man" lettering

GI: Nausea, vomiting, diarrhea, anorexia, pancreatitis, cramps, constipation, increased appetite, increased weight, **cholestatic jaundice, hepatic adenoma**

GU: Amenorrhea, cervical erosion, breakthrough bleeding, dysmenorrhea, vaginal candidiasis, breast changes, *gynecomastia, testicular atrophy, impotence,* **increased risk of breast cancer, endometrial cancer,** changes in libido

INTEG: Rash, urticaria, acne, hirsutism, alopecia, oily skin, seborrhea, purpura, melasma

META: Folic acid deficiency, hypercalcemia, hyperglycemia

Contraindications: Pregnancy (X), breast cancer, thromboembolic disorders, reproductive cancer, genital bleeding (abnormal, undiagnosed), lactation

Precautions: Hypertension, asthma, blood dyscrasias, gallbladder disease, CHF, diabetes mellitus, bone disease, depression, migraine headache, seizure disorders, renal/hepatic disease, family history of cancer of breast or reproductive tract, smoking

PHARMACOKINETICS

PO/INJ/TD: Degraded in liver; excreted in urine; crosses placenta; excreted in breast milk

INTERACTIONS

Increase: action of corticosteroids

Increase: toxicity—cycloSPORINE, dantrolene

Decrease: action of anticoagulants, oral hypoglycemics, tamoxifen

Decrease: estradiol action—anticonvulsants, barbiturates, phenylbutazone, rifampin, calcium

Drug/Herb

• Altered estrogen effect: black cohosh, DHEA

Increase: estrogen effect—alfalfa, hops

Decrease: estrogen effect—saw palmetto

Drug/Food

Increase: estrogen level—grapefruit juice

Drug/Lab Test

Increase: BSP retention test, PBI, T_4, serum sodium, platelet aggregation, thyroxine-binding globulin (TBG), prothrombin, factors VII, VIII, IX, X, triglycerides

Decrease: Serum folate, serum triglyceride, T_3 resin uptake test, glucose tolerance test, antithrombin III, pregnanediol, metyrapone test

False positive: LE prep, ANA

NURSING CONSIDERATIONS

Assess:

• Blood glucose of diabetic patient, hyperglycemia may occur

• Weight daily, notify prescriber of weekly weight gain >5 lb; if increase, diuretic may be ordered

• B/P q4h, watch for increase caused by H_2O and sodium retention

• I&O ratio; decreasing urinary output, increasing edema, report changes

• Hepatic studies, including AST, ALT, bilirubin, alk phos baseline, periodically

• Hypertension, cardiac symptoms, jaundice, hypercalcemia

• Mental status: affect, mood, behavioral changes, aggression

• Female patient for intact uterus, if so, progesterone should be added to estrogen therapy to decrease risk of endometrial cancer

Administer:

• Titrated dose; use lowest effective dose

• IM inj deeply in large muscle mass

PO route

• With food or milk to decrease GI symptoms

Transdermal route

• Apply to trunk of body 2 ×/wk; press firmly and hold in place for 10 sec to ensure good contact

• On intermittent cycle schedule: 3 wk on, then 1 wk off; if patch falls off, reapply

Vaginal route

• Use applicator provided

Evaluate:

• Therapeutic response: reversal of menopause symptoms or decrease in tumor size in prostatic, breast cancer

Teach patient/family:

• To weigh weekly, report gain >5 lb

⚠ To report breast lumps, vaginal bleeding, edema, jaundice, dark urine, clay-colored stools, dyspnea, headache, blurred vision, abdominal pain, numbness or stiffness in legs, chest pain, tenderness, redness, and swelling in extremities; male to report impotence or gynecomastia

---

Rarely Used

estramustine
(ess-tra-muss'teen)
Emcyt
Func. class.: Antineoplastic

Uses: Metastatic prostate cancer

DOSAGE AND ROUTES

• *Adult:* **PO** 10-16 mg/kg in 3-4 divided doses/day; treatment may continue for ≥3 mo or 600 mg/m^2/day in 3 divided doses

Contraindications: Pregnancy (D), hypersensitivity to estradiol, thromboembolic disorders

---

estrogens, conjugated
Cenestin, C.E.S. ♣, Congest, Premarin

estrogens, conjugated synthetic B
Enjuvia
Func. class.: Estrogen, hormone

Do not confuse:

Premarin/Provera

Action: Needed for adequate functioning of female reproductive system; affects release of pituitary gonadotropins, inhibits ovulation, adequate calcium use in bone

Uses: Vasomotor symptoms (menopause), inoperable breast cancer, prostatic cancer, abnormal uterine bleeding,

hypogonadism, primary ovarian failure, prevention of osteoporosis

DOSAGE AND ROUTES

Estrogens conjugated

Vasomotor symptoms (menopause)
• *Adult:* **PO** 0.3-1.25 mg daily 3 wk on, 1 wk off

Prevention of osteoporosis
• *Adult:* **PO** 0.625 mg daily or in cycle

Atrophic vaginitis
• *Adult:* **VAG CREAM** 2-4 g daily × 21 days, off 7 days, repeat

Prostatic cancer
• *Adult:* **PO** 1.25-2.5 mg tid

Advanced inoperable breast cancer
• *Adult:* **PO** 10 mg tid × 3 mo or longer

Abnormal uterine bleeding
• *Adult:* **IV/IM** 25 mg, repeat in 6-12 hr

Castration/primary ovarian failure
• *Adult:* **PO** 1.25 mg daily, 3 wk on, 1 wk off

Hypogonadism
• *Adult:* **PO** 2.5 mg bid-tid × 20 days/mo

Estrogens conjugated synthetic B

Vasomotor symptoms (menopause)
• *Adult:* **PO** 0.625 mg daily initially; may increase based on response

Available forms: Tabs 0.3, 0.625, 0.9, 1.25, 2.5 mg; inj 25 mg/vial; vag cream 0.625 mg/g; *synthetic B:* tabs 0.625, 1.25 mg

SIDE EFFECTS

CNS: Dizziness, headache, migraine, depression, **seizures**

CV: Hypotension, thrombophlebitis, edema, **thromboembolism, stroke, pulmonary embolism, myocardial infarction**

EENT: Contact lens intolerance, increased myopia, astigmatism

GI: Nausea, vomiting, diarrhea, anorexia, pancreatitis, cramps, constipation, increased appetite, increased weight, **cholestatic jaundice, hepatic adenoma**

GU: Amenorrhea, cervical erosion, breakthrough bleeding, dysmenorrhea, vaginal candidiasis, breast changes, *gynecomastia, testicular atrophy, impotence,* in-

---

creased risk of breast cancer, endometrial cancer, libido changes

INTEG: Rash, urticaria, acne, hirsutism, alopecia, oily skin, seborrhea, purpura, melasma

META: Folic acid deficiency, hypercalcemia, hyperglycemia

Contraindications: Pregnancy (X), thromboembolic disorders, reproductive cancer, genital bleeding (abnormal, undiagnosed), lactation

Precautions: Hypertension, asthma, blood dyscrasias, gallbladder disease, CHF, diabetes mellitus, bone disease, depression, migraine headache, seizure disorders, hepatic disease, renal disease, family history of cancer of breast or reproductive tract, smoking

PHARMACOKINETICS

PO/IV/IM: Degraded in liver, excreted in urine, crosses placenta, excreted in breast milk

INTERACTIONS

Increase: toxicity—cycloSPORINE, dantrolene

Increase: action of corticosteroids

Decrease: action of estrogens—anticonvulsants, barbiturates, phenylbutazone, rifampin

Decrease: action of anticoagulants, oral hypoglycemics, tamoxifen

Drug/Herb

• Altered estrogen effect—black cohosh, DHEA

Increase: estrogen effect—alfalfa, hops

Decrease: estrogen effect—saw palmetto

Drug/Food

Increase: estrogen level—grapefruit juice

Drug/Lab Test

Increase: BSP retention test, PBI, T_4, serum sodium, platelet aggregation, thyroxine-binding globulin (TBG), prothrombin, factors VII, VIII, IX, X, triglycerides

Decrease: Serum folate, serum triglyceride, T_3 resin uptake test, glucose tolerance test, antithrombin III, pregnanediol, metyrapone test

False positive: LE prep, antinuclear antibodies

NURSING CONSIDERATIONS

Assess:

• Blood glucose if diabetic patient, hyperglycemia may occur

• Weight daily; notify prescriber of weekly weight gain >5 lb; if increase, diuretic may be ordered

• B/P q4h; watch for increase caused by H_2O and Na retention

• I&O ratio; be alert for decreasing urinary output, increasing edema

• Hepatic studies: AST, ALT, bilirubin, alk phos

• Hypertension, cardiac symptoms, jaundice, hypercalcemia

• Mental status: affect, mood, behavioral changes, aggression

• Female patient for intact uterus, if so, progesterone should be added to estrogen therapy to decrease risk of endometrial cancer

Administer:

• Titrated dose, use lowest effective dose

IM route

• IM reconstitute after withdrawing >5 ml of air from container and inject sterile diluent on vial side, rotate to dissolve; give inj deep in large muscle mass

• With food or milk to decrease GI symptoms (PO)

Vaginal route

• Use applicator provided

IV, direct route

• IV, after reconstituting as for IM, inject into distal port of running IV line of D_5W, 0.9% NaCl, LR at 5 mg/min or less

Y-site compatibilities: Heparin/hydrocortisone, potassium chloride, vit B/C

Evaluate:

• Therapeutic response: absence of breast engorgement, reversal of menopause symptoms, or decrease in tumor size in prostatic cancer

Teach patient/family:
• To avoid breastfeeding, since drug is excreted in breast milk
• To weigh weekly, report gain >5 lb
⚠ To report breast lumps, vaginal bleeding, edema, jaundice, dark urine, clay-colored stools, dyspnea, headache, blurred vision, abdominal pain, leg pain and redness, numbness or stiffness in legs, chest pain; male to report impotence or gynecomastia
• To avoid sunlight or wear sunscreen; burns may occur
• To notify prescriber if pregnancy is suspected

---

etanercept (R)
(eh-tan'er-sept)
Enbrel
Func. class.: Antirheumatic agent (disease modifying) (DMARDs)
Chem. class.: Anti-TNF agent

Action: Binds tumor necrosis factor (TNF), which is involved in immune and inflammatory reactions
Uses: Acute, chronic rheumatoid arthritis that has not responded to other disease-modifying agents, polyarticular course juvenile rheumatoid arthritis (JRA), ankylosing spondylitis, plaque psoriasis, psoriatic arthritis
Unlabeled uses: Crohn's disease

DOSAGE AND ROUTES
Rheumatoid/psoriatic arthritis, ankylosing spondylitis
• *Adult:* SUBCUT 50 mg qwk
• *Child 4-17 yr:* SUBCUT 0.8 mg/kg/wk, max 25 mg 1 dose
Plaque psoriasis
• *Adult:* SUBCUT 50 mg 2 ×/wk
Available forms: Powder for inj: 25 mg; inj 50 mg/ml

SIDE EFFECTS
CNS: Headache, asthenia, dizziness
GI: Abdominal pain, dyspepsia
HEMA: Pancytopenia
INTEG: Rash, *inj site reaction*

RESP: Pharyngitis, cough, URI, non-URI, sinusitis, *rhinitis*
SYST: **Serious infections, sepsis, death, malignancies**
Contraindications: Hypersensitivity, sepsis, active infections
Precautions: Pregnancy (B), lactation, children <4 yr, geriatric, malignancies, latex allergy

PHARMACOKINETICS
Elimination half-life 115 hr, 60% absorbed SUBCUT

INTERACTIONS
• Do not give concurrently with vaccines, immunizations should be brought up to date before treatment
• Avoid use with anakinra, cyclophosphamide

NURSING CONSIDERATIONS
Assess:
• Pain, stiffness, ROM, swelling of joints before, during and after treatment
• For inj site pain, swelling, usually occurs after 2 inj (4-5 days)
Administer:
• After reconstituting 1 ml of supplied diluent, slowly inject diluent into vial, swirl contents, do not shake, sol should be clear/colorless, do not use if cloudy or discolored
• Do not admix with other sol or medications, do not use filter
• May be injected SUBCUT into upper arm, abdomen, or thigh, rotate inj sites
Evaluate:
• Therapeutic response: decreased inflammation, pain in joints
Teach patient/family:
• That drug must be continued for prescribed time to be effective
• To use caution when driving; dizziness may occur
• Not to receive live vaccinations during treatment
• About self-administration if appropriate: inj should be made in thigh, abdo-

men, upper arm; rotate sites at least 1 in from old site
• To notify prescriber of possible infection (upper respiratory or other)

ethambutol (R)
(e-tham'byoo-tole)
Etibi ♣, Myambutol
Func. class.: Antitubercular
Chem. class.: Diisopropylethylene diamide derivative

Do not confuse:
ethambutol/Ethmozine
Action: Inhibits RNA synthesis, decreases tubercle bacilli replication
Uses: Pulmonary tuberculosis, as an adjunct, other mycobacterial infections

DOSAGE AND ROUTES
• *Adult and child >13 yr:* **PO** 15-25 mg/kg/day as a single dose or 50 mg/kg 2 ×/wk or 25-30 mg/kg 3 ×/wk
Renal disease
• CCr 10-50 ml/min dose q24-36h; CCr <10 ml/min dose q48h
Retreatment
• *Adult:* **PO** 25 mg/kg/day as single dose × 2 mo with at least 1 other drug, then decrease to 15 mg/kg/day as single dose, max 2.5 g/day
• *Child:* **PO** 15 mg/kg/day
Available forms: Tabs 100, 400 mg

SIDE EFFECTS
CNS: Headache, confusion, fever, malaise, dizziness, *disorientation,* hallucinations
EENT: Blurred vision, optic neuritis, photophobia, decreased visual acuity
GI: Abdominal distress, anorexia, nausea, vomiting
INTEG: Dermatitis, pruritus, **toxic epidermal necrolysis**
META: Elevated uric acid, acute gout, impaired hepatic function
MISC: **Thrombocytopenia,** joint pain, bloody sputum, **anaphylaxis**
Contraindications: Hypersensitivity, optic neuritis, child <13 yr

Precautions: Pregnancy (B), lactation, renal disease, diabetic retinopathy, cataracts, ocular defects, hepatic and hematopoietic disorders

PHARMACOKINETICS
PO: Peak 2-4 hr, half-life 3 hr; metabolized in liver; excreted in urine (unchanged drug/inactive metabolites, unchanged drug in feces)

INTERACTIONS
• Delayed absorption of ethambutol: aluminum salts
• Neurotoxicity: other neurotoxics

NURSING CONSIDERATIONS
Assess:
• Hepatic studies qwk × 2 wk, then q2mo: ALT, AST, bilirubin
• Signs of anemia: Hct, Hgb, fatigue
• Mental status often: affect, mood, behavioral changes; psychosis may occur
• Hepatic status: decreased appetite, jaundice, dark urine, fatigue
• C&S, including sputum, before treatment
• Visual status: decreased activity, altered color perception
Administer:
• With meals to decrease GI symptoms
• Antiemetic if vomiting occurs
• After C&S is completed; qmo to detect resistance
• 2 hr before antacids
Evaluate:
• Therapeutic response: decreased symptoms of TB, decrease in acid-fast bacteria
Teach patient/family:
• To avoid alcohol products
• That compliance with dosage schedule, duration is necessary
• That scheduled appointments must be kept or relapse may occur
• To report any visual changes, rash, hot, swollen, painful joints, numbness or tingling of extremities to prescriber

Side effects: *italics* = common; **bold** = life-threatening

Rarely Used

ethosuximide (Rx)
(eth-oh-sux'i-mide)
Zarontin
Func. class.: Anticonvulsant

Uses: Absence seizures, partial seizures, tonic-clonic seizures

DOSAGE AND ROUTES
• *Adult and child >6 yr:* **PO** 250 mg bid initially; may increase by 250 mg q4-7d, max 2 g/day
• *Child 3-6 yr:* **PO** 250 mg/day or 125 mg bid; may increase by 250 mg q4-7d
Contraindications: Hypersensitivity

etidronate (Rx)
(eh-tih-droe'nate)
Didronel, Didronel IV
Func. class.: Bone resorption inhibitor
Chem. class.: Bisphosphonate

Do not confuse:
etidronate/etretinate/etomidate
Action: Decreases bone resorption and new bone development (accretion)
Uses: Paget's disease, heterotopic ossification, hypercalcemia of malignancy

DOSAGE AND ROUTES
Paget's disease
• *Adult:* **PO** 5-10 mg/kg/day, 2 hr before meals with water, not to exceed 20 mg/kg/day, max 6 mo or 11-20 mg/kg/day for max of 3 mo
Heterotopic ossification
• *Adult:* **PO** 20 mg/kg daily × 2 wk, then 10 mg/kg/day for 10 wk, total 12 wk
Hypercalcemia
• *Adult:* **IV** 7.5 mg/kg/day × 3 days, then **PO** 20 mg/kg/day
Heterotopic ossification/hip replacement
• *Adult:* **PO** 20 mg/kg/day × 4 wk before and 3 mo after surgery (4 mo total)

Available forms: Tabs 200, 400 mg; inj 50 mg/ml

SIDE EFFECTS
GI: Nausea, constipation; metallic taste (IV), diarrhea
GU: **Nephrotoxicity**
MISC: Dyspnea, low magnesium, phosphorus, alopecia
MS: Bone pain, hypocalcemia, decreased mineralization of nonaffected bones
Contraindications: Pathologic fractures, clinically overt osteomalacia, severe renal disease with creatinine >5 mg/dl
Precautions: Pregnancy (C), renal disease, lactation, restricted vit D, calcium for children, enterocolitis

PHARMACOKINETICS
Absorbed poorly (PO), not metabolized; excreted in urine/feces; therapeutic response: 1-3 mo

INTERACTIONS
Increase: protime—warfarin
Decrease: absorption—calcium, aluminum, magnesium antacids/supplements, iron products
Drug/Food
• Dairy products: decreased absorption

NURSING CONSIDERATIONS
Assess:
• I&O ratio; check for decreased output in renal patients
• BUN, creatinine, uric acid, phosphate chloride, albumin, pH, urine calcium, magnesium, alk phos, urinalysis; calcium should be kept at 9-10 mg/dl, vit D 50-135 international units/dl
• Muscle spasm, laryngospasm, paresthesias, facial twitching, colic; may indicate hypocalcemia
• Nutritional status, diet for sources of vit D (milk, some seafood), calcium (dairy products, dark green vegetables), phosphates—adequate intake is necessary
• Persistent nausea or diarrhea

⚠ Safety alert   *"Tall Man" lettering

Administer:

PO route

• Drug therapy should not last longer than 6 mo

• On empty stomach with water 2 hr before meals

IV route

• IV after diluting in 250 ml or more 0.9% NaCl; give over 2 hr or longer

• Food, especially high in calcium; vitamins with mineral supplements or antacids high in metals should not be given within 2 hr of dose

Evaluate:

• Therapeutic response: management of bone deficiencies, Paget's disease

Teach patient/family:

• To avoid OTC products

• That therapeutic response may take 1-3 mo; effects persist for months after drug is discontinued

• That adequate intake of calcium, vit D is necessary

• To report sudden onset of unexplained pain, restricted mobility, heat over bone; hypercalcemic relapse

---

Rarely Used

etomidate (℞)

(e-tom′i-date)

Amidate

Func. class.: General anesthetic

Uses: Induction of general anesthesia

DOSAGE AND ROUTES

• *Adult and child >10 yr:* **IV** 0.2-0.6 mg/kg over ½-1 min

Contraindications: Hypersensitivity, labor/delivery

⚠ High Alert

etoposide (℞)

(e-toe-poe′side)

VePesid, VP-16

etoposide phosphate

Etopophos

Func. class.: Antineoplastic—miscellaneous

Chem. class.: Semisynthetic podophyllotoxin

E

Do not confuse:

VePesid/Versed

Action: Inhibits mitotic activity through metaphase to mitosis; also inhibits cells from entering mitosis, depresses DNA, RNA synthesis, cell cycle specific S and G_2

Uses: Leukemias, testicular cancer, lymphomas, small cell carcinoma of the lung

Unlabeled uses: Lymphomas

DOSAGE AND ROUTES

Testicular cancer

• *Adult:* **IV** 50-100 mg/m^2/day × 5 days given q3-5wk or 200-250 mg/m^2/wk, or 125-140 mg/m^2/day 3 × wk, q5wk

Small cell carcinoma of the lung

• *Adult:* **PO** 70 mg/m^2/day × 4 days, given q3-4wk, **IV** 35 mg/m^2/day × 4 days, up to 50 mg/m^2 daily × 5 day q3-4 wk

Available forms: Inj 20 mg/ml; caps 50 mg

SIDE EFFECTS

CNS: Headache, *fever,* peripheral neuropathy, paresthesias, confusion

CV: Hypotension, **MI, dysrhythmias**

GI: Nausea, vomiting, anorexia, **hepatotoxicity,** dyspepsia, diarrhea, constipation

GU: **Nephrotoxicity**

HEMA: **Thrombocytopenia, leukopenia, myelosuppression, anemia**

INTEG: Rash, alopecia, phlebitis at IV site, radiation recall

RESP: **Bronchospasm,** pleural effusion

SYST: **Anaphylaxis**

Contraindications: Pregnancy (D),

---

lactation, hypersensitivity, bone marrow depression, severe renal/hepatic disease, bacterial infection, viral infection
Precautions: Renal/hepatic disease, children, gout

PHARMACOKINETICS

Half-life 7 hr, metabolized in liver; excreted in urine; crosses placental barrier

INTERACTIONS

Increase: bone marrow depression—other antineoplastics, radiation
Increase: adverse reactions—live virus vaccines

NURSING CONSIDERATIONS
Assess:
• CBC, differential, platelet count weekly; withhold drug if WBC is <1000 or platelet count is <50,000; notify prescriber
• Renal studies: BUN, serum uric acid, urine CCr, electrolytes before, during therapy
• I&O ratio; report fall in urine output to <30 ml/hr; check blood pressure bid and report any significant decrease
• Monitor temp q4h; may indicate beginning infection
• Hepatic studies before, during therapy (bilirubin, AST, ALT, LDH) as needed or monthly
• Bleeding: hematuria, guaiac stools, bruising or petechiae, mucosa or orifices q8h
• Effects of alopecia on body image; discuss feelings about body changes
• Jaundice of skin and sclera, dark urine, clay-colored stools, itchy skin, abdominal pain, fever, diarrhea
• B/P q15 min during inf, if systolic reading <90 mm Hg, discontinue inf and notify prescriber
• Buccal cavity q8h for dryness, sores or ulceration, white patches, oral pain, bleeding, dysphagia
• Local irritation, pain, burning, discoloration at inj site
⚠ Symptoms indicating severe allergic reaction: rash, pruritus, urticaria, purpuric skin lesions, itching, flushing
⚠ Symptoms of anaphylaxis: flushing, restlessness, coughing, difficulty breathing
• Frequency of stools, characteristics: cramping, acidosis; signs of dehydration: rapid respirations, poor skin turgor, decreased urine output, dry skin, restlessness, weakness
Administer:
• Antiemetic 30-60 min before giving drug and prn to prevent vomiting
• Allopurinol or sodium bicarbonate to maintain uric acid levels, alkalinization of urine
• Antispasmodic, epINEPHrine, corticosteroids, antihistamines for reactions
IV route (VePesid)
• Using cytotoxic handling procedures
• After diluting 100 mg/250 ml or more D_5W or NaCl to 0.2-0.4 mg/ml, infuse over 30-60 min; phosphate may be given over 5 min-3½ hr; may dilute further to 0.1 mg/ml in 0.9% NaCl, D_5W
Additive compatibilities: Carboplatin, cisplatin, cytarabine, floxuridine, fluorouracil, hydrOXYzine, ifosfamide, ondansetron
Y-site compatibilities: Allopurinol, amifostine, aztreonam, cladribine, DOXOrubicin liposome, fludarabine, granisetron, melphalan, ondansetron, paclitaxel, piperacillin/tazobactam, sargramostim, sodium bicarbonate, teniposide, thiotepa, vinorelbine
Intermittent IV INF route (Etopophos)
• Reconstitute each vial with 5 or 10 ml of D_5W, 0.9% NaCl for a concentration of 20 mg/ml or 10 mg/ml, respectively; may give diluted or undiluted to concentration of as little as 0.1 mg/ml
Perform/provide:
• Liquid diet: carbonated beverages, Jell-O; dry toast or crackers may be added if patient is not nauseated or vomiting
• Increase fluid intake to 2-3 L/day to prevent urate deposits, calculi formation
• Diet low in purines: organ meats (kid-

ney, liver), dried beans, peas to maintain alkaline urine
• Nutritious diet with iron, vitamin supplements

Evaluate:
• Therapeutic response: decreased tumor size, spread of malignancy

Teach patient/family:
• To report any complaints or side effects to nurse or prescriber
• To report any changes in breathing or coughing
• That hair may be lost during treatment; a wig or hairpiece may make patient feel better; tell patient that new hair may be different in color, texture
• That metallic taste may occur
• To report symptoms of infection
• Avoid immunizations
• Avoid crowds or persons with known infections
• Use reliable contraception; avoid breastfeeding

exemestane (Ŗ)
(ex-em'eh-stane)
Aromasin
Func. class.: Antineoplastic
Chem. class.: Aromatase inhibitor

Action: Lowers serum estradiol concentrations; many breast cancers have strong estrogen receptors
Uses: Advanced breast carcinoma not responsive to other therapy (postmenopausal)

DOSAGE AND ROUTES
• *Adult:* **PO** 25 mg daily after meals
Available forms: Tabs 25 mg

SIDE EFFECTS
CNS: Headache, depression, insomnia, anxiety, fatigue
CV: Hypertension
GI: Nausea, vomiting, diarrhea, constipation, abdominal pain, *hot flashes,* increased appetite
HEMA: Lymphopenia
RESP: Cough, *dyspnea*

Contraindications: Pregnancy (D), lactation, hypersensitivity, premenopausal women
Precautions: Children, geriatric, renal/hepatic disease

PHARMACOKINETICS
Half-life 24 hr, excreted in feces, urine

INTERACTIONS
Decrease: exemestane action—CYP3A4 inducers, estrogens

NURSING CONSIDERATIONS
Assess:
• B/P, hypertension may occur
Administer:
• With meals at same time of day
Perform/provide:
• Liquid diet, if needed, including cola, gelatin; dry toast or crackers may be added if patient is not nauseated or vomiting
• Nutritious diet with iron, vitamin supplements as ordered
Evaluate:
• Therapeutic response: decreased tumor size, spread of malignancy
Teach patient/family:
• To report any complaints, side effects to prescriber
• That hot flashes are reversible after discontinuing treatment
• To use reliable contraception; do not breastfeed

exenatide (Ŗ)
(ex-en'a-tide)
Byetta
Func. class.: Antidiabetic
Chem. class.: Incretin mimetic

Action: Binds and activates known human GLP-1 receptor, mimics natural physiology for self-regulating glycemic control
Uses: Type 2 diabetes mellitus given in combination with metformin or a sulfonylurea

DOSAGE AND ROUTES

• *Adult:* **SUBCUT** 5 mcg bid 1 hr before morning and evening meal; may increase to 10 mcg bid after 1 mo of therapy

Available forms: Inj 250 mcg/ml pen injector

SIDE EFFECTS

CNS: Headache, dizziness, feeling jittery, restlessness, weakness

ENDO: **Hypoglycemia**

GI: Nausea, vomiting, diarrhea, dyspepsia, anorexia, gastroesophageal reflux, weight loss

Contraindications: Hypersensitivity

Precautions: Pregnancy (C), geriatric, severe renal/hepatic/GI disease

PHARMACOKINETICS

Peak 2.1 hr, elimination by glomerular filtration

INTERACTIONS

• May increase the effect of acetaminophen

• Do not use with erythromycin, metoclopramide

Increase: exenatide action

Increase: hypoglycemia—ACE inhibitors, corticosteroids, disopyramide, anabolic steroids, androgens, fibric acid derivatives, alcohol

Increase: hyperglycemia—phenothiazines

Decrease: action of digoxin, lovastatin, acetaminophen (elixir)

Decrease: hypoglycemia—niacin, dextrothyroxine, thiazide diuretics, triamterene, estrogens, progestins, oral contraceptives, MAOIs

NURSING CONSIDERATIONS

Assess:

• Fasting blood, glucose, A1c levels, postprandial glucose during treatment to determine diabetes control

• Hypo/hyperglycemic reaction that can occur soon after meals; for severe hypoglycemia give IV $D_{50}W$, then IV dextrose solution

Administer:

• Drug 1 hr before meals; if patient is NPO, may need to hold dose to prevent hypoglycemia

Perform/provide:

• Storage in refrigerator

Evaluate:

• Therapeutic response: decrease in polyuria, polydipsia, polyphagia, clear sensorium, improving A1c, weight; absence of dizziness, stable gait

Teach patient/family:

• The symptoms of hypo/hyperglycemia, what to do about each; to have glucagon emergency kit available; to carry a glucose source (candy, sugar cube) to treat hypoglycemia

• That drug must be continued on daily basis; explain consequences of discontinuing drug abruptly

• That diabetes is a lifelong illness; drug will not cure disease

• That all food in diet plan must be eaten to prevent hypoglycemia

• To carry emergency ID with prescriber and medications

• To continue weight control, dietary restrictions, exercise, hygiene

• That regular blood glucose monitoring and A1c testing is needed

• To notify prescriber if pregnant or intend to become pregnant

• To read "Information for the Patient" and "Pen User Manual"

---

ezetimibe (R)

(ehz-eh-tim'bee)

Zetia

Func. class.: Antilipemic; cholesterol absorption inhibitor

Action: Inhibits absorption of cholesterol by the small intestine

Uses: Hypercholesterolemia, homozygous familial hypercholesterolemia (HoFH), homozygous sitosterolemia

DOSAGE AND ROUTES

• *Adult:* **PO** 10 mg daily; may be given with HMG-CoA reductase inhibitor at same

---

time; may be given with bile acid sequestrant; give ezetimibe 2 hr before or 4 hr
after the bile acid sequestrant
Available forms: Tabs 10 mg

SIDE EFFECTS

CNS: Fatigue, dizziness, headache
GI: Diarrhea, abdominal pain
MISC: Chest pain
MS: Myalgias, arthralgias, back pain
RESP: Pharyngitis, sinusitis, cough, URI
Contraindications: Hypersensitivity,
severe hepatic disease
Precautions: Pregnancy (C), lactation,
children, hepatic disease

PHARMACOKINETICS

Metabolized in small intestine, liver, excreted in feces 78%, urine 11%

INTERACTIONS

Increase: action of ezetimibe—fibric
acid derivatives, cycloSPORINE
Decrease: action of ezetimibe—
antacids, cholestyramine
Drug/Herb
Increase: effect—glucomannan
Decrease: effect—gotu kola

NURSING CONSIDERATIONS

Assess:
• Lipid levels, LFTs baseline and periodi-
cally during treatment
Administer:
• Without regard to meals
Evaluate:
• Therapeutic response: decreased cho-
lesterol
Teach patient/family:
• That compliance is needed
• That risk factors should be decreased:
high-fat diet, smoking, alcohol consump-
tion, absence of exercise
• To notify prescriber if pregnancy is sus-
pected or planned

⚠ High Alert

**factor IX complex
(human) (R)**
Alpha-Nine SD, Benefix,
Konyne 80, Mononine,
Profilnine/Alpha Nine,
Proplex SX-T, Proplex T
Func. class.: Hemostatic
Chem. class.: Factors II, VII, IX, X

F

Action: Causes an increase in blood levels of clotting factors II, VII, IX, X; factor
IX (human) has IX activity
Uses: Hemophilia B (Christmas disease),
factor IX deficiency, anticoagulant reversal, control of bleeding in patients with
factor VIII inhibitors, reversal of overdose of anticoagulants in emergencies

DOSAGE AND ROUTES

*Factor IX complex (human) bleeding
in hemophilia B*
• *Adult and child:* **IV** establish 25% of
normal factor IX or 60-75 units/kg, then
10-20 units/kg/day 1-2 ×/wk
*Prophylaxis for bleeding in hemo-
philia B*
• *Adult and child:* **IV** 10-20 units/kg 1-2
×/wk
*Bleeding in hemophilia A/inhibitors
of factor VIII (Proplex T, Konyne
80)*
• *Adult and child:* **IV** 75 units/kg, repeat in 12 hr
Oral anticoagulant reversal
• *Adult and child:* **IV** 15 units/kg
*Factor VII deficiency (use Proplex T
only)*
• *Adult and child:* **IV** 0.5 units/kg ×
weight (kg) × desired factor IX increase
(% of normal); repeat q4-6h if needed
*Factor IX (human) minor-moderate
hemorrhage*
Use only Alpha Nine, Alpha-Nine SD
• *Adult and child:* **IV** dose to increase
factor IX level to 20%-30% in one dose

Serious hemorrhage
• *Adult and child:* **IV** dose to increase factor IX to 30%-50% as daily inf
Minor hemorrhage (mononine only)
• *Adult and child:* **IV** dose to increase factor IX to 15%-25% (20-30 units/kg), repeat in 24 hr if needed
Major hemorrhage
• *Adult and child:* **IV** dose to increase factor IX to 25%-50% (75 units/kg) q18-30h × 10 days or less
Available forms: Inj (number of units noted on label)

SIDE EFFECTS

CNS: Headache, dizziness, malaise, paresthesia, *lethargy, chills, fever, flushing*
CV: Hypotension, tachycardia, *MI,* **venous thrombosis, pulmonary embolism**
GI: Nausea, vomiting, abdominal cramps, jaundice, **viral hepatitis**
HEMA: **Thrombosis, hemolysis, AIDS, DIC**
INTEG: Rash, flushing, *urticaria*
RESP: **Bronchospasm**
Contraindications: Hypersensitivity to mouse/hamster protein, hepatic disease, DIC, elective surgery, mild factor IX deficiency
Precautions: Pregnancy (C), neonates/infants

PHARMACOKINETICS

IV: Half-life factor VII–3-6 hr, factor IX–24-36 hr; rapidly cleared from plasma

INTERACTIONS

• Incompatible with protein products
A *Increase:* thrombosis risk—aminocaproic acid; do not administer
Decrease: effect of warfarin

NURSING CONSIDERATIONS

Assess:
• Blood studies (coagulation factors assays by % normal: 5% prevents spontaneous hemorrhage, 30%-50% for surgery, 80%-100% for severe hemorrhage)

• Increased B/P, pulse
• For bleeding q15-30min, immobilize and apply ice to affected joints
• I&O; if urine becomes orange or red, notify prescriber
• Allergic or pyrogenic reaction: fever, chills, rash, itching, slow inf rate if not severe
A DIC: bleeding, ecchymosis, hypersensitivity, changes in coagulation tests
• For tingling sensation; if present, rate should be reduced
Administer:
• Hepatitis B vaccine before administration
• IV after warming to room temperature 3 ml/min or less, with plastic syringe only; do not admix
• After dilution with provided diluent, 50 units/ml or 25 units/ml; do not exceed 10 ml/min; decrease rate if fever, headache, flushing, tingling occur
• After crossmatch if patient has blood type A, B, AB, to determine incompatibility with factor
Perform/provide:
• Storage of reconstituted sol for 3 hr at room temperature or up to 2 yr refrigeration (powder); check expiration date
Evaluate:
• Therapeutic response: prevention of hemorrhage
Teach patient/family:
• To report any signs of bleeding: gums, under skin, urine, stools, emesis
• The risk of viral hepatitis, AIDS; to be tested q2-3mo for HIV, even though risk is low
• That immunization for hepatitis B may be given first
• To carry emergency ID identifying disease; avoid salicylates, NSAIDs; inform other health professionals of condition

---

A Safety alert   *"Tall Man" lettering

famciclovir (℞)
(fam-cy'clo-veer)
Famvir
Func. class.: Antiviral
Chem. class.: Guanosine nucleoside

Action: Inhibits DNA polymerase and viral DNA synthesis by conversion of this guanosine nucleoside to penciclovir

Uses: Treatment of acute herpes zoster (shingles), genital herpes; recurrent mucocutaneous herpes simplex virus (HSV) in HIV patients

Unlabeled uses: Initial episodes of herpes genitalis

DOSAGE AND ROUTES
Herpes zoster
• *Adult:* PO 500 mg q8h for 7 days
Renal dose
• *Adult:* PO CCr ≥60 ml/min, 500 mg q8h; 40-59 ml/min, 500 mg q12h; 20-39 ml/min, 500 mg q24h
Recurrent herpes simplex virus
• *Adult:* PO 125 mg q12h × 5 days
Renal dose
• *Adult:* PO CCr <39 ml/min 125 mg q24h × 5 days
Suppression of recurrent herpes simplex virus
• *Adult:* PO 250 mg q12h up to 1 yr
Renal dose
• *Adult:* PO CCr 20-39 ml/min 125 mg q12h × 5 days; CCr <20 ml/min 125 mg q24h × 5 days
Genital herpes (recurrent)
• *Adult:* PO 125 mg bid × 5 days; begin treatment at first sign of recurrence
Suppression of recurrent genital herpes
• *Adult:* PO 250 mg bid for up to a year
Herpes genitalis initial episodes (unlabeled)
• *Adult:* PO 25 mg tid × 7-10 days
Available forms: Tabs 125, 250, 500 mg

SIDE EFFECTS
CNS: Headache, fatigue, dizziness, paresthesia, somnolence, fever
GI: Nausea, vomiting, diarrhea, constipation, abdominal pain, anorexia
GU: Decreased sperm count
INTEG: Pruritus
MS: Back pain, arthralgia
RESP: Pharyngitis, sinusitis
Contraindications: Hypersensitivity to this drug, penciclovir
Precautions: Pregnancy (B), renal disease, hypersensitivity to acyclovir, ganciclovir, lactation

PHARMACOKINETICS
Unknown

INTERACTIONS
Decrease: renal excretion—theophylline, probenecid, digoxin
Decrease: metabolism—cimetidine

NURSING CONSIDERATIONS
Assess:
• For number, distribution of lesions; burning, itching, pain, which are early symptoms of herpes infection
• Renal studies: urine CCr, BUN before and during treatment if decreased renal function; dose may have to be lowered
• Bowel pattern before, during treatment; diarrhea may occur
• Posttherapeutic neuralgia during and after treatment
Administer:
• With or without meals; absorption does not appear to be lowered when taken with food
• As soon as diagnosed; in herpes zoster within 72 hr
Evaluate:
• Therapeutic response: decreased size, spread of lesions
Teach patient/family:
• How to recognize beginning infection
• How to prevent spread of infection; that this medication does not prevent the spread to others, that condoms should be used

• The reason for medication, expected results
• That women with genital herpes should have yearly Pap smears, cervical cancer is more likely

---

famotidine (OTC, ℞)

(fa-moe'ti-deen)
Maximum Strength Pepcid, Mylanta AR, Pepcid, Pepcid AC, Pepcid AC Acid Controller, Pepcid RPD
Func. class.: H$_2$-histamine receptor antagonist

Action: Competitively inhibits histamine at histamine H$_2$-receptor site, decreasing gastric secretion while pepsin remains at a stable level
Uses: Short-term treatment of active duodenal ulcer, maintenance therapy for duodenal ulcer, Zollinger-Ellison syndrome, multiple endocrine adenomas, gastric ulcers; gastroesophageal reflux disease, heartburn
Unlabeled uses: GI disorders in those taking NSAIDs; urticaria; prevention of stress ulcers, aspiration pneumonitis, inactivation of oral pancreatic enzymes in pancreatic disorders

DOSAGE AND ROUTES

Active ulcer
• *Adult:* **PO** 40 mg daily at bedtime × 4-8 wk, then 20 mg daily at bedtime if needed (maintenance); **IV** 20 mg q12h if unable to take **PO**
• *Child 1-16 yr:* 0.5 mg/kg/day at bedtime or divided bid, max 40 mg daily
Hypersecretory conditions
• *Adult:* **PO** 20 mg q6h; may give 160 mg q6h if needed; **IV** 20 mg q12h if unable to take **PO**
• *Child 1-16 yr:* 1 mg/kg/day divide bid, max 40 mg bid
Heartburn relief/prevention
• *Adult:* **PO** 10 mg with water or 1 hr before eating

Paclitaxel hypersensitivity reactions
• *Adult:* **IV** 20 mg ½ hr prior to infusion
Renal disease
• *Adult:* **PO** CCr <10 ml/min 20 mg at bedtime or increase interval of usual dose to 36-48 hr
Available forms: Tabs 10, 20, 40 mg; gel cap 10 mg; powder for oral susp 40 mg/5 ml; inj 10 mg/ml, 20 mg/50 ml 0.9% NaCl; orally disintegrating tabs (RPD) 20, 40 mg; chew tabs 10 mg

SIDE EFFECTS

CNS: Headache, dizziness, paresthesia, depression, anxiety, somnolence, insomnia, fever
CV: **Dysrhythmias**
EENT: Taste change, tinnitus, orbital edema
GI: Constipation, nausea, vomiting, anorexia, cramps, abnormal hepatic enzymes, diarrhea
HEMA: **Thrombocytopenia, aplastic anemia**
INTEG: Rash
MS: Myalgia, arthralgia
Contraindications: Hypersensitivity
Precautions: Pregnancy (B), lactation, children <12 yr, severe renal/hepatic disease, geriatric

PHARMACOKINETICS

PO: Onset 30-60 min, duration 6-12 hr, peak 1-3 hr, absorption 50%
IV: Onset immediate, peak 30-60 min, duration 8-15 hr, plasma protein-binding 15%-20%; metabolized in liver 30% (active metabolites), 70% excreted by kidneys, half-life 2½-3½ hr

INTERACTIONS

Decrease: absorption—ketoconazole
Decrease: famotidine absorption—antacids

NURSING CONSIDERATIONS

Assess:
• For epigastric pain, adominal pain, frank or occult blood in emesis, stools
• Blood counts during therapy; watch for

---

decreasing platelets; if low, therapy may have to be discontinued and restarted after hematologic recovery

• For bleeding, hematuria, hematuresis, occult blood in stools; abdominal pain

• Blood dyscrasias (thrombocytopenia): bruising, fatigue, bleeding, poor healing

Administer:

• Antacids 1 hr before or 2 hr after famotidine; may be given with foods or liquids

• After shaking oral suspension

IV, direct route

• After diluting 2 ml of drug (10 mg/ml) in 0.9% NaCl to total volume of 5-10 ml; inject over 2 min to prevent hypotension

IV Intermittent INF route

• After diluting 20 mg (2 ml) of drug in 100 ml of LR, 0.9% NaCl, D_5W, $D_{10}W$; run over 15-30 min

Additive compatibilities: Cefazolin, flumazenil, vancomycin

Y-site compatibilities: Acyclovir, allopurinol, amifostine, aminophylline, amphotericin, ampicillin, ampicillin/sulbactam, amrinone, amsacrine, atropine, aztreonam, bretylium, calcium gluconate, cefazolin, cefoperazone, cefotaxime, cefotetan, cefoxitin, ceftazidime, ceftizoxime, ceftriaxone, cefuroxime, cephalothin, cephapirin, chlorproMAZINE, cisatracurium, cisplatin, cladribine, cyclophosphamide, cytarabine, dexamethasone, dextran 40, digoxin, diphenhydrAMINE, DOBUTamine, DOPamine, DOXOrubicin, DOXOrubicin liposome, droperidol, enalaprilat, epINEPHrine, erythromycin, esmolol, filgrastim, fluconazole, fludarabine, folic acid, gentamicin, granisetron, haloperidol, heparin, hydrocortisone, hydromorphone, hydrOXYzine, imipenem/cilastatin, insulin (regular), isoproterenol, labetalol, lidocaine, lorazepam, magnesium sulfate, melphalan, meperidine, methotrexate, methylPREDNISolone, metoclopramide, mezlocillin, midazolam, morphine, nafcillin, nitroglycerin, nitroprusside, norepinephrine, ondansetron, oxacillin, paclitaxel, perphenazine, phenylephrine, phenytoin, phytonadione, piperacillin, potassium chloride/phosphate, procainamide, propofol, remifentanil, sar-

gramostim, sodium bicarbonate, teniposide, theophylline, thiamine, thiotepa, ticarcillin, ticarcillin/clavulanate, verapamil, vinorelbine

Perform/provide:

• Storage in cool environment (oral); IV sol is stable for 48 hr at room temperature; do not use discolored sol; discard unused oral sol after 1 mo

• Increase in bulk and fluids in the diet to prevent constipation

Evaluate:

• Therapeutic response: decreased abdominal pain

Teach patient/family:

• That drug must be continued for prescribed time in prescribed method to be effective; do not double dose

• To report bleeding, bruising, fatigue, malaise, since blood dyscrasias occur

• About possibility of decreased libido, reversible after discontinuing therapy

• To avoid irritating foods, alcohol, aspirin, and extreme temperature of foods that may irritate GI system

• That smoking should be avoided; diminishes effectiveness of drug

• To avoid tasks requiring alertness; dizziness, drowsiness may occur

---

fat emulsions (Ŗ)

Intralipid 10%, Intralipid 20%, Liposyn II 10%, Liposyn II 20%, Liposyn III 10%, Liposyn III 20%, Soyacal 20%

Func. class.: Caloric

Chem. class.: Fatty acid, long chain; nutritional supplement

Action: Needed for energy, heat production; consist of neutral triglycerides, primarily unsaturated fatty acids

Uses: Increase calorie intake, fatty acid deficiency, prevention

DOSAGE AND ROUTES

Deficiency

• *Adult and child:* IV 8%-10% of required calorie intake (intralipid)

Adjunct to TPN
• *Adult:* **IV** 1 ml/min over 15-30 min (10%) or 0.5 ml/min over 15-30 min (20%); may increase to 500 ml over 4-8 hr if no adverse reactions occur; not to exceed 2.5 g/kg
• *Child:* **IV** 0.1 ml/min over 10-15 min (10%) or 0.05 ml/min over 10-15 min (20%); may increase to 1 g/kg over 4 hr if no adverse reactions occur; not to exceed 4 g/kg

Prevention of deficiency
• **Adult: IV** 500 ml 2 ×/wk (10%), given 1 ml/min for 30 min, not to exceed 500 ml over 6 hr
• *Child:* **IV** 5-10 ml/kg/day (10%), given 0.1 ml/min for 30 min, not to exceed 100 ml/hr

Available forms: Inj 10% (50, 100, 200, 250, 500 ml), 20% (50, 100, 200, 250, 500 ml)

SIDE EFFECTS

CNS: Dizziness, headache, drowsiness, **focal seizures**
CV: **Shock**
GI: Nausea, vomiting, **hepatomegaly**
HEMA: **Hyperlipemia, hypercoagulation, thrombocytopenia, leukopenia, leukocytosis**
RESP: Dyspnea, **fat in lung tissue**

Contraindications: Hypersensitivity to this product or eggs, soybeans, legumes; hyperlipemia, lipid necrosis, acute pancreatitis accompanied by hyperlipemia, hyperbilirubinemia of the newborn; renal insufficiency, hepatic damage

Precautions: Pregnancy (C), severe hepatic disease, diabetes mellitus, thrombocytopenia, gastric ulcers, premature/term newborns, sepsis

NURSING CONSIDERATIONS

Assess:
• Triglycerides, free fatty acid levels, platelet counts daily to prevent fat overload, thrombocytopenia
• Hepatic studies: AST, ALT, Hct, Hgb; notify prescriber if abnormal
• Nutritional status: calorie count by dietitian; monitor weight daily

Administer:
IV Intermittent INF route
• At 10% (1 ml/min); 20% (0.5 ml/min) initially × 15-30 min, may increase 10% (120 ml/hr); 20% (62.5 ml/hr) if no adverse reaction; do not give more than 500 ml on first day
• After changing IV tubing at each infusion: infection may occur with old tubing
• With inf pump at prescribed rate; do not use in-line filter sized for lipid emulsion; clogging will occur

Additive compatibilities: Chloramphenicol, cimetidine, cycloSPORINE, diphenhydrAMINE, famotidine, heparin, hydrocortisone, multivitamins, nizatidine, penicillin G potassium

Y-site compatibilities: Ampicillin, cefamandole, cefazolin, cefoxitin, cephapirin, clindamycin, digoxin, DOPamine, erythromycin, furosemide, gentamicin, IL-2, isoproterenol, kanamycin, lidocaine, norepinephrine, oxacillin, penicillin G potassium, ticarcillin, tobramycin

Perform/provide:
• Do not use mixed sol if separated or oily looking

Evaluate:
• Therapeutic response: increased weight

Teach patient/family:
• The reason for use of lipids

Rarely Used

felbamate (℞)
(fell′ba-mate)
Felbatol
Func. class.: Anticonvulsant

Uses: Partial seizures, with or without generalization in adults; partial and generalized seizures in children with Lennox-Gastaut syndrome

DOSAGE AND ROUTES

Adjunctive therapy
• *Adult and child >14 yr:* **PO** add 1.2 g/day in 3-4 divided doses; reduce other anticonvulsants (valproic acid, phenytoin, carbamazepine and derivatives) by

20% to control plasma concentrations; may increase felbamate 1.2 g/day increments qwk, up to 3.6 g/day

Monotherapy

• *Adult:* **PO** 1.2 g/day in 3-4 divided doses; titrate with close supervision; increase dose by 600-mg increments q2wk to 3.6 g/day if needed

Lennox-Gastaut syndrome adjunctive therapy

• *Child 2-14 yr:* **PO** add 15 mg/kg/day in 3-4 divided doses; reduce other anticonvulsants (valproic acid, phenytoin, carbamazepine and derivatives) by 20% to control plasma concentrations; may increase felbamate 15 mg/kg/day qwk up to 45 mg/day

Contraindications: Hypersensitivity to this drug, other carbamates, history of blood dyscrasia, aplastic anemia, hepatic disease

---

felodipine (℞)

(fe-loe′-di-peen)
Plendil, Renedil ✦
Func. class.: Antihypertensive, calcium channel blocker, antianginal
Chem. class.: Dihydropyridine

Do not confuse:
Plendil/pindolol/Pletal/Prilosec/Prinivil

Action: Inhibits calcium ion influx across cell membrane, resulting in inhibition of excitation/contraction

Uses: Essential hypertension, alone or with other antihypertensives, angina pectoris, Prinzmetal's angina (vasospastic)

DOSAGE AND ROUTES

• *Adult:* **PO** 5 mg daily initially, usual range 5-10 mg daily; max 10 mg daily; do not adjust dosage at intervals of <2 wk

• *Geriatric:* **PO** 2.5 mg daily

Hepatic disease

• **PO** 2.5-5 mg, max 10 mg/day

Available forms: Ext rel tabs 2.5, 5, 10 mg

SIDE EFFECTS

CNS: Headache, fatigue, drowsiness, dizziness, anxiety, depression, nervousness, insomnia, light-headedness, paresthesia, tinnitus, psychosis, somnolence

CV: **Dysrhythmia,** edema, **CHF,** hypotension, palpitations, **MI, pulmonary edema,** tachycardia, syncope, AV block, angina

GI: Nausea, vomiting, diarrhea, gastric upset, constipation, increased LFTs, dry mouth

GU: Nocturia, polyuria

HEMA: Anemia

INTEG: Rash, pruritus

MISC: Flushing, sexual difficulties, cough, nasal congestion, shortness of breath, wheezing, epistaxis, respiratory infection, chest pain, **Stevens-Johnson syndrome,** gingival hyperplasia

Contraindications: Hypersensitivity, sick sinus syndrome, 2nd- or 3rd-degree heart block, hypotension <90 mm Hg systolic

Precautions: Pregnancy (C), CHF, hepatic injury, lactation, children, renal disease, geriatric

PHARMACOKINETICS

Peak plasma levels 2.5-5 hr; highly protein bound, >99% metabolized in liver, 0.5% excreted unchanged in urine; elimination half-life 11-16 hr

INTERACTIONS

Increase: bradycardia, CHF—β-blockers, digoxin, phenytoin, disopyramide

Increase: toxicity—ketoconazole, erythromycin, itraconazole, propranolol

Increase: hypotension—fentanyl, nitrates, alcohol, quinidine

Decrease: antihypertensive effects—NSAIDs

Drug/Herb

Increase: toxicity, death—aconite

Increase: antihypertensive effect—barberry, betony, black catechu, black cohosh, bloodroot, broom, burdock, cat's

---

claw, dandelion, ginseng, ginkgo, golden-seal, Irish moss, Jamaican dogwood, kelp, khella, mistletoe, parsley

Increase or decrease: antihypertensive effect—astragalus, cola tree

Decrease: antihypertensive effect—coltsfoot, guarana, khat, licorice, St. John's wort, yohimbine

Drug/Food

Increase: felodipine level—grapefruit juice

NURSING CONSIDERATIONS

Assess:

• I&O, weight daily; for CHF: weight gain, crackles, dyspnea, edema, jugular venous distention

• Renal, hepatic studies

• Cardiac status: B/P, pulse, respiration; ECG periodically

• For angina pain: location, duration, intensity; ameliorating, aggravating factors

Administer:

• Swallow whole; do not break, crush, or chew ext rel products

• Once daily without regard to meals

Evaluate:

• Therapeutic response: decreased B/P, decreased anginal attacks, increase in activity tolerance

Teach patient/family:

• To avoid hazardous activities until stabilized on drug, dizziness is no longer a problem

• To avoid OTC drugs, alcohol, unless directed by a prescriber, to limit caffeine consumption

• The importance of complying with all areas of medical regimen: diet, exercise, stress reduction, drug therapy

• That tablets may appear in stools, but are insignificant

• To report dyspnea, palpitations, irregular heart beat, swelling of extremities, nausea, vomiting, severe dizziness, severe headache

• To change positions slowly to prevent orthostatic hypotension

• To obtain correct pulse, to contact prescriber if pulse is <50 bpm

• To use protective clothing, sunscreen to prevent photosensitivity

Treatment of overdose: Atropine for AV block, vasopressor for hypotension

---

fenofibrate (℞)

(fen-oh-fee'brate)
Antara, Lofibra, Tricor, Triglide
Func. class.: Antilipemic
Chem. class.: Fibric acid derivative

Action: Increases lipolysis and elimination of triglyceride-rich particles from plasma by activating lipoprotein lipase, resulting in triglyceride change in size and composition of LDL leading to rapid breakdown of LDL; mobilizes triglycerides from tissue; increases excretion of neutral sterols

Uses: Hypercholesterolemia, types IV, V hyperlipidemia that do not respond to other treatment and are at risk for pancreatitis, Fredrickson type IIa, IIb, hypertriglyceridemia

Unlabeled uses: Polymetabolic syndrome X

DOSAGE AND ROUTES

Hypertriglyceridemia

• *Adult:* **PO** (Antara) 43-130 mg/day; (Lofibra) 67-200 mg/day; (Tricor) 48-145 mg/day; (Triglide) 50-160 mg/day

Primary hypercholesterolemia/ mixed hyperlipidemia

• *Adult:* **PO** (Antara) 130 mg/day; (Lofibra) 200 mg/day; (Tricor) 145 mg/day; (Triglide) 160 mg/day

Renal dose (geriatric)

• *Adult:* **PO** (Antara) 43 mg/day; (Lofibra) 67 mg/day; (Tricor) 48 mg/day

Available forms: Tabs (Triglide) 50, 160 mg; (Tricor) 48, 145 mg; micronized cap (Antara) 45, 87, 130 mg; (Lofibra) 67, 134, 200 mg

SIDE EFFECTS

CNS: Fatigue, weakness, drowsiness, dizziness, insomnia, depression, vertigo

CV: Angina, **dysrhythmias,** hypertension

⚠ Safety alert   *"Tall Man" lettering

GI: Nausea, vomiting, dyspepsia, increased liver enzymes, flatulence, hepatomegaly, gastritis

GU: Dysuria, proteinuria, oliguria, urinary frequency

HEMA: Anemia, leukopenia, ecchymosis

INTEG: Rash, urticaria, pruritus

MISC: Polyphagia, weight gain

MS: Myalgias, arthralgias, myopathy

RESP: Pharyngitis, bronchitis, cough

Contraindications: Hypertensivity, severe renal/hepatic disease, primary biliary cirrhosis, preexisting gallbladder disease

Precautions: Pregnancy (C), peptic ulcer, lactation, pancreatitis, renal/hepatic disease, geriatric

PHARMACOKINETICS

Peak 6-8 hr; protein binding 99%, converted to fenofibric acid, metabolized in liver, excreted in urine (60%), half-life 20 hr

INTERACTIONS

• Nephrotoxicity: cycloSPORINE
• Avoid use with HMG-CoA reductase inhibitors, rhabdomyolysis may occur

Increase: anticoagulant effects—oral anticoagulants

Decrease: absorption of fenofibrate—bile acid sequestrants

Drug/Herb

Increase: effect—glucomannan

Decrease: effect—gotu kola

Drug/Food

Increase: absorption

NURSING CONSIDERATIONS

Assess:

• Lipid levels, LFTs baseline and periodically during treatment, CPK if muscle pain occurs, CBC, Hct, Hgb; PT with anticoagulant therapy

• Pancreatitis, cholelithiasis renal failure, rhabdomyolyis (when combined with HMG Co-A reductase inhibitors), myositis, drug should be discontinued

Administer:

• Drug with meals; may increase q4-8wk

Evaluate:

• Therapeutic response: decreased triglycerides

Teach patient/family:

• That compliance is needed
• That risk factors should be decreased: high-fat diet, smoking, alcohol consumption, absence of exercise
• To notify prescriber if pregnancy is suspected or planned
• To report GU symptoms: decreased libido, impotence, dysuria, proteinuria, oliguria, hematuria
• To notify prescriber of muscle pain, weakness, fever, fatigue; epigastric pain

fenoldopam (Ŗ)
(feh-nahl′doh-pam)
Corlopam
Func. class.: Antihypertensive, vasodilator

Action: Agonist at D_1-like dopamine receptors; binds to α_2-adrenoceptors; increases renal blood flow

Uses: Hypertensive crisis, malignant hypertension

Unlabeled uses: Prevention of contrast agent–associated nephrotoxicity

DOSAGE AND ROUTES

• *Adult:* **IV** 0.01-1.6 mcg/kg/min
• *Child:* **CONT IV** 0.2 mcg/kg/min with effects within 5 min; may increase dose to 0.3-0.5 mcg/kg/min q20-30min depending on response

Available forms: Inj conc 10 mg/ml in single-use ampules; inj 10 mg/ml

SIDE EFFECTS

CNS: Headache, anxiety, dizziness, insomnia

CV: **Hypotension,** ST-T-wave changes, angina pectoris, tachycardia, palpitations, **MI, ischemic heart disease, flushing**

GI: Nausea, vomiting, constipation, diarrhea

HEMA: **Leukocytosis,** bleeding

INTEG: Sweating

META: Increased BUN, glucose, LDH, creatinine, hypokalemia

Contraindications: Hypersensitivity, sulfite sensitivity

Precautions: Pregnancy (B), tachycardia, lactation, children, intraocular pressure, hypokalemia

PHARMACOKINETICS

Adult: Onset 5 min, duration 15-30 min, elimination half-life 5 min, steady state 20 min, crosses placenta, conjugated in the liver

Child 1 mo-12 yr: Elimination half-life 3-5 min

INTERACTIONS

Increase: hypotension—avoid use with β-blockers

Drug/Herb

Increase: toxicity, death—aconite

Increase: antihypertensive effect—barberry, betony, black catechu, black cohosh, bloodroot, broom, burdock, cat's claw, dandelion, goldenseal, Irish moss, Jamaican dogwood, kelp, khella, mistletoe, parsley

Increase or decrease: antihypertensive effect—astragalus, cola tree

Decrease: antihypertensive effect—coltsfoot, guarana, khat, licorice

NURSING CONSIDERATIONS

Assess:

• B/P, HR q5min until stabilized, then q1h × 2 hr, then q4h, pulse, jugular venous distention q4h ECG; expect tachycardia (dose-dependent)

• Electrolytes, blood studies: K, Na, Cl, CO_2, CBC, serum glucose

• IV site for extravasation

Administer:

• To patient in recumbent position; keep in that position for 1 hr after administration

Adult

• After diluting contents of ampules in 0.9% NaCl, or 5% dextrose inj (40 mcg/ml); then add 4 ml of conc (40 mg of drug/1000 ml); 2 ml of conc (20 mg

of drug/500 ml); 1 ml of conc (10 mg of drug/250 ml); do not admix

Child

• Use infusion pump

• After dilution 3 ml (30 mg)/500 ml (60 mcg/ml); 1.5 ml (15 mg)/250 ml (60 mcg/ml); 0.6 ml (6 mg)/100 ml (60 mcg/ml)

Perform/provide:

• Diluted sol is stable in normal light/temperature for 24 hr

Evaluate:

• Therapeutic response: decreased B/P

Teach patient/family:

• To report dyspnea, chest pain, bleeding, pain at inj site

• Reason for medication and expected results

Rarely Used

fenoprofen (℞)

(fen-oh-proe'fen)

Fenoprofen, Nalfon

Func. class.: Nonsteroidal antiinflammatory/nonopioid analgesic

Uses: Mild to moderate pain, osteoarthritis, rheumatoid arthritis, acute gout, arthritis, inflammation

DOSAGE AND ROUTES

Pain

• *Adult:* **PO** 200 mg q4-6h prn

Arthritis

• *Adult:* **PO** 300-600 mg qid, not to exceed 3.2 g/day

Contraindications: Hypersensitivity, asthma, severe renal/hepatic disease

⚠ High Alert

fentanyl (℞)

(fen'ta-nill)
Actiq, Fentanyl, Fentanyl
Oralet, Sublimaze
Func. class.: Opioid analgesic
Chem. class.: Synthetic phenylpiperidine

Controlled Substance Schedule II
Do not confuse:
fentanyl/Sufenta

Action: Inhibits ascending pain pathways in CNS, increases pain threshold, alters pain perception by binding to opiate receptors

Uses: Preoperatively, postoperatively; adjunct to general anesthetic, adjunct to regional anesthesia; Fentanyl Oralet—anesthesia as premedication, conscious sedation; Actiq—breakthrough cancer pain

DOSAGE AND ROUTES

Anesthetic
• *Adult:* IV 25-100 mcg (0.7-2 mcg/kg) q2-3 min prn
Anesthesia supplement
• *Adult and child >12 yr:* **IM/IV** 2-20 mcg/kg **IV INF** 0.025-0.25 mcg/kg/min
Induction and maintenance
• *Adult:* **IV BOL** 5-40 mcg/kg
• *Child 2-12 yr:* **IV** 2-3 mcg/kg
Preoperatively
• *Adult and child >12 yr:* **IM/IV** 0.05-0.1 mg q30-60min before surgery
Postoperatively
• *Adult and child >12 yr:* **IM/IV** 0.05-0.1 mg q1-2h prn
Sedation/analgesia
• *Adult and child >12 yr:* **IV** 0.5-1 mcg/kg/dose; may repeat after 30-60 min
• *Child 1-12 yr:* **IV BOL** 1-2 mcg/kg/dose; may repeat after 30-60 min intervals; **CONT IV** 1-5 mcg/kg/hr after IV bol dose
• *Neonates:* **IV BOL** 0.5-3 mcg/kg/dose; **CONT IV** 0.5-2 mcg/kg/hr after IV bol

Fentanyl Oralet
• *Adult:* Transmucosal 5 mcg/kg = fentanyl IM 0.75-1.25 mcg/kg, do not exceed 5 mcg/kg
• *Child:* Transmucosal may need doses of 5-15 mcg/kg; must be watched continuously for hypoventilation
Actiq
• *Adult:* Transmucosal 200 mcg, redose if needed 15 min after completion of 1st dose, do not give more than 2 doses during titration period
Available forms: Inj 0.05 mg/ml; lozenges 100, 200, 300, 400 mcg; lozenges on a stick 200, 400, 600, 800, 1200, 1600 mcg

SIDE EFFECTS

CNS: Dizziness, delirium, euphoria
CV: **Bradycardia, arrest,** hypotension or hypertension
EENT: Blurred vision, miosis
GI: Nausea, vomiting
GU: Urinary retention
INTEG: Rash, diaphoresis
MS: Muscle rigidity
RESP: **Respiratory depression, arrest, laryngospasm**
Contraindications: Hypersensitivity to opiates, myasthenia gravis
Precautions: Pregnancy (C), geriatric, respiratory depression, increased intracranial pressure, seizure disorders, severe respiratory disorders, cardiac dysrhythmias, lactation

PHARMACOKINETICS

IM: Onset 7-8 min, peak 30 min, duration 1-2 hr
IV: Onset 1 min, peak 3-5 min, duration ½-1 hr; metabolized by liver; excreted by kidneys; crosses placenta; excreted in breast milk; half-life 1½-6 hr; 80% bound to plasma proteins

INTERACTIONS

Increase: with other CNS depressants—alcohol, opioids, sedative/hypnotics, antipsychotics, skeletal muscle relaxants

Drug/Herb
Increase: anticholinergic effect—corkwood
Increase: action—Jamaican dogwood, kava, lavender, mistletoe, nettle, pokeweed, poppy, senega, valerian
Drug/Lab Test
Increase: Amylase, lipase

NURSING CONSIDERATIONS
Assess:
• VS after parenteral route; note muscle rigidity, drug history, hepatic and renal function tests
• CNS changes: dizziness, drowsiness, hallucinations, euphoria, LOC, pupil reaction
• Allergic reactions: rash, urticaria
• Respiratory dysfunction: respiratory depression, character, rate, rhythm; notify prescriber if respirations are <10/min
Administer:
• By inj (IM, IV); give slowly to prevent rigidity
• Must have emergency equipment available, opioid antagonists, O_2; to be used by only those trained; (IV) products to be used in OR, ER, ICU
Transmucosal route
• Remove foil just before administration; instruct patient to place under tongue and suck, not chew (Oralet); place between cheek and lower gum, moving it back and forth and suck, not chew (Actiq); all products not used or partially used should be flushed down the toilet
IV route
• IV undiluted by anesthesiologist or diluted with 5 ml or more sterile H_2O or 0.9% NaCl given through Y-tube or 3-way stopcock at 0.1 mg or less/1-2 min
Additive compatibilities: Bupivacaine
Solution compatibilities: D_5W, 0.9% NaCl
Syringe compatibilities: Atracurium, atropine, bupivacaine/ketamine, butorphanol, chlorproMAZINE, cimetidine, clonidine/lidocaine, diphenhyDRINATE, diphenhydrAMINE, droperidol, heparin, hydromorphone, hydrOXYzine, meperidine, metoclopramide, midazolam, morphine, pentazocine, perphenazine, prochlorperazine, promazine, promethazine, ranitidine, scopolamine
Y-site compatibilities: Amphotericin B cholesteryl, atracurium, cisatracurium, diltiazem, DOBUTamine, DOPamine, enalaprilat, epINEPHrine, esmolol, etomidate, furosemide, heparin, hydrocortisone, hydromorphone, labetalol, lorazepam, midazolam, milrinone, morphine, nafcillin, niCARdipine, nitroglycerin, norepinephrine, pancuronium, potassium chloride, propofol, ranitidine, remifentanil, sargramostim, thiopental, vecuronium, vit B/C
Perform/provide:
• Storage in light-resistant area at room temperature
Teach patient/family:
• Coughing, turning, deep breathing for postoperative patients
• Safety measures: side rails, night-light, call bell within reach
Evaluate:
• Therapeutic response: induction of anesthesia, breakthrough cancer pain

---

⚠ High Alert

fentanyl transdermal (℞)
Duragesic
Func. class.: Opioid analgesic
Chem. class.: Synthetic phenylpiperidine

Controlled Substance Schedule II
Action: Inhibits ascending pain pathways in CNS, increases pain threshold, alters pain perception by binding to opiate receptors
Uses: Management of chronic pain for those requiring opioid analgesia

DOSAGE AND ROUTES
• *Adult:* 25 mcg/hr; may increase until pain relief occurs; apply patch to flat surface on upper torso and wear for 72 hr; apply new patch on different site for continued relief

---

⚠ Safety alert   *"Tall Man" lettering

Available forms: Patch 12.5, 25, 50, 75, 100 mcg/hr

SIDE EFFECTS

CNS: Dizziness, delirium, euphoria, lightheadedness, sedation, dysphoria, agitation, anxiety, confusion, headache, depression

CV: Bradycardia, **cardiac arrest,** hypotension or hypertension, facial flushing, chills, chest pain, dysrhythmias

EENT: Blurred vision, miosis

GI: Nausea, vomiting, diarrhea, cramps, anorexia, constipation, dyspepsia

GU: Urinary retention, urgency, dysuria, frequency, oliguria

INTEG: Sweating, pruritus, rash, erythema, papules

MS: Asthenia

RESP: **Respiratory depression, laryngospasm, bronchospasm,** depresses cough, hypoventilation, dyspnea, hiccups, apnea

Contraindications: Hypersensitivity to opiates, myasthenia gravis, children <12 yr, patient <18 yr with weight <110 lb

Precautions: Pregnancy (C), geriatric, respiratory depression, increased intracranial pressure, seizure disorders, severe respiratory disorders, cardiac dysrhythmias, fever

INTERACTIONS

Increase: with other CNS depressants—alcohol, opioids, sedative/hypnotics, antipsychotics, skeletal muscle relaxants

Drug/Herb

Increase: anticholinergic effect—corkwood

Increase: action—Jamaican dogwood, kava, lavender, mistletoe, nettle, pokeweed, poppy, senega, valerian

Drug/Lab Test

Increase: Amylase, lipase

NURSING CONSIDERATIONS

Assess:

• Pain control; check for duration, site, character of pain, fever; use pain and sedation scoring

• CNS changes: dizziness, drowsiness, hallucinations, euphoria, LOC, pupil reaction; ongoing use may lead to dependence

• Allergic reactions: rash, urticaria

• VS: B/P, pulse respirations; respiratory depression, character, rate, rhythm; notify prescriber if respirations are <10/min

• Bowel function, severe constipation may occur

Administer:

• q72h for continuous pain relief; dosage is adjusted after at least two applications, apply to clean, dry skin, press firmly

• Give short-acting analgesics until patch takes effect (8-12 hr); when reducing dosage or switching to alternate IV treatment, withdraw gradually; serum levels drop gradually, give ½ the equianalgesic dose of new analgesic 12-18 hr after removal as ordered

Perform/provide:

• Safety measures: side rails, night-light, call bell within reach

Evaluate:

• Therapeutic response: decreased pain

Teach patient/family:

• To avoid activities that require alertness

• That excessive heat may increase absorption

• That excessive perspiration may alter adhesiveness

• To dispose of patch by placing sticky sides together and flushing in toilet

• That patient may need to clip hair before applying to ensure adhesion

Side effects: *italics* = common; **bold** = life-threatening

ferrous fumarate (℞)

Femiron, Feostat, Feostat Drops, Hemocyte, Ircon, Nephro-Fer, Novofumar ✦, Palafer ✦, Span-FF

ferrous gluconate (℞)

Fergon, Fertinic ✦, Novoferrogluc ✦

ferrous sulfate (℞)

Apo-Ferrous Sulfate ✦, ED-IN-SOL, Feosol, Fer-gen-sol, Fer-Iron Drops, Fero-Grad, Mol-Iron

ferrous sulfate, dried (℞)

Fe^{50}, Feosol, Feratab, Novoferrosulfa ✦, PMS-Ferrous Sulfate, Slow Fe

ferric gluconate complex (℞)

Ferrlecit

carbonyl iron

(kar'bo-nil)

Feosol

iron polysaccharide

Hytinic, Niferex, Nu-Iron, Nu-Iron 150

Func. class.: Hematinic
Chem. class.: Iron preparation

Action: Replaces iron stores needed for red blood cell development, energy and O_2 transport, utilization; fumarate contains 33% elemental iron; gluconate, 12%; sulfate, 20%; iron, 30%; ferrous sulfate exsiccated

Uses: Iron deficiency anemia, prophylaxis for iron deficiency in pregnancy

DOSAGE AND ROUTES

Fumarate
• *Adult:* **PO** 200 mg daily-qid
• *Child 2-12 yr:* **PO** 3 mg/kg/day (elemental iron) tid-qid
• *Child 6 mo-2 yr:* **PO** up to 6 mg/kg/day (elemental iron) tid-qid

• *Infant:* **PO** 10-25 mg/day (elemental iron) in 3-4 divided doses, max 15 mg/day

Gluconate
• *Adult:* **PO** 200-600 mg daily-tid
• *Child 6-12 yr:* **PO** 300-900 mg daily
• *Child <6 yr:* **PO** 100-300 mg daily

Sulfate
• *Adult:* **PO** 0.75-1.5 g/day in divided doses tid
• *Child 6-12 yr:* **PO** 600 mg/day in divided doses

Pregnancy
• *Adult:* **PO** 300-600 mg/day in divided doses

Complex
• *Adult:* **IV INF** (125 mg) 10 ml/100 ml of NaCl for inj given over 1 hr

Iron polysaccharide
• *Adult:* **PO** 100-200 mg tid
• *Child:* **PO** 4-6 mg/kg/day in 3 divided doses

Available forms: *Fumarate:* tabs 63, 195, 200, 324, 325 mg; chewable tabs 100 mg; cont rel tabs 300 mg; oral susp 100 mg/5 ml, 45 mg/0.6 ml; *gluconate:* tabs 300, 320, 325 mg; caps 86, 325, 435 mg; film-coated tabs 300 mg; elix 300 mg/5 ml; *sulfate:* tabs 195, 300, 325 mg; enteric-coated tabs 325 mg; ext rel tabs, time-rel caps, 525 mg; *dried:* tabs 200 mg; ext rel tabs 160 mg; ext rel caps 160 mg; *complex:* inj 62.5 mg/5 ml (12.5 mg/ml); *iron polysaccharide:* tabs 50 mg; caps 150 mg; sol 100 mg/5 ml

SIDE EFFECTS

GI: Nausea, constipation, epigastric pain, black and red tarry stools, vomiting, diarrhea
INTEG: Temporarily discolored tooth enamel and eyes
Contraindications: Hypersensitivity, ulcerative colitis/regional enteritis, hemosiderosis/hemochromatosis, peptic ulcer disease, hemolytic anemia, cirrhosis
Precautions: Pregnancy (B) (ferric gluconate complex), (C) (iron dextran, oral products), anemia (long term)

PHARMACOKINETICS

PO: Excreted in feces, urine, skin, breast milk; enters bloodstream; bound to transferrin; crosses placenta

INTERACTIONS

Increase: action of iron preparation—ascorbic acid, chloramphenicol

Decrease: absorption of penicillamine, levodopa, methyldopa, fluoroquinolones, L-thyroxine, tetracycline

Decrease: absorption of iron preparations—antacids, H₂-antagonists, proton pump inhibitors, cholestyramine, vit E

Drug/Herb

• Forms insoluble complex: black catechu

Increase: iron effect—anise

Decrease: iron absorption—allspice, bilberry, condurango, elderberry, eyebright (PO), gentian, ground ivy, hawthorn, horse chestnut, lady mantle, lemon balm, marshmallow, meadowsweet, mistletoe, motherwort, nettle, oak bark, plantain, poplar, prickly ash, raspberry, sage, tea made with artichoke, valerian

Drug/Food

Decrease: absorption—dairy products, caffeine, eggs

Drug/Lab Test

False positive: Occult blood

NURSING CONSIDERATIONS

Assess:

• Blood studies: Hct, Hgb, reticulocytes, bilirubin before treatment, at least monthly; iron studies (Fe, TIBC, ferritin)

⚠ Toxicity: nausea, vomiting, diarrhea (green, then tarry stools), hematemesis, pallor, cyanosis, shock, coma

• Elimination; if constipation occurs, increase water, bulk, activity

• Nutrition: amount of iron in diet (meat, dark green leafy vegetables, dried beans, dried fruits, eggs)

• Cause of iron loss or anemia, including salicylates, sulfonamides, antimalarials, quinidine

Administer:

• Swallow tabs whole; not to break, crush, or chew unless labeled as chewable

• Between meals for best absorption; may give with juice; do not give with antacids or milk, delay at least 1 hr; if GI symptoms occur, give after meals even if absorption is decreased; eggs, milk products, chocolate, caffeine interfere with absorption

• Liquid through plastic straw to avoid discoloration of tooth enamel; dilute thoroughly

• At least 1 hr before bedtime, since corrosion may occur in stomach; ferrous gluconate is less GI irritating than ferrous sulfate

• For <6 mo for anemia

Perform/provide:

• Storage in tight, light-resistant container

Evaluate:

• Therapeutic response: improvement in Hct, Hgb, reticulocytes; decreased fatigue, weakness

Teach patient/family:

• That iron will change stools black or dark green

• That iron poisoning may occur if increased beyond recommended level

• To keep out of reach of children

• Not to substitute one iron salt for another; elemental iron content differs (e.g., 300 mg ferrous fumarate contains about 100 mg elemental iron; 300 mg ferrous gluconate contains only about 30 mg elemental iron)

• To avoid reclining position for 15-30 min after taking drug to avoid esophageal corrosion

• To follow diet high in iron

Treatment of overdose: Induce vomiting; give eggs, milk until lavage can be done

F

fexofenadine (Rx)

(fex-oh-fi′na-deen)

Allegra

Func. class.: Antihistamine

Chem. class.: Piperidine, peripherally selective

Do not confuse:

Allegra/Viagra

Action: Acts on blood vessels, GI, respiratory system by competing with histamine for H_1-receptor site; decreases allergic response by blocking pharmacologic effects of histamine

Uses: Rhinitis, allergy symptoms, chronic idiopathic urticaria

DOSAGE AND ROUTES

• *Adult and child >12 yr:* 60 mg bid or 180 mg daily

• *Child 6-11 yr:* **PO** 30 mg bid

Renal dose

• *Adult and child ≥12 yr:* **PO** CCr <80 ml/min 60 mg daily

Available forms: Tabs 30, 60, 180 mg; caps 60 mg

SIDE EFFECTS

CNS: Headache, stimulation, drowsiness, sedation, fatigue, confusion, blurred vision, tinnitus, restlessness, tremors, paradoxical excitation in children or geriatric

CV: Hypotension, palpitations, bradycardia, tachycardia, **dysrhythmias** (rare)

GI: Nausea, diarrhea, abdominal pain, vomiting, constipation

GU: Frequency, dysuria, urinary retention, impotence

HEMA: **Hemolytic anemia, thrombocytopenia, leukopenia, agranulocytosis, pancytopenia**

INTEG: Rash, eczema, photosensitivity, urticaria

RESP: Thickening of bronchial secretions, dry nose, throat

Contraindications: Hypersensitivity, newborn or premature infants, lactation, severe hepatic disease

Precautions: Pregnancy (C), geriatric, children, respiratory disease, narrow-angle glaucoma, prostatic hypertrophy, bladder neck obstruction, asthma

PHARMACOKINETICS

Well absorbed; onset 1 hr; peak 2-3 hr; duration 12-24 hr; 80% excreted in urine; half-life 14.5 hr, increased in renal disease

INTERACTIONS

Decrease: effect—magnesium-aluminum-containing antacids

Drug/Food

Decrease: absorption—apple, orange, grapefruit juice

Drug/Lab Test

False negative: Skin allergy tests

NURSING CONSIDERATIONS

Assess:

• Allergy: itchy, runny, watery eyes; congested nose; before and during treatment

• I&O ratio: be alert for urinary retention, frequency, dysuria, especially geriatric; drug should be discontinued if these occur

• Respiratory status: rate, rhythm, increase in bronchial secretions, wheezing, chest tightness

Administer:

• With food or milk to decrease GI symptoms; caps/tabs should not be given with juice

Perform/provide:

• Storage in tight, light-resistant container

Evaluate:

• Therapeutic response: absence of running or congested nose or rashes

Teach patient/family:

• All aspects of drug use; to notify prescriber if confusion, sedation, hypotension occur

• To avoid driving, other hazardous activity if drowsiness occurs

⚠ Safety alert   *"Tall Man" lettering

- To avoid alcohol, other CNS depressants
- Not to exceed recommended dose; dysrhythmias may occur

Treatment of overdose: Lavage, diazepam, vasopressors, barbiturates (short acting)

---

filgrastim (℞)

(fill-grass'stim)

G-CSF, granulocyte colony stimulator, Neupogen

Func. class.: Biologic modifier
Chem. class.: Granulocyte colony-stimulating factor

Action: Stimulates proliferation and differentiation of neutrophils

Uses: To decrease infection in patients receiving antineoplastics that are myelosuppressive; to increase WBC in patients with drug-induced neutropenia; bone marrow transplantation

Unlabeled uses: Neutropenia in HIV infection, aplastic anemia, ganciclovir-induced neutropenia, zidovudine-induced neutropenia

DOSAGE AND ROUTES

After myelosuppressive chemotherapy

- *Adult and child:* **IV/SUBCUT** 5 mcg/kg/day in a single dose × 14 days; may increase by 5 mcg/kg in each cycle; give daily for up to 2 wk until the absolute neutrophil count (ANC) is 10,000/mm³; response to G-CSF is much greater with **SUBCUT** than **IV** therapy

After bone marrow transplantation

- *Adult:* **IV/SUBCUT** 10 mcg/kg/day as an **INF (IV)** over 4 hr or 24 hr, begin 24 hr after chemotherapy and 24 hr after bone marrow transplantation

Peripheral blood progenitor cell collection/therapy

- *Adult:* 10 mcg/kg/day as a bolus or **CONT INF** × 4 days or more before leukapheresis, continue to last leukapheresis; may alter dose if WBC >100,000 cells/mm³

Severe neutropenia (chronic), idiopathic/cyclical

- *Adult:* **SUBCUT** 5 mcg/kg daily-bid

Available forms: Inj 300 mcg/ml

SIDE EFFECTS

CNS: Fever

GI: Nausea, vomiting, diarrhea, mucositis, anorexia

HEMA: **Thrombocytopenia,** excessive leukocytosis

INTEG: Alopecia, exacerbation of skin conditions, urticaria

MS: Osteoporosis, skeletal pain

OTHER: Chest pain

RESP: Respiratory distress syndrome, wheezing

Contraindications: Hypersensitivity to proteins of *E. coli*

Precautions: Pregnancy (C), lactation, cardiac conditions, children, myeloid malignancies, radiation therapy, sepsis, sickle cell disease

PHARMACOKINETICS

IV: Onset 5-60 min, peak 24 hr, duration up to a week

SUBCUT: Onset 5-60 min, peak 2-8 hr, duration up to a week

INTERACTIONS

Increase: adverse reactions—do not use this drug concomitantly with antineoplastics

Drug/Lab Test

Increase: Uric acid, LDH, alk phos

NURSING CONSIDERATIONS

Assess:

- Blood studies: CBC, platelet count before treatment and twice weekly; neutrophil counts may be increased for 2 days after therapy
- B/P, respirations, pulse before and during therapy
- Bone pain, give mild analgesics
- CBC with differential platelets

Administer:

- Using single-use vials; after dose is withdrawn, do not reenter vial

---

- No earlier than 24 hr after antineoplastics, bone marrow infusion
- Do not shake; may warm to room temperature before using; discard any product left out for >6 hr
- For 2 wk or until ANC is 10,000/mm³ after the expected chemotherapy neutrophil nadir

SUBCUT route
- May divide into 2 inj if amount to be given is >1 ml

CONT IV INF route
- Dilute in D₅W to a conc of >15 mcg/ml, vial is for one-time use; give over 15-30 min (chemotherapy); over 4-24 hr (bone marrow transplantation); do not use 0.9% NaCl to dilute drug

Y-site compatibilities: Acyclovir, allopurinol, amikacin, aminophylline, ampicillin, ampicillin/sulbactam, aztreonam, bleomycin, bumetanide, buprenorphine, butorphanol, calcium gluconate, carboplatin, carmustine, cefazolin, cefotetan, ceftazidime, chlorproMAZINE, cimetidine, cisplatin, cyclophosphamide, cytarabine, dacarbazine, DAUNOrubicin, dexamethasone, diphenhydrAMINE, DOXOrubicin, doxycycline, droperidol, enalaprilat, famotidine, floxuridine, fluconazole, fludarabine, gallium, ganciclovir, granisetron, haloperidol, hydrocortisone, hydromorphone, hydrOXYzine, idarubicin, ifosfamide, leucovorin, lorazepam, mechlorethamine, melphalan, meperidine, mesna, methotrexate, metoclopramide, miconazole, minocycline, mitoxantrone, morphine, nalbuphine, netilmicin, ondansetron, plicamycin, potassium chloride, promethazine, ranitidine, sodium bicarbonate, streptozocin, ticarcillin, ticarcillin/clavulanate, tobramycin, trimethoprim-sulfamethoxazole, vancomycin, vinBLAStine, vinCRIStine, vinorelbine, zidovudine

Perform/provide:
- Storage in refrigerator; do not freeze; may store at room temperature up to 6 hr
- Avoid shaking

Evaluate:
- Therapeutic response: absence of infection

Teach patient/family:
- The technique for self-administration: dose, side effects, disposal of containers and needles; provide instruction sheet

finasteride (℞)
(fin-ass'te-ride)
Propecia, Proscar
Func. class.: Hormone, androgen inhibitor, hair stimulant
Chem. class.: 5-α-Reductase inhibitor

Do not confuse:
Proscar/ProSom/Prozac
Action: Inhibits 5-α-reductase and reduction in DHT; DHT induces androgenic effects by binding to androgen receptors in the cell nuclei of the prostate gland, liver, skin; prevents development of BHP
Uses: Symptomatic benign prostatic hyperplasia (Proscar); male-pattern baldness (Propecia)

DOSAGE AND ROUTES
BPH
- *Adult:* **PO** 5 mg daily × 6-12 mo
Male pattern baldness
- *Adult:* **PO** 1 mg daily
Available forms: (Propecia) tabs 1 mg, (Proscar) 5 mg

SIDE EFFECTS
GU: Impotence, decreased libido, decreased volume of ejaculate
Contraindications: Pregnancy (X), hypersensitivity, children, women who are pregnant or may become pregnant should not handle tabs
Precautions: Large residual urinary volume, severely diminished urinary flow, hepatic function abnormalities

PHARMACOKINETICS
Bioavailability 63%, readily absorbed from GI tract, plasma protein binding 90%; metabolized in the liver; excreted in urine (metabolites) 39%, feces (57%); crosses blood-brain barrier; peak 1-2 hr, duration 24 hr

INTERACTIONS

Decrease: finasteride effect—theophylline, adrenergic bronchodilators, anticholinergics

Drug/Lab Test

Decrease: PSA levels (finasteride)

NURSING CONSIDERATIONS

Assess:
• BPH: urinary patterns, residual urinary volume, severely diminished urinary flow
• PSA levels and digital rectal exam prior to initiating therapy and periodically thereafter
• Hepatic studies prior to treatment; extensively metabolized in liver

Administer:
• Without regard to meals
• For a minimum of 6 mo; not all patients will respond

Perform/provide:
• Storage <86° F (30° C); protect from light; keep container tightly closed

Evaluate:
• Therapeutic response: increased urinary flow, decreased postvoiding dribbling, frequency, nocturia or hair growth within 3-6 mo

Teach patient/family:
⚠ Pregnant women or women who may become pregnant should not touch crushed tabs or come into contact with semen of a patient taking this drug; may adversely affect developing male fetus
• That volume of ejaculate may be decreased during treatment; impotence and decreased libido may also occur
• Propecia results may not occur for 3 mo
• Proscar results may not occur for 6-12 mo

flavocoxid (℞)

(flav-uh-kox'id)
Limbrel
Func. class.: Analgesic, nonopioid
Chem. class.: Flavanoid

Action: Exhibits antiinflammatory, analgesic properties, thought to be due to inhibition of prostaglandin synthesis via inhibition of cyclooxygenase

Uses: For dietary management of osteoarthritis

DOSAGE AND ROUTES
• *Adult:* **PO** 250 mg q12h
Available forms: Cap 250 mg

SIDE EFFECTS
MISC: Hypertension, increase in varicose veins, psoriasis
MS: Fluid accumulation in the knees
Contraindications: Hypersensitivity
Precautions: Pregnancy (UK), lactation, children <18 yr, history of stomach ulcers

PHARMACOKINETICS
Metabolism primarily via glucuronidation and sulfation

INTERACTIONS
• Unknown

NURSING CONSIDERATIONS
Assess:
• For pain of rheumatoid arthritis, osteoarthritis; check ROM, inflammation of joints, characteristics of pain
Administer:
• 1 hr before or after meals
Evaluate:
• Therapeutic response: decreased pain, inflammation in arthritic conditions
Teach patient/family:
• That drug does not take the place of other drugs, including corticosteroids for osteoarthritis
• To notify prescriber if pregnancy is planned or suspected

Rarely Used

flavoxate (R)
(fla-vox′ate)
Func. class.: Spasmolytic

Uses: Relief of nocturia, incontinence, suprapubic pain, dysuria, frequency associated with urologic conditions (symptomatic only)

DOSAGE AND ROUTES
• *Adult and child >12 yr:* **PO** 100-200 mg tid-qid
Contraindications: Hypersensitivity, GI obstruction, GI hemorrhage, GU obstruction

flecainide (R)
(flek-ay′nide)
Tambocor
Func. class.: Antidysrhythmic (Class IC)

Action: Decreases conduction in all parts of the heart, with greatest effect on His-Purkinje system, which stabilizes cardiac membrane
Uses: Life-threatening ventricular dysrhythmias, sustained ventricular tachycardia, supraventricular tachydysrhythmias, paroxysmal atrial fibrillation/flutter associated with disabling symptoms
Unlabeled uses: Atrial fibrillation, single dose

DOSAGE AND ROUTES
PSVTT/PAF
• *Adult:* **PO** 50 mg q12h; may increase q4d by 50 mg q12h to desired response, max 300 mg/day
Life-threatening ventricular dysrhythmias
• *Adult:* **PO** 100 mg q12h; may increase by 50 mg q12h q4d, max 400 mg/day
Renal dose
• *Adult:* **PO** CCr <35 ml/min dose 50%-75%

Available forms: Tabs 50, 100, 150 mg

SIDE EFFECTS
CNS: Headache, dizziness, involuntary movement, confusion, psychosis, restlessness, irritability, paresthesias, ataxia, flushing, somnolence, depression, anxiety, malaise, fatigue, asthenia, tremors
CV: Hypotension, bradycardia, angina, PVCs, **heart block, cardiovascular collapse, arrest,** dysrhythmias, **CHF, fatal ventricular tachycardia**
EENT: Tinnitus, *blurred vision,* hearing loss
GI: Nausea, vomiting, anorexia, constipation, abdominal pain, flatulence, change in taste
GU: Impotence, decreased libido, polyuria, urinary retention
HEMA: Leukopenia, thrombocytopenia
INTEG: Rash, urticaria, edema, swelling
RESP: Dyspnea, **respiratory depression**
Contraindications: Hypersensitivity, severe heart block, cardiogenic shock, nonsustained ventricular dysrhythmias, frequent PVCs, non–life-threatening dysrhythmias
Precautions: Pregnancy (C), lactation, children, renal/hepatic disease, CHF, respiratory depression, myasthenia gravis

PHARMACOKINETICS
PO: Peak 3 hr; half-life 12-27 hr; metabolized by liver; excreted unchanged by kidneys (10%); excreted in breast milk

INTERACTIONS
Increase: of both drugs—propranolol
Increase: CV depressant action—β-blockers, disopyramide, verapamil
Increase: flecainide level—amiodarone, cimetidine, ritonavir
Increase: digoxin level—digoxin
Increase or decrease: effect—urinary, alkalinizing agents, acidifying agents
Drug/Herb
Increase: toxicity, death—aconite
Increase: effect—aloe, broom, chronic

buckthorn use, cascara sagrada (chronic use), Chinese rhubarb, figwort, fumitory, goldenseal, kudzu, licorice

Increase: serotonin effect—horehound
Decrease: effect—coltsfoot
Drug/Lab Test
Increase: CPK

NURSING CONSIDERATIONS
Assess:
• I&O, daily weight
⚠ CHF: edema, weight gain, dyspnea, jugular vein distention, crackles
• For hypokalemia, hyperkalemia before administration; correct electrolytes
• Blood levels: trough (0.2-1 mcg/ml)
• B/P, ECG or Holter monitor continuously for fluctuations; watch for QRS widening, prolongation of QT and PR
• CNS effects: dizziness, confusion, psychosis, paresthesias, convulsions; drug should be discontinued
• Increased respiration, increased pulse; drug should be discontinued
Administer:
• Reduced dosage as soon as dysrhythmia is controlled
• May give with meals for GI upset
• May adjust dose q4 day
Evaluate:
• Therapeutic response: decreased dysrhythmias
Teach patient/family:
• To change position slowly from lying or sitting to standing to minimize orthostatic hypotension
• To take as prescribed, not to skip or double dose
• To avoid hazardous activities that require alertness until response is known
• To carry emergency ID with disorder, medications taken
• To notify all health care providers of treatment
Treatment of overdose: O_2, artificial ventilation, ECG, DOPamine for circulatory depression, diazepam or thiopental for convulsions, treat ventricular dysrhythmias

Rarely Used
floxuridine (℞)
(flox-yoor′i-deen)
Floxuridine, FUDR
Func. class.: Antineoplastic, antimetabolite

Uses: GI adenocarcinoma metastatic to liver; cancer of breast, head, neck, liver, brain, gallbladder, bile duct

DOSAGE AND ROUTES
• *Adult:* **INTRAARTERIAL** by cont inf 0.1-0.6 mg/kg/day × 1-6 wk; **HEPATIC ARTERY INJ** 0.4-0.6 mg/kg/day × 1-6 wk
Contraindications: Pregnancy (D), hypersensitivity, myelosuppression, poor nutritional status, serious infections, lactation

fluconazole (℞)
(floo-kon′a-zole)
Diflucan
Func. class.: Antifungal, systemic
Chem class: Triazole derivative

Do not confuse:
Diflucan/Diprivan
Action: Inhibits ergosterol biosynthesis, causes direct damage to fungal membrane phospholipids
Uses: Oropharyngeal candidiasis, chronic mucocutaneous candidiasis, systemic, vaginal, urinary candidiasis, cryptococcal meningitis, prevention of candidiasis in bone marrow transplant

DOSAGE AND ROUTES
Vaginal candidiasis
• *Adult:* **PO** 150 mg as a single dose
Serious fungal infections
• *Adult:* **PO/IV** 50-400 mg initially, then 200 mg daily for 4 wk
• *Child:* 6-12 mg/kg/day
Oropharyngeal candidiasis
• *Adult:* **PO/IV** 200 mg initially, then 100 mg daily for at least 2 wk
• *Child:* **PO/IV** 3 mg/kg/day

Prevention of candidiasis in bone marrow transplant
• *Adult:* **PO/IV** 400 mg daily
Renal disease
• *Adult:* **PO/IV** CCr 11-50 ml/min dose 50%

Available forms: Tabs 50, 100, 150, 200 mg; inj 2 mg/ml; powder for oral susp 50, 200 mg/ml

SIDE EFFECTS

CNS: Headache
GI: Nausea, vomiting, diarrhea, cramping, flatus, increased AST, ALT, **hepatotoxicity**
INTEG: **Stevens-Johnson syndrome**
Contraindications: Hypersensitivity to this drug or azoles
Precautions: Pregnancy (C), renal/hepatic disease, lactation

PHARMACOKINETICS

Peak 2-4 hr, bioavailability (PO) >90%, excreted unchanged in urine 80%, metabolized by CYP3A enzyme system at dose >200 mg/day

INTERACTIONS

Increase: hypoglycemia—oral antidiabetics
Increase: anticoagulation—warfarin
Increase: plasma concentrations—cycloSPORINE, phenytoin, theophylline, rifabutin, tacrolimus
Increase: effect of zidovudine
Decrease: effect of oral contraceptives
Drug/Herb
Increase: nephrotoxicity—gossypol

NURSING CONSIDERATIONS

Assess:
• For infection: clearing of CSF and other culture during treatment, obtain C&S baseline and throughout, drug may be started as soon as culture is taken
⚠ For hepatotoxicity: increasing AST, ALT, periodically alk phos, bilirubin
Administer:
PO route
• Shake oral susp before each use

IV route
• After diluting according to package directions; run at 200 mg/hr or less; do not use plastic containers in connections; check for bag leaks
• Using an infusion pump check for extravasation and necrosis q2h
• Do not use if cloudy or precipitated
• Do not admix; do not refrigerate
Y-site compatibilities: Acyclovir, aldesleukin, allopurinol, amifostine, amikacin, aminophylline, ampicillin/sulbactam, aztreonam, benztropine, cefazolin, cefepime, cefotetan, cefoxitin, chlorproMAZINE, cimetidine, cisatracurium, dexamethasone, diphenhydrAMINE, DOBUTamine, DOPamine, DOXOrubicin liposome, droperidol, famotidine, filgrastim, fludarabine, foscarnet, gallium, ganciclovir, gentamicin, granisetron, heparin, hydrocortisone, immune globulin, leucovorin, lorazepam, melphalan, meperidine, meropenem, metoclopramide, metronidazole, midazolam, morphine, nafcillin, nitroglycerin, ondansetron, oxacillin, paclitaxel, pancuronium, penicillin G potassium, phenytoin, piperacillin/tazobactam, prochlorperazine, promethazine, propofol, ranitidine, remifentanil, sargramostim, tacrolimus, teniposide, theophylline, thiotepa, ticarcillin/clavulanate, tobramycin, vancomycin, vecuronium, vinorelbine, zidovudine
Perform/provide:
• Storage protected from moisture and light, diluted sol is stable 24 hr, do not freeze
Evaluate:
• Therapeutic response: decreasing oral candidiasis, fever, malaise, rash; negative C&S for infection organism
Teach patient/family:
• That long-term therapy may be needed to clear infection
• That medication may be taken with food to reduce GI effects
• To notify prescriber of nausea, vomiting, diarrhea, jaundice, anorexia, clay-colored stools, dark urine
• Use alternative method of contraception while taking this drug

fludarabine (℞)

(floo-dar'a-been)
Fludara
Func. class.: Antineoplastic, antimetabolite

Uses: Chronic lymphocytic leukemia, non-Hodgkin's lymphoma

DOSAGE AND ROUTES

• *Adult:* **IV** 25 mg/m² over 30 min daily × 5 days, may repeat q28d; reconstitute with 2 ml of sterile water for inj; dissolution should occur in <15 sec
Contraindications: Pregnancy (D), hypersensitivity, lactation

fludrocortisone (℞)

(floo-droe-kor'ti-sone)
Florinef
Func. class.: Corticosteroid, synthetic
Chem. class.: Mineralocorticoid

Action: Promotes increased reabsorption of sodium and loss of potassium, water, hydrogen from distal renal tubules
Uses: Adrenal insufficiency, salt-losing adrenogenital syndrome
Unlabeled uses: Renal tubular acidosis (type IV), idiopathic orthostatic hypotension

DOSAGE AND ROUTES

• *Adult:* **PO** 100-200 mcg daily
• *Child:* **PO** 50-100 mcg/day
Idiopathic hypotension (unlabeled)
• *Adult:* **PO** 50-100 mcg/day
Available forms: Tabs 100 mcg (0.1 mg)

SIDE EFFECTS

CNS: Flushing, sweating, headache, paralysis, dizziness
CV: Hypertension, **circulatory collapse, thrombophlebitis, embolism,** tachycardia, **CHF,** edema
ENDO: Weight gain, adrenal suppression
META: Hypokalemia
MISC: Hypersensitivity
MS: Fractures, osteoporosis, weakness
Contraindications: Hypersensitivity, acute glomerulonephritis, amebiasis, psychoses, Cushing's syndrome, fungal infections, child <2 yr
Precautions: Pregnancy (C), osteoporosis, CHF, lactation, child >2 yr, hypertension, diabetes

PHARMACOKINETICS

PO: Peak 1.5 hr, half-life 3.5 hr, metabolized by liver, excreted in urine

INTERACTIONS

Increase: B/P—sodium-containing food or medication
Decrease: fludrocortisone action—barbiturates, rifampin, phenytoin
Decrease: potassium levels—thiazides, potassium-wasting drugs, loop diuretics, amphotericin B, piperacillin, mezlocillin
Drug/Herb
Increase: Hypokalemia—aloe, buckthorn, cascara sagrada, Chinese rhubarb, senna
Increase: Corticosteroid effect—aloe, licorice, perilla
Drug/Lab Test
Increase: Potassium, sodium
Decrease: Hct

NURSING CONSIDERATIONS

Assess:
• Weight daily; notify prescriber of weekly gain >5 lb
• I&O ratio; be alert for decreasing urinary output, increasing edema
• B/P q4h, pulse; notify prescriber if chest pain occurs
• Potassium depletion: paresthesias, fatigue, nausea, vomiting, depression, polyuria, dysrhythmias, weakness
• Electrolytes: sodium, potassium, chloride, hypokalemia is common

---

Administer:
- Titrated dose; use lowest effective dose
- With food or milk to decrease GI symptoms

Perform/provide:
- Assistance with ambulation in patient with bone tissue disease to prevent fractures

Evaluate:
- Therapeutic response: correction of adrenal insufficiency

Teach patient/family:
- That emergency ID as steroid user should be carried
- Not to discontinue this medication abruptly
- To notify health care provider of muscle cramps, weight gain, edema, nausea, infection, trauma, stress
- Not to breastfeed while taking this medication

---

flumazenil (R)
(flu-maz′e-nill)
Anexate ♦, Romazicon
Func. class.: Antidote: Benzodiazepine receptor antagonist
Chem. class.: Imidazobenzodiazepine derivative

Action: Antagonizes actions of benzodiazepines on CNS, competitively inhibits activity at benzodiazepine recognition site on GABA/benzodiazepine receptor complex

Uses: Reversal of sedative effects of benzodiazepines

DOSAGE AND ROUTES

Reversal of conscious sedation or in general anesthesia
- *Adult:* **IV** 0.2 mg given over 15 sec; wait 45 sec, then give 0.2 mg if consciousness does not occur; may be repeated at 60-sec intervals prn (max 3 mg/hr)
- *Child:* **IV** 10 mcg (0.01 mg)/kg; cumulative dose of 1 mg or less

Management of suspected benzodiazepine overdose
- *Adult:* **IV** 0.2 mg given over 30 sec; wait 30 sec, then give 0.3 mg over 30 sec if consciousness does not occur; further doses of 0.5 mg can be given over 30 sec at intervals of 1 min up to cumulative dose of 3 mg
- *Child:* **IV** 100 mcg (0.1 mg)/kg; cumulative dose of 1 mg or less

Available forms: Inj 0.1 mg/ml

SIDE EFFECTS

CNS: Dizziness, agitation, emotional lability, confusion, **seizures,** somnolence
CV: Hypertension, palpitations, cutaneous vasodilation, **dysrhythmias,** bradycardia, tachycardia, chest pain
EENT: Abnormal vision, blurred vision, tinnitus
GI: Nausea, vomiting, hiccups
SYST: Headache, inj site pain, increased sweating, fatigue, rigors

Contraindications: Hypersensitivity to this drug or benzodiazepines, serious cyclic antidepressant overdose, patients given benzodiazepine for control of life-threatening condition

Precautions: Pregnancy (C), lactation, children, geriatric, status epilepticus, head injury, labor/delivery, renal/hepatic disease, hypoventilation, panic disorder, drug and alcohol dependency, ambulatory patients

PHARMACOKINETICS

Terminal half-life 41-79 min; metabolized in liver

INTERACTIONS

- Toxicity: mixed drug overdosage
- Antagonize action of benzodiazepines, zaleplon, zolpidem

NURSING CONSIDERATIONS

Assess:
- Cardiac status using continuous monitoring
- For seizures; protect patient from in-

---

jury; most likely those that have withdrawals from sedatives

• GI symptoms: nausea, vomiting; place in side-lying position to prevent aspiration

• Allergic reactions: flushing, rash, urticaria, pruritus

Administer:

• Check airway and IV access before administration

IV, direct route

• Give undiluted or diluted with 0.9% NaCl, D₅W, LR, give over 15 sec into running IV

Additive compatibilities: Aminophylline, cimetidine, DOBUTamine, DOPamine, famotidine, heparin, lidocaine, procainamide, ranitidine

Solution compatibilities: D₅W

Evaluate:

• Therapeutic response: decreased sedation, respiratory depression, toxicity

Teach patient/family:

• That amnesia may continue

• Not to engage in hazardous activities for 18-24 hr after discharge

• Not to take any alcohol or nonprescription drugs for 18-24 hr

---

flunisolide nasal agent
See Appendix C

---

fluocinolone topical
See Appendix C

---

fluoride (PO) (℞)
(floor′ide)
Fluor-A-Day ✦, Fluoride Loz, Fluoritab, Flura-Loz, Karidium, Luride, Pediaflor, Pharmaflur, Phos-Flur, Solu-Flur ✦

fluoride (TOP) (℞)
ACT, Fluorigard, Fluorinse, Gel Kam, Gel-Tin, Karigel, MouthKote, Stop, Thera-Flur
Func. class.: Trace elements
Chem. class.: Fluoride ion

Action: Needed for hard tooth enamel and for resistance to periodontal disease; reduces acid production by dental bacteria

Uses: Prevention of dental caries, osteoporosis

DOSAGE AND ROUTES

Prevention of dental caries

• *Adult and child >12 yr:* **TOP** 10 ml 0.2% sol daily after brushing teeth, rinse mouth for >1 min with sol

• *Child 6-12 yr:* **TOP** 5 ml 0.2% sol

• *Child >3 yr:* **PO** 1 mg daily

• *Child <3 yr:* **PO** 0.5 mg daily

Mild-moderate osteoporosis

• *Adult:* **PO** slow rel fluoride 25 mg, given as calcium citrate 400 mg bid

Available forms: Chew tabs 0.5, 1 mg; tabs 1 mg; effervescent tabs 10 mg; drops 0.125, 0.25, 0.5 mg/drop; rinse supplements 0.2 mg/ml, rinse 0.01%, 0.02%, 0.04%, 0.09%; gel 0.1%, 0.5%; lozenges 1 mg; sol 0.2 mg/ml; honey-wax, slow rel sodium fluoride tab

SIDE EFFECTS

ACUTE OVERDOSE: **Black tarry stools, bloody vomit, diarrhea, decreased respiration, increased salivation, watery eyes**

CHRONIC OVERDOSE: **Hypocalcemia and tetany, respiratory arrest, sores in mouth, constipation, loss of appetite, nausea, vomiting, weight loss,**

discoloration of teeth (white, black, brown)

Contraindications: Pregnancy (UK), hypersensitivity

Precautions: Child <6 yr

PHARMACOKINETICS

PO: Excreted in urine and feces; crosses placenta, breast milk

INTERACTIONS

Drug/Food
• Avoid use with dairy products

NURSING CONSIDERATIONS

Assess:
• For mottling of teeth during treatment

Administer:
• Drops after meals with fluids or undiluted tabs; may be chewed; do not swallow whole; may be given with water or juice; avoid milk

Evaluate:
• Therapeutic response: absence of dental caries

Teach patient/family:
• To monitor children using gel or rinse; not to be swallowed
• Not to drink, eat, or rinse mouth for at least ½ hr
• Not to use during pregnancy
• To apply after brushing and flossing at bedtime
• To store out of children's reach

---

fluorometholone ophthalmic
See Appendix C

⚠ High Alert

fluorouracil (℞)
(flure-oh-yoor'a-sil)
Adrucil, Efudex, Fluoroplex, 5-FU

Func. class.: Antineoplastic, antimetabolite

Chem. class.: Pyrimidine antagonist

Do not confuse:
fluorouracil/flucytosine

Action: Inhibits DNA, RNA synthesis; interferes with cell replication by competitively inhibiting thymidylate production, S phase of cell cycle–specific, a vesicant

Uses: *Systemic:* Cancer of breast, colon, rectum, stomach, pancreas; *topical:* multiple actinic keratoses, superficial basal cell carcinomas

DOSAGE AND ROUTES

Advanced colorectal cancer
• *Adult:* **IV** 370 mg/m^2 given after leucovorin or 425 mg/m^2 given after leucovorin daily × 5 days; repeat q4-5wk

Other cancer
• *Adult:* **IV** 12 mg/kg/day × 4 days, not to exceed 800 mg/day; may repeat with 6 mg/kg on days 6, 8, 10, 12; maintenance is 10-15 mg/kg/wk as a single dose, not to exceed 1 g/wk

Actinic/solar keratoses
• *Adult:* **TOP** 1% cream/sol 1-2 ×/day or 2-5% sol for hands

Superficial basal cell carcinoma
• *Adult:* **TOP** 5% sol or cream 2 ×/day × 3-12 wk

Available forms: Inj 50 mg/ml; cream 1%, 5%; sol 1%, 2%, 5%

SIDE EFFECTS

Systemic use
CNS: Lethargy, malaise, weakness, acute cerebellar dysfunction
CV: Myocardial ischemia, angina
EENT: Epistaxis
GI: Anorexia, stomatitis, diarrhea, nausea, vomiting, **hemorrhage,** enteritis glossitis

---

HEMA: **Thrombocytopenia, leukopenia, myelosuppression, anemia, agranulocytosis**

INTEG: Rash, fever, photosensitivity

Contraindications: Pregnancy (D), hypersensitivity, myelosuppression, poor nutritional status, serious infections, major surgery within 1 month, lactation

Precautions: Renal/hepatic disease, bone marrow depression, angina, children

PHARMACOKINETICS

Half-life 20 hr terminal; metabolized in the liver; excreted in the urine; crosses blood-brain barrier

INTERACTIONS

Increase: toxicity, bone marrow depression—radiation or other antineoplastics

Decrease: antibody response—live virus vaccines

Drug/Lab Test

Increase: AST, ALT, LDH, serum bilirubin, Hct, Hgb, WBC, platelets, 5-HIAA

Decrease: Albumin

NURSING CONSIDERATIONS

Assess:
• CBC, differential, platelet count daily (IV); withhold drug if WBC is <3500/mm³ or platelet count is <100,000/mm³; notify prescriber of these results; drug should be discontinued; nadir of leukopenia within 2 wk, recovery 1 mo

• Renal studies: BUN, serum uric acid, urine CCr, electrolytes before, during therapy

• Hepatic studies before, during therapy: bilirubin, alk phos, AST, ALT, LDH; before and during therapy

• Bleeding: hematuria, guaiac, bruising or petechiae, mucosa or orifices q8h

• Inflammation of mucosa, breaks in skin; buccal cavity q8h for dryness, sores or ulceration, white patches, oral pain, bleeding, dysphagia

• GI symptoms: frequency of stools, cramping, intractable vomiting, stomatitis

Administer:
• Antiemetic 30-60 min before giving drug to prevent vomiting and for several days thereafter

Topical route
• Wear gloves when applying; may use with a loose dressing; use a plastic or wooden applicator

IV route
• Prepared in biologic cabinet using gloves, gown, mask; use cytoxic handling procedures

• Undiluted; may inject through Y-tube or 3-way stopcock; give over 1-3 min; may be diluted in NS, D₅W, given over 2-8 hr as IV INF

Additive compatibilities: Bleomycin, cephalothin, cyclophosphamide, etoposide, floxuridine, hydromorphone, ifosfamide, methotrexate, mitoxantrone, prednisoLONE, vinCRIStine

Solution compatibilities: Amino acids 4.25%/D₂₅, D₅/LR, D₃.₃/0.3 NaCl, D₅W, 0.9% NaCl, TPN #23

Syringe compatibilities: Bleomycin, cisplatin, cyclophosphamide, furosemide, heparin, leucovorin, methotrexate, metoclopramide, mitomycin, vinBLAStine, vinCRIStine

Y-site compatibilities: Allopurinol, amifostine, aztreonam, bleomycin, cefepime, cisplatin, cyclophosphamide, DOXOrubicin, DOXOrubicin liposome, fludarabine, furosemide, granisetron, heparin, hydrocortisone, leucovorin, mannitol, melphalan, methotrexate, metoclopramide, mitomycin, paclitaxel, piperacillin/tazobactam, potassium chloride, propofol, sargramostim, teniposide, thiotepa, vinBLAStine, vinCRIStine, vit B/C

Perform/provide:
• Strict asepsis, protective isolation if WBC levels are low

• Changing of IV site q48h

• Rinsing of mouth tid-qid with water, club soda; brushing of teeth bid-tid with soft brush or cotton-tipped applicator for

stomatitis; use unwaxed dental floss, give ice chips for mucositis
• Nutritious diet with iron, vitamin supplements, low fiber, few dairy products, especially when combined with radiotherapy as ordered
Evaluate:
• Therapeutic response: decreased tumor size, spread of malignancy
Teach patient/family:
• To avoid crowds, persons with known infections
• To avoid foods with citric acid, hot or rough texture if stomatitis is present; to drink adequate fluids
• To report stomatitis: any bleeding, white spots, ulcerations in mouth; tell patient to examine mouth daily, report symptoms; viscous lidocaine may be used
• To report signs of infection: fever, sore throat, flulike symptoms
• To report signs of anemia: fatigue, headache, faintness, shortness of breath, irritability
• To report bleeding: avoid use of razors, commercial mouthwash
• To avoid use of aspirin products or NSAIDs
• To use contraception during therapy (men and women); avoid breastfeeding (topical use)
• Not to receive vaccinations during therapy
• To use sunscreen or stay out of the sun to prevent photosensitivity
• About hair loss, explore use of wigs or other products until hair regrowth occurs
• To apply topically only to affected areas, being careful around mouth, nose, eyes

fluoxetine (℞)
(floo-ox'eh-teen)
Prozac, Prozac Weekly, Sarafem
Func. class.: Antidepressant, SSRI (selective serotonin reuptake inhibitor)

Do not confuse:
Prozac/Proscar/ProSom/Prilosec
Sarafem/Serophene
Action: Inhibits CNS neuron uptake of serotonin but not of norepinephrine
Uses: Major depressive disorder, obsessive-compulsive disorder (OCD), bulimia nervosa; *Sarafem:* premenstrual dysphoric disorder (PMDD)
Unlabeled uses: Alcoholism, anorexia nervosa, ADHD, bipolar II affective disorder, borderline personality disorder, cataplexy, narcolepsy, kleptomania, migraine, obesity, posttraumatic stress disorder, schizophrenia, Tourette's syndrome, trichotillomania, levodopa-induced dyskinesia, social phobia, premenstrual dysphoric disorder

DOSAGE AND ROUTES
Bulimia nervosa
• *Adult:* **PO** 60 mg/day in AM
Depression/obsessive-compulsive disorder
• *Adult:* **PO** 20 mg daily in AM; after 4 wk if no clinical improvement is noted, dose may be increased to 20 mg bid in AM, PM, not to exceed 80 mg/day; **PO** weekly
• *Geriatric:* **PO** 5-10 mg/day, increase as needed
• *Child 5-18 yr:* **PO** 5-10 mg/day, max 20 mg/day
Premenstrual dysphoric disorder (Sarafem)
• *Adult:* **PO** 20 mg daily, may be taken daily week before menses
ADHD (unlabeled)
• *Adult:* **PO** 20-60 mg/day
Alcoholism (unlabeled)
• *Adult:* **PO** 20-80 mg/day

Anorexia nervosa (unlabeled)
• *Adult:* **PO** 10 mg every other day-20 mg/day

Bipolar II affective disorder (unlabeled)
• *Adult:* **PO** 10 mg every other day-20 mg/day

Borderline personality disorder (unlabeled)
• *Adult:* **PO** 20 mg/day

Kleptomania (unlabeled)
• *Adult:* **PO** 60-80 mg/day

Migraine, chronic daily headaches (unlabeled)
• *Adult:* **PO** 10-80 mg/day

Narcolepsy (unlabeled)
• *Adult:* **PO** 20-40 mg/day

Posttraumatic stress disorder (unlabeled)
• *Adult:* **PO** 10-80 mg/day

Schizophrenia (unlabeled)
• *Adult:* **PO** 20-60 mg/day

Available forms: Caps 10, 20, 40 mg; tabs 10, 20 mg; oral sol 20 mg/5 ml; del rel caps (Prozac Weekly) 90 mg

SIDE EFFECTS

CNS: Headache, nervousness, insomnia, drowsiness, anxiety, tremor, dizziness, fatigue, sedation, poor concentration, abnormal dreams, agitation, **seizures,** apathy, euphoria, hallucinations, delusions, psychosis

CV: Hot flashes, palpitations, angina pectoris, **hemorrhage,** hypertension, **tachycardia,** first-degree AV block, **bradycardia, MI, thrombophlebitis**

EENT: Visual changes, ear/eye pain, photophobia, tinnitus

GI: Nausea, diarrhea, dry mouth, anorexia, dyspepsia, constipation, cramps, vomiting, taste changes, flatulence, decreased appetite

GU: Dysmenorrhea, decreased libido, urinary frequency, UTI, amenorrhea, cystitis, impotence, urine retention

INTEG: Sweating, rash, pruritus, acne, alopecia, urticaria

MS: Pain, arthritis, twitching

RESP: Infection, pharyngitis, nasal congestion, sinus headache, sinusitis, cough, dyspnea, bronchitis, asthma, hyperventilation, pneumonia

SYST: Asthenia, viral infection, fever, allergy, chills

Contraindications: Hypersensitivity

Precautions: Pregnancy (B), lactation, children, geriatric, diabetes mellitus

PHARMACOKINETICS

PO: Peak 6-8 hr; metabolized in liver; excreted in urine; terminal half-life 2-3 days; steady state 28-35 days, protein binding 94%

INTERACTIONS

• Paradoxical worsening of OCD: busPIRone

• Do not use with thioridazine, or within 5 wk of discontinuing fluoxetine

⚠ Do not use MAOIs with or 14 days prior to fluoxetine

Increase: side effects—highly protein-bound drugs

Increase: effect—haloperidol

Increase: half-life of diazepam

Increase: levels or toxicity of carbamazepine, lithium, digoxin, warfarin, phenytoin

Increase: levels of tricyclics, phenothiazines

Increase: CNS depression—alcohol, antidepressants, opioids, sedatives

Decrease: fluoxetine effect—cyproheptadine

Drug/Herb

⚠ Do not use together; increased risk of serotonin syndrome: St. John's wort, SAM-e

Increase: anticholinergic effect—corkwood, jimsonweed

Increase: CNS effect—hops, kava, lavender

Drug/Lab Test

Increase: Serum bilirubin, blood glucose, alk phos

Decrease: VMA, 5-HIAA

False increase: Urinary catecholamines

Side effects: *italics* = common; **bold** = life-threatening

NURSING CONSIDERATIONS
Assess:
- Mental status: mood, sensorium, affect, suicidal tendencies, increase in psychiatric symptoms, depression, panic; monitor for seizures, seizure potential is increased
- Appetite in bulimia nervosa, weight daily, increase nutritious foods in diet, watch for bingeing and vomiting
- Allergic reactions: itching, rash urticaria, drug should be discontinued, may need to give antihistamine
- B/P (lying/standing), pulse q4h; if systolic B/P drops 20 mm Hg, hold drug, notify prescriber; take vital signs q4h in patients with cardiovascular disease
- Blood studies: CBC, leukocytes, differential, cardiac enzymes if patient is receiving long-term therapy; check platelets; bleeding can occur
- Hepatic studies: AST, ALT, bilirubin, creatinine
- Weight qwk; appetite may decrease with drug
- ECG for flattening of T wave, bundle branch, AV block, dysrhythmias in cardiac patients
- Alcohol consumption; if alcohol is consumed, hold dose until AM

Administer:
- With food or milk for GI symptoms
- Crushed if patient is unable to swallow medication whole (tab only)
- Dosage at bedtime if oversedation occurs during the day; may take entire dose at bedtime; geriatric may not tolerate once/day dosing
- Gum, hard candy, frequent sips of water for dry mouth
- Prozac weekly on the same day each week

Perform/provide:
- Storage at room temperature; do not freeze
- Assistance with ambulation during therapy, since drowsiness, dizziness occur
- Safety measures primarily in geriatric
- Checking to see if PO medication swallowed

Evaluate:
- Therapeutic response: decreased depression, symptoms of OCD

Teach patient/family:
- That therapeutic effect may take 1-4 wk
- To use caution in driving, other activities requiring alertness because of drowsiness, dizziness, blurred vision
- To use sunscreen to prevent photosensitivity
- To avoid alcohol ingestion, other CNS depressants
- To notify prescriber if pregnant or plan to become pregnant or breastfeed
- To change positions slowly, orthostatic hypotension may occur
- To avoid all OTC drugs unless approved by prescriber

---

fluphenazine decanoate (℞)
(floo-fen′a-zeen)
Modecate ✦, Modecate Concentrate ✦, Prolixin Decanoate

fluphenazine enanthate (℞)
Moditen Enanthate ✦, Prolixin Enanthate

fluphenazine hydrochloride (℞)
Apo-Fluphenazine ✦, Moditen HCL ✦, Moditen HCl-H.P ✦, Permitil ✦, Prolixin
Func. class.: Antipsychotic
Chem. class.: Phenothiazine, piperazine

Do not confuse:
Prolixin/Proloid

Action: Depresses cerebral cortex, hypothalamus, limbic system, which control activity and aggression; blocks neurotransmission produced by dopamine at synapse; exhibits strong α-adrenergic and anticholinergic blocking action; mechanism for antipsychotic effects is unclear

Uses: Psychotic disorders, schizophrenia

fluphenazine decanoate 477

DOSAGE AND ROUTES

Decanoate
- *Adult and child >16 yr:* **SUBCUT/IM** 12.5-25 mg q1-3wk, may increase slowly
- *Child 12-16 yr:* **IM/SUBCUT** 6.25-18.75 mg, then repeat q1-3wk, then increase slowly, max 25 mg
- *Child 5-12 yr:* **IM/SUBCUT** 3.125-12.5 mg, then repeat q1-3wk, increase slowly

Enanthate
- *Adult:* **IM/SUBCUT** 25 mg q1-3wk, max 100 mg/dose

HCI
- *Adult:* **PO** 2.5-10 mg, in divided doses q6-8h, not to exceed 20 mg daily; **IM** initially 1.25 mg, then 2.5-10 mg in divided doses q6-8h
- *Child:* **PO** 0.25-3.5 mg daily in divided doses q4-6h, max 10 mg/daily

Available forms: *Decanoate:* inj 25 mg/ml; *enanthate:* inj 25 mg/ml; *HCI:* tabs 1, 2.5, 5, 10 mg; elix 2.5 mg/5 ml; inj 2.5 ml

SIDE EFFECTS

CNS: EPS: pseudoparkinsonism, akathisia, dystonia, tardive dyskinesia, drowsiness, headache, **seizures, neuroleptic malignant syndrome**

CV: Orthostatic hypotension, hypertension, **cardiac arrest,** ECG changes, **tachycardia**

EENT: Blurred vision, glaucoma, dry eyes

GI: Dry mouth, nausea, vomiting, anorexia, constipation, diarrhea, jaundice, weight gain, **paralytic ileus, hepatitis,** cholecystic jaundice

GU: Urinary retention, urinary frequency, enuresis, impotence, amenorrhea, gynecomastia

HEMA: Anemia, **leukopenia, leukocytosis, agranulocytosis, aplastic anemia, thrombocytopenia**

INTEG: Rash, photosensitivity, dermatitis

RESP: **Laryngospasm,** dyspnea, **respiratory depression**

Contraindications: Hypersensitivity, circulatory collapse, hepatic damage, cerebral arteriosclerosis, coronary disease, severe hypertension/hypotension, blood dyscrasias, coma, brain damage, narrow-angle glaucoma, bone marrow depression, alcohol and barbiturate withdrawal

Precautions: Pregnancy (C), lactation, seizure disorders, hypertension, hepatic/cardiac disease, geriatric, child <12 yr

PHARMACOKINETICS

PO/IM (HCI): Onset 1 hr, peak 2-4 hr, duration 6-8 hr, half-life 3.5-4 days

IM/SUBCUT (enanthate): Onset 24-72 hr, duration 1-3 wk

IM/SUBCUT (decanoate): Onset 1-3 days; peak 1-2 days, duration over 4 wk; single-dose half-life 6.8-9.6 days, multiple dose 14.3 days

Metabolized by liver; excreted in urine (metabolites); crosses placenta; enters breast milk; protein binding >90%

INTERACTIONS

Increase: sedation—other CNS depressants, alcohol, barbiturate anesthetics

Increase: toxicity—epINEPHrine

Increase: anticholinergic effects—anticholinergics

Decrease: effects of levodopa, lithium

Decrease: fluphenazine effects—smoking, barbiturates

Drug/Herb

Increase: EPS—betel palm, kava

Increase: anticholinergic effect—henbane leaf

Increase: action—cola tree, hops, kava, nettle, nutmeg

Drug/Lab Test

Increase: LFTs, cardiac enzymes, cholesterol, blood glucose, prolactin, bilirubin, cholinesterase

Decrease: Hormones (blood and urine)

False positive: Pregnancy tests, PKU urinary steroids, 17-OHCS

NURSING CONSIDERATIONS

Assess:
- Swallowing of PO medication; check for hoarding, giving of medication to other patients

- I&O ratio; palpate bladder if low urinary output occurs, urinary retention may be the cause
- Bilirubin, CBC, LFTs monthly
- Urinalysis is recommended before and during prolonged therapy
- Affect, orientation, LOC, reflexes, gait, coordination, sleep pattern disturbances
- B/P standing and lying; take pulse and respirations q4h during initial treatment; establish baseline before starting treatment; report drops of 30 mm Hg
- Dizziness, faintness, palpitations, tachycardia on rising
- EPS including akathisia (inability to sit still, no pattern to movements), tardive dyskinesia (bizarre movements of jaw, mouth, tongue, extremities), pseudoparkinsonism (rigidity, tremors, pill rolling, shuffling gait)
- Constipation, urinary retention daily; if these occur, increase bulk, H_2O in diet

Administer:
- Elixir with juice, milk, or uncaffeinated drinks
- Antiparkinsonian agent if EPS occur
- IM inj into large muscle mass; to minimize postural hypotension, give inj and have patient remain seated or recumbent for ½ hr
- Use dry needle, or solution will become cloudy; use 21G or larger due to viscosity

Syringe compatibilities: Benztropine, diphenhydrAMINE, hydrOXYzine

Perform/provide:
- Decreased sensory input by dimming lights, avoiding loud noises
- Supervised ambulation until stabilized on medication; do not involve in strenuous exercise; fainting is possible; patient should not stand still for long periods
- Increased fluids to prevent constipation
- Sips of water, candy, gum for dry mouth
- Storage in tight, light-resistant container in cool environment

Evaluate:
- Therapeutic response: decrease in emotional excitement, hallucinations, delusions, paranoia, reorganization of patterns of thought, speech

Teach patient/family:
- That orthostatic hypotension occurs often; to rise from sitting or lying position gradually; avoid hazardous activities until stabilized on medication
- To avoid hot tubs, hot showers, tub baths, since hypotension may occur; that in hot weather, heat stroke may occur; take extra precautions to stay cool
- ⚠ To avoid abrupt withdrawal of this drug, or EPS may result; drug should be withdrawn slowly
- To avoid OTC preparations (cough, hay fever, cold) unless approved by prescriber; serious drug interactions may occur; avoid use with alcohol, CNS depressants; increased drowsiness may occur
- To use a sunscreen to prevent burns
- About importance of compliance with drug regimen
- About EPS and necessity for meticulous oral hygiene, since oral candidiasis may occur
- To report sore throat, malaise, fever, bleeding, mouth sores; if these occur, CBC should be drawn and drug discontinued
- That urine may turn pink to reddish-brown

Treatment of overdose: Lavage; if orally ingested, provide an airway; *do not induce vomiting*

flurandrenolide topical
See Appendix C

flurazepam (℞)

(flure-az′e-pam)
Apo-Flurazepam ✤, Dalmane,
flurazepam, Novoflupam ✤,
Somnol ✤

Func. class.: Sedative/hypnotic
Chem. class.: Benzodiazepine derivative

**Controlled Substance Schedule IV
(USA), Targeted (CDSA IV)
(Canada)**

Do not confuse:
flurazepam/temazepam

Action: Produces CNS depression at the limbic, thalamic, hypothalamic levels of CNS; may be mediated by neurotransmitter γ-aminobutyric acid (GABA); results are sedation, hypnosis, skeletal muscle relaxation, anticonvulsant activity, anxiolytic action

Uses: Insomnia, short term

DOSAGE AND ROUTES

• *Adult:* **PO** 15-30 mg at bedtime; may repeat dose once if needed
• *Geriatric:* **PO** 15 mg at bedtime; may increase if needed
Available forms: Caps 15, 30 mg

SIDE EFFECTS

CNS: Lethargy, drowsiness, daytime sedation, dizziness, confusion, lightheadedness, headache, anxiety, irritability, complex sleep related reactions: sleep driving, sleep eating
CV: Chest pain, pulse changes, palpitations
GI: Nausea, vomiting, diarrhea, heartburn, abdominal pain, constipation
HEMA: **Leukopenia, granulocytopenia** (rare)
MISC: Physical, psychological dependence
Contraindications: Pregnancy (UK), hypersensitivity to benzodiazepines, lactation, intermittent porphyria, uncontrolled pain
Precautions: Anemia, renal/hepatic disease, suicidal individuals, drug abuse, geriatric, psychosis, child <15 yr

PHARMACOKINETICS

PO: Onset 15-45 min, duration 7-8 hr; metabolized by liver; excreted by kidneys (inactive/active metabolites); crosses placenta; excreted in breast milk; half-life 47-100 hr

INTERACTIONS

Increase: flurazepam effects—cimetidine, disulfiram, probenicid, isoniazid, oral contraceptives, fluoxetine, ketoconazole, propranolol, valproic acid
Increase: CNS depression—alcohol, CNS depressants
Decrease: flurazepam effect—rifampin, barbiturates, theophylline
Drug/Herb
Increase: sedative effect—catnip, chamomile, clary, cowslip, kava, lavender, mistletoe, nettle, pokeweed, poppy, Queen Anne's lace, senega, valerian
Increase: hypotension—black cohosh
Drug/Lab Test
Increase: AST, ALT, serum bilirubin
Decrease: RAI uptake
False increase: Urinary 17-OHCS

NURSING CONSIDERATIONS

Assess:
• Mental status: mood, sensorium, affect, memory (long, short), physical, psychological dependence or tolerance
• Type of sleep problem: falling asleep, staying asleep
Administer:
• After removal of cigarettes to prevent fires
• After trying conservative measures for insomnia
• ½-1 hr before bedtime for sleeplessness
• Caps may be opened and mixed with food
Perform/provide:
• Assistance with ambulation after receiving dose
• Safety measures: night-light, call bell within easy reach
• Checking to see if PO medication has been swallowed

Side effects: *italics* = common; **bold** = life-threatening

• Storage in tight container in cool environment

Evaluate:
• Therapeutic response: ability to sleep at night, decreased amount of early morning awakening if taking drug for insomnia

Teach patient/family:
• To avoid driving or other activities requiring alertness until drug is stabilized
• To avoid alcohol ingestion or CNS depressants; serious CNS depression may result
• That effects may take 2 nights for benefits to be noticed
• Alternative measures to improve sleep: reading, exercise several hr before bedtime, warm bath, warm milk, TV, self-hypnosis, deep breathing
• That hangover is common in geriatric

Treatment of overdose: Lavage, activated charcoal; monitor electrolytes, VS

flurbiprofen ophthalmic
See Appendix C

flutamide (℞)
(floo′-ta-mide)
Apo-Flutamide ✦, Eulexin, Novo-Flutamide ✦
Func. class.: Antineoplastic, hormone
Chem. class.: Antiandrogen

Action: Interferes with androgen uptake in the nucleus or androgen activity in target tissues; arrests tumor growth in androgen-sensitive tissue (i.e., prostate gland)
Uses: Metastatic prostatic carcinoma, stage D_2 in combination with LHRH agonistic analogs (leuprolide)

DOSAGE AND ROUTES
• *Adult:* **PO** 250 mg q8h, for a daily dosage of 750 mg
Available forms: Caps 125, 250 ✦ mg

SIDE EFFECTS
CNS: Hot flashes, drowsiness, confusion, depression, anxiety, paresthesia
GI: Diarrhea, nausea, vomiting, increased levels in hepatic studies, **hepatitis,** anorexia, **hepatotoxicity**
GU: Decreased libido, impotence, gynecomastia
HEMA: **Leukopenia, thrombocytopenia, hemolytic anemia**
INTEG: Irritation at site, rash, photosensitivity
MISC: Edema, neuromuscular and pulmonary symptoms, hypertension
Contraindications: Pregnancy (D), hypersensitivity

PHARMACOKINETICS
Rapidly and completely absorbed; excreted in urine and feces as metabolites; half-life 6 hr, geriatric half-life 8 hr; 94% bound to plasma proteins

INTERACTIONS
Increase: PT—warfarin
Decrease: flutamide action—LHRH analog (leuprolide)

NURSING CONSIDERATIONS
Assess:
⚠ Hepatic studies: AST, ALT, alk phos, which may be elevated; if LFTs are elevated, drug may need to be discontinued; monitor CBC, bilirubin, creatinine
• For CNS symptoms, including drowsiness, confusion, depression, anxiety
Administer:
• Do not break, crush, or chew caps
• Flutamide must be taken with leuprolide; do not change dosing
Evaluate:
• Therapeutic response: decrease in prostatic tumor size, decrease in spread of cancer
Teach patient/family:
• To report side effects: decreased libido, impotence, breast enlargement, hot flashes, diarrhea

- To report nausea, vomiting, yellow eyes or skin, dark urine, clay-colored stools, hepatotoxicity may be the cause
- Notify of yellow, green urine discoloration
- Avoid sun exposure, tanning beds

---

fluticasone (℞)

(floo-tic´a-sone)

Flonase, Flovent HFA, Flovent Diskus ✦

Func. class: Corticosteroids, inhalation; antiasthmatic

Action: Decreases inflammation by inhibiting mast cells, macrophages, and leukotrienes; antiinflammatory, and vasoconstrictor properties

Uses: Prevention of chronic asthma during maintenance treatment in those requiring oral corticosteroids; nasal symptoms of seasonal/perennial, and allergic/nonallergic rhinitis

DOSAGE AND ROUTES

Prevention of chronic asthma during maintenance treatment in those requiring oral corticosteroids

Flovent HFA

- *Adult and child ≥12 yr:* **INH** 88-440 mcg bid (in those previously taking bronchodilators, alone); **INH** 88-220 mcg bid, max 440 mcg bid (in those previously taking inhaled corticosteroids); **INH** 440 mcg bid, max 880 mcg bid (in those previously taking oral corticosteroids)

Flovent Diskus ✦

- *Adult and child ≥12 yr:* **INH** 100 mcg bid, max 500 mcg (in those previously taking bronchodilators, alone); **INH** 100-250 mcg bid, max 500 mcg bid (in those previously taking inhaled corticosteroids); **INH** 500-1000 mcg bid, max 1000 mcg bid (in those previously taking oral corticosteroids)
- *Child 4-11 yr:* **INH** Initially 50 mcg bid, max 100 mcg bid (in those previously taking bronchodilators alone or inhaled corticosteroids)

Nasal symptoms of seasonal/perennial rhinitis

Flonase

- *Adult:* **NASAL SPRAY** 2 sprays (100 mcg) in each nostril daily or 1 spray (50 mcg) in each nostril bid; when symptoms are controlled, decrease to 1 spray (50 mcg) in each nostril every day
- *Adolescent and child ≥4 yr:* **NASAL SPRAY** 1 spray (50 mcg) in each nostril daily; may increase to 2 sprays (100 mcg) in each nostril daily; max 2 sprays in each nostril daily

Available forms: Nasal spray 50 mcg/metered spray; oral inhalation aerosol 44, 110, 220 mcg; oral inhalation powder 50, 100, 250 mcg

SIDE EFFECTS

CNS: Fever, headache, nervousness, dizziness, migraines

EENT: Pharyngitis, sinusitis, rhinitis, laryngitis, hoarseness, dry eyes, cataracts, nasal discharge, epistaxis

GI: Diarrhea, abdominal pain, nausea, vomiting, *oral candidiasis*, gastroenteritis

GU: UTI

INTEG: Urticaria, dermatitis

META: Hyperglycemia, growth retardation in children, cushingoid features

MISC: Influenza, **eosinophilic conditions, angioedema, Churg-Strauss syndrome**

MS: Osteoporosis, muscle soreness, joint pain

RESP: Upper respiratory infection, dyspnea, cough, bronchitis, **bronchospasm**

Contraindications: Hypersensitivity, primary treatment in status asthmaticus

Precautions: Pregnancy (C), lactation, active infections, glaucoma, diabetes, immunocompromised patients

PHARMACOKINETICS

Absorption 30% aerosol, 13.5% powder; protein binding 91%, metabolized in the liver after absorption in lung, half-life 7.8 hr, <5% excreted in urine and feces

---

Nasal INH: Onset 12 hr, peak several days, duration 1-2 wk

Oral INH: Onset 24 hr, peak several days, duration 1-2 wk

INTERACTIONS

Increase: fluticasone levels—CYP450 3A4 inhibitors (ketoconazole)

Drug/Lab Test

Increase: Urine/serum glucose

NURSING CONSIDERATIONS

Assess:

• Respiratory status: lung sounds, pulmonary function tests during and several months after change from systemic to inhalation corticosteroids

• Withdrawal symptoms from oral corticosteroids: depression, pain in joints, fatigue

⚠ Adrenal insufficiency: nausea, weakness, fatigue, hypotension, hypoglycemia, anorexia; may occur when changing from systemic to inhalation corticosteroids; may be life-threatening

• Growth rate in children

• Adrenal function tests periodically: hypothalamic–pituitary-adrenal axis suppression in long-term treatment

Administer:

• Give at 1 min intervals

• Decrease dose to lowest effective dose after desired effect, decrease dose at 2-4 wk intervals

Teach patient/family:

• To use bronchodilator first before using inhalation, if taking both

• Not to use for acute asthmatic attack; for acute asthma, may require oral corticosteroids

• To avoid smoking, smoke-filled rooms, those with URIs, those not immunized against chickenpox or measles

---

fluticasone nasal agent
See Appendix C

---

fluticasone topical
See Appendix C

---

fluvastatin (Ŗ)
(flu'vah-stay-tin)
Lescol, Lescol XL
Func. class.: Antilipidemic
Chem. class.: HMG-CoA reductase inhibitor

Action: Inhibits HMG-CoA reductase enzyme, which reduces cholesterol synthesis

Uses: As an adjunct in primary hypercholesterolemia (types Ia, Ib), coronary atherosclerosis in CAD; to reduce the risk of undergoing coronary revascularization in patients with CAD

DOSAGE AND ROUTES

• *Adult:* **PO** 20-40 mg daily in PM initially, usual range 20-80 mg, max 80 mg; may be given in 2 doses (40 mg AM, 40 mg PM); dosage adjustments may be made in 4 wk intervals or more

Available forms: Caps 20, 40 mg; ext rel tab 80 mg

SIDE EFFECTS

CNS: Headache, dizziness, insomnia

EENT: Lens opacities

GI: Abdominal pain, cramps, nausea, constipation, diarrhea, dyspepsia, flatus, **hepatic dysfunction,** pancreatitis

HEMA: **Thrombocytopenia, hemolytic anemia, leukopenia**

INTEG: Rash, pruritus

MISC: Fatigue, influenza, photosensitivity

MS: Myalgia, **myositis, rhabdomyolysis,** *arthritis, arthralgia*

RESP: Upper respiratory infection, rhinitis, cough, pharyngitis, sinusitis

Contraindications: Pregnancy (X), hypersensitivity, lactation, active hepatic disease

Precautions: Past hepatic disease, alcoholism, severe acute infections, trauma, hypotension, uncontrolled seizure disorders, severe metabolic disorders, electrolyte imbalance

PHARMACOKINETICS

Peak response 3-4 wk, metabolized in liver, highly protein bound, excreted primarily in feces, half-life <1 hr

INTERACTIONS

Increase: effects of warfarin, digoxin

Increase: myalgia, myositis—cycloSPORINE, gemfibrozil, niacin, erythromycin, clofibrate; azole antiinfectives

Increase: effects of fluvastatin—alcohol, cimetidine, ranitidine, omeprazole, saquinavir

Decrease: fluvastatin effect—rifampin

Drug/Herb

Increase: effect—glucomannan

Decrease: effect—gotu kola, St. John's wort

Drug/Food

• Grapefruit juice: possible increased toxicity

Decrease: absorption—oat bran, high fat

NURSING CONSIDERATIONS

Assess:

• Fasting lipid profile (cholesterol, LDL, HDL, TG) q8wk, then q3-6mo when stable

• Hepatic studies q1-2mo during the first 1½ yr of treatment; AST, ALT, LFTs may be increased

• Renal studies in patients with compromised renal system: BUN, I&O ratio, creatinine

⚠ For muscle pain, tenderness; obtain baseline CPK if elevated; if these occur, drug should be discontinued

Administer:

• Do not break, crush, or chew ext rel tabs

• Bile acid sequestrant should be given at least 2 hr before or after fluvastatin

Perform/provide:

• Storage in cool environment in tight container protected from light

Evaluate:

• Therapeutic response: decrease in LDL, VLDL, total cholesterol; increased HDL, decreased triglycerides

Teach patient/family:

• That blood work will be necessary during treatment, to take as prescribed

• To report severe GI symptoms, headache, muscle pain, weakness, tenderness

• That previously prescribed regimen will continue: low-cholesterol diet, exercise program, smoking cessation

• To report suspected pregnancy, not to use during pregnancy

• To use sunscreen or stay out of sun to prevent photosensitivity

• To notify all health care providers of drugs taken

---

fluvoxamine (℞)

(flu-vox'a-meen)

Luvox

Func. class.: Antidepressant SSRI (selective serotonin reuptake inhibitor)

Do not confuse:

Luvox/Levoxyl

Action: Inhibits CNS neuron uptake of serotonin but not of norepinephrine

Uses: Obsessive-compulsive disorder

Unlabeled uses: Depression, bulimia nervosa, panic disorder, social phobia

DOSAGE AND ROUTES

• *Adult:* **PO** 50 mg at bedtime, increase by 50 mg at 4-7 day intervals, max 300 mg, doses over 100 mg should be divided

• *Child 8-17 yr:* **PO** 25 mg at bedtime, increase by 25 mg/day q4-7d, max 200 mg/day, doses over 50 mg should be divided

Hepatic dose/geriatric

• *Adult:* **PO** 25 mg at bedtime, may titrate upward slowly

Available forms: Tabs 25, 50, 100 mg

Side effects: *italics* = common; **bold** = life-threatening

SIDE EFFECTS

CNS: Headache, drowsiness, dizziness, seizures, sleep disorders, insomnia
GI: Nausea, anorexia, constipation, **hepatotoxicity,** *vomiting, diarrhea,* dry mouth
GU: Decreased libido
INTEG: Rash, sweating
Contraindications: Hypersensitivity
Precautions: Pregnancy (C), lactation, children, geriatric

PHARMACOKINETICS

Crosses blood-brain barrier, 77% protein binding, metabolism by the liver, terminal half-life 16.9 hr, peak 2-8 hr

INTERACTIONS

⚠ Fatal reaction—MAO inhibitors
Increase: CNS depression—alcohol, barbiturates, benzodiazepines
Increase: fluvoxamine, toxicity levels—tricyclics, clozapine
Increase: metabolism, decrease effects—smoking
Decrease: metabolism, increase action of propranolol, diazepam, lithium, theophylline, carbamazepine, warfarin
Drug/Herb
⚠ *Increase:* effect, possible fatal reaction—St. John's wort
Increase: anticholinergic effect—corkwood, jimsonweed
Increase: CNS effect—hops, kava, lavender

NURSING CONSIDERATIONS

Assess:
• Hepatic studies: AST, ALT, bilirubin
• Mental status: mood, sensorium, affect, suicidal tendencies; increase in psychiatric symptoms: depression, panic, obsessive-compulsive symptoms
• Constipation; most likely in geriatric
⚠ For toxicity: nausea, vomiting, diarrhea, syncope, increased pulse, seizures
Administer:
• With food, milk for GI symptoms

Perform/provide:
• Storage at room temperature; do not freeze
Evaluate:
• Therapeutic response: decrease in depression
Teach patient/family:
• That therapeutic effects may take 2-3 wk
• To use caution in driving, other activities requiring alertness because of drowsiness, dizziness that may occur
• Not to use other CNS depressants, alcohol, barbiturates, benzodiazepines, St. John's wort, kava
• To notify prescriber if pregnancy is suspected or planned
• To notify prescriber of allergic reaction
• To increase bulk in diet if constipation occurs, especially geriatric

---

folic acid (vit B₉) (OTC)
(foe'lik a'sid)
Apo-Folic ✦, Folate, Folvite, Novofolacid ✦, Vitamin B₉
Func. class.: Vit B complex group

Action: Needed for erythropoiesis; increases RBC, WBC, platelet formation in megaloblastic anemias
Uses: Megaloblastic or macrocytic anemia caused by folic acid deficiency; hepatic disease, alcoholism, hemolysis, intestinal obstruction, pregnancy

DOSAGE AND ROUTES
RDA
• *Adult and child ≥14 yr:* **PO** 200 mcg
• *Adult (pregnant/lactating):* **PO** 400 mcg/day
• *Child 9-13 yr:* **PO** 300 mcg
• *Child 4-8 yr:* **PO** 200 mcg
• *Child 1-3 yr:* **PO** 150 mcg
• *Infant 6 mo-1 yr:* **PO** 80 mcg
• *Neonates and infants <6 mo:* **PO** 65 mcg

⚠ Safety alert   *"Tall Man" lettering

Megaloblastic/macrocytic anemia due to folic acid or nutritional deficiency
- *Pregnant:* **PO** 600 mcg
- *Lactating:* **PO** 500 mcg

Therapeutic dose
- *Adult and child:* **PO/IM/SUBCUT/IV** up to 1 mg daily

Maintenance dose
- *Adult and child >4 yr:* **PO/IM/IV/SUBCUT** 0.4 mg/day
- *Pregnant and lactating:* **PO/IM/IV/SUBCUT** 0.8 mg/day
- *Child <4 yr:* **PO/IM/IV/SUBCUT** up to 0.3 mg/day
- *Infant:* **PO/IM/IV/SUBCUT** up to 0.1 mg/day

Prevention of neural tube defects during pregnancy
- *Adult:* **PO** 0.4 mg daily

Prevention of megaloblastic anemia during pregnancy
- *Adult:* **PO/IM/SUBCUT** up to 1 mg/day during pregnancy

Tropical sprue
- *Adult:* **PO** 3-15 mg daily

Available forms: Tabs 0.1, 0.4, 0.8, 1, 5 mg; inj 5, 10 mg/ml

SIDE EFFECTS

INTEG: Flushing
RESP: **Bronchospasm**
Contraindications: Hypersensitivity, anemias other than megaloblastic/macrocytic anemia, vit B$_{12}$ deficiency anemia, uncorrected pernicious anemia
Precautions: Pregnancy (A)

PHARMACOKINETICS

PO: Peak ½-1 hr; bound to plasma proteins; excreted in breast milk; metabolized by liver; excreted in urine (small amounts)

INTERACTIONS

Increase: need for folic acid—estrogen, hydantoins, carbamazepine, glucocorticoids
Decrease: folate levels—methotrexate, sulfonamides, sulfasalazine

Decrease: phenytoin levels, fosphenytoin, may increase seizures

NURSING CONSIDERATIONS
Assess:
- For fatigue, dyspnea, weakness, dyspnea that are signs of megaloblastic anemia
- Hgb, Hct, and reticulocyte count
- Nutritional status: bran, yeast, dried beans, nuts, fruits, fresh vegetables, asparagus
- Drugs currently taken: estrogen, carbamazepine, glucocorticoids, hydantoins; these drugs may cause increased folic acid use by body and contribute to a deficiency

Administer:
IV route
- Direct undiluted 5 mg or less/1 min or more; or may be added to most IV sol or TPN

Solution compatibilities: D$_{20}$W
Y-site compatibilities: Famotidine
Perform/provide:
- Storage in light-resistant container

Evaluate:
- Therapeutic response: increased weight, oriented, well-being; absence of fatigue; increase in reticulocyte count within 5 days of beginning treatment

Teach patient/family:
- To take drug exactly as prescribed; periodic lab work is required
- To alter nutrition to include high-folic-acid foods: organ meats, vegetables, fruit
- That urine will turn bright yellow
- To notify prescriber of allergic reaction

F

fondaparinux (R)
(fon-dah-pair'ih-nux)
Arixtra
Func. class.: Anticoagulant, antithrombotic
Chem. class.: Synthetic, selective factor Xa inhibitor

Do not confuse:

Arixtra/Anti-Xa

Action: Acts by antithrombin III (ATIII)-mediated selective inhibition of factor Xa; neutralization of factor Xa interrupts blood coagulation and inhibits thrombin formation; does not inactivate thrombin (activated factor II) or affect platelets

Uses: Prevention of deep-vein thrombosis, pulmonary emboli in hip and knee replacement, hip fracture or abdominal surgery

DOSAGE AND ROUTES

Deep vein thrombosis/PE

• *Adult <50 kg:* **SUBCUT** 5 mg daily × 5 days or more until INR is 2-3; may give warfarin within 72 hr of fondaparinux

• *Adult 50-100 kg:* **SUBCUT** 7.5 mg daily × 5 days or more until INR is 2-3; may give warfarin within 72 hr of fondaparinux

• *Adult >100 kg:* **SUBCUT** 10 mg daily × 5 days or more until INR is 2-3; may give warfarin within 72 hr of fondaparinux

Prevention of deep vein thrombosis

• *Adult:* **SUBCUT** 2.5 mg daily, given 6 hr after surgery; continue for 5-9 days; hip surgery up to 32 days; abdominal surgery up to 24 days

Available forms: Inj 2.5 mg/0.5 ml, 5 mg/0.4 ml, 7.5 mg/0.6 ml, 10 mg/0.8 ml prefilled syringes

SIDE EFFECTS

CNS: Fever, confusion, headache, dizziness, *insomnia*

GI: Nausea, vomiting, diarrhea, dyspepsia, *constipation,* increased AST, ALT

GU: UTI, urinary retention

HEMA: Anemia, minor bleeding, purpura, hematoma, **thrombocytopenia, major bleeding (intracranial, cerebral, retroperitoneal hemorrhage), postoperative hemorrhage**

INTEG: Increased wound drainage, bullous eruption, local reaction—*rash,* pruritus, inj site bleeding

META: Hypokalemia

OTHER: Hypotension, pain, *edema*

Contraindications: Hypersensitivity to this drug; hemophilia, leukemia with bleeding, peptic ulcer disease, hemorrhagic stroke, surgery, thrombocytopenic purpura, weight <50 kg, severe renal disease (CCr <30 ml/min), active major bleeding, bacterial endocarditis

Precautions: Pregnancy (B), alcoholism, hepatic disease (severe), blood dyscrasias, heparin-induced thrombocytopenia, uncontrolled, severe hypertension, subacute bacterial endocarditis, acute nephritis, lactation, geriatric, children, mild to moderate renal disease

PHARMACOKINETICS

Rapidly, completely absorbed; peak steady state 3 hr; distributed primarily in blood, does not bind to plasma proteins except 94% to ATIII; metabolism unknown; eliminated unchanged in urine in 72 hr in normal renal function

INTERACTIONS

• Do not mix with other drugs or infusion fluids

Increase: risk of bleeding—salicylates, NSAIDs, abciximab, eptifibatide, tirofiban, clopidogrel, dipyridamole, quinidine, valproic acid

Drug/Herb

Increase: risk of bleeding—agrimony, alfalfa, angelica, anise, basil, bay, bilberry, black haw, bogbean, bromelain, buchu, chondroitin, cinchona bark, dong quai, fenugreek, feverfew, garlic, ginger, ginkgo, ginseng, horse chestnut, Irish moss, kelp, kelpware, khella, lovage, lungwort, meadowsweet, motherwort, mugwort, nettle, papaya, parsley (large amounts), pau d'arco, pineapple, poplar, prickly ash, saf-

---

⚠ Safety alert   *"Tall Man" lettering

flower, saw palmetto, tonka bean, turmeric, wintergreen, yarrow
Decrease: anticoagulant effect—chamomile, coenzyme Q10, flax, glucomannan, goldenseal, guar gum

NURSING CONSIDERATIONS

Assess:
• Blood studies (Hct, CBC, coagulation studies, platelets, occult blood in stools), thrombocytopenia may occur; if platelets <100,000/mm^3, treatment should be discontinued
• For bleeding: gums, petechiae, ecchymosis, black tarry stools, hematuria; decreased Hct, notify prescriber
• For neurologic symptoms in patients who have received spinal anesthesia
• For risk of hemorrhage if coadministering with other drugs that may cause bleeding
• For hypersensitivity: rash, fever, chills; notify prescriber

Administer:
• Alone; do not mix with other drugs or solutions; cannot be used interchangeably (unit to unit) with other anticoagulants
• For 5-9 days
• Only after screening patient for bleeding disorders
• SUBCUT only; do not give IM; do not give earlier than 6 hr after surgery

SUBCUT route
• Check for discolored sol or sol with particulate; if present, do not give
• Administer 6-8 hr after surgery
• Administer to recumbent patient, rotate inj sites (left/right anterolateral, left/right posterolateral abdominal wall)
• Wipe surface of inj site with alcohol swab, twist plunger cap and remove, remove rigid needle guard by pulling straight off needle, do not aspirate, do not expel air bubble from surface
• Insert whole length of needle into skinfold held with thumb and forefinger
• When drug is injected, a soft click may be felt or heard
• Give at same time each day to maintain steady blood levels; observe inj site

• Avoid all IM inj that may cause bleeding

⚠ Administer only this drug when ordered; not interchangeable with heparin

Perform/provide:
• Storage at 25° C (77° F); do not freeze

Evaluate:
• Therapeutic response: Prevention of deep vein thrombosis

Teach patient/family:
• To use soft-bristle toothbrush to avoid bleeding gums, to use electric razor
• To report any signs of bleeding: gums, under skin, urine, stools
• To avoid OTC drugs containing aspirin

---

formoterol (℞)
(for-moh′ter-ahl)
Foradil Aerolizer
Func. class.: Bronchodilator
Chem. class.: β-Adrenergic agonist

Do not confuse:
Foradil/Toradol

Action: Has β_1 and β_2 action; relaxes bronchial smooth muscle and dilates the trachea and main bronchi by increasing levels of cAMP, which relaxes smooth muscles; causes increased contractility and heart rate by acting on β-receptors in heart

Uses: Maintenance, treatment of asthma, COPD, prevention of exercise-induced bronchospasm

DOSAGE AND ROUTES

Maintenance, treatment of asthma
• *Adult and child ≥5 yr:* **INH** AM and PM long-term 1 cap (12 mcg) q12h using aerolizer inhaler
Maintenance of COPD
• *Adult:* **INH** 12 mcg q12h
Prevention of exercise-induced bronchospasm
• *Adult and child ≥12 yr:* **INH** prn occasionally 1 cap (12 mcg) at least 15 min before exercise

---

Available form: INH powder in cap 12 mcg

SIDE EFFECTS

CNS: Tremors, anxiety, insomnia, headache, dizziness, stimulation
CV: Palpitations, tachycardia, hypertension
GI: Nausea, vomiting, xerostomia
RESP: Bronchial irritation, dryness of oropharynx, **bronchospasms** (overuse)
Contraindications: Hypersensitivity to sympathomimetics, narrow-angle glaucoma
Precautions: Pregnancy (C), cardiac disorders, hyperthyroidism, diabetes mellitus, prostatic hypertrophy, geriatric, hypertension

PHARMACOKINETICS

INH: Onset 15 min, peak 1-3 hr, duration 12 hr
Metabolized in liver, lungs, GI tract; half-life 10 hr

INTERACTIONS

⚠ *Increase:* serious dysrhythmias—MAOIs, tricyclics
Increase: effects of both drugs—other sympathomimetics
Decrease: action when used with β-blockers

NURSING CONSIDERATIONS

Assess:
• Respiratory function: B/P, pulse, lung sounds; note sputum color, character; respiratory function tests prior to and during treatment
• I&O ratio; check for urinary retention, frequency, hesitancy
• For paresthesias and coldness of extremities; peripheral blood flow may decrease

Administer:
• Place cap in aerolizer inhaler; the cap is punctured; do not wash aerolizer inhaler
• Pull off cover, twist mouthpiece to open, push buttons in; make sure the four pins are visible; remove cap from blister pack, place cap in chamber; twist to close, press (a click will be heard), release, patient should exhale, place inhaler in mouth, inhale rapidly

Perform/provide:
• Storage at room temperature, protection from heat, moisture

Evaluate:
• Therapeutic response: ease of breathing

Teach patient/family:
• To rinse mouth after use
• Correct use of inhaler; review package insert with patient; to avoid getting aerosol in eyes
• About all aspects of drug; to avoid smoking, smoke-filled rooms, persons with respiratory infections

Treatment of overdose: Administration of a β-blocker

---

fosamprenavir (℞)
(fos-am-pren′a-veer)
Lexiva
Func. class.: Antiretroviral
Chem. class.: Protease inhibitor

Action: A prodrug of amprenavir; inhibits human immunodeficiency virus (HIV) protease, which prevents maturation of the infectious virus
Uses: HIV-1 infection in combination with antiretrovirals

DOSAGE AND ROUTES

Therapy-naïve patients
• *Adult:* **PO** 1400 mg bid without ritonavir or fosamprenavir 1400 mg daily and ritonavir 200 mg daily or fosamprenavir 700 mg bid and ritonavir 100 mg bid
Protease experienced patients (PI)
• *Adult:* **PO** 700 mg bid and ritonavir 100 mg bid
Combination with efavirenz
• *Adult:* **PO** Add another 100 mg/day of ritonavir for a total of 300 mg/day when all three drugs are given

---

Hepatic dose
• *Adult:* **PO** (Child-Pugh 5-8) 700 mg bid, (Child-Pugh 9-12) do not use
Available forms: Tabs 700 mg (equivalent to 600 mg amprenavir)

SIDE EFFECTS
CNS: Headache, fatigue, depression, oral paresthesia
GI: Nausea, diarrhea, vomiting, abdominal pain
INTEG: Rash, pruritus
MISC: Redistribution or accumulation of body fat, hyperglycemia, **Stevens-Johnson syndrome**
Contraindications: Hypersensitivity to protease inhibitors
Precautions: Pregnancy (C), hepatic disease, hemolytic anemia, diabetes, sulfa sensitivity, lactation, geriatric

PHARMACOKINETICS
A prodrug of amprenavir, peak 1½-4 hr, 90% protein binding, metabolized in the liver by cytochrome P4503AY (CYP3A4), excretion of unchanged drug is minimal, half-life 7.7 hr

INTERACTIONS
• May affect coagulation: warfarin
• Avoid use with rifampin, delavirdine, H₂ receptor antagonists, proton-pump inhibitors, carbamazepine, phenobarbital, phenytoin because may lose virologic response and possibly lead to resistance to fosamprenavir
⚠ Serious life-threatening reactions: amiodarone, calcium channel blockers, lidocaine, pimozide, ergots, midazolam, triazolam, flecainide, propafenone
Increase: effect—rifabutin, ketoconazole, itraconazole, sildenafil, vardenafil
Increase: toxicity—HMG-CoA reductase inhibitors
Decrease: effect of oral contraceptives, methadone
Decrease: fosamprenavir levels—nevirapine, antacids, efavirenz, saquinavir, ranitidine, carbamazepine, phenytoin

Drug/Herb
• Avoid use with—St. John's wort
Drug/Lab Test
Increase: Serum glucose, AST, ALT, triglycerides

NURSING CONSIDERATIONS
Assess:
• Bowel pattern before, during treatment, monitor hydration
• Skin eruptions, rash, urticaria, itching; allergy to sulfonamides, cross sensitivity may occur
• Viral load, CD4 cell counts baseline and throughout treatment
⚠ Stevens-Johnson syndrome; skin reactions, report immediately
Administer:
• Without regard to food
Teach patient/family:
• To avoid taking with other medications unless directed by provider
• That drug does not cure, but does manage symptoms and does not prevent transmission of HIV to others
• To use nonhormonal form of birth control while taking this drug
• If dose is missed, take as soon as remembered up to 1 hr before next dose; do not double dose
• Not to alter dose or stop therapy without talking to physician
• Advise physician if they have sulfa allergy
• To report all medications including herbal supplements to physician
• That patients receiving phosphodiesterase type 5 inhibitors may be at increased risk for PDE5 inhibitor adverse effects

foscarnet (℞)
(foss-kar'net)
Foscavir
Func. class.: Antiviral
Chem. class.: Inorganic pyrophosphate organic analog

Action: Antiviral activity is produced by selective inhibition at the pyrophosphate binding site on virus-specific DNA polymerases and reverse transcriptases at concentrations that do not affect cellular DNA polymerases

Uses: Treatment of CMV retinitis, HSV infections, used with ganciclovir for relapsing patients

DOSAGE AND ROUTES

CMV retinitis
• *Adult:* **IV INF** 60 mg/kg given over at least 1 hr, q8h × 2-3 wk initially, then 90-120 mg/kg/day over 2 hr, usually give with at least 750-1000 ml **NS** daily
HSV
• *Adult:* **IV** 40 mg/kg q8-12h × 2-3 wk
Renal dose
• *Adult:* **IV**
Male:

$$\frac{140 - age}{serum\ creatinine \times 72} = CCr$$

Female: 0.85 × above value
Dose based on table provided in package insert

Available forms: Inj 6000 mg/250 ml, 12,000 mg/500 ml (24 mg/ml)

SIDE EFFECTS

CNS: Fever, dizziness, *headache*, **seizures**, *fatigue*, neuropathy, tremor, ataxia, dementia, stupor, EEG abnormalities, vertigo, **coma**, abnormal gait, hypertonia, EPS, hemiparesis, **paralysis**, hyperreflexia, paraplegia, **tetany**, hyporeflexia, neuralgia, neuritis, **cerebral edema**, *paresthesia*, depression, *confusion*, *anxiety*, insomnia, somnolence, amnesia, hallucinations, agitation
CV: Hypertension, palpitations, ECG abnormalities, 1st-degree AV block, nonspecific ST-T segment changes, hypotension, cerebrovascular disorder, cardiomyopathy, **cardiac arrest,** bradycardia, dysrhythmias
EENT: Visual field defects, vocal cord paralysis, speech disorders, taste perversion, eye pain, conjunctivitis, tinnitus, otitis
GI: Nausea, vomiting, diarrhea, anorexia, abdominal pain, constipation, dysphagia, rectal hemorrhage, dry mouth,

melena, flatulence, ulcerative stomatitis, pancreatitis, enteritis, enterocolitis, glossitis, proctitis, stomatitis, increased amylases, gastroenteritis, **pseudomembranous colitis,** duodenal ulcer, **paralytic ileus, esophageal ulceration,** abnormal A-G ratio, increased AST, ALT, cholecystitis, **hepatitis,** dyspepsia, tenesmus, hepatosplenomegaly, jaundice
GU: **Acute renal failure,** decreased CCr and increased serum creatinine, **glomerulonephritis, toxic nephropathy, nephrosis, renal tubular disorders, pyelonephritis, uremia, hematuria, albuminuria,** dysuria, polyuria
HEMA: Anemia, **granulocytopenia, leukopenia, thrombocytopenia,** platelet abnormalities, **thrombosis, pulmonary embolism, coagulation disorders, decreased prothrombin, hypochromic anemia, pancytopenia, hemolysis, leukocytosis,** lymphadenopathy, epistaxis, lymphopenia
INTEG: Rash, sweating, pruritus, skin ulceration, seborrhea, skin discoloration, alopecia, acne, dermatitis, pain/inflammation at inj site, facial edema, dry skin, urticaria
MS: Arthralgia, myalgia
RESP: Coughing, dyspnea, pneumonia, sinusitis, pharyngitis, **pulmonary infiltration,** stridor, **pneumothorax, hemoptysis, bronchospasm,** bronchitis, **respiratory depression, pleural effusion, pulmonary hemorrhage,** rhinitis
SYST: Hypokalemia, hypocalcemia, hypomagnesemia; increased alk phos, LDH, BUN; acidosis, hypophosphatemia, hyperphosphatemia, dehydration, glycosuria, increased CPK, hypervolemia, infection, **sepsis, death, ascites,** hyponatremia, hypochloremia, hypercalcemia
Contraindications: Hypersensitivity, CCr <0.4 ml/min/kg
Precautions: Pregnancy (C), lactation, children, geriatric, renal disease, seizure disorders, electrolyte/mineral imbalances, severe anemia

▲ Safety alert   *"Tall Man" lettering

PHARMACOKINETICS

14%-17% plasma protein bound, half-life 2-8 hr in normal renal function

INTERACTIONS

Increase: nephrotoxicity—aminoglycosides, amphotericin B
Increase: hypocalcemia—pentamidine

NURSING CONSIDERATIONS

Assess:

General

• Renal, hepatic studies: BUN, creatinine, AST, ALT

• I&O ratio, urine pH, serum creatinine baseline, 3 ×/wk during initial therapy, then 2 ×/wk thereafter; CCr baseline, throughout treatment; if CCr <0.4 ml/min/kg, discontinue

• Blood counts q2wk; watch for decreasing granulocytes, Hgb; if low, therapy may have to be discontinued and restarted after hematologic recovery; blood transfusions may be required

• Lesions in HSV

• Electrolytes and minerals (Ca, P, Mg, Na, K); watch closely for tetany during first administration

• GI symptoms: nausea, vomiting, diarrhea; severe symptoms may necessitate discontinuing drug

⚠ Blood dyscrasias (anemia, granulocytopenia); bruising, fatigue, bleeding, poor healing

• Allergic reactions: flushing, rash, urticaria, pruritus

CMV retinitis

• Culture should be done prior to treatment (blood, urine, throat); a negative culture does not rule out CMV

• Ophthalmic exam should confirm diagnosis

Administer:

• Increased fluids before and during drug administration to induce diuresis and minimize renal toxicity

IV Intermittent INF route

• Using inf device, at no more than 1 mg/kg/min; do not give by rapid or bolus IV; give by CVP or peripheral vein; standard 24 mg/ml sol may be used without dilution if using by CVP; dilute the 24 mg/ml sol to 12 mg/ml with D₅W or NS if using peripheral vein

Y-site compatibilities: Aldesleukin, amikacin, aminophylline, ampicillin, aztreonam, benzquinamide, cefazolin, cefoperazone, cefoxitin, ceftazidime, ceftizoxime, ceftriaxone, cefuroxime, chloramphenicol, cimetidine, clindamycin, dexamethasone, DOPamine, erythromycin, fluconazole, flucytosine, furosemide, gentamicin, heparin, hydrocortisone, hydromorphone, hydrOXYzine, imipenem-cilastatin, metoclopramide, metronidazole, miconazole, morphine, nafcillin, oxacillin, penicillin G potassium, phenytoin, piperacillin, ranitidine, ticarcillin/clavulanate, tobramycin

Perform/provide:

• Regular ophthalmologic exams

• Close monitoring during therapy for tingling, numbness, paresthesias; if these occur, stop infusion, obtain lab sample for electrolytes

Evaluate:

• Therapeutic response: improvement in CMV retinitis

Teach patient/family:

• To call prescriber if sore throat, swollen lymph nodes, malaise, fever occur, since other infections may occur

• To report perioral tingling, numbness in extremities, and paresthesias

• That serious drug interactions may occur if OTC products are ingested; check first with prescriber

• That drug is not a cure but will control symptoms

fosinopril (℞)

(foss'in-oh-pril)
Monopril
Func. class.: Antihypertensive
Chem. class.: Angiotensin-converting enzyme (ACE) inhibitor

Do not confuse:

Monopril/minoxidil/Accupril/Monoket

Action: Selectively suppresses renin-angiotensin-aldosterone system; inhibits ACE; prevents conversion of angiotensin I to angiotensin II; results in dilation of arterial, venous vessels

Uses: Hypertension, alone or in combination with thiazide diuretics, systolic CHF

DOSAGE AND ROUTES

CHF

• *Adult:* **PO** 10 mg daily, then up to 40 mg/day increased over several wk; use lower dose in those diuresed before fosinopril

Hypertension

• *Adult:* **PO** 10 mg daily initially, then 20-40 mg/day divided bid or daily, max 80 mg/day

Available forms: Tabs 10, 20, 40 mg

SIDE EFFECTS

CNS: Insomnia, paresthesia, headache, dizziness, fatigue, memory disturbance, tremor, mood change

CV: Hypotension, chest pain, palpitations, angina, orthostatic hypotension, dysrhythmias, tachycardia

GI: Nausea, constipation, vomiting, diarrhea

GU: **Proteinuria,** increased BUN, creatinine, decreased libido

HEMA: Decreased Hct, Hgb; **eosinophilia, leukopenia, neutropenia**

INTEG: **Angioedema,** rash, flushing, sweating, photosensitivity, pruritus

META: Hyperkalemia

MS: Arthralgia, myalgia

RESP: Cough, sinusitis, dyspnea, **bronchospasm**

Contraindications: Pregnancy (D) 2nd/3rd trimester, hypersensitivity to ACE inhibitors, lactation, children

Precautions: Impaired hepatic function, hypovolemia, blood dyscrasias, CHF, COPD, asthma, geriatric, angioedema, hyperkalemia, renal artery stenosis, renal disease

PHARMACOKINETICS

PO: Peak 3 hr; serum protein binding 97%; half-life 11.5-14 hr; metabolized by liver (metabolites excreted in urine, feces)

INTERACTIONS

Increase: hypersensitivity reactions—allopurinol

Increase: hypotension—diuretics, other antihypertensives, ganglionic blockers, adrenergic blockers, phenothiazines, nitrates, acute alcohol ingestion

Increase: toxicity—vasodilators, hydrALAZINE, prazosin, potassium-sparing diuretics, sympathomimetics, digoxin, lithium

Decrease: absorption—antacids

Decrease: antihypertensive effect—indomethacin, NSAIDs, salicylates

Drug/Herb

⚠ *Increase:* fatal hypokalemia—arginine

Increase: severe photosensitivity—St. John's wort

Increase: antihypertensive effect—hawthorn, pill-bearing spurge

Decrease: antihypertensive effect—pineapple, yohimbe

Drug/Lab Test

Increase: AST, ALT, alk phos, glucose, bilirubin, uric acid

False-positive: Urine acetone

Positive: ANA titer

NURSING CONSIDERATIONS

Assess:

• Blood studies: neutrophils, decreased platelets; obtain WBC with diff baseline and qmo × 6 mo, then q2-3 mo × 1 yr; if neutrophils <1000/mm³, discontinue

⚠ Safety alert   *"Tall Man" lettering

(recommended in collagen-vascular disease)

• B/P, orthostatic hypotension, syncope
• Renal studies: protein, BUN, creatinine; increased levels may indicate nephrotic syndrome
• Baselines in renal, hepatic studies before therapy begins
• Potassium levels, although hyperkalemia rarely occurs
• Edema in feet, legs daily, weigh daily in CHF
• Allergic reactions: rash, fever, pruritus, urticaria; drug should be discontinued if antihistamines fail to help

Administer:
• May be taken without regard to meals

Perform/provide:
• Storage in tight container at 86° F (30° C) or less
• Supine position for severe hypotension

Evaluate:
• Therapeutic response: decrease in B/P

Teach patient/family:
• Not to discontinue drug abruptly
• Not to use OTC products (cough, cold, allergy) unless directed by prescriber; not to use salt substitutes containing potassium without consulting prescriber
• The importance of complying with dosage schedule, even if feeling better
• To rise slowly to sitting or standing position to minimize orthostatic hypotension
• To notify prescriber of mouth sores, sore throat, fever, swelling of hands or feet, irregular heartbeat, chest pain
• To report excessive perspiration, dehydration, vomiting, diarrhea; may lead to fall in B/P
• That drug may cause dizziness, fainting, light-headedness during first few days of therapy
• That drug may cause skin rash or impaired perspiration
• How to take B/P; normal readings for age-group
• To notify prescriber if pregnancy is planned or suspected

Treatment of overdose: 0.9% NaCl IV inf, hemodialysis

---

fosphenytoin (Ⓡ)
(foss-fen′i-toy-in)
Cerebyx
Func. class.: Anticonvulsant
Chem. class.: Hydantoin

Action: Inhibits spread of seizure activity in motor cortex by altering ion transport; increases AV conduction
Uses: Generalized tonic-clonic seizures; status epilepticus

F

DOSAGE AND ROUTES

All doses in PE (phenytoin sodium equivalent)
Status epilepticus
• *Adult and child >1 mo:* **IV** 15-18 mg PE/kg
• *Neonate:* **IV** 15-20 mg PE/kg
Nonemergency/maintenance dosing
• *Adult and adolescent >16 yr:* **IM/IV** 10-20 mg PE/kg 10 mg dose; 4-6 mg PE/kg/day (maintenance); start maintenance 12 hr after loading dose; give in 2-3 divided doses
• *Child 10-16 yr:* **IM/IV** 6-7 mg PE/kg/day
• *Child 7-9 yr:* **IM/IV** 7-8 mg PE/kg/day
• *Child 4-6 yr:* **IM/IV** 7.5-9 mg PE/kg/day
• *Child 6 mo-3 yr:* **IM/IV** 8-10 mg PE/kg/day
• *Infant:* **IM/IV** 5 mg PE/kg/day
• *Neonate:* **IM/IV** 5-8 mg PE/kg/day

Available forms: Inj 150 mg (100 mg phenytoin equiv), 750 mg (500 mg phenytoin equiv)

SIDE EFFECTS

CNS: Drowsiness, dizziness, insomnia, paresthesias, depression, suicidal tendencies, aggression, headache, confusion
CV: Hypotension, **ventricular fibrillation**
EENT: Nystagmus, diplopia, blurred vision
GI: Nausea, vomiting, diarrhea, constipation, anorexia, weight loss, hepatitis, jaundice, gingival hyperplasia
HEMA: **Agranulocytosis, leukopenia,**

aplastic anemia, thrombocytopenia, megaloblastic anemia
INTEG: Rash, lupus erythematosus, **Stevens-Johnson syndrome,** hirsutism
SYST: Hyperglycemia

Contraindications: Pregnancy (D), hypersensitivity, psychiatric conditions, bradycardia, SA and AV block, Stokes-Adams syndrome
Precautions: Allergies, renal/hepatic disease, lactation, myocardial insufficiency

PHARMACOKINETICS

Metabolized by liver, excreted by kidneys

INTERACTIONS

Increase: fosphenytoin level—cimetidine, amiodarone, chloramphenicol, estrogens, H$_2$ antagonists, phenothiazines, salicylates, sulfonamides, tricyclics
Decrease: fosphenytoin effects—alcohol (chronic use), antihistamines, antacids, antineoplastics, rifampin, folic acid, carbamazepine, theophylline
Drug/Herb
Increase: anticonvulsant effect—ginkgo
Decrease: anticonvulsant effect—ginseng, santonica, valerian
Drug/Lab Test
Increase: Glucose, alk phos
Decrease: Dexamethasone, metyrapone test serum, PBI, urinary steroids

NURSING CONSIDERATIONS
Assess:
• Drug level: toxic level 30-50 mcg/ml, wait at least 2 hr after dose before testing
• Blood studies: CBC, platelets q2wk until stabilized, then qmo × 12 mo, then q3mo; discontinue drug if neutrophils <1600/mm^3; serum calcium albumin, phosphorus
• Mental status: mood, sensorium, affect, memory (long, short)
• Seizure activity including type, location, duration, and character; provide seizure precaution

• Renal studies: urinalysis, BUN, urine creatinine
• Hepatic studies: ALT, AST, bilirubin, creatinine
• Allergic reaction: red, raised rash; if this occurs, drug should be discontinued
• For toxicity: bone marrow depression, nausea, vomiting, ataxia, diplopia, cardiovascular collapse, slurred speech, confusion
• Respiratory depression; rate, depth, character of respirations
⚠ Blood dyscrasias: fever, sore throat, bruising, rash, jaundice
• Continuous monitoring of ECG, B/P, respiratory function
• Rash, discontinue as soon as rash develops, serious adverse reactions such as Stevens-Johnson syndrome can occur
Administer:
IV route
• Dilute in D$_5$ or 0.9% NaCl to 1.5-25 mg PE/ml, give <150 mg PE/min
IV, direct route
• Dilute product in D$_5$W or 0.9% NaCl (1.5-25 mg PE/ml); give at a rate of <150 mg PE/min (adult) or <3 mg PE/kg/min
Y-site compatibilities: Esmolol, famotidine, foscarnet, lorazepam
Additive compatibilities: Potassium chloride
Solution compatibilities: D$_5$W, D$_{10}$W, amino acid inj 10%, D$_5$LR, D$_5$/0.9% NaCl, Plasmalyte A, LR, sterile water for inj
Evaluate:
• Therapeutic response: decrease in severity of seizures
Teach patient/family:
• The reason for and expected outcome of treatment
• Not to use machinery or engage in hazardous activity, as drowsiness, dizziness may occur
• To carry emergency ID denoting drug use, name of prescriber
• To notify prescriber of rash, bleeding, bruising, slurred speech, jaundice of skin or eyes, joint pain, nausea, vomiting, severe headaches
• To keep all medical appointments, including lab work, physical assessment

---

⚠ Safety alert   *"Tall Man" lettering

• To notify prescriber if pregnancy is planned, suspected
• To use contraception while using this product

frovatriptan (R)
(froh-vah-trip′tan)
Frova
Func. class.: Antimigraine agent
Chem. class.: 5-HT$_1$-Receptor agonist

Action: Binds selectively to the vascular 5-HT$_{1B}$, 5-HT$_{1D}$ receptor subtypes, exerts antimigraine effect; binds to benzodiazepine receptor sites, causes vasoconstriction in cranium

Uses: Acute treatment of migraine with or without aura

DOSAGE AND ROUTES

• *Adult:* **PO** 2.5 mg, a 2nd dose may be taken after ≥2 hr; max 3 tabs (7.5 mg/day)
Available form: Tabs 2.5 mg

SIDE EFFECTS

CNS: Hot/cold sensation, paresthesia, *dizziness,* headache, fatigue
CV: Flushing, chest pain, palpitation
GI: Dry mouth, dyspepsia, abdominal pain, diarrhea, vomiting
MS: Skeletal pain

Contraindications: Hypersensitivity, angina pectoris, history of MI, documented silent ischemia, Prinzmetal's angina, ischemic heart disease; concurrent ergotamine-containing preparations; uncontrolled hypertension; basilar or hemiplegic migraine; ischemic bowel disease; peripheral vascular disease, severe hepatic disease, prophylactic migraine treatment

Precautions: Pregnancy (C), postmenopausal women, men >40 yr, risk factors for coronary artery disease, hypercholesterolemia, obesity, diabetes, impaired hepatic function, lactation, children, geriatric, seizure disorder

PHARMACOKINETICS

Onset of pain relief 2-3 hr, terminal half-life 25-29 hr, protein binding 15%, metabolized liver CYP450 1A2 enzyme system

INTERACTIONS

Increase: frovatriptan levels—CYP1A2 inhibitors (cimetidine, ciprofloxacin, erythromycin), estrogen, propranolol, oral contraceptives
Increase: toxicity—SSRIs, other serotonin agonists (dextromethorphan, tramadol, antidepressants)
Drug/Herb
Increase: effect—butterbur

NURSING CONSIDERATIONS

Assess:
• Migraine symptoms: aura, unable to view light
• B/P; signs/symptoms of coronary vasospasms
• For stress level, activity, recreation, coping mechanisms
• Ingestion of tyramine-containing foods (pickled products, beer, wine, aged cheese), food additives, preservatives, colorings, artificial sweeteners, chocolate, caffeine, which may precipitate these types of headaches

Administer:
• Swallow tabs whole; do not break, crush, or chew
• 2 days/wk or less; rebound headache may occur

Perform/provide:
• Quiet, calm environment with decreased stimulation from noise, bright light, excessive talking

Evaluate:
• Therapeutic response: decrease in frequency, severity of migraine

Teach patient/family:
• To report any side effects to prescriber
• To use contraception while taking drug; inform prescriber if pregnant or intend to become pregnant
• Consult prescriber if breastfeeding

fulvestrant (Ᵽ)

(full-vess'trant)
Faslodex
Func. class.: Antineoplastic
Chem. class.: Antiestrogen hormone

Action: Inhibits cell division by binding to cytoplasmic estrogen receptors

Uses: Advanced breast carcinoma in estrogen-receptor-positive patients (usually postmenopausal)

DOSAGE AND ROUTES

• *Adult:* **IM** 250 mg qmo
Available forms: Inj 50 mg/ml

SIDE EFFECTS

CNS: Headache, depression, dizziness, insomnia, paresthesia, anxiety
GI: Nausea, vomiting, anorexia, constipation, diarrhea, abdominal pain
INTEG: Rash, sweating, hot flashes, inj site pain
MS: Bone pain, arthritis, back pain
RESP: Pharyngitis, dyspnea, cough
Contraindications: Pregnancy (D), hypersensitivity, lactation, children
Precautions: Hepatic disease

PHARMACOKINETICS

Half-life 40 days, metabolized by CYP3A4, excretion feces 90%

NURSING CONSIDERATIONS

Assess:
• For side effects, report to prescriber
Administer:
IM route
• IM 5 ml as a single inj or 2, 2.5 ml inj; give slowly in buttock
• Antiemetic 30-60 min before giving drug to prevent vomiting prn
Perform/provide:
• Liquid diet, if needed, including cola, gelatin; dry toast or crackers may be added if patient is not nauseated or vomiting
• Nutritious diet with iron, vitamin supplements as ordered
• Store in refrigerator, protect from light

Evaluate:
• Therapeutic response: decreased tumor size, spread of malignancy
Teach patient/family:
• To report any complaints, side effects to prescriber
• To report vaginal bleeding immediately
• That tumor flare—increase in size of tumor, increased bone pain—may occur and will subside rapidly; may take analgesics for pain
• That premenopausal women must use mechanical birth control because ovulation may be induced; do not breastfeed

furosemide (Ᵽ)

(fur-oh'se-mide)
Apo-Furosemide ✣,
Furoside ✤, Lasix, Lasix
Special ✤, Myrosemide ✤,
Novosemide ✤, Uritol ✤
Func. class.: Loop diuretic
Chem. class.: Sulfonamide derivative

Do not confuse:
furosemide/torsemide
Lasix/Luvox/Lomotil/Lanoxin
Action: Inhibits reabsorption of sodium and chloride at proximal and distal tubule and in the loop of Henle
Uses: Pulmonary edema; edema in CHF, hepatic disease, nephrotic syndrome, ascites, hypertension
Unlabeled uses: Hypercalcemia in malignancy

DOSAGE AND ROUTES

Edema
• *Adult:* **PO** 20-80 mg/day in AM; may give another dose in 6 hr up to 600 mg/day; **IM/IV** 20-40 mg, increased by 20 mg q2h until desired response
• *Child:* **PO/IM/IV** 2 mg/kg; may increase by 1-2 mg/kg/q6-8h up to 6 mg/kg
Acute pulmonary edema
• *Adult:* **IV** 40 mg given over several min, repeated in 1 hr; increase to 80 mg if needed

---

Ⓐ Safety alert   *"Tall Man" lettering

Hypertensive crisis/acute renal failure
• *Adult:* **IV** 100-200 mg over 1-2 min
Antihypercalcemia
• *Adult:* **IM/IV** 80-100 mg q1-4h or **PO** 120 mg daily or divided bid
• *Child:* **IM/IV** 25-50 mg, repeat q4h if needed
Available forms: Tabs 20, 40, 80 mg; oral sol 8 mg/ml, 10 mg/ml; inj 10 mg/ml

SIDE EFFECTS

CNS: Headache, fatigue, weakness, vertigo, paresthesias
CV: Orthostatic hypotension, chest pain, ECG changes, **circulatory collapse**
EENT: **Loss of hearing,** ear pain, tinnitus, blurred vision
ELECT: Hypokalemia, hypochloremic alkalosis, hypomagnesemia, hyperuricemia, hypocalcemia, hyponatremia, metabolic alkalosis
ENDO: Hyperglycemia
GI: Nausea, diarrhea, dry mouth, vomiting, anorexia, cramps, oral, gastric irritations, pancreatitis
GU: Polyuria, **renal failure,** glycosuria
HEMA: **Thrombocytopenia, agranulocytosis, leukopenia, neutropenia, anemia**
INTEG: Rash, pruritus, purpura, **Stevens-Johnson syndrome,** sweating, photosensitivity, urticaria
MS: Cramps, stiffness
Contraindications: Hypersensitivity to sulfonamides, anuria, hypovolemia, infants, lactation, electrolyte depletion
Precautions: Pregnancy (C), diabetes mellitus, dehydration, severe renal disease, cirrhosis, ascites

PHARMACOKINETICS

PO: Onset 1 hr, peak 1-2 hr, duration 6-8 hr; absorbed 70%
IV: Onset 5 min, peak ½ hr, duration 2 hr (metabolized by the liver 30%); excreted in urine, some as unchanged drug, feces; crosses placenta; excreted in breast milk; half-life ½-1 hr

INTERACTIONS

Increase: toxicity—lithium, nondepolarizing skeletal muscle relaxants, digoxin
Increase: hypotensive action of antihypertensives, nitrates
Increase: ototoxicity—aminoglycosides, cisplatin, vancomycin
Drug/Herb
• Severe photosensitivity: St. John's wort
Increase: diuretic effect—aloe, cucumber, dandelion, khella, horsetail, pumpkin, Queen Anne's lace
Drug/Lab Test
Interference: GTT

NURSING CONSIDERATIONS

Assess:
• Signs of metabolic alkalosis: drowsiness, restlessness
• Signs of hypokalemia: postural hypotension, malaise, fatigue, tachycardia, leg cramps, weakness
• Rashes, temp elevation daily
• Confusion, especially in geriatric; take safety precautions if needed
• Hearing, including tinnitus and hearing loss, when giving high doses for extended periods
• Weight, I&O daily to determine fluid loss; effect of drug may be decreased if used daily
• Rate, depth, rhythm of respiration, effect of exertion, lung sounds
• B/P lying, standing; postural hypotension may occur
• Electrolytes (K, Na, Cl); include BUN, blood glucose, CBC, serum creatinine, blood pH, ABGs, uric acid, calcium, magnesium
• Skin turgor, edema, condition of mucous membranes in mouth and nose
• Glucose in urine if patient is diabetic
• Allergies to sulfonamides, thiazides
Administer:
• In AM to avoid interference with sleep if using drug as a diuretic
• Potassium replacement if potassium <3 mg/dl

- PO with food if nausea occurs; absorption may be decreased slightly; tabs may be crushed

IV route
- Undiluted; may be given through Y-tube or 3-way stopcock; give 20 mg or less/min; may be added to NS or D_5W if large doses are required and given as IV inf, max 4 mg/min; use infusion pump

Additive compatibilities: Amikacin, aminophylline, ampicillin, atropine, bumetanide, calcium gluconate, cefamandole, cefoperazone, cefuroxime, cimetidine, cloxacillin, dexamethasone, diamorphine, digoxin, epINEPHrine, heparin, isosorbide, kanamycin, lidocaine, meropenem, morphine, nitroglycerin, penicillin G, potassium chloride, ranitidine, scopolamine, sodium bicarbonate, theophylline, tobramycin, verapamil

Syringe compatibilities: Bleomycin, cisplatin, cyclophosphamide, fluorouracil, heparin, leucovorin, methotrexate, mitomycin

Y-site compatibilities: Allopurinol, amifostine, amikacin, amphotericin B cholesteryl, aztreonam, bleomycin, cefepime, cisplatin, cladribine, cyclophosphamide, cytarabine, docetaxel, DOXOrubicin liposome, epINEPHrine, fentanyl, fludarabine, fluorouracil, foscarnet, granisetron, heparin, hydrocortisone, hydromorphone, indomethacin, kanamycin, leucovorin, linezolid, lorazepam, melphalan, meropenem, methotrexate, mitomycin, nitroglycerin, norepinephrine, paclitaxel, piperacillin/tazobactam, potassium chloride, propofol, ranitidine, remifentanil, sargramostim, tacrolimus, teniposide, thiotepa, tobramycin, tolazoline, vit B/C

Perform/provide:
- Increased fluid intake 2-3 L/day unless contraindicated

Evaluate:
- Therapeutic response: improvement in edema of feet, legs, sacral area (CHF); increase urine output, decreased B/P; decreased calcium levels (hypercalcemia)

Teach patient/family:
- To discuss the need for a high-potassium diet or potassium replacement with prescriber
- To rise slowly from lying or sitting position; orthostatic hypotension may occur
- To recognize adverse reactions that may occur: muscle cramps, weakness, nausea, dizziness
- Regarding entire regimen, including exercise, diet, stress relief for hypertension
- To take with food or milk for GI symptoms
- To use sunscreen or protective clothing to prevent photosensitivity
- To take early in day to prevent sleeplessness
- To avoid OTC medication unless directed by prescriber

Treatment of overdose: Lavage if taken orally; monitor electrolytes; administer dextrose in saline; monitor hydration, CV, renal status

gabapentin (℞)
(gab′a-pen-tin)
Gabarone, Neurontin
Func. class.: Anticonvulsant

Do not confuse:
Neurontin/Noroxin/Neoral

Action: Mechanism unknown; may increase seizure threshold; structurally similar to GABA; gabapentin binding sites in neocortex, hippocampus

Uses: Adjunct treatment of partial seizures, with or without generalization in patients >12 yr; adjunct in partial seizures in children 3-12 yr, postherpetic neuralgia

Unlabeled uses: Tremors in multiple sclerosis, neuropathic pain, bipolar disorder, migraine prophylaxis, diabetic neuropathy

DOSAGE AND ROUTES
- *Adult and child >12 yr:* **PO** 900-1800 mg/day in 3 divided doses; may titrate by giving 300 mg on first day, 300 mg bid on second day, 300 mg tid on third day; may

increase to 1800 mg/day by adding 300 mg on subsequent days

• *Child 5-12 yr:* **PO** 10-15 mg/kg/day in 3 divided doses, initially titrate dose upward over approximately 3 days; 25-35 mg/kg/day; all given in 3 divided doses; rect 200 mg as single dose

• *Child 3-4 yr:* **PO** 10-15 mg/kg/day in 3 divided doses, initially titrate dose upward over approximately 3 days; 40 mg/kg/day; all given in 3 divided doses; rect 200 mg as single dose

Postherpetic neuralgia

• *Adult:* **PO** 300 mg on day 1, 600 mg/day divided bid on day 2, 900 mg/day divided tid, may titrate to 1800 mg divided tid if needed

Renal dose

• *Adult and child >12 yr:* CCr 30-60 ml/min 300 mg bid, CCr 15-30 ml/min 300 mg daily, CCr <15 ml/min 125 mg daily

Available forms: Caps 100, 300, 400 mg; tabs 600, 800 mg; oral sol 250 mg/5 ml

SIDE EFFECTS

CNS: Drowsiness, confusion, dizziness, fatigue, anxiety, somnolence, ataxia, amnesia, abnormal thinking, unsteady gait, *depression;* 3-12 yr old, emotional lability, aggression, thought disorder, hyperkinesia

CV: Vasodilation, peripheral edema, hypotension

EENT: Dry mouth, blurred vision, *diplopia,* nystagmus

GI: Constipation, increased appetite, dental abnormalities, nausea, vomiting

GU: Impotence, bleeding, *UTI*

HEMA: **Leukopenia,** decreased WBC

INTEG: Pruritus, abrasion

MS: Myalgia

RESP: Rhinitis, pharyngitis, cough

Contraindications: Hypersensitivity to this drug

Precautions: Pregnancy (C), renal disease, lactation, children <12 yr, geriatric, hemodialysis

PHARMACOKINETICS

Largely unbound to plasma proteins; not metabolized; excreted in urine (unchanged); elimination half-life 5-7 hr; prolonged to 130 hr in ESRD

INTERACTIONS

Increase: CNS depression—alcohol, sedatives, antihistamines, all other CNS depressants

Decrease: gabapentin levels—antacids

Drug/Herb

Increase: CNS depression—chamomile, hops, kava, skullcap, valerian

Drug/Lab Test

[*False-positive:* Urinary protein using Ames N-multistix SG

NURSING CONSIDERATIONS

Assess:

• Seizures: aura, location, duration, activity at onset

• Pain: location, duration, characteristics if using for chronic pain

• Renal studies: urinalysis, BUN, urine creatinine q3mo

• Description of seizures; location, duration, characteristics

• Mental status: mood, sensorium, affect, behavioral changes; if mental status changes, notify prescriber

• Eye problems, need for ophthalmic exam before, during, after treatment (slit lamp, funduscopy, tonometry)

Administer:

• Do not crush or chew caps; caps may be opened and contents put in applesauce or dissolved in juice

• 2 hr apart when giving antacids

• Give without regard to meals

• Gradually withdraw over 7 days, abrupt withdrawal may precipitate seizures

Perform/provide:

• Storage at room temperature away from heat and light

• Hard candy, frequent rinsing of mouth, gum for dry mouth

• Assistance with ambulation during early part of treatment; dizziness occurs

Side effects: *italics* = common; **bold** = life-threatening

G

- Seizure precautions: padded side rails; move objects that may harm patient
- Increased fluids, bulk in diet for constipation

Evaluate:
- Therapeutic response: decreased seizure activity; decrease in chronic pain

Teach patient/family:
- To carry emergency ID stating patient's name, drugs taken, condition, prescriber's name and phone number
- To avoid driving, other activities that require alertness: dizziness, drowsiness may occur
- Not to discontinue medication quickly after long-term use, taper over ≥1 wk; withdrawal-precipitated seizures may occur, not to double doses if dose is missed, take if 2 hr or more before next dose
- To notify prescriber if pregnancy planned or suspected, avoid breastfeeding

Treatment of overdose: Lavage, VS

---

galantamine (℞)
(gah-lan'tah-meen)
Razadyne, Razadyne ER
Func. class.: Anti-Alzheimer agent, cholinesterase inhibitor

Action: May enhance cholinergic functioning by increasing acetylcholine

Uses: Mild to moderate dementia of Alzheimer's disease

DOSAGE AND ROUTES

- *Adult:* **PO** 4 mg bid with morning and evening meals; after 4 wk or more may increase to 8 mg bid; may increase to 12 mg bid after another 4 wk, usual dose 16-24 mg/day in 2 divided doses; **EXT REL** 8 mg/day in AM; may increase to 16 mg/day after 4 wk, and 24 mg/day after another 4 wk

Hepatic dose
- *Adult, Child-Pugh 7-9:* **PO** max 16 mg/day
- *Adult, Child-Pugh 10-15:* **PO** avoid use

Renal dose
- *Adult, moderate renal impairment:* **PO** max 16 mg/day
- *Adult, CCr <9 ml/min:* **PO** avoid use

Available forms: Tabs 4, 8, 12 mg; ext rel tabs 8, 16, 24 mg; oral sol 4 mg/ml

SIDE EFFECTS

CNS: Tremors, insomnia, depression, dizziness, headache, somnolence, fatigue
CV: Bradycardia, anemia, hematuria, chest pain
GI: Nausea, vomiting, anorexia, abdominal distress, flatulence, diarrhea
GU: Urinary incontinence, bladder outflow obstruction, hematuria
META: Weight decrease
MS: Asthenia, anemia
RESP: URI, rhinitis

Contraindications: Hypersensitivity to this drug

Precautions: Pregnancy (B), renal/hepatic/respiratory disease, seizure disorder, peptic ulcer, asthma, lactation, children

PHARMACOKINETICS

Rapidly and completely absorbed, metabolized by CYP450 enzyme, excreted via kidneys; clearance is lower in the geriatric, hepatic disease; clearance is 20% lower in females, elimination half-life 7 hr

INTERACTIONS

- Synergistic effect: cholinomimetics, other cholinesterase inhibitors

Increase: galantamine bioavailability—cimetidine, paroxetine, ketoconazole, erythromycin, quinidine, amitriptyline, fluvoxamine

Drug/Herb
- Cholinergic antagonism: jimsonweed, scopolia

Increase: effect—pill-bearing spurge

NURSING CONSIDERATIONS

Assess:
- Hepatic studies: AST, ALT, alk phos, LDH, bilirubin, CBC

- For severe GI effects: nausea, vomiting, anorexia, weight loss
- B/P, respiration during initial treatment
- Mental status: affect, mood, behavioral changes, depression, memory, attention, confusion

Administer:
- With meals; take with morning and evening meal (immediate rel); morning (ext rel)
- Dose increase after minimum of 4 wk at prior dose
- Ext rel product can be opened and sprinkled on food

Perform/provide:
- Assistance with ambulation during beginning therapy
- Complete suicide assessment

Evaluate:
- Therapeutic response: decreased confusion

Teach patient/family:
- Correct procedure for giving oral solution, using instruction sheet provided
- To notify prescriber of severe GI effects
- To report hypo/hypertension

---

gallium (℞)
(gal'ee-um)
Ganite
Func. class.: Electrolyte modifier
Chem. class.: Hypocalcemic drug

Action: Lowers serum calcium levels by inhibiting calcium resorption from bone
Uses: Cancer-related hypercalcemia

DOSAGE AND ROUTES
- *Adult:* **IV** 100-200 mg/m² daily × 5 days; infuse over 24 hr, rest period of 2-4 wk between courses

Available forms: Inj 25 mg/ml

SIDE EFFECTS
CV: Tachycardia, hypotension
EENT: Blurred vision, optic neuritis, hearing loss
GI: Nausea, vomiting, diarrhea, constipation, mucositis, metallic taste

GU: **Nephrotoxicity,** increased BUN, creatinine
HEMA: **Anemia, leukopenia, thrombocytopenia**
META: Hypophosphatemia, hypocalcemia, decreased serum bicarbonate

Contraindications: Hypersensitivity, hypocalcemia, renal failure, severe renal disease (specific gravity >2.5 mg/dl)
Precautions: Pregnancy (C), lactation, children, mild renal disease, dehydration

PHARMACOKINETICS
IV: Onset 12-48 hr, peak 5 days, duration 4-14 days, excreted by kidneys

INTERACTIONS
Increase: nephrotoxicity—aminoglycosides, amphotericin B, cisplatin, foscarnet, ganciclovir, vancomycin

NURSING CONSIDERATIONS
Assess:
- Renal status: BUN, creatinine, urine output; if creatinine level is 2.5 mg/dl or more, drug should be discontinued
- Monitor calcium, phosphate, bicarbonate, since all levels may be decreased and supplements of phosphate may be needed
- For hypercalcemia: nausea, vomiting, fatigue, weakness, thirst, dehydration, dysrhythmias, change in mental status
- For hypocalcemia: dysrhythmias; paresthesia; twitching; colic; laryngospasm; Trousseau's, Chvostek's sign; tremors
- For hypophosphatemia: confusion, decreased reflexes, joint stiffness and pain, portal hypotension

Administer:

IV route
- Adequate hydration with IV saline, 2 L/day during treatment
- After dilution of dose/1 L 0.9% NaCl or D₅W, run over 24 hr, use infusion pump

Y-site compatibilities: Acyclovir, allopurinol, amifostine, aminophylline, ampicillin/sulbactam, aztreonam, cefazolin, ceftazidime, ceftriaxone, cimetidine, ciprofloxacin, cladribine, cyclophosphamide, dexamethasone, diphenhydrAMINE,

G

filgrastim, fluconazole, furosemide, granisetron, heparin, hydrocortisone, ifosfamide, magnesium sulfate, mannitol, melphalan, meperidine, mesna, methotrexate, metoclopramide, ondansetron, piperacillin, piperacillin/tazobactam, potassium chloride, ranitidine, sodium bicarbonate, teniposide, thiotepa, ticarcillin/clavulanate, trimethoprim-sulfamethoxazole, vancomycin, vinorelbine

Perform/provide:
• Storage of solution 48 hr at room temperature, 1 wk in refrigerator

Evaluate:
• Therapeutic response: decreased serum calcium levels

Teach patient/family:
• To follow dietary guidelines given by prescriber, including avoiding calcium (dairy products, broccoli) and vit D (fortified milk, grain products, fish oil)

Rarely Used

galsulfase (℞)
(gal-sul'face)
Naglazyme
Func. class.: Miscellaneous drug

Uses: Mucopolysaccharidosis VI (MPS VI); Maroteaux-Lamy syndrome

DOSAGE AND ROUTES
• *Adult and child ≥5 yr:* **IV** 1 mg/kg infused over ≥4 hr once per week
Contraindications: Hypersensitivity

ganciclovir (℞)
(gan-sye'kloe-vir)
Cytovene, Vitrasert
Func. class.: Antiviral
Chem. class.: Synthetic nucleoside analog

Do not confuse:
Cytovene/Cytosar
Action: Inhibits replication of herpesviruses, competitively inhibits human CMV DNA polymerase and is incorporated resulting in termination of DNA elongation

Uses: Cytomegalovirus (CMV) retinitis in immunocompromised persons, including those with AIDS, after indirect ophthalmoscopy confirms diagnosis, prophylaxis CVM in transplantation
Unlabeled uses: CMV pneumonia in organ transplant patients, CMV gastroenteritis in patients with IBS, CMV pneumonitis

DOSAGE AND ROUTES
Renal dose
• *Adult:* **PO/IV** Reduce dose in CCr <70 ml/min
Prevention of CMV
• *Adult:* **IV** 5 mg/kg/dose over 1 hr q12h × 1-2 wk, then 5 mg/kg/day 7 day/wk, then 6 mg/kg/day × 5 days/wk; **PO** 1000 mg tid
Induction treatment
• *Adult:* **IV** 5 mg/kg/dose given over 1 hr, q12h × 2-3 wk
Maintenance treatment
• *Adult:* **IV INF** 5 mg/kg given over 1 hr, daily × 7 days/wk; or 6 mg/kg daily × 5 days/wk; **PO** 1000 mg tid with food or 500 mg q3h while awake for 6 doses; **INTRAVITREAL** 4.5 mg implant
Available forms: Powder for inj 500 mg/vial; caps 250, 500 mg; implant, intraviteral 4.5 mg

SIDE EFFECTS
CNS: Fever, chills, **coma,** *confusion,* abnormal thoughts, dizziness, bizarre dreams, *headache,* psychosis, tremors, somnolence, *paresthesia, weakness,* **seizures**
CV: Dysrhythmia, hyper/hypotension
EENT: Retinal detachment in CMV retinitis
GI: Abnormal LFTs, nausea, vomiting, anorexia, diarrhea, abdominal pain, **hemorrhage**
GU: **Hematuria,** *increased creatinine,* BUN
HEMA: **Granulocytopenia, thrombocytopenia, irreversible neutropenia, anemia,** eosinophilia
INTEG: Rash, alopecia, *pruritus,* urticaria, pain at site, phlebitis, **Stevens-Johnson syndrome**
RESP: Dyspnea

A Safety alert   *"Tall Man" lettering

Contraindications: Hypersensitivity to acyclovir or ganciclovir, absolute neutrophil count <500, platelet count <25,000
Precautions: Pregnancy (C), preexisting cytopenias, renal function impairment, lactation, children <6 mo, geriatric

PHARMACOKINETICS

Half-life 3-4½ hr; excreted by kidneys (unchanged); crosses blood-brain barrier, CSF

INTERACTIONS

⚠ Severe granulocytopenia: zidovudine, antineoplastics, radiation; do not give together
Increase: ganciclovir toxicity—adriamycin, amphotericin B, cycloSPORINE, dapsone, DOXOrubicin, flucytosine, pentamidine, probenecid, trimethoprimsulfamethoxazole combinations, vinBLAStine, vinCRIStine, or other nucleoside analogs
Increase: seizures—imipenem/cilastatin
Decrease: ganciclovir renal clearance—probenecid
Decrease: didanosine effect—ganciclovir

NURSING CONSIDERATIONS

Assess:
• CMV retinitis: culture should be completed before starting treatment (urine, blood, throat), ophthalmic exam
• Infection: increased temp, sore throat, chills, fever; report to prescriber
• For leukopenia/neutropenia/thrombocytopenia: WBCs, platelets q2d during 2 ×/day dosing and then q1wk
• For leukopenia with daily WBC count in patients with prior leukopenia with other nucleoside analogs or for whom leukopenia counts are <1000 cells/mm^3 at start of treatment
• Serum creatinine or CCr ≥q2wk
Administer:
PO route
• With food

IV route
• Mixed in biologic cabinet, using gown, gloves, mask; use cytotoxic handling procedures
Intermittent INF route
• IV after diluting 500 mg/10 ml sterile H_2O for inj (50 mg/ml); shake; further dilute in 100 ml D_5W, 0.9% NaCl, LR, Ringer's and run over 1 hr; use infusion pump, in-line filter
• Slowly; do not give by bolus IV, IM, SUBCUT inj
• Using reconstituted sol within 12 hr; do not refrigerate or freeze; infusion solution is stable for 14 days when refrigerated
Y-site compatibilities: Allopurinol, amphotericin B cholesteryl, cisplatin, cyclophosphamide, DOXOrubicin liposome, enalaprilat, etoposide, filgrastim, fluconazole, gatifloxacin, granisetron, linezolid, melphalan, methotrexate, paclitaxel, propofol, remifentanil, tacrolimus, teniposide, thiotepa
Evaluate:
• Therapeutic response: decreased symptoms, or prevention of CMV
Teach patient/family:
• That drug does not cure condition, that regular blood tests, ophthalmologic exams are necessary
• That major toxicities may necessitate discontinuing drug
• To use contraception during treatment and that infertility may occur; should use barrier contraception for 90 days after treatment
• To take PO with food
⚠ To report infection: fever, chills, sore throat; blood dyscrasias: bruising, bleeding, petechiae
• To avoid crowds, persons with respiratory infections
• To use sunscreen to prevent burns

Side effects: *italics* = common; **bold** = life-threatening

ganirelix (R)
Antagon
Func. class.: Gonadotropin-releasing hormone antagonist
Chem. class.: Synthetic decapeptide

Action: Inhibitor of pituitary gonadotropin secretion; initially increases LH and FSH, induces a rapid suppression of gonadotropin secretion

Uses: For inhibition of premature LH surges in women undergoing controlled ovarian hyperstimulation

DOSAGE AND ROUTES
• *Adult:* **SUBCUT** 250 mcg daily during early to mid-follicular phase, continue until the day of hCG administration
Available forms: Inj 250 mcg/0.5 ml

SIDE EFFECTS
CNS: Headache
ENDO: Ovarian hyperstimulation syndrome, abdominal pain (GYN)
GI: Nausea
GU: Spotting, breakthrough bleeding
INTEG: Pain on inj
SYST: **Fetal death**
Contraindications: Pregnancy (X), hypersensitivity, latex allergy, lactation

PHARMACOKINETICS
Excreted in feces/urine, half-life 13-16 hr, metabolized to metabolites, protein binding 82%

NURSING CONSIDERATIONS
Assess:
• For suspected pregnancy, drug should not be used
• For latex allergy, drug should not be used
Administer:
• SUBCUT using abdomen, around navel or upper thigh, swab inj area with disinfectant, clean a 2-in circle and allow to dry, pinch up area between thumb and finger, insert needle at 45°-90° to surface, if positioned correctly, no blood will be drawn back into syringe, if blood is drawn into syringe, reposition needle without removing it
Perform/provide:
• Protection from light
Evaluate:
• Therapeutic response: pregnancy
Teach patient/family:
• To report abdominal pain, vaginal bleeding

gatifloxacin ophthalmic
See Appendix C

gefitinib (R)
(ge-fi'tye-nib)
Iressa
Func. class.: Antineoplastic—miscellaneous
Chem. class.: Epidermal growth factor receptor inhibitor

Action: Not fully understood; inhibits intracellular phosphorylation of cell surface receptors associated with epidermal growth factor receptors
Uses: Advanced/metastatic non–small cell lung cancer (NSCLC) in those that have not responded to platinum or docetaxel products

DOSAGE AND ROUTES
• *Adult:* **PO** 250 mg daily
CYP3A4 inducers concurrently (such as rifampin or phenytoin)
• *Adult:* **PO** 500 mg daily
Available forms: Tabs 250 mg

SIDE EFFECTS
GI: Nausea, diarrhea, vomiting, anorexia, **pancreatitis,** mouth ulceration
INTEG: Rash, pruritus, *acne, dry skin,* **toxic epidermal neurolysis, angioedema**
MISC: Peripheral edema, amblyopia, conjunctivitis, eye pain, corneal erosion/ulcer

RESP: **Interstitial lung disease,** cough, dyspnea
Contraindications: Pregnancy (D), hypersensitivity, lactation, children
Precautions: Renal/hepatic/ocular, pulmonary disorders, geriatric

PHARMACOKINETICS

Slowly absorbed, excreted in feces (86%), urine (<4%); elimination half-life 48 hr, metabolism by CYP3A4

INTERACTIONS

Increase: gefitinib concentrations—ketoconazole, itraconazole, erythromycin, clarithromycin
Increase: plasma concentration of warfarin, metoprolol
Decrease: gefitinib levels—phenytoin, rifampin, cimetidine, ranitidine, sodium bicarbonate
Herb/Drug
Decrease: gefitinib levels—St. John's wort

NURSING CONSIDERATIONS

Assess:
⚠ Pulmonary changes: lung sounds, cough, dyspnea; interstitial lung disease may occur, may be fatal; discontinue therapy if confirmed
• Ocular changes: eye irritation, corneal erosion/ulcer, aberrant eyelash growth
⚠ Pancreatitis: abdominal pain, levels of amylase, lipase
⚠ Toxic epidermal necrosis, angioedema
• GI symptoms: frequency of stools, if diarrhea is poorly tolerated, therapy may be discontinued for up to 14 days
Administer:
• Without regard to food; avoid grapefruit juice
Evaluate:
• Therapeutic response: decreased non–small cell lung cancer cells
Teach patient/family:
⚠ To report adverse reactions immediately: SOB, severe abdominal pain, ocular changes, skin eruptions

• Reason for treatment, expected results
• Use contraception during treatment; avoid breastfeeding
• Avoid persons with infections

---

gemcitabine (R)

(jem-sit′a-been)
Gemzar
Func. class.: Antineoplastic—miscellaneous
Chem. class.: Nucleoside analog

Do not confuse:
Gemzar/Zinecard
Action: Exhibits antitumor activity by killing cells undergoing DNA synthesis (S-phase) and blocking G1/S-phase boundary
Uses: Adenocarcinoma of the pancreas (nonresectable stage II, III, or metastatic stage IV); non–small cell lung cancer (stage IIIA or B, IV); in combination with cisplatin for inoperable, advanced, or metastatic non–small cell lung cancer; advanced breast cancer in combination with paclitaxel

DOSAGE AND ROUTES

Pancreatic carcinoma
• *Adult:* **IV** 1000 mg/m^2 given over ½ hr qwk × 7 wk, then 1 wk rest period; subsequent cycles should be infused once qwk × 3 wk out of every 4 wk
Non–small cell lung cancer
• *Adult:* **IV** (4-wk schedule) 1000 mg/m^2 given over ½ hr on days 1, 8, 15, of each 28-day cycle; give cisplatin **IV** 100 mg/m^2 on day 1 after gemcitabine
• *Adult:* **IV** (3-wk schedule) 1250 mg/m^2 given over ½ hr on days 1, 8 of each 21-day cycle; give cisplatin 100 mg/m^2 after the inf of gemcitabine on day 1
Advanced breast cancer
• *Adult:* **IV** 1250 mg/m^2 on days 1 and 8 of a 21-day cycle; give paclitaxel on day 1
Available forms: Lyophilized powder for inj 20 mg/ml

SIDE EFFECTS

GI: Diarrhea, nausea, vomiting, anorexia, constipation, stomatitis

GU: Proteinuria, hematuria

HEMA: **Leukopenia, anemia, neutropenia, thrombocytopenia**

INTEG: Irritation at site, rash, alopecia

OTHER: Dyspnea, fever, **hemorrhage,** infection, flulike symptoms, paresthesia

Contraindications: Pregnancy (D), hypersensitivity, lactation

Precautions: Children, geriatric, myelosuppression, irradiation, renal/hepatic disease

PHARMACOKINETICS

Half-life 42-79 min, crosses placenta

INTERACTIONS

Increase: bleeding—NSAIDs, alcohol, salicylates

Increase: myelosuppression, diarrhea—other antineoplastics, radiation

Decrease: antibody response—live virus vaccines

Drug/Lab Test

Increase: BUN, AST, ALT, alk phos, bilirubin, creatinine

NURSING CONSIDERATIONS

Assess:

• CBC, differential, platelet count before each dose; absolute granulocyte count >1000, platelets >100,000, give complete dose; absolute granulocyte count 500-1000, platelets 50,000-100,000, give 75%; absolute granulocyte count <500, platelets <50,000, do not give

• Blood dyscrasias: bruising, bleeding, petechiae

• I&O, nutritional intake; food preferences: list likes, dislikes

• Renal, hepatic studies before and during treatment; may increase AST, ALT, alk phos, bilirubin, BUN, creatinine

• Buccal cavity q8h for dryness, sores/ulceration, white patches, oral pain, bleeding, dysphagia

• GI symptoms: frequency of stools; cramping

• Signs of dehydration: rapid respirations, poor skin turgor, decreased urine output, dry skin, restlessness, weakness

Administer:

IV route

• Prepare in biologic cabinet using gown, mask, gloves; use cytotoxic handling procedures

• After reconstituting with 0.9% NaCl 5 ml/200 mg vial of drug or 25 ml/1 g of drug, shake = 40 mg/ml may be further diluted with 0.9% NaCl to conc as low as 0.1 mg/ml; discard unused portions, give over ½ hr, do not admix

Y-site compatibilities: Amifostine, amikacin, aminophylline, ampicillin, aztreonam, bleomycin, bumetanide, butorphanol, calcium gluconate, cefoxitin, ceftazidime, ceftizoxime, ceftriaxone, chlorproMAZINE, cimetidine, ciprofloxacin, cisplarin, clindamycin, cyclophosphamide, cytarabine, dactinomycin, DAUNOrubicin, diphenhydrAMINE, DOBUTamine, docetaxel, DOPamine, DOXOrubicin, droperidol, enalaprilat, etoposide, famotidine, floxuridine, fluconazole, fludarabine, fluorouracil, gentamicin, granisetron, haloperidol, heparin, hydrocortisone, hydromorphone, idarubicin, ifosfamide, leucovorin, linezolid, lorazepam, mannitol, meperidine, mesna, metoclopramide, metronidazole, minocycline, mitoxantrone, morphine, nalbuphine, ondansetron, paclitaxel, promethazine, ranitidine, streptozocin, teniposide, thiotepa, ticarcillin, tobramycin, topotecan, trimethoprim/sulfamethoxazole, vancomycin, vinBLAStine, vinCRIStine, vinorelbine, zidovudine

Perform/provide:

• Increased fluid intake to 2-3 L/day to prevent dehydration, unless contraindicated

• Changing of IV site q48h

• Rinsing of mouth tid-qid with water, club soda; brushing of teeth bid-tid with soft brush or cotton-tipped applicator for stomatitis; use unwaxed dental floss

• Nutritious diet with iron, vitamin supplement, low fiber, few dairy products

---

Evaluate:
• Therapeutic response: decrease in tumor size, decrease in spread of cancer

Teach patient/family:
• To avoid foods with citric acid or hot or rough texture if stomatitis is present; to drink adequate fluids
• To avoid use with NSAIDs, alcohol, salicylates
• To report stomatitis; any bleeding, white spots, ulcerations in mouth; tell patient to examine mouth daily, report symptoms
• To report signs of anemia: fatigue, headache, faintness, shortness of breath, irritability; hematuria, dysuria
• To use contraception during therapy and for 4 mo after
• Not to receive vaccinations during treatment

gemfibrozil (R)
(jem-fi'broe-zil)
gemfibrozil, Lopid
Func. class.: Antilipemic
Chem. class.: Fibric acid derivative

Do not confuse:
Lopid/Levbid/Slo-bid
Action: Inhibits biosynthesis of VLDL, decreases triglycerides, increases HDL
Uses: Type IIb, IV, V hyperlipidemia as adjunct with diet therapy

DOSAGE AND ROUTES
• *Adult:* **PO** 600 mg bid 30 min before AM, PM meal
Available forms: Tabs 600 mg; caps 300 mg ✦

SIDE EFFECTS
CNS: Fatigue, vertigo, headache, paresthesia, dizziness, somnolence
GI: Dyspepsia, diarrhea, abdominal pain, nausea, vomiting
HEMA: **Leukopenia, anemia, eosinophilia, thrombocytopenia**
INTEG: Rash, urticaria, pruritus
MISC: Taste perversion
Contraindications: Severe renal/hepatic disease, preexisting gallbladder disease, primary biliary cirrhosis, hypersensitivity
Precautions: Pregnancy (C), monitor hematologic and hepatic function, lactation

PHARMACOKINETICS
PO: Peak 1-2 hr; plasma protein binding >90%; half-life 1½ hr; 70% excreted in urine as conjugate; <2% excreted unchanged; metabolized in liver (minimal)

INTERACTIONS
Increase: hypoglycemic effect—sulfonylureas
Increase: anticoagulant properties—oral anticoagulants
Increase: risk of myositis, myalgia—HMG-CoA reductase inhibitors
Decrease: effect of cycloSPORINE
Drug/Herb
Increase: effect—glucomannan
Decrease: effect—gotu kola
Drug/Lab Test
Increase: LFTs, CPK, BSP, thymol turbidity, glucose
Decrease: Hgb, Hct, WBC

NURSING CONSIDERATIONS
Assess:
• Triglycerides, cholesterol; if lipids increase, drug should be discontinued; LDL, VLDL baseline and periodically
• Renal, hepatic studies, CBC, blood glucose if patient is on long-term therapy; if LFTs increase, therapy should be discontinued
• Bowel pattern daily; watch for increasing diarrhea (common)
Administer:
• 30 min before morning and evening meals
Evaluate:
• Therapeutic response: decreased cholesterol, triglyceride levels, HDL, cholesterol ratios improved
Teach patient/family:
• That compliance is needed for positive results; do not double or skip dose

Side effects: *italics* = common; **bold** = life-threatening

- That risk factors should be decreased: high-fat diet, smoking, alcohol consumption, absence of exercise
- To notify prescriber of diarrhea, nausea, vomiting, chills, fever, sore throat, muscle cramps, abdominal cramps, severe flatulence
- That drug may be discontinued if no improvement in 3 mo

---

gemifloxacin (Rx)
(gem-ah-flox'a-sin)
Factive
Func. class.: Antiinfective
Chem. class.: Fluoroquinolone

Action: Inhibits DNA gyrase, which is an enzyme involved in replication, transcription, and repair of bacterial DNA

Uses: Acute bacterial exacerbation of chronic bronchitis caused by *Streptococcus pneumoniae, Haemophilus influenzae, Haemophilus parainfluenzae, Moraxella catarrhalis*; community-acquired pneumonia caused by *Streptococcus pneumoniae* including multi-drug resistant strains, *H. influenzae, M. catarrhalis, Mycoplasma pneumoniae, Chlamydia pneumoniae, Klebsiella pneumoniae*

DOSAGE AND ROUTES
- *Adult:* **PO** 320 mg/day × 5-10 days depending on type of infection
Renal dose
- *Adult:* **PO** CCr ≤40 ml/min 160 mg q24hr
Available forms: Tabs 320 mg

SIDE EFFECTS
CNS: Dizziness, headache, somnolence, depression, insomnia, nervousness, confusion, agitation, **seizures**
CV: QT prolongation, vasodilation
EENT: Visual disturbances
GI: Diarrhea, *nausea,* vomiting, anorexia, flatulence, heartburn, dry mouth; increased AST, ALT; constipation, abdominal pain, oral thrush, glossitis, stomatitis, **pseudomembranous colitis**

INTEG: Rash, pruritus, urticaria, *photosensitivity*
SYST: **Anaphylaxis, Stevens-Johnson syndrome**
Contraindications: Hypersensitivity to quinolones
Precautions: Pregnancy (C), hypokalemia, hypomagnesium, lactation, children, geriatric, renal disease, seizure disorders, excessive exposure to sunlight, psychosis, increased intracranial pressure, history of arrhythmias, history of QT interval prolongation, dysrhythmias

PHARMACOKINETICS
PO: Peak 1-2 hr, half-life 6-8 hr; excreted in urine as active drug, metabolites

INTERACTIONS
Increase: toxicity of gemifloxacin—probenecid
⚠ ***Decrease:*** effect of antidysrhythmias (amiodarone, procainamide, quinidine, sotalol, disopyramide), tricyclics; result in life-threatening arrhythmias, QT prolongation
Decrease: absorption antacids containing aluminum, magnesium, sucralfate, zinc, iron, give 4 hr before meals or 2 hr after meals
Drug/Herb
- Do not use acidophilus with antiinfectives; separate by several hours

NURSING CONSIDERATIONS
Assess:
- Renal, hepatic studies: BUN, creatinine, AST, ALT; I&O ratio
- CNS symptoms: insomnia, vertigo, headache, agitation, confusion
⚠ Allergic reactions and anaphylaxis: rash, flushing, urticaria, pruritus, chills, fever, joint pain; may occur a few days after therapy begins; epINEPHrine and resuscitation equipment should be available for anaphylactic reaction
- Bowel pattern daily, if severe diarrhea occurs, drug should be discontinued
- For overgrowth of infection: perineal itching, fever, malaise, redness, pain,

---

swelling, drainage, rash, diarrhea, change in cough, sputum
• For tendon pain, if present, discontinue use

Administer:
• 4 hr before or 2 hr after antacids, iron, calcium, zinc products

Evaluate
• Therapeutic response: negative C&S, absence of signs/symptoms of infection

Teach patient/family:
• May take with or without food
• That fluids must be increased to 2 L/day to avoid crystallization in kidneys
• That if dizziness or light-headedness occurs, perform activities with assistance
• To complete full course of drug therapy
• To contact prescriber if adverse reactions occur
• To avoid iron- or mineral-containing supplements or antacids within 4 hr before and 2 hr after dosing
• That photosensitivity may occur and sunscreen should be used
• To use frequent rinsing of mouth, sugarless candy or gum for dry mouth
• To avoid other medication unless approved by prescriber

⚠ High Alert

gemtuzumab (℞)
(gem-tue-zue′mab)
Mylotarg
Func. class.: Antineoplastic—miscellaneous
Chem. class.: Monoclonal antibody

Action: Composed of recombinant humanized IgG_4 kappa antibody, binds to CD33 antigen that is released in myeloid cells
Uses: Acute myeloid leukemia (AML) in patients with first relapse who are 60 yr or older

DOSAGE AND ROUTES
• *Adult:* **IV** 9 mg/m^2 as a 2 hr inf; before giving inf, give diphenhydrAMINE 50 mg **PO,** acetaminophen 650-1000 mg **PO** 1 hr prior to inf; then use acetaminophen 650-1000 mg q1-4h prn
Available forms: Powder for inj, lyophilized 5 mg

SIDE EFFECTS
CNS: Dizziness, insomnia, depression
CV: Hypertension, hemorrhage, tachycardia, hypotension
GI: Anorexia, diarrhea, constipation, nausea, stomatitis, vomiting
GU: Hematuria, **vaginal hemorrhage**
INTEG: Rash, herpes simplex, local reaction, petechiae
META: Hypokalemia, hypomagnesemia
MISC: Fever, myalgias, headache, chills
RESP: Cough, pneumonia, epistaxis, rhinitis

Contraindications: Pregnancy (D), hypersensitivity, severe myelosuppression, lactation
Precautions: Children, severe renal/hepatic disease

PHARMACOKINETICS
Half-life 45 and 100 hr, respectively

NURSING CONSIDERATIONS
Assess:
• For symptoms of infection; chills, fever, headache, may be masked by drug fever
• CNS reaction: LOC, mental status, dizziness, confusion
• Cardiac status: lung sounds; ECG before and during treatment, especially in those with cardiac disease
• Bone marrow depression: bruising, bleeding, blood in stools, urine, sputum, emesis

Administer:
• Do not give IV push or bolus
• Protect from light; use biologic safety hood; allow to come to room temp
• Reconstitute each vial with 5 ml sterile water for inj using sterile syringes; swirl each vial; check for discoloration or particulate matter; give over 2 hr; use a separate line with 1.2 micron terminal filter

---

Perform/provide:
• Storage of reconstituted sol for ≤8 hr in refrigerator

Evaluate:
• Therapeutic response: decrease in size, number of lesions

Teach patient/family:
• To take acetaminophen for fever
• To avoid hazardous tasks, since confusion, dizziness may occur; avoid prolonged sunlight, use sunscreen
• To report signs of infection: sore throat, fever, diarrhea, vomiting
• To avoid immunizations
• To avoid crowds, people with known infections

---

gentamicin (℞)

(jen-ta-mye'sin)
Cidomycin ✦, Garamycin, gentamicin sulfate, G-Mycin, Jenamicin
Func. class.: Antiinfective
Chem. class.: Aminoglycoside

Do not confuse:
Garamycin/kanamycin

Action: Interferes with protein synthesis in bacterial cell by binding to ribosomal subunit, causing misreading of genetic code; inaccurate peptide sequence forms in protein chain, causing bacterial death

Uses: Severe systemic infections of CNS, respiratory, GI, urinary tract, bone, skin, soft tissues caused by susceptible strains of *Pseudomonas aeruginosa, Proteus, Klebsiella, Serratia, Escherichia coli, Enterobacter, Citrobacter, Staphylococcus, Shigella, Salmonella, Acinetobacter, Bacillus anthracis,* acute PID

DOSAGE AND ROUTES

Severe systemic infections
• *Adult:* IV INF 3-6 mg/kg/day in divided doses q8h; dilute in 50-200 ml 0.9% NaCl or D₅W given over 30 min-1 hr; **IM** 3 mg/kg/day in divided doses q8h
• *Child:* **IV/IM** 2-2.5 mg/kg q8h

• *Neonate and infant:* **IV/IM** 2.5 mg/kg q8-12h
• *Neonate <1 wk:* **IV** 2.5 mg/kg q12-24h

Once daily dosing/extended interval dosing (unlabeled)
• *Adult:* **IV** 4-7 mg/kg/q24h, adjust according to levels

Renal dose
• *Adult:* **IV/IM** 1-1.7 mg/kg initially, then adjust according to renal function studies

Available forms: Inj 10, 40 mg/ml; premixed inj 40, 60, 70, 80, 100 mg/50 ml; 40, 60, 80, 90, 100, 120, 160, 180 mg/ml

SIDE EFFECTS

CNS: Confusion, depression, numbness, tremors, **seizures,** muscle twitching, **neurotoxicity,** dizziness, vertigo
CV: Hypotension, hypertension, palpitations
EENT: **Ototoxicity,** *deafness,* visual disturbances, tinnitus
GI: Nausea, vomiting, anorexia; increased ALT, AST, bilirubin; hepatomegaly, **hepatic necrosis,** splenomegaly
GU: **Oliguria, hematuria, renal damage, azotemia, renal failure, nephrotoxicity,** proteinuria
HEMA: **Agranulocytosis, thrombocytopenia, leukopenia, eosinophilia,** anemia
INTEG: **Rash,** burning, urticaria, dermatitis, alopecia

Contraindications: Severe renal disease, hypersensitivity

Precautions: Pregnancy (C), neonates, mild renal disease, hearing deficits, myasthenia gravis, lactation, geriatric, Parkinson's disease

PHARMACOKINETICS

IM: Onset rapid, peak 1-2 hr
IV: Onset immediate; peak 1-2 hr; plasma half-life 1-2 hr, infants 6-7 hr; duration 6-8 hr
Not metabolized; excreted unchanged in urine; crosses placental barrier

---

INTERACTIONS

Increase: ototoxicity, neurotoxicity, nephrotoxicity—other aminoglycosides, amphotericin B, polymyxin, vancomycin, ethacrynic acid, furosemide, mannitol, methoxyflurane, cisplatin, cephalosporins, penicillins, cidofovir, acyclovir

Increase: effects—nondepolarizing neuromuscular blockers

Drug/Herb

• Do not use acidophilus with antiinfectives; separate by several hours

NURSING CONSIDERATIONS

Assess:

• Weight before treatment; calculation of dosage is usually based on ideal body weight, but may be calculated on actual body weight

• I&O ratio, urinalysis daily for proteinuria, cells, casts; report sudden change in urine output; toxicity is increased in patients with decreased renal function if high doses are given

• VS during infusion; watch for hypotension, change in pulse

• IV site for thrombophlebitis, including pain, redness, swelling, q30min, change site if needed; discontinue, apply warm compresses to site

• Serum peak, drawn at 30-60 min after IV inf or 60 min after IM inj, and trough level drawn just before next dose; blood level should be 2-4 times bacteriostatic level; peak = 4-12 mcg/ml, trough = 1-2 mcg/ml

• Urine pH if drug is used for UTI; urine should be kept alkaline

• Renal impairment by securing urine for CCr testing, BUN, serum creatinine; lower dosage should be given in renal impairment (CCr <80 ml/min)

• Eighth cranial nerve dysfunction by audiometric testing; also ringing, roaring in ears, vertigo; assess hearing before, during, after treatment

• Dehydration: high specific gravity, decrease in skin turgor, dry mucous membranes, dark urine

• Overgrowth of infection including fever, malaise, redness, pain, swelling, perineal itching, diarrhea, stomatitis, change in cough or sputum

• C&S before starting treatment to identify infecting organism

• Vestibular dysfunction: nausea, vomiting, dizziness, headache; drug should be discontinued if severe

• Injection sites for redness, swelling, abscesses; use warm compresses at site

Administer:

• IM inj in large muscle mass; rotate inj sites

• Drug in evenly spaced doses to maintain blood level

IV route

• After diluting in 50-200 ml NS or D₅W; sol concentration should be 1 mg/ml or less; decrease vol of diluent in child; maintain 0.1% sol run over ½-1 hr (adults) or up to 2 hr (children); flush IV line with NS or D₅W after administration

Additive compatibilities: Atracurium, aztreonam, bleomycin, cefoxitin, cimetidine, ciprofloxacin, fluconazole, meropenem, methicillin, metronidazole, ofloxacin, penicillin G sodium, ranitidine, verapamil

Syringe compatibilities: Clindamycin, methicillin, penicillin G sodium

Y-site compatibilities: Acyclovir, amifostine, amiodarone, amsacrine, atracurium, aztreonam, cefpirome, ciprofloxacin, cyclophosphamide, cytarabine, diltiazem, enalaprilat, esmolol, famotidine, filgrastim, fluconazole, fludarabine, foscarnet, granisetron, hydromorphone, IL-2, insulin, labetalol, lorazepam, magnesium sulfate, melphalan, meperidine, meropenem, midazolam, morphine, multivitamins, ondansetron, paclitaxel, pancuronium, perphenazine, sargramostim, tacrolimus, teniposide, theophylline, thiotepa, tolazine, vecuronium, vinorelbine, vit B/C, zidovudine

Perform/provide:

• Adequate fluids of 2-3 L/day, unless contraindicated, to prevent irritation of tubules

---

- Supervised ambulation, other safety measures with vestibular dysfunction

Evaluate:
- Therapeutic response: absence of fever, draining wounds, negative C&S after treatment

Teach patient/family:
- To report headache, dizziness, symptoms of overgrowth of infection, renal impairment
- To report loss of hearing, ringing, roaring in ears, or feeling of fullness in head

gentamicin ophthalmic
See Appendix C

gentamicin topical
See Appendix C

glatiramer (℞)
(glah-tear′a-meer)
Copaxone
Func. class.: Multiple sclerosis agent

Action: Unknown, may modify the immune responses responsible for multiple sclerosis (MS)

Uses: Reduction of the frequency of relapses in patients with relapsing-remitting MS

DOSAGE AND ROUTES
- *Adult:* **SUBCUT** 20 mg/day

Available forms: Inj, premixed 20 mg/ml

SIDE EFFECTS

CNS: Anxiety, hypertonia, tremor, vertigo, speech disorder, *agitation,* confusion

CV: Migraine, palpitations, syncope, tachycardia, vasodilation, chest pain

EENT: Ear pain, blurred vision

GI: Nausea, vomiting, diarrhea, anorexia, gastroenteritis

GU: Urinary urgency, dysmenorrhea, vaginal moniliasis

HEMA: Ecchymosis, lymphadenopathy

INTEG: Pruritus, rash, sweating, urticaria, erythema

META: Edema, weight gain

MS: Arthralgia, back pain, neck pain

RESP: Bronchitis, dyspnea, laryngismus, rhinitis

Contraindications: Hypersensitivity to this drug or mannitol

Precautions: Pregnancy (B), immune disorders, renal disease, lactation, child <18 yr

PHARMACOKINETICS
May be hydrolyzed locally, may reach regional lymph nodes

NURSING CONSIDERATIONS

Assess:
- Blood, renal, hepatic studies: prior to treatment
- For CNS symptoms: anxiety, confusion, vertigo
- GI status: diarrhea, vomiting, abdominal pain, gastroenteritis
- Cardiac status: tachycardia, palpitations, vasodilation, chest pain

Administer:

SUBCUT route
- Using a sterile syringe/needle to transfer the supplied diluent into the vial; rotate vial gently; do not shake; withdraw medication using a syringe with 27G needle; administer SUBCUT into hip, thigh, arm; discard unused portion
- Use SUBCUT route only; do not give IM or IV
- Do not use sol that contains precipitate or is discolored
- Use immediately

Evaluate:
- Therapeutic response: decreased symptoms of MS

Teach patient/family:
- Give written, detailed instructions about the drug; provide initial and return demonstrations on inj procedure; give information on use and disposal of drug, inj

site reaction (hives, rash, irritation, severe pain, flushing, chest pain)
• That blurred vision, sweating may occur
• That irregular menses, dysmenorrhea, or metrorrhagia as well as breast pain may occur; use contraception during treatment
• That if pregnancy is suspected, or if nursing, notify prescriber
• Not to change dosing or to stop taking drug without advice of prescriber
• Immediate post inj reaction: flushing, chest pain, palpitations, anxiety, dyspnea, laryngeal constriction, urticaria, does not usually require treatment

glimepiride
(glye-me′pi-ride)
Amaryl
glipiZIDE (℞)
(glip-i′zide)
Glucotrol, Glucotrol XL
Func. class.: Antidiabetic
Chem. class.: Sulfonylurea (2nd generation)

Do not confuse:
glipiZIDE/Glucotrol/glyBURIDE
Action: Causes functioning β-cells in pancreas to release insulin, leading to drop in blood glucose levels; may improve insulin binding to insulin receptors or increase the number of insulin receptors with prolonged administration; may also reduce basal hepatic glucose secretion; not effective if patient lacks functioning β-cells
Uses: Type 2 diabetes mellitus

DOSAGE AND ROUTES
Glimepiride
• *Adult:* PO 1-2 mg daily, then increase q1-2wk up to 8 mg/day
• *Geriatric:* PO 1 mg/day; may increase if needed
Renal dose
• *Adult:* PO CCr <20 ml/min, 1 mg daily

with breakfast, may titrate upward as needed
GlipiZIDE
• *Adult:* PO 5 mg initially, then increase to desired response; max 40 mg/day in divided doses or 15 mg/dose
• *Geriatric:* PO 2.5 mg/day; may increase if needed
Hepatic disease
• *Adult:* PO 2.5 mg initially, then increase to desired response; max 40 mg/day in divided doses or 15 mg/dose
Available forms: *Glimepiride:* tabs 1, 2, 4 mg; *glipiZIDE:* tabs, scored; 5, 10 mg ext rel tab (XL) 5, 10 mg

SIDE EFFECTS
CNS: Headache, weakness, dizziness, drowsiness, tinnitus, fatigue, vertigo
ENDO: **Hypoglycemia**
GI: **Hepatotoxicity, cholestatic jaundice,** nausea, vomiting, diarrhea, heartburn
HEMA: **Leukopenia, thrombocytopenia, agranulocytosis, aplastic anemia;** increased AST, ALT, alk phos; **pancytopenia, hemolytic anemia**
INTEG: Rash, allergic reactions, pruritus, urticaria, eczema, photosensitivity, erythema
Contraindications: Hypersensitivity to sulfonylureas, type 1/juvenile diabetes, diabetic ketoacidosis
Precautions: Pregnancy (C), geriatric, cardiac disease, severe renal/hepatic disease, thyroid disease

PHARMACOKINETICS
PO: Completely absorbed by GI route, onset 1-1½ hr, peak 1-3 hr, duration 10-24 hr, half-life 2-4 hr; metabolized in liver; excreted in urine; 90%-95% is plasma protein bound

INTERACTIONS
• May mask symptoms of hypoglycemia: β-blockers
Increase: action of digoxin, glycosides
Increase: hypoglycemic effects—insulin, MAOIs, cimetidine, chloramphenicol,

guanethidine, methyldopa, NSAIDs, salicylates, probenecid, androgens, anticoagulants, clofibrate, fenfluramine, fluconazole, gemfibrozil, histamine H_2 antagonists, magnesium salts, phenylbutazone, sulfinpyrazone, sulfonamides, tricyclics, urinary acidifiers

Decrease: thiazide diuretics, rifampin, isoniazid, cholestyramine, diazoxide, hydantoins, urinary alkalinizers, charcoal

Drug/Herb

Increase: antidiabetic effect—alfalfa, aloe, basil, bay, bilberry, bitter melon, black catechu, buchu, burdock, coriander, dandelion, eyebright (po), garlic, glucomannan, glucosamine, goat's rue, gymnema, horehound, horse chestnut, jambul, myrrh, myrtle

Increase: glucose tolerance—karela

Increase or decrease: hypoglycemic effect—chromium, fenugreek, ginseng, coenzyme Q10

Decrease: hypoglycemic effect—broom, buchu, dandelion, glucosamine, juniper

Decrease: antidiabetic effect—bee pollen, blue cohosh, broom, chromium, elecampane, eucalyptus, gotu kola

Drug/Lab Test

Increase: AST, ALT, LDH, BUN, creatinine

NURSING CONSIDERATIONS

Assess:
• Hypo/hyperglycemic reaction that can occur soon after meals; for severe hypoglycemia give IV $D_{50}W$, then IV dextrose solution
• Blood, A1c levels during treatment to determine diabetes control
• CBC baseline and throughout treatment

Administer:
• Do not break, crush, or chew ext rel tabs; may crush tabs and mix with fluids if unable to swallow whole
• Drug 30 min before meals; if patient is NPO, may need to hold dose to prevent hypoglycemia

Perform/provide:
• Storage in tight, light-resistant container at room temperature

Evaluate:
• Therapeutic response: decrease in polyuria, polydipsia, polyphagia, clear sensorium, absence of dizziness, stable gait

Teach patient/family:
• Not to drink alcohol; explain disulfiram reaction (nausea, headache, cramps, flushing, hypoglycemia)
• To check for symptoms of cholestatic jaundice: dark urine, pruritus, yellow sclera; prescriber should be notified
• The symptoms of hypo/hyperglycemia, what to do about each; to have glucagon emergency kit available, carry sugar packets
• That drug must be continued on daily basis; explain consequences of discontinuing drug abruptly
• To take drug in morning to prevent hypoglycemic reactions at night
• To use sunscreen or stay out of the sun to prevent photosensitivity
• To avoid OTC medications unless ordered by prescriber
• That diabetes is a lifelong illness; drug will not cure disease
• That all food in diet plan must be eaten to prevent hypoglycemia
• To carry emergency ID with prescriber and medications
• To test using blood glucose meter while on this drug
• To continue weight control, dietary restrictions, exercise, hygiene
• Ext rel tab may appear in stool

Treatment of overdose: Glucose 25 g IV via dextrose 50% solution 50 ml or 1 mg glucagon

---

*glyBURIDE (R)

(glye'byoor-ide)
Apo-Glyburide ✦, DiaBeta ✦,
Euglucon ✦, Gen-Glybe ✦,
Glynase PresTab, Micronase,
Novo-Glyburide ✦,
Nu-Glyburide ✦
Func. class.: Antidiabetic
Chem. class.: Sulfonylurea (2nd
generation)

Do not confuse:
glyBURIDE/Glucotrol/glipiZIDE
DiaBeta/Zebeta

Action: Causes functioning β-cells in pancreas to release insulin, leading to drop in blood glucose levels; may improve insulin binding to insulin receptors and increase number of insulin receptors with prolonged administration; may also reduce basal hepatic glucose secretion; not effective if patient lacks functioning β-cells

Uses: Type 2 diabetes mellitus

DOSAGE AND ROUTES

DiaBeta/Micronase
• *Adult:* PO 1.25-5 mg initially, then increased to desired response at weekly intervals up to 20 mg/day
• *Geriatric:* PO 1.25 mg initially, then increased to desired response; max 20 mg/day, maintenance 1.25-20 mg/daily
Glynase PresTab (micronized)
• *Adult:* PO 1.5-3 mg/day initially, may increase by 1.5 mg/wk, max 12 mg/day
• *Geriatric:* PO 0.75-3 mg/day, may increase by 1.5 mg/wk
Available forms: Tabs (DiaBeta) 1.25, 2.5, 5 mg; (Glynase PresTab) 1.5, 3, 6 mg

SIDE EFFECTS

CNS: *Headache, weakness,* paresthesia, tinnitus, fatigue, vertigo
ENDO: **Hypoglycemia**
GI: Nausea, fullness, heartburn, **hepatotoxicity, cholestatic jaundice,** vomiting, diarrhea

HEMA: **Leukopenia, thrombocytopenia, agranulocytosis, aplastic anemia,** increased AST, ALT, alk phos
INTEG: Rash, allergic reactions, pruritus, urticaria, eczema, photosensitivity, erythema
MS: Joint pain
Contraindications: Hypersensitivity to sulfonylureas, juvenile or type 1 diabetes, diabetic ketoacidosis
Precautions: Pregnancy (B), geriatric, cardiac disease, severe renal/hepatic disease, thyroid disease, severe hypoglycemic reactions

PHARMACOKINETICS

PO: Completely absorbed by GI route; onset 2-4 hr, peak 4 hr, duration 24 hr; half-life 10 hr; metabolized in liver; excreted in urine, feces (metabolites); crosses placenta; 99% is plasma protein bound

INTERACTIONS

• Mask symptoms of hypoglycemia: decrease-blockers
Increase: level—digoxin
Increase: hypoglycemic effects—insulin, MAOIs, oral anticoagulants, chloramphenicol, guanethidine, methyldopa, NSAIDs, salicylates, probenecid, androgens, fenfluramine, fluconazole, gemfibrozil, histamine H_2 antagonists, magnesium salts, phenylbutazone, sulfinpyrazone, sulfonamides, tricyclics, urinary acidifiers
Decrease: both drugs' effect—diazoxide
Decrease: glyBURIDE action—thiazide diuretics, rifampin, isoniazid, cholestyramine, hydantoins, urinary alkalinizers, charcoal
Drug/Herb
Increase: antidiabetic effect—alfalfa, aloe, basil, bay, bilberry, bitter melon, black catechu, buchu, burdock, coriander, dandelion, eyebright (po), garlic, glucomannan, glucosamine, goat's rue, gymnema, horehound, horse chestnut, jambul, myrrh, myrtle
Increase: glucose tolerance: karela

Increase or decrease: hypoglycemic effect—chromium, coenzyme Q10, fenugreek, ginseng
Decrease: antidiabetic effect—bee pollen, blue cohosh, broom, chromium, elecampane, eucalyptus, gotu kola
Decrease: hypoglycemic effect—broom, buchu, dandelion, glucosamine, juniper

Drug/Lab Test
Increase: AST, ALT, LDH, BUN, creatinine

NURSING CONSIDERATIONS

Assess:
• Hypo/hyperglycemic reaction that can occur soon after meals; for severe hypoglycemia, give IV $D_{50}W$, then IV dextrose sol
• Blood glucose; A1c levels during treatment
• CBC baseline and throughout treatment

Administer:
• With breakfast, hold dose if NPO to avoid hypoglycemia

Perform/provide:
• Storage in tight container in cool environment

Evaluate:
• Therapeutic response: decrease in polyuria, polydipsia, polyphagia, clear sensorium, absence of dizziness, stable gait

Teach patient/family:
• To check for symptoms of cholestatic jaundice: dark urine, pruritus, jaundiced sclera; if these occur, notify prescriber
• To use a blood glucose meter for testing while on this drug
• The symptoms of hypo/hyperglycemia, what to do about each
• That drug must be continued on daily basis; explain consequences of discontinuing drug abruptly
• To take drug in morning to prevent hypoglycemic reactions at night
• To avoid OTC medications unless ordered by prescriber
• That diabetes is a lifelong illness; drug will not cure disease
• That all food included in diet plan must be eaten to prevent hypoglycemia; to have

glucagon emergency kit, sugar packets available
• To use sunscreen or stay out of the sun to prevent photosensitivity
• To carry an emergency ID with prescriber and medications

Treatment of overdose: Glucose 25 g IV via dextrose 50% sol, 50 ml or 1 mg glucagon

---

Rarely Used

glycerin (OTC)
(gli′ser-in)
Fleet Babylax, Glycerin USP, Glycerol, Osmoglyn, Sani-Supp
Func. class.: Laxative, hyperosmotic

Uses: Constipation, intraocular pressure reduction

DOSAGE AND ROUTES

Laxative
• *Adult and child >6 yr:* **RECT SUPP** 3 g; **ENEMA** 5-15 ml
• *Child <6 yr:* **RECT SUPP** 1-1.5 g; **ENEMA** 2-5 ml

Intraocular pressure reduction
• *Adult:* **PO** 1-1.5 g/kg once, then may be given 500 mg/kg q6h
• *Child:* **PO** 1-1.5 g/kg once, then 500 mg/kg 4-8 hr after first dose

Contraindications: Hypersensitivity

---

glycopyrrolate (Rx)
(glye-koe-pye′roe-late)
glycopyrrolate, Robinul, Robinul-Forte
Func. class.: Cholinergic blocker, antispasmodic
Chem. class.: Quaternary ammonium compound

Action: Inhibits the action of acetylcholine at receptor sites in parasympathetic nervous system, which controls secretions, free acids in stomach

---

Uses: Decreased secretions before surgery, reversal of neuromuscular blockade, peptic ulcer disease, irritable bowel syndrome, bradycardia, drooling

DOSAGE AND ROUTES
Preoperatively
• *Adult:* **IM** 4 mcg/kg ½-1 hr before surgery, max 0.1 mg
• *Child >2 yr:* **IM** 4 mcg/kg 30-60 min before procedure
• *Child <2 yr:* **IM** 4-9 mcg/kg
Intraoperative
• *Adult:* **IV** 0.1 mg; may repeat q2-3 min prn
• *Child:* **IM/IV** 4 mcg/kg q2-3min prn; max 0.1 mg/dose
Reversal of neuromuscular blockade
• *Adult and child:* **IV** 200 mcg for each 1 mg of neostigmine or 5 mg **IV** of pyridostigmine simultaneously
GI disorders
• *Adult:* **PO** 1-2 mg bid-tid; **IM/IV** 100-200 mcg tid-qid, titrated to patient response
Antidysrhythmic
• *Adult:* **IV** 100 mcg, may repeat q2min
• *Child:* **IV** 4.4 mcg/kg, may repeat q2min, max 100 mcg
Secretion control
• *Child:* **PO** 40-100 mcg/kg/dose tid-qid; **IM/IV** 4-10 mcg/kg/dose q3-4h; max 0.2 mg/dose or 0.8 mg/24 hr
Available forms: Tabs 1, 2 mg; inj 200 mcg (0.2 mg)/ml

SIDE EFFECTS
CNS: Confusion, anxiety, restlessness, irritability, delusions, hallucinations, headache, sedation, depression, incoherence, dizziness, lethargy, flushing, weakness
CV: Palpitations, tachycardia, postural hypotension, paradoxical bradycardia
EENT: Blurred vision, photophobia, dilated pupils, difficulty swallowing, increased intraocular pressure, mydriasis, cycloplegia
GI: Dryness of mouth, constipation, nausea, vomiting, abdominal distress, paralytic ileus, altered taste perception

GU: Urinary hesitancy, retention, impotence
INTEG: Urticaria, allergic reactions
MISC: Suppression of lactation, nasal congestion, decreased sweating
SYST: **Anaphylaxis**

Contraindications: Hypersensitivity, narrow-angle glaucoma, myasthenia gravis, GI/GU obstruction, child <3 yr, tachycardia, myocardial ischemia, hepatic disease, ulcerative colitis, toxic megacolon, prostatic hypertrophy
Precautions: Pregnancy (B), geriatric, lactation, renal disease, CHF, pulmonary disease, hyperthyroidism

PHARMACOKINETICS
PO: Peak 1 hr, duration 8-12 hr
IM: Peak 30-45 min, duration 2-7 hr
IV: Peak 10-15 min, duration 2-7 hr; excreted in urine (50%) (unchanged); half-life 1-2 hr

INTERACTIONS
Increase: anticholinergic effect—alcohol, antihistamines, phenothiazines, amantadine, tricyclics
Decrease: glycopyrrolate absorption—antacids, antidiarrheals

NURSING CONSIDERATIONS
Assess:
• I&O ratio; retention commonly causes decreased urinary output
• Urinary hesitancy, retention: palpate bladder if retention occurs
• Constipation; increase fluids, bulk, exercise if this occurs
• Mental status: affect, mood, CNS depression, worsening of mental symptoms during early therapy
Administer:
• Parenteral dose with patient recumbent to prevent postural hypotension
• Parenteral dose slowly; keep in bed for at least 1 hr after dose; monitor VS
• After checking dose carefully; even slight overdose may lead to toxicity
• With or after meals to prevent GI upset; may give with fluids other than water

IV route

• Undiluted, give through a Y-tube or 3-way stopcock; give 0.2 mg or less over 1-2 min

Syringe compatibilities: Atropine, benzquinamide, chlorproMAZINE, cimetidine, codeine, diphenhydrAMINE, droperidol, droperidol/fentanyl, hydromorphone, hydrOXYzine, levorphanol, lidocaine, meperidine, meperidine/promethazine, midazolam, morphine, nalbuphine, neostigmine, oxymorphone, procaine, prochlorperazine, promazine, promethazine, pyridostigmine, ranitidine, scopolamine, triflupromazine, trimethobenzamide

Solution compatibilities: D$_5$W, 0.9% NaCl, Ringer's, D$_5$/0.45% NaCl

Perform/provide:

• Storage at room temperature

Evaluate:

• Therapeutic response: decreased secretions; decreased pain in GI disorders; reversal of neuromuscular blockers

Teach patient/family:

• Hard candy, frequent drinks, sugarless gum to relieve dry mouth, use good oral hygiene

• Not to discontinue this drug abruptly; to taper off over 1 wk; to take PO ½-1 hr ac

• To avoid driving, other hazardous activities; drowsiness, blurred vision may occur

• To avoid OTC medication: cough, cold preparations with alcohol, antihistamines unless directed by prescriber

• To avoid hot temperatures, since sweating is decreased, heat stroke is possible

• To change positions slowly to prevent orthostatic hypotension

• To notify prescriber of eye pain, blurred vision, light sensitivity

goserelin (℞)
(goe'se-rel-lin)
Zoladex
Func. class.: Gonadotropin-releasing hormone, antineoplastic (hormone)
Chem. class.: Synthetic decapeptide analog of LHRH

Action: Inhibitor of pituitary gonadotropin secretion; initially increases LH and FSH, with increases in testosterone, reduction in sex steroid levels (substitute serum testosterone levels)

Uses: Advanced prostate cancer stage B2-C (10.8 mg), endometriosis, advanced breast cancer, endometrial thinning (3.6 mg)

DOSAGE AND ROUTES

• *Adult:* **SUBCUT** 3.6 mg q28days or 10.8 mg q12wk

Endometrial thinning

• *Adult:* **SUBCUT** 1-2 depot inj, usually 1 depot, surgery performed at 4 wk, if 2 depots, surgery performed 2-4 wk after 2nd depot

Available forms: Depot inj 3.6, 10.8 mg

SIDE EFFECTS

CNS: Headaches, **spinal cord compression,** *anxiety, depression, dizziness, insomnia, lethargy*

CV: **Dysrhythmia, cerebrovascular accident,** hypertension, **MI,** chest pain, **CHF**

ENDO: Gynecomastia, breast tenderness, hot flashes

GI: Nausea, vomiting, constipation, diarrhea, ulcer

GU: Spotting, breakthrough bleeding, decreased libido, renal insufficiency, urinary obstruction, urinary tract infection, *impotence*

INTEG: Rash, pain on inj

MS: Osteoneuralgia

RESP: COPD, URI

Contraindications: Pregnancy (D) (breast cancer), (X) (endometriosis), lactation, nondiagnosed vaginal bleeding; hypersensitivity to LHRH, LHRH-agonist analogs, children

PHARMACOKINETICS

Peak serum concentrations in 14-28 days; half-life 4½ hr

INTERACTIONS

Drug/Lab Test

Increase: Alk phos, estradiol, FSH, LH, testosterone levels

Decrease: Testosterone levels, progesterone

NURSING CONSIDERATIONS

Assess:

• I&O ratios; palpate bladder for distention in urinary obstruction

• For relief of bone pain (back pain), change in motor function

• Acid phosphatase PSA baseline and periodically

Administer:

Depot

• SUBCUT using implant, inserted by qualified person into upper subcutaneous tissue in abdominal wall q28d or q12wk (10.8 mg)

Evaluate:

• Therapeutic response: more normal levels of PSA, acid phosphatase, alk phosphatase; testosterone level of <25 ng/dl

Teach patient/family:

• That gynecomastia and postmenopausal symptoms may occur but will decrease after treatment is discontinued

• That bone pain may increase, then decrease

• To notify prescriber of difficulty urinating, hot flashes

• To keep appointments

• Not to breastfeed, use effective nonhormonal contraception

---

granisetron (Ŗ)
(grane-iss'e-tron)
Kytril
Func. class.: Antiemetic
Chem. class.: 5-HT₃ receptor antagonist

Action: Prevents nausea, vomiting by blocking serotonin peripherally, centrally, and in the small intestine

Uses: Prevention of nausea, vomiting associated with cancer chemotherapy including high-dose cisplatin

Unlabeled uses: Acute nausea, vomiting following surgery

DOSAGE AND ROUTES

Nausea, vomiting in chemotherapy

• *Adult and child ≥2 yr:* **IV** 10 mcg/kg over 5 min, 30 min before the start of cancer chemotherapy

• *Adult:* **PO** 1 mg bid, give first dose 1 hr before chemotherapy and next dose 12 hr after first

Nausea, vomiting in radiation therapy

• *Adult:* **PO** 2 mg daily 1 hr prior to radiation

Available forms: Inj 1 mg/ml; tab 1 mg

SIDE EFFECTS

CNS: Headache, asthenia, anxiety, dizziness

CV: Hypertension

GI: Diarrhea, *constipation,* increased AST, ALT, *nausea*

HEMA: **Leukopenia,** anemia, **thrombocytopenia**

MISC: Rash, **bronchospasm**

Contraindications: Hypersensitivity

Precautions: Pregnancy (B), lactation, children, geriatric, ondansetron hypersensitivity

PHARMACOKINETICS

Metabolized in liver to an active metabolite, half-life 10-12 hr

---

INTERACTIONS

Increase: EPS—antipsychotics

NURSING CONSIDERATIONS

Assess:
• For absence of nausea, vomiting during chemotherapy
• Hypersensitive reaction: rash, bronchospasm

Administer:

IV, direct route
• Dilute in 0.9% NaCl for inj or D$_5$W (20-50 ml); give over 5-15 min; ½ hr before chemotherapy

Additive compatibilities: Dexamethasone, methylPREDNISolone

Solution compatibilities: D$_5$W, 0.9% NaCl

Y-site compatibilities: Acyclovir, allopurinol, amifostine, amikacin, aminophylline, amphotericin B cholesteryl, ampicillin, ampicillin/sulbactam, amsacrine, aztreonam, bleomycin, bumetanide, buprenorphine, butorphanol, calcium gluconate, carboplatin, carmustine, cefazolin, cefepime, cefonicid, cefoperazone, cefotaxime, cefotetan, cefoxitin, ceftazidime, ceftizoxime, ceftriaxone, cefuroxime, chlorproMAZINE, cimetidine, ciprofloxacin, cisplatin, cladribine, clindamycin, cyclophosphamide, cytarabine, dacarbazine, dactinomycin, DAUNOrubicin, dexamethasone, diphenhydrAMINE, DOBUTamine, DOPamine, DOXOrubicin, DOXOrubicin liposome, doxycycline, droperidol, enalaprilat, etoposide, famotidine, filgrastim, fluconazole, fluorouracil, floxuridine, fludarabine, furosemide, gallium, ganciclovir, gentamicin, haloperidol, heparin hydrocortisone, hydromorphone, hydrOXYzine, idarubicin, ifosfamide, imipenem-cilastatin, leucovorin, lorazepam, magnesium sulfate, melphalan, meperidine, mesna, methotrexate, methylPREDNISolone, metoclopramide, metronidazole, mezlocillin, miconazole, minocycline, mitomycin, mitoxantrone, morphine, nalbuphine, netilmicin, ofloxacin, paclitaxel, piperacillin, piperacillin/tazobactam, plicamycin, potassium chloride, prochlorperazine, promethazine, propofol, ranitidine, sargramostim, sodium bicarbonate, streptozocin, teniposide, thiotepa, ticarcillin, ticarcillin/clavulanate, tobramycin, trimethoprim-sulfamethoxazole, vancomycin, vinBLAStine, vinCRIStine, vinorelbine, zidovudine

Perform/provide:
• Storage at room temperature for 24 hr after dilution

Evaluate:
• Therapeutic response: absence of nausea, vomiting during cancer chemotherapy

Teach patient/family:
• To report diarrhea, constipation, rash, changes in respirations
• That headache requiring an analgesic is common

Rarely Used

griseofulvin microsize (℞)

(gris-ee-oh-ful′vin)
Fulvicin-U/F, Grifulvin V, Grisactin, Grisovin-FP ✤

griseofulvin ultramicrosize (℞)

Fulvicin P/G, Grisactin Ultra, Gris-PEG
Func. class.: Antifungal

Uses: Mycotic infections: tinea corporis, tinea pedis, tinea cruris, tinea barbae, tinea capitis, tinea unguium if caused by *Epidermophyton, Microsporum, Trichophyton*

DOSAGE AND ROUTES

• *Adult:* **PO** 500-1000 mg daily in single or divided doses (microsize), 125-165 mg bid (ultramicrosize) or 250-330 mg daily; may need 500-660 mg in divided doses for severe infections
• *Child:* **PO** 10 mg/kg/day or 30 mg/m^2/day (microsize) or 5 mg/kg/day (ultramicrosize)

Contraindications: Hypersensitivity, porphyria, hepatic disease, lupus erythematosus

---

guaifenesin (OTC, ℞)
(gwye-fen'e-sin)
AllFen Jr., Altarussin, Benylin-E ♣, Calmylin Expectorant ♣, Diabetic Tussin, Ganidin NR, guaifenesin, Guaifenesin NR, Guiatuss, Hytuss, Hytuss 2X, Mucinex, Naldecon Senior EX, Organidin NR, Respa-GF, Resyl ♣, Robitussin, Scot-Tussin Expectorant, Siltussin DAS, Siltussin SA
Func. class.: Expectorant

Action: Acts as an expectorant by stimulating a gastric mucosal reflex to increase the production of lung mucus

Uses: Productive and nonproductive cough

DOSAGE AND ROUTES

• *Adult and child ≥12 yr:* **PO** 200-400 mg q4h, not to exceed 2.4 g/day; **EXT REL** (Mucinex) 600-1200 mg q12h, max 2.4 g/day
• *Child 6-12 yr:* **PO** 100-200 mg q4h; **EXT REL** 600 mg q12h
• *Child 2-6 yr:* **PO** 50-100 mg q4h; max 600 mg/day
• *Child 6 mo-<2 yr:* **PO** 25-50 mg q4h, max 300 mg/day, individualized

Available forms: Tabs 100, 200, 400 mg; caps 200 mg; oral sol 100, 200 mg/5 ml; ext rel tabs (Mucinex) 600, 1200 mg; syrup 100 mg/5 ml

SIDE EFFECTS

CNS: Drowsiness, headache, dizziness
GI: Nausea, anorexia, vomiting
Contraindications: Hypersensitivity; chronic, persistent cough
Precautions: Pregnancy (C)

PHARMACOKINETICS

Half-life 1 hr, excreted urine (metabolites)

NURSING CONSIDERATIONS

Assess:
• Cough: type, frequency, character, including sputum; fluids should be increased to 2 L/day
Administer:
• Do not break, crush, chew ext rel tabs
• Scot-Tussin is not recommended for child <2 yr, Naldecon Senior EX, Mucinex is not recommended in child <12 yr
Perform/provide:
• Storage at room temperature
• Increased fluids, room humidification to liquefy secretions
Evaluate:
• Therapeutic response: absence of cough
Teach patient/family:
• To avoid driving, other hazardous activities if drowsiness occurs (rare)
• To avoid smoking, smoke-filled room, perfumes, dust, environmental pollutants, cleansers
• To consult health provider if cough lasts >7 days

Rarely Used

guanfacine (℞)
(gwahn'fa-seen)
Func. class.: Antihypertensive

Uses: Hypertension in individual using a thiazide diuretic or other antihypertensive
Unlabeled uses: Heroin withdrawal

DOSAGE AND ROUTES

• *Adult:* **PO** 1 mg/day at bedtime; may increase dose in 3-4 wk to 2 mg/day, max 4 mg daily
Contraindications: Hypersensitivity

---

halcinonide topical
See Appendix C

haloperidol (℞)
(hal-oh-pehr'ih-dol)
Apo-Haloperidol ✤, Haldol,
Novo-Peridol ✤, Peridol ✤
haloperidol decanoate (℞)
Haldol Decanoate,
Haldol LA ✤
haloperidol lactate (℞)
Haldol, Haldol Concentrate,
Haloperidol Intensol
Func. class.: Antipsychotic, neuro-leptic
Chem. class.: Butyrophenone

Do not confuse:
haloperidol/Halotestin
Haldol/Stadol

Action: Depresses cerebral cortex, hypothalamus, limbic system, which control activity and aggression; blocks neurotransmission produced by dopamine at synapse; exhibits strong α-adrenergic, anticholinergic blocking action; mechanism for antipsychotic effects unclear

Uses: Psychotic disorders, control of tics, vocal utterances in Gilles de la Tourette's syndrome, short-term treatment of hyperactive children showing excessive motor activity, prolonged parenteral therapy in chronic schizophrenia, control of severe nausea and vomiting in chemotherapy, organic mental syndrome with psychotic features, hiccups (short-term), emergency sedation of severely agitated or delirious patients

Unlabeled uses: Nausea, vomiting in chemotherapy, surgery

DOSAGE AND ROUTES
Psychosis
• *Adult:* **PO** 0.5-5 mg bid or tid initially depending on severity of condition; dose is increased to desired dose, max 100 mg/day; **IM** (lactate) 2-5 mg q4-8h or bid-tid
• *Geriatric:* **PO/IM** 0.25-0.5 mg daily-bid, titrate q3-4 days by 0.25-0.5 mg/dose
• *Child 3-12 yr:* **PO/IM** (lactate) 0.05-0.15 mg/kg/day
• *Adult:* **IM** (decanoate) initial dose is 10-15 mg × daily oral dose at 4 wk interval; do not administer **IV**; not to exceed 100 mg
Chronic schizophrenia
• *Adult:* **IM** (decanoate) 50-100 mg q4wk
• *Child 3-12 yr:* **PO/IM** 0.05-0.15 mg/kg/day
Tics/vocal utterances
• *Adult:* **PO** 0.5-5 mg bid or tid, increased until desired response occurs
• *Child 3-12 yr:* **PO** 0.05-0.075 mg/kg/day
Hyperactive children
• *Child 3-12 yr:* **PO** 0.05-0.075 mg/kg/day
Available forms: Tabs 0.5, 1, 2, 5, 10, 20 mg; *lactate:* conc 2 mg/ml; inj 5 mg/ml, *decanoate:* 50 mg base/ml, 100 mg base/ml

SIDE EFFECTS
CNS: EPS: pseudoparkinsonism, akathisia, dystonia, tardive dyskinesia, drowsiness, headache, **seizures, neuroleptic malignant syndrome,** confusion
CV: Orthostatic hypotension, hypertension, **cardiac arrest,** ECG changes, **tachycardia**
EENT: Blurred vision, glaucoma, dry eyes
GI: Dry mouth, nausea, vomiting, anorexia, constipation, diarrhea, jaundice, weight gain, **ileus, hepatitis**
GU: Urinary retention, dysuria, urinary frequency, enuresis, impotence, amenorrhea, gynecomastia

INTEG: Rash, photosensitivity, dermatitis
RESP: **Laryngospasm,** dyspnea, **respiratory depression**

Contraindications: Hypersensitivity, blood dyscrasias, coma, child <3 yr, brain damage, bone marrow depression, alcohol and barbiturate withdrawal states, Parkinson's disease, angina, epilepsy, urinary retention, narrow-angle glaucoma

Precautions: Pregnancy (C), lactation, seizure disorders, hypertension, hepatic/cardiac disease, geriatric

PHARMACOKINETICS

PO: Onset erratic, peak 2-6 hr, half-life 24 hr

IM: Onset 15-30 min, peak 15-20 min, half-life 21 hr

IM (Decanoate): Peak 4-11 days, half-life 3 wk

Metabolized by liver; excreted in urine, bile; crosses placenta; enters breast milk

INTERACTIONS

Increase: oversedation—other CNS depressants, alcohol, barbiturate anesthetics

Increase: toxicity—epINEPHrine, lithium

Increase: both drugs' effects—β-adrenergic blockers, alcohol

Increase: anticholinergic effects—anticholinergics

Decrease: effects—lithium, levodopa

Decrease: haloperidol effects—phenobarbital, carbamazepine

Drug/Herb

• Antagonist action: jimsonweed, scopolia

Increase: action—chamomile, cola tree, hops, kava, nettle, nutmeg, skullcap, valerian

Increase: EPS—betel palm, kava

Drug/Lab Test

Increase: LFTs, cardiac enzymes, cholesterol, blood glucose, prolactin, bilirubin, PBI, cholinesterase, alk phos

Decrease: Hormones (blood, urine), PT
False positive: Pregnancy tests, PKU
False negative: Urinary steroids

NURSING CONSIDERATIONS

Assess:

• Swallowing of PO medication; check for hoarding or giving of medication to other patients

• I&O ratio; palpate bladder if low urinary output occurs

• Bilirubin, CBC, LFTs monthly

• Urinalysis is recommended before and during prolonged therapy

• Affect, orientation, LOC, reflexes, gait, coordination, sleep pattern disturbances

• B/P standing and lying; take pulse and respirations q4h during initial treatment; establish baseline before starting treatment; report drops of 30 mm Hg

• Dizziness, faintness, palpitations, tachycardia on rising

• EPS including akathisia (inability to sit still, no pattern to movements), tardive dyskinesia (bizarre movements of jaw, mouth, tongue, extremities), pseudoparkinsonism (rigidity, tremors, pill rolling, shuffling gait)

• Skin turgor daily

⚠ For neuroleptic malignant syndrome: hyperthermia, muscle rigidity, altered mental status, increased CPK, seizures, hyper/hypotension, tachycardia, notify prescriber immediately

• Constipation, urinary retention daily; if these occur, increase bulk, water in diet

Administer:

• Reduced dose to geriatric

• Antiparkinsonian agent, to be used if EPS occurs

• Avoid use with CNS depressants

PO route

• Oral liquid: use calibrated dropper; do not mix in coffee or tea

• PO with food or milk

IM route

• IM inj into large muscle mass, use 21G, 2-in needle; give no more than 3 ml/inj site; patient should remain recumbent for ½ hr

Side effects: *italics* = common; **bold** = life-threatening

IV route
- Give undiluted for psychotic episode at 5 mg/min
- Give by intermittent inf after dilution in 30-50 ml of D_5W, run over ½ hr

Solution compatibilities: D_5W

Syringe compatibilities: Hydromorphone, sufentanil

Y-site compatibilities: Amifostine, amsacrine, aztreonam, cimetidine, cisatracurium, cladribine, DOBUTamine, DOPamine, DOXOrubicin liposome, famotidine, filgrastim, fludarabine, granisetron, lidocaine, lorazepam, melphalan, midazolam, nitroglycerin, norepinephrine, ondansetron, paclitaxel, phenylephrine, propofol, remifentanil, sufentanil, tacrolimus, teniposide, theophylline, thiotepa, vinorelbine

Perform/provide:
- Decreased sensory input by dimming lights, avoiding loud noises
- Supervised ambulation until stabilized on medication; do not involve in strenuous exercise program because fainting is possible; patient should not stand still for long periods
- Increased fluids, fiber to prevent constipation
- Sips of water, sugarless candy, gum for dry mouth
- Storage in tight, light-resistant container

Evaluate:
- Therapeutic response: decrease in emotional excitement, hallucinations, delusions, paranoia, reorganization of patterns of thought, speech, improvement in specific behaviors

Teach patient/family:
- That orthostatic hypotension occurs often and to rise from sitting or lying position gradually
- To avoid hazardous activities until stabilized on medication
- To remain lying down after IM inj for at least 30 min
- To avoid hot tubs, hot showers, tub baths, since hypotension may occur
- To avoid abrupt withdrawal of this drug, or EPS may result; drug should be withdrawn slowly

- To avoid OTC preparations (cough, hay fever, cold) unless approved by prescriber, since serious drug interactions may occur; avoid use with alcohol; increased drowsiness may occur
- To use a sunscreen to prevent burns
- Regarding compliance with drug regimen
- About EPS and necessity for meticulous oral hygiene, since oral candidiasis may occur
- To report impaired vision, jaundice, tremors, muscle twitching
- That in hot weather, heat stroke may occur; take extra precautions to stay cool

Treatment of overdose: Activated charcoal, lavage if orally ingested; provide an airway; do not induce vomiting

> **⚠ High Alert**
>
> **heparin (℞)**
> (hep'a-rin)
> Calcilean ✦, Calciparine ✦,
> Hepalean ✦, Heparin Leo ✦,
> heparin sodium, Hep-Lock,
> Hep-Lock U/P
> *Func. class.:* Anticoagulant, antithrombotic

Do not confuse:
heparin/Hespan

Action: Prevents conversion of fibrinogen to fibrin and prothrombin to thrombin by enhancing inhibitory effects of antithrombin III

Uses: Prevention of deep-vein thrombosis, pulmonary emboli, myocardial infarction, open heart surgery, disseminated intravascular clotting syndrome, atrial fibrillation with embolization, as an anticoagulant in transfusion and dialysis procedures, prevention of DVT/PE, to maintain patency of indwelling venipuncture devices; diagnosis, treatment of disseminated intravascular coagulation (DIC)

⚠ Safety alert   *"Tall Man" lettering

DOSAGE AND ROUTES

Deep vein thrombosis/MI
• *Adult:* **IV BOL** 5000-7000 units q4h then titrated to PTT or ACT level; **IV INF** after bolus dose, then 1000 units/hr titrated to PTT or ACT level
• *Child:* **IV INF** 50 units/kg, maintenance 100 units/kg q4h or 20,000 units/m² daily

Anticoagulation
• *Adult:* **SUBCUT** 5000 units IV then 10,000-20,000 units, then 8,000-10,000 units q8h or 15,000-20,000 units q12h **Intermittent IV BOL** 10,000 units, then 5000-10,000 units q4-6h; **CONT IV INF** 5000 units (35-70 units/kg), then 20,000-40,000 units given over 24 hr
• *Child >1 yr:* **Intermittent IV BOL** 50-100 units/kg, then 50-100 units/kg q4h; **CONT INF** 75 units/kg, then 20 units/kg/hr, adjust to maintain aPTT at 60-85 sec
• *Neonates, infants <1 yr:* **CONT IV INF** 75 units/kg, then 28 units/kg/h, adjust to maintain aPTT at 60-85 sec

Cardiovascular surgery
• *Adult:* **IV INF** 150-300 units/kg
• *Child, infants, neonates:* **IA** 100 units/kg in artery prior to cardiac catheter

Prophylaxis for DVT/PE
• *Adult:* **SUBCUT** 5000 units q8-12h

Heparin flush
• *Adult and child:* **IV** 10-100 units/ml

Arterial line patency
• *Neonate:* **IA** 0.5-2 units/ml

Available forms: Sol for inj 10, 100, 1000, 5000, 7500, 10,000, 20,000, 40,000 units/ml; premixed 1000 units/500 ml, 2000 units/1000 ml, 12,500 units/250 ml, 25,000 units/250 ml, 25,000 units/500 ml; arterial line neonates IA 0.5-2 units/ml; lock flush preparations 10 units/ml

SIDE EFFECTS

CNS: Fever, chills, headache
GU: **Hematuria**
HEMA: **Hemorrhage, thrombocytopenia, anemia**
INTEG: Rash, dermatitis, urticaria, pruri-
tus, delayed transient alopecia, hematoma, cutaneous necrosis (SUBCUT)
SYST: **Anaphylaxis**

Contraindications: Hypersensitivity, hemophilia, leukemia with bleeding, peptic ulcer disease, severe thrombocytopenic purpura, severe renal/hepatic disease, blood dyscrasias, severe hypertension, subacute bacterial endocarditis, acute nephritis

Precautions: Pregnancy (C), alcoholism, geriatric, children, hyperlipidemia, diabetes, renal disease

PHARMACOKINETICS

IV: Peak 5 min, duration 2-6 hr
SUBCUT: Onset 20-60 min, duration 8-12 hr, well absorbed
Half-life 1½ hr, excreted in urine, 95% bound to plasma proteins, does not cross placenta or alter breast milk; removed from the system via the lymph and spleen, partially metabolized in kidney, liver, excreted in urine (<50% unchanged)

INTERACTIONS

• Resistance to heparin: streptokinase
Increase: diazepam action
Increase: heparin action—oral anticoagulants, salicylates, dextran, NSAIDs, platelet inhibitors, cephalosporins, penicillins, ticlopidine, dipyridamole
Decrease: corticosteroids action
Decrease: heparin action—digoxin, tetracyclines, antihistamines

Drug/Herb
Increase: risk of bleeding—agrimony, alfalfa, angelica, anise, basil, bay, bilberry, black haw, bogbean, bromelain, buchu, chamomile, chondroitin, cinchona bark, dong quai, fenugreek, feverfew, garlic, ginger, ginkgo, ginseng, horse chestnut, Irish moss, kelp, kelpware, khella, lovage, lungwort, meadowsweet, motherwort, mugwort, nettle, papaya, parsley (large amts), pau d'arco, pineapple, poplar, prickly ash, safflower, saw palmetto, tonka bean, turmeric, wintergreen, yarrow

H

Decrease: anticoagulant effect—coenzyme Q10, flax, glucomannan, goldenseal, guar gum

Drug/Lab Test

Increase: ALT, AST, INR, PT, PTT, potassium

Decrease: Platelets, triglycerides, cholesterol, plasma free fatty acids

NURSING CONSIDERATIONS

Assess:

⚠ Bleeding: gums, petechiae, ecchymosis, black tarry stools, hematuria, epistaxis, decrease in Hct, B/P; may indicate bleeding, hemorrhage

• Blood studies (Hct, occult blood in stools) q3mo

• Partial prothrombin time, which should be 1.5-2 × control; for continuous IV inf, check aPTT baseline 6 hr after initiation and 6 hr after any dose change; use aPTT for dosing adjustments; once 2 therapeutic aPTT has been measured, check aPTT daily

• Platelet count q2-3d; thrombocytopenia may occur on 4th day of treatment

• Hypersensitivity: rash, chills, fever, itching; report to prescriber

Administer:

• Cannot be used interchangeably (unit for unit) with LMWHS or heparinoids

• At same time each day to maintain steady blood levels

• Do not mistake heparin sodium injection 10,000 units/ml and HEP-Lock U/P 10 units/ml; they have similar blue labeling

• SUBCUT deep with 25G ⅜-in needle; do not massage area or aspirate when giving SUBCUT inj; give in abdomen between pelvic bones, rotate sites; do not pull back on plunger, leave in for 10 sec; apply gentle pressure for 1 min

• Changing needles is not recommended

• Avoiding all IM inj that may cause bleeding, hematoma

IV route

• Diluted in 0.9% NaCl, dextrose, Ringer's sol and given by direct, intermittent, or continuous infusion; give 1000 units or less over 1 min; then 5000 units or less over 1 min; infusion may run from 4-24 hr; use infusion pump

• When drug is added to inf sol for cont IV, invert container at least 6 times to ensure adequate mixing

• Blood after adding 7500 units/100 ml NaCl inj, add 6-8 ml of this sol/100 ml of whole blood

Additive compatibilities: Aminophylline, amphotericin, ascorbic acid, bleomycin, calcium gluconate, cefepime, chloramphenicol, clindamycin, colistimethate, dimenhyDRINATE, DOPamine, enalaprilat, esmolol, floxacillin, fluconazole, flumazenil, furosemide, hydrocortisone, isoproterenol, lidocaine, lincomycin, magnesium sulfate, meropenem, methyldopate, methylPREDNISolone, metronidazole/sodium bicarbonate, nafcillin, norepinephrine, octreotide, penicillin G, potassium chloride, promazine, ranitidine, sodium bicarbonate, verapamil, vit B/C

Syringe compatibilities: Aminophylline, amphotericin B, ampicillin, atropine, azlocillin, bleomycin, cefamandole, cefazolin, cefoperazone, cefotaxime, cefoxitin, chloramphenicol, cimetidine, cisplatin, clindamycin, cyclophosphamide, diazoxide, digoxin, dimenhyDRINATE, DOBUTamine, DOPamine, epINEPHrine, fentanyl, fluorouracil, furosemide, leucovorin, lidocaine, lincomycin, methotrexate, metoclopramide, mitomycin, moxalactam, nafcillin, naloxone, neostigmine, nitroglycerin, norepinephrine, pancuronium, penicillin G, phenobarbital, piperacillin, sodium nitroprusside, succinylcholine, trimethoprim-sulfamethoxazole, verapamil, vinCRIStine

Y-site compatibilities: Acyclovir, aldesleukin, allopurinol, amifostine, aminophylline, ampicillin, ampicillin/sulbactam, atracurium, atropine, aztreonam, betamethasone, bleomycin, calcium gluconate, cefazolin, cefotetan, ceftazidime, ceftriaxone, chlordiazepoxide, chlorproMAZINE, cimetidine, cisplatin, cladribine, clindamycin, conjugated estrogens, cyanocobalamin, cyclophosphamide, cytarabine, dexamethasone, digoxin, diphenhydrAMINE,

DOPamine, DOXOrubicin liposome, edrophonium, enalaprilat, epINEPHrine, esmolol, ethacrynate, etoposide, famotidine, fentanyl, fluconazole, fludarabine, fluorouracil, foscarnet, furosemide, gallium, gemcitabine, granisetron, hydrALAZINE, hydrocortisone, hydromorphone, insulin (regular), isoproterenol, kanamycin, leucovorin, linezolid, lidocaine, lorazepam, magnesium sulfate, melphalan, menadiol, meperidine, meropenem, methotrexate, methoxamine, methyldopa, methylergonovine, metoclopramide, metronidazole, midazolam, milrinone, minocycline, mitomycin, morphine, nafcillin, neostigmine, nitroglycerin, nitroprusside, norepinephrine, ondansetron, oxacillin, oxytocin, paclitaxel, pancuronium, penicillin G potassium, pentazocine, phytonadione, piperacillin, piperacillin/tazobactam, potassium chloride, prednisoLONE, procainamide, prochlorperazine, propofol, propranolol, pyridostigmine, ranitidine, remifentanil, sargramostim, scopolamine, sodium bicarbonate, streptokinase, succinylcholine, tacrolimus, theophylline, thiopental, thiotepa, ticarcillin, ticarcillin/clavulanate, tirofiban, trimethobenzamide, trimethaphan, vecuronium, vinBLAStine, vinorelbine, warfarin, zidovudine

Perform/provide:

• Storage at room temperature

Evaluate:

• Therapeutic response: decrease of deep vein thrombosis, PTT 1.5-2.5 × control, free flowing IV

Teach patient/family:

• To avoid OTC preparations that may cause serious drug interactions unless directed by prescriber

• That drug may be held during active bleeding (menstruation), depending on condition

• To use soft-bristle toothbrush to avoid bleeding gums, avoid contact sports, use electric razor, avoid IM inj

• To carry emergency ID identifying drug taken

• To report to prescriber any signs of bleeding: gums, under skin, urine, stools

• To report to prescriber any signs of hypersensitivity: rash, chills, fever, itching

Treatment of overdose: Withdraw drug, protamine 1 mg protamine/100 units heparin

hepatitis B immune globulin (℞)

BayHep B, Nabi-HB

Func. class.: Immune globulin

Action: Provides passive immunity to hepatitis B

Uses: Prevention of hepatitis B virus in exposed patients, including passive immunity in neonates born to HBsAg-positive mother

DOSAGE AND ROUTES

• *Adult and child:* IM 0.06 ml/kg (usual 3-5 ml) within 7 days of exposure; repeat 28 days after exposure, if patient wishes not to receive the hepatitis B vaccine

Neonates born to hepatitis B surface antigen—positive persons

• *Neonate:* IM 0.5 ml within 12 hr of birth

Available forms: Inj 1, 4, 5 ml vials; neonatal syringe 0.5 ml

SIDE EFFECTS

CNS: Headache, dizziness, fever

GI: Nausea, vomiting

INTEG: Soreness at inj site, urticaria, erythema, swelling

SYST: Induration, **anaphylaxis, angioedema**

Contraindications: Hypersensitivity to immune globulins, coagulation disorders

Precautions: Pregnancy (C), hemophilia, geriatric, lactation, children; active infection, IgA deficiency

INTERACTIONS

• Do not use within 3 months of hepatitis B immune globulin: MMR, varicella, or rotavirus vaccines

NURSING CONSIDERATIONS

Assess:

• For history of allergies, skin conditions (eczema, psoriasis, dermatitis), reactions to vaccinations

• For skin reactions: rash, induration, urticaria

⚠ For anaphylaxis: inability to breathe, bronchospasm, hypotension, wheezing, diaphoresis, fever, flushing

Administer:

• After rotating vial; do not shake

• Only with epINEPHrine 1:1000 on unit to treat laryngospasm

• In deltoid for better absorption (adult)

Perform/provide:

• Written record of immunization

• Comfort measures

Evaluate:

• Prevention of hepatitis B

Teach patient/family:

• That discomfort may occur at site

• To report any rash, wheezing, inability to breathe immediately

---

hetastarch (℞)
(het′a-starch)
Hespan
Func. class.: Plasma expander
Chem. class.: Synthetic polymer

Do not confuse:

Hespan/heparin

Action: Similar to human albumin, which expands plasma volume by colloidal osmotic pressure

Uses: Plasma volume expander, leukapheresis, hypovolemia

DOSAGE AND ROUTES

• *Adult:* **IV INF** 500-1000 ml (30-60 g), total dose not to exceed 1500 ml/day, not to exceed 20 ml/kg/hr (hemorrhagic shock)

Leukapheresis

• *Adult:* **IV INF** 250-700 ml infused at 1:8 ratio with whole blood, may be repeated 2/wk up to 10 treatments

Renal dose

• *Adult:* **IV** CCr <10 ml/min give initial dose, but reduce subsequent doses by 25%-50%

Available forms: 6% hetastarch/0.9% NaCl inj

SIDE EFFECTS

CNS: Headache

EENT: Periorbital edema

GI: Nausea, vomiting

HEMA: Decreased Hct, platelet function, increased bleeding/coagulation times, increased sed rate, DIC

INTEG: Rash, urticaria, pruritus, chills, fever, flushing, peripheral edema

RESP: Wheezing, dyspnea, **bronchospasm, pulmonary edema**

SYST: **Anaphylaxis, angioedema**

Contraindications: Hypersensitivity, severe bleeding disorders, renal failure, CHF (severe), anuria, oliguria, intracranial bleeding

Precautions: Pregnancy (C), hepatic disease, pulmonary edema

PHARMACOKINETICS

IV: Expands blood volume 1-2× amount infused, excreted in urine

INTERACTIONS

Increase: sodium, water retention—fludrocortisone

Drug/Lab Test

False increase: Bilirubin

NURSING CONSIDERATIONS

Assess:

• VS q5min × 30 min; CVP during infusion (5-10 cm H_2O normal range), PCWP

• Monitor CBC with differential, Hgb, Hct, PT, PTT, platelet count, clotting time during treatment; Hct may drop; do not allow to drop >30% by vol

• Urine output q1h, watch for increase in urinary output (common); if output does not increase, decrease or discontinue infusion

• I&O ratio and specific gravity, urine osmolarity; if specific gravity is very low, re-

---

nal clearance is low; drug should be discontinued
- Allergy: rash, urticaria, pruritus, wheezing, dyspnea, bronchospasm; drug should be discontinued immediately

A For circulatory overload: increased pulse, respirations, dyspnea, wheezing, chest tightness, chest pain
- For dehydration after infusion: decreased output, fever, poor skin turgor, increased specific gravity, dry skin

Administer:

IV route
- INF undiluted, run at 20 ml/kg/hr (1.2 g/kg); reduced rate in septic shock, burns

Additive compatibilities: Cloxacillin, fosphenytoin

Y-site compatibilities: Cimetidine, diltiazem, enalaprilat
- Storage at room temperature; discard unused portion, do not freeze, do not use if turbid or deep brown or if precipitate forms

Evaluate:
- Therapeutic response: increased plasma volume

Teach patient/family:
- When to notify prescriber

---

homatropine ophthalmic
See Appendix C

---

*hydrALAZINE (R)
(hye-dral'a-zeen)
Apresoline, hydrALAZINE HCl, Novo-Hylazin ♣
Func. class.: Antihypertensive, direct-acting peripheral vasodilator
Chem. class.: Phthalazine

Do not confuse:
hydrALAZINE/hydrOXYzine
Apresoline/allopurinol

Action: Vasodilates arteriolar smooth muscle by direct relaxation; reduction in blood pressure with reflex increases in heart rate, stroke volume, cardiac output

Uses: Essential hypertension; severe essential hypertension
Unlabeled uses: CHF

DOSAGE AND ROUTES

Hypertension
- *Adult:* PO 10 mg qid 2-4 days, then 25 mg for rest of first wk, then 50 mg qid individualized to desired response, not to exceed 300 mg daily
- *Child:* PO 0.75-1 mg/kg/day in 4 divided doses, max 25 mg/dose

Hypertensive crisis
- *Adult:* IV BOL 10-20 mg q4-6h, administer PO as soon as possible; IM 10-50 mg q4-6h
- *Child:* IV BOL 0.1-0.6 mg/kg q4-6h; IM 0.1-0.6 mg/kg q4-6h

CHF
- *Adult:* PO 10-25 mg tid, max 75 mg tid
Available forms: Inj 20 mg/ml; tabs 10, 25, 50, 100 mg

SIDE EFFECTS

CNS: Headache, tremors, dizziness, anxiety, peripheral neuritis, depression, fever, chills
CV: Palpitations, reflex tachycardia, angina, **shock,** rebound hypertension
GI: Nausea, vomiting, anorexia, diarrhea, constipation, paralytic ileus
GU: Urinary retention
HEMA: **Leukopenia, agranulocytosis,** anemia, **thrombocytopenia**
INTEG: Rash, pruritus, urticaria
MISC: Nasal congestion, muscle cramps, *lupuslike symptoms,* flushing, edema, dyspnea

Contraindications: Hypersensitivity to hydrALAZINEs, mitral valvular rheumatic heart disease, dissecting aortic aneurysm
Precautions: Pregnancy (C), CVA, advanced renal disease, geriatric, coronary artery disease, lactation, hepatic disease, systemic lupus erythematosus

PHARMACOKINETICS

PO: Onset 20-30 min, peak 1-2 hr, duration 6-12 hr
IM: Onset 10-30 min, peak 1 hr, duration 2-12 hr

IV: Onset 5-30 min, peak 10-80 min, duration 2-12 hr

Half-life 2-8 hr; metabolized by liver; 12%-14% excreted in urine, protein binding 89%

INTERACTIONS

Increase: severe hypotension—MAOIs

Increase: tachycardia, angina—sympathomimetics (epINEPHrine, norepinephrine)

Increase: hypotension—other antihypertensives, alcohol

Increase: effects of β-blockers

Decrease: hydrALAZINE effects—indomethacin

Drug/Herb

Increase: toxicity, death—aconite

Increase: antihypertensive effect—barberry, betony, black catechu, black cohosh, bloodroot, broom, burdock, cat's claw, dandelion, goldenseal, hawthorn, Irish moss, Jamaican dogwood, kelp, khella, mistletoe, parsley

Increase or decrease: antihypertensive effect—astragalus, cola tree

Decrease: antihypertensive effect—coltsfoot, guarana, khat, licorice, yohimbine

NURSING CONSIDERATIONS

Assess:

• B/P q5min × 2 hr, then q1h × 2 hr, then q4h

• Pulse, jugular venous distention q4h

• Electrolytes, blood studies: K, Na, Cl, CO_2, CBC, serum glucose

• Weight daily, I&O

• LE prep, ANA titer before starting therapy and during treatment; assess for fever, joint pain, rash, sore throat (lupus-like symptoms); notify prescriber

• Edema in feet, legs daily

• Skin turgor, dryness of mucous membranes for hydration status

• Crackles, dyspnea, orthopnea

• IV site for extravasation, rate

• Fever, joint pain, tachycardia, palpitations, headache, nausea

• Mental status: affect, mood, behavior, anxiety; check for personality changes

Administer:

• Give with meals (PO) to enhance absorption

• To recumbent patient, keep for 1 hr after administration

IV route

• IV undiluted; give through Y-tube or 3-way stopcock, give each 10 mg ≤min

Additive compatibilities: DOBUTamine

Y-site compatibilities: Heparin, hydrocortisone, potassium chloride, verapamil, vit B/C

Solution compatibilities: D_5LR, D_5W, $D_{10}W$, $D_{10}LR$ 0.45% NaCl, 0.9% NaCl, Ringer's, LR

Evaluate:

• Therapeutic response: decreased B/P

Teach patient/family:

• To take with food to increase bioavailability (PO)

• To avoid OTC preparations unless directed by prescriber

• To notify prescriber if chest pain, severe fatigue, fever, muscle or joint pain occurs

• To rise slowly to prevent orthostatic hypotension

• To notify prescriber if pregnancy is suspected

Treatment of overdose: Administer vasopressors, volume expanders for shock; if PO, lavage or give activated charcoal, digitalization

hydrochlorothiazide (Ᵽ)

(hye-droe-klor-oh-thye′a-zide)
Apo-Hydrol ✤, Esidrix, HCTZ, Hydro-Chlor, hydrochlorothiazide, Hydro-D, HydroDIURIL, Microzide, Neo-Codema ✤, Novohydrazide ✤, Oretic, Urozide ✤

Func. class.: Thiazide diuretic, antihypertensive
Chem. class.: Sulfonamide derivative

Action: Acts on distal tubule and ascending limb of loop of Henle by increasing excretion of water, sodium, chloride, potassium

Uses: Edema, hypertension, diuresis, CHF; edema in corticosteroid, estrogen, NSAIDs, idiopathic lower extremity edema therapy

DOSAGE AND ROUTES

- *Adult:* **PO** 12.5-100 mg/day
- *Geriatric:* **PO** 12.5 mg/day, initially
- *Child >6 mo:* **PO** 1-2 mg/kg/day in divided doses
- *Child <6 mo:* **PO** up to 3 mg/kg/day in divided doses

Available forms: Tabs 25, 50, 100 mg; caps 12.5 mg; oral sol 10 mg/5 ml, 100 mg/ml

SIDE EFFECTS

CNS: Drowsiness, paresthesia, depression, headache, *dizziness, fatigue, weakness,* fever
CV: Irregular pulse, orthostatic hypotension, palpitations, volume depletion, allergic myocarditis
EENT: Blurred vision
ELECT: Hypokalemia, hypercalcemia, hyponatremia, hypochloremia, hypomagnesemia
GI: Nausea, vomiting, anorexia, constipation, diarrhea, cramps, pancreatitis, GI irritation, **hepatitis**

GU: Urinary frequency, polyuria, **uremia, glucosuria,** hyperuricemia
HEMA: **Aplastic anemia, hemolytic anemia, leukopenia, agranulocytosis, thrombocytopenia, neutropenia**
INTEG: Rash, urticaria, purpura, photosensitivity, alopecia, erythema multiforme
META: Hyperglycemia, hyperuricemia, increased creatinine, BUN

Contraindications: Hypersensitivity to thiazides or sulfonamides, anuria, renal decompensation, hypomagnesemia
Precautions: Pregnancy (B), hypokalemia, renal/hepatic disease, lactation, gout, COPD, LE, diabetes mellitus, hyperlipidemia, CCr <25 ml/min

PHARMACOKINETICS

PO: Onset 2 hr, peak 4 hr, duration 6-12 hr, half-life 6-15 hr; excreted unchanged by kidneys; crosses placenta; enters breast milk

INTERACTIONS

Increase: hyperglycemia, hyperuricemia, increased antihypertensives—diazoxide
Increase: hypokalemia—glucocorticoids, amphotericin B
Increase: toxicity—lithium, nondepolarizing skeletal muscle relaxants, cardiac glycosides
Increase: renal failure risk—NSAIDs
Increase: effects—loop diuretics
Decrease: antidiabetics effects
Decrease: thiazides absorption—cholestyramine, colestipol
Drug/Herb
- Severe photosensitivity: St. John's wort
Increase: hypokalemia—aloe, buckthorn, cascara sagrada, Chinese rhubarb, gossypol, licorice, nettle, senna
Increase: diuretic effect—cucumber, dandelion, ginkgo, horsetail, khella, licorice, nettle, pumpkin, Queen Anne's lace
Drug/Lab Test
Increase: BSP retention, amylase, parathyroid test
Decrease: PBI, PSP

H

Side effects: *italics* = common; **bold** = life-threatening

NURSING CONSIDERATIONS

Assess:

- Weight, I&O daily to determine fluid loss; effect of drug may be decreased if used daily
- Rate, depth, rhythm of respiration, effect of exertion
- B/P lying, standing; postural hypotension may occur
- Electrolytes: K, Mg, Na, Cl; include BUN, blood glucose, CBC, serum creatinine, blood pH, ABGs, uric acid, Ca; renal function
- Glucose in urine if patient is diabetic
- Signs of metabolic alkalosis: drowsiness, restlessness
- Signs of hypokalemia: postural hypotension, malaise, fatigue, tachycardia, leg cramps, weakness, dehydration
- Rashes, temp daily
- Confusion, especially in geriatric; take safety precautions if needed

Administer:

- In AM to avoid interference with sleep if using drug as a diuretic
- Potassium replacement if potassium <3 mg/dl
- With food; if nausea occurs, absorption may be decreased slightly

Evaluate:

- Therapeutic response: improvement in edema of feet, legs, sacral area daily, decreased B/P

Teach patient/family:

- To increase fluid intake to 2-3 L/day unless contraindicated; to rise slowly from lying or sitting position
- To notify prescriber of muscle weakness, cramps, nausea, dizziness
- That drug may be taken with food or milk
- To use sunscreen for photosensitivity
- That blood glucose may be increased in diabetics
- To take early in day to avoid nocturia
- To avoid alcohol; avoid OTC meds unless approved by prescriber

Treatment of overdose: Lavage if taken orally; monitor electrolytes; administer dextrose in saline; monitor hydration, CV, renal status

---

hydrocodone (℞)

(hye-droe-koe′done)
Hycodan, Robidone ✦
Tussigon

hydrocodone/ acetaminophen

Anexsia, Bancap HC, Ceta-Plus, Co-Gesic, Dolacet, Dolagesic, Duocet, Hycomed, Hyco-Pap, Hydrocet, Hydrogesic, Lorcet, Lortab, Norco, Onset, Pancet, Panlor, Polygesic, Stagesic, T-Gesic, Ugesic, Vanacet, Vandone, Vicodin, Zydone

hydrocodone/aspirin

Alor, Azdone, Damason-P, Lortab ASA, Panasal

hydrocodone/ ibuprofen

Vicoprofen
Func. class.: Antitussive opioid analgesic, nonopioid analgesic

---

Controlled Substance Schedule III
Do not confuse:
hydrocodone/hydrocortisone
Hycodan/Vicodin
Action: Acts directly on cough center in medulla to suppress cough; binds to opiate receptors in CNS to reduce pain
Uses: Hyperactive and nonproductive cough, mild pain

DOSAGE AND ROUTES

Analgesic

- *Adult:* **PO** 2.5-10 mg q3-6h prn
- *Child:* **PO** 0.15-0.2 mg/kg q3-6h

Antitussive

- *Adult:* **PO** 5 mg q4-6 hr prn

Available forms: *Hydrocodone:* tabs 5 mg (Hycodan); syr 5 mg/ml (Hycodan, Robidone ✦); *hydrocodone/acetamin-*

---

ophen: tabs 2.5 mg hydrocodone/500 mg acetaminophen (Lortab 2.5/500), 5 mg hydrocodone/400 mg acetaminophen (Zydone), 5 mg hydrocodone/500 mg acetaminophen (Anexsia 5/500, Co-Gesic, Dolacet, Hydrocet, Hydrogesic, Hy-Phen, Lorcet, Lortab 5/500, Maragesic-H, Panacet 5/500, Stagesic, T-Gesic, Vicodin); 7.5 mg hydrocodone/400 mg acetaminophen (Zydone), 7.5 mg hydrocodone/500 mg acetaminophen (Lortab 7.5/500, 7.5 mg hydrocodone/650 mg acetaminophen (Anexsia 7.5/650, Lorcet Plus), 7.5 mg hydrocodone/750 mg acetaminophen (Vicodin ES), 10 mg hydrocodone/325 acetaminophen (Norco), 10 mg hydrocodone/500 mg acetaminophen (Lortab 10/500), 10 mg hydrocodone/650 mg acetaminophen (Lorcet 10/650, Vicodin HP), 10 mg hydrocodone/660 acetaminophen (Anexsia 10/660); caps 5 mg hydrocodone/500 mg acetaminophen (Bancap HC, Dolacet, Hydrocet, Hydrogesic, Lorcet-HD, Maragesic-H, Stagesic, T-Gesic, Zydone); elixir or oral solution 2.5 mg hydrocodone/167 mg acetaminophen/5 ml; *hydrocodone/aspirin:* tabs 5 mg hydrocodone/500 mg aspirin (Alor 5/500, Azdone, Damason-P, Lortab ASA, Panasal 5/500); *hydrocodone/ibuprofen:* tabs 7.5 mg hydrocodone/200 mg ibuprofen (Vicoprofen)

SIDE EFFECTS

CNS: Drowsiness, dizziness, lightheadedness, confusion, headache, sedation, euphoria, dysphoria, weakness, hallucinations, disorientation, mood changes, dependence, **seizures**

CV: Palpitations, tachycardia, bradycardia, change in B/P, **circulatory depression,** syncope

EENT: Tinnitus, blurred vision, miosis, diplopia

GI: Nausea, vomiting, anorexia, constipation, cramps, dry mouth

GU: Increased urinary output, dysuria, urinary retention

INTEG: Rash, urticaria, flushing, pruritus

RESP: **Respiratory depression**

Contraindications: Hypersensitivity, addiction (opioid)

Precautions: Pregnancy (C), addictive personality, lactation, increased intracranial pressure, MI (acute), severe heart disease, respiratory depression, renal/hepatic disease

PHARMACOKINETICS

Onset 10-20 min, duration 4-6 hr, half-life 3½-4½ hr; metabolized in liver; excreted in urine; crosses placenta

INTERACTIONS

Increase: CNS depression—alcohol, opioids, sedative/hypnotics, phenothiazines, skeletal muscle relaxants, general anesthetics, tricyclics

Increase: severe reactions—MAOIs

Drug/Herb

Increase: CNS depression—Jamaican dogwood, lavender, mistletoe, nettle, pokeweed, poppy, senega, valerian

Increase: anticholinergic effect—corkwood

Drug/Lab Test

Increase: Amylase, lipase

NURSING CONSIDERATIONS

Assess:

• Pain: intensity, type, location, and other characteristics

• CNS changes: dizziness, drowsiness, hallucinations, euphoria, LOC, pupil reaction

• Allergic reactions: rash, urticaria

• Cough and respiratory dysfunction: respiratory depression, character, rate, rhythm; notify prescriber if respirations are <10/min

• Need for pain medication, physical dependence

Administer:

• Do not break, crush, or chew tabs; only scored tabs can be broken

• With antiemetic after meals if nausea or vomiting occurs

Perform/provide:

• Storage in light-resistant area at room temperature

• Assistance with ambulation

Side effects: *italics* = common; **bold** = life-threatening

- Safety measures: night-light, call bell within easy reach

Evaluate:
- Therapeutic response: decrease in pain or cough

Teach patient/family:
- To report any symptoms of CNS changes, allergic reactions
- That physical dependency may result when used for extended periods
- That withdrawal symptoms may occur: nausea, vomiting, cramps, fever, faintness, anorexia
- To avoid driving, other hazardous activities, drowsiness occurs
- To avoid other CNS depressants, will enhance sedating properties of this drug

Treatment of overdose: Naloxone HCl (Narcan) 0.2-0.8 mg IV, O$_2$, IV fluids, vasopressors

---

hydrocortisone (℞)
(hy-dro-kor'tih-sone)
Cortef, Cortenema, Hydrocortone

hydrocortisone acetate (℞)
Cortifoam, Hydrocortone Acetate

hydrocortisone cypionate (℞)
Cortef

hydrocortisone sodium phosphate (℞)
Hydrocortone Phosphate

hydrocortisone sodium succinate (℞)
A-hydroCort, Solu-Cortef
Func. class.: Corticosteroid
Chem. class.: Short-acting glucocorticoid

Do not confuse:
hydrocortisone/hydrocodone
Action: Decreases inflammation by suppression of migration of polymorphonuclear leukocytes, fibroblasts, reversal of increased capillary permeability, and lysosomal stabilization
Uses: Severe inflammation, septic shock, adrenal insufficiency, ulcerative colitis, collagen disorders

DOSAGE AND ROUTES

Adrenal insufficiency/inflammation
- *Adult:* **PO** 5-30 mg bid-qid; **IM/IV** 100-250 mg (succinate), then 50-100 mg **IM** as needed; **IM/IV** 15-240 mg q12h (phosphate)

Shock
- *Adult:* **IM/IV** 500 mg-2 g q2-6h (succinate)
- *Child:* **IM/IV** 0.186-1 mg/kg bid-tid (succinate)

Colitis
- *Adult:* **ENEMA** 100 mg nightly for 21 days

Available forms: Tabs 5, 10, 20 mg; inj 25, 50 mg/ml; enema 100 mg/60 ml; *acetate:* inj 25 ✤, 50 mg/ml ✤, enema 10% aerosol foam; supp 25 mg; *cypionate:* oral susp 10 mg/5 ml; *phosphate:* inj 50 mg/ml; *succinate:* inj 100 mg ✤, 250 mg ✤, 500 mg ✤, 1000 mg/vial ✤

SIDE EFFECTS

CNS: Depression, flushing, sweating, headache, mood changes
CV: Hypertension, **circulatory collapse, thrombophlebitis, embolism,** tachycardia, edema
EENT: Fungal infections, increased intraocular pressure, blurred vision
GI: Diarrhea, nausea, abdominal distention, **GI hemorrhage,** increased appetite, **pancreatitis**
HEMA: **Thrombocytopenia**
INTEG: Acne, poor wound healing, ecchymosis, petechiae
MS: Fractures, osteoporosis, weakness
Contraindications: Psychosis, hypersensitivity, idiopathic thrombocytopenia (IM), acute glomerulonephritis, amebiasis, fungal infections, nonasthmatic bronchial disease, child <2 yr, AIDS, TB
Precautions: Pregnancy (C), lactation, diabetes mellitus, glaucoma, osteoporosis, seizure disorders, ulcerative colitis,

---

⚠ Safety alert   *"Tall Man" lettering

CHF, myasthenia gravis, renal disease, esophagitis, peptic ulcer

PHARMACOKINETICS

PO: Onset 1-2 hr, peak 1 hr, duration 1-1½ days
IM/IV: Onset 20 min, peak 4-8 hr, duration 1-1½ days
RECT: Onset 3-5 days
Metabolized by liver, excreted in urine (17-OHCS, 17-KS), crosses placenta

INTERACTIONS

• Risk of GI bleeding: salicylates, NSAIDs
Increase: side effects—alcohol, amphotericin B, Digoxin, cycloSPORINE, diuretics
Decrease: hydrocortisone action—cholestyramine, colestipol, barbiturates, rifampin, epHEDrine, phenytoin, theophylline
Decrease: anticoagulant effects, anticonvulsants, antidiabetics, toxoids, vaccines
Drug/Herb
Increase: hypokalemia—aloe, buckthorn, cascara sagrada, Chinese rhubarb, senna
Increase: corticosteroid effect—aloe, licorice, perilla
Drug/Lab Test
Increase: Cholesterol, sodium, blood glucose, uric acid, calcium, urine glucose
Decrease: Ca, K, T_4, T_3, thyroid ^{131}I uptake test, urine 17-OHCS, 17-KS
False negative: Skin allergy tests

NURSING CONSIDERATIONS

Assess:
• Potassium, blood glucose, urine glucose while on long-term therapy; hypokalemia and hyperglycemia
• Weight daily, notify prescriber of weekly gain >5 lb
• B/P q4h, pulse; notify prescriber of chest pain
• I&O ratio; be alert for decreasing urinary output, increasing edema
• Plasma cortisol levels during long-term therapy (normal level: 138-635 nmol/L SI units when drawn at 8 AM)
• Infection: increased temp, WBC, even

after withdrawal of medication; drug masks infection
• Potassium depletion: paresthesias, fatigue, nausea, vomiting, depression, polyuria, dysrhythmias, weakness
• Edema, hypertension, cardiac symptoms
• Mental status: affect, mood, behavioral changes, aggression
Administer:
• Daily dose in AM for better results
• IM inj deep in large muscle mass; rotate sites; avoid deltoid; use 21G needle
• In one dose in AM to prevent adrenal suppression; avoid SUBCUT administration; may damage tissue
• With food or milk for GI symptoms (PO)
• Rectal: telling patient to retain for 20 min if possible
IV route
• Phosphate: IV undiluted or added to dextrose or saline inj and given by inf; give 25 mg or less/min
• Succinate: IV in mix-o-vial, or reconstitute 250 mg or less/2 ml bacteriostatic H_2O for inj; mix gently; give direct IV over 1 min or more; may be further diluted in 100, 250, 500, or 1000 ml of D_5W, D_5 0.9%, NaCl 0.9% given over ordered rate
Sodium phosphate preparations
Additive compatibilities: Amikacin, amphotericin B, bleomycin, cephapirin, metaraminol, sodium bicarbonate, verapamil
Syringe compatibilities: Metoclopramide
Y-site compatibilities: Allopurinol, amifostine, aztreonam, cefepime, cladribine, famotidine, filgrastim, fluconazole, fludarabine, granisetron, melphalan, ondansetron, paclitaxel, piperacillin/tazobactam, teniposide, thiotepa, vinorelbine
Sodium succinate preparations
Additive compatibilities: Amikacin, aminophylline, amphotericin B, calcium chloride, calcium gluconate, cephalothin, cephapirin, chloramphenicol, clindamycin, cloxacillin, corticotropin, DAUNOrubicin, diphenhydrAMINE, DOPamine, erythromycin, floxacillin, lidocaine, magnesium sulfate, mephenter-

H

mine, metronidazole/sodium bicarbonate, mitomycin, mitoxantrone, netilmicin, netilmicin/potassium chloride, norepinephrine, penicillin G potassium/sodium, piperacillin, polymyxin B, potassium chloride, sodium bicarbonate, theophylline, thiopental, vancomycin, verapamil, vit B/C

Syringe compatibilities: Metoclopramide, thiopental

Y-site compatibilities: Acyclovir, allopurinol, amifostine, aminophylline, amphotericin B cholesteryl, ampicillin, amrinone, amsacrine, atracurium, atropine, aztreonam, betamethasone, calcium gluconate, cefepime, cefmetazole, cephalothin, cephapirin, chlordiazepoxide, chlorproMAZINE, cisatracurium, cladribine, cyanocobalamin, cytarabine, dexamethasone, digoxin, diphenhydrAMINE, DOPamine, DOXOrubicin liposome, droperidol, edrophonium, enalaprilat, epiNEPHrine, esmolol, estrogens conjugated, ethacrynate, famotidine, fentanyl, fentanyl/droperidol, filgrastim, fludarabine, fluorouracil, foscarnet, furosemide, gallium, granisetron, heparin, hydrALAZINE, insulin (regular), isoproterenol, kanamycin, lidocaine, lorazepam, magnesium sulfate, melphalan, menadiol, meperidine, methicillin, methoxamine, methylergonovine, minocycline, morphine, neostigmine, norepinephrine, ondansetron, oxacillin, oxytocin, paclitaxel, pancuronium, penicillin G potassium, pentazocine, phytonadione, piperacillin/tazobactam, prednisolone, procainamide, prochlorperazine, propofol, propranolol, pyridostigmine, remifentanil, scopolamine, sodium bicarbonate, succinylcholine, tacrolimus, teniposide, theophylline, thiotepa, trimethaphan, trimethobenzamide, vecuronium, vinorelbine

Perform/provide:
• Assistance with ambulation in patient with bone tissue disease to prevent fractures

Evaluate:
• Therapeutic response: ease of respirations, decreased inflammation

Teach patient/family:
• That emergency ID as steroid user should be carried
• To notify prescriber if therapeutic response decreases; dosage adjustment may be needed; of signs of infection
• Not to discontinue abruptly, or adrenal crisis can result; drug should be tapered off
• To avoid OTC products: salicylates, alcohol in cough products, cold preparations unless directed by prescriber
• About cushingoid symptoms of adrenal insufficiency: nausea, anorexia, fatigue, dizziness, dyspnea, weakness, joint pain

---

hydrocortisone topical
See Appendix C

⚠ High Alert

hydromorphone (℞)
(hye-droe-mor'fone)
Dilaudid, Dilaudid HP,
hydromorphone HCl,
Hydrostat IR,
PMS-Hydromorphone
Func. class.: Opiate analgesic
Chem. class.: Semisynthetic phenanthrene

Controlled Substance Schedule II
Do not confuse:
hydromorphone/meperidine/morphine
Dilaudid/Demerol
Action: Inhibits ascending pain pathways in CNS, increases pain threshold, alters pain perception
Uses: Moderate to severe pain, nonproductive cough

DOSAGE AND ROUTES
Analgesic
• *Adult:* **PO** 1-6 mg q4-6h prn; **IM/SUBCUT/IV** 2-4 mg q4-6h; **RECT** 3 mg q4-6h prn
• *Geriatric:* **PO** 1-2 mg q4-6h

⚠ Safety alert   *"Tall Man" lettering

- *Child:* **PO** 0.03-0.08 mg/kg q4-6h, max 5 mg/dose

Antitussive

- *Adult:* **PO** 1 mg q3-4h prn

Available forms: Inj 1, 2, 3, 4, 10 mg/ml; tabs 1, 2, 3, 4, 8 mg; supp 3 mg; oral sol 5 mg/5 ml; syrup 1 mg/5 ml

SIDE EFFECTS

CNS: Drowsiness, dizziness, confusion, headache, sedation, euphoria, mood changes, **seizures**

CV: Palpitations, bradycardia, change in B/P, hypotension, tachycardia

EENT: Tinnitus, blurred vision, miosis, diplopia

GI: Nausea, vomiting, anorexia, constipation, cramps, dry mouth

GU: Increased urinary output, dysuria, urinary retention

INTEG: Rash, urticaria, bruising, flushing, diaphoresis, pruritus

RESP: **Respiratory depression**

Contraindications: Hypersensitivity, addiction (opiate)

Precautions: Pregnancy (C), addictive personality, lactation, increased intracranial pressure, MI (acute), severe heart disease, respiratory depression, renal/hepatic disease, child <18 yr

PHARMACOKINETICS

Onset 15-30 min, peak ½-1 hr, duration 4-5 hr; metabolized by liver; excreted by kidneys; crosses placenta; excreted in breast milk, half-life 2-3 hr

INTERACTIONS

Increase: with other CNS depressants—alcohol, opiates, sedative/hypnotics, antipsychotics, skeletal muscle relaxants

⚠ *Increase:* severe reactions—MAOIs

Drug/Herb

Increase: action—chamomile, hops, Jamaican dogwood, kava, lavender, mistletoe, nettle, pokeweed, poppy, senega, skullcap, valerian

Increase: anticholinergic effect—corkwood

Drug/Lab Test

Increase: Amylase

NURSING CONSIDERATIONS

Assess:

- Respiratory dysfunction: respiratory depression, character, rate, rhythm; notify prescriber if respirations are <10/min
- I&O ratio; check for decreasing output; may indicate urinary retention
- CNS changes: dizziness, drowsiness, hallucinations, euphoria, LOC, pupil reaction
- Bowel function, constipation
- Allergic reactions: rash, urticaria
- Need for pain medication, physical dependence
- Pain control, sedation by scoring on 0-10 scale, ATC dosing is best for pain control

Administer:

- With antiemetic if nausea, vomiting occur
- When pain is beginning to return; determine interval by response
- Rotate inj sites when giving SUBCUT

IV route

- Direct, diluted with 5 ml sterile H$_2$O or NS; give through Y-connector or 3-way stopcock; give 2 mg or less/3-5 min
- IV INF: Dilute each 0.1-1 mg/ml NS (0.1-1 mg/ml), deliver by opioid syringe infusor; may be diluted in D$_5$W, D$_5$/NaCl, 0.45% NaCl, or NS for larger amounts and delivery through an infusion pump

Additive compatibilities: Bupivacaine, fluorouracil, midazolam, ondansetron, promethazine, verapamil

Solution compatibilities: D$_5$W, D$_5$/0.45% NaCl, D$_5$/0.9% NaCl, D$_5$/LR, D$_5$/Ringer's sol, 0.45% NaCl, 0.9% NaCl, Ringer's and lactated Ringer's sol

Syringe compatibilities: Atropine, bupivacaine, ceftazidime, chlorproMAZINE, cimetidine, dimenhyDRINATE, diphenhydrAMINE, fentanyl, glycopyrrolate, haloperidol, hydrOXYzine, lorazepam, midazolam, pentazocine, pentobarbital, prochlorperazine, promethazine, ranitidine, scopolamine, tetracaine, thiethylperazine, trimethobenzamide

Y-site compatibilities: Acyclovir, allopurinol, amifostine, amikacin, amsacrine, aztreonam, cefamandole, cefazolin, cefepime, cefmetazole, cefoperazone, cefotaxime, cefoxitin, ceftazidime, ceftizoxime, cefuroxime, cephalothin, cephapirin, chloramphenicol, cisatracurium, cisplatin, cladribine, clindamycin, cyclophosphamide, cytarabine, diltiazem, DOBUTamine, DOPamine, DOXOrubicin, DOXOrubicin liposome, doxycycline, epINEPHrine, erythromycin lactobionate, famotidine, fentanyl, filgrastim, fludarabine, foscarnet, furosemide, gentamicin, granisetron, heparin, kanamycin, labetalol, lorazepam, magnesium sulfate, melphalan, methotrexate, metronidazole, mezlocillin, midazolam, milrinone, morphine, moxalactam, nafcillin, niCARdipine, nitroglycerin, norepinephrine, ondansetron, oxacillin, paclitaxel, penicillin G potassium, piperacillin, piperacillin/tazobactam, propofol, ranitidine, remifentanil, teniposide, thiotepa, ticarcillin, tobramycin, trimethoprim-sulfamethoxazole, vancomycin, vecuronium, vinorelbine

Perform/provide:
• Storage in light-resistant area at room temperature
• Assistance with ambulation
• Safety measures: side rails, night-light, call bell within easy reach

Evaluate:
• Therapeutic response: decrease in pain

Teach patient/family:
• To report any symptoms of CNS changes, allergic reactions
• That physical dependency may result when used for extended periods
• That withdrawal symptoms may occur: nausea, vomiting, cramps, fever, faintness, anorexia
• To avoid driving, other hazardous activities, drowsiness occurs

Treatment of overdose: Naloxone HCl (Narcan) 0.2-0.8 mg IV, O$_2$, IV fluids, vasopressors

hydromorphone/guaifenesin/alcohol (℞)
(hye-droe-mor′fone)
Dilaudid Cough Syrup
Func. class.: Antitussive, opioid
Chem. class.: Phenanthrene derivative

Controlled Substance Schedule II
Do not confuse:
hydromorphone/meperidine/morphine
Action: Increases respiratory tract fluid by decreasing surface tension, adhesiveness, which increases removal of mucus; analgesic, antitussive suppresses the cough reflex by a direct central action
Uses: Cough

DOSAGE AND ROUTES
• *Adult:* **PO** 1 mg q3-4h prn
Available forms: Syr 1 mg/5 ml

SIDE EFFECTS
CNS: Dizziness, drowsiness
CV: Hypotension
GI: Nausea, constipation, vomiting, anorexia
INTEG: Urticaria, rash
RESP: **Respiratory depression**
Contraindications: Hypersensitivity, increased intracranial pressure, status asthmaticus
Precautions: Pregnancy (C), hypothyroidism, Addison's disease, CNS depression, brain tumor, renal/hepatic disease, COPD, psychosis, alcoholism, seizure disorders, lactation

PHARMACOKINETICS
Metabolized by liver; half-life 2-4 hr

INTERACTIONS
Increase: CNS depression—barbiturates, opioids, antipsychotics, antidepressants
Drug/Herb
Increase: anticholinergic effect—corkwood
Increase: sedative effect—chamomile, hops, Jamaican dogwood, lavender, mis-

tletoe, nettle, pokeweed, poppy, senega, skullcap, valerian

NURSING CONSIDERATIONS

Assess:
• VS, cardiac status, including hypotension
• Respiratory rate, depth
• Cough: type, frequency, character, including sputum

Administer:
• Decreased dose to geriatric patients; metabolism may be slowed

Perform/provide:
• Storage at room temperature
• Increased fluids, bulk, exercise to decrease constipation

Evaluate:
• Therapeutic response: absence of cough

Teach patient/family:
• To avoid driving, other hazardous activities until patient stabilized on medication if drowsiness occurs
• To avoid alcohol, other CNS depressants; will enhance sedating properties of this drug
• May be taken with food for GI upset
• Physical dependency may result when used for extended periods of time

---

hydroxychloro-quine (℞)

(hye-drox-ee-klor'oh-kwin)
Plaquenil
Func. class.: Antimalarial, antirheumatic (DMARDs)
Chem. class.: 4-Aminoquinoline derivative

Action: Inhibits parasite replications, transcription of DNA to RNA by forming complexes with DNA in parasite
Uses: Malaria caused by *Plasmodium vivax, P. malariae, P. ovale, P. falciparum* (some strains); SLE, rheumatoid arthritis

DOSAGE AND ROUTES

Malaria
• *Adult:* **PO** suppression or prevention 200 mg qwk, begin 1-2 wk before travel, continue 4 wk after returning; treatment 400 mg, then 200 mg at 6, 24, 48 hr after 1st dose
• *Child:* **PO** suppression or prevention 5 mg/kg qwk, begin 1-2 wk before travel, continue 4 wk after returning; treatment 10 mg/kg, then 5 mg/kg at 6, 18, 24 hr after 1st dose

Lupus erythematosus
• *Adult:* **PO** 400 mg daily-bid; length depends on patient response; maintenance 200-400 mg daily

Rheumatoid arthritis
• *Adult:* **PO** 400-600 mg daily for 4-12 wk; then 200-300 mg daily after good response
• *Child:* **PO** 3-5 mg/kg/day max 400 mg/day

Available forms: Tabs 200 mg

SIDE EFFECTS

CNS: Headache, stimulation, fatigue, irritability, **seizures,** bad dreams, dizziness, confusion, psychosis, decreased reflexes
CV: Hypotension, heart block, **asystole with syncope**
EENT: Blurred vision, corneal changes, retinal changes, difficulty focusing, tinnitus, vertigo, deafness, photophobia, corneal edema
GI: Nausea, vomiting, anorexia, diarrhea, cramps
HEMA: **Thrombocytopenia, agranulocytosis, leukopenia, aplastic anemia**
INTEG: Pruritus, pigmentation changes, skin eruptions, lichen planus–like eruptions, eczema, **exfoliative dermatitis,** alopecia

Contraindications: Hypersensitivity, retinal field changes, children (long term)
Precautions: Pregnancy (C), blood dyscrasias, severe GI disease, neurologic dis-

H

Side effects: *italics* = common; **bold** = life-threatening

ease, alcoholism, hepatic disease, G6PD deficiency, psoriasis, eczema, lactation

PHARMACOKINETICS

PO: Peak 1-2 hr, half-life 3-5 days; metabolized in liver; excreted in urine, feces, breast milk; crosses placenta

INTERACTIONS

Increase: digoxin levels
Increase: antibody titer—rabies vaccine
Decrease: hydroxychloroquine action—Mg or Al compounds

NURSING CONSIDERATIONS

Assess:
• For SLE, malaria symptoms before and daily
• For rheumatoid arthritis: pain, swelling, ROM, temperature of joints
• Ophthalmic exam baseline and q6mo if long-term treatment or drug dosage >150 mg/day
• Hepatic studies qwk: AST, ALT, bilirubin, if on long-term treatment
• Blood studies: CBC, platelets; WBC, RBC, platelets may be decreased; if severe, drug should be discontinued
• For decreased reflexes: knee, ankle
• ECG during therapy: watch for depression of T waves, widening of QRS complex
• Allergic reactions: pruritus, rash, urticaria
• Blood dyscrasias: malaise, fever, bruising, bleeding (rare)
• For ototoxicity (tinnitus, vertigo, change in hearing); audiometric testing should be done before, after treatment
⚠ For toxicity: blurring vision, difficulty focusing, headache, dizziness, knee, ankle reflexes; drug should be discontinued immediately
Administer:
• Tabs may be crushed and mixed with food, fluids
• Take with food or milk; at same time each day to maintain drug level
• For malaria prophylaxis should be started 2 wk prior to exposure and 4-6 wk after leaving exposure area

Perform/provide:
• Storage in tight, light-resistant container at room temperature; keep inj in cool environment
Evaluate:
• Therapeutic response: decreased symptoms of malaria, SLE, rheumatoid arthritis
Teach patient/family:
• To use sunglasses in bright sunlight to decrease photophobia
• That urine may turn rust or brown
• To report hearing, visual problems, fever, fatigue, bruising, bleeding, which may indicate blood dyscrasias
Treatment of overdose: Induce vomiting; gastric lavage; administer barbiturate (ultrashort acting), vasopressor, ammonium chloride; tracheostomy may be necessary

---

hydroxyurea (℞)
(hye-drox′ee-yoo-ree-ah)
Droxia, Hydrea
Func. class.: Antineoplastic, antimetabolite
Chem. class.: Synthetic urea analog

Action: Acts by inhibiting DNA synthesis without interfering with RNA or protein synthesis; incorporates thymidine into DNA, causing direct damage to DNA strands; S phase specific of cell cycle
Uses: Melanoma, chronic myelocytic leukemia, recurrent or metastatic ovarian cancer, squamous cell carcinoma of the head and neck, sickle cell anemia, psoriasis

DOSAGE AND ROUTES

Solid tumors
• *Adult:* **PO** 80 mg/kg as a single dose q3d or 20-30 mg/kg as a single dose daily
In combination with radiation
• *Adult:* **PO** 80 mg/kg as a single dose q3d; should be started 7 days before irradiation
Resistant chronic myelocytic leukemia
• *Adult:* **PO** 20-30 mg/kg/day as a single daily dose

⚠ Safety alert   *"Tall Man" lettering

Sickle cell anemia
• *Adult:* PO 15 mg/kg/day, may increase by 5 mg/kg/day, max 35 mg/kg/day
Renal disease
• CCr 10-50 ml/min dose 50%; CCr <10 ml/min dose 20%
Available forms: Caps 200, 300, 400, 500 mg

SIDE EFFECTS

CNS: Headache, confusion, hallucinations, dizziness, **seizures**
CV: Angina, ischemia
GI: Nausea, vomiting, anorexia, diarrhea, stomatitis, constipation
GU: Increased BUN, uric acid, creatinine, temporary renal function impairment
HEMA: **Leukopenia, anemia, thrombocytopenia, megaloblastic erythropoiesis**
INTEG: *Rash,* urticaria, pruritus, dry skin, facial erythema
MISC: Fever, chills, malaise
Contraindications: Pregnancy (D), hypersensitivity, leukopenia (<2500/mm^3), thrombocytopenia (<100,000/mm^3), anemia (severe), lactation
Precautions: Renal disease (severe)

PHARMACOKINETICS

Readily absorbed when taken orally, peak level in 2 hr; degraded in liver; excreted in urine, almost totally eliminated in 24 hr; readily crosses blood-brain barrier, eliminated as CO_2

INTERACTIONS

Increase: toxicity—radiation or other antineoplastics
Drug/Lab Test
Increase: Renal studies

NURSING CONSIDERATIONS

Assess:
• CBC, differential, platelet count qwk; withhold drug if WBC is <2500/mm^3 or platelet count is <100,000/mm^3; notify prescriber; drug should be discontinued
• Renal studies: BUN, serum uric acid, urine CCr, electrolytes before, during therapy

• I&O ratio; report fall in urine output to <30 ml/hr
• Monitor temp q4h; fever may indicate beginning infection
• Hepatic studies before, during therapy: bilirubin, alk phos, AST, ALT, LDH; prn or qmo
• B/P q3-4h; check for chest pain; angina, ischemia may occur
• Bleeding: hematuria, guaiac, bruising or petechiae, mucosa or orifices q8h
• Food preferences; list likes, dislikes
• Inflammation of mucosa, breaks in skin
• Buccal cavity q8h for dryness, sores or ulceration, white patches, oral pain, bleeding, dysphagia
• Symptoms indicating severe allergic reaction: rash, urticaria, itching, flushing
• Neurotoxicity: headaches, hallucinations, convulsions, dizziness
Administer:
• Do not crush or chew caps; caps can be opened and contents mixed with water
• Allopurinol or $NaHCO_3$ concurrently to prevent high uric acid levels; extra fluids
• Antiemetic 30-60 min before giving drug and prn
• Antibiotics for prophylaxis of infection
• Transfusion for anemia
Perform/provide:
• Rinsing of mouth tid-qid with water, club soda; brushing of teeth bid-tid with soft brush or cotton-tipped applicators for stomatitis; use unwaxed dental floss
• Nutritious diet with iron, vitamin supplements as ordered
Evaluate:
• Therapeutic response: decreased tumor size, spread of malignancy
Teach patient/family:
• To report signs of infection: elevated temp, sore throat, flulike symptoms
• To report signs of anemia: fatigue, headache, faintness, shortness of breath, irritability
• To report bleeding: avoid use of razors, commercial mouthwash
• To avoid use of aspirin products, ibuprofen
• To avoid foods with citric acid, hot or rough texture if stomatitis is present

- To report stomatitis: any bleeding, white spots, ulcerations in the mouth; tell patient to examine mouth daily, report symptoms
- That contraceptive measures are recommended during therapy
- To notify prescriber of fever, chills, sore throat, nausea, vomiting, anorexia, diarrhea, bleeding, bruising; may indicate blood dyscrasias

---

*hydrOXYzine (℞)

(hye-drox'i-zeen)
Apo-Hydroxyzine ✿, Atarax, hydroxyzine, Hyzine-50, Multi-pax ✿, Novohydroxyzine ✿, Vistaril
Func. class.: Antianxiety/antihistamine/sedative-hypnotic, antiemetic
Chem. class.: Piperazine derivative

Do not confuse:
hydrOXYzine/hydrALAZINE
Atarax/amoxicillin/Ativan
Vistaril/Versed

Action: Depresses subcortical levels of CNS, including limbic system, reticular formation; competes with H_1-receptor sites

Uses: Anxiety preoperatively, postoperatively to prevent nausea, vomiting, to potentiate opioid analgesics; sedation; pruritus

DOSAGE AND ROUTES

- *Adult:* **PO** 25-100 mg tid-qid, max 600 mg/day
- *Geriatric:* **PO** 10 mg tid-qid (pruritus)
- *Child >6 yr:* **PO** 50-100 mg/day in divided doses
- *Child <6 yr:* **PO** 50 mg/day in divided doses

Preoperatively/postoperatively
- *Adult:* **IM** 25-100 mg q4-6h
- *Child:* **IM** 0.5-1.1 mg/kg q4-6h

Pruritus
- *Adult:* **PO** 25 mg tid-qid

Antiemetic
- *Adult:* **IM** 25-100 mg/dose q4-6h prn

Available forms: Tabs 10, 25, 50, 100 mg; caps 10, 25, 50, 100 mg; oral susp 25 mg/5 ml; inj 25, 50 mg/ml

SIDE EFFECTS

CNS: Dizziness, drowsiness, confusion, headache, tremors, fatigue, depression, **seizures**
CV: Hypotension
GI: Dry mouth, increased appetite, nausea, diarrhea, weight gain
Contraindications: Pregnancy (1st trimester), hypersensitivity to this drug or cetirizine, lactation, acute asthma
Precautions: Pregnancy (C) (2nd/3rd trimester), geriatric, debilitated, hepatic disease, renal disease, narrow-angle glaucoma, COPD, prostatic hypertrophy

PHARMACOKINETICS

PO: Onset 15-30 min, duration 4-6 hr, half-life 3 hr, metabolized by liver, excreted by kidneys

INTERACTIONS

Increase: CNS depressant effect—barbiturates, opioids, analgesics, alcohol
Increase: anticholinergic effects—phenothiazines, quinidine, disopyramide, antihistamines, antidepressants, atropine, haloperidol
Drug/Herb
Increase: anticholinergic effect—corkwood, henbane leaf, jimsonweed, scopolia
Increase: sedative action—chamomile, cowslip, hops, Jamaican dogwood, kava, khat, Queen Anne's lace, senega, skullcap, valerian

NURSING CONSIDERATIONS

Assess:
- B/P (lying, standing), pulse; if systolic B/P drops 20 mm Hg, hold drug, notify prescriber
- Mental status: mood, sensorium, affect, anxiety, behavior, increased sedation

---

⚠ Safety alert   *"Tall Man" lettering

Administer:

PO route

• With food or milk for GI symptoms (PO)

• Crushed if patient is unable to swallow medication whole

• Gum, hard candy, frequent sips of water for dry mouth

IM route

• By Z-track inj in large muscle for IM to decrease pain, chance of necrosis, never give IV/SUBCUT

Additive compatibilities: Cisplatin, cyclophosphamide, cytarabine, dimenhyDRINATE, etoposide, lidocaine, mesna, methotrexate, nafcillin

Syringe compatibilities: Atropine, atropine/meperidine, benzquinamide, bupivacaine, butorphanol, chlorproMAZINE, cimetidine, codeine, diphenhydrAMINE, doxapram, droperidol, fentanyl, fluphenazine, glycopyrrolate, hydromorphone, lidocaine, meperidine, meperidine/atropine, methotrimeprazine, metoclopramide, midazolam, morphine, nalbuphine, oxymorphone, pentazocine, perphenazine, procaine, prochlorperazine, promazine, promethazine, scopolamine, sufentanil, thiothixene

Perform/provide:

• Assistance with ambulation during beginning therapy, since drowsiness/dizziness occurs

• Safety measures, including side rails

• Checking to see if PO medication has been swallowed

Evaluate:

• Therapeutic response: decreased anxiety

Teach patient/family:

• That medication is not to be used for everyday stress or used longer than 4 mo

• To avoid OTC preparations (cold, cough, hay fever) unless approved by prescriber

• To avoid driving, activities that require alertness

• To avoid alcohol ingestion, psychotropic medications

• Not to discontinue medication quickly after long-term use

• To rise slowly or fainting may occur

Treatment of overdose: Lavage if orally ingested; VS, supportive care; IV norepinephrine for hypotension

---

hyoscyamine (℞)

(hye-oh-sye'a-meen)

Anaspaz, A-Spas S/L, Cystospaz, Donnamar, ED-SPAZ, Gastrosed, Levsin, Levsinex, NuLev Timecaps

Func. class.: Anticholinergic/antispasmodics

Chem. class.: Belladonna alkaloid

Action: Inhibits muscarinic actions of acetylcholine at postganglionic parasympathetic neuroeffector sites, reduces rigidity, tremors, hyperhidrosis of parkinsonism

Uses: Treatment of peptic ulcer disease in combination with other drugs; other GI disorders, other spastic disorders, IBS, urinary incontinence

DOSAGE AND ROUTES

• *Adult:* **PO/SL** 0.125-0.25 mg tid-qid before meals, at bedtime; **TIME REL** 0.375-0.75 q12h; **IM/SUBCUT/IV** 0.25-0.5 mg q6h

• *Child 2-12 yr:* **PO** (orally disintegrating tabs) 0.0625-0.125 mg (½-1 tab) q4h, max 6×/day

• *Child 34-36 kg:* **PO** 125-187 mcg q4h prn

• *Child 22.7-33 kg:* **PO** 94-125 mcg q4h prn

• *Child 13.6-22.6 kg:* **PO** 63 mcg q4h prn

• *Child 9.1-13.5 kg:* **PO** 31.3 mcg q4h prn

• *Child 6.8-9 kg:* **PO** 25 mg q4h prn

• *Child 4.5-6.7 kg:* **PO** 18.8 mcg q4h prn

• *Child 3.4-4.4 kg:* **PO** 15.6 mcg q4h prn

• *Child 2.3-3.3 kg:* **PO** 12.5 mcg q4h prn

Available forms: Tabs 0.125, 0.15 mg; time rel caps 0.375 mg; time rel tabs 0.375 ml; sol 0.125 mg/ml; elix 0.125 mg/5 ml; inj 0.5 mg/ml

SIDE EFFECTS

CNS: Confusion, stimulation in geriatric, headache, insomnia, dizziness, drowsiness, anxiety, weakness, hallucination

CV: Palpitations, tachycardia

EENT: Blurred vision, photophobia, mydriasis, cycloplegia, increased ocular tension

GI: Dry mouth, constipation, paralytic ileus, heartburn, nausea, vomiting, dysphagia, absence of taste

GU: Urinary hesitancy, retention, impotence

INTEG: Urticaria, rash, pruritus, anhidrosis, fever, allergic reactions

Contraindications: Hypersensitivity to anticholinergics, narrow-angle glaucoma, GI obstruction, myasthenia gravis, paralytic ileus, GI atony, toxic megacolon, prostatic hypertrophy

Precautions: Pregnancy (C), hyperthyroidism, coronary artery disease, dysrhythmias, CHF, ulcerative colitis, hypertension, hiatal hernia, renal/hepatic disease, urinary retention, geriatric

PHARMACOKINETICS

PO: Duration 4-6 hr; metabolized by liver; excreted in urine; half-life 3.5 hr

INTERACTIONS

Increase: anticholinergic effect—amantadine, tricyclics, MAOIs, H_1-antihistamines

Decrease: hyoscyamine effect—antacids

Decrease: effect of phenothiazines, levodopa, ketoconazole

Drug/Herb

Increase: constipation—black catechu

Increase: anticholinergic effect—butterbur, jimsonweed

Decrease: anticholinergic effect—jaborandi tree, pill-bearing spurge

NURSING CONSIDERATIONS

Assess:

• VS, cardiac status: checking for dysrhythmias, increased rate, palpitations

• I&O ratio; check for urinary retention or hesitancy

• GI complaints: pain, nausea, vomiting, anorexia

Administer:

• Do not break, crush, or chew time rel caps

• ½ hr before meals for better absorption

• Decreased dose to geriatric patients; metabolism may be slowed

• Gum, hard candy, frequent rinsing of mouth for dryness of oral cavity

Perform/provide:

• Storage in tight container protected from light

• Increased fluids, bulk, exercise to decrease constipation

Evaluate:

• Therapeutic response: absence of epigastric pain, bleeding, nausea, vomiting

Teach patient/family:

• To avoid driving, other hazardous activities until stabilized on medication

• To avoid alcohol or other CNS depressants; will enhance sedating properties of this drug

• To avoid hot environments; heat stroke may occur; drug suppresses perspiration

• To use sunglasses when outside to prevent photophobia; may cause blurred vision

---

ibritumomab tiuxetan (℞)

(ee-brit-u-moe'mab)

Zevalin

Func. class.: Antineoplastic—miscellaneous

Chem. class.: Monoclonal antibody

Action: High affinity for indium-111, yttrium-90; induces CD20 + B-cell lines

Uses: Non-Hodgkin's lymphoma, B-cell NHL

DOSAGE AND ROUTES

• *Adult:* **IV INF** 250 mg/m^2 at a rate of 50 mg/hr; if hypersensitivity does not occur, increase rate by 50 mg/hr q$^1/_2$h, max 400 mg/hr; slow/interrupt inf if hypersensitivity occurs

Available forms: Inj 3.2 mg/2 ml

SIDE EFFECTS

CV: **Cardiac dysrhythmias**
GI: Nausea, vomiting, anorexia, abdominal pain, diarrhea
GU: **Renal failure**
HEMA: **Leukopenia, neutropenia, thrombocytopenia,** anemia
INTEG: Irritation at site, rash, **fatal mucocutaneous infections (rare)**
OTHER: Fever, chills, asthenia, headache, angioedema, hypotension, myalgia, **bronchospasm, hemorrhage,** infections, cough, dyspnea, dizziness, anxiety
SYST: **Stevens-Johnson syndrome**
Contraindications: Pregnancy (D), hypersensitivity to this agent or murine proteins
Precautions: Lactation, children, geriatric, cardiac conditions, immunizations after therapy

PHARMACOKINETICS

Half-life 30 hr

NURSING CONSIDERATIONS

Assess:
⚠ For signs of fatal infusion reaction: hypoxia, pulmonary infiltrates, ARDS, MI, ventricular fibrillation, cardiogenic shock; most fatal infusion reactions occur with first infusion; potentially fatal
• Biodistribution: 1st image 2-24 hr, 2nd image 48-72 hr, 3rd image 90-120 hr (optimal)
⚠ For signs of severe mucocutaneous reactions: Stevens-Johnson syndrome, lichenoid dermatitis, toxic epidermal lysis; occur 1-13 wk after drug was given
⚠ Tumor lysis syndrome: acute renal failure requiring hemodialysis, hyperkalemia, hypocalcemia, hyperuricemia, hyperphosphatemia

• CBC, differential, platelet count weekly; withhold drug if WBC is < 3500/mm^3, or platelet count <100,000/mm^3; notify prescriber of these results; drug should be discontinued
• GI symptoms: frequency of stools
• Signs of dehydration: rapid respirations, poor skin turgor, decreased urine output, dry skin, restlessness, weakness

Administer:
• Do not use as bolus or IV direct

IV INF route
• See manufacturer's product labeling for preparation

Perform/provide:
• Increased fluid intake to 2-3 L/day to prevent dehydration, unless contraindicated
• Emergency equipment nearby with epINEPHrine, antihistamines, corticosteroids
• Changing of IV site q48h
• Nutritious diet with iron, vitamin supplement, low fiber, few dairy products
• Storage of vials at 36°-46° F, do not freeze

Evaluate:
• Therapeutic response: decrease in tumor size, decrease in spread of cancer

Teach patient/family:
• To report adverse reactions
• To use contraception during and for 12 months after therapy

Side effects: *italics* = common; **bold** = life-threatening

ibuprofen (OTC, ℞)

(eye-byoo-proe′fen)
Actiprofen ✤, Advil, Advil
Liqui-Gels, Advil Migraine,
Apo-Ibuprofen ✤, Bayer
Select Ibuprofen Pain Relief,
Children's Advil, Children's
Motrin, Excedrin IB, Genpril,
Haltran, ibuprofen, IBU-TAB,
Infant's Motrin, Junior
Strength Advil, Medipren,
Menadol, Midol Maximum
Strength Cramp Formula,
Motrin, Motrin IB, Motrin
Junior Strength, Motrin
Migraine Pain, Novoprofen ✤,
Nu-Ibuprofen, Nuprin,
PediaCare Children's Fever,
Pediatric Advil drops,
PediaCare Fever

Func. class.: Nonsteroidal antiinflammatory, antipyretic, nonopioid
analgesics

Chem. class.: Propionic acid derivative

Do not confuse:

Nuprin/Lupron

Action: Inhibits prostaglandin synthesis
by decreasing enzyme needed for biosynthesis; analgesic, antiinflammatory, antipyretic

Uses: Rheumatoid arthritis, osteoarthritis, primary dysmenorrhea, gout, dental
pain, musculoskeletal disorders, fever

DOSAGE AND ROUTES

Analgesic
• *Adult:* PO 200-400 mg q4-6h, not to
exceed 3.2 g/day
• *Child:* PO 4-10 mg/kg/dose q6-8h

Antipyretic
• *Child 6 mo-12 yr:* PO 5 mg/kg (temp
<102.5° F or 39.2° C), 10 mg/kg, (temp
>102.5° F), may repeat q4-6h, max 40
mg/kg/day

Antiinflammatory
• *Adult:* PO 300-800 mg tid-qid, max 3.2
g/day
• *Child:* PO 30-40 mg/kg/day in 3-4 divided doses, max 50 mg/kg/day

Available forms: Tabs 100, 200, 300,
400, 600, 800 mg; cap, liq gels 200 mg;
oral susp 100 mg/2.5 ml, 100 mg/5 ml;
liq 100 mg/5 ml; chew tabs 50, 100 mg;
drops 50 mg/1.25 ml

SIDE EFFECTS

CNS: Headache, dizziness, drowsiness, fatigue, tremors, confusion, insomnia, anxiety, depression
CV: Tachycardia, peripheral edema, palpitations, dysrhythmias, **CV thrombotic
events, MI, stroke**
EENT: Tinnitus, hearing loss, blurred vision
GI: Nausea, *anorexia,* vomiting, diarrhea,
jaundice, **hepatitis,** constipation, flatulence, cramps, dry mouth, peptic ulcer,
GI bleeding, ulceration
GU: **Nephrotoxicity:** dysuria, hematuria, oliguria, azotemia
HEMA: **Blood dyscrasias,** increased
bleeding time
INTEG: Purpura, rash, pruritus, sweating,
urticaria, **nectrotizing fasciitis**
SYST: **Anaphylaxis, Stevens-Johnson
syndrome**

Contraindications: Hypersensitivity,
asthma, severe renal/hepatic disease,
avoid in 2nd/3rd trimester of pregnancy,
perioperative pain in CABG

Precautions: Pregnancy (B) 1st trimester, lactation, children, bleeding disorders, GI disorders, cardiac disorders, hypersensitivity to other antiinflammatory
agents, geriatric, CHF, CCr <25 ml/min

PHARMACOKINETICS

Well absorbed (PO)

PO: Onset ½ hr; peak 1-2 hr, half-
life 2-4 hr, metabolized in liver (inactive metabolites), excreted in urine
(inactive metabolites), 90%-99%
plasma protein binding, does not enter breast milk

🅐 Safety alert   *"Tall Man" lettering

INTERACTIONS

Increase: bleeding risk—cefotetan, valproic acid, thrombolytics, antiplatelets, warfarin

Increase: blood dyscrasias possibility—antineoplastics, radiation

Increase: toxicity—digoxin, lithium, oral anticoagulants, cycloSPORINE, probenecid

Increase: GI reactions—aspirin, corticosteroids, NSAIDs, alcohol

Increase: hypoglycemia—oral antidiabetics, insulin

Decrease: effect of antihypertensives, thiazides, furosemide

Decrease: ibuprofen action—aspirin

Drug/Herb

Increase: bleeding risk—arnica, chamomile, clove, dong quai, fenugreek, feverfew, garlic, ginger, ginkgo, ginseng *(Panax)*

Increase: gastric irritation—arginine, gossypol

Increase: NSAID effect—bearberry, bilberry

Increase: bleeding risk—bogbean, chondroitin

NURSING CONSIDERATIONS

Assess:

• Renal, hepatic, blood studies: BUN, creatinine, AST, ALT, Hgb, before treatment, periodically thereafter

• Pain: note type, duration, location, and intensity with ROM 1 hr after administration

• Audiometric, ophthalmic exam before, during, after treatment; for eye, ear problems: blurred vision, tinnitus; may indicate toxicity

• Fever: temp before and 1 hr after administration

• Cardiac status: edema (peripheral), tachycardia, palpitations; monitor B/P, pulse for character, quality, rhythm especially in patients with cardiac disease/geriatric

• For history of peptic ulcer disorder; asthma, aspirin, hypersensitivity, check closely for hypersensitivity reactions

Administer:

• With food, milk, or antacid to decrease GI symptoms; however, taking on empty stomach best facilitates absorption; if nausea and vomiting occur/persist, notify prescriber

Perform/provide:

• Storage at room temperature

Evaluate:

• Therapeutic response: decreased pain, stiffness in joints; decreased swelling in joints; ability to move more easily; reduction in fever or menstrual cramping

Teach patient/family:

• To report blurred vision, ringing, roaring in ears; may indicate toxicity; eye and hearing tests should be done during long-term therapy

• To avoid driving, other hazardous activities if dizziness or drowsiness occurs

⚠ To report change in urinary pattern, increased weight, edema, increased pain in joints, fever, blood in urine; indicate nephrotoxicity

• That therapeutic inflammatory effects may take up to 1 mo

⚠ To avoid alcohol, NSAIDs, salicylates; bleeding may occur

• To use sunscreen to prevent photosensitivity

⚠ High Alert

ibutilide (℞)
(eye-byoo'tih-lide)
Corvert
Func. class.: Antidysrhythmic (Class III)

Action: Prolongs duration of action potential and effective refractory period

Uses: For rapid conversion of atrial fibrillation/flutter including within 1 wk of coronary artery bypass or valve surgery

---

DOSAGE AND ROUTES
Atrial fibrillation flutter
• *Adult ≥60 kg:* **IV INF** 1 vial (1 mg) given over 10 min, may repeat same dose in 10 min
• *Adult <60 kg:* **IV INF** 0.01 mg/kg given over 10 min, may repeat same dose in 10 min
Atrial fibrillation/flutter after cardiac surgery
• *Adult ≥60 kg:* **IV INF** 0.5 mg; may repeat 1 time
• *Adult <60 kg:* **IV INF** 0.005 mg/kg; may repeat 1 time
Available forms: Inj 0.1 mg/ml

SIDE EFFECTS
CNS: Headache
CV: Hypotension, bradycardia, **sinus arrest, CHF, dysrhythmias,** hypertension, extrasystoles, ventricular tachycardia, bundle branch block, AV block, palpitations, supraventricular extrasystoles, syncope
GI: Nausea

Contraindications: Hypersensitivity
Precautions: Pregnancy (C), sinus node dysfunction, 2nd- or 3rd-degree AV block, electrolyte imbalances, bradycardia, lactation, children <18 yr, renal/hepatic disease, geriatric

PHARMACOKINETICS
Elimination half-life in 6 hr; metabolized by liver, excreted by kidneys

INTERACTIONS
• Prodysrhythmia: phenothiazines, tricyclics, tetracyclics, antidepressants, H₁-receptor antagonists, antihistamines
• Masking of cardiotoxicity: digoxin
• Do not use within 5 hr of ibutilide: Class Ia antidysrhythmics (disopyramide, quinidine, procainamide), Class III agents (amiodarone, sotalol)
Drug/Herb
Increase: toxicity, death—aconite
Increase: effect—aloe, broom, chronic buckthorn use, cascara sagrada (chronic use), Chinese rhubarb, figwort, fumitory, goldenseal, kudzu, licorice

Increase: serotonin effect—horehound
Decrease: effect—coltsfoot

NURSING CONSIDERATIONS
Assess:
• ECG continuously to determine drug effectiveness, measure PR, QRS, QT intervals, check for PVCs, other dysrhythmias, discontinue if atrial fibrillation/flutter ceases
• I&O ratio; electrolytes: K, Na, Cl
• Hepatic studies: AST, ALT, bilirubin, alk phos
• For dehydration or hypovolemia
• For rebound hypertension after 1-2 hr
• Cardiac rate, respiration: rate, rhythm, character, chest pain
Administer:
IV route
• Undiluted or diluted in 50 ml 0.9% NaCl, or D₅W (0.017 mg/ml) give over 10 min
• Solution is stable for 48 hr refrigerated or 24 hr, room temperature
• Do not admix with other solution, drugs
• Reduce dosage slowly with ECG monitoring
Evaluate:
• Therapeutic response: decrease in atrial fibrillation/flutter
Teach patient/family:
• To report side effects immediately
• Reason for medication

⚠ High Alert

idarubicin (℞)
(eye-dah-roob'ih-sin)
Idamycin, Idamycin PFS
Func. class.: Antineoplastic, antibiotic
Chem. class.: Anthracycline glycoside

Do not confuse:
idarubicin/DOXOrubicin
Idamycin/Adriamycin
Action: Inhibits DNA synthesis by binding to DNA, a vesicant derived from dau-

---

norubicin by binding to DNA, which causes strand splitting; cell cycle specific (S phase)
Uses: Used in combination with other antineoplastics for acute myelocytic leukemia in adults
Unlabeled uses: Breast cancer, solid tumors

DOSAGE AND ROUTES

• *Adult:* **IV** 12 mg/m^2/day × 3 days in combination with extarabine (induction)
Renal/hepatic dose
• *Adult:* **IV** Reduce dose, if bilirubin is >5 mg/dl, do not administer
Available forms: Inj 1 mg/ml

SIDE EFFECTS

CNS: Fever, chills, *headache*
CV: **Dysrhythmias, CHF, pericarditis, myocarditis,** peripheral edema, angina, **MI**
GI: Nausea, vomiting, abdominal pain, mucositis, diarrhea, **hepatotoxicity**
GU: **Nephrotoxicity**
HEMA: **Thrombocytopenia, leukopenia, anemia**
INTEG: Rash, extravasation, dermatitis, *reversible alopecia,* urticaria, thrombophlebitis and tissue necrosis at inj site
Contraindications: Pregnancy (D), hypersensitivity, lactation, myelosuppression
Precautions: Renal/hepatic disease, gout, bone marrow depression, children, preexisting CV disease

PHARMACOKINETICS

Half-life 22 hr; metabolized by liver; crosses placenta; excreted in bile, urine (primarily as metabolites)

INTERACTIONS

Increase: toxicity—other antineoplastics or radiation
Decrease: antibody response—live virus vaccines
Drug/Lab Test
Increase: Uric acid

NURSING CONSIDERATIONS

Assess:

• CBC, differential, platelet count weekly; withhold drug if WBC is <4000/mm^3 or platelet count is <75,000/mm^3; notify prescriber of these results
• Blood, urine, uric acid levels
• Renal studies: BUN, serum uric acid, urine CCr, electrolytes before, during therapy
• I&O ratio; report fall in urine output to <30 ml/hr
• Monitor temp q4h; fever may indicate beginning infection
• Hepatic studies before, during therapy: bilirubin, AST, ALT, alk phos prn or qmo; check for jaundice of skin, sclera, dark urine, clay-colored stools, itchy skin, abdominal pain, fever, diarrhea
• Cardiac toxicity: CHF, dysrythmias, cardiomyopathy; cardiac studies should be done before and periodically during treatment: ECG, chest x-ray
• ECG: watch for ST-T wave changes, low QRS and T, possible dysrhythmias (sinus tachycardia, heart block, PVCs)
• Bleeding: hematuria, guaiac stools, bruising or petechiae, mucosa or orifices q8h
• Effects of alopecia on body image; discuss feelings about body changes
• Inflammation of mucosa, breaks in skin
• Buccal cavity q8h for dryness, sores, ulceration, white patches, oral pain, bleeding, dysphagia
• Local irritation, pain, burning at inj site
• GI symptoms: frequency of stools, cramping
• Acidosis, signs of dehydration: rapid respirations, poor skin turgor, decreased urine output, dry skin, restlessness, weakness

Administer:

• Allopurinol or sodium bicarbonate to reduce uric acid levels, alkalinization of urine
• Transfusion for anemia
• Hydrocortisone for extravasation; apply ice compress after stopping infusion

---

Side effects: *italics* = common; **bold** = life-threatening

IV, direct route
• Do not give IM/SUBCUT
• Use cytotoxic handling procedures after preparing in biologic cabinet wearing gown, gloves, mask
• Antiemetic 30-60 min before giving drug and 6-10 hr after treatment to prevent vomiting
• After reconstituting 5 mg vial with 5 ml 0.9% NaCl (1 mg/1 ml); give over 10-15 min through Y-tube or 3-way stopcock of inf of D₅ or NS; discard unused portion
Solution compatibilities: D₃.₃/0.3% NaCl, D₅/0.9% NaCl, D₅W, LR, 0.9% NaCl
Y-site compatibilities: Amifostine, amikacin, aztreonam, cimetidine, cladribine, cyclophosphamide, cytarabine, diphenhydrAMINE, droperidol, erythromycin, filgrastim, granisetron, imipenem/cisplatin, magnesium sulfate, mannitol, melphalan, metoclopramide, potassium chloride, ranitidine, sargramostim, thiotepa, vinorelbine
Perform/provide:
• Strict hand-washing technique, gloves, protective clothing
• Liquid diet: carbonated beverages, gelatin may be added if patient is not nauseated or vomiting
• Increase fluid intake to 2-3 L/day to prevent urate and calculi formation
• Rinsing of mouth tid-qid with water, club soda; brushing of teeth tid-qid with soft brush or cotton-tipped applicators for stomatitis; use unwaxed dental floss
• Storage at room temperature for 3 days after reconstituting or 7 days refrigerated
Evaluate:
• Therapeutic response: decreased tumor size, spread of malignancy
Teach patient/family:
• To report any complaints, side effects to nurse or prescriber
• That hair may be lost during treatment and wig or hairpiece may make patient feel better; tell patient that new hair may be different in color, texture
• To avoid foods with citric acid, hot or rough texture
• To report any bleeding, white spots, ul-

cerations in mouth; tell patient to examine mouth daily
• That urine may be red-orange for 48 hr
• To use contraception during treatment with this drug and for ≥4 mo after treatment

idursulfase
See Appendix A—Selected New Drugs

⚠ High Alert

ifosfamide (℞)
(i-foss'fa-mide)
Ifex
Func. class.: Antineoplastic alkylating agent
Chem. class.: Nitrogen mustard

Action: Alkylates DNA, RNA, inhibits enzymes that allow synthesis of amino acids in proteins; also responsible for cross-linking DNA strands; activity is not cell cycle stage specific
Uses: Testicular cancer, soft tissue sarcoma, Ewing's sarcoma, non-Hodgkin's lymphoma, lung, pancreatic sarcoma

DOSAGE AND ROUTES
• *Adult:* **IV** 1.2 g/m²/day × 5 days, repeat course q3wk, given with mesna
Available forms: Inj 1, 3 g vials

SIDE EFFECTS
CNS: Facial paresthesia, fever, malaise, somnolence, confusion, depression, hallucinations, dizziness, disorientation, **seizures, coma,** cranial nerve dysfunction
GI: Nausea, vomiting, anorexia, **hepatotoxicity,** stomatitis, constipation, diarrhea
GU: **Hematuria, nephrotoxicity, hemorrhagic cystitis,** dysuria, urinary frequency

HEMA: **Thrombocytopenia, leukopenia, anemia**

INTEG: Dermatitis, alopecia, pain at inj site

Contraindications: Pregnancy (D), hypersensitivity, bone marrow suppression

Precautions: Renal disease, lactation, children

PHARMACOKINETICS

Metabolized by liver; saturation occurs at high doses; excreted in urine; half-life 7-15 hr

INTERACTIONS

Increase: myelosuppression—other antineoplastics, radiation

Increase: toxicity—barbiturates, allopurinol

Decrease: antibody response—live virus vaccines

NURSING CONSIDERATIONS

Assess:

• Hepatic studies before, during therapy (bilirubin, AST, ALT, LDH) as needed or monthly

• CBC, differential, platelet count weekly; withhold drug if WBC <2000 or platelet count <50,000; notify prescriber

• Monitor temp q4h (may indicate beginning infection)

• Blood dyscrasias (anemia, granulocytopenia); bruising, fatigue, bleeding, poor healing

• Allergic reactions: dermatitis, exfoliative dermatitis, pruritus, urticaria

• I&O ratio; monitor for hematuria; hemorrhagic cystitis can occur; increase fluids to 3 L/day

• Neurologic symptoms: hallucinations, confusion, disorientation, drug should be discontinued

• Bleeding: hematuria, guaiac, bruising or petechiae, mucosa or orifices q8h

• Jaundice of skin, sclera, dark urine, clay-colored stools, itchy skin, abdominal pain, fever, diarrhea

Administer:

• Antiemetic 30-60 min before giving drug to prevent vomiting

• Antibiotics for prophylaxis of infection

• Always give with mesna to prevent ifosfamide-induced hemorrhagic cystitis

IV route

• After diluting 1 g/20 ml sterile or bacteriostatic H_2O for inj with parabens or benzyl only; shake; may be diluted further with D_5W, LR, NS, sterile H_2O for inj; 1 g/20 ml = 50 mg/ml; 1 g/50 ml = 20 mg/ml; 1 g/200 ml = 5 mg/ml; give over ≥30 min; may also give as cont inf over 72 hr

Additive compatibilities: Carboplatin, cisplatin, etoposide, fluorouracil, mesna

Syringe compatibilities: Mesna

Y-site compatibilities: Allopurinol, amifostine, amphotericin B cholesteryl, aztreonam, DOXOrubicin liposome, filgrastim, fludarabine, gallium, granisetron, melphalan, ondansetron, paclitaxel, piperacillin/tazobactam, propofol, sargramostim, sodium bicarbonate, teniposide, thiotepa, vinorelbine

Perform/provide:

• Storage of powder at room temperature

• Increase fluid intake to 3 L/day to prevent hemorrhagic cystitis

• Warm compresses at inj site for inflammation

Evaluate:

• Therapeutic response: decrease in size and spread of tumor

Teach patient/family:

• To notify prescriber of sore throat, swollen lymph nodes, malaise, fever; other infections may occur

• Not to have vaccinations during treatment

• That hair may be lost during treatment; a wig or hairpiece may make the patient feel better; new hair may be different in color, texture

• To report signs of anemia: fatigue, headache, faintness, shortness of breath, irritability

Side effects: *italics* = common; **bold** = life-threatening

• To report bleeding; avoid use of razors, commercial mouthwash
• To avoid use of aspirin products, NSAIDs, ibuprofen, hemorrhage can occur
• To use contraceptive measures during therapy
• To avoid crowds, those with infections
• To report confusion, hallucinations, extreme drowsiness, numbness, tingling; avoid alcohol use for ≥4 mo after treatment

---

imatinib (R̶)
(im-ah-tin′ib)
Gleevec
Func. class.: Antineoplastic—miscellaneous
Chem. class.: Protein-tyrosine kinase inhibitor

Action: Inhibits Bcr-Abl tyrosine kinase created in chronic myeloid leukemia (CML)

Uses: Treatment of chronic myeloid leukemia (CML) in blast cell crisis or chronic failure after treatment failure with interferon alfa; gastrointestinal stromal tumors (GIST)

DOSAGE AND ROUTES

CML, *chronic phase*
• *Adult:* **PO** 400 mg/day
• *Child:* **PO** 260 mg/m^2/day

Hepatic dose
• *Adult:* **PO** 300 mg daily, may increase to 400 mg dialy
• *Child ≥3 yr:* **PO** 200 mg/m^2/day; may increase to 260 mg/m^2/day in 1-2 divided doses

CML, *accelerated phase/blast crisis*
• *Adult:* **PO** 600 mg/day

GIST
• *Adult:* **PO** 400 or 600 mg/day
Available forms: Tabs 100, 400 mg

SIDE EFFECTS

CNS: **CNS hemorrhage,** headache, dizziness, insomnia
CV: Hemorrhage

GI: Nausea, **hepatotoxicity, vomiting, dyspepsia,** GI hemorrhage, *anorexia, abdominal pain*
HEMA: **Neutropenia, thrombocytopenia, bleeding**
INTEG: Rash, pruritus
META: Fluid retention, hypokalemia, edema
MISC: Fatigue, epistaxis, pyrexia, night sweats, increased weight
MS: Cramps, pain, arthralgia, myalgia
RESP: Cough, dyspnea, nasopharyngitis, pneumonia, URI
Contraindications: Pregnancy (D), hypersensitivity
Precautions: Lactation, children, geriatric

PHARMACOKINETICS

Well absorbed (98%) (PO), protein binding 95%, metabolized by CYP3A4, excreted in feces, small amount in urine; peak 2-4 hr, duration 24 hr (imatinib), 40 hr (metabolite), half-life 18 hr

INTERACTIONS

Increase: hepatotoxicity—acetaminophen
Increase: imatinib concentrations—ketoconazole, itraconazole, erythromycin, clarithromycin
Increase: plasma concentrations of simvastatin, calcium channel blockers
Increase: plasma concentration of warfarin; avoid use with warfarin, use low-molecular-weight anticoagulants instead
Decrease: imatinib concentrations—dexamethasone, phenytoin, carbamazepine, rifampin, phenobarbital
Drug/Herb
Decrease: imatinib concentration—St. John's wort

NURSING CONSIDERATIONS

Assess:
• ANC and platelets; in chronic phase if ANC <1 × 10^9/L and/or platelets <50 × 10^9/L, stop until ANC >1.5 × 10^9/L and platelets >75 × 10^9/L; in accelerated

---

phase/blast crisis if ANC $<0.5 \times 10^9$/L and/or platelets $<10 \times 10^9$/L, determine whether cytopenia is related to biopsy/aspirate, if not, reduce dose by 200 mg, if cytopenia continues, reduce dose by another 100 mg; if cytopenia continues for 4 wk, stop drug until ANC $\geq 1 \times 10^9$/L

• For renal toxicity: if bilirubin $>3 \times$ IULN, withhold imatinib until bilirubin levels return to $<1.5 \times$ IULN

• For hepatotoxicity: monitor LFTs, before treatment and qmo; if liver transaminases $>5 \times$ IULN, withhold imatinib until transaminase levels return to $<2.5 \times$ IULN

• CBC, differential, platelet count weekly; withhold drug if WBC is <3500/mm^3, or platelet count $<100,000$/mm^3; notify prescriber of these results; drug should be discontinued

• Signs of fluid retention, edema: weigh, monitor lung sounds, assess for edema, some fluid retention is dose dependent

Administer:
• With meal and large glass of water, to decrease GI symptoms, doses of 800 mg should be given 400 mg bid

Perform/provide:
• Nutritious diet with iron, vitamin supplement, low fiber, few dairy products
• Storage at 25° C (77° F)

Evaluate:
• Therapeutic response: decrease in leukemic cells or size of tumor

Teach patient/family:
• To report adverse reactions immediately: SOB, swelling of extremities, bleeding
• Reason for treatment, expected result

---

imipenem/cilastatin (Ŗ)
(i-me-pen'em sye-la-stat'in)
Primaxin IM, Primaxin IV
Func. class.: Antiinfective—miscellaneous
Chem. class.: Carbapenem

Do not confuse:
imipenem/Omnipen
Primaxin/Premarin

Action: Interferes with cell wall replication of susceptible organisms; osmoti-cally unstable cell wall swells, bursts from osmotic pressure; addition of cilastatin prevents renal inactivation that occurs with high urinary concentrations of imipenem

Uses: Serious infections caused by gram-positive: *Streptococcus pneumoniae,* group A β-hemolytic streptococci, *Staphylococcus aureus,* enterococcus; gram-negative: *Klebsiella, Proteus, Escherichia coli, Acinetobacter, Serratia, Pseudomonas aeruginosa, Salmonella, Shigella, Haemophilus influenzae, Listeria* sp.

DOSAGE AND ROUTES
• *Adult:* IV 250-500 mg q6-8h; severe infections may require 1 g q8h; may give **IM** q12h (total daily **IM** dosage >1500 mg not recommended); mild to moderate infections
• *Child:* IV 60-100 mg/kg/day in divided doses, max 4 g/day; IM 10-15 mg/kg q6h
Renal dose
• *Adult:* IV CCr 30-70 ml/min give 50% dose q6-8h; CCr 20-30 ml/min give 40% dose q8-12h; CCr 5-20 ml/min give 25% dose q12h
Available forms: Inj 250, 500 mg (IV); inj 500, 750 mg (IM)

SIDE EFFECTS
CNS: Fever, somnolence, **seizures,** confusion, dizziness, weakness, myoclonia
CV: Hypotension, palpitations, tachycardia
GI: Diarrhea, nausea, vomiting, **pseudomembranous colitis, hepatitis,** glossitis
HEMA: **Eosinophilia, neutropenia,** decreased Hgb, Hct
INTEG: Rash, urticaria, pruritus, pain at injection site, phlebitis, erythema at injection site
RESP: Chest discomfort, dyspnea, hyperventilation
SYST: **Anaphylaxis, Stevens-Johnson syndrome**
Contraindications: Hypersensitivity, IM hypersensitivity to local anesthetics of the amide type
Precautions: Pregnancy (C), lactation, geriatric, hypersensitivity to penicillins,

Side effects: *italics* = common; **bold** = life-threatening

seizure disorders, renal disease, children, head trauma

PHARMACOKINETICS

IV: Onset immediate, peak ½-1 hr, half-life 1 hr; 70%-80% excreted unchanged in urine

INTERACTIONS

Increase: imipenem plasma levels—probenecid
Increase: antagonistic effect—β-lactam antibiotics
Increase: seizure risk—ganciclovir, theophylline, aminophylline, cycloSPORINE
Drug/Herb
• Do not use acidophilus with antiinfectives; separate by several hours
Drug/Lab Test
Increase: AST, ALT, LDH, BUN, alk phos, bilirubin, creatinine
False-positive: Direct Coombs' test

NURSING CONSIDERATIONS
Assess:
• For infection: increased temp, WBC, characteristics of wounds, sputum, urine culture or stool culture
• Sensitivity to penicillin—may have sensitivity to this drug
• Renal disease: lower dose may be required
• Bowel pattern daily; if severe diarrhea occurs, drug should be discontinued; may indicate pseudomembranous colitis
⚠ Allergic reactions, anaphylaxis: rash, urticaria, pruritus, wheezing, laryngeal edema; may occur few days after therapy begins; have epINEPHrine, antihistamine, emergency equipment available
• Overgrowth of infection: perineal itching, fever, malaise, redness, pain, swelling, drainage, rash, diarrhea, change in cough, sputum
Administer:
• After C&S is taken
IM route
• Reconstitute 500 mg/2 ml; or 750 mg/3 ml lidocaine without epINEPHrine; shake

IV route
• After reconstitution of 250 or 500 mg with 10 ml of diluent and shake; add to at least 100 ml of same inf sol
• 250-500 mg over 20-30 min; 1 g over 40-60 min; give through Y-tube or 3-way stopcock; do not give by IV bolus or if cloudy

Y-site compatibilities: Acyclovir, amifostine, aztreonam, cefepime, cisatracurium, diltiazem, famotidine, fludarabine, foscarnet, granisetron, idarubicin, insulin (regular), melphalan, methotrexate, ondansetron, propofol, remifentanil, tacrolimus, teniposide, thiotepa, vinorelbine, zidovudine

Evaluate:
• Therapeutic response: negative C&S; absence of signs and symptoms of infection

Teach patient/family:
⚠ To report severe diarrhea; may indicate pseudomembranous colitis
⚠ To report sore throat, bruising, bleeding, joint pain; may indicate blood dyscrasias (rare)

Treatment of anaphylaxis: EpINEPHrine, antihistamines; resuscitate if needed

---

imipramine (℞)
(im-ip′ra-meen)
Apo-Imipramine ✦, imipramine HCl ✦, Impril ✦, Norfranil, Novo Pramine ✦, Tipramine, Tofranil, Tofranil PM
Func. class.: Antidepressant, tricyclic
Chem. class.: Dibenzazepine, tertiary amine

Do not confuse:
imipramine/desipramine

Action: Blocks reuptake of norepinephrine, serotonin into nerve endings, increasing action of norepinephrine, serotonin in nerve cells
Uses: Depression, enuresis in children

Unlabeled uses: Chronic pain, migraine headaches, cluster headaches as adjunct, incontinence

DOSAGE AND ROUTES

• *Adult:* **PO/IM** 75-100 mg/day in divided doses, may increase by 25-50 mg to 200 mg, not to exceed 300 mg/day; may give daily dose at bedtime
• *Geriatric:* **PO** 25 mg at bedtime, may increase to 100 mg/day in divided doses
• *Child:* **PO** 25-75 mg/day
Enuresis
• *Child 6-12 yr:* **PO** 10 mg at bedtime, max 50 mg
Available forms: Tabs 10, 25, 50, 75 mg; inj 25 mg/2 ml (12.5 mg/ml); caps 75, 100, 125, 150 mg

SIDE EFFECTS

CNS: Dizziness, drowsiness, confusion, **seizures,** headache, anxiety, tremors, stimulation, weakness, insomnia, nightmares, EPS (geriatric), increased psychiatric symptoms, paresthesia
CV: Orthostatic hypotension, ECG changes, tachycardia, hypertension, palpitations, **dysrhythmias**
EENT: Blurred vision, tinnitus, mydriasis
GI: Diarrhea, dry mouth, nausea, vomiting, **paralytic ileus;** increased appetite; cramps, epigastric distress, jaundice, **hepatitis,** stomatitis, constipation, taste change
GU: Retention, **acute renal failure**
HEMA: **Agranulocytosis, thrombocytopenia, eosinophilia, leukopenia**
INTEG: Rash, urticaria, sweating, pruritus, photosensitivity
Contraindications: Hypersensitivity to tricyclics, recovery phase of MI, convulsive disorders, prostatic hypertrophy
Precautions: Pregnancy (C), suicidal patients, severe depression, increased intraocular pressure, narrow-angle glaucoma, urinary retention, hepatic/cardiac disease, hyperthyroidism, electroshock therapy, elective surgery, geriatric, lactation

PHARMACOKINETICS

PO: Steady state 2-5 days; metabolized by liver; excreted in urine, breast milk, feces; crosses placenta; half-life 6-20 hr

INTERACTIONS

⚠ Hyperpyretic crisis, seizures, hypertensive episode: MAOIs, clonidine
⚠ *Increase:* toxicity: SSRIs, avoid concurrent use
Increase: effects of direct-acting sympathomimetics (epINEPHrine), alcohol, barbiturates, benzodiazepines, CNS depressants
Decrease: effects of guanethidine, clonidine, indirect-acting sympathomimetics (epHEDrine)
Drug/Herb
Increase: anticholinergic effect—belladonna, corkwood, henbane, jimsonweed, scopolia
Increase: imipramine action—chamomile, hops, kava, lavender, skullcap, valerian
Increase: hypertension—yohimbe
Increase: serotonin syndrome—SAM-e, St. John's wort
Drug/Lab Test
Increase: Serum bilirubin, alk phos, blood glucose
Decrease: 5-HIAA, VMA, urinary catecholamines

NURSING CONSIDERATIONS

Assess:
• B/P (lying, standing), pulse q4h; if systolic B/P drops 20 mm Hg, hold drug, notify prescriber; take vital signs q4h in patients with cardiovascular disease
• Blood studies: CBC, leukocytes, differential, cardiac enzymes if patient is receiving long-term therapy
• Hepatic studies: AST, ALT, bilirubin
• Weight qwk; appetite may increase with drug
⚠ ECG for flattening of T wave, bundle branch block, AV block, dysrhythmias in cardiac patients
• EPS primarily in geriatric: rigidity, dystonia, akathisia

Side effects: *italics* = common; **bold** = life-threatening

• Mental status: mood, sensorium, affect, suicidal tendencies, increase in psychiatric symptoms: depression, panic
• Urinary retention, constipation; constipation is more likely to occur in children, geriatric
⚠ Withdrawal symptoms: headache, nausea, vomiting, muscle pain, weakness, diarrhea, insomnia, restlessness; not usual unless drug is discontinued abruptly
• Alcohol consumption; if alcohol is consumed, hold dose until morning

Administer:
• Not to break, crush, or chew caps
• Increased fluids, bulk in diet for constipation, urinary retention
• With food or milk for GI symptoms
• Dosage at bedtime if oversedation occurs during day; may take entire dose at bedtime; geriatric may not tolerate once/day dosing
• Sugarless gum, hard candy, or frequent sips of water for dry mouth
• In IM route after running warm water over ampule to dissolve crystals

Syringe compatibilities: Doxapram
Y-site compatibilities: Cladribine

Perform/provide:
• Storage in tight container at room temperature; do not freeze
• Assistance with ambulation during beginning therapy, since drowsiness/dizziness, orthostatic hypotension occurs
• Safety measures, primarily in geriatric

Evaluate:
• Therapeutic response: decreased depression, enuresis, pain

Teach patient/family:
• That therapeutic effects may take 2-3 wk
• That drug is dispensed in small amounts because of suicide potential, especially in beginning of therapy
• To use caution in driving, other activities requiring alertness because of drowsiness, dizziness, blurred vision
• To report urinary retention immediately
• To avoid alcohol ingestion, other CNS depressants during treatment
• Not to discontinue medication quickly

after long-term use; may cause nausea, headache, malaise
• To wear sunscreen or large hat, since photosensitivity occurs
• To rise slowly, orthostatic hypotension may occur

Treatment of overdose: ECG monitoring; induce emesis; lavage, activated charcoal; administer anticonvulsant

---

immune globulin IM
gamma globulin, IG, IGIM
Bay Gam

immune globulin IV (IGIV) (℞)
Carimune NF, Flebogamma 5%, Gamimune N, Gammagard S/D, gamma globulin, Gammar-P IV, Gamunex, Iveegam, Octagam, Panglobulin NF, Polygam, Polygam S/D, Sandoglobulin, Venoglobulin-I, Venoglobulin-S

Func. class.: Immune serum
Chem. class.: IgG

Action: Provides passive immunity to hepatitis A, measles, varicella, rubella, immune globulin deficiency; contains gamma globulin antibodies (IgG)

Uses: Immunodeficiency syndrome, B-cell chronic lymphocytic leukemia, Kawasaki syndrome, bone marrow transplantation, pediatric HIV infection, agammaglobulinemia, hepatitis A, B exposure, measles exposure, measles vaccine complications, purpura, rubella exposure, chickenpox exposure

Unlabeled uses: IV posttransfusion purpura, Guillain-Barré syndrome, chronic inflammatory demyelinating polyneuropathy

DOSAGE AND ROUTES
Primary immunodeficiency
• *Adult and child:* IV (Carimune NF, Panglobulin NF) 200 mg/kg qmo, max 300 mg/kg qmo or give more frequently

if needed; **IV** (Gamimune N) 100-200 mg/kg qmo, max 400 mg/kg; **IV** (Gammagard S/D) 200-400 mg qmo, minimum 100 mg/kg qmo; **IV** (Gamunex) 300-600 mg/kg q3-4wk; **IV** (Iveegam EN) 200 mg/kg qmo, max 800 mg/kg; **IV** (Octagam) 300-600 mg/kg q3-4wk; **IV** (Polygam S/D) 200-400 mg/kg qmo

Hepatitis A exposure (IGIM)
• *Adult and child:* **IM** 0.02-0.04 ml/kg

Chickenpox exposure (IGIM)
• *Adult and child:* **IM** 0.6-1.2 ml/kg as soon as exposed

Measles (postexposure)(IGIM)
• *Adult and child:* **IM** 0.25 ml/kg within 6 days

B-cell chronic lymphocytic leukemia (CLL)(IGIV) (Gammagard S/D, Polygam S/D)
• *Adult:* **IV** 400 mg/kg q3-4wk

Idiopathic thrombocytopenia, purpura
• *Adult and child:* **IV** 0.4 g/kg/day × 5 days or 1 g/kg/day × 1-2 days

Kawasaki syndrome to prevent coronary artery aneurysm (IGIV) (Iveegam, Venoglobulin-S, Gammagard S/D, Polygam S/D)
• *Adult and child:* **IV** (Iveegam, Venoglobulin-S 5% or 10%) 2000 mg/kg over 10-12 hr, may repeat; **IV** (Gammagard S/D) 1 g/kg as single dose

Bone marrow transplantation (IGIV) (Gamimune N)
• *Adults >20 yr:* **IV** 500 mg/kg 5% or 10% sol on days 2, 7 before transplant, then qwk for 90 days thereafter

Pediatric HIV (IGIV) (Gamimune N)
• *Child:* **IV** 400 mg/kg 5% or 10% sol q28days

Available forms: *IM:* Inj 2-, 10-ml vial (Bay Gam); *IV:* 5%, 10% sol (Gamimune N, Venoglobulin-S); powder for inj 1-, 3-, 6-, 12-g vials (Carimune NF; 50 mg protein/ml in 2.5-, 5-, 10-g vials (Gammagard S/D); 1-, 2.5-, 5-, 10-g vials (Gammar-P IV); 500 mg, 1-, 2.5-, 5-g vials (Iveegam); 6-, 12-g vials (Panglobulin); 2.5-, 5-, 10-g vials (Polygam S/D);

sol for inj 1-, 2.5-, 5-, 10-, 20-g vials (Gamunex)

SIDE EFFECTS
CNS: Headache, fatigue, malaise
GI: Abdominal pain
INTEG: Pain at inj site, rash, pruritus, chills
MS: Arthralgia, chest pain
SYST: Lymphadenopathy, **anaphylaxis**
Contraindications: Hypersensitivity
Precautions: Pregnancy (C)

INTERACTIONS
• Do not administer live virus vaccines within 3 mo of this drug

NURSING CONSIDERATIONS
Assess:
• For exposure date: this drug should be given within 6 days of measles, 7 days of hepatitis B, 14 days of hepatitis A
• For anaphylaxis: diaphoresis, wheezing, chest tightness, hypotension
Administer:
• IM ≤3 ml in one site, use large muscle mass
• Only with epINEPHrine 1:1000, resuscitative equipment available
• Only within 2 wk of exposure to hepatitis A
• Immune globulin should not be given SUBCUT, IV, or intradermally
IV route
• Gamimune N: IV undiluted or dilute with D₅; give 0.01 ml/kg/min; may increase to 0.02-0.04 ml/kg/min
• Sandoglobulin: IV diluted with provided diluent; give 0.5-1 ml/min × 15-30 min; may increase to 1.5-2.5 ml/min
• Venoglobulin-I: (50 mg/ml sol) give 0.01-0.02 ml/kg/min; if no adverse reaction in ½ hr, increase to 0.04 ml/kg/min, store at room temperature
• Gammagard: reconstitute with sterile H₂O for inj (50 mg protein/ml); give 0.5 ml/kg/hr, may increase to 4 ml/kg/hr, use infusion set provided
• Gammar-IV: give 0.01 ml/kg/min (50 mg/ml sol) × 15-30 min, may increase to 0.02 ml/kg/min, may increase to 0.03-0.06 ml/kg/min

Y-site compatibilities: Fluconazole, sargramostim
Perform/provide:
• Storage at 36°-46° F (2°-8° C)
Evaluate:
• Prevention of infection, increased platelets
Teach patient/family:
• That passive immunity is temporary
• The treatment of anaphylaxis: epINEPHrine, diphenhydrAMINE, O₂, vasopressors, corticosteroids

⚠ High Alert

inamrinone (℞)
(in-am′rih-nohn)
Inocor
Func. class.: Inotropic
Chem. class.: Bipyrimidine derivative

Do not confuse:
inamrinone/amiodarone
Action: Positive inotropic agent with vasodilator properties; reduces preload and afterload by direct relaxation of vascular smooth muscle, increases cardiac output
Uses: Short-term management of CHF that has not responded to other medication (diuretics, other vasodilators); can be used with digoxin

DOSAGE AND ROUTES
• *Adult and child:* IV **BOL** 0.75 mg/kg given over 2-3 min; start inf of 5-10 mcg/kg/min; may give another bol 30 min after start of therapy, max 10 mg/kg total daily dose
• *Infant:* IV 3-4.5 mg/kg in divided doses, then give by inf 10 mcg/kg/min
• *Neonate:* IV 3-4.5 mg/kg in divided doses, then give by inf 3-5 mcg/kg/min
Available forms: Inj 5 mg/ml

SIDE EFFECTS
CV: **Dysrhythmias,** *hypotension,* chest pain

GI: Nausea, vomiting, anorexia, abdominal pain, **hepatotoxicity (rare), ascites,** jaundice, hiccups
HEMA: **Thrombocytopenia**
INTEG: Allergic reactions, burning at inj site
RESP: Pleuritis, **pulmonary densities, hypoxemia**
Contraindications: Hypersensitivity to this drug or bisulfites, severe aortic disease, severe pulmonic valvular disease, acute MI
Precautions: Pregnancy (C), lactation, children, renal/hepatic disease, atrial flutter/fibrillation, geriatric, asthma

PHARMACOKINETICS
IV: Onset 2-5 min, peak 10 min, duration variable; half-life 4-6 hr, metabolized in liver, excreted in urine as drug and metabolites 60%-90%

INTERACTIONS
• Excessive hypotension: antihypertensives, disopyramide
• Additive effect: cardiac glycosides
Drug/Herb
Increase: amrinone action—aloe, buckthorn, cascara sagrada, senna
Drug/Lab Test
Increase: Hepatic enzymes
Decrease: Serum K

NURSING CONSIDERATIONS
Assess:
• B/P and pulse q5min during infusion; if B/P drops 30 mm Hg, stop infusion and call prescriber
• Electrolytes: K, S, Cl, Ca; renal studies: BUN, creatinine; blood studies: platelet count; monitor fluid status (CVP) in geriatric
• ALT, AST, bilirubin daily
• I&O ratio and weight daily; diuresis should increase with continuing therapy
⚠ If platelets are <150,000/mm³, drug is usually discontinued and another drug started
• Extravasation; change site q48h

Administer:
IV route
• Solution should be clear yellow
• Do not mix directly with dextrose solutions; chemical reaction occurs over 24 hr; precipitate forms if inamrinone and furosemide come in contact
• May inject into running dextrose infusion through Y-connector or directly into tubing; may give undiluted over 2-3 min or dilute with 0.9%, 0.45% NaCl to 1-3 mg/ml, run at prescribed rate by continuous infusion
• By infusion pump for doses other than bolus
• Potassium supplements if ordered for potassium levels <3.0, correct before using amrinone

Syringe compatibilities: Propranolol, verapamil

Y-site compatibilities: Aminophylline, atropine, bretylium, calcium chloride, cimetidine, cisatracurium, digoxin, DOBUTamine, DOPamine, epINEPHrine, famotidine, hydrocortisone, isoproterenol, lidocaine, metaraminol, methylPREDNISolone, nitroglycerin, nitroprusside, norepinephrine, phenylephrine, potassium chloride, propofol, propranolol, remifentanil, verapamil

Evaluate:
• Therapeutic response: increased cardiac output, decreased PCWP, adequate CVP, decreased dyspnea, fatigue, edema, ECG

Teach patient/family:
• That burning may occur at IV site
• To report adverse reactions promptly
• Not to breastfeed unless approved by prescriber

Treatment of overdose: Discontinue drug, support circulation

indapamide (R)
(in-dap′a-mide)
indapamide, Lozide ✤ Lozol
Func. class.: Diuretic—thiazide-like, antihypertensive
Chem. class.: Indoline

Action: Acts on proximal section of distal renal tubule by inhibiting reabsorption of sodium; may act by direct vasodilation caused by blocking of calcium channels
Uses: Edema of CHF, hypertension, diuresis

DOSAGE AND ROUTES
Edema
• *Adult:* **PO** 2.5 mg daily in AM; may be increased to 5 mg daily if needed
Antihypertensive
• *Adult:* **PO** 1.25-5 mg daily; may increase to 5 mg/day over 8 wk
Available forms: Tabs 1.25, 2.5 mg

SIDE EFFECTS
CNS: Headache, dizziness, fatigue, weakness, nervousness, agitation, extremity numbness, depression
CV: Orthostatic hypotension, volume depletion, palpitations, dysrhythmias, PVCs
EENT: Blurred vision, nasal congestion, increased intraocular pressure
ELECT: Hypochloremic alkalosis, hypomagnesemia, hyperuricemia, hypercalcemia, hyponatremia, hypokalemia, hyperglycemia
GI: Nausea, diarrhea, dry mouth, vomiting, anorexia, cramps, constipation, abdominal pain
GU: Polyuria, nocturia, urinary frequency, impotence
INTEG: Rash, pruritus
MS: Cramps
Contraindications: Hypersensitivity, anuria, hepatic coma
Precautions: Pregnancy (B), hypokalemia, dehydration, ascites, hepatic disease, severe renal disease, lactation, CCr <25 ml/min (not effective)

PHARMACOKINETICS

Well absorbed (PO), widely distributed, metabolized by liver, excreted by kidney (small amounts); onset 1-2 hr, peak 2 hr, duration up to 36 hr; excreted in urine, feces; half-life 14-18 hr

INTERACTIONS

Increase: hyperglycemia—diazoxide

Increase: toxicity of muscle relaxants, steroids, lithium, digoxin

Decrease: hypokalemia—steroids, amphotericin B, other diuretics

Decrease: effects—antidiabetics, antigout agents, anticoagulants

Decrease: absorption—cholestyramine, colestipol

Decrease: hypotensive effect—indomethacin, NSAIDs

Drug/Herb

• Severe photosensitivity: St. John's wort

Increase: hypokalemia—aloe, buckthorn, cascara sagrada, Chinese cucumber, licorice, senna

Increase: diuretic effect—aloe, cucumber, dandelion, horsetail, pumpkin, Queen Anne's lace

Drug/Lab Test

Increase: Calcium, parathyroid test glucose, uric acid

NURSING CONSIDERATIONS

Assess:

• Weight daily, I&O daily to determine fluid loss; effect of drug may be decreased if used daily

• Rate, depth, rhythm of respiration, effect of exertion

• B/P lying, standing; postural hypotension may occur

• Electrolytes: K, Mg, Na, Cl: include BUN, CBC, serum creatinine, blood pH, ABGs, uric acid, Ca, glucose

• Signs of metabolic alkalosis, hypokalemia

• Rashes, fever daily; allergy to sulfa products

• Confusion, especially in geriatric; take safety precautions if needed

• Hydration: skin turgor, thirst, dry mucous membranes

Administer:

• In AM to avoid interference with sleep

• With food, if nausea occurs; absorption may be decreased slightly

Evaluate:

• Therapeutic response: improvement in edema of feet, legs, sacral area daily, decreased B/P

Teach patient/family:

• Diet high in potassium; to rise slowly from lying or sitting position

• To recognize adverse reactions: muscle cramps, weakness, nausea, dizziness

• To take with food or milk for GI symptoms

• To take early in day to prevent nocturia

• To notify prescriber if urinary output decreases; daily weight

Treatment of overdose: Lavage if taken orally; monitor electrolytes, administer IV fluids; monitor hydration, CV, renal status

indinavir (℞)

(en-den'a-veer)

Crixivan

Func. class.: Antiretroviral

Chem. class.: Protease inhibitor

Do not confuse:

indinavir/Denavir

Action: Inhibits human immunodeficiency virus (HIV-1) protease; this prevents maturation of virus

Uses: HIV-1 in combination with other antiretrovirals

Unlabeled uses: Prevention of HIV-1 after exposure

DOSAGE AND ROUTES

• Reduce dose in mild/moderate hepatic impairment and ketoconazole coadministration

• *Adult:* **PO** 800 mg q8h; if given with ddI, give 1 hr apart on empty stomach

Available forms: Caps 100, 200, 333, 400 mg

SIDE EFFECTS

CNS: Headache, insomnia, dizziness, somnolence
GI: Diarrhea, abdominal pain, nausea, vomiting, anorexia, dry mouth
GU: Nephrolithiasis
INTEG: Rash
MS: Pain
OTHER: Asthenia, **insulin-resistant hyperglycemia,** hyperlipidemia, **ketoacidosis,** lipodystrophy
Contraindications: Hypersensitivity
Precautions: Pregnancy (C), lactation, children, renal/hepatic disease, history of renal stones, diabetes, hypercholesterolemia

PHARMACOKINETICS

Terminal half-life 1-2 hr, 60% protein binding, metabolized liver, excreted 20% unchanged in urine

INTERACTIONS

⚠ Life-threatening dysrhythmias: ergots, midazolam, rifampin, triazolam
Increase: myopathy—atorvastatin, lovastatin, simvastatin
Increase: indinavir levels—ketoconazole, delavirdine, itraconazole
Increase: levels of both drugs—clarithromycin, zidovudine
Increase: levels of isoniazid, oral contraceptives
Decrease: indinavir levels—rifamycins, fluconazole, nevirapine, efavirenz
Decrease: of both drugs—anticonvulsants
Drug/Herb
Decrease: indinavir levels—St. John's wort; avoid concurrent use
Drug/Food
Decrease: indinavir absorption—grapefruit juice, high-fat, high-protein foods
Drug/Lab Test
Increase: AST, ALT, amylase, total bilirubin

NURSING CONSIDERATIONS

Assess:
• For complaints of lower back, flank pain, indicates kidney stones
• Signs of infection, anemia, the presence of other sexually transmitted diseases
• Hepatic studies: ALT, AST; total bilirubin, amylase, all may be elevated
• Viral load, CD4 during treatment
• Bowel pattern before, during treatment; if severe abdominal pain with bleeding occurs, drug should be discontinued; monitor hydration
• Skin eruptions; rash, urticaria, itching
• Allergies before treatment, reaction of each medication; place allergies on chart
Administer:
• Do not break, crush, or chew caps
• With water, 1 hr before or 2 hr after meals; may be given with other liquids or small meal; do not give with high-fat, high-protein meals
• Dosage adjustment will need to be considered when given with efavirenz
• Water to 1.5 L/day minimum to prevent nephrolithiasis
Teach patient/family:
• To take as prescribed; if dose is missed, take as soon as remembered up to 1 hr before next dose; do not double dose
• That drug must be taken in equal intervals around the clock to maintain blood levels for duration of therapy
⚠ That hyperglycemia may occur; watch for increased thirst, weight loss, hunger, dry, itchy skin; notify prescriber
• To increase fluids to prevent kidney stones, if stone formation occurs, treatment may need to be interrupted
• That drug does not cure AIDS, only controls symptoms; not to donate blood

indomethacin (℞)
(in-doe-meth'a-sin)
Apo-Indomethacin ✦
Indameth ✦, Indocid ✦,
Indocin, Indocin IV, Indocin
PDA ✦, Indocin SR,
indomethacin, Indomethacin
Extended-Release,
Indomethacin SR,
Novomethacin ✦, Nu-Indo ✦
Func. class.: Nonsteroidal antiin-
flammatory drug (NSAID), antirheu-
matic
Chem. class.: Propionic acid deriva-
tive

Action: Inhibits prostaglandin synthesis
by decreasing enzyme needed for biosynthesis; analgesic, antiinflammatory, antipyretic
Uses: Rheumatoid arthritis, ankylosing
spondylitis, osteoarthritis, bursitis, tendinitis, acute gouty arthritis; closure of patent ductus arteriosus in premature infants (IV)

DOSAGE AND ROUTES
Arthritis/antiinflammatory
• *Adult:* **PO** 25-50 mg bid; may increase
by 25 mg/day qwk, not to exceed 200 mg/
day; **SUS REL** 75 mg daily, may increase
to 75 mg bid
Acute arthritis
• *Adult:* **PO** 100 mg intially, then 50 mg
tid; use only for acute attack, then reduce
dose
Patent ductus arteriosus
Longer or repeated treatment courses may
be necessary for very premature infants
• *Infant <2 days:* **IV** 0.2 mg/kg, then
0.1 mg/kg × 2 doses after 12, 24 hr
• *Infant 2-7 days:* **IV** 0.2 mg/kg, then
0.2 mg/kg × 2 doses after 12, 24 hr
• *Infant >7 days:* **IV** 0.2 mg/kg, then
0.25 mg/kg × 2 doses after 12, 24 hr
Available forms: Caps 25, 50 mg; sus
rel caps 75 mg; oral susp 25 mg/5 ml; inj
1-mg vial

SIDE EFFECTS
CNS: Dizziness, drowsiness, fatigue, tremors, confusion, insomnia, anxiety, depression, headache
CV: Tachycardia, peripheral edema, palpitations, dysrhythmias, hypertension, **CV
thrombotic events, MI, stroke**
EENT: Tinnitus, hearing loss, blurred vision
GI: Nausea, anorexia, *vomiting,* diarrhea,
jaundice, **cholestatic hepatitis,** *constipation,* flatulence, cramps, dry mouth,
peptic ulcer, **ulceration, perforation**,
GI bleeding
GU: **Nephrotoxicity: dysuria, hematuria, oliguria, azotemia**
HEMA: **Blood dyscrasias,** prolonged
bleeding
INTEG: Purpura, rash, pruritus, sweating
Contraindications: Pregnancy (X)
2nd/3rd trimester, hypersensitivity,
asthma, severe renal/hepatic disease, ulcer disease, perioperative pain in CABG
Precautions: Pregnancy (B) 1st trimester, lactation, children, bleeding disorders, GI disorders, cardiac disorders, hypersensitivity to other antiinflammatory
agents, depression

PHARMACOKINETICS
PO: Onset 1-2 hr, peak 3 hr, duration
4-6 hr; metabolized in liver, kidneys;
excreted in urine, bile, feces; crosses
placenta; excreted in breast milk; 99%
plasma protein binding

INTERACTIONS
Increase: hyperkalemia—potassium-
sparing diuretics
Increase: toxicity—lithium, methotrexate, cycloSPORINE, zidovudine
Increase: effect of digoxin, penicillamine,
phenytoin, aminoglycosides
Increase: bleeding risk—anticoagulants,
abciximab, cefamandole, cefoperazone,
cefotetan, clopidogrel, eptifibatide, plicamycin, ticlopidine, tirofiban, valproic acid,
thrombolytics, aspirin
Decrease: effect of antihypertensives

Drug/Herb
Increase: bleeding risk—anise, arnica, bogbean, chamomile, chondroitin, clove, dong quai, feverfew, garlic, ginger, ginkgo, ginseng (*Panax*)
Increase: gastric irritation—arginine, gossypol
Increase: NSAIDs effect—bearberry, bilberry

NURSING CONSIDERATIONS
Assess:
• Arthritis symptoms: ROM, pain, swelling before and 2 hr after treatment
• Patent ductus arteriosus: respiratory rate, character, heart sounds
• Renal, hepatic, blood studies: BUN, creatinine, AST, ALT, Hgb, before treatment, periodically thereafter; if renal function has decreased, do not give subsequent doses
• For eye, ear problems: blurred vision, tinnitus; may indicate toxicity; audiometric, ophthalmic exam before, during, after treatment if on long-term therapy
• For confusion, mood changes, hallucinations, especially in geriatric
• For asthma, nasal polyps, aspirin sensitivity, may develop hypersensitivity to indomethacin
Administer:
PO route
• Do not break, crush, or chew sus rel cap or reg caps.
• With food to decrease GI symptoms and prevent ulcerations
• Shake susp, do not mix with other liquids
IV route
• After diluting 1-2 mg/ml or more NS or sterile H$_2$O for inj without preservative; 5-10 sec to avoid dramatic shift in cerebral blood flow
Y-site compatibilities: Furosemide, insulin (regular), potassium chloride, sodium bicarbonate, sodium nitroprusside
Perform/provide:
• Storage at room temperature
Evaluate:
• Therapeutic response: decreased pain, stiffness in joints, decreased swelling in joints, ability to move more easily

Teach patient/family:
• To report blurred vision, ringing, roaring in ears; may indicate toxicity
• To avoid driving, other hazardous activities if dizziness, drowsiness occurs
• To report change in urine pattern, increased weight, edema, increased pain in joints, fever, blood in urine; indicate nephrotoxicity; to report mood changes: anxiety, depression
• That therapeutic antiinflammatory effects may take up to 1 mo
• To avoid alcohol, NSAIDs, salicylates; bleeding may occur

infliximab
(in-fliks'ih-mab)
Remicade
Func. class.: Monoclonal antibody

Action: Monoclonal antibody that neutralizes the activity of tumor necrosis factor alpha (TNF α) found in Crohn's disease; decreased infiltration of inflammatory cells
Uses: Crohn's disease, fistulizing (moderate-severe); rheumatoid arthritis given with methotrexate
Unlabeled uses: Plaque psoriasis, ankylosing spondylitis, ulcerative colitis, psoriatic arthritis, psoriasis, Behçet's syndrome, uveitis, juvenile arthritis

DOSAGE AND ROUTES
Crohn's disease (moderate-severe)
• *Adult:* **IV INF** 5 mg/kg × 1
Crohn's disease (fistulizing)
• *Adult:* **IV INF** 5 mg/kg initially, then repeat dose 2 wk, 6 wk after 1st dose
Rheumatoid arthritis
• *Adult:* **IV** 3 mg/kg initially and q2, 6, 8wk thereafter given with methotrexate
Available forms: Powder for inj 100 mg

SIDE EFFECTS
CNS: Headache, dizziness, depression, vertigo, fatigue, anxiety, fever, **seizures,** *chills, flulike symptoms*

CV: Chest pain, hyper/hypotension, **tachycardia,** CHF

GI: Nausea, vomiting, abdominal pain, stomatitis, constipation, dyspepsia, flatulence

GU: Dysuria, urinary frequency

HEMA: **Anemia**

INTEG: Rash, dermatitis, urticaria, dry skin, sweating, flushing, hematoma, pruritus

MS: Myalgia, back pain, arthralgia

RESP: URI, pharyngitis, bronchitis, cough, dyspnea, sinusitis

SYST: **Anaphylaxis, fatal infections, sepsis, malignancies, immunogenicity**

Contraindications: Hypersensitivity to murines, moderate to severe CHF (NYHA Class III/IV)

Precautions: Pregnancy (B), lactation, children, geriatric

PHARMACOKINETICS

Distributed to vascular compartment, half-life 9.5 days

INTERACTIONS

• Do not administer live vaccines concurrently

NURSING CONSIDERATIONS
Assess:
• For rheumatoid arthritis, ROM, pain
• GI symptoms: nausea, vomiting, abdominal pain
• Periodic blood counts (CBC)
• CV status: B/P, pulse, chest pain

⚠ Allergic reaction, anaphylaxis: rash, dermatitis, urticaria, dyspnea, hypotension, fever, chills; discontinue if severe, administer epINEPHrine, corticosteroids, antihistamines; assess for allergies to murine proteins before starting therapy

⚠ Fatal infections: discontinue if infection occurs, do not administer to patients with active infections

• Identify TB before beginning treatment, a TB test should be obtained, if present, TB should be treated prior to receiving infliximab

Administer:
IV INF route
• Give immediately after reconstitution; reconstitute each vial with 10 ml of sterile water for inj; further dilute total dose/250 ml of 0.9% NaCl inj to a total conc of 0.4-4 mg/ml; use 21G or smaller needle for reconstitution; direct sterile water at glass wall of vial; gently swirl; do not shake; may foam; allow to stand for 5 min, give within 3 hr
• Give over ≥2 hr, use polyethylene-lined infusion with in-line, sterile, low-protein-bind filter
• Do not admix

Perform/provide:
• Refrigerated storage, do not freeze

Evaluate:
• Therapeutic response: absence of fever, mucus in stools

Teach patient/family:
• Not to breastfeed while taking this drug
• To notify prescriber of GI symptoms, hypersensitivity reactions
• Not to operate machinery, drive if dizziness, vertigo occur

⚠ High Alert

INSULINS

Rapid Acting
insulin glulisine (℞)
Apidra
insulin aspart (℞)
Novolog
insulin lispro (℞)
Humalog

Short Acting
insulin, regular (OTC)
Humulin R ✦ Novolin R, Novolin R PenFill, Novolin R Prefilled
insulin, regular concentrated (℞)
regular (concentrated)

Intermediate Acting
insulin, isophane suspension (NPH) (otc)
Humulin N, Novolin N, Novolin N PenFill, Novolin N Prefilled
insulin, zinc suspension (Lente) (otc)
Novolin GE Lente ✤, Novolin L

Long Acting
insulin detemir (℞)
Levemir
insulin glargine (℞)
Lantus

Mixtures
insulin, isophane suspension and regular insulin (℞)
Humulin 70/30, Humalin 30/70 ✤, Novolin 70/30, Novolin 70/30 PenFill, Novolin 70/30 Prefilled, Novolin ge 30/70 ✤
isophane insulin suspension (NPH) and insulin mixtures (℞)
Humulin 50/50, Novolin 50/50
insulin lispro mixture (℞)
Humalog Mix 75/25
insulin aspart mixture (℞)
Novolog Mix 70/30

Func. class.: Antidiabetic, pancreatic hormone

Chem. class.: Modified structures of endogenous human insulin

Do not confuse:
Lantus/lente
Novolin 70/30 PenFill/Novolin 70/30 Prefilled

Action: Decreases blood glucose; by transport of glucose into cells and the conversion of glucose to glycogen, indirectly increases blood pyruvate and lactate, decreases phosphate and potassium; insulin may be human (processed by recombinant DNA technologies)

Uses: Type 1 diabetes mellitus, type 2 diabetes mellitus, gestational diabetes, insulin lispro may be used in combination with sulfonylureas in children >3 yr

DOSAGE AND ROUTES
Insulin glulisine
• *Adult:* **SUBCUT** dosage individualized, give within 15 min before or 20 min after starting a meal

Insulin aspart
• *Adult and child ≥6 yr:* 0.5-1 unit/kg/day divided in treatment, meal-related, highly individualized

Insulin lispro
• *Adult:* **SUBCUT** 15 min ac

Human regular
• *Adult:* **SUBCUT** ½-1 ac

Insulin, isophane suspension
• *Adult:* **SUBCUT** dosage individualized by blood, urine glucose; usual dose 7-26 units; may increase by 2-10 units/day if needed

Insulin detemir
• *Adult:* **SUBCUT** 1 or 2 times daily; if 1 time, give with evening meal

Insulin glargine
• *Adult and child ≥ 6 yr:* **SUBCUT** 10 international units daily, range 2-100 international units/day

Regular insulin (ketoacidosis)
• *Adult:* **IV** 5-10 units, then 5-10 units/hr until desired response, then switch to **SUBCUT** dose; **IV/inf** 2-12 units (50 units/500 ml of normal saline)
• *Child:* **IV** 0.1 units/kg

Replacement
• *Adult and child:* **SUBCUT** 0.5-1 units/kg/day qid given 30 min before meals
• *Adolescent:* **SUBCUT** 0.8-1.2 mg/kg/

day; this dosage is used during rapid growth

Available forms: *NPH* Inj 100 units/ml; *regular* inj 100 units/ml, cartridges 100 units/ml; *zinc susp* 100 units/ml; *insulin analog* inj 100 units/ml; *insulin zinc suspension, (lente)* inj 100 units/ml; *isophane insulin* inj 100 units/ml, cartridges 100 units/ml; *insulin lispro* 100 units/ml, 1.5-ml cartridges; *insulin glulisine* inj 100 units/ml; *insulin glargine* inj 100 units/ml; *insulin detemir* inj 100 units/ml in 10 vials, 3-ml cartridges; Flex Pen solution for inj 100 units/ml

SIDE EFFECTS

EENT: Blurred vision, dry mouth
INTEG: Flushing, rash, urticaria, warmth, *lipodystrophy,* lipohypertrophy, swelling, redness
META: Hypoglycemia, rebound hyperglycemia (Somogyi effect 12-72 hr or longer)
SYST: **Anaphylaxis**

Contraindications: Hypersensitivity to protamine
Precautions: Pregnancy (B) lispro, (C) all others

PHARMACOKINETICS

Rapid acting
Insulin glulisine: Onset 15-30 min, peak ½-1½ hr, duration, 3-4 hr
Insulin aspart: Onset 10-20 min, peak 1-3 hr, duration 3-5 hr
Insulin lispro: Onset 15-30 min, peak ½-1½ hr, duration 3-4 hr

Short acting
Insulin regular: Onset 30 min, peak 2.5-5 hr, duration up to 6 hr

Intermediate acting
Insulin, isophane suspension (NPH): Onset 1.5-4 hr, peak 4-12 hr, duration up to 24 hr
Insulin, zinc suspension (Lente): Onset 3-4 hr, peak 6-12 hr, duration 12-18 hr

Long acting
Insulin detemir: Onset 0.8-2 hr, peak unknown, duration up to 24 hr

Insulin glargine: Onset 5 hr, no peak identified, duration ≥24 hr

Mixtures
Insulin, isophane suspension and regular insulin (70/30): Onset 10-20 min, peak 2.4 hr, duration up to 24 hr
Insophane insulin suspension (NPH) and insulin mixtures (50/50): Onset ½-1 hr, peak dual, duration 10-16 hr

INTERACTIONS

Increase: hypoglycemia—salicylate, alcohol, β-blockers, anabolic steroids, fenfluramine, phenylbutazone, sulfinpyrazone, guanethidine, oral hypoglycemics, MAOIs, tetracycline
Decrease: hypoglycemia—thiazides, thyroid hormones, oral contraceptives, corticosteroids, estrogens, DOBUTamine, epINEPHrine

Drug/Herb
Increase: antidiabetic effect—alfalfa, aloe, basil, bay, bilberry, bitter melon, black catechu, buchu, burdock, coriander, dandelion, eyebright (po), fenugreek, garlic, ginseng, glucomannan, glucosamine, goat's rue, gymnema, horehound, horse chestnut, jambul, myrrh, myrtle
Increase: glucose tolerance—karela
Increase: hypoglycemics—aceitilla, adiantum agrimony, aloe gel, banana flowers/roots, banyan stembark, bilberry, bitter melon, broom, bugleweed, burdock, carob, cumin, damiana, dandelion, eucalyptus, fenugreek, fo-ti, garlic, goat's rue, guar gum, horse chestnut, jambue, juniper, konjac, maitake, onion, psyllium, reishi
Decrease or increase: hypoglycemic effect—chromium
Decrease: hypoglycemic effect—annato, cocoa seeds, coffee seeds, cola seeds, guarana, ma huang, yerba maté, rosemary
Decrease: antidiabetic effect—bee pollen, blue cohosh, broom, chromium, elecampane, eucalyptus, gotu kola

Drug/Lab Test
Increase: VMA
Decrease: Potassium, calcium
Interference: LFTs, thyroid function studies

NURSING CONSIDERATIONS
Assess:
• Fasting blood glucose, 2 hr PP (80-150 mg/dl, normal fasting level; 70-130 mg/dl, normal 2 hr level); also A1c may be drawn to identify treatment effectiveness q3mo
• Urine ketones during illness; insulin requirements may increase during stress, illness, surgery
• For hypoglycemic reaction that can occur during peak time (sweating, weakness, dizziness, chills, confusion, headache, nausea, rapid weak pulse, fatigue, tachycardia, memory lapses, slurred speech, staggering gait, anxiety, tremors, hunger)
• For hyperglycemia: acetone breath, polyuria, fatigue, polydipsia, flushed, dry skin, lethargy
Administer:
SUBCUT route
• After warming to room temperature by rotating in palms to prevent injecting cold insulin; use only insulin syringes with markings or syringe matching units/ml; rotate inj sites within one area: abdomen, upper back, thighs, upper arm, buttocks; keep record of sites
• Increased dosages if tolerance occurs
• Premixed insulins and NPH are cloudy suspensions
• Regular human insulin, rapid-acting analogs, and long-acting analogs are clear; do not use if cloudy, thick, or discolored
IV route
⚠ When regular insulin is administered IV, monitor glucose, potassium often to prevent fatal hypoglycemia, hypokalemia
• IV direct, undiluted via vein, Y-site, 3-way stopcock; give at 50 units/min or less
• By cont inf after diluting with IV sol and run at prescribed rate; use IV inf pump for correct dosing; give reduced dose at serum glucose level of 250 mg/100 ml

Additive compatibilities: Bretylium, cimetidine, lidocaine, meropenem, ranitidine, verapamil
Syringe compatibilities: Metoclopramide
Y-site compatibilities: Amiodarone, ampicillin, ampicillin/sulbactam, aztreonam, cefazolin, cefotetan, DOBUTamine, esmolol, famotidine, gentamicin, heparin, heparin/hydrocortisone, imipenem/cilastatin, indomethacin, magnesium sulfate, meperidine, meropenem, midazolam, morphine, nitroglycerin, oxytocin, pentobarbital, potassium chloride, propofol, ritodrine, sodium bicarbonate, sodium nitroprusside, tacrolimus, terbutaline, ticarcillin, ticarcillin/clavulanate, tobramycin, vancomycin, vit B/C
Perform/provide:
• Store at room temperature for <1 mo (some insulins); keep away from heat and sunlight; refrigerate all other supply; NPH, premixed insulins are cloudy; regular, rapid-acting analogs, long-acting analogs are clear; do not freeze—IV route, regular only
Evaluate:
• Therapeutic response: decrease in polyuria, polydipsia, polyphagia, clear sensorium, absence of dizziness, stable gait
Teach patient/family:
• That blurred vision occurs; not to change corrective lens until vision is stabilized 1-2 mo
• To keep insulin, equipment available at all times; carry a glucagon kit, candy, or lump sugar to treat hypoglycemia
• That drug does not cure diabetes but controls symptoms
• To carry emergency ID as diabetic
• To recognize hypoglycemia reaction: headache, tremors, fatigue, weakness
• To recognize hyperglycemia reaction: frequent urination, thirst, fatigue, hunger
• The dosage, route, mixing instructions, if any diet restrictions, disease process
• The symptoms of ketoacidosis: nausea, thirst, polyuria, dry mouth, decreased B/P, dry, flushed skin, acetone breath, drowsiness, Kussmaul respirations

• That a plan is necessary for diet, exercise; all food on diet should be eaten; exercise routine should not vary
• About blood glucose testing; make sure patient is able to determine glucose level
• To avoid OTC drugs unless directed by prescriber

Treatment of overdose: Glucose 25 g IV, via dextrose 50% sol, 50 ml or glucagon 1 mg

---

⚠ High Alert

insulin, inhaled (℞)
Exubera
Func. class.: Antidiabetic, pancreatic hormone, inhaled
Chem. class.: Exogenous unmodified insulin

Action: Decreases blood glucose; by transport of glucose into cells and the conversion of glucose to glycogen, indirectly increases blood pyruvate and lactate, decreases phosphate and potassium; processed by recombinant DNA technologies

Uses: Adult patients with type 1 or type 2 diabetes mellitus

DOSAGE AND ROUTES

• *Adult:* **INH** insert dose in handheld inhalation device and inhale 10 min before meal

Available forms: Inhaled, dry powder 1, 3 mg unit dose blisters (3 of the 1 mg blister packs is not equal to 1, 3 mg blister pack)

SIDE EFFECTS

EENT: Blurred vision, dry mouth, cough
GI: Nausea, vomiting, weight gain
META: Hypoglycemia, insulin resistance
RESP: **Bronchospasm,** laryngitis, dyspnea, epistaxis, rhinitis, sinusitis
SYST: **Anaphylaxis,** antibody formation

Contraindications: Hypersensitivity; poorly controlled, unstable lung disease; smokers; those who have quit smoking within the last 6 mo, diabetic ketoacidosis, hyperosmolar hyperglycemic state

(HHs), hypoglycemia, mannitol hypersensitivity

Precautions: Pregnancy (C); chronic lung disorders (asthma, bronchitis, emphysema); renal/hepatic disease; cystic fibrosis

PHARMACOKINETICS

INH: Onset 10-20 min, peak 49 min, range 30-90 min, duration 6 hr, mean bioavailability is 10% of regular insulin (SUBCUT)

INTERACTIONS

Increase: hypoglycemia—salicylate, alcohol, β-blockers, anabolic steroids, sulfinpyrazone, guanethidine, oral hypoglycemics, MAOIs, ACE inhibitors, fibric acid derivatives
Decrease: hypoglycemia—thiazides, thyroid hormones, oral contraceptives, corticosteroids, estrogens, atypical psychotics, progestins

NURSING CONSIDERATIONS

Assess:
• Fasting blood glucose, 2 hr PP (80-150 mg/dl, normal fasting level; 70-130 mg/dl, normal 2 hr level); also A1c may be drawn to identify treatment effectiveness
• For hypoglycemic reaction that can occur during peak time (sweating, weakness, dizziness, chills, confusion, headache, nausea, rapid weak pulse, fatigue, tachycardia, memory lapses, slurred speech, staggering gait, anxiety, tremors, hunger)
• For hyperglycemia: acetone breath, polyuria, fatigue, polydipsia, flushed, dry skin, lethargy

Administer:
• 10 min before meal
• 1 mg and 3 mg blisters are used in combination, consecutive inhalation of 3 (1 mg blisters) is associated with 30%-40% greater insulin exposure than 1 (3 mg blister); they are not interchangeable
• SUBCUT regular insulin 3 units = 1 mg Exubera (1 blister pack)

⚠ Safety alert   *"Tall Man" lettering

Evaluate:
• Therapeutic response: decrease in polyuria, polydipsia, polyphagia, clear sensorium, absence of dizziness, stable gait; improving A1c

Teach patient/family:
• That if blurred vision occurs, not to change corrective lens until vision is stabilized 1-2 mo
• To keep insulin, equipment available at all times
• That drug does not cure diabetes but controls symptoms
• To carry emergency ID as diabetic
• To recognize hypoglycemia reaction: headache, tremors, fatigue, weakness
• The dosage, route, mixing instructions, if any diet restrictions, disease process
• To carry candy or lump sugar to treat hypoglycemia
• The symptoms of ketoacidosis: nausea, thirst, polyuria, dry mouth, decreased B/P, dry, flushed skin, acetone breath, drowsiness, Kussmaul respirations
• That a plan is necessary for diet, exercise; all food on diet should be eaten; exercise routine should not vary
• About blood glucose testing; make sure patient is able to determine glucose level in order to self monitor
• To avoid OTC drugs unless directed by prescriber

Treatment of overdose: Glucose 25 g IV, via dextrose 50% sol, 50 ml or glucagon 1 mg

---

interferon alfa-2a (recombinant)
Roferon-A

interferon alfa-2b (recombinant)
a-2-interferon, Intron A

Func. class.: Antineoplastic—miscellaneous
Chem. class.: Protein product

Do not confuse:
Roferon-A/Imferon

Action: Antiviral action inhibits viral replication by reprogramming virus; antitumor action suppresses cell proliferation; immunomodulating action phagocytizes target cells; may also inhibit virus replication in virus-infested cells

Uses: Hairy cell leukemia in persons >18 yr, condylomata acuminata, malignant melanoma, AIDS (use phase II with zidovudine), chronic hepatitis B, C

Unlabeled uses: Bladder tumors, carcinoid tumors, non-Hodgkin's lymphoma, essential thrombocytopenia, cytomegaloviruses, herpes simplex, Kaposi's sarcoma, HPV-associated diseases

DOSAGE AND ROUTES

alfa-2a
Hairy cell leukemia
• *Adult:* **SUBCUT/IM** 3 million international units/day × 16-24 wk, then 3 million international units 3 ×/wk maintenance

Condylomata acuminata
• 1 million international units/lesion 3 ×/wk × 3 wk

alfa-2b
Chronic hepatitis B
• *Adult:* 3 million international units/3 ×/wk × 18-24 mo **SUBCUT/IM** as 5 million international units/day or 10 million international units/3 ×/wk × 16 wk

Hairy cell leukemia
• 2 million international units/m² 3 ×/wk; if severe adverse reactions occur, dose should be skipped or reduced by ½

Kaposi's sarcoma
• *Adult:* **SUBCUT/IM** 30 million international units/m² 3 ×/wk

Available forms: *alfa-2a:* inj 3, 6, 36 million international units/ml; *alfa-2b:* inj 3, 5, 10, 18, 25 million units/vial, powder for inj 5, 10, 18, 25, 50 million units/vial

SIDE EFFECTS

CNS: Dizziness, confusion, numbness, paresthesias, hallucinations, **seizures, coma,** amnesia, anxiety, mood changes, depression, somnolence, paranoia, irritability

CV: Edema, hypotension, hypertension,

---

chest pain, palpitations, dysrhythmias, **CHF, MI, CVA,** tachycardia, syncope

GI: Weight loss, taste changes, nausea, anorexia, diarrhea, xerostomia

GU: Impotence

HEMA: **Neutropenia, thrombocytopenia**

INTEG: Rash, dry skin, itching, alopecia, flushing, photosensitivity

MISC: Flulike syndrome; fever, fatigue, myalgias, headache, chills

Contraindications: Hypersensitivity

Precautions: Pregnancy (C), severe hypotension, dysrhythmia, tachycardia, lactation, children, severe renal/hepatic disease, seizure disorder

PHARMACOKINETICS

Half-life (interferon alfa-2a) 3.7-8.5 hr, peak 3-4 hr; half-life (interferon alfa-2b) 2-7 hr, peak 6-8 hr

INTERACTIONS

Increase: theophylline levels—aminophylline

Increase: neutropenia—zidovudine

Drug/Lab Test

Interference: AST, ALT, LDH, alk phos, WBC, platelets, granulocytes, creatinine

NURSING CONSIDERATIONS

Assess:

• For symptoms of infection; chills, fever, headache; may be masked by drug fever

• CNS reaction: LOC, mental status, dizziness, confusion, paresthesia, slurred speech, anxiety, depression, paranoia, hallucinations

• Cardiac status: lung sounds; ECG before and during treatment, especially in those with cardiac disease; MI, CHF, CVA may occur

• Bone marrow depression: bruising, bleeding, blood in stools, urine, sputum, emesis

• Mental status: depression, suicidal thoughts, hallucinations, amnesia

• CBC with diff before and during treatment, nadirs of leukopenia/thrombocytopenia occurs in 18-19 days (alfa-2a);

recovery is in 3-4 wk; if granulocytes <750/mm^3 or platelets <50,000/mm^2, reduce by 50%; if granulocytes <500/mm^3 or platelets <30,000/mm^2 discontinue

Administer:

alfa-2a

• SUBCUT/IM after reconstituting 18 million units/3 ml of diluent provided (6 million units/ml)

• 36 million units/ml is used for Kaposi's sarcoma only

alfa-2b

• IM/SUBCUT after reconstituting 3-5 million international units/1 ml, 10 million international units/2 ml, 25 million international units/5 ml, of diluent provided, mix gently

• Intralesional after reconstituting 10 million international units/1 ml bacteriostatic water for inj; no more than 5 lesions can safely be treated at a time

• At bedtime to minimize side effects

• Acetaminophen as ordered to alleviate fever and headache

Perform/provide:

• Reconstituted sol must be used within 30 days

• Increased fluid intake to 2-3 L/day

Evaluate:

• Therapeutic response: decrease in size, number of lesions

Teach patient/family:

• To take acetaminophen for fever

• To avoid hazardous tasks, since confusion, dizziness may occur; avoid prolonged sunlight, use sunscreen

• That brands of this drug should not be changed; each form is different, with different doses

• That fatigue is common; activity may have to be altered; to take at bedtime to minimize flulike symptoms

• Not to become pregnant while taking drug; possible mutagenic effects

• To report signs of infection: sore throat, fever, diarrhea, vomiting, sore or white patches in mouth

• That impotence may occur during treatment but is temporary

• That emotional lability is common; notify prescriber if severe or incapacitating

---

interferon alfacon-1 (R)

(in-ter-feer'on al'fa-kon)
Infergen
Func. class.: Recombinant type 1 interferon

Action: Induces biologic responses and has antiviral, antiproliferative, and immunomodulatory effects

Uses: Chronic hepatitis C infections in those 18 yr and older with compensated liver disease who have anti-HCV antibodies or HCV RNA

Unlabeled uses: Hairy cell leukemia when used with G-CSF

DOSAGE AND ROUTES

• *Adult:* SUBCUT 9 mcg as a single inj 3 ×/wk × 24 wk
Available forms: Inj 9 mcg/0.3 ml, 15 mcg/0.5 ml

SIDE EFFECTS

CNS: Depression, headache, fatigue, fever, rigors, insomnia, dizziness
CV: Hypertension, palpitation
EENT: Tinnitus, earache, conjunctivitis, eye pain
GI: Abdominal pain, nausea, diarrhea, anorexia, dyspepsia, vomiting, constipation, flatulence, hemorrhoids, decreased salivation
GU: Dysmenorrhea, vaginitis, menstrual disorders
HEMA: **Granulocytopenia, thrombocytopenia, leukopenia,** ecchymosis
INTEG: Alopecia, pruritus, rash, erythema, dry skin
MS: Back, limb, neck skeletal pain
PSYCH: Nervousness, depression, anxiety, lability, abnormal thinking
RESP: Pharyngitis, upper respiratory infection, cough, sinusitis, rhinitis, respiratory tract congestion, epistaxis, dyspnea, bronchitis
Contraindications: Hypersensitivity to alpha interferons, or products from *Escherichia coli*

Precautions: Pregnancy (C), thyroid disorders, myelosuppression, hepatic/cardiac disease, lactation, children <18 yr, seizure disorder

PHARMACOKINETICS
Peak 24-36 hr

INTERACTIONS
• None known

NURSING CONSIDERATIONS
Assess:
• For past or present history of depression, seizures; use with caution in these disorders
• Platelet counts, heme concentration, ANC, serum creatinine concentration, albumin, bilirubin, TSH, T$_4$
• For myelosuppression: hold dose if neutrophil count is <500 × 10^6/L or if platelets are <50 × 10^9/L
• For hypersensitivity: discontinue immediately if hypersensitivity occurs
Evaluate:
• Therapeutic response: decreased chronic hepatitis C signs/symptoms
Teach patient/family:
• Provide patient or family member with written, detailed information about drug

interferon alfa-n 3 (R)

(in-ter-feer'on)
Alferon N
Func. class.: Antineoplastic, antiviral
Chem. class.: Human interferon α-protein

Action: Binds interferon to membrane receptors on cell surface with high specificity; this produces protein synthesis, inhibition of virus replication, suppression of cell proliferation, increased phagocytosis

Uses: Condylomata acuminata (venereal/genital warts), papillomavirus

Unlabeled uses: Adenovirus, coronavirus, encephalomyocarditis virus, hepatitis B virus, hepatitis C infection/virus, hepatitis D, herpes simplex type 1 and 2, HIV, HTLV-I, poliovirus, rhinovirus, varicella-zoster virus, variola virus, vesicular stomatitis virus

DOSAGE AND ROUTES
External condylomata acuminata
• *Adult:* 0.05 ml (250,000 international units) per wart, given 2 ×/wk × 8 wk; not to exceed 0.5 ml (2.5 million international units); inject into base of wart
Chronic hepatitis C (unlabeled)
• *Adult:* **SUBCUT/IM** 3-6 million international units 3 ×/wk
Available forms: Inj 5 m international units/L ml vial with 3.3 mg/ml phenol and 1 mg/ml human albumin

SIDE EFFECTS
CNS: Fever, headache, sweating, vasovagal reaction, chills, fatigue, dizziness, insomnia, sleepiness, depression
CV: Chest pain, hypotension
GI: Nausea, vomiting, heartburn, diarrhea, constipation, anorexia, stomatitis, dry mouth
INTEG: Pain at inj site, pruritus
MS: Myalgias, arthralgia, back pain, flulike symptoms
Contraindications: Hypersensitivity to this product, egg protein, IgG, neomycin, murine protein
Precautions: Pregnancy (C), lactation, children, CHF, angina (unstable), COPD, diabetes mellitus with ketoacidosis, hemophilia, pulmonary embolism, thrombophlebitis, bone marrow depression, seizure disorder

PHARMACOKINETICS
Unable to detect

INTERACTIONS
Drug/Lab Test
Interference: AST, ALT, LDH, alk phos, WBC, platelets, granulocytes, creatinine

NURSING CONSIDERATIONS
Assess:
• For symptoms of infection; may be masked by drug fever

• CNS reaction: LOC, mental status, dizziness, confusion, insomnia, depression
• For body image disturbance
Administer:
• Acetaminophen to alleviate fever and headache
Perform/provide:
• Storage of reconstituted sol for 1 mo in refrigerator
• Increased fluid intake to 2-3 L/day
Evaluate:
• Therapeutic response: decrease in wart size
Teach patient/family:
• To avoid hazardous tasks, since confusion, dizziness may occur
• That brands of this drug should not be changed; each form is different, with different doses
• That fatigue is common; activity may have to be altered
• Not to become pregnant while taking drug; possible mutagenic effects
• To report signs of infection: sore throat, fever, diarrhea, vomiting
• To recognize the signs of hypersensitivity: liver, urticaria, wheezing, dyspnea; notify prescriber immediately

interferon beta-1a
(in-ter-feer'on)
Avonex, Rebif
interferon beta-1b (℞)
Betaseron
Func. class.: Multiple sclerosis agent, immune modifier
Chem. class.: Interferon, *Escherichia coli* derivative

Action: Antiviral, immunoregulatory; action not clearly understood; biologic response modifying properties mediated through specific receptors on cells, inducing expression of interferon-induced gene products
Uses: Ambulatory patients with relapsing-remitting multiple sclerosis

Unlabeled uses: May be useful in treatment of AIDS, AIDS-related Kaposi's sarcoma, malignant melanoma, metastatic renal cell carcinoma, cutaneous T cell lymphoma, acute non-A, non-B hepatitis

DOSAGE AND ROUTES

Interferon beta-1a
• *Adult:* IM 30 mcg qwk
Interferon beta-1b
Relapsing-remitting multiple sclerosis
• *Adult:* SUBCUT 0.25 mg (8 international units) every other day
Available forms: *beta-1a:* 33 mcg (6.6 million international units/vial); *beta-1b:* powder for inj 0.3 mg (9.6 m international units)

SIDE EFFECTS

CNS: Headache, fever, pain, chills, mental changes, depression, hypertonia, **suicide attempts, seizures**
CV: Migraine, palpitations, hypertension, tachycardia, peripheral vascular disorders
EENT: Conjunctivitis, blurred vision
GI: Diarrhea, constipation, vomiting, abdominal pain
GU: Dysmenorrhea, irregular menses, metrorrhagia, cystitis, breast pain
HEMA: **Decreased lymphocytes, ANC, WBC;** *lymphadenopathy*
INTEG: Sweating, inj site reaction
MS: Myalgia, **myasthenia**
RESP: Sinusitis, dyspnea

Contraindications: Hypersensitivity to natural or recombinant interferon-β or human albumin, hamster protein
Precautions: Pregnancy (C), lactation, child <18 yr, chronic progressive MS, depression, mental disorders, seizure disorder, latex allergy

PHARMACOKINETICS

beta-1a: Onset up to 12 hr, peak 48 hr, duration 4 days, half-life 8-6 hr
beta-1b: Onset rapid, peak 2-8 hr, duration unknown, half-life 8 min-4.3 hr

INTERACTIONS

Increase: myelosuppression—antineoplastics
Decrease: clearance of zidovudine
Drug/Herb
• Change in immunomodulation: astragalus, echinacea, melatonin

NURSING CONSIDERATIONS

Assess:
• Blood, renal, hepatic studies: CBC, differential, platelet counts, BUN, creatinine ALT, urinalysis; if absolute neutrophil count <750/mm^3, or if AST/ALT is 10 × normal, drug is discontinued
• CNS symptoms: headache, fatigue, depression
• GI status: diarrhea or constipation, vomiting, abdominal pain
• Cardiac status: increased B/P, tachycardia
• Mental status: depression, depersonalization, suicidal thoughts, insomnia
• For multiple sclerosis symptoms
Administer:
• Acetaminophen for fever, headache
• SUBCUT only; products are not interchangeable
Interferon beta-1a
• Reconstitute with 1.1-ml diluent, swirl, give within 6 hr
Interferon beta-1b
• Reconstitute by injecting diluent provided (1.2 ml) into vial; swirl (8 m international units/ml); use 27G needle for inj
Perform/provide:
• Storage in refrigerator; do not freeze
Evaluate:
• Therapeutic response: decreased symptoms of multiple sclerosis
Teach patient/family:
• To provide patient or family member with written, detailed information about the drug
• That blurred vision, sweating may occur
• That female patients may experience irregular menses, dysmenorrhea, or metrorrhagia as well as breast pain

- To use sunscreen to prevent photosensitivity
- To notify prescriber if pregnancy is suspected
- Inj technique and care of equipment
- To notify prescriber of increased temp, chills, muscle soreness, fatigue

---

interferon gamma-1b (℞)

(in-ter-feer'on)

Actimmune

Func. class.: Biologic response modifier

Chem. class.: Lymphokine, interleukin type

Action: Species-specific protein synthesized in response to viruses, effects; can mediate killing of *Staphylococcus aureus, Toxoplasma gondii, Leishmania donovani, Listeria monocytogenes, Mycobacterium avium intracellulare;* enhances oxidative metabolism of macrophages, enhances antibody-dependent cellular cytotoxicity

Uses: Serious infections associated with chronic granulomatous disease, osteoporosis

Unlabeled uses: Osteoporosis, *Mycobacterium avium* complex (MAC), ovarian cancer, pulmonary fibrosis

DOSAGE AND ROUTES

- *Adult:* **SUBCUT** 50 mcg/m^2 (1.5 million units/m^2) for patients with surface area >0.5 m^2; 1.5 mcg/kg/dose for patient with surface area <0.5 m^2; give Monday, Wednesday, Friday for 3 ×/wk dosing

Available forms: Inj 100 mcg (3 million units)/single-dose vial

SIDE EFFECTS

CNS: Headache, fatigue, depression, fever, chills

GI: Nausea, anorexia, abdominal pain, weight loss, diarrhea, vomiting

INTEG: Rash, pain at inj site

MS: Myalgia, arthralgia

Contraindications: Hypersensitivity to interferon-γ, *Escherichia coli*-derived products

Precautions: Pregnancy (C), cardiac disease, seizure disorders, CNS disorders, myelosuppression, lactation, children

PHARMACOKINETICS

SUBCUT: Dose absorbed 89%, elimination half-life 5.9 hr, peak 7 hr

INTERACTIONS

- May interfere with fosphenytoin, phenytoin, warfarin

Increase: myelosuppression—other myelosuppressive agents

Increase: level of theophylline, aminophylline

NURSING CONSIDERATIONS

Assess:

- Blood, renal, hepatic studies: CBC, differential, platelet counts, BUN, creatinine, ALT, urinalysis
- CNS symptoms: headache, fatigue, depression

Administer:

- At bedtime to minimize adverse reactions; administer acetaminophen for fever, headache
- 50% of dose if severe reactions occur or discontinue treatment until reactions subside
- In right and left deltoid and anterior thigh
- Warm to room temperature before use; do not leave at room temperature over 12 hr (unopened vial)

Perform/provide:

- Storage in refrigerator upon receipt; do not freeze; do not shake

Evaluate:

- Therapeutic response: decreased serious infections, improvement in existing infections and inflammatory conditions

Teach patient/family:

- The method of administration if family members will be giving medication
- Provide patient or family member with written, detailed information about drug

---

ipratropium (℞)

(i-pra-troe′pee-um)
Atrovent HFA
Func. class.: Anticholinergic, bronchodilator
Chem. class.: Synthetic quaternary ammonium compound

Do not confuse:
Atrovent/Alupent

Action: Inhibits interaction of acetylcholine at receptor sites on the bronchial smooth muscle, resulting in decreased cGMP and bronchodilation

Uses: COPD; rhinorrhea in children 6-11 yr (nasal spray)

DOSAGE AND ROUTES

• *Adult:* 1-4 **INH** 4 × day, not to exceed 24 **INH**/24 hr; sol 250-500 mcg (1 unit dose) given 3-4 ×/day
• *Child:* **INH** 1-2 inhalations q6-8h; **NEB** 125-250 mcg q4-6h
• *Child 5-12 yr:* **NASAL** 1 spray in each nostril

Available forms: Aerosol 18 mcg/actuation; nasal spray 0.03%, 0.06%; sol for inh 0.0125% ♣, 0.02%

SIDE EFFECTS

CNS: Anxiety, dizziness, headache, nervousness
CV: Palpitation
EENT: Dry mouth, blurred vision
GI: Nausea, vomiting, cramps
INTEG: Rash
RESP: Cough, worsening of symptoms, **bronchospasms**

Contraindications: Hypersensitivity to this drug, atropine, soya lecithin

Precautions: Pregnancy (B), lactation, children <12 yr, narrow-angle glaucoma, prostatic hypertrophy, bladder neck obstruction

PHARMACOKINETICS

Half-life 2 hr; does not cross blood-brain barrier

INTERACTIONS

Increase: toxicity—other bronchodilators (INH)
Increase: anticholinergic action—phenothiazines, antihistamines, disopyramide

Drug/Herb
Increase: constipation—black catechu
Increase: anticholinergic effect—butterbur, jimsonweed
Increase: bronchodilator effect—green tea (large amts), guarana
Decrease: anticholinergic effect—jaborandi tree, pill-bearing spurge

NURSING CONSIDERATIONS

Assess:
• For palpitations; if severe, drug may have to be changed
• For tolerance over long-term therapy; dose may have to be increased or changed
• Atropine sensitivity; may also be sensitive to this product
• Respiratory status: rate, rhythm, auscultate breath sounds prior to and after administration

Administer:
Nebulizer
• Use sol in nebulizer with a mouthpiece rather than a face mask

Nasal spray
• Priming pump initially requires 7 actuations of the pump, priming again is not necessary if used regularly

Perform/provide:
• Storage at room temperature
• Hard candy, frequent drinks, sugarless gum to relieve dry mouth

Evaluate:
• Therapeutic response: ability to breathe adequately

Teach patient/family:
• That compliance is necessary with number of inhalations/24 hr or overdose may occur; spacer device in the geriatric
• To shake before using
• The correct method of inhalation and cleaning of equipment daily

---

Side effects: *italics* = common; **bold** = life-threatening

irbesartan (R)

(er-be-sar'tan)
Avapro
Func. class.: Antihypertensive
Chem. class.: Angiotensin II receptor
blocker (Type AT_1)

Do not confuse:
Avapro/Anaprox

Action: Blocks the vasoconstrictor and aldosterone-secreting effects of angiotensin II; selectively blocks the binding of angiotensin II to the AT_1 receptor found in tissues

Uses: Hypertension, alone or in combination; nephropathy in type 2 diabetic patients

Unlabeled uses: Heart failure

DOSAGES AND ROUTES

Hypertension
• *Adult:* **PO** 150 mg daily; may be increased to 300 mg daily

Neuropathy in type 2 diabetic patients
• *Adult:* **PO** maintenance dose 300 mg daily, start 75 mg daily
• *Child 13-16 yr:* **PO** 150 mg daily, may increase to 300 mg daily
• *Child 6-12 yr:* **PO** 75 mg daily, may increase to 150 mg daily

Volume- and salt-depleted patients
• *Adult:* **PO** 75 mg daily

Available forms: Tabs 75, 150, 300 mg

SIDE EFFECTS

CNS: Dizziness, anxiety, headache, fatigue
CV: Hypotension
GI: Diarrhea, dyspepsia
MISC: Edema, chest pain, rash, tachycardia, UTI, **angioedema,** hyperkalemia
RESP: Cough, upper respiratory infection, sinus disorder, pharyngitis, rhinitis
Contraindications: Pregnancy (D) 2nd/3rd trimester, hypersensitivity
Precautions: Pregnancy (C) 1st trimester, hypersensitivity to ACE inhibitors; lactation, children, geriatric, hepatic/renal disease; renal artery stenosis

PHARMACOKINETICS

Peak 1.5-2 hr, extensively metabolized, half-life 11-15 hr, highly bound to plasma proteins, excreted in urine and feces, protein binding 90%

INTERACTIONS

Increase: hyperkalemia: potassium-sparing diuretics, potassium salt substitutes
Increase: irbesartan—CYP2C9 inhibitors
Decrease: antihypertensive effect—NSAIDs
Drug/Herb
Increase: toxicity, death—aconite
Increase: antihypertensive effect—barberry, betony, black catechu, black cohosh, bloodroot, broom, burdock, cat's claw, dandelion, goldenseal, hawthorn, Irish moss, Jamaican dogwood, kelp, khella, mistletoe, parsley
Increase or decrease: antihypertensive effect—astragalus, cola tree
Decrease: antihypertensive effect—coltsfoot, guarana, khat, licorice, yohimbine

NURSING CONSIDERATIONS

Assess:
• B/P, pulse q4h; note rate, rhythm, quality
• Electrolytes: K, Na, Cl
• Baselines in renal, hepatic studies before therapy begins
• Edema in feet, legs daily
• Skin turgor, dryness of mucous membranes for hydration status
Administer:
• Without regard to meals
Evaluate:
• Therapeutic response: decreased B/P
Teach patient/family:
• To comply with dosage schedule, even if feeling better
• That drug may cause dizziness, fainting; light-headedness may occur

• To rise slowly to sitting or standing position to minimize orthostatic hypotension

• To notify prescriber if pregnancy is suspected

⚠ High Alert

irinotecan (R̠)
(ear-een-oh-tee'kan)
Camptosar
Func. class.: Antineoplastic hormone
Chem. class.: Topoisomerase inhibitor

Action: Cytotoxic by producing damage to double-strand DNA during DNA synthesis

Uses: Metastatic carcinoma of the colon or rectum, or 1st-line treatment in combination with 5-FU and leucovorin for metastatic colon or rectal carcinomas

DOSAGE AND ROUTES
Single agent
• *Adult:* IV 125 mg/m^2 given over 1½ hr qwk × 4 wk, then 2-wk rest period, may be repeated; 4 wk or 2 wk off; dosage adjustments may be made to 150 mg/m^2 (high) or 50 mg/m^2 (low); adjustments should be made in increments of 25-50 mg/m^2 depending on patient's tolerance

Combination dosage schedules
• *Regimen 1:* irinotecan 75-125 mg/m^2, leucovorin 20 mg/m^2, 5-FU 300-500 mg/m^2 depending on dosing levels
• *Regimen 2:* irinotecan 120-180 mg/m^2, leucovorin 200 mg/m^2, 5-FU BOL 240-400 mg/m^2, 5-FU infusion 360-600 mg/m^2

Hepatic dose
• *Adult:* IV 100 mg/m^2 qwk × 4 wk, then 2-wk rest, may repeat cycle or 300 mg/m^2 q3wk, dose may be adjusted up or down
Available forms: Inj 20 mg/ml

SIDE EFFECTS
CNS: Fever, headache, chills, dizziness
CV: Vasodilation
GI: **Severe diarrhea,** nausea, vomiting, anorexia, constipation, cramps, flatus, stomatitis, dyspepsia, **hepatotoxicity**
HEMA: **Leukopenia, anemia, neutropenia**
INTEG: Irritation at site, rash, sweating, alopecia
MISC: Edema, asthenia, weight loss
RESP: Dyspnea, increased cough, rhinitis
Contraindications: Pregnancy (D), hypersensitivity
Precautions: Lactation, children, geriatric, myelosuppression, irradiation

PHARMACOKINETICS
Rapidly and completely absorbed; excreted in urine and bile as metabolites; half-life 10 hr, bound to plasma proteins 30%-68%

INTERACTIONS
Increase: myelosuppression, diarrhea—other antineoplastics, radiation
Increase: lymphocytopenia—dexamethasone
Increase: akathisia—prochlorperazine
Increase: dehydration—diuretics

NURSING CONSIDERATIONS
Assess:
• For CNS symptoms: fever, headache, chills, dizziness
• CBC, differential, platelet count weekly; withhold drug if WBC is <2000/mm^3, or platelet count <100,000/mm^3, Hgb ≤9 g/dl, neutrophil ≤1000/mm^3; notify prescriber of these results; drug should be discontinued and colony-stimulating factor given
• Buccal cavity q8h for dryness, sores or ulceration, white patches, oral pain, bleeding, dysphagia
⚠ GI symptoms: frequency of stools; cramping; severe life-threatening diarrhea may occur with fluid and electrolyte imbalances
• Signs of dehydration: rapid respira-

tions, poor skin turgor, decreased urine output, dry skin, restlessness, weakness
• Bone marrow depression: bruising, bleeding, blood in stools, urine, sputum, emesis

Administer:
• Antiemetics and dexamethasone 10 mg at least ½ hr before antineoplastics
• Use cytotoxic handling procedure after preparing in biologic cabinet using gloves, mask, gown
• Early diarrhea and other cholinergic symptoms can be treated with atropine
• Late diarrhea must be treated promptly with loperimide; late diarrhea can be life-threatening

IV route
• By intermittent inf after diluting with 0.9% NaCl or D_5 (0.12-1.1 mg/ml); give over 1½ hr
• Do not admix with other solutions or medications
• Stable for 24 hr at room temperature; 48 hr, refrigerated

Perform/provide:
• Increased fluid intake to 2-3 L/day to prevent dehydration, unless contraindicated
• Changing of IV site q48h
• Rinsing of mouth tid-qid with water, club soda; brushing of teeth bid-tid with soft brush or cotton-tipped applicator for stomatitis; use unwaxed dental floss
• Nutritious diet with iron, vitamin supplement, low fiber, few dairy products

Evaluate:
• Therapeutic response: decrease in tumor size, decrease in spread of cancer

Teach patient/family:
• To avoid foods with citric acid or hot or rough texture if stomatitis is present; to drink adequate fluids
• To report stomatitis; any bleeding, white spots, ulcerations in mouth; tell patient to examine mouth daily, report symptoms
• To report signs of anemia: fatigue, headache, faintness, shortness of breath, irritability
• To use contraception during therapy
• To avoid salicylates, NSAIDs, alcohol; bleeding may occur

• About alopecia, that when hair grows back, it will be different texture, thickness
• To avoid vaccinations while taking this drug
⚠ To report diarrhea that occurs 24 hr after administration, severe dehydration can occur rapidly

Treatment of overdose: Induce vomiting, provide supportive care, prevent dehydration

---

iron dextran (℞)

DexFerrum, Imferon, InFeD
Func. class.: Hematinic
Chem. class.: Ferric hydroxide complex with dextran

Do not confuse:
Imferon/Imuran
Imferon/Roferon-A

Action: Iron is carried by transferrin to the bone marrow, where it is incorporated into hemoglobin

Uses: Iron deficiency anemia

DOSAGE AND ROUTES
• *Adult and child:* IM 0.5 ml as a test dose by Z-track, then no more than the following per day:
• *Adult <50 kg:* IM 100 mg
• *Adult >50 kg:* IM 250 mg
• *Child <5-9 kg:* IM 50 mg
• *Infant <5 kg:* IM 25 mg
• *Adult:* IV 0.5 ml (25 mg) test dose, then 100 mg daily after 2-3 days; give 25 mg test dose, wait 5 min, then infuse over 6-12 hr or use equation that follows:

$$0.3 \times wt\ (lb) \times \frac{100\text{-Hgb (g/dl)} \times 100}{14.8} = mg\ iron$$

<30 lb (66 kg) should be given 80% of above formula dose

Available forms: Inj 50 mg/ml (2-ml, 10-ml vials)

SIDE EFFECTS
CNS: Headache, paresthesia, dizziness, shivering, weakness, **seizures**

CV: Chest pain, **shock,** hypotension, tachycardia
GI: Nausea, vomiting, metallic taste, abdominal pain
HEMA: **Leukocytosis**
INTEG: Rash, pruritus, urticaria, fever, sweating, chills, brown skin discoloration, pain at inj site, necrosis, sterile abscesses, phlebitis
OTHER: **Anaphylaxis**
RESP: Dyspnea

Contraindications: Hypersensitivity, all anemias excluding iron deficiency anemia, hepatic disease

Precautions: Pregnancy (C), acute renal disease, children, asthma, lactation, rheumatoid arthritis (IV), infants <4 mo

PHARMACOKINETICS

IM: Excreted in feces, urine, bile, breast milk; crosses placenta; most absorbed through lymphatics; can be gradually absorbed over weeks/months from fixed locations

INTERACTIONS

Increase: toxicity—oral iron; do not use
Decrease: reticulocyte response—chloramphenicol
Drug/Lab Test
False increase: Serum bilirubin
False decrease: Serum calcium
False positive: ^{99m}Tc diphosphate bone scan, iron test (large doses >2 ml)

NURSING CONSIDERATIONS

Assess:
• Observe for 1 hr after test dose
• Blood studies: Hct, Hgb, reticulocytes, transferrin, plasma iron concentrations, ferritin, total iron-binding, bilirubin before treatment, at least monthly
• Allergy: anaphylaxis, rash, pruritus, fever, chills, wheezing; notify prescriber immediately, keep emergency equipment available
• Cardiac status: anginal pain, hypotension, tachycardia
• Nutrition: amount of iron in diet (meat,

dark green leafy vegetables, dried beans, dried fruits, eggs)
• Cause of iron loss or anemia, including use of salicylates, sulfonamides
• Toxicity: nausea, vomiting, diarrhea, fever, abdominal pain (early symptoms), cyanotic-looking lips, nailbeds, seizures, CV collapse (late symptoms)
Administer:
• D/C oral iron before parenteral; give only after test dose of 25 mg by preferred route; wait at least 1 hr before giving remaining portion
• IM deeply in large muscle mass; use Z-track method and a 19-20G 2-3-in needle; ensure needle is long enough to place drug deep in muscle; change needles after withdrawing drug and before injecting to prevent skin, tissue staining
⚠ Only with epINEPHrine available in case of anaphylactic reaction during dose
IV route
• IV after flushing with 10 ml 0.9% NaCl; give undiluted; may be diluted in 50-250 ml NS for infusion; give 1 ml (50 mg) or less over 1 min or more; flush line after use with 10 ml 0.9% NaCl; patient should remain recumbent for ½-1 hr
• IV injection requires single-dose vial without preservative; verify on label IV use is approved
Additive compatibilities: Netilmicin
Solution compatibility: TPN #211
Perform/provide:
• Storage at room temperature in cool environment
• Recumbent position 30 min after IV inj to prevent orthostatic hypotension
• Therapeutic response: increased serum iron levels, Hct, Hgb
Teach patient/family:
• That iron poisoning may occur if increased beyond recommended level; not to take oral iron preparation
• That delayed reaction may occur 1-2 days after administration and last 3-4 days (IV), 3-7 days (IM); report fever, chills, malaise, muscle, joint aches, nausea, vomiting, backache
Treatment of overdose: Discontinue drug, treat allergic reaction, give diphen-

hydramine or epINEPHrine as needed, give iron-chelating drug in acute poisoning

iron sucrose (℞)
Venofer
Func. class.: Hematinic
Chem. class.: Ferric hydroxide complex with dextran

Action: Iron is carried by transferrin to the bone marrow, where it is incorporated into hemoglobin
Uses: Iron deficiency anemia
Unlabeled uses: Dystrophic epidermolysis bullosa (DEB)

DOSAGE AND ROUTES
• *Adult:* IV 5 ml (100 mg of elemental iron) given during dialysis, most will need 1000 mg of elemental iron over 10 dialysis sessions
Available forms: Inj 20 mg/ml

SIDE EFFECTS
CNS: Headache, dizziness
CV: Chest pain, hypotension, hypertension, hypervolemia
GI: Nausea, vomiting, abdominal pain
INTEG: Rash, pruritus, urticaria, fever, sweating, chills
OTHER: **Anaphylaxis**
RESP: Dyspnea, pneumonia, cough
Contraindications: Hypersensitivity, all anemias excluding iron deficiency anemia, iron overload
Precautions: Pregnancy (B), lactation, geriatric, children

PHARMACOKINETICS
Excreted in urine, half-life 6 hr

INTERACTIONS
Increase: toxicity—oral iron; do not use

NURSING CONSIDERATIONS
Assess:
• Blood studies: Hct, Hgb, reticulocytes, transferrin, plasma iron concentrations, ferritin, total iron-binding, bilirubin before treatment, at least monthly
• Allergy: anaphylaxis, rash, pruritus, fever, chills, wheezing; notify prescriber immediately, keep emergency equipment available
• Cardiac status: hypotension, hypertension, hypervolemia
• Toxicity: nausea, vomiting, diarrhea, fever, abdominal pain (early symptoms), cyanotic-looking lips, nailbeds, seizures, CV collapse (late symptoms)
Administer:
⚠ Only with epINEPHrine available in case of anaphylactic reaction during dose
IV route
• Give directly in dialysis line by slow inj or inf; give by slow inj at 1 ml/min (5 min/vial); inf dilute each vial exclusively in a maximum of 100 ml of 0.9% NaCl, give at rate of 100 mg of iron/15 min, discard unused portions
Perform/provide:
• Storage at room temperature in cool environment, do not freeze
• Therapeutic response: increased serum iron levels, Hct, Hgb
Teach patient/family:
• That iron poisoning may occur if increased beyond recommended level; not to take oral iron preparation
Treatment of overdose: Discontinue drug, treat allergic reaction, give diphenhydrAMINE or epINEPHrine as needed, give iron-chelating drug in acute poisoning

isoflurophate ophthalmic
See Appendix C

isoniazid (R)

(eye-soe-nye'a-zid)
INH, isoniazid, Isotamine ✿,
Laniazid, Nydrazid,
PMS-Isoniazid ✿
Func. class.: Antitubercular
Chem. class.: Isonicotinic acid hydrazide

Action: Bactericidal interference with lipid, nucleic acid biosynthesis
Uses: Treatment, prevention of TB

DOSAGE AND ROUTES

• *Adult:* **PO/IM** 300 mg/day or 15 mg/kg 2-3 ×/wk, max 900 mg 2-3 ×/wk
• *Child and infant:* **PO/IM** 10-20 mg/kg daily in 1-2 divided doses max 300 mg/day or 20-40 mg/kg, max 900 mg 2-3 ×/wk
Available forms: Tabs 50, 100, 300 mg; inj 100 mg/ml; powder, syr 50 mg/5 ml

SIDE EFFECTS

CNS: Peripheral neuropathy, dizziness, memory impairment, **toxic encephalopathy, seizures,** psychosis, slurred speech
EENT: Blurred vision, optic neuritis
GI: **Nausea,** *vomiting,* epigastric distress, **jaundice, fatal hepatitis**
HEMA: **Agranulocytosis, hemolytic, aplastic anemia, thrombocytopenia, eosinophilia, methemoglobinemia**
Hypersensitivity: Fever, skin eruptions, lymphadenopathy, vasculitis
MISC: Dyspnea, B_6 deficiency, pellagra, hyperglycemia, metabolic acidosis, gynecomastia, rheumatic syndrome, SLE-like syndrome
Contraindications: Hypersensitivity, acute hepatic disease
Precautions: Pregnancy (C), renal/hepatic disease, diabetic retinopathy, cataracts, ocular defects, child <13 yr

PHARMACOKINETICS

PO: Peak 1-2 hr, duration 6-8 hr
IM: Peak 45-60 min
Metabolized in liver; excreted in urine (metabolites); crosses placenta; excreted in breast milk

INTERACTIONS

Increase: toxicity—tyramine foods, alcohol, cycloSERINE, ethionamide, rifampin, carbamazepine, warfarin, phenytoin, benzodiazepines, meperidine
Decrease: absorption—aluminum antacids
Decrease: effectiveness of BCG vaccine, ketoconazole
Drug/Food
• Do not give with high-tyramine foods

NURSING CONSIDERATIONS

Assess:
• Hepatic studies qwk: ALT, AST, bilirubin; increased test results may indicate hepatitis
• Mental status often: affect, mood, behavioral changes; psychosis may occur
• Hepatic status: decreased appetite, jaundice, dark urine, fatigue
• For paresthesia in hands, feet
Administer:
• PO with meals to decrease GI symptoms; better to take on empty stomach 1 hr before or 2 hr after meals
• Antiemetic if vomiting occurs
• After C&S is completed; qmo to detect resistance
• IM deep in large muscle mass; massage; rotate inj site; warm inj to room temperature to dissolve crystals
Evaluate:
• Therapeutic response: decreased symptoms of TB
Teach patient/family:
• That compliance with dosage schedule, duration is necessary, not to skip or double dose
• That scheduled appointments must be kept or relapse may occur
⚠ To avoid alcohol while taking drug, may increase risk of hepatic injury

---

✿ Canada only   Side effects: *italics* = common; **bold** = life-threatening

• That if diabetic, use blood glucose monitor to obtain correct result

⚠ To report weakness, fatigue, loss of appetite, nausea, vomiting, jaundice of skin or eyes, tingling/numbness of hands/feet

Treatment of overdose: Pyridoxine

Rarely Used

isoproterenol (℞)
(eye-soe-proe-ter′e-nole)
Aerolone, Dispos-a-Medisoproterenol HCl, Isoproterenol HCl, Isuprel, Isuprel Glossets, Isuprel Mistometer, Medihaler-Iso, Vapo-Iso
Func. class.: β-Adrenergic agonist

Uses: Bronchospasm, asthma, heart block, ventricular dysrhythmias, shock

DOSAGE AND ROUTES

Asthma, bronchospasm
• *Adult:* **SL** 10-20 mg q6-8h, max 60 mg/day; **INH** 1 puff, may repeat in 2-5 min, maintenance 1-2 puffs 4-6 ×/day; **IV** 10-20 mcg during anesthesia
• *Child:* **SL** 5-10 mg q6-8h; **INH** 1 puff, may repeat in 2-5 min, maintenance 1-2 puffs 4-6 ×/day

Shock
• *Adult:* **IV INF** 0.5-5 mcg/min 1 mg/500 ml D₅W, titrate to B/P, CVP, hourly urine output

Contraindications: Hypersensitivity to sympathomimetics, narrow-angle glaucoma, tachydysrhythmias, angina

isosorbide dinitrate (℞)
(eye-soe-sor′bide)
Apo-ISDN ✣, Cedocard-SR ✣, Coronex ✣, Dilatrate-SR, ISDN, Iso-Bid, Isonate, Isorbid, Isordil, Isosorbide dinitrate, Isotrate, Novasorbide ✣, Sorbitrate

isosorbide mononitrate
(eye-soe-sor′bide)
Imdur, ISMO, Isotrate ER, Monoket
Func. class.: Antianginal, vasodilator
Chem. class.: Nitrate

Do not confuse:
Monoket/Monopril
Imdur/Imuran/Inderal/K-Dur

Action: Relaxation of vascular smooth muscle, which leads to decreased preload, after-load, which is responsible for decreasing left ventricular end-diastolic pressure, systemic vascular resistance and reducing cardiac O₂ demand

Uses: Treatment, prevention of chronic stable angina pectoris, diffuse esophageal spasm

DOSAGE AND ROUTES

Isosorbide dinitrate
• *Adult:* **PO** 5-40 mg qid; **SL,** buccal 2.5-5 mg, may repeat q5-10 min × 3 doses; **CHEW TAB** 5-10 mg prn or q2-3h as prophylaxis; **SUS REL** 40-80 mg q8-12h

Isosorbide mononitrate
• *Adult:* **PO** ISMO, Monoket: 10-20 mg bid, 7 hr apart; Imdur: initiate at 30-60 mg/day as a single dose, increase q3d as needed, may increase to 120 mg daily, max 240 mg/day

Available forms: *Isosorbide dinitrate:* sus rel caps (SR) 40 mg; tabs 5, 10, 20, 30, 40 mg; SL tabs 2.5, 5, 10 mg; chew tabs 5, 10 mg; *isosorbide mononitrate:* tabs (ISMO, Monoket) 10, 20 mg; ext rel (Imdur, ER) 30, 60, 120 mg

---

SIDE EFFECTS

CNS: Vascular headache, flushing, dizziness, weakness, faintness
CV: Postural hypotension, tachycardia, **collapse,** syncope, palpitations
GI: Nausea, vomiting, diarrhea
INTEG: Pallor, sweating, rash
MISC: Twitching, hemolytic anemia, **methemoglobinemia**

Contraindications: Hypersensitivity to this drug or nitrates, severe anemia, increased intracranial pressure, cerebral hemorrhage, acute MI

Precautions: Pregnancy (C), postural hypotension, lactation, children, MI, CHF, severe renal/hepatic disease

PHARMACOKINETICS

Mononitrate
SUS REL: Duration 6-8 hr
Dinitrate
PO: Onset 15-30 min, duration 4-6 hr
SUS REL: Onset up to 4 hr, duration 6-8 hr
SL: Onset 2-5 min, duration 1-4 hr
CHEW TAB: Onset 3 min, duration ½-3 hr
Metabolized by liver, excreted in urine as metabolites (80%-100%)

INTERACTIONS

⚠ Fatal hypotension: sildenafil, tadalafil, vardenafil
Increase: hypotension—β-blockers, diuretics, antihypertensives, alcohol, calcium channel blockers, phenothiazines
Drug/Herb
Decrease: antianginal effect—blue cohosh

NURSING CONSIDERATIONS

Assess:
• Pain: duration, time started, activity being performed, character
• B/P, pulse, respirations during beginning therapy
• Tolerance if taken over long period
• Headache, light-headedness, decreased B/P; may indicate a need for decreased dosage

Administer:
• Do not break, crush, or chew sus rel caps, SL tabs
• After checking expiration date
• PO with 8 oz H_2O on empty stomach
• SL tabs should be placed under the tongue until dissolved

Evaluate:
• Therapeutic response: decrease or prevention of anginal pain

Teach patient/family:
• To leave tabs in original container
• To avoid alcohol products
• That drug may cause headache, but tolerance usually develops; taking with meals may reduce or eliminate headache
• That drug may be taken before stressful activity (exercise, sexual activity)
• That SL may sting when drug comes in contact with mucous membranes
• To avoid hazardous activities if dizziness occurs
• The importance of complying with complete medical regimen
• To make position changes slowly to prevent orthostatic hypotension

Rarely Used

isotretinoin (℞)
(eye-soe-tret′i-noyn)
Accutane, Amnesteem, Claravis, Sotret
Func. class.: Antiacne agent, retinoid

Uses: Severe recalcitrant cystic acne

DOSAGE AND ROUTES

• *Adult:* **PO** 0.5-2 mg/kg/day in 2 divided doses × 15-20 wk; if relapse occurs, repeat after 2 mo off drug
Contraindications: Pregnancy (X), hypersensitivity, inflamed skin

Side effects: *italics* = common; **bold** = life-threatening

isradipine (℞)

(is-ra'di-peen)
DynaCirc, DynaCirc CR
Func. class.: Antihypertensive, anti-anginal (calcium channel blocker)
Chem. class.: Dihydropyridine

Do not confuse:

DynaCirc/Dynabac/Dynacin

Action: Inhibits calcium ion influx across cell membrane during cardiac depolarization; produces relaxation of coronary vascular smooth muscle, peripheral vascular smooth muscle; dilates coronary vascular arteries

Uses: Essential hypertension, angina pectoris, vasospastic angina

DOSAGE AND ROUTES

• *Adult:* **PO** 2.5 mg bid; increase at 2-4 wk intervals up to 10 mg bid or 5 mg daily; **CONT REL** 5 mg daily; increase q2-4 wk; max 20 mg daily

Available forms: Caps 2.5, 5 mg, cont rel tabs (CR) 5, 10 mg

SIDE EFFECTS

CNS: Headache, fatigue, dizziness, fainting, sleep disturbances, weakness, depression, drowsiness
CV: Peripheral edema, tachycardia, hypotension, chest pain, **dysrhythmias,** syncope
GI: Nausea, vomiting, diarrhea, gastric upset, constipation, **hepatitis,** abdominal pain, distention, dry mouth
GU: Nocturia, urinary frequency
HEMA: **Leukopenia**
INTEG: Rash, pruritus, urticaria
MISC: Flushing

Contraindications: Sick sinus syndrome, 2nd- or 3rd-degree heart block, hypotension less than 90 mm Hg systolic, hypersensitivity

Precautions: Pregnancy (C), CHF, hypotension, lactation, children, renal/hepatic disease, geriatric

PHARMACOKINETICS

Metabolized in liver; metabolites excreted in urine, feces; secreted in breast milk; peak plasma levels at 1.5 hr immediate rel, 7-18 hr cont rel; half-life 8 hr; protein binding 95%

INTERACTIONS

Increase: additive/synergistic effect—β-blockers
Increase: bradycardia, conduction defects—disopyramide
Increase: hypotension—nitrates, fentanyl, other antihypertensives
Increase: serum conc of isradipine—cimetidine, ranitidine, CYP3A4 inducers
Decrease: serum conc of isradipine—rifampin, CYP3A4 inhibitors
Decrease: conc—fluvastatin, lovastatin
Decrease: antihypertensive action—NSAIDs, salicylates
Drug/Herb
Increase: toxicity, death—aconite
Increase: antihypertensive effect—barberry, betony, black catechu, black cohosh, bloodroot, broom, burdock, cat's claw, dandelion, ginkgo, ginseng, goldenseal, hawthorn, Irish moss, Jamaican dogwood, kelp, khella, mistletoe, parsley
Increase or decrease: antihypertensive effect—astragalus, cola tree
Decrease: antihypertensive effect—coltsfoot, guarana, khat, licorice, St. John's wort, yohimbine

NURSING CONSIDERATIONS

Assess:

• I&O ratio, daily weight, watch for CHF: edema, dyspnea, weight gain, crackles, jugular vein distention
• Renal, hepatic studies, electrolytes prior to and during treatment
• Cardiac status: B/P, pulse, respiration, ECG; assess anginal pain, precipitating, ameliorating factors

Administer:

• Do not break, crush, or chew cont rel tabs
• Without regard to meals

⚠ Safety alert   *"Tall Man" lettering

Evaluate:
• Therapeutic response: decreased anginal pain, decreased B/P

Teach patient/family:
• To avoid hazardous activities until stabilized on drug, dizziness is no longer a problem
• To limit caffeine consumption
• To avoid OTC drugs unless directed by prescriber
• The importance of compliance in all areas of regimen: diet, exercise, stress reduction, drug therapy
• To notify prescriber of irregular heartbeat, shortness of breath, swelling of feet and hands, pronounced dizziness, constipation, nausea, hypotension

Treatment of overdose: Defibrillation, β-agonists, IV calcium inotropic agents, diuretics, atropine for AV block, vasopressor for hypotension

---

itraconazole (R)

(it-ra-con'a-zol)

Sporanox

Func. class.: Antifungal, systemic
Chem. class.: Triazole derivative

Action: Alters cell membranes and inhibits several fungal enzymes

Uses: Systemic candidiasis, chronic mucocandidiasis, oral thrush, candiduria, histoplasmosis, chromomycosis, paracoccidioidomycosis, blastomycosis (pulmonary and extrapulmonary), aspergillosis onychomycosis

Unlabeled uses: Dermatomycosis, chromoblastomycosis, coccidioidomycosis, pityriasis versicolor, sebopsoriasis, vaginal candidiasis, cryptococcus, subcutaneous mycoses, dimorphic infections, leishmaniasis, fungal keratitis, alternariosis, zygomycosis

DOSAGE AND ROUTES

Dose varies with type of infection
• *Adult:* **PO** 200 mg daily with food; may increase to 400 mg daily if needed; life-threatening infections may require a loading dose of 200 mg tid × 3 days; **IV** 200

mg bid × 4 doses, then 200 mg daily, give each dose over 1 hr; maintenance **PO** 200-400 mg/day
• *Child:* **PO** 3-5 mg/kg/day

Available forms: Caps 100 mg; oral sol 10 mg/ml; inj 10 mg/ml

SIDE EFFECTS

CNS: Headache, dizziness, insomnia, somnolence, depression
CV: Hypertension
GI: Nausea, vomiting, anorexia, diarrhea, cramps, abdominal pain, flatulence, **GI bleeding, hepatotoxicity**
GU: Gynecomastia, impotence, decreased libido
INTEG: Pruritus, fever, *rash,* **toxic epidermal necrolysis**
MISC: Edema, fatigue, malaise, hypokalemia, tinnitus, **rhabdomyolysis**

Contraindications: Hypersensitivity, fungal meningitis, onychomycosis or dermatomycosis in cardiac dysfunction
Precautions: Pregnancy (C), hepatic/cardiac disease, achlorhydria or hypochlorhydria (drug-induced), children, lactation

PHARMACOKINETICS

PO: Peak 3-5 hr, half-life 21 hr; metabolized in liver; excreted in bile, feces; requires acid pH for absorption; distributed poorly to CSF; highly protein bound; inhibits CYP4503A4

INTERACTIONS

⚠ Life-threatening CV reactions: pimozide, quinidine, dofetilide
Increase: tinnitus, hearing loss—quinidine
Increase: hepatotoxicity—other hepatotoxic drugs
Increase: edema—calcium channel blockers
Increase: severe hypoglycemia—oral hypoglycemics
Increase: sedation—triazolam, oral midazolam
Increase: levels, toxicity—busPIRone, busulfan, clarithromycin, cycloSPORINE,

Side effects: *italics* = common; **bold** = life-threatening

diazepam, digoxin, felodipine, indinavir, isradipine, niCARdipine, niFEDipine, nimodipine, phenytoin, quinidine, ritonavir, saquinavir, tacrolimus, warfarin

Decrease: effect of oral contraceptives

Decrease: itraconazole action—antacids, H_2-receptor antagonists, rifamycins, didanosine

Drug/Herb

• Nephrotoxicity: gossypol

Drug/Food

• Food increases absorption

NURSING CONSIDERATIONS

Assess:

• For type of infection, may begin treatment prior to obtaining results

• For infection: temp, WBC, sputum, baseline and periodically

• I&O ratio, potassium levels

• Hepatic studies (ALT, AST, bilirubin) if on long-term therapy

• For allergic reaction: rash, photosensitivity, urticaria, dermatitis

⚠ For hepatotoxicity: nausea, vomiting, jaundice, clay-colored stools, fatigue

Administer:

• In the presence of acid products only; do not use alkaline products or antacids within 2 hr of drug; may give coffee, tea, acidic fruit juices

PO route

• Swallow caps whole; do not break, crush, or chew caps

• Oral sol: patient should swish in mouth vigorously, use on empty stomach

• Give caps after full meal to ensure absorption

• Oral sol and caps are not interchangeable on an mg/mg basis

IV route

• After adding full contents 25-50 ml bag of 0.9% NaCl mix, use infusion pump, give at a rate of 1 ml/min, flush line with 0.9% NaCl after infusion; do not use by bolus

Perform/provide:

• Storage in tight container at room temperature, do not freeze

Evaluate:

• Therapeutic response: decreased fever, malaise, rash, negative C&S for infecting organism

Teach patient/family:

• That long-term therapy may be needed to clear infection (1 wk-6 mo depending on infection)

• To avoid hazardous activities if dizziness occurs

• To take 2 hr before administration of other drugs that increase gastric pH (antacids, H_2-blockers, omeprazole, sucralfate, anticholinergics); to notify health care provider of all medications taken; to take after a full meal (caps), on empty stomach (oral sol)

• The importance of compliance with drug regimen, to use alternative method of contraceptive

• To notify prescriber of GI symptoms, signs of hepatic dysfunction (fatigue, nausea, anorexia, vomiting, dark urine, pale stools)

Rarely Used

kanamycin (℞)

(kan-a-mye'sin)

kanamycin sulfate, Kantrex

Func. class.: Antiinfective

Chem. class.: Aminoglycoside

Uses: Severe systemic infections of CNS; respiratory, GI, urinary tract; bone, skin, soft tissues caused by *Escherichia coli, Acinetobacter, Proteus, Klebsiella pneumoniae, Pseudomonas aeruginosa, Serratia marcescens;* also used as adjunct in hepatic coma, peritonitis, preoperatively to sterilize bowel; decreases ammonia-producing bacteria in bowel and intraperitoneally after fecal spill during surgery

DOSAGE AND ROUTES

Severe systemic infections

• *Adult and child:* **IV INF** 15 mg/kg/day in divided doses q8-12h; diluted 500 mg/200 ml of NS or D_5W given over 30-60

---

min, not to exceed 1.5 g/day; **IM** 15 mg/kg/day in divided doses q8-12h, not to exceed 1.5 g/day, irrigation not to exceed 1.5 g/day; **NEB/INH** 250 mg qid

Preoperative bowel sterilization

• *Adult:* **PO** 1 g qh × 4 doses, then q6h × 36-72 hr

Renal dose

• *Adult:* **IM/IV** 7.5 mg/kg, may increase or decrease dose based on renal status

Contraindications: Pregnancy (D), bowel obstruction, severe renal disease, hypersensitivity

---

ketoconazole (℞)
(kee-toe-koe′na-zole)
Nizoral
Func. class.: Antifungal
Chem. class.: Imidazole derivative

Do not confuse:
Nizoral/Nasarel/Neoral

Action: Alters cell membrane permeability and inhibits several fungal enzymes leading to cell death

Uses: Systemic candidiasis, chronic mucocandidiasis, oral thrush, candiduria, coccidioidomycosis, histoplasmosis, chromomycosis, para-coccidioidomycosis, blastomycosis; tinea cruris, tinea corporis, tinea versicolor, *Pityrosporum ovale*

Unlabeled uses: Cushing's syndrome, advanced prostatic cancer

DOSAGE AND ROUTES

• *Adult:* **PO** 200-400 mg daily for 1-2 wk (candidiasis), 6 wk (other infections); 400 mg tid (prostate cancer—unlabeled)
• *Child >2 yr:* **PO:** 3.3-6.6 mg/kg/day as single daily dose

Available forms: Tabs 200 mg; oral susp 100 mg/5 ml ✦

SIDE EFFECTS

CNS: Headache, dizziness, somnolence
GI: Nausea, vomiting, anorexia, diarrhea, abdominal pain, **hepatotoxicity**
GU: Gynecomastia, impotence

HEMA: **Thrombocytopenia, leukopenia, hemolytic anemia**
INTEG: Pruritus, fever, chills, photophobia, rash, dermatitis, purpura, urticaria
SYST: **Anaphylaxis**

Contraindications: Hypersensitivity, lactation, fungal meningitis; coadministration with terfenadine or drugs that prolong QTc interval

Precautions: Pregnancy (C), renal/hepatic disease, achlorhydria (drug-induced), children <2 yr, other hepatotoxic agents including terfenadine, other drugs metabolized by CYP450

PHARMACOKINETICS

PO: Peak 1-2 hr, half-life 2 hr, terminal 8 hr; metabolized in liver; excreted in bile, feces; requires acid pH for absorption; distributed poorly to CSF; highly protein bound

INTERACTIONS

• Ketoconazole may decrease theophylline effect
• Inhibited metabolism: paclitaxel
Increase: hepatotoxicity—other hepatotoxic drugs, alcohol
Increase: anticoagulant effect—warfarin, anticoagulants
Decrease: CYP 4503A4 pathway, toxicity: alfentanil, alprazolam, amprenavir, atorvastatin, calcium channel blockers, carbamazepine, cerivastatin, clarithromycin, corticosteroids, cyclophosphamide, cycloSPORINE, donepezil, erythromycin, fentanyl, ifosfamide, indinavir, lovastatin, midazolam, nelfinavir, nisoldipine, quinidine, ritonavir, saquinavir, sildenafil, simvastatin, sufentanil, tamoxifen, triazolam, vinBLAStine, vinca alkaloids, vinCRIStine, zolpidem
Decrease: action of ketoconazole—antacids, H₂-receptor antagonists, anticholinergics, phenytoin, isoniazid, rifampin, ddI, gastric acid pump inhibitors
Decrease: effect of oral contraceptives
Drug/Herb
Increase: nephrotoxicity—gossypol
Decrease: ketoconazole action—yew

NURSING CONSIDERATIONS

Assess:

• For infection symptoms before and after treatment

• Hepatic studies (ALT, AST, bilirubin) if on long-term therapy

• For allergic reaction: rash, photosensitivity, urticaria, dermatitis

⚠ For hepatotoxicity: nausea, vomiting, jaundice, clay-colored stools, fatigue

Administer:

• In the presence of acid products only; do not use alkaline products, proton pump inhibitors, H$_2$-antagonists, antacids within 2 hr of drug; may give coffee, tea, acidic fruit juices, cola

• With food to decrease GI symptoms

• With HCl if achlorhydria is present; dissolve tab/4 ml of aqueous sol 0.2 N hydrochloric acid; use straw to avoid contact; rinse with water afterward and swallow

Perform/provide:

• Storage in tight container at room temperature

Evaluate:

• Therapeutic response: decreased fever, malaise, rash, negative C&S for infecting organism, absence of scaling

Teach patient/family:

• That long-term therapy may be needed to clear infection (1 wk-6 mo depending on infection)

• To avoid hazardous activities if dizziness occurs

• To take 2 hr before administration of other drugs that increase gastric pH (antacids, H$_2$-blockers, omeprazole, sucralfate, anticholinergics)

• The importance of compliance with drug regimen

⚠ To notify prescriber of GI symptoms, signs of hepatic dysfunction (fatigue, nausea, anorexia, vomiting, dark urine, pale stools)

• Use sunglasses to prevent photophobia

• To use alternative method of contraception while taking this drug

---

ketoconazole topical
See Appendix C

---

ketoprofen (otc, ℞)
(ke-toe-proe'fen)
Apo-Keto ✦, Apo-Keto-E ✦, ketoprofen, Orudis-E ✦, Orudis-KT, Orudis-SR ✦, Rhodis ✦

Func. class.: Nonsteroidal antiinflammatory drug (NSAID), antirheumatic

Chem. class.: Propionic acid derivative

Action: Inhibits prostaglandin synthesis by decreasing enzyme needed for biosynthesis; analgesic, antiinflammatory, antipyretic

Uses: Mild to moderate pain, osteoarthritis, rheumatoid arthritis, dysmenorrhea; OTC relief of minor aches, pains

DOSAGE AND ROUTES

Antiinflammatory

• *Adult:* **PO** 150-300 mg in divided doses tid-qid, not to exceed 300 mg/day or **EXT REL** 200 mg daily

Analgesic

• *Adult:* **PO** 25-50 mg q6-8h

Available forms: Caps 50, 75 mg; ext rel cap 200 mg; tabs 12.5 mg

SIDE EFFECTS

CNS: Dizziness, drowsiness, fatigue, tremors, confusion, insomnia, anxiety, depression, headache

CV: Tachycardia, peripheral edema, palpitations, dysrhythmias, hypertension

EENT: Tinnitus, hearing loss, blurred vision

GI: Nausea, anorexia, vomiting, diarrhea, jaundice, **hepatitis,** constipation, flatulence, cramps, dry mouth, peptic ulcer, **GI bleeding**

GU: **Nephrotoxicity: dysuria, hematuria, oliguria, azotemia**

HEMA: **Blood dyscrasias**

⚠ Safety alert   ✦ "Tall Man" lettering

INTEG: Purpura, rash, pruritus, sweating
SYST: **Anaphylaxis**
Contraindications: Avoid in 2nd/3rd trimester, hypersensitivity, asthma, severe renal/hepatic disease, ulcer disease
Precautions: Pregnancy (B) 1st trimester, lactation, children, bleeding disorders, GI disorders, cardiac disorders, hypersensitivity to other antiinflammatory agents, geriatric

PHARMACOKINETICS

PO: Peak 2 hr, half-life 2-4 hr; metabolized in liver; excreted in urine (metabolites); excreted in breast milk; 99% plasma protein binding

INTERACTIONS

Increase: hypoglycemia—insulin, sulfonylureas
Increase: toxicity—cycloSPORINE, lithium, methotrexate, phenytoin, alcohol
Increase: bleeding risk—cefamandole, cefoperazone, cefotetan, clopidogrel, eptifibatide, plicamycin, thrombolytics, ticlopidine, tirofiban, valproic acid, warfarin
Increase: ketoprofen levels—aspirin, probenecid
Increase: adverse GI reactions—aspirin, corticosteroids, NSAIDs, alcohol
Increase: hematologic toxicity—radiation
Decrease: effect of diuretics, antihypertensives

Drug/Herb

Increase: bleeding risk—anise, arnica, bogbean, chondroitin chamomile, clove, dong quai, feverfew, garlic, ginger, ginkgo, ginseng *(Panax)*
Increase: gastric irritation—arginine, gossypol
Increase: NSAIDs effect—bearberry, bilberry

Drug/Lab Test

Increase: Potassium, BUN, alk phos, AST, ALT, LDH, creatinine, bleeding time
Decrease: Blood glucose, HCT, Hgb, platelets, CCr, leukocyte
Interference: Urine albumin, 17 KS, 17-hydroxycorticosteroid, bilirubin

NURSING CONSIDERATIONS

Assess:

• For pain: type, location, intensity, ROM before and 1-2 hr after treatment
• Renal, hepatic, blood studies: BUN, creatinine, AST, ALT, Hgb, before treatment, periodically thereafter
⚠ For aspirin sensitivity, asthma; these patients may be more likely to develop hypersensitivity to NSAIDs
• Audiometric, ophthalmic exam before, during, after treatment
• For eye, ear problems: blurred vision, tinnitus; may indicate toxicity
• For GI bleeding: blood in sputum, emesis, stools

Administer:

• Do not break, crush, or chew ext rel caps
• With food to decrease GI symptoms; however, taking on empty stomach best facilitates absorption

Perform/provide:

• Storage at room temperature

Evaluate:

• Therapeutic response: decreased pain, stiffness in joints, decreased swelling in joints, ability to move more easily; decreased fever

Teach patient/family:

• To report blurred vision, ringing, roaring in ears; may indicate toxicity
• To avoid driving, other hazardous activities if dizziness, drowsiness occurs, especially elderly
• To report change in urine pattern, increased weight, edema, increased pain in joints, fever, blood in urine; indicate nephrotoxicity; rash, itching, blurred vision, ringing in the ears, flulike symptoms
• That therapeutic effects may take up to 1 mo, to take with 8 oz of water and sit upright for ½ hr after administration to prevent GI irritation
• To avoid aspirin, alcohol, steroids, acetaminophen or other medications, supplements unless approved by prescriber
• To wear sunscreen to prevent photosensitivity

ketorolac (R)
(kee-toe′role-ak)
Toradol
Func. class.: Nonsteroidal antiinflammatory/nonopioid analgesic
Chem. class.: Acetic acid

Do not confuse:
Toradol/Tegretol/Foradil/Inderal/
Torecan/tramadol

Action: Inhibits prostaglandin synthesis by decreasing an enzyme needed for biosynthesis; analgesic, antiinflammatory, antipyretic effects

Uses: Mild to moderate pain; seasonal allergic conjunctivitis (ophth)

DOSAGE AND ROUTES
• *Adult <65 yr:* **PO** 20 mg then 10 mg q4-6h prn, max 40 mg/day
• *Adult >65 yr, renal disease, <50 kg:* **PO** 10 mg q4-6h prn, max 40 mg/day
• *Adult <65 yr:* **IM** (single dose) 60 mg **IV** 30 mg; **IM** (multiple dosing) 15 mg q6h, max 60 mg/day × 5 day combined either **PO/IM/IV**
• *Adult >65 yr, renal disease, <50 kg:* **IM** single dose 30 mg; **IV** 15 mg **IM/IV** (multiple dosing) 15 mg q6h, max 60 mg/day × 5 days combined either **PO/IM/IV**
Available forms: Inj 15, 30 mg/ml (prefilled syringes); tab 10 mg

SIDE EFFECTS
CNS: Dizziness, *drowsiness,* tremors
CV: Hypertension, flushing, syncope, pallor, edema, vasodilation
EENT: Tinnitus, hearing loss, blurred vision
GI: Nausea, anorexia, vomiting, diarrhea, constipation, flatulence, cramps, dry mouth, peptic ulcer, **GI bleeding, perforation**, taste change
GU: **Nephrotoxicity: dysuria, hematuria, oliguria, azotemia**
HEMA: **Blood dyscrasias,** prolonged bleeding
INTEG: Purpura, rash, pruritus, sweating

Contraindications: Hypersensitivity, asthma, severe renal/hepatic disease, peptic ulcer disease, L&D, lactation, CV bleeding

Precautions: Pregnancy (C), children, bleeding disorders, GI disorders, cardiac disorders, hypersensitivity to other antiinflammatory agents, geriatric, CCr <25 ml/min

PHARMACOKINETICS
PO: Peak 2-3 hr, duration 4-6 hr
IM: Peak 50 min, half-life 6 hr, enters breast milk, <50% metabolized by liver, excreted by kidneys

INTERACTIONS
Increase: toxicity—methotrexate, lithium, cycloSPORINE
Increase: bleeding risk—anticoagulants, cefamandole, cefoperazone, cefotetan, clopidogrel, eptifibatide, plicamycin, salicylates, ticlopidine, tirofiban, thrombolytics, valproic acid
Increase: renal impairment—ACE inhibitors
⚠ *Increase:* ketorolac levels—aspirin, other NSAIDs, contraindicated
Increase: GI effects—steroids, alcohol, aspirin, NSAIDs, potassium products
Decrease: effects—antihypertensives, diuretics
Drug/Herb
Increase: gastric irritation—arginine, gossypol
Increase: NSAIDs effect—bearberry, bilberry
Increase: bleeding risk—anise, arnica, bogbean, chamomile, chondroitin, clove, dong quai, feverfew, garlic, ginger, ginkgo, ginseng *(Panax)*
Drug/Lab Test
Increase: AST, ALT, LDH, alk phos, bleeding time, BUN, creatinine, potassium
Decrease: Blood glucose, Hct/Hgb, platelets

⚠ Safety alert   *"Tall Man" lettering

NURSING CONSIDERATIONS

Assess:

• Patients with aspirin sensitivity, asthma; may be more likely to develop hypersensitivity to NSAIDs, monitor for hypersensitivity

• For pain: type, location, intensity, ROM before and 1 hr after treatment

• Renal, hepatic, blood studies: BUN, creatinine, AST, ALT, Hgb before treatment, periodically thereafter; check for dehydration

• Bleeding times; check for bruising, bleeding; test for occult blood in urine

• For eye, ear problems: blurred vision, tinnitus (may indicate toxicity)

⚠ Hepatic dysfunction: jaundice, yellow sclera and skin, clay-colored stools

• Audiometric, ophthalmic exam before, during, after treatment

• GI bleeding: blood in sputum, emesis, stools

Administer:

• IM/IV for 5 days or less; continue therapy with PO

• IM inj deeply in large muscle mass

IV route

• Give undiluted over ≥15 sec

Solution compatibility: D₅W, 0.9% NaCl, LR, D₅, plasmalate

Syringe compatibilities: Sufentanil

Y-site compatibilities: Cisatracurium, remifentanil, sufentanil

Perform/provide:

• Storage at room temperature

Evaluate:

• Therapeutic response: decreased pain, stiffness, swelling in joints, ability to move more easily

Teach patient/family:

• To report blurred vision or ringing, roaring in ears (may indicate toxicity)

• To avoid driving, other hazardous activities if dizziness or drowsiness occurs

• To report change in urine pattern, weight increase, edema, pain increase in joints, fever, blood in urine (indicates nephrotoxicity)

• To avoid alcohol, salicylates, other NSAIDs, acetaminophen

ketorolac ophthalmic
See Appendix C

ketotifen ophthalmic
See Appendix C

kunecatechins
See Appendix A—Selected New Drugs

labetalol (℞)
(la-bet′a-lole)
Normodyne, Trandate
Func. class.: Antihypertensive, antianginal
Chem. class.: α/β-Blocker

Do not confuse:
Trandate/Tridrate

Action: Produces decreases in B/P without reflex tachycardia or significant reduction in heart rate through mixture of α-blocking, β-blocking effects; elevated plasma renins are reduced

Uses: Mild to moderate hypertension; treatment of severe hypertension (IV)

Unlabeled uses: Hypertension in patients with pheochromocytoma, hypertension in clonidine withdrawal

DOSAGE AND ROUTES

Hypertension

• *Adult:* **PO** 100 mg bid; may be given with a diuretic; may increase to 200 mg bid after 2 days; may continue to increase q1-3d; max 2400 mg/day in divided doses

Hypertensive crisis

• *Adult:* **IV INF** 200 mg/160 ml D₅W, run at 2 mg/min or 1.6 ml/min; stop inf at desired response, repeat q6-8h as needed; **IV BOL** 20-80 mg over 2 min, may repeat 20-80 mg q10min, not to exceed 300 mg

Available forms: Tabs 100, 200, 300 mg; inj 5 mg/ml in 20-ml amps

SIDE EFFECTS

CNS: Dizziness, mental changes, drowsiness, fatigue, headache, catatonia, depression, anxiety, nightmares, paresthesias, lethargy

CV: Orthostatic hypotension, bradycardia, **CHF,** chest pain, **ventricular dysrhythmias,** AV block, scalp tingling

EENT: Tinnitus, visual changes, sore throat, double vision, dry, burning eyes

GI: Nausea, vomiting, diarrhea, dyspepsia, taste distortion

GU: Impotence, dysuria, ejaculatory failure

HEMA: **Agranulocytosis, thrombocytopenia, purpura** (rare)

INTEG: Rash, alopecia, urticaria, pruritus, fever

RESP: **Bronchospasm,** dyspnea, wheezing

Contraindications: Hypersensitivity to β-blockers, cardiogenic shock, heart block (2nd or 3rd degree), sinus bradycardia, CHF, bronchial asthma

Precautions: Pregnancy (C), major surgery, lactation, diabetes mellitus, renal disease, thyroid disease, COPD, well-compensated heart failure, CAD, nonallergic bronchospasm, geriatric, hepatic disease, peripheral vascular disease

PHARMACOKINETICS

PO: Onset ½-2 hr, peak 1-4 hr, duration 8-24 hr

IV: Onset 5 min, peak 15 min, duration 2-4 hr

Half-life 2.5-8 hr; metabolized by liver (metabolites inactive); excreted in urine; crosses placenta; excreted in breast milk; protein binding 50%

INTERACTIONS

• Do not use within 2 wk of MAOIs

Increase: myocardial depression—hydantoins, general anesthetics, verapamil

Increase: hypotension—diuretics, other antihypertensives, cimetidine, nitroglycerin, alcohol

Decrease: effects—sympathomimetics, lidocaine, indomethacin, theophylline, β-blockers, bronchodilators, xanthines

Decrease: labetalol effect—glutethimide

Decrease: antihypertensive effect—NSAIDs, salicylates

Drug/Herb

Increase: toxicity, death—aconite

Increase: antihypertensive effect—barberry, betony, black catechu, black cohosh, bloodroot, broom, burdock, cat's claw, dandelion, goldenseal, hawthorn, Irish moss, Jamaican dogwood, kelp, khella, mistletoe, parsley

Increase or decrease: antihypertensive effect—astragalus, cola tree

Decrease: antihypertensive effect—coltsfoot, guarana, khat, licorice, yohimbine

Drug/Lab Test

Increase: ANA titer, blood glucose, alk phos, LDH, AST, ALT, BUN, potassium, triglyceride, uric acid

False increase: Urinary catecholamines

NURSING CONSIDERATIONS

Assess:

⚠ I&O, weight daily; fluid overload: weight gain, jugular venous distention, edema, crackles in lungs

• B/P during beginning treatment, periodically thereafter; pulse q4h; note rate, rhythm, quality

• Apical/radial pulse before administration; notify prescriber of any significant changes

• Baselines in renal, hepatic studies before therapy begins

• Edema in feet, legs daily

• Skin turgor, dryness of mucous membranes for hydration status

Administer:

• PO before meals, at bedtime; tab may be crushed or swallowed whole, give with meals to increase absorption

• Reduced dosage in renal dysfunction

IV route

• Undiluted or diluted in LR, D₅W, D₅ in 0.2%, 0.9%, 0.33% NaCl or Ringer's inj, give undiluted 20 mg or less/2 min; inf is titrated to patient response; 200 mg of drug/160 ml sol = 1 mg/ml; 300 mg of drug/240 ml sol = 1 mg/ml; 200 mg of drug/250 ml sol = 2 mg/3 ml; use infusion pump

• Keeping patient recumbent during and for 3 hr after administration, monitor VS q5-15min

Solution compatibilities: D₅R, D₅LR, D₂½/0.45% NaCl, D₅/0.2% NaCl, D₅/0.33% NaCl, D₅/0.9% NaCl, D₅W, Ringer's, LR

Y-site compatibilities: Amikacin, aminophylline, amiodarone, ampicillin, butorphanol, calcium gluconate, cefazolin, ceftazidime, ceftizoxime, chloramphenicol, cimetidine, clindamycin, diltiazem, DOBUTamine, DOPamine, enalaprilat, epINEPHrine, erythromycin, esmolol, famotidine, fentanyl, gentamicin, hydromorphone, lidocaine, lorazepam, magnesium sulfate, meperidine, metronidazole, midazolam, milrinone, morphine, niCARdipine, nitroglycerin, norepinephrine, nitroprusside, oxacillin, penicillin G potassium, piperacillin, potassium chloride, potassium phosphate, propofol, ranitidine, sodium acetate, tobramycin, trimethoprim-sulfamethoxazole, vancomycin, vecuronium

Perform/provide:

• Storage in dry area at room temperature; do not freeze

Evaluate:

• Therapeutic response: decreased B/P after 1-2 wk

Teach patient/family:

• Not to discontinue drug abruptly; taper over 2 wk; may cause precipitate angina

• Not to use OTC products containing α-adrenergic stimulants (nasal decongestants, OTC cold preparations) unless directed by prescriber

• To report bradycardia, dizziness, confusion, depression, fever

• To take pulse at home, advise when to notify prescriber

• To avoid alcohol, smoking, sodium intake

• To comply with weight control, dietary adjustments, modified exercise program

• To carry emergency ID to identify drug, allergies

• To avoid hazardous activities if dizziness is present

• To report symptoms of CHF: difficulty breathing, especially on exertion or when lying down, night cough, swelling of extremities

• To take medication at bedtime to prevent effect of orthostatic hypotension, to rise slowly

• To wear support hose to minimize effects of orthostatic hypotension

Treatment of overdose: Lavage, IV atropine for bradycardia, IV theophylline for bronchospasm, digitalis, O₂, diuretic for cardiac failure; hemodialysis is useful for removal, hypotension; administer vasopressor (norepinephrine)

---

lactulose (Ŗ)

(lak′tyoo-lose)
Cephulac, Cholac, Chronulac, Constilac, Constulose, Duphalac, Enulose, Evalose, Heptalac, Kristalose, Lactulax ✤, Lactulose PSE, Portalac

Func. class.: Laxative; ammonia detoxicant (hyperosmotic)
Chem. class.: Lactose synthetic derivative

Action: Prevents absorption of ammonia in colon; increases water in stool

Uses: Chronic constipation, portal-systemic encephalopathy in patients with hepatic disease

DOSAGE AND ROUTES

Constipation

• *Adult:* **PO** 15-30 ml daily (10-20 g) may increase to 60 ml/day prn

• *Child* (unlabeled): **PO** 7.5 ml daily

Encephalopathy

• *Adult:* **PO** 30-45 ml tid or qid until stools are soft; **RETENTION ENEMA** 300 ml diluted

• *Child:* (unlabeled) **PO** 40-90 ml/day in divided doses given 2-4 ×/day

• *Infant:* (unlabeled) **PO** 2.5-10 ml/day in divided doses

---

Side effects: *italics* = common; **bold** = life-threatening

Available forms: Syr 10 g/15 ml; single-use packets (Kristalose) 10, 20 g

SIDE EFFECTS

GI: Nausea, vomiting, anorexia, abdominal cramps, diarrhea, flatulence, distention, belching

Contraindications: Hypersensitivity, low-galactose diet

Precautions: Pregnancy (B), lactation, diabetes mellitus, geriatric, debilitated patients

PHARMACOKINETICS

Metabolized in intestine, excreted by kidneys; onset 1-2 days, peak unknown, duration unknown

INTERACTIONS

Drug/Herb
• Do not use with other laxatives
Increase: laxative action—flax, senna
Decrease: lactulose effects—neomycin, other oral antiinfectives

NURSING CONSIDERATIONS

Assess:
• Stool: amount, color, consistency
• Blood ammonia level (30-70 mg/100 ml); may decrease ammonia level by 25%-50%
• Blood, urine electrolytes if drug is used often; may cause diarrhea, hypokalemia, hyponatremia
• I&O ratio to identify fluid loss
• Cause of constipation; determine whether fluids, bulk, or exercise is missing from lifestyle, constipating drugs
• Cramping, rectal bleeding, nausea, vomiting; if these symptoms occur, drug should be discontinued
• Clearing of confusion, lethargy, restlessness, irritability if portal-systemic encephalopathy

Administer:
PO route
• With 8 oz fruit juice, water, milk to increase palatability of oral form

Rectal route
• Retention enema by diluting 300 ml lactose/700 ml of water; administer by rectal balloon catheter
• Increased fluids to 2 L/day; do not give with other laxatives; if diarrhea occurs, reduce dosage

Evaluate:
• Therapeutic response: decreased constipation, decreased blood ammonia level, clearing of mental state

Teach patient/family:
• Not to use laxatives long-term
• To dilute with water or fruit juice to counteract sweet taste
• To store in cool environment; do not freeze
• To take on an empty stomach for rapid action
• To report diarrhea; may indicate overdose

lamivudine (℞)
(lam-i-voo′deen)
Epivir, Epivir-HBV, 3TC
Func. class.: Antiretroviral
Chem. class.: Nucleoside reverse transcriptase inhibitor

Do not confuse:
lamivudine/lamotrigine
Action: Inhibits replication of HIV virus by incorporating into cellular DNA by viral reverse transcriptase, thereby terminating cellular DNA chain
Uses: HIV-1 infection in combination with other antiretrovirals; chronic hepatitis B (Epivir-HBV)
Unlabeled uses: Prophylaxis of HIV—postexposure with indinavir and zidovudine

DOSAGE AND ROUTES
HIV
• *Adult and child >12 yr:* **PO** 150 mg bid or 300 mg daily
• *Child 3 mo-12 yr:* **PO** 4 mg/kg bid, max 150 mg bid

Renal dose
• *Adult:* **PO** CCr 30-49 ml/min 150 mg daily; CCr 15-29 ml/min 150 mg 1st dose, then 100 mg daily; CCr 5-14 ml/min 150 mg daily, then 50 mg daily; CCr <5 ml/min, 50 mg 1st dose, then 25 mg daily

Chronic hepatitis B
• *Adult:* **PO** 100 mg daily

Available forms: (Epivir) oral sol 10 mg/ml; tabs 150, 300 mg; (Epivir-HBV) oral sol 5 mg/ml; tabs 100 mg

SIDE EFFECTS

CNS: Fever, headache, malaise, dizziness, insomnia, depression, fatigue, chills, **seizures**

EENT: Taste change, hearing loss, photophobia

GI: Nausea, vomiting, diarrhea, anorexia, cramps, dyspepsia, **hepatomegaly with steatosis, pancreatitis**

HEMA: **Neutropenia, anemia, thrombocytopenia**

INTEG: Rash

MS: Myalgia, arthralgia, pain

RESP: Cough

SYST: **Lactic acidosis, anaphylaxis, Stevens-Johnson syndrome**

Contraindications: Hypersensitivity

Precautions: Pregnancy (C), granulocyte count <1000/mm^3 or Hgb <9.5 g/dl, lactation, children, renal disease, severe hepatic dysfunction, pancreatitis, geriatric

PHARMACOKINETICS

Rapidly absorbed, distributed to extravascular space, excreted unchanged in urine, protein binding <36%, terminal half-life 5-7 hr

INTERACTIONS

• May decrease both drugs: zalcitabine
Increase: lamivudine level—trimethoprim-sulfamethoxazole
Increase: level—zidovudine

Drug/Lab Test
Increase: ALT, bilirubin
Decrease: Hgb, neutrophil, platelet count

NURSING CONSIDERATIONS

Assess:
• Blood counts q2wk; watch for neutropenia, thrombocytopenia, Hgb, CD4, viral load; if low, therapy may have to be discontinued and restarted after hematologic recovery; blood transfusions may be required
• Hepatic studies: AST, ALT, bilirubin; amylase, lipase, triglycerides, CD4, viral load periodically during treatment
• Children for pancreatitis: abdominal pain, nausea, vomiting
⚠ Lactic acidosis, severe hepatomegaly with steatosis: obtain baseline LFTs, if elevated discontinue treatment; discontinue even if LFTs are normal if lactic acidosis, severe hepatomegaly develop

Administer:
• PO daily or bid, without regard to meals

Perform/provide:
• With other antiretrovirals only
• Storage in cool environment; protect from light

Evaluate:
• Blood dyscrasias: bruising, fatigue, bleeding, poor healing

Teach patient/family:
• That GI complaints, insomnia resolve after 3-4 wk of treatment
• That drug is not a cure for HIV, but will control symptoms
• To notify prescriber of sore throat, swollen lymph nodes, malaise, fever; other infections may occur
• That patient is still infective, may pass HIV virus on to others
• That follow-up visits must be continued since serious toxicity may occur; blood counts must be done q2wk
• That drug must be taken as prescribed, even if patient feels better
• That other drugs may be necessary to prevent other infections
• That drug may cause fainting or dizziness

lamotrigine (Ŗ)
(la-moe'tri-geen)
Lamictal, Lamictal Chewable
Dispersible
Func. class.: Anticonvulsant, misc.
Chem. class.: Phenyltriazine

Do not confuse:
lamotrigine/lamivudine
Lamictal/Lomotil/Lamisil

Action: Unknown, may inhibit voltage-sensitive sodium channels

Uses: Adjunct in the treatment of partial seizures; children with Lennox-Gastaut syndrome, bipolar disorder

Unlabeled uses: Generalized tonic-clonic, absence, atypical absence and myoclonic seizures

DOSAGE AND ROUTES

Seizures: Monotherapy
• *Adult:* **PO** 50 mg/day for wk 1-2, then increase to 100 mg divided bid for wk 3-4; maintenance, 300-500 mg/day
• *Child:* **PO** 2 mg/kg/day in 2 divided doses × 2 wk, then 10 mg/kg/day, max 15 mg/kg/day or 400 mg/day

Seizures: Multiple therapy
• *Adult:* **PO** 25 mg every other day wk 1-4, then 150 mg/day in divided doses
• *Child:* **PO** 0.1-0.2 mg/kg/day initially, then increase q2wk as needed to 2 mg/kg/day or 150 mg/day

Hepatic dose
• *Adult, Child-Pugh grade B:* **PO** Reduce by 50%
• *Adult, Child-Pugh grade C:* **PO** Reduce by 75%

Bipolar disorder
• *Adult:* **PO** wk 1-2 25 mg daily; wk 3-4 50 mg daily; wk 5 100 mg daily; wk 6-7 200 mg daily; for patients taking valproic acid: wk 1-2 12 mg every other day, wk 3-4 25 mg daily; wk 5 50 mg daily; wk 6 100 mg daily; wk 7 100 mg daily

Available forms: Tabs 25, 100, 150, 200 mg; chew dispersible tabs 2, 5, 25 mg

SIDE EFFECTS

CNS: Dizziness, ataxia, *headache,* fever, insomnia, tremor, depression, anxiety
EENT: Nystagmus, *diplopia, blurred vision*
GI: Nausea, vomiting, anorexia, abdominal pain, **hepatotoxicity**
GU: Dysmenorrhea
INTEG: **Rash (potentially life-threatening),** alopecia, photosensitivity
SYST: **Stevens-Johnson syndrome**
Contraindications: Hypersensitivity
Precautions: Pregnancy (C), lactation, child <16 yr, renal/hepatic/cardiac disease, geriatric, severe depression, suicidal, blood dyscrasias

PHARMACOKINETICS

Half-life varies depending on dose; rapidly, completely absorbed; metabolized by slucuronic acid conjunction

INTERACTIONS

Decrease: metabolic clearance of lamotrigine—valproic acid
Decrease: lamotrigine serum concentration—carbamazepine, rifamycins, oral contraceptives, acetaminophen, phenytoin, primodone, phenobarbital, oxcarbazepine, succinimides

Drug/Herb
Increase: anticonvulsant effect—ginkgo
Decrease: anticonvulsant effect—ginseng, santonica

NURSING CONSIDERATIONS

Assess:
• For seizure activity: duration, type, intensity, halo before seizure
⚠ For rash (Stevens-Johnson syndrome or toxic epidermal necrolysis) in pediatric patients, drug should be discontinued at first sign of rash

Administer:
• Chewable dispersible tabs; swallow whole, chew, or dispersed in water or diluted fruit juice; if chewed, drink a small amount of water

Evaluate:
• Therapeutic response: decrease in severity of seizures

Teach patient/family:
• To take PO doses divided with or after meals to decrease adverse effects, not to discontinue drug abruptly; seizures may occur
• To avoid hazardous activities until stabilized on drug
• To carry emergency ID, to notify prescriber of skin rash or increased seizure activity, to use sunscreen and protective clothing if photosensitivity occurs
• To notify prescriber if pregnant or intend to become pregnant

---

lansoprazole (R)

(lan-so-prey´zole)
Prevacid, Prevacid IV,
Prevacid SoluTab
Func. class.: Antiulcer, proton pump inhibitor
Chem. class.: Benzimidazole

Do not confuse:
Prevacid/Pravachol/Prinivil

Action: Suppresses gastric secretion by inhibiting hydrogen/potassium ATPase enzyme system in gastric parietal cell; characterized as gastric acid pump inhibitor, since it blocks final step of acid production

Uses: Gastroesophageal reflux disease (GERD), severe erosive esophagitis, poorly responsive systemic GERD, pathologic hypersecretory conditions (Zollinger-Ellison syndrome, systemic mastocytosis, multiple endocrine adenomas); possibly effective for treatment of duodenal, gastric ulcers, maintenance of healed duodenal ulcers

DOSAGE AND ROUTES

NG tube
• *Adult:* Use intact granules mixed in 40 ml of apple juice and injected through **NG** tube, then flush with apple juice

Duodenal ulcer
• *Adult:* **PO** 15 mg daily before eating for 4 wk, then 15 mg daily to maintain healing of ulcers; associated with *Helicobacter pylori*—30 mg lansoprazole, 500 mg clarithromycin, 1 g amoxicillin bid × 14 days or 30 mg lansoprazole, 1 g amoxicillin tid × 14 days

Erosive esophagitis
• *Adult:* **IV** 30 mg over 30 min or for up to 7 days; switch to PO as soon as patient can tolerate, for 6-8 wk

Pathologic hypersecretory conditions
• *Adult:* **PO** 60 mg daily, may give up to 90 mg bid, administer doses of >120 mg/day in divided doses

GERD/esophagitis
• *Child 1-11 yr (>30 kg):* **PO** 30 mg daily ≤12 wk
• *Child 1-11 yr (≤30 kg):* **PO** 15 mg daily ≤12 wk

Available forms: Del rel caps 15, 30 mg; granules for oral susp 15, 30 mg/packet; orally disintegrating tabs 15, 30 mg; lyophilized powder for IV inj 30 mg/vial

SIDE EFFECTS

CNS: Headache, dizziness, confusion, agitation, amnesia, depression
CV: Chest pain, angina, tachycardia, bradycardia, palpitations, **CVA**, hypertension/hypotension, **MI, shock**, vasodilation
EENT: Tinnitus, taste perversion, deafness, eye pain, otitis media
GI: Diarrhea, abdominal pain, vomiting, nausea, constipation, flatulence, acid regurgitation, anorexia, irritable colon
GU: **Hematuria**, glycosuria, impotence, kidney calculus, breast enlargement
HEMA: **Hemolysis**, anemia
INTEG: Rash, urticaria, pruritus, alopecia
META: Weight gain/loss, gout
RESP: Upper respiratory infections, cough, epistaxis, asthma, bronchitis, dyspnea

Contraindications: Hypersensitivity
Precautions: Pregnancy (B), lactation, children

Side effects: *italics* = common; **bold** = life-threatening

PHARMACOKINETICS

Absorption after granules leave stomach—>80%; plasma half-life 1½-2 hr; protein binding 97%; extensively metabolized in liver; excreted in urine, feces; clearance decreased in the geriatric, renal/hepatic impairment

INTERACTIONS

• Delayed lansoprazole absorption: sucralfate

Decrease: absorption of ketoconazole, itraconazole, iron, indinivir, calcium carbonate

NURSING CONSIDERATIONS

Assess:
• GI system: bowel sounds q8h, abdomen for pain, swelling, anorexia
• Hepatic studies: AST, ALT, alk phos during treatment

Administer:
• Swallow caps whole before eating; do not crush or chew caps; caps may be opened and contents sprinkled on food

Evaluate:
• Therapeutic response: absence of epigastric pain, swelling, fullness

Teach patient/family:
• To report severe diarrhea; drug may have to be discontinued
• That diabetic patient should know that hypoglycemia may occur
• To avoid hazardous activities; dizziness may occur
• To avoid alcohol, salicylates, ibuprofen; may cause GI irritation

---

Rarely Used

lanthanum (℞)
(lan'-tha-num)
Fosrenol
Func. class.: Phosphate binder

Uses: End-stage renal disease

DOSAGE AND ROUTES

• *Adult:* **PO** 750-1500 mg daily in divided doses with meals; titrate dose

q2-3wk until an acceptable phosphate level is reached; tablets should be chewed completely before swallowing; intact tablets should not be swallowed
Contraindications: Hypophosphatemia, hypersensitivity

Rarely Used

laronidase (℞)
(lah-rah'nih-daze)
Aldurazyme
Func. class.: Miscellaneous agent

Uses: Mucopolysaccharidosis I (MPSI), patients with Hurler and Hurler-Scheie forms of MPSI

DOSAGE AND ROUTES

• *Adult:* **IV INF** 0.58 mg/kg qwk; pretreat with antipyretic and/or antihistamines 1 hr prior to **IV INF**
Contraindications: Hypersensitivity

---

latanoprost ophthalmic
See Appendix C

---

leflunomide (℞)
(leh-floo'noh-mide)
Arava
Func. class.: Antirheumatic (DMARDs)
Chem. class.: Immune modulator, pyrimidine synthesis inhibitor

Action: Inhibits an enzyme involved in pyrimidine synthesis and has antiproliferative, antiinflammatory effect
Uses: Rheumatoid arthritis, to reduce disease process and symptoms
Unlabeled uses: Juvenile rheumatoid arthritis

DOSAGE AND ROUTES

Rheumatoid arthritis
• *Adult:* **PO** loading dose 100 mg/day × 3 days, maintenance 20 mg/day,

---

may be decreased to 10 mg/day if not well tolerated

Juvenile rheumatoid arthritis (unlabeled)
• *Adolescent and child >40 kg:* **PO** 20 mg
• *Adolescent and child 20-40 kg:* **PO** 15 mg
• *Adolescent and child 10-19.9 kg:* **PO** 10 mg

Available forms: Tabs 10, 20, 100 mg

SIDE EFFECTS

CNS: Headache, dizziness, insomnia, depression, paresthesia, anxiety, migraine, neuralgia
CV: Palpitations, hypertension, chest pain, angina pectoris, peripheral edema
EENT: Pharyngitis, oral candidiasis, stomatitis, dry mouth, blurred vision
GI: Nausea, anorexia, vomiting, constipation, flatulence, diarrhea, elevated LFTs, **hepatotoxicity**
HEMA: Anemia, ecchymosis, hyperlipidemia
INTEG: Rash, pruritus, alopecia, acne, hematoma, herpes infections
RESP: Pharyngitis, rhinitis, bronchitis, cough, respiratory infection, pneumonia, sinusitis

Contraindications: Pregnancy (X), hypersensitivity, lactation, jaundice, lactase deficiency, hepatic disease
Precautions: Renal disorders, vaccinations, infection, alcoholism, children, immunosuppression

PHARMACOKINETICS

PO: metabolized in liver to active metabolite, excreted in urine

INTERACTIONS

Increase: NSAIDs effect—NSAIDs
Increase: leflunomide side effects—hepatotoxic agents, methotrexate
Increase: rifampin levels—rifampin
Decrease: antibody response—live virus vaccines
Decrease: leflunomide effect—activated charcoal, cholestyramine

NURSING CONSIDERATIONS

Assess:
• Arthritic symptoms: ROM, mobility, swelling of joints baseline and during treatment
• Hepatic studies: if ALT elevations are > twofold ULN, reduce dose to 10 mg/day

Administer:
• With food for GI upset
• To eliminate drug: give cholestyramine 8 g tid × 11 days, check levels

Evaluate:
• Therapeutic response: decreased inflammation, pain in joints

Teach patient/family:
• That drug must be continued for prescribed time to be effective
• To take with food, milk, or antacids to avoid GI upset
• To use caution when driving; drowsiness, dizziness may occur
• To take with a full glass of water to enhance absorption
• To avoid pregnancy while taking this drug; not to breastfeed while taking this drug; men should also discontinue drug and begin leflunomide removal protocol if a pregnancy is planned
• That hair may be lost, review alternatives
• To avoid vaccinations during treatment (live virus)

⚠ High Alert

lepirudin (℞)
(lep-ih-roo'din)
Refludan
Func. class.: Anticoagulant
Chem. class.: Thrombin inhibitor, hirudin

Action: Direct inhibitor of thrombin that is highly specific
Uses: Anticoagulation in those with heparin-induced thrombocytopenia and other thromboembolic conditions
Unlabeled uses: Adjunct therapy in unstable angina, acute MI without ST eleva-

Side effects: *italics* = common; **bold** = life-threatening

tion, prevention of deep vein thrombosis, percutaneous coronary intervention

DOSAGE AND ROUTES

- *Adult:* IV 0.4 mg/kg over 15-20 sec; then 0.15 mg/kg/hr as a cont inf for 2-10 days or longer

Concomitant use with thrombolytic therapy

- *Adult:* IV BOLUS 0.2 mg/kg initially
- *Adult:* CONT IV INF 0.1 mg/kg/hr

Renal dose

- *Adult:* IV BOLUS 0.2 mg/kg over 15-20 sec, then if CCr 45-60 ml/min 0.075 mg/kg/hr, CCr 30-44 ml/min 0.045 mg/kg/hr, CCr 15-29 ml/min 0.0225 mg/kg/hr

Available forms: Powder for inj 50 mg

SIDE EFFECTS

CNS: Fever, **intracranial bleeding**
CV: **Heart failure, pericardial effusion, ventricular fibrillation**
GI: GI bleeding, abnormal LFTs
GU: **Hematuria,** abnormal kidney function, vaginal bleeding
HEMA: **Hemorrhage, thrombocytopenia**
INTEG: Allergic skin reactions
RESP: Pneumonia
SYST: **Multiorgan failure, sepsis, anaphylaxis**

Contraindications: Hypersensitivity to hirudins
Precautions: Pregnancy (B), intracranial bleeding, lactation, children, hepatic disease, recent major surgery, hemorrhagic diathesis bacterial endocarditis, severe uncontrolled hypertension, advanced renal disease, recent active peptic ulcer, recent CVA, stroke, intracerebral surgery, geriatric, women

PHARMACOKINETICS

May be metabolized by the release of amino acids during catabolism; 50% unchanged in urine

INTERACTIONS

Increase: bleeding risk—warfarin derivatives, thrombolytics, NSAIDs, plicamy-cin, cefamandole, cefotetan, cefoperazone, aspirin, clopidogrel, dipyridamole, eptifibatide, ticlopidine, tirofiban, valproic acid

Drug/Herb
Increase: risk of bleeding—agrimony, alfalfa, angelica, anise, basil, bay, bilberry, black haw, bogbean, bromelain, buchu, chondroitin, cinchona bark, dong quai, fenugreek, feverfew, garlic, ginger, ginkgo, ginseng, horse chestnut, Irish moss, kelp, kelpware, khella, lovage, lungwort, meadowsweet, motherwort, mugwort, nettle, papaya, parsley (large amts), pau d'arco, pineapple, poplar, prickly ash, safflower, saw palmetto, tonka bean, turmeric, wintergreen, yarrow
Decrease: anticoagulant effect—chamomile, coenzyme Q10, flax, glucomannan, goldenseal, guar gum

NURSING CONSIDERATIONS

Assess:
- Obtain baseline in aPTT before treatment; do not start treatment if aPTT ratio ≥2.5, then aPTT 4 hr after initiation of treatment and at least daily thereafter; if aPTT above target, stop inf for 2 hr, then restart at 50%, take aPTT in 4 hr; if below target, increase inf rate by 20%, take aPTT in 4 hr, do not exceed inf rate of 0.21 mg/kg/hr without checking for coagulation abnormalities
- aPTT, which should be 1.5-2.5 × control

⚠ Bleeding gums, petechiae, ecchymosis, black tarry stools, hematuria/epistaxis, B/P, vaginal bleeding and possible hemorrhage
- Fever, skin rash, urticaria

Administer:
- Avoiding all IM inj
- After reconstitution and further dilution under sterile conditions; use water for inj or 0.9% NaCl; for further dilution 0.9% NaCl or D$_5$; for rapid and complete reconstitution, inject 1 ml of diluent into vial and shake gently; use immediately; warm to room temp before use

IV BOLUS route
• Reconstitute each vial with 1 ml sterile water or 0.9% NaCl; shake gently; transfer content of vial into 10-ml syringe and dilute to a volume of 10 ml with sterile water for inj, D_5W, or 0.9% NaCl, final conc 5 mg/ml

IV INF route
• Reconstitute 2 vials with 1 ml each of sterile water for inj, or 0.9% NaCl; transfer contents into infusion bag containing 250 or 500 ml 0.9% NaCl or D_5W for a conc 0.2 mg/ml or 0.4 mg/ml respectively; infuse at 0.15 mg/kg/hr; use infusion pump

Evaluate:
• Therapeutic response: anticoagulation

Teach patient/family:
• To use soft-bristle toothbrush to avoid bleeding gums, avoid contact sports, use electric razor, avoid IM inj
• To report any signs of bleeding: gums, under skin, urine, stools

---

letrozole (℞)
(let′tro-zohl)
Femara
Func. class.: Antineoplastic, non-steroidal aromatase inhibitor

Action: Binds to the heme group of aromatase; inhibits conversion of androgens to estrogens to reduce plasma estrogen levels; 30% of breast cancers decrease in size when deprived of estrogen

Uses: Early, advanced, or metastatic breast cancer in post-menopausal women

Unlabeled uses: Ovulation stimulation

DOSAGE AND ROUTES
• *Adult:* **PO** 2.5 mg daily
Available forms: Tabs 2.5 mg

SIDE EFFECTS
CNS: Headache, lethargy, somnolence, dizziness, depression, anxiety
CV: **Angina, MI, CVA, thromboembolic events,** hypertension

GI: Nausea, vomiting, anorexia, **hepatotoxicity,** constipation, heartburn, diarrhea
GU: **Endometrial cancer, vaginal bleeding, endometrial proliferation disorders**
INTEG: Rash, pruritus, alopecia, sweating, hot flashes
MISC: Hot flashes, night sweats, **second malignancies**
MS: Arthralgia, arthritis, bone fracture, myalgia, osteoporosis
RESP: Dyspnea, cough

Contraindications: Pregnancy (D), hypersensitivity
Precautions: Hepatic disease, respiratory disease

PHARMACOKINETICS
Metabolized in liver, excreted in urine

INTERACTIONS
• None known

NURSING CONSIDERATIONS
Assess:
• Monitor temp q4h; may indicate beginning infection
• Hepatic studies before, during therapy (bilirubin, AST, ALT, LDH) as needed or monthly
• Jaundiced skin, sclera, dark urine, clay-colored stools, itchy skin, abdominal pain, fever, diarrhea

Administer:
• Without regard to meals; use a small glass of water

Perform/provide:
• Liquid diet, including cola, Jell-O; dry toast or crackers as ordered may be added if patient is not nauseated or vomiting
• Nutritious diet with iron and vitamin supplements as ordered

Evaluate:
• Therapeutic response: decrease in size of tumor

Teach patient/family:
• To report allergic reactions (rash; hives; difficulty breathing; tightness in chest; swelling on mouth, face, lips, tongue)
• That dizziness, drowsiness may occur and to avoid driving or operating heavy machinery

leucovorin (Ŗ)

(loo-koe-vor'in)
citrovorum factor, folinic acid, leucovorin calcium
Func. class.: Vitamin, folic acid/methotrexate antagonist antidote
Chem. class.: Tetrahydrofolic acid derivative

Do not confuse:
leucovorin/Leukeran/leukine
folinic acid/folic acid

Action: Needed for normal growth patterns; prevents toxicity during antineoplastic therapy by protecting normal cells
Uses: Megaloblastic or macrocytic anemia caused by folic acid deficiency, overdose of folic acid antagonist, methotrexate toxicity, toxicity caused by pyrimethamine or trimethoprim, pneumocystosis, toxoplasmosis

DOSAGE AND ROUTES
Megaloblastic anemia caused by enzyme deficiency
• *Adult and child:* **PO/IV/IM** up to 6 mg/day
Megaloblastic anemia caused by deficiency of folate
• *Adult and child:* **IM** 1 mg or less daily until adequate response
Methotrexate toxicity
• *Adult and child:* **PO/IM/IV** normal elimination given 6 hr after dose of methotrexate (10 mg/m²) until methotrexate is <10⁻⁸ M; CCr is >50% above prior level or methotrexate level is 5×10 at 24 hr, or at 48-hr level is $>9 \times 10$ M, give leucovorin 100 mg/m² q3h until level drops to <10 M

Pyrimethamine toxicity
• *Adult and child:* **PO/IM** 5-15 mg daily
Trimethoprim toxicity
• *Adult and child:* **PO/IM** 400 mg daily
Advanced colorectal cancer
• *Adult:* **IV** 200 mg/m², then 5-FU 370 mg/m²; or leucovorin 20 mg/m², then 5-FU 425 mg/m²; give daily × 5 days q4-5wk

Available forms: Tabs 5, 10, 15, 25 mg; inj 3, 5 mg/ml; powder for inj 10 mg/ml

SIDE EFFECTS
HEMA: Thrombocytosis (intraarterial)
INTEG: Rash, pruritus, erythema, urticaria
RESP: Wheezing
Contraindications: Hypersensitivity, anemias other than megaloblastic not associated with vit B_{12} deficiency
Precautions: Pregnancy (C)

INTERACTIONS
Increase: metabolism of phenobarbital, hydantoins
Increase: toxicity—fluorouracil
Decrease: folate levels—chloramphenicol

NURSING CONSIDERATIONS
Assess:
• CCr, creatinine before leucovorin rescue and daily to detect nephrotoxicity; methotrexate level
• I&O; watch for nausea and vomiting
• Other drugs taken: alcohol, hydantoins, trimethoprim may cause increased folic acid use by body
Administer:
• Within 1 hr of folic acid antagonist
IM route
• No reconstitution needed
• Treatment of megaloblastic anemia uses IM dosing
IV route
• For IV reconstitute 50 mg/5 ml bacteriostatic or sterile H₂O for inj (10 mg/ml) or (100 mg/10 ml); use immediately if sterile H₂O is used
• Give by direct IV over 160 mg/min or less (16 ml of 10 mg/ml sol/min)

⚠ Safety alert   *"Tall Man" lettering

• Give by intermittent inf after diluting in 100-500 ml of 0.9% NaCl, D5W, D10W, LR, Ringer's sol

Additive compatibilities: Cisplatin, cisplatin/floxuridine, floxuridine

Syringe compatibilities: Bleomycin, cisplatin, cyclophosphamide, DOXOrubicin, fluorouracil, furosemide, heparin, methotrexate, metoclopramide, mitomycin, vinBLAStine, vinCRIStine

Y-site compatibilities: Amifostine, aztreonam, bleomycin, cefepime, cisplatin, cladribine, cyclophosphamide, DOXOrubicin, DOXOrubicin liposome, filgrastim, fluconazole, fluorouracil, furosemide, granisetron, heparin, methotrexate, metoclopramide, mitomycin, piperacillin/tazobactam, tacrolimus, teniposide, thiotepa, vinBLAStine, vinCRIStine

Perform/provide:

• Increase fluid intake if used to treat folic acid inhibitor overdose

• Protection from light and heat

Evaluate:

• Therapeutic response: increased weight; improved orientation, well-being; absence of fatigue; reversal of toxicity (methotrexate, folic acid antagonist overdose)

Teach patient/family:

• For leucovorin rescue have patient drink 3 L fluid daily of rescue

• For folic acid deficiency eat folic acid rich foods: bran, yeast, dried beans, nuts, fresh, green leafy vegetables

• To take drug exactly as prescribed

• To notify prescriber of side effects

• To report signs of hyposensitivity reaction immediately

⚠ High Alert

leuprolide (℞)
(loo-proe'lide)
Eligard, Lupron Depo Ped, Lupron, Lupron Depot, Lupron Depot-3 month, Lupron Depot-4 month, Viadur
Func. class.: Antineoplastic hormone
Chem. class.: Gonadotropin-releasing hormone

Do not confuse:

Lupron/Nuprin/Lopurin

Action: Causes initial increase in circulating levels of LH, FSH; continuous administration results in decreased LH, FSH; in men, testosterone is reduced to castrate levels; in premenopausal women, estrogen is reduced to menopausal levels

Uses: Metastatic prostate cancer (inj implant), management of endometriosis, central precocious puberty, uterine leiomyomata (fibroids)

DOSAGE AND ROUTES

Prostate cancer

• *Adult:* SUBCUT 1 mg/day; IM 7.5 mg/dose qmo; Viadur implant (72 mg) qyr; or IM 22.5 mg q3mo; or IM 30 mg q4mo

Endometriosis/fibroids

• *Adult:* IM 3.75 mg qmo or 11.25 q3mo or 30 mg q4mo

Central precocious puberty

• *Child:* SUBCUT 50 mcg/kg/day; may increase by 10 mcg/kg/day as needed

• *Child >37.5 kg:* IM 15 mg q4wk

• *Child 25-37.5 kg:* IM 11.25 mg q4wk

• *Child ≤25 kg:* 7.5 mg q4wk

Available forms: Inj 5 mg/ml; powder for inj, lyophilized 7.5 mg; microspheres for inj, lyophilized 3.75, 7.5, 11.25, 15, 22.5, 30 mg; implant 72 mg; depot 7.5, 22.5, 30, 45 mg; depot 3.75, 11.25 mg

SIDE EFFECTS

CV: **MI, pulmonary emboli, dysrhythmias**

GI: Anorexia, diarrhea, **GI bleeding**

GU: Edema, hot flashes, impotence, decreased libido, amenorrhea, vaginal dryness, gynecomastia

Contraindications: Pregnancy (X), hypersensitivity to GnRH or analogs, thromboembolic disorders, lactation, undiagnosed vaginal bleeding

Precautions: Edema, hepatic disease, CVA, MI, seizures, hypertension, diabetes mellitus

PHARMACOKINETICS

SUBCUT: Onset 1-2 wk, peak 2-4 wk; absorbed rapidly (SUBCUT), slowly (IM depot); half-life 3 hr

INTERACTIONS

Increase: antineoplastic action—flutamide, megestrol

NURSING CONSIDERATIONS

Assess:

• For symptoms of endometriosis (lower abdominal pain)/fibroids (pelvic pain, excessive vaginal bleeding, bloating) before, during, and after treatment

• For central precocious puberty (CPP) if treatment is for this condition; secondary S_4 characteristics to child <9 yr, estradiol/testosterone levels, GnRH test, tomography of head, adrenal steroids, chorionic gonadotropin, wrist x-ray, height, weight

• Hepatic studies before, during therapy (bilirubin, AST, ALT, LDH) as needed or monthly, PSA in prostate cancer

• Pituitary gonadotropic and gonadal function during therapy and 4-8 wk after therapy is decreased

• Worsening of signs and symptoms; normal during beginning therapy

• Fatigue, increased pulse, pallor, lethargy; edema in feet, joints; stomach pain

⚠ Symptoms indicating severe allergic reaction: rash, pruritus, urticaria, purpuric skin lesions, itching, flushing

Administer:

• IM/SUBCUT using syringe and drug packaged together; give deep in large muscle mass; rotate sites

• Use depot IM only

• Monthly: reconstitute single-use vial with 1 ml of diluent; if multiple vials used, withdraw 0.5 ml and inject into each vial (1 ml); withdraw all and inject

• 3-month: reconstitute microspheres using 1.5 ml of diluent and inject in vial; shake, withdraw, and inject

• 12-month: insert into upper arm; at the end of 12 months, implant must be removed

Perform/provide:

• Nutritious diet with iron, vitamin supplements as ordered

• Storage in tight container at room temperature

Evaluate:

• Therapeutic response: decreased tumor size and spread of malignancy, decrease in lesions, pain in endometriosis, fibroids, correction of CPP

Teach patient/family:

• To notify prescriber if menstruation continues; menstruation should stop

• To use a nonhormonal method of contraception during therapy

• That bone pain will disappear after 1 wk

• To report any complaints, side effects to nurse or prescriber; hot flashes may occur; record weight, report gain of >2 lb/day

• How to prepare, give; to rotate sites for SUBCUT inj

• To keep accurate records of dose

• That tumor flare may occur: increase in size of tumor, increased bone pain, will subside rapidly; may take analgesics for pain; premenopausal women must use mechanical birth control; ovulation may be induced

• Do not breastfeed while taking this drug

• Voiding problems may increase in beginning of therapy, but will decrease in several weeks

---

⚠ Safety alert   *"Tall Man" lettering

levalbuterol (R)

(lev-al-byoo'ter-ole)

Xopenex

Func. class.: Bronchodilator, adrenergic β_2-agonist

Action: Causes bronchodilation by action on β_2 (pulmonary) receptors by increasing levels of cAMP, which relaxes smooth muscle; produces bronchodilation, CNS, cardiac stimulation, as well as increased diuresis and gastric acid secretion

Uses: Treatment or prevention of bronchospasm (reversible obstructive airway disease)

DOSAGE AND ROUTES

• *Adult and child ≥12 yr:* **INH** 0.63 mg tid, q6-8h by nebulization, may increase 1.25 mg q8h
• *Child 6-11 yr:* **INH** 0.31 mg tid by nebulization, max 0.63 mg tid
Available forms: Sol, inh 0.63 mg, 1.25 mg/3 ml

SIDE EFFECTS

CNS: Tremors, anxiety, insomnia, headache, dizziness, stimulation, *restlessness,* hallucinations, flushing, irritability
CV: Palpitations, tachycardia, hypertension, angina, hypotension, dysrhythmias
EENT: Dry nose, irritation of nose and throat
GI: Heartburn, nausea, vomiting
INTEG: Rash
META: Hypokalemia, hyperglycemia
MS: Muscle cramps
RESP: Cough

Contraindications: Hypersensitivity to sympathomimetics, tachydysrhythmias, severe cardiac disease
Precautions: Pregnancy (C), lactation, cardiac disorders, hyperthyroidism, diabetes mellitus, hypertension, prostatic hypertrophy, narrow-angle glaucoma, seizures, renal disease

PHARMACOKINETICS

Metabolized in the liver and tissues; crosses placenta, breast milk, blood-brain barrier; half-life 3.3-4 hr
INH: Onset 5-15 min, peak 1-1½ hr, duration 6-8 hr

INTERACTIONS

Increase: action of aerosol bronchodilators
Increase: levalbuterol action—tricyclics, MAOIs, other adrenergics
Decrease: levalbuterol action—other β-blockers
Drug/Herb
Increase: stimulation—black/green tea, coffee, cola nut, guarana, yerba maté

NURSING CONSIDERATIONS
Assess:
• Respiratory function: vital capacity, forced expiratory volume, ABGs, lung sounds, heart rate and rhythm (baseline); character of sputum: color, consistency, amount
• For evidence of allergic reactions, paradoxical bronchospasm
Administer:
• By nebulization q6-8h; wait at least 1 min between inhalation of aerosols
Evaluate:
• Therapeutic response: absence of dyspnea, wheezing after 1 hr, improved airway exchange, improved ABGs
Teach patient/family:
• Not to use OTC medications; excess stimulation may occur
• To avoid getting aerosol in eyes; blurring may result
• To avoid smoking, smoke-filled rooms, persons with respiratory infections
⚠ That paradoxic bronchospasm may occur and to stop drug immediately, contact prescriber
• To limit caffeine products such as chocolate, coffee, tea, and colas or herbs such as cola nut, guarana, yerba maté
Treatment of overdose: Administer a β_1-adrenergic blocker

levetiracetam (R)

(lev-eh-teer-ass'eh-tam)
Keppra
Func. class.: Anticonvulsant

Action: Unknown, may inhibit nerve impulses by limiting influx of sodium ions across cell membrane in motor cortex
Uses: Adjunctive therapy in partial-onset seizures

DOSAGE AND ROUTES

• *Adult:* **PO** 500 mg bid, may increase by 1000 mg/day q2wk max 3000 mg/day
Available forms: Tabs 250, 500, 750 mg; oral sol 100 mg/ml

SIDE EFFECTS

CNS: Dizziness, somnolence, asthenia
HEMA: Lowered Hct, Hgb, RBC, infection
MISC: Infection, abdominal pain, pharyngitis
Contraindications: Hypersensitivity
Precautions: Pregnancy (C), renal/cardiac disease, psychosis, lactation, children, geriatric

PHARMACOKINETICS

Rapidly absorbed, not protein bound, excreted via kidneys 66% unchanged; half-life 6-8 hr, longer in geriatric

NURSING CONSIDERATIONS

Assess:
• Renal studies: urinalysis, BUN, urine creatinine q3mo
• Blood studies: RBC, Hct, Hgb
• Description of seizures
• Mental status: mood, sensorium, affect, behavioral changes; if mental status changes, notify prescriber
Administer:
• Swallow tab whole; do not break, crush, or chew
• With food, milk to decrease GI symptoms (rare)
Perform/provide:
• Storage at room temperature
• Assistance with ambulation during early part of treatment; dizziness occurs
Evaluate:
• Therapeutic response: decreased seizure activity, document on patient's chart
Teach patient/family:
• To carry emergency ID stating patient's name, drugs taken, condition, prescriber's name, phone number
• Use oral sol; if swallowing is a problem, measure oral sol in medicine cup or dropper, don't use teaspoon
• To notify prescriber if pregnant or intend to become pregnant
• To avoid driving, other activities that require alertness
• Not to discontinue medication quickly after long-term use, withdrawal seizure may occur

levobetaxolol ophthalmic

See Appendix C

levobunolol ophthalmic

See Appendix C

Rarely Used

levobupivacaine (R)

(lee-voh-bu-piv'ah-kane)
Chirocaine
Func. class.: Local anesthetic

Uses: Local, regional anesthesia, surgical anesthesia, pain management, continuous epidural analgesia

DOSAGE AND ROUTES

• Varies with route of anesthesia
Contraindications: Hypersensitivity, children <12 yr, geriatric, severe hepatic disease

---

A Safety alert   *"Tall Man" lettering

levocabastine ophthalmic
See Appendix C

levodopa (℞)
(lee'voe-doe-pa)
Dopar, Larodopa, L-Dopa
Func. class.: Antiparkinson agent
Chem. class.: Dopamine agonist

Do not confuse:
L-dopa/levodopa/methyldopa
Action: Decarboxylation to dopamine, which increases dopamine levels in brain
Uses: Parkinson's disease

DOSAGE AND ROUTES
• *Adult:* **PO** 0.5-1 g daily divided bid-qid with meals; may increase by up to 0.75 g q3-7d not to exceed 8 g/day unless closely supervised
Available forms: Caps 100, 250, 500 mg; tabs 100, 250, 500 mg

SIDE EFFECTS
CNS: Involuntary choreiform movements, hand tremors, fatigue, headache, anxiety, twitching, numbness, weakness, confusion, agitation, insomnia, nightmares, psychosis, hallucination, hypomania, severe depression, dizziness
CV: Orthostatic hypotension, tachycardia, hypertension, palpitation
EENT: Blurred vision, diplopia, dilated pupils
GI: Nausea, vomiting, anorexia, abdominal distress, dry mouth, flatulence, dysphagia, bitter taste, diarrhea, constipation
HEMA: **Hemolytic anemia, leukopenia, agranulocytosis**
INTEG: Rash, sweating, alopecia
MISC: Urinary retention, incontinence, weight change, dark urine
Contraindications: Hypersensitivity, narrow-angle glaucoma, undiagnosed skin lesions

Precautions: Pregnancy (C), renal/hepatic/cardiac disease, respiratory disease, MI with dysrhythmias, convulsions, peptic ulcer, asthma, endocrine disease, affective disorders, psychosis, lactation, children <12 yr, peptic ulcer

PHARMACOKINETICS
PO: Peak 1-3 hr, excreted in urine (metabolites)

INTERACTIONS
⚠ Hypertensive crisis: MAOIs
Increase: levodopa effects—antacids
Decrease: levodopa effects—anticholinergics, hydantoins, papaverine, pyridoxine
Drug/Herb
Increase: parkinsonian symptoms—kava
Decrease: levodopa action, increase EPS—Indian snakeroot
Drug/Food
Decrease: levodopa absorption—high-protein foods
Drug/Lab Test
Decrease: VMA
False positive: Urine ketones, urine glucose, Coombs' test
False negative: Urine glucose (glucose oxidase)
False increase: Uric acid, urine protein

NURSING CONSIDERATIONS
Assess:
• Renal, hepatic studies: AST, ALT, alk phos, LDH, bilirubin, CBC, BUN, protein-bound iodine
• Involuntary movements in parkinsonism: akinesia, tremors, staggering gait, muscle rigidity, drooling
⚠ Levodopa toxicity: mental, personality changes, hallucinations, increased twitching, grimacing, tongue protrusion, GI side effects
• B/P, respiration during initial treatment; hypo/hypertension should be reported
• Mental status: affect, mood, behavioral changes, depression; complete suicide assessment

Administer:
• Drug until NPO before surgery
• Adjust dosage to patient response
• With meals; limit protein taken with drug
• Only after MAOIs have been discontinued for 2 wk

Perform/provide:
• Assistance with ambulation during beginning therapy, orthostatic hypotension may occur
• Testing for diabetes mellitus, acromegaly if on long-term therapy

Evaluate:
• Therapeutic response: decrease in akathisia, increased mood

Teach patient/family:
• That therapeutic effects may take several weeks to a few months
• To change positions slowly to prevent orthostatic hypotension
• To report side effects: twitching, eye spasms; indicate overdose
• To use drug exactly as prescribed; if drug is discontinued abruptly, parkinsonian crisis may occur
• That urine, sweat may darken
• To avoid vit B_6 preparations, vitamin-fortified foods containing B_6; these foods can reverse effects of levodopa

---

levofloxacin (R)
(lee-voh-floks′a-sin)
Levaquin
Func. class.: Antiinfective
Chem. class.: Fluoroquinolone

Action: Interferes with conversion of intermediate DNA fragments into high-molecular-weight DNA in bacteria; DNA gyrase inhibitor; inhibits topoisomerase IV

Uses: Acute sinusitis, acute chronic bronchitis, community-acquired pneumonia, uncomplicated skin infections, complicated UTI, cellulitis, PID, prostatitis, inhalational anthrax (postexposure), acute pyelonephritis caused by *Streptococcus pneumoniae, Haemophilus influenzae, Haemophilis parainfluenzae, Moraxella catarrhalis, Escherichia coli, Serratia marcescens, Klebsiella pneumoniae, Chlamydia pneumoniae, Legionella pneumophilia, Mycoplasma pneumoniae, Enterococcus faecalis, Staphylococcus epidermidis, Staphylococcus pyogenes*

Unlabeled uses: Gonococcal infections, disseminated; PID

DOSAGE AND ROUTES

Acute bacterial exacerbation of chronic bronchitis
• *Adult:* **PO/IV** 500 mg q24h × 7 days
Acute bacterial sinusitis
Adult: **PO** 500 mg q24h × 10-14 days or 750 mg q24h × 5 days
Acute pyelonephritis
• *Adult:* **PO** 250 mg q24h × 10 days
Chronic bacterial prostitis
• *Adult:* **PO** 500 mg q24h × 28 days
Postexposure inhalational anthrax
• *Adult:* **PO/IV** 500 mg q24h × 60 days
Pneumonia, community acquired
• *Adult:* **PO/IV** 500 mg q24h × 7-14 days or 750 mg q24h × 5 days
Pneumonia, nosocomial
• *Adult:* **PO/IV** 750 mg q24h × 7-14 days
SSSI, complicated
• *Adult:* **PO/IV** 750 mg q24h × 7-14 days
SSSI, uncomplicated
• *Adult:* **PO** 500 mg q24h × 7-10 days
UTI, complicated
• *Adult:* **PO/IV** 250 mg q24h × 10 days
UTI, uncomplicated
• *Adult:* **PO** 250 mg q24h × 3 days
Gonococcal infection, disseminated (unlabeled)
• *Adult:* **IV** 250 mg q24h × 24-48 hr, then **PO** 500 mg/day × 7 days
PID (unlabeled)
• *Adult:* **IV** 500 mg q24h × 14 days
Renal disease
• *Adult:* **PO/IV** CCr 20-49 ml/min initial 500 mg, then 250 mg, q24h; CCr 10-19 ml/min 250 or 500 mg, depending on condition; then 250 mg q48h

Available forms: Single-use vials 500, 750 mg; premixed flexible containers 250 mg/50 ml D_5W, 500 mg/100 ml D_5W, 750 mg/150 ml D_5W; tabs 250, 500, 750 mg

---

SIDE EFFECTS

CNS: Headache, dizziness, *insomnia,* anxiety, **seizures,** encephalopathy, paresthesia

CV: Chest pain, palpitations, vasodilation, QT prolongation

EENT: Dry mouth, visual impairment

GI: Nausea, flatulence, *vomiting,* diarrhea, abdominal pain, **pseudomembranous colitis**

GU: Vaginitis, crystalluria

HEMA: Eosinophilia, **hemolytic anemia,** lymphopenia

INTEG: Rash, pruritus, *photosensitivity,* epidermal necrolysis

MISC: Hypoglycemia, hypersensitivity, tendon rupture

RESP: Pneumonitis

SYST: **Anaphylaxis, multisystem organ failure, Stevens-Johnson syndrome**

Contraindications: Hypersensitivity to quinolones, photosensitivity

Precautions: Pregnancy (C), lactation, children

PHARMACOKINETICS

Metabolized in liver, excreted in urine unchanged, half-life 6-8 hr

INTERACTIONS

• Do not use with magnesium in the same IV line

Increase: CNS stimulation, seizures—NSAIDs, foscarnet

Increase: bleeding risk—warfarin

Decrease: levofloxacin absorption—antacids containing aluminum, magnesium; sucralfate, zinc, iron, calcium

Decrease: clearance of theophylline, toxicity may result

Drug/Herb

• Do not use acidophilus with antiinfectives; separate by several hours

Increase: antiinfective effect—cola tree

Drug/Lab Test

Decrease: Glucose, lymphocytes

NURSING CONSIDERATIONS

Assess:

• For previous sensitivity reaction

• For signs and symptoms of infection: characteristics of sputum, WBC >10,000/mm^3, fever; obtain baseline information before and during treatment

• C&S before beginning drug therapy to identify if correct treatment has been initiated

⚠ For allergic reactions and anaphylaxis: rash, urticaria, pruritus, chills, fever, joint pain; may occur a few days after therapy begins; epINEPHrine and resuscitation equipment should be available for anaphylactic reaction

• Bowel pattern daily; if severe diarrhea occurs, drug should be discontinued

⚠ For overgrowth of infection: perineal itching, fever, malaise, redness, pain, swelling, drainage, rash, diarrhea, change in cough, sputum

• For cardiac function, watch for QT prolongation; for tendon pain, renal function

Administer:

• PO 4 hr before or 2 hr after antacids, iron, calcium, zinc

• Not to use theophylline with this product; toxicity may result

IV route

• Only by slow IV infusion over 60-90 min

• Discard any unused sol in the single-dose vial

• Using premix, tear outer wrap at notch and remove sol container; check for leaks; close control clamps; remove cover from port at bottom of container; insert pin into port with a twist; suspend container from hanger; squeeze and release drip chamber to proper fluid level; open flow control to expel air, close clamp; regulate rate with flow control clamps

Solution compatibilities: 0.9% NaCl, D$_5$W, D$_5$/0.9% NaCl, D$_5$LR, D$_5$/0.45% NaCl, sodium lactate, plasma-lyte 56/D$_5$W

Perform/provide:

• Increase fluid intake to 2 L/day to prevent crystalluria

Evaluate:

• Therapeutic response: absence of signs/symptoms of infection (WBC <10,000/mm^3, temp WNL)

Teach patient/family:

• To contact prescriber if vaginal itching, loose, foul-smelling stools, furry tongue occur (may indicate superinfection); report itching, rash, pruritus, urticaria

• To notify prescriber of diarrhea with blood or pus

• To take 4 hr before or 2 hr after antacids, iron, calcium, zinc products

• To complete full course of therapy

• To avoid hazardous activities until response is known

• To use frequent rinsing of mouth, sugarless candy or gum for dry mouth

• To avoid other medication unless approved by prescriber

• To prevent sun exposure or use sunscreen to prevent phototoxicity

---

levofloxacin ophthalmic

See Appendix C

---

levothyroxine (T₄) (R)

(lee-voe-thye-rox′een)
Eltroxin ✦, Levo-T, Levothroid, levothyroxine sodium, Levoxyl, PMS-Levothyroxine Sodium ✦, Synthroid, T₄
Func. class.: Thyroid hormone
Chem. class.: Levoisomer of thyroxine

Do not confuse:
Synthroid/Symmetrel

Action: Increases metabolic rate, controls protein synthesis, increases cardiac output, renal blood flow, O_2 consumption, body temp, blood volume, growth, development at cellular level, exact mechanism unknown

Uses: Hypothyroidism, myxedema coma, thyroid hormone replacement, thyrotoxicosis, congenital hypothyroidism, some types of thyroid cancer

DOSAGE AND ROUTES

Severe hypothyroidism

• *Adult:* **PO** 50 mcg/day, increase by 25 mcg/day every 6-8 wks, average dose 100-200 mcg/day; max 200 mcg/day **IM/IV** 50-100 mcg/day as a single dose or 50% of usual oral dosage

• *Child >12 yr:* **PO** 2-3 mcg/kg/day as a single dose AM

• *Child 6-12 yr:* **PO** 4-5 mcg/kg/day as a single dose AM

• *Child 1-5 yr:* **PO** 5-6 mcg/kg/day as a single dose AM

• *Child 6-12 mo:* **PO** 6-8 mcg/kg/day as a single dose AM

• *Child to 6 mo:* **PO** 8-10 mcg/kg/day as a single dose AM

Myxedema coma

• *Adult:* **IV** 200-500 mcg, may increase by 100-300 mcg after 24 hr; place on oral medication as soon as possible

Available forms: Powder for inj 200, 500 mcg/vial; tabs 0.025, 0.05, 0.075, 0.088, 0.1, 0.112, 0.125, 0.137, 0.15, 0.175, 0.2, 0.3 mg

SIDE EFFECTS

CNS: Anxiety, insomnia, tremors, headache, **thyroid storm**

CV: Tachycardia, palpitations, angina, dysrhythmias, hypertension, **cardiac arrest**

GI: Nausea, diarrhea, increased or decreased appetite, cramps

MISC: Menstrual irregularities, weight loss, sweating, heat intolerance, fever, alopecia

Contraindications: Adrenal insufficiency, recent MI, thyrotoxicosis, hypersensitivity to beef, alcohol intolerance (inj only)

Precautions: Pregnancy (A), geriatric, angina pectoris, hypertension, ischemia, cardiac disease, lactation, diabetes

---

⚠ Safety alert   *"Tall Man" lettering

PHARMACOKINETICS

PO: Onset 3-5 days, peak 6-8 wk, duration 1-3 wk

IV: Onset 6-8 hr, peak 24 hr, duration unknown

Half-life euthyroid 6-7 days; hypothyroid 9-10 days; hyperthyroid 3-4 days; distributed throughout body tissues

INTERACTIONS

Increase: cardiac insufficiency risk—epINEPHrine products

Increase: effects of anticoagulants, sympathomimetics, tricyclics

Decrease: levothyroxine absorption—cholestyramine, colestipol, ferrous sulfate

Decrease: effects of digitalis drugs, insulin, hypoglycemics

Decrease: levothyroxine effects—estrogens, SSRIs

Drug/Herb

Decrease: thyroid hormone effect—agar, bugleweed carnitine, kelpware, soy, spirulina

Drug/Lab Test

Increase: CPK, LDH, AST, blood glucose

Decrease: Thyroid function tests

NURSING CONSIDERATIONS

Assess:

• B/P, pulse periodically during treatment
• Weight daily in same clothing, using same scale, at same time of day
• Height, growth rate of a child
• T$_3$, T$_4$, FTIs, which are decreased; radioimmunoassay of TSH, which is increased; radio uptake, which is increased if patient is on too low a dose of medication
• PT may require decreased anticoagulant; check for bleeding, bruising
• Increased nervousness, excitability, irritability, which may indicate too high dose of medication, usually after 1-3 wk of treatment
• Cardiac status: angina, palpitation, chest pain, change in VS

Administer:

• IV after diluting with provided diluent 0.5 mg/5 ml; shake; give through Y-tube or 3-way stopcock; give 0.1 mg or less over 1 min; do not add to IV inf; 0.1 mg = 1 ml
• Considered to be incompatible in syringe with all other drugs
• In AM if possible as a single dose to decrease sleeplessness; at same time each day to maintain drug level; take on empty stomach
• Only for hormone imbalances; not to be used for obesity, male infertility, menstrual conditions, lethargy
• Lowest dose that relieves symptoms; lower dose to the geriatric and in cardiac diseases
• Crushed and mixed with water; nonsoy formula, or breast milk for infants/children

Perform/provide:

• Storage in tight, light-resistant container; sol should be discarded if not used immediately
• Withdrawal of medication 4 wk before RAIU test

Evaluate:

• Therapeutic response: absence of depression; increased weight loss, diuresis, pulse, appetite; absence of constipation, peripheral edema, cold intolerance; pale, cool, dry skin; brittle nails, alopecia, coarse hair, menorrhagia, night blindness, paresthesias, *syncope, stupor, coma,* rosy cheeks

Teach patient/family:

• That hair loss will occur in child, is temporary
• To report excitability, irritability, anxiety, which indicate overdose
• Not to switch brands unless approved by prescriber
• That drug may be discontinued after giving birth, thyroid panel evaluated after 1-2 mo
• That hypothyroid child will show almost immediate behavior/personality change
• That drug is not to be taken to reduce weight

- To avoid OTC preparations with iodine; read labels
- To avoid iodine food, iodized salt, soybeans, tofu, turnips, high-iodine seafood, some bread
- That drug is not a cure but controls symptoms and treatment is lifelong

---

⚠ High Alert

lidocaine (parenteral) (℞)
(lye'doe-kane)
LidoPen Auto-Injector,
Xylocaine, Xylocard ✤
Func. class.: Antidysrhythmic (Class Ib)
Chem. class.: Aminoacyl amide

Action: Increases electrical stimulation threshold of ventricle, His-Purkinje system, which stabilizes cardiac membrane, decreases automaticity

Uses: Ventricular tachycardia, ventricular dysrhythmias during cardiac surgery, myocardial infarction, digoxin toxicity, cardiac catheterization

DOSAGE AND ROUTES
- *Adult:* **IV BOL** 50-100 mg (1 mg/kg) over 2-3 min, repeat q3-5min, not to exceed 300 mg in 1 hr; begin **IV INF; IV INF** 20-50 mcg/kg/min; **IM** 200-300 mg (4.3 mg/kg) in deltoid muscle, may repeat in 1-1½ hr if needed

CHF, reduced hepatic function
- *Geriatric:* **IV BOL** give ½ adult dose
- *Child:* **IV BOL** 1 mg/kg, then **IV INF** 30 mcg/kg/min

Available forms: IV INF 0.2% (2 mg/ml), 0.4% (4 mg/ml), 0.8% (8 mg/ml); IV ad 4% (40 mg/ml), 10% (100 mg/ml), 20% (200 mg/ml); IV dir 1% (10 mg/ml), 2% (20 mg/ml); IM 10% 300 mg/ml

SIDE EFFECTS
CNS: Headache, dizziness, involuntary movement, confusion, tremor, drowsiness, euphoria, **seizures**

CV: Hypotension, bradycardia, **heart block, cardiovascular collapse, arrest**
EENT: Tinnitus, blurred vision
GI: Nausea, vomiting, anorexia
INTEG: Rash, urticaria, edema, swelling
MISC: Febrile response, phlebitis at inj site
RESP: Dyspnea, **respiratory depression**

Contraindications: Hypersensitivity to amides, severe heart block, supraventricular dysrhythmias, Adams-Stokes syndrome, Wolff-Parkinson-White syndrome
Precautions: Pregnancy (B), lactation, children, renal/hepatic disease, CHF, respiratory depression, malignant hyperthermia, geriatric, myasthenia gravis, weight <50 kg

PHARMACOKINETICS
IV: Onset 2 min, duration 20 min
IM: Onset 5-15 min, duration 1½ hr; half-life 8 min, 1-2 hr (terminal); metabolized in liver; excreted in urine; crosses placenta

INTERACTIONS
Increase: neuromuscular blockade—neuromuscular blockers, tubocurarine
Increase: lidocaine effects—cimetidine, phenytoin, propranolol, metoprolol
Decrease: lidocaine effects—barbiturates
Drug/Herb
Increase: lidocaine action—aloe, buckthorn, cascara sagrada, senna
Increase: toxicity, death—aconite
Increase: effect—aloe, broom, chronic buckthorn use, cascara sagrada (chronic use), Chinese rhubarb, figwort, fumitory, goldenseal, kudzu, licorice
Increase: serotonin effect—horehound
Decrease: effect—coltsfoot
Drug/Lab Test
Increase: CPK

NURSING CONSIDERATIONS
Assess:
⚠ ECG continuously to determine increased PR or QRS segments; if these develop, discontinue or reduce rate; watch

---

for increased ventricular ectopic beats; may have to rebolus, B/P

• IV infusion rate using infusion pump; run at less than 4 mg/min

• Blood levels (therapeutic level: 1.5-5 mcg/ml)

• I&O ratio, electrolytes (K, Na, Cl)

A Malignant hyperthermia: tachypnea, tachycardia, changes in B/P, increased temp

• Respiratory status: rate, rhythm, lung fields for crackles, watch for respiratory depression; lung fields, bilateral crackles may occur in CHF patient; increased respiration, increased pulse; drug should be discontinued

• CNS effects: dizziness, confusion, psychosis, paresthesias, convulsions; drug should be discontinued

Administer:

• IM inj in deltoid; aspirate to avoid intravascular administration; check site daily for infiltration or extravasation

IV route

• Bolus undiluted (1%, 2% only) give 50 mg or less over 1 min or dilute 1 g/250-500 ml of D₅W; titrate to patient response; use infusion pump; pediatric inf is 120 mg of lidocaine/100 ml D₅W; 1-2.5 ml/kg/hr = 20-50 mcg/kg/min; use only 1%, 2% sol for IV bol

Additive compatibilities: Alteplase, aminophylline, amiodarone, atracurium, bretylium, calcium chloride, calcium gluceptate, calcium gluconate, chloramphenicol, chlorothiazide, cimetidine, dexamethasone, digoxin, diphenhydrAMINE, DOBUTamine, DOPamine, epHEDrine, erythromycin lactobionate, floxacillin, flumazenil, furosemide, heparin, hydrocortisone, hydrOXYzine, insulin (regular), mephentermine, metaraminol, nafcillin, nitroglycerin, penicillin G potassium, pentobarbital, phenylephrine, potassium chloride, procainamide, prochlorperazine, promazine, ranitidine, sodium bicarbonate, sodium lactate, theophylline, verapamil, vit B/C

Solution compatibilities: D₅W, D₅/0.9% NaCl, D₅/0.45% NaCl, D₅/LR, LR, 0.9% NaCl, 0.45% NaCl

Syringe compatibilities: Cloxacillin, glycopyrrolate, heparin, hydrOXYzine, methicillin, metoclopramide, milrinone, moxalactam, nalbuphine

Y-site compatibilities: Alteplase, amiodarone, amrinone, cefazolin, ciprofloxacin, cisatracurium, diltiazem, DOBUTamine, DOPamine, enalaprilat, etomidate, famotidine, haloperidol, heparin, heparin/hydrocortisone, labetalol, meperidine, morphine, nitroglycerin, nitroprusside, potassium chloride, propofol, remifentanil, streptokinase, theophylline, vit B/C, warfarin

Evaluate:

• Therapeutic response: decreased dysrhythmias

Teach patient/family:

• The use of automatic lidocaine injection device if ordered for personal use

Treatment of overdose: O₂, artificial ventilation, ECG; administer DOPamine for circulatory depression, diazepam or thiopental for convulsions; decrease drug if needed

L

---

lidocaine topical
See Appendix C

---

lindane (R)
(lin′dane)
GBH ♣, G-Well, Hexit ♣, Kwell, lindane, PMS-Lindane ♣, Scabene, Thionex
Func. class.: Scabicide, pediculicide
Chem. class.: Chlorinated hydrocarbon (synthetic)

Action: Stimulates nervous system of arthropods, resulting in seizures, death of organism

Uses: Scabies, lice (head/pubic/body), nits

DOSAGE AND ROUTES
Lice

• *Adult and child:* **CREAM/LOTION** wash area with soap, water; remove visi-

---

Side effects: *italics* = common; **bold** = life-threatening

ble crusts; apply to skin surfaces; remove with soap, water in 8-12 hr; may reapply in 1 wk if needed; shampoo using 30 ml: work into lather, rub for 5 min, rinse, dry with towel; comb with fine-toothed comb to remove nits; most require 1 oz, max 2 oz

Scabies
• *Adult and child:* **TOP** apply 1% cream/lotion to skin, neck to bottom of feet, toes; repeat in 1 wk prn; most require 1 oz, max 2 oz

Available forms: Lotion, shampoo, cream (1%)

SIDE EFFECTS

CNS: Tremors, **seizures, CNS toxicity,** stimulation, dizziness (chronic inhalation of vapors), anxiety, insomnia

CV: **Ventricular fibrillation** (chronic inhalation of vapors)

GI: *Nausea, vomiting, diarrhea,* liver damage (inhalation of vapors)

GU: **Kidney damage** (chronic inhalation of vapors)

HEMA: **Aplastic anemia** (chronic inhalation of vapors), myelosuppression

INTEG: Pruritus, rash, irritation, contact dermatitis

Contraindications: Hypersensitivity; premature neonate; patients with known seizure disorders; inflammation of skin, abrasions, or skin breaks, Norwegian (crusted) scabies

Precautions: Pregnancy (C), avoid contact with eyes, children <10 yr, infants, lactation

INTERACTIONS
• Oils may increase absorption; if an oil-based hair dressing is used, shampoo, rinse, dry hair before applying lindane shampoo

NURSING CONSIDERATIONS
Assess:
• Head, hair for lice and nits before and after treatment; if scabies are present check all skin surfaces
• Identify source of infection: school, family, sexual contacts

Administer:
• To body areas, scalp only; do not apply to face, lips, mouth, eyes, any mucous membrane, anus, or meatus
• Topical corticosteroids as ordered to decrease contact dermatitis
• Antihistamines
• Lotions of menthol or phenol to control itching
• Topical antibiotics for infection

Perform/provide:
• Isolation until areas on skin, scalp have cleared and treatment is completed
• Removal of nits by using a fine-toothed comb rinsed in vinegar after treatment; use gloves

Evaluate:
• Therapeutic response: decreased crusts, nits, brownish trails on skin, itching papules in skin folds, decreased itching after several weeks

Teach patient/family:
• To wash all inhabitants' clothing, using insecticide; preventive treatment may be required of all persons living in same house, using lotion or shampoo to decrease spread of infection; use rubber gloves when applying drug
• That itching may continue for 4-6 wk
• That drug must be reapplied if accidently washed off, or treatment will be ineffective
• Not to apply to face; if accidental contact with eyes occurs, flush with water
• Instruct patient to remove after specified time to prevent toxicity
• To treat sexual contacts simultaneously
• To check for CNS toxicity: dizziness, cramps, anxiety, nausea, vomiting, seizures

Treatment of ingestion: Gastric lavage, saline laxatives, IV diazepam (Valium) for convulsions

linezolid (℞)

(line-zoe'lide)
Zyvox
Func. class.: Broad-spectrum antiinfective
Chem. class.: Oxazolidinone

Action: Inhibits protein synthesis by interfering with translation; binds to bacterial 23S ribosomal RNA of the 50S subunit preventing formation of the bacterial translation process in primarily gram-positive organisms

Uses: Vancomycin-resistant *Enterococcus faecium* infections, nosocomial pneumonia, uncomplicated or complicated skin and skin structure infections, community-acquired pneumonia

DOSAGE AND ROUTES

Vancomycin-resistant Enterococcus faecium *infections*
• *Adult:* **IV/PO** 600 mg q12h × 14-28 days; max 1200 mg/day
Nosocomial pneumonia/complicated skin infections/community-acquired pneumonia/concurrent bacterial infection
• *Adult:* **IV/PO** 600 mg q12h × 10-14 days; max 1200 mg/day
• *Child: birth-11 yr:* **PO** 10 mg/kg q8h × 10-14 days
Uncomplicated skin infections
• *Adult:* **PO** 400 mg q12h × 10-14 days; max 1200 mg/day
• *Adolescent:* **PO** 600 mg q12h × 10-14 days; max 1200 mg/day
• *Infant preterm <7 days old:* **PO** 10 mg/kg q12h × 10-14 days
Available forms: Tabs 600 mg; oral sus 100 mg/5 ml; inj 2 mg/ml

SIDE EFFECTS

CNS: Headache, dizziness
GI: Nausea, diarrhea, **pseudomembranous colitis,** increased ALT, AST, *vomiting,* taste change, tongue color change
HEMA: **Myelosuppression**

MISC: Vaginal moniliasis, fungal infection, oral moniliasis, **lactic acidosis**
Contraindications: Hypersensitivity
Precautions: Pregnancy (C), lactation, children, thrombocytopenia, bone marrow suppression

PHARMACOKINETICS

Rapidly and extensively absorbed, protein binding 31%, metabolized by oxidation of the morpholine ring

INTERACTIONS

⚠ Do not use with MAOIs or those that possess MAOI-like action (furazolidone, isoniazid, INH, procarbazine); hypertensive crisis may occur
⚠ *Increase:* hypertensive crisis, seizures, coma—amoxapine, maprotiline, mirtazapine, trazodone, cyclobenzaprine, tricyclics
⚠ *Increase:* hypertensive crisis—levodopa
Increase: effects of adrenergic agents, serotonergic agents
Drug/Herb
• Do not use acidophilus with antiinfectives; separate by several hours
• Avoid use with green tea
Drug/Food
• Tyramine foods: avoid, increased pressor response

NURSING CONSIDERATIONS
Assess:
• CBC with differential weekly, assess for myelosuppression (anemias, leukopenia, pancytopenia, thrombocytopenia)
• For serotonin syndrome
• CNS symptoms: headache, dizziness
• Hepatic studies: AST, ALT
• Allergic reactions: fever, flushing, rash, urticaria, pruritus
⚠ For pseudomembranous colitis, product should be discontinued
• For lactic acidosis: nausea, vomiting, low bicarbonate levels

Administer:
PO route
- With or without food
- Store reconstituted oral suspension at room temperature, use within 3 wk

IV route
- 30-120 min; do not use IV infusion bag in series connections; do not use with additives in sol; do not use with another drug, administer separately

Y-site compatibilities: acyclovir, alfentanil, amikacin, aminophylline, ampicillin, aztreonam, bretylium, buprenorphine, butorphanol, calcium gluconate, carboplatin, cefazolin, cefoperazone, cefotetan, cefoxitin, ceftazidine, ceftizoxime, cefuroxime, cimetidine, ciprofloxacin, cisatracurium, cisplatin, clindamycin, cyclophosphamide, cycloSPORINE, cytarabine, digoxin, furosemide, ganciclovir, gemcitabine, gentamicin, heparin, hydromorphone, ifosfamide, labetalol, leucovorin, levofloxacin, lidocaine, lorazepam, magnesium sulfate, mannitol, meperidine, meropenem, mesna, methotrexate, methylPREDNISolone, metoclopramide, metronidazole, midazolam, minocycline, mitoxantrone, morphine, nalbuphine, naloxone, nitroglycerin, ofloxacin, ondansetron, paclitaxel, pentobarbital, phenobarbital, piperacillin, potassium chloride, prochlorperazine, promethazine, propranolol, ranitidine, remifentanil, sufentanil, theophylline, ticarcillin, tobramycin, vancomycin, vecuronium, verapamil, vinCRIStine, zidovudine

Solution compatibilities: D₅, 0.9% NaCl, LR

Evaluate:
- Therapeutic response: decreased symptoms of infection, blood cultures negative

Teach patient/family:
- If dizziness occurs, to ambulate, perform activities with assistance
- To complete full course of drug therapy
- To contact prescriber if adverse reaction occurs
- To inform prescriber if SSRIs or cold products, decongestants are being used
- To inform prescriber if there is a history of hypertension
- To avoid large amounts of high-tyramine foods, drinks (provide list)

---

liothyronine (T₃) (℞)
(lye-oh-thye′roe-neen)
Cytomel, ʟ-triiodothyronine, T₃, liothyronine sodium, Triostat
Func. class.: Thyroid hormone
Chem. class.: Synthetic T₃

Action: Increases metabolic rates, cardiac output, O₂ consumption, body temp, blood volume, growth, development at cellular level; exact mechanism unknown
Uses: Hypothyroidism, myxedema coma, thyroid hormone replacement, congenital hypothyroidism, nontoxic goiter, T₃ suppression test

DOSAGE AND ROUTES
- *Adult:* **PO** 25 mcg daily, increased by 12.5-25 mcg q1-2wk until desired response, maintenance dose 25-75 mcg daily, max 100 mcg/day
- *Geriatric:* **PO** 5 mcg/day, increase by 5 mcg/day q1-2wk, maintenance 25-75 mcg/day

Congenital hypothyroidism
- *Child >3 yr:* **PO** 50-100 mcg daily
- *Child <3 yr:* **PO** 5 mcg daily, increased by 5 mcg q3-4d titrated to response, maintenance 20 mcg/day

Myxedema, severe hypothyroidism
- *Adult:* **PO** 25-50 mcg then may increase by 5-10 mcg q1-2wk; maintenance dose 50-100 mcg daily

Myxedema coma/precoma
- *Adult:* **IV** 25-50 mcg initially, 5 mcg in geriatric, 10-20 mcg in cardiac disease; give doses q4-12h

Nontoxic goiter
- *Adult:* **PO** 5 mcg daily, increased by 12.5-25 mcg q1-2wk; maintenance dose 75 mcg daily

---

⚠ Safety alert   *"Tall Man" lettering

Suppression test
• *Adult:* PO 75-100 mcg daily × 1 wk; radioactive ¹³¹I is given before and after 1-wk dose

Available forms: Tabs 5, 25, 50 mcg; inj 10 mcg/ml

SIDE EFFECTS

CNS: Insomnia, tremors, headache, **thyroid storm**

CV: Tachycardia, palpitations, angina, dysrhythmias, hypertension, **cardiac arrest**

GI: Nausea, diarrhea, increased or decreased appetite, cramps

MISC: Menstrual irregularities, weight loss, sweating, heat intolerance, fever, alopecia

Contraindications: Adrenal insufficiency, myocardial infarction, thyrotoxicosis

Precautions: Pregnancy (A), geriatric, angina pectoris, hypertension, ischemia, cardiac disease, lactation, diabetes

PHARMACOKINETICS

PO/IV: Peak 12-48 hr, duration 72 hr, half-life 1-2 days

INTERACTIONS

Increase: effects of anticoagulants, sympathomimetics, tricyclics, amphetamines, decongestants, vasopressors

Decrease: absorption of liothyronine—cholestyramine, colestipol

Decrease: effects of digoxin, insulin, hypoglycemics

Decrease: effects of liothyronine—estrogens

Drug/Herb
Decrease: thyroid hormone effect—agar, bugleweed, carnitine, kelpware, soy, spirulina

Drug/Lab Test
Increase: CPK, LDH, AST, PBI, blood glucose

Decrease: Thyroid function tests

NURSING CONSIDERATIONS

Assess:
• B/P, pulse, periodically during treatment
• Weight daily in same clothing, using same scale, at same time of day
• Height, growth rate of child
• T₃, T₄, which are decreased; radioimmunoassay of TSH, which is increased; radio uptake, which is increased if patient is on too low a dose of medication
• PT may require decreased anticoagulant; check for bleeding, bruising
• Increased nervousness, excitability, irritability, which may indicate too high a dose of medication, usually after 1-3 wk of treatment
• Cardiac status: angina, palpitation, chest pain, change in VS

Administer:
• In AM if possible as a single dose to decrease sleeplessness
• At same time each day to maintain drug level
• Only for hormone imbalances; not to be used for obesity, male infertility, menstrual conditions, lethargy
• Lowest dose that relieves symptoms
• Liothyronine after discontinuing other thyroid preparation

Perform/provide:
• Removal of medication 4 wk before RAIU test

Evaluate:
• Therapeutic response: absence of depression; increased weight loss, diuresis, pulse, appetite; absence of constipation, peripheral edema, cold intolerance; pale, cool, dry skin; brittle nails, alopecia, coarse hair, menorrhagia, night blindness, paresthesia, syncope, stupor, coma, rosy cheeks

Teach patient/family:
• That hair loss will occur in child but is temporary
• To report excitability, irritability, anxiety, which indicates overdose
• Not to switch brands unless approved by prescriber

• That hypothyroid child will show almost immediate behavior/personality change
• That drug is not to be taken to reduce weight
• To avoid OTC preparations with iodine; read labels
• To avoid iodine food, iodized salt, soybeans, tofu, turnips, high iodine seafood, some bread
• That drug controls symptoms but does not cure; treatment is lifelong

---

liotrix (R)
(lye'oh-trix)
Thyrolar, T_3/T_4
Func. class.: Thyroid hormone
Chem. class.: Levothyroxine/liothyronine (synthetic T_4, T_3)

Do not confuse:
Thyrolar/Thyrar
Action: Increases metabolic rates, cardiac output, O_2 consumption, body temp, blood volume, growth, development at cellular level, exact mechanism unknown
Uses: Hypothyroidism, thyroid hormone replacement

DOSAGE AND ROUTES

• *Adult:* **PO** a single dose of Thyrolar ¼ or ½, adjust as needed at 2-wk intervals
• *Geriatric:* **PO** ¼ tab, initially, adjust q6-8 wks
Available forms: Tabs: Levothyroxine 12.5 mcg/liothyronine 3.1 mcg; levothyroxine 25 mcg/liothyronine 6.25 mcg (Thyrolar-½); levothyroxine 50 mcg/liothyronine 12.5 mcg (Thyrolar-1); levothyroxine 100 mcg/liothyronine 25 mcg (Thyrolar-2); levothyroxine 150 mcg/liothyronine 37.5 mcg (Thyrolar-3)

SIDE EFFECTS

CNS: Insomnia, tremors, headache, **thyroid storm**
CV: Tachycardia, palpitations, angina, dysrhythmias, hypertension, **cardiac arrest**

GI: Nausea, diarrhea, increased or decreased appetite, cramps
MISC: Menstrual irregularities, weight loss, sweating, heat intolerance, fever
Contraindications: Adrenal insufficiency, myocardial infarction, thyrotoxicosis
Precautions: Pregnancy (A), geriatric, angina pectoris, hypertension, ischemia, cardiac disease, lactation, diabetes

PHARMACOKINETICS

PO (T_4): Onset unknown, peak 1-3 wk, duration 1-3 wk; terminal half-life 6-7 days
PO (T_3): Onset unknown, peak 24-72 hr, duration 72 hr, terminal half-life 1-2 days

INTERACTIONS

Increase: effects of amphetamines, decongestants, vasopressors, anticoagulants, sympathomimetics, tricyclics, catecholamines
Decrease: absorption of liotrix—cholestyramine, colestipol
Decrease: effects of digoxin, insulin, hypoglycemics
Decrease: effects of liotrix—estrogens
Drug/Herb
Decrease: thyroid hormone effect—agar, bugleweed, carnitine, kelpware, soy, spirulina
Drug/Lab Test
Increase: CPK, LDH, AST, PBI, blood glucose
Decrease: Thyroid function tests

NURSING CONSIDERATIONS

Assess:
• B/P, pulse periodically during treatment
• Weight daily in same clothing, using same scale, at same time of day
• Height, growth rate of child
• T_3, T_4, FTIs, which are decreased; radioimmunoassay of TSH, which is increased; radio uptake, which is increased if patient is on too low a dose of medication
• PT may require decreased anticoagulant; check for bleeding, bruising

---

▲ Safety alert   *"Tall Man" lettering

• Increased nervousness, excitability, irritability, which may indicate too high dose of medication, usually after 1-3 wk of treatment

• Cardiac status: angina, palpitation, chest pain, change in VS

Administer:

• In AM if possible as a single dose to decrease sleeplessness

• At same time each day to maintain drug level

• Only for hormone imbalances; not to be used for obesity, male infertility, menstrual conditions, lethargy

• Lowest dose that relieves symptoms

Perform/provide:

• Withdrawal of medication 4 wk before RAIU test

• Storage in airtight, light-resistant container

Evaluate:

• Therapeutic response: absence of depression; increased weight loss, diuresis, pulse, appetite; absence of constipation, peripheral edema, cold intolerance; pale, cool, dry skin; brittle nails, coarse hair, menorrhagia, night blindness, paresthesias, syncope, stupor, coma, rosy cheeks

Teach patient/family:

• That hair loss will occur in child, is temporary

• To report excitability, irritability, chest pain, increased pulse rate, palpitations, excessive sweating, heat intolerance, nervousness, anxiety, which indicate overdose

• Not to switch brands unless approved by prescriber

• That hypothyroid child will show almost immediate behavior/personality change

• That drug is not to be taken to reduce weight

• To avoid OTC preparations with iodine; read labels

• To avoid iodine food, iodized salt, soybeans, tofu, turnips, high iodine seafood, some bread

• That drug does not cure, but controls symptoms, treatment is lifelong

lisinopril (℞)

(lyse-in'oh-pril)
Prinivil, Zestril

Func. class.: Antihypertensive, angiotensin-converting enzyme (ACE) inhibitor

Chem. class.: Enalaprilat lysine analog

Do not confuse:

lisinopril/Risperdal
Prinivil/Plendil/Proventil/Prilosec

Action: Selectively suppresses renin-angiotensin-aldosterone system; inhibits ACE, preventing conversion of angiotensin I to angiotensin II

Uses: Mild to moderate hypertension, adjunctive therapy of systolic CHF, acute MI

DOSAGE AND ROUTES

Hypertension

• *Adult:* PO 10-40 mg daily; may increase to 80 mg daily if required

• *Geriatric:* PO 2.5-5 mg/day, increase q7d

CHF

Adult: PO 5 mg initially with diuretics/digoxin, range 5-40 mg

Available forms: Tabs 2.5, 5, 10, 20, 30, 40 mg

SIDE EFFECTS

CNS: Vertigo, depression, **stroke,** insomnia, paresthesias, headache, *fatigue,* asthenia, dizziness

CV: Chest pain, hypotension

EENT: Blurred vision, nasal congestion

GI: Nausea, vomiting, anorexia, constipation, flatulence, GI irritation, diarrhea

GU: **Proteinuria, renal insufficiency,** sexual dysfunction, impotence

INTEG: Rash, pruritus

MISC: Muscle cramps, hyperkalemia

RESP: Dry cough, dyspnea

SYST: **Angioedema**

Contraindications: Pregnancy (D) 2nd/3rd trimesters, hypersensitivity, angioedema

Precautions: Pregnancy (C) 1st trimester, lactation, renal disease, hyperkalemia, renal artery stenosis, CHF

PHARMACOKINETICS

Onset 1 hr, peak 6-8 hr, duration 24 hr, excreted unchanged in urine, half-life 12 hr

INTERACTIONS

• Hyperkalemia: potassium salt substitutes, potassium-sparing diuretics, potassium supplements, cycloSPORINE
• Possible toxicity: lithium, digoxin

Increase: hypotensive effect—diuretics, other hypertensives, probenecid, phenothiazines, nitrates, acute alcohol ingestion
Increase: hypersensitivity—allopurinol
Decrease: lisinopril effects—aspirin, indomethacin, NSAIDs

Drug/Herb
Increase: toxicity, death—aconite
Increase: antihypertensive effect—barberry, betony, black catechu, black cohosh, bloodroot, broom, burdock, cat's claw, dandelion, goldenseal, hawthorn, Irish moss, Jamaican dogwood, kelp, khella, mistletoe, parsley
Increase or decrease: antihypertensive effect—astragalus, cola tree
Decrease: antihypertensive effect—coltsfoot, guarana, khat, licorice, yohimbine

Drug/Food
• High-potassium diet (bananas, orange juice, avocados, nuts, spinach) should be avoided; hyperkalemia may occur

Drug/Lab Test
Interference: Glucose/insulin tolerance tests, ANA titer

NURSING CONSIDERATIONS

Assess:
⚠ Blood studies, platelets; WBC with diff baseline and periodically q3mo; if neutrophils <1000/mm^3, discontinue treatment (recommended in collagen-vascular disease)
• B/P, pulse q4h; note rate, rhythm, quality

• Electrolytes: K, Na, Cl
• Apical/pedal pulse before administration; notify prescriber of any significant changes
• Baselines in renal, hepatic studies before therapy begins and periodically LFTs, uric acid and glucose may be increased
• Edema in feet, legs daily, weight daily in CHF
• Skin turgor, dryness of mucous membranes for hydration status
• Symptoms of CHF: edema, dyspnea, wet crackles

Administer:
• Severe hypotension may occur after 1st dose of this medication; may be prevented by reducing or discontinuing diuretic therapy 3 days before beginning lisinopril therapy

Evaluate:
• Therapeutic response: decreased B/P, CHF symptoms

Teach patient/family:
• Not to discontinue drug abruptly
• To rise slowly to sitting or standing position to minimize orthostatic hypotension
• To avoid increasing potassium in the diet

Treatment of overdose: Lavage, IV atropine for bradycardia, IV theophylline for bronchospasm, digitalis, O_2, diuretic for cardiac failure

---

lithium (℞)

(li'thee-um)
Carbolith ✚, Duralith ✚, Eskalith, Eskalith-CR, lithium carbonate, Lithizine ✚, Lithonate, Lithotabs
Func. class.: Antimanic, antipsychotic
Chem. class.: Alkali metal ion salt

Action: May alter sodium, potassium ion transport across cell membrane in nerve, muscle cells; may balance biogenic amines of norepinephrine, serotonin in

CNS areas involved in emotional responses

Uses: Bipolar disorders (manic phase), prevention of bipolar manic-depressive psychosis

DOSAGE AND ROUTES
• *Adult:* **PO** 300-600 mg tid, maintenance 300 mg tid or qid; **SLOW REL TABS** 300 mg bid; dose should be individualized to maintain blood levels at 0.5-1.5 mEq/L
• *Geriatric:* **PO** 300 mg bid, increase q7 days by 300 mg to desired dose
• *Child:* **PO** 15-20 mg (0.4-0.5 mEq/kg/day in 2-3 divided doses, increase as needed, do not exceed adult doses)
Renal dose
• *Adult:* **PO** CCr 10-50 ml/min 50%-75% of dose; CCr <10 ml/min 25%-50% of dose
Available forms: Caps 150, 300, 600 mg; tabs 300 mg; ext rel tabs 300, 450 mg; syr 300 mg/5 ml (8 mEq/5 ml); slow rel caps 150, 300 mg ♣

SIDE EFFECTS
CNS: Headache, drowsiness, dizziness, tremors, twitching, ataxia, **seizure,** slurred speech, restlessness, confusion, stupor, memory loss, clonic movements, fatigue
CV: Hypotension, ECG changes, **dysrhythmias, circulatory collapse,** edema
EENT: Tinnitus, blurred vision
ENDO: Hyponatremia, hypothyroidism, goiter, hyperglycemia, hyperthyroidism
GI: Dry mouth, anorexia, nausea, vomiting, diarrhea, incontinence, abdominal pain, metallic taste
GU: **Polyuria, glycosuria, proteinuria, albuminuria,** urinary incontinence, polydipsia
HEMA: **Leukocytosis**
INTEG: Drying of hair, alopecia, rash, pruritus, hyperkeratosis, acneiform lesions, folliculitis
MS: Muscle weakness
Contraindications: Pregnancy (D), hepatic disease, brain trauma, OBS, lactation, children <12 yr, schizophrenia, severe cardiac disease, severe renal disease, severe dehydration
Precautions: Geriatric, thyroid disease, seizure disorders, diabetes mellitus, systemic infection, urinary retention

PHARMACOKINETICS
PO: Onset rapid, peak ½-4 hr, half-life 18-36 hr depending on age; crosses blood-brain barrier; 80% of filtered lithium is reabsorbed by the renal tubules, excreted in urine; crosses placenta; enters breast milk; well absorbed by oral method

INTERACTIONS
• Neurotoxicity: haloperidol, thioridazine
Increase: hypothyroid effects—antithyroid agents, calcium iodide, potassium iodide, iodinated glycerol
Increase: effects of neuromuscular blocking agents, phenothiazines
Increase: renal clearance—sodium bicarbonate, acetaZOLAMIDE, mannitol, aminophylline
Increase: toxicity—indomethacin, diuretics, nonsteroidal antiinflammatories, losartan
Increase: lithium effect/toxicity—carbamazepine, fluoxetine, methyldopa, NSAIDs, thiazide diuretics, probenecid
Decrease: lithium effects—theophyllines, urea, urinary alkalinizers
Drug/Herb
Increase: lithium effects, increase toxicity—broom, buchu, dandelion, goldenrod, horsetail, juniper, nettle, parsley
Decrease: lithium levels—black/green tea, coffee, cola nut, guarana, plantain, yerba maté
Drug/Food
• Significant changes in sodium intake will alter lithium excretion
Drug/Lab Test
Increase: Potassium excretion, urine glucose, blood glucose, protein, BUN
Decrease: VMA, T_3, T_4, PBI, ^{131}I

NURSING CONSIDERATIONS
Assess:
• Weight daily; check for and report edema in legs, ankles, wrists
• Sodium intake; decreased sodium intake with decreased fluid intake may lead to lithium retention; increased sodium and fluids may decrease lithium retention
• Skin turgor at least daily
• Urine for albuminuria, glycosuria, uric acid during beginning treatment, q2mo thereafter
• Neurologic status: LOC, gait, motor reflexes, hand tremors
• Serum lithium levels qwk initially, then q2mo (therapeutic level: 0.5-1.5 mEq/L)
Administer:
• Do not break, crush, or chew caps, ext rel tabs
• Reduced dose to geriatric
• With meals to avoid GI upset
• Adequate fluids (2-3 L/day) to prevent dehydration during initial treatment, 1-2 L/day during maintenance
Evaluate:
• Therapeutic response: decrease in excitement, manic phase
Teach patient/family:
• The symptoms of minor toxicity: vomiting, diarrhea, poor coordination, fine motor tremors, weakness, lassitude; major toxicity: coarse tremors, severe thirst, tinnitus, diluted urine
• To monitor urine specific gravity, emphasize need for follow-up care to determine lithium levels; monitor lithium levels to ensure effective levels and treatment
• That contraception is necessary, since lithium may harm fetus
• Not to operate machinery until lithium levels are stable
• That beneficial effects may take 1-3 wk
• About drugs that interact with lithium (provide list) and discuss need for adequate stable intake of salt and fluids
Treatment of overdose: Induce emesis or lavage, maintain airway, respiratory function; dialysis for severe intoxication

---

Iodoxamide ophthalmic
See Appendix C

---

lomustine (℞)
(loe-mus′teen)
CCNU, CeeNU
Func. class.: Antineoplastic alkylating agent
Chem. class.: Nitrosourea

Action: Responsible for crosslinking DNA strands, which leads to cell death; activity is not cell cycle phase specific
Uses: Hodgkin's disease, lymphomas, melanomas, multiple myeloma; brain, lung, bladder, kidney, colon cancer
Unlabeled uses: Brain, breast, renal, GI tract, bronchogenic carcinoma; melanomas

DOSAGE AND ROUTES
• *Adult:* **PO** 130 mg/m^2 as a single dose q6wk; titrate dose to WBC; do not give repeat dose unless WBC >4000/mm^3, platelet count >100,000/mm^3
Available forms: Caps 10, 40, 100 mg

SIDE EFFECTS
GI: Nausea, vomiting, anorexia, stomatitis, **hepatotoxicity**
GU: **Azotemia, renal failure**
HEMA: **Thrombocytopenia, leukopenia, myelosuppression, anemia**
RESP: **Fibrosis, pulmonary infiltrate**
Contraindications: Pregnancy (D), hypersensitivity, leukopenia, thrombocytopenia, lactation, ''blastic'' phase of CML
Precautions: Radiation therapy

PHARMACOKINETICS
Metabolized in liver, excreted in urine; half-life 16-48 hr; 50% protein bound; crosses blood-brain barrier; appears in breast milk

---

INTERACTIONS
• Lomustine potentiation: succinylcholine
Increase: bleeding—aspirin, anticoagulants
Increase: toxicity—barbiturates, phenytoin, chloral hydrate
Increase: lomustine metabolism—phenobarbital
Increase: bone marrow depression—allopurinol
Drug/Lab Test
False positive: Cytology tests for breast, bladder, cervix, lung

NURSING CONSIDERATIONS
Assess:
• CBC, differential, platelet count qwk; withhold drug if WBC <4000/mm³ or platelet count <100,000/mm³; notify prescriber
• Pulmonary function tests, chest x-ray films before, during therapy; chest film should be obtained q2wk during treatment
• Renal studies: BUN, serum uric acid, urine CCr before, during therapy
• I&O ratio; report fall in urine output of 30 ml/hr
• Monitor temp q4h (may indicate beginning infection); no rectal temps
• Hepatic studies before, during therapy (bilirubin, AST, ALT, LDH) as needed or monthly
• Bleeding: hematuria, guaiac, bruising or petechiae, mucosa or orifices q8h
• Dyspnea, crackles, unproductive cough, chest pain, tachypnea
• Food preferences; list likes, dislikes
• Jaundiced skin and sclera, dark urine, clay-colored stools, itchy skin, abdominal pain, fever, diarrhea
• Inflammation of mucosa, breaks in skin
• Buccal cavity q8h for dryness, sores or ulceration, white patches, oral pain, bleeding, dysphagia
• Local irritation, pain, burning, discoloration at inj site
⚠ Symptoms indicating severe allergic reaction: rash, pruritus, urticaria, purpuric skin lesions, itching, flushing

Administer:
• Antiemetic 30-60 min before giving drug to prevent vomiting
• Antibiotics for prophylaxis of infection
Perform/provide:
• Storage in tight container at room temperature
• Strict medical asepsis, protective isolation if WBC levels are low
• Deep-breathing exercises with patient tid-qid; place in semi-Fowler's position
• Rinsing of mouth tid-qid with water, club soda; brushing of teeth bid-tid with soft brush or cotton-tipped applicators for stomatitis; use unwaxed dental floss
Evaluate:
• Therapeutic response: decreased tumor size, spread of malignancy
Teach patient/family:
• About protective isolation
• To report any changes in breathing or coughing
• To avoid foods with citric acid, hot or rough texture if buccal inflammation is present
• To report any bleeding, white spots, or ulcerations in mouth to prescriber; tell patient to examine mouth daily
• To report signs of infection: fever, sore throat, flulike symptoms
• To use effective contraception, avoid breastfeeding
• To report signs of anemia: fatigue, headache, faintness, shortness of breath, irritability
• To avoid use of razors, commercial mouthwash
• To avoid use of all OTC medications
• To take entire dose at one time

loperamide (otc, ℞)
(loe-per'a-mide)
loperamide solution,
Imodium, Imodium A-D,
Imodium A-D Caplet,
loperamide, Kaopectate II
Caplets, Maalox Antidiarrheal
Caplets, Neo-Diaral, Pepto
Diarrhea Control
Func. class.: Antidiarrheal
Chem. class.: Piperidine derivative

Action: Direct action on intestinal muscles to decrease GI peristalsis; reduces volume, increases bulk, electrolytes not lost

Uses: Diarrhea (cause undetermined), travelers' diarrhea, chronic diarrhea, to decrease amount of ileostomy discharge

DOSAGE AND ROUTES
• *Adult:* **PO** 4 mg, then 2 mg after each loose stool, max 16 mg/day
• *Child 9-11 yr:* **PO** 2 mg, then 1 mg after each loose stool, max 6 mg/24 hr
• *Child 2-5 yr:* **PO** 1 mg then 0.1 mg/kg after each loose stool, max 4 mg/24 hr
Available forms: Caps 2 mg; liq 1 mg/5 ml; tabs 2 mg

SIDE EFFECTS
CNS: Dizziness, drowsiness, fatigue, fever
GI: Nausea, *dry mouth, vomiting, constipation,* abdominal pain, anorexia, **toxic megacolon**
INTEG: Rash

Contraindications: Hypersensitivity, severe ulcerative colitis, pseudomembranous colitis, acute diarrhea associated with *Escherichia coli*

Precautions: Pregnancy (B), lactation, children <2 yr, hepatic disease, dehydration, bacterial disease

PHARMACOKINETICS
PO: Onset ½-1 hr, duration 4-5 hr, half-life 7-14 hr; metabolized in liver; excreted in feces as unchanged drug; small amount in urine

INTERACTIONS
Increase: CNS depression—alcohol, antihistamines, analgesics, opioids, sedative/hypnotics
Drug/Herb
Increase: CNS depression—chamomile, hops, kava, skullcap, valerian
Increase: antidiarrheal effect—nutmeg

NURSING CONSIDERATIONS
Assess:
• Stools: volume, color, characteristics
• Electrolytes (K, Na, Cl) if on long-term therapy
• Skin turgor q8h if dehydration is suspected
• Bowel pattern before; for rebound constipation
• Response after 48 hr; if no response, drug should be discontinued
• Dehydration, CNS problems in children
• Abdominal distention, toxic megacolon; may occur in ulcerative colitis
Administer:
• Do not break, crush, or chew caps
• For 48 hr only
• Do not mix oral sol with other sols
Perform/provide:
• Storage in tight container
Evaluate:
• Therapeutic response: decreased diarrhea
Teach patient/family:
• To avoid OTC products unless directed by prescriber
• That ileostomy patient may take this drug for extended time
• That if drowsiness occurs, not to operate machinery
• To use hard candy, sips of water for dry mouth

loracarbef
See cephalosporins—2nd generation

loratadine (otc, R)

(lor-a'ti-deen)
Alavert, Children's Loratadine,
Children's ND Non-Drowsy
Allergy, Claritin, Claritin Non-
Drowsy Allergy, Claritin
Reditabs, Clear-Atadine,
Dimetapp, Tavist ND
Func. class.: Antihistamine, 2nd
generation
Chem. class.: Selective histamine
(H_1)-receptor antagonist

Action: Binds to peripheral histamine receptors, providing antihistamine action without sedation

Uses: Seasonal rhinitis, chronic idiopathic urticaria for those ≥2 yr

DOSAGE AND ROUTES

• *Adult and child ≥6 yr:* **PO** 10 mg daily
• *Child 2-5 yr:* **PO** 5 mg daily
Renal dose
• *Adult:* **PO** 10 mg every other day (CCr <30 ml/min)
Hepatic dose
• *Adult:* **PO** 10 mg every other day
Available forms: Tabs 10 mg; rapid-disintegrating tabs 10 mg; orally disintegrating tabs 10 mg; syr 1 mg/ml; susp 5 mg/ml

SIDE EFFECTS

CNS: Sedation (more common with increased doses), headache
Contraindications: Hypersensitivity, acute asthma attacks, lower respiratory tract disease
Precautions: Pregnancy (B), increased intraocular pressure, bronchial asthma

PHARMACOKINETICS

Onset 1-3 hr, peak 8-10 hr, duration 24 hr, metabolized in liver to active metabolites, excreted in urine, active metabolite deslovatadine half-life 20 hr

INTERACTIONS

Increase: antihistamine effects—MAOIs

Increase: CNS depressant effects—alcohol, antidepressants, other antihistamines, sedative/hypnotics
Increase: loratadine level—cimetidine, ketoconazole, macrolides (clarithromycin, erythromycin)
Drug/Herb
Increase: CNS depression—chamomile, hops, Jamaican dogwood, kava, khat, senega, skullcap, valerian
Increase: anticholinergic effect—corkwood, henbane leaf
Drug/Lab Test
False negative: Skin allergy tests (discontinue antihistamine 3 days before testing)

NURSING CONSIDERATIONS

Assess:
• Allergy: hives, rash, rhinitis; monitor respiratory status
Administer:
• Rapid-disintegrating tabs by placing on tongue, then swallow after disintegrated with or without water
• Use within 6 mo of opening pouch and immediately after opening blister pack
• On empty stomach daily
Perform/provide:
• Storage in tight container at room temperature
• Increased fluids to 2 L/day to decrease secretions
Evaluate:
• Therapeutic response: absence of running or congested nose, other allergy symptoms
Teach patient/family:
• To avoid driving, other hazardous activities if drowsiness occurs
• To use sunscreen or stay out of the sun to prevent photosensitivity
• To avoid use of other CNS depressants
• To increase fluids to 2 L/day to decrease secretions

lorazepam (℞)

(lor-a′ze-pam)
Apo-Lorazepam ✣, Ativan,
lorazepam, Novo-Lorazem ✦,
Nu-Loraz ✦

Func. class.: Sedative, hypnotic;
antianxiety
Chem. class.: Benzodiazepine

Controlled Substance Schedule IV
Do not confuse:

lorazepam/alprazolam/clonazepam

Action: Potentiates the actions of GABA,
especially in system and reticular formation

Uses: Anxiety, irritability in psychiatric
or organic disorders, preoperatively, insomnia, adjunct in endoscopic procedures

Unlabeled uses: Antiemetic prior to
chemotherapy, status epilepticus, rectal
use

DOSAGE AND ROUTES

Anxiety
• *Adult:* **PO** 2-6 mg/day in divided doses,
max 10 mg/day
• *Geriatric:* **PO** 0.5-1 mg/day in divided
doses; or 0.5-1 mg at bedtime
• *Child:* **PO** 0.05 mg/kg/dose, q4-8h
Insomnia
• *Adult:* **PO** 2-4 mg at bedtime; only min-
imally effective after 2 wk continuous ther-
apy
• *Geriatric:* **PO** 1-2 mg initially
Preoperatively
• *Adult:* **IM** 50 mcg/kg 2 hr prior to sur-
gery; **IV** 44 mcg/kg 15-20 min prior to
surgery, max 2 mg 15-20 min prior to
surgery
• *Child:* **IV** 0.05 mg/kg
Status epilepticus
• *Neonate:* **IV** 0.05 mg/kg
• *Child:* **IV** 0.1 mg/kg up to 4 mg/dose;
RECTAL (unlabeled) 0.05-0.1 mg × 2;
wait 7 min before giving 2nd dose
Available forms: Tabs 0.5, 1, 2 mg;
inj 2, 4 mg/ml; conc oral sol 2 mg/ml

SIDE EFFECTS

CNS: Dizziness, drowsiness, confusion,
headache, anxiety, tremors, stimulation,
fatigue, depression, insomnia, hallucinations, weakness, unsteadiness
CV: Orthostatic hypotension, **ECG
changes, tachycardia,** hypotension; **apnea, cardiac arrest (IV, rapid)**
EENT: Blurred vision, tinnitus, mydriasis
GI: Constipation, dry mouth, nausea, vomiting, anorexia, diarrhea
INTEG: Rash, dermatitis, itching
Contraindications: Pregnancy (D),
hypersensitivity to benzodiazepines,
narrow-angle glaucoma, psychosis, lactation, history of drug abuse, COPD
Precautions: Geriatric, debilitated,
renal/hepatic disease, child <12 yr

PHARMACOKINETICS

PO: Onset ½ hr, peak 1-6 hr, duration 24-48 hr
IM: Onset 15-30 min, peak 1-1½ hr,
duration 24-48 hr
IV: Onset 5-15 min, peak unknown,
duration 24-48 hr
Metabolized by liver; excreted by kidneys; crosses placenta, breast milk; half-
life 14 hr

INTERACTIONS

Increase: lorazepam effects—CNS de-
pressants, alcohol, disulfiram, oral con-
traceptives
Decrease: lorazepam effects—valproic
acid
Drug/Herb
Increase: hypotension—black cohosh
Increase: CNS depression—catnip,
chamomile, clary, cowslip, hops, kava,
lavender, mistletoe, nettle, pokeweed,
poppy, Queen Anne's lace, senega, skull-
cap, valerian
Drug/Lab Test
Increase: AST, ALT, serum bilirubin
Decrease: RAIU
False increase: 17-OHCS

NURSING CONSIDERATIONS
Assess:
• B/P (lying, standing), pulse; if systolic B/P drops 20 mm Hg, hold drug, notify prescriber; respirations q5-15min if given IV
• Blood studies: CBC during long-term therapy; blood dyscrasias have occurred rarely
• Hepatic studies: AST, ALT, bilirubin, creatinine, LDH, alk phos
• Mental status: mood, sensorium, affect, sleeping pattern, drowsiness, dizziness
• Physical dependency, withdrawal symptoms: headache, nausea, vomiting, muscle pain, weakness, tremors, convulsions, after long-term, excessive use
⚠ Suicidal tendencies
Administer:
• With food or milk for GI symptoms
• Crushed if patient is unable to swallow medication whole
• Sugarless gum, hard candy, frequent sips of water for dry mouth
• Deep into large muscle mass (IM inj)
IV route
• Prepare immediately before use, short stability time
• IV after diluting in equal vol sterile H_2O, 5% dextrose or 0.9% NaCl for inj; give through Y-tube or 3-way stopcock; give at 2 mg or less over 1 min

Syringe compatibilities: Cimetidine, hydromorphone
Y-site compatibilities: Acyclovir, albumin, allopurinol, amifostine, amikacin, amoxicillin, amoxicillin/clavulanate, amphotericin B cholesteryl, amsacrine, atracurium, bumetanide, cefepime, cefotaxime, ciprofloxacin, cisatracurium, cisplatin, cladribine, clonidine, cyclophosphamide, cytarabine, dexamethasone, diltiazem, DOBUTamine, DOPamine, DOXOrubicin, DOXOrubicin liposome, epINEPHrine, erythromycin, etomidate, famotidine, fentanyl, filgrastim, fluconazole, fludarabine, furosemide, gentamicin, granisetron, haloperidol, heparin, hydrocortisone, hydromorphone, ketanserin, labetalol, melphalan, methotrexate, metronidazole, midazolam, milrinone, morphine, niCARdipine, nitroglycerin, norepinephrine, paclitaxel, pancuronium, piperacillin, piperacillin/tazobactam, potassium chloride, propofol, ranitidine, remifentanil, tacrolimus, teniposide, thiotepa, trimethoprim-sulfamethoxazole, vancomycin, vecuronium, vinorelbine, zidovudine

Perform/provide:
• Assistance with ambulation during beginning therapy, since drowsiness/dizziness occurs
• Check to see if PO medication has been swallowed
• Refrigerate parenteral form
Evaluate:
• Therapeutic response: decreased anxiety, restlessness, insomnia
Teach patient/family:
• That drug may be taken with food
• Not to use drug for everyday stress or longer than 4 mo unless directed by prescriber
• Not to take more than prescribed amount; may be habit forming
• To avoid OTC preparations (cough, cold, hay fever) unless approved by prescriber
• To avoid driving, activities that require alertness, since drowsiness may occur
• To avoid alcohol ingestion, other psychotropic medications, unless directed by prescriber
• Not to discontinue medication abruptly after long-term use
• To rise slowly or fainting may occur, especially geriatric
• That drowsiness may worsen at beginning of treatment
• To use birth control if child-bearing age
Treatment of overdose: Lavage, VS, supportive care, flumazenil

---

Side effects: *italics* = common; **bold** = life-threatening

losartan (℞)

(lo-zar'tan)
Cozaar
Func. class.: Antihypertensive
Chem. class.: Angiotensin II receptor
(type AT_1)

Do not confuse:
losartan/valsartan
Cozaar/Zocor

Action: Blocks the vasoconstrictor and aldosterone-secreting effects of angiotensin II; selectively blocks the binding of angiotensin II to the AT_1 receptor found in tissues

Uses: Hypertension, alone or in combination, nephropathy in type 2 diabetes, hypertension with left ventricular hypertrophy

DOSAGE AND ROUTES

Hypertension
• *Adult:* **PO** 50 mg daily alone or 25 mg daily when used in combination with diuretic; maintenance 25-100 mg daily

Hepatic dose
• *Adult:* **PO** 25 mg daily as starting dose

Hypertension with left ventricular hypertrophy
• *Adult:* **PO** 50 mg daily, add hydrochlorothiazide 12.5 mg/day and/or increase losartan to 100 mg daily, then increase hydrochlorothiazide to 25 mg daily

Nephropathy in type 2 diabetic patients
• *Adult:* **PO** 50 mg daily, may increase to 100 mg daily

Available forms: Tabs 25, 50, 100 mg

SIDE EFFECTS

CNS: Dizziness, insomnia, anxiety, confusion, abnormal dreams, migraine, tremor, vertigo, headache
CV: Angina pectoris, 2nd-degree AV block, **cerebrovascular accident,** hypotension, **myocardial infarction,** *dysrhythmias*
EENT: Blurred vision, burning eyes, conjunctivitis

GI: Diarrhea, dyspepsia, anorexia, constipation, dry mouth, flatulence, gastritis, vomiting
GU: Impotence, nocturia, urinary frequency, UTI, **renal failure**
HEMA: Anemia
INTEG: Alopecia, dermatitis, dry skin, flushing, photosensitivity, rash, pruritus, sweating, **angioedema**
META: Gout
MS: Cramps, myalgia, pain, stiffness
RESP: Cough, upper respiratory infection, congestion, dyspnea, bronchitis

Contraindications: Pregnancy (D) 2nd/3rd trimesters, hypersensitivity

Precautions: Pregnancy (C) 1st trimester; hypersensitivity to ACE inhibitors; lactation, children, geriatric, hepatic disease, angioedema, renal artery stenosis

PHARMACOKINETICS

Peak 1-4 hr, extensively metabolized, half-life 2 hr, metabolite 6-9 hr, excreted in urine and feces, protein binding 98.7%

INTERACTIONS

Increase: lithium toxicity—lithium
Increase: antihypertensive effect—fluconazole
Increase: hyperkalemia—potassium sparing diuretics, potassium supplements, ACE inhibitors
Decrease: antihypertensive effect—NSAIDs, phenobarbital, rifamycin, salicylates

Drug/Herb
Increase: toxicity, death—aconite
Increase: antihypertensive effect—barberry, betony, black catechu, black cohosh, bloodroot, broom, burdock, cat's claw, dandelion, goldenseal, hawthorn, Irish moss, Jamaican dogwood, kelp, khella, mistletoe, parsley
Increase or decrease: antihypertensive effect—astragalus, cola tree
Decrease: antihypertensive effect—coltsfoot, guarana, khat, licorice, yohimbine

NURSING CONSIDERATIONS

Assess:

• B/P with position changes, pulse q4h; note rate, rhythm, quality

• Electrolytes: K, Na, Cl

• Baselines in renal, hepatic studies before therapy begins

• Edema in feet, legs daily

• Skin turgor, dryness of mucous membranes for hydration status

Administer:

• Without regard to meals

Evaluate:

• Therapeutic response: decreased B/P

Teach patient/family:

• To avoid sunlight or wear sunscreen if in sunlight; photosensitivity may occur

• To comply with dosage schedule, even if feeling better

• To notify prescriber of mouth sores, fever, swelling of hands or feet, irregular heartbeat, chest pain

• That excessive perspiration, dehydration, vomiting, diarrhea may lead to fall in blood pressure; consult prescriber if these occur

• That drug may cause dizziness, fainting; light-headedness may occur

• To rise slowly to sitting or standing position to minimize orthostatic hypotension

• To use contraception while taking this product

---

loteprednol ophthalmic
See Appendix C

---

lovastatin (℞)
(loh-vah-stat′in)
Altocor, Altoprev, Mevacor
Func. class.: Antilipemic
Chem. class.: HMG-CoA reductase inhibitor

Do not confuse:
lovastatin/Lotensin
Action: Inhibits HMG-CoA reductase enzyme, which reduces cholesterol synthesis

Uses: As an adjunct in primary hypercholesterolemia (types IIa, IIb), atherosclerosis, primary and secondary prevention of coronary events

DOSAGE AND ROUTES

• *Adult:* **PO** 20 mg daily with evening meal; may increase to 20-80 mg/day in single or divided doses, not to exceed 80 mg/day; dosage adjustments should be made qmo, reduce dose in renal disease; **EXT REL** 20-60 mg daily at bedtime

Available forms: Tabs 10, 20, 40 mg; ext rel tab (Altocor) 10, 20, 40, 60 mg

SIDE EFFECTS

CNS: Dizziness, headache, tremor, insomnia, paresthesia

EENT: Blurred vision, lens opacities

GI: Flatus, nausea, constipation, diarrhea, dyspepsia, abdominal pain, heartburn, **hepatic dysfunction,** vomiting, acid regurgitation, dry mouth, dysgeusia

HEMA: **Thrombocytopenia, hemolytic anemia, leukopenia**

INTEG: Rash, pruritus, photosensitivity

MS: Muscle cramps, myalgia, **myositis, rhabdomyolysis,** leg, shoulder or localized pain

Contraindications: Pregnancy (X), hypersensitivity, lactation, active hepatic disease

Precautions: Past hepatic disease, alcoholism, severe acute infections, trauma, hypotension, uncontrolled seizure disorders, severe metabolic disorders, electrolyte imbalances, visual disorder, children

PHARMACOKINETICS

PO: Peak 2-4 hr; peak response 4-6 wk; metabolized in liver (metabolites); highly protein bound; excreted in urine 10%, feces 83%; crosses placenta, excreted in breast milk; half-life 3-4 hr

---

Side effects: *italics* = common; **bold** = life-threatening

INTERACTIONS

Increase: myalgia, myositis—azole antifungals, clarithromycin, clofibrate, cycloSPORINE, dalfopristin, danazol, diltiazem, erythromycin, gemfibrozil, niacin, protease inhibitors, quinupristin, telithromycin, verapamil

Increase: bleeding—warfarin

Increase: effects of digoxin

Decrease: effects of lovastatin—bile acid sequestrants, exonatide, bosentan

Drug/Herb

Increase: effect—glucomannan

Decrease: effect—gotu kola, St. John's wort

Drug/Food

• Possible toxicity: grapefruit juice

Increase: levels of lovastatin with food, must be taken with food

Decrease: absorption—oat bran

Drug/Lab Test

Increase: CPK, LFTs

NURSING CONSIDERATIONS

Assess:

• Diet, obtain diet history including fat, cholesterol in diet

• Fasting cholesterol, LDL, HDL, triglycerides periodically during treatment

• Hepatic studies q1-2mo during the first 1½ yr of treatment; AST, ALT, LFTs may increase

• Renal function in patients with compromised renal system: BUN, creatinine, I&O ratio

⚠ For muscle pain, tenderness, obtain CPK baseline and if these occur, drug may need to be discontinued

Administer:

• In evening with meal; if dose is increased, take with breakfast and evening meal

Perform/provide:

• Storage in cool environment in airtight, light-resistant container

Evaluate:

• Therapeutic response: cholesterol at desired level after 8 wk

Teach patient/family:

• To report suspected pregnancy

• That blood work and ophthalmic exam will be necessary during treatment

• To report blurred vision, severe GI symptoms, dizziness, headache, muscle pain, weakness

• To use sunscreen or stay out of the sun to prevent photosensitivity

• That previously prescribed regimen will continue: low-cholesterol diet, exercise program, smoking cessation

• That drug should be taken with food

---

loxapine (Ŗ)

(lox′a-peen)

Loxapac ♣, loxapine succinate ♣, Loxitane, Loxitane IM, Loxitane-C

Func. class.: Antipsychotic, neuroleptic

Chem. class.: Dibenzoxazepine

Do not confuse:

Loxitane/Soriatane

Action: Depresses cerebral cortex, hypothalamus, limbic system, which control activity and aggression; blocks neurotransmission produced by dopamine at synapse; exhibits strong α-adrenergic, anticholinergic blocking action; mechanism for antipsychotic effects is unclear

Uses: Psychotic disorders, nonpsychotic symptoms associated with dementia

Unlabeled uses: Depression, anxiety

DOSAGE AND ROUTES

• *Adult:* **PO** 10 mg bid-qid initially, may be rapidly increased depending on severity of condition, maintenance 60-100 mg/day; **IM** 12.5-50 mg q4-6h or more until desired response, then start **PO** form

• *Geriatric:* **PO** 5-10 mg daily-bid, increase q4-7d by 5-10 mg, max 125 mg

Available forms: Caps 5, 10, 25, 50 mg; tabs 5, 10, 25, 50 mg; conc 25 mg/ml; inj 50 mg/ml

SIDE EFFECTS

CNS: EPS: pseudoparkinsonism, akathisia, dystonia, tardive dyskinesia, drows-

---

⚠ Safety alert   *"Tall Man" lettering

iness, headache, **seizures,** confusion, **neuroleptic malignant syndrome**
CV: Orthostatic hypotension, **cardiac arrest,** ECG changes, tachycardia
EENT: Blurred vision, glaucoma
GI: Dry mouth, nausea, vomiting, anorexia, constipation, diarrhea, jaundice, weight gain
GU: Urinary retention, urinary frequency, enuresis, impotence, amenorrhea, gynecomastia
HEMA: **Anemia, leukopenia, leukocytosis, agranulocytosis**
INTEG: Rash, photosensitivity, dermatitis
RESP: **Laryngospasm,** dyspnea, **respiratory depression**
Contraindications: Hypersensitivity, blood dyscrasias, coma, brain damage, bone marrow depression, alcohol and barbiturate withdrawal states, severe CNS depression, narrow-angle glaucoma
Precautions: Pregnancy (C), lactation, seizure disorders, hepatic/cardiac disease, prostatic hypertrophy, cardiac conditions, child <16 yr, geriatric

PHARMACOKINETICS

PO: Onset 20-30 min, peak 2-4 hr, duration 12 hr
IM: Onset 15-30 min, peak 15-20 min, duration 12 hr
Metabolized by liver; excreted in urine; crosses placenta; enters breast milk; initial half-life 5 hr; terminal half-life 19 hr

INTERACTIONS

• Toxicity: epINEPHrine
Increase: EPS—other antipsychotics
Increase: CNS depression—MAOIs, antidepressants, alcohol
Decrease: effects—guanadrel, guanethidine
Drug/Herb
Increase: CNS depression—chamomile, cola tree, hops, kava, nettle, nutmeg, skullcap, valerian
Increase: EPS—betel palm, kava

NURSING CONSIDERATIONS

Assess:
• Mental status before initial administration
• Swallowing of PO medication; check for hoarding or giving of medication to other patients
• I&O ratio; palpate bladder if low urinary output occurs, urinary retention may be the cause
• Bilirubin, CBC, LFTs qmo
• Urinalysis is recommended before and during prolonged therapy
• Affect, orientation, LOC, reflexes, gait, coordination, sleep pattern disturbances
• B/P standing and lying; take pulse and respirations q4h during initial treatment; establish baseline before starting treatment; report drops of 30 mm Hg
• Dizziness, faintness, palpitations, tachycardia on rising
• EPS including akathisia (inability to sit still, no pattern to movements), tardive dyskinesia (bizarre movements of the jaw, mouth, tongue, extremities), pseudoparkinsonism (rigidity, tremors, pill rolling, shuffling gait)
⚠ For neuroleptic malignant syndrome: muscle rigidity, increased CPK, altered mental status, hyperthermia
• Constipation, urinary retention daily; if these occur, increase bulk, water in diet
Administer:
• Reduced dose to geriatric
• Antiparkinsonian agent if EPS symptoms occur
PO route
• Concentrate mixed in orange or grapefruit juice
IM route
• IM inj into large muscle mass
Perform/provide:
• Decreased sensory input by dimming lights, avoiding loud noises
• Supervised ambulation until stabilized on medication; do not involve in strenuous exercise program because fainting is possible; patient should not stand still for long periods

Side effects: *italics* = common; **bold** = life-threatening

- Increased fluids to prevent constipation
- Sips of water, candy, gum for dry mouth
- Storage in airtight, light-resistant container

Evaluate:
- Therapeutic response: decrease in emotional excitement, hallucinations, delusions, paranoia; reorganization of patterns of thought, speech

Teach patient/family:
- That orthostatic hypotension may occur and to rise from sitting or lying position gradually
- To remain lying down after IM injection for at least 30 min
- To avoid hot tubs, hot showers, tub baths, as hypotension may occur; that in hot weather heat stroke may occur; take extra precautions to stay cool
- To avoid abrupt withdrawal of this drug, or EPS may result; drug should be withdrawn slowly
- To avoid OTC preparations (cough, hay fever, cold) unless approved by prescriber; serious drug interactions may occur; avoid use with alcohol, CNS depressants; increased drowsiness may occur
- To avoid hazardous activities until stabilized on medication
- To use sunscreen during sun exposure to prevent burns
- About necessity for meticulous oral hygiene, since oral candidiasis may occur
- To report impaired vision, jaundice, tremors, muscle twitching

Treatment of overdose: Lavage if orally ingested; provide an airway

lubiprostone (℞)
(loo-bee-pros'-tone)
Amitiza
Func. class.: Gastrointestinal agent —miscellaneous

Action: Locally acting chloride channel activator, enhances a chloride rich intestinal fluid secretion without altering other electrolytes; increases motility in the intestine, increasing softening and passage of stool

Uses: Chronic idiopathic constipation

DOSAGE AND ROUTES
- *Adult:* **PO** 24 mcg bid with food

Available forms: Caps 24 mcg

SIDE EFFECTS
CNS: Headache, dizziness, depression, fatigue, insomnia
CV: Hypertension, chest pain
GI: Nausea, abdominal pain, eructation, abdominal distention, constipation, diarrhea, dry mouth, dyspepsia, flatulence, gastroenteritis viral, gastroesophageal reflux disease, vomiting, fecal incontinence, fecal urgency
GU: UTI
MISC: Chest pain, peripheral edema, influenza, pyrexia, viral infection
MS: Back pain, arthralgia, muscle cramps, pain in extremities
RESP: Bronchitis, cough, dyspnea, nasopharyngitis, sinusitis, URI

Contraindications: Hypersensitivity, GI obstruction

Precautions: Pregnancy (C), lactation, children, diarrhea, inflammatory bowel disease

PHARMACOKINETICS
Peak 1.14 hr; 94% protein binding; half-life 0.9-1.4 hr; metabolism rapid, extensively in stomach, jejunum

INTERACTIONS
Decrease: effect by antidiarrheals and anticholinergics

NURSING CONSIDERATIONS
Assess:
- GI symptoms: nausea, abdominal pain
- Periodically need for continued treatment

Administer:
- With foods, bid

Perform/provide:
- Store at room temperature

⚠ Safety alert   *"Tall Man" lettering

Evaluate:
• Therapeutic response: decreased constipation

Teach patient/family:
• To notify prescriber of GI symptoms, diarrhea, hypersensitivity reactions

---

lymphocyte immune globulin (antithymocyte) (℞)
Atgam, Thymoglobulin
Func. class.: Immune globulins—immunosuppressant

Action: Produces immunosuppression by inhibiting the function of lymphocytes (T)

Uses: Organ transplants to prevent rejection, aplastic anemia

Unlabeled uses: Multiple sclerosis; myasthenia gravis; immunosuppressant in liver, bone marrow, heart, and other organ transplants; pure red-cell aplasia; scleroderma

DOSAGE AND ROUTES
Renal allograft
• *Adult:* **IV** 10-30 mg/kg/day
• *Child:* **IV** 5-25 mg/kg/day

Delay of renal allograft rejection
• *Adult:* **IV** 15 mg/kg/day × 14 days, then every other day × 14 days for a total of 21 doses in 28 days

Aplastic anemia
• *Adult:* **IV** 10-20 mg/kg/day × 8-14 days
Available forms: Inj 50 mg horse gamma globulin/ml

SIDE EFFECTS
Renal transplant
CNS: Fever, chills, headache, dizziness, weakness, faintness, **seizures**
CV: Chest pain, hyper/hypotension, tachycardia
GI: Diarrhea, nausea, vomiting, epigastric pain, **GI bleeding**
INTEG: Rash, pruritus, urticaria, wheal
SYST: **Anaphylaxis**

Aplastic anemia
CNS: Fever, chills, headache, **seizures,** lightheadedness, encephalitis, postviral encephalopathy
CV: Bradycardia, myocarditis, irregularity
GI: Nausea, LFTs abnormality
Contraindications: Hypersensitivity
Precautions: Pregnancy (C), severe renal/hepatic disease, lactation, children

PHARMACOKINETICS
Onset rapid, half-life 5-7 days

INTERACTIONS
• None known

NURSING CONSIDERATIONS
Assess:
• For infection; if infection occurs, evaluation will be needed to continue therapy
• Renal studies: BUN, creatinine at least monthly during treatment, 3 mo after treatment
• Hepatic studies: alk phos, AST, ALT, bilirubin

Administer:
• Do not infuse <4 hr; usually given over 4-8 hr

Aplastic anemia
• Skin testing must be completed prior to treatment; use intradermal inj of 0.1 ml of a 1:1000 dilution (5 mcg horse IgG) in 0.9% NaCl, if a wheal or rash >10 mm or both, use caution during inf
• Dilute in saline sol before inf; invert IV bag so undiluted drug does not contact the air inside; concentration should not be >1 mg/ml; do not shake
• Keep emergency equipment nearby for severe allergic reaction

Evaluate:
• Therapeutic response: absence of rejection; hematologic recovery (aplastic anemia)

Teach patient/family:
• To report fever, chills, sore throat, fatigue, since serious infections may occur
• To use contraceptive measures during treatment, for 12 wk after ending therapy

mafenide topical
See Appendix C

magaldrate (OTC)
(mag'al-drate)
Losopan ♣, Lowsium,
Riopan, Riopan Extra
Strength ♣
Func. class.: Antacid
Chem. class.: Aluminum/magnesium
hydroxide

Action: Neutralizes gastric acidity; drug is dissolved in gastric contents; combination of aluminum, magnesium
Uses: Antacid, peptic ulcer disease (adjunct), duodenal, gastric ulcers, reflux esophagitis, hyperacidity, indigestion, heartburn

DOSAGE AND ROUTES
• *Adult:* **SUSP** 5-10 ml (400-800 mg) with H_2O between meals, at bedtime, not to exceed 100 ml/day
Available forms: Susp 540 mg/5 ml, liquid 540 mg/5 ml

SIDE EFFECTS
GI: Constipation, diarrhea
META: Hypermagnesemia, hypophosphatemia
Contraindications: Hypersensitivity to this drug or aluminum
Precautions: Pregnancy (C), geriatric, fluid restriction, decreased GI motility, GI obstruction, dehydration, renal disease, sodium-restricted diets

PHARMACOKINETICS
PO: Duration 60 min

INTERACTIONS
Increase: action when taken in large amounts—quinidine, flecainide, amphetamines
Decrease: absorption of anticholinergics, chlordiazepoxide, cimetidine, corticosteroids, fluoroquinolones, iron salts, isoniazid, ketoconazole, phenothiazines, phenytoin, salicylates, tetracyclines
Decrease: action when taken in large amounts—salicylates

NURSING CONSIDERATIONS
Assess:
• GI status: location of pain, intensity, characteristics, heartburn, hematemesis
• Serum magnesium levels with impaired renal function; calcium, phosphate, potassium if using long term; may increase calcium, decrease phosphate
• Constipation: increase bulk in diet if needed
Administer:
• Laxatives or stool softeners if constipation occurs
• After shaking; give between meals and bedtime
Evaluate:
• Therapeutic response: absence of pain, decreased acidity
Teach patient/family:
• To separate enteric-coated drugs and antacid by 2 hr
• To notify prescriber immediately of coffee-ground emesis, emesis with frank blood, black tarry stools

Rarely Used
magnesium salicylate (OTC, ℞)
Doan's Pills, Magan, Mobidin
Func. class.: Nonopioid analgesic, nonsteroidal antiinflammatory

Uses: Mild to moderate pain or fever including arthritis, juvenile rheumatoid arthritis

DOSAGE AND ROUTES
Arthritis
• *Adult:* **PO** not to exceed 4.8 g/day in divided doses
Pain/fever
• *Adult:* **PO** 600 mg qid or 1160 mg tid

Contraindications: Pregnancy (D) 1st trimester, hypersensitivity to salicylates, GI bleeding, bleeding disorders, children <12 yr, vit K deficiency

---

magnesium salts
(mag-nee′zee-um)

magnesium chloride (Ŗ)
Chloromag, Slo-Mag

magnesium citrate (oтc)
Citrate of Magnesia, Citroma, CitroMag ♣

magnesium gluconate (oтc)
Almoate, Magonate, magtrate OTC

magnesium oxide (oтc)
Mag-Ox 400, Maox, Uro-Mag

magnesium hydroxide (oтc)
Phillips' Magnesia Tablets, Phillips' Milk of Magnesia, MOM

magnesium sulfate (oтc, Ŗ)
epsom salts; magnesium sulfate (IV)—**HIGH ALERT**
Func. class.: Electrolyte; anticonvulsant; saline laxative, antacid

---

Action: Increases osmotic pressure, draws fluid into colon, neutralizes HCl
Uses: Constipation, bowel preparation before surgery or exam, anticonvulsant in preeclampsia, eclampsia (magnesium sulfate), electrolyte

DOSAGE AND ROUTES
Laxative
• *Adult:* **PO** 30-60 ml at bedtime (Milk of Magnesia), 300 mg
• *Adult and child >6 yr:* **PO** 15 g in 8 oz H_2O (magnesium sulfate); **PO** 10-20 ml (Concentrated Milk of Magnesia); **PO** 5-10 oz at bedtime (magnesium citrate)
• *Child 2-6 yr:* 5-15 ml/day (Milk of Magnesia)
Prevention of magnesium deficiency
• *Adult and child ≥10 yr:* **PO** male: 350-400 mg/day; female: 280-300 mg/day; lactation: 335-350 mg/day; pregnancy 320 mg/day
• *Child 8-10 yr:* **PO** 170 mg/day
• *Child 4-7 yr:* **PO** 120 mg/day
• *Infant and child to 4 yr:* 40-80 mg/day
Magnesium sulfate deficiency
• *Adult:* **PO** 200-400 mg in divided doses tid-qid; **IM** 1 g q6h × 4 doses; **IV** 5 g (severe)
• *Child 6-12 yr:* 3-6 mg/kg/day in divided doses tid-qid
Pre-eclampsia/eclampsia magnesium sulfate
• *Adult:* **IM/IV** 4-5 g **IV inf;** with 5 g **IM** in each gluteus, then 5 g q4h or 4 g **IV INF,** then 1-2 g/hr **CONT INF,** max 40 g/day or 20 g/48 hr in severe renal disease
Available forms: *Chloride:* sus rel tabs 535 mg (64 mg Mg) enteric tabs 833 mg (100 mg Mg); *citrate:* oral sol 240, 296, 300 ml bottles (77 mEq/100 ml); *oxide:* tabs 400 mg; caps 140 mg; *hydroxide:* liq 400 mg/5 ml; conc liq 800 mg/5 ml; chew tabs 300, 600 mg; *sulfate:* powder for oral; bulk packages; epsom salts, bulk packages; inj 10%, 12.5%, 25%, 50%

SIDE EFFECTS
CNS: Muscle weakness, flushing, sweating, confusion, sedation, depressed reflexes, **flaccid paralysis,** hypothermia
CV: Hypotension, heart block, **circulatory collapse**
GI: Nausea, vomiting, anorexia, cramps
META: Electrolyte, fluid imbalances
RESP: Respiratory depression
Contraindications: Hypersensitivity, abdominal pain, nausea/vomiting, obstruction, acute surgical abdomen, rectal bleeding
Precautions: Pregnancy (A); (B) (magnesium sulfate), renal/cardiac disease

M

Side effects: *italics* = common; **bold** = life-threatening

636   mannitol

PHARMACOKINETICS

PO: Onset 3-6 hr
IM: Onset 1 hr, duration 4 hr
IV: Duration ½ hr
Excreted by kidney, effective anticonvulsant serum levels 2.5-7.5 mEq/L

INTERACTIONS

Increase: effect of neuromuscular blockers
Decrease: absorption of tetracyclines, aminoquinolones, nitrofurantoin

NURSING CONSIDERATIONS

Assess:
• I&O ratio; check for decrease in urinary output
• Cause of constipation; lack of fluids, bulk, exercise
• Cramping, rectal bleeding, nausea, vomiting; drug should be discontinued
⚠ Magnesium toxicity: thirst, confusion, decrease in reflexes

Administer:
PO route
• With 8 oz H_2O
• Refrigerate magnesium citrate before giving
• Shake susp before using as antacid at least 2 hr after meals

IM route (magnesium sulfate)
• Give deeply in gluteal site

IV route (magnesium sulfate)
• Only when calcium gluconate available for magnesium toxicity

IV, direct route
• IV undiluted 1.5 ml of 10% sol over 1 min
• May dilute to 20% sol, infuse over 3 hr
• IV at less than 150 mg/min; circulatory collapse may occur
• Use infusion pump

Additive compatibilities: Cephalothin, chloramphenicol, cisplatin, heparin, hydrocortisone, isoproterenol, meropenem, methyldopate, norepinephrine, penicillin G potassium, potassium phosphate, verapamil

Y-site compatibilities: Acyclovir, aldesleukin, amifostine, amikacin, ampicil-

lin, aztreonam, cefazolin, cefoperazone, cefotaxime, cefoxitin, cephalothin, cephapirin, chloramphenicol, cisatracurium, DOBUTamine, doxycycline, DOXOrubicin liposome, enalaprilat, erythromycin, esmolol, famotidine, fludarabine, gallium, gentamicin, granisetron, heparin, hydromorphone, idarubicin, insulin, kanamycin, labetalol, meperidine, metronidazole, minocycline, morphine, moxalactam, nafcillin, ondansetron, oxacillin, paclitaxel, penicillin G potassium, piperacillin, piperacillin/tazobactam, potassium chloride, propofol, remifentanil, sargramostim, thiotepa, ticarcillin, tobramycin, trimethoprim-sulfamethoxazole, vancomycin, vit B complex/C

Evaluate:
• Therapeutic response: decreased constipation

Teach patient/family:
• Not to use laxatives for long-term therapy; bowel tone will be lost
• That chilling helps the taste of magnesium citrate
• To shake suspension well
• To not give at bedtime as a laxative; may interfere with sleep
• To give citrus fruit after administering to counteract unpleasant taste

---

mannitol (℞)
(man′i-tole)
mannitol, Osmitrol, Resectisol
Func. class.: Diuretic, osmotic
Chem. class.: Hexahydric alcohol

Action: Acts by increasing osmolarity of glomerular filtrate, which inhibits reabsorption of water and electrolytes and increases urinary output

Uses: Edema, promote systemic diuresis in cerebral edema, decrease intraocular pressure, improve renal function in acute renal failure, chemical poisoning

---

⚠ Safety alert   *"Tall Man" lettering

DOSAGE AND ROUTES

Test dose
• *Adult and child:* IV 0.2 g/kg over 3-5 min

Intraocular pressure/intracranial pressure
• *Adult:* IV 0.25-2 g/kg 15%-25% sol over 30-60 min
• *Child:* IV 1-2 g/kg (30-60 g/m^2) as 15%-20% sol run over 2-6 hr

Edema, oliguria, renal failure
• *Adult:* IV 50-100 g/24 hr as a 5%-25% sol, adjusted to maintain output of 30-50 mg/hr
• *Child:* IV 0.25-2 g/kg (60 g/m^2) as a 15%-20% sol over 2-6 hr

Diuresis in drug intoxication
• *Adult:* IV 50-200 g as a 5%-25% sol, titrated to maintain urine flow of 100-500 ml/hr
• *Child:* IV up to 2 g/kg (60 g/m^2) as a 5%-10% sol

Available forms: Inj 5%, 10%, 15%, 20%; GU irrigation: 5%

SIDE EFFECTS

CNS: Dizziness, headache, **seizures, rebound increased ICP,** confusion
CV: Edema, thrombophlebitis, hypotension, hypertension, **tachycardia,** angina-like chest pains, fever, chills, **CHF circulatory overload**
EENT: Loss of hearing, blurred vision, nasal congestion, decreased intraocular pressure
ELECT: Fluid, electrolyte imbalances, *acidosis,* electrolyte loss, dehydration, hyper/hypokalemia
GI: Nausea, vomiting, dry mouth, diarrhea
GU: Marked diuresis, urinary retention, thirst
RESP: Pulmonary congestion

Contraindications: Active intracranial bleeding, hypersensitivity, anuria, severe pulmonary congestion, edema, severe dehydration, progressive heart, renal failure

Precautions: Pregnancy (C), dehydration, severe renal disease, CHF, lactation, electrolyte imbalances

PHARMACOKINETICS

IV: Onset 30-60 min for diuresis, ½-1 hr for intraocular pressure, 25 min for cerebrospinal fluid; duration 4-6 hr for intraocular pressure, 3-8 hr for cerebrospinal fluid; excreted in urine, half-life 100 min

INTERACTIONS

Drug/Food
• Potassium foods: increased hyperkalemia

Drug/Lab Test
Interference: Inorganic phosphorus, ethylene glycol

NURSING CONSIDERATIONS

Assess:
• Weight, I&O daily to determine fluid loss; effect of drug may be decreased if used daily; output qh prn
• Rate, depth, rhythm of respiration, effect of exertion
• B/P lying, standing; postural hypotension may occur
• Electrolytes: K, Na, Cl; include BUN, CBC, serum creatinine, blood pH, ABGs, CVP, PAP
• Signs of metabolic acidosis: drowsiness, restlessness
• Signs of hypokalemia: postural hypotension, malaise, fatigue, tachycardia, leg cramps, weakness, or hyperkalemia
• Rashes, temp daily
• Confusion, especially in geriatric; take safety precautions if needed
• Hydration including skin turgor, thirst, dry mucous membranes
• For blurred vision, pain in eyes, before and during treatment (increased intraocular pressure); neurologic checks, intracranial pressure during treatment (increased intracranial pressure)

M

Side effects: *italics* = common; **bold** = life-threatening

Administer:
IV route
• In 15%-25% sol with filter; give over ½-1½ hr; rapid infusion may worsen CHF; warm in hot water and shake to dissolve crystals
• Test dose in severe oliguria, 0.2 g/kg over 3-5 min; if no urine increase, give second test dose; if no response, reassess patient
Irrigation
• 100 ml of 25%/900 ml of sterile water for inj (2.5% sol)
Additive compatibilities: Amikacin, bretylium, cefamandole, cefoxitin, cimetidine, cisplatin, DOPamine, fosphenytoin, furosemide, gentamicin, metoclopramide, nizatidine, ofloxacin, ondansetron, sodium bicarbonate, tobramycin, verapamil
Y-site compatibilities: Allopurinol, amifostine, amphotericin B cholesteryl, aztreonam, cisatracurium, cladribine, docetaxel, etoposide, fludarabine, fluorouracil, gatifloxacin, gemcitabine, idarubicin, linezolid, melphalan, ondansetron, paclitaxel, piperacillin, propofol, remifentanil, sargramostim, teniposide, thiotepa, vinorelbine
Evaluate:
• Therapeutic response: improvement in edema of feet, legs, sacral area daily if medication is being used in CHF; decreased intraocular pressure, prevention of hypokalemia, increased excretion of toxic substances; decreased ICP
Teach patient/family:
• To rise slowly from lying or sitting position
• The reason for and method of treatment
• To report signs of electrolyte imbalance; confusion
Treatment of overdose: Discontinue infusion; correct fluid, electrolyte imbalances; hemodialysis; monitor hydration, CV, renal function

---

mebendazole (℞)
(me-ben′da-zole)
Vermox
Func. class.: Anthelmintic
Chem. class.: Carbamate

Action: Inhibits glucose uptake, degeneration of cytoplasmic microtubules in the cell; interferes with absorption, secretory function

Uses: Pinworms, roundworms, hookworms, whipworms, thread-worms, pork tapeworms, dwarf tapeworms, beef tapeworms, hydatid cyst

DOSAGE AND ROUTES
• *Adult and child >2 yr:* **PO** 100 mg as a single dose (pinworms) or bid × 3 days (whipworms, roundworms, or hookworms); course may be repeated in 3 wk if needed
Available forms: Chew tabs 100 mg

SIDE EFFECTS
CNS: Dizziness, fever, headache
GI: Transient diarrhea, abdominal pain, nausea, vomiting
Contraindications: Hypersensitivity
Precautions: Pregnancy (C) (1st trimester), child <2 yr, lactation, Crohn's disease, hepatic disease, IBD, ulcerative colitis

PHARMACOKINETICS
PO: Peak ½-7 hr; excreted in feces primarily (metabolites), small amount in urine (unchanged); highly bound to plasma proteins 95%

INTERACTIONS
Decrease: mebendazole effect—carbamazepine, hydantoins
Drug/Food
Increase: absorption—high-fat meal

⚠ Safety alert   *"Tall Man" lettering

NURSING CONSIDERATIONS
Assess:
• Stools during entire treatment; specimens must be sent to lab while still warm, also 1-3 wk after treatment is completed
• For allergic reaction: rash (rare)
• For diarrhea during expulsion of worms; avoid self-contamination with patient's feces
• For infection in other family members, since infection from person to person is common
• Blood studies: AST, ALT, alk phos, BUN, CBC during treatment

Administer:
• May be crushed, chewed, swallowed whole, mixed with food
• PO after meals to avoid GI symptoms, since absorption is not altered by food
• Second course after 3 wk if needed; usually recommended

Perform/provide:
• Storage in tight container

Evaluate:
• Therapeutic response: expulsion of worms and 3 negative stool cultures after completion of treatment

Teach patient/family:
• Proper hygiene after BM, including hand-washing technique; tell patient to avoid putting fingers in mouth; clean fingernails
• That infected person should sleep alone; do not shake bed linen, change bed linen daily, wash in hot water, change and wash undergarments daily
• To clean toilet daily with disinfectant (green soap solution)
• The need for compliance with dosage schedule, duration of treatment
• To wear shoes, wash all fruits and vegetables well before eating; use commercial fruit/vegetable cleaner
• That all members of the family should be treated (pinworms)

mecasermin (R)
(mec-a'sir-men)
Increlex
Func. class.: Biologic response modifier; insulin-like growth factor

Action: Stimulates growth; IGF-1 is the principal hormonal mediator of statural growth; GH binds to its receptor in the liver and other tissues

Uses: Growth failure in children with severe primary insulin-like growth factor-1 (IGF-1) deficiency (primary IGFD) or with growth hormone (GH) gene deletion who have developed neutralizing antibodies to GH

Unlabeled uses: ALS

DOSAGE AND ROUTES
• *Child:* **SUBCUT** 0.04 mg/kg (40 mcg/kg) bid; if well tolerated for 1 wk, may increase by 0.04 mg/kg/dose, max 0.12 mg/kg bid

Available forms: Inj 10 mg/ml

SIDE EFFECTS
CNS: Headache, **seizures,** dizziness, cardiac valvulopathy
CV: Cardiac murmur
EENT: Ear pain, otitis media, abnormal tympanometry, papilledema, visual impairment
ENDO: **Hypoglycemia, ketosis, hypothyroidism**
GU: Vomiting
HEMA: Thymus hypertrophy
META: Hypoglycemic
MISC: Bruising, lipohypertrophy, hypersensitivity reactions
MS: Arthralgia, joint pain
RESP: Snoring, tonsillar hypertrophy, **apnea**
SYST: **Antibodies to growth hormone**

Contraindications: Hypersensitivity, benzyl alcohol, closed epiphyses, active/suspected neoplasia, IV use
Precautions: Pregnancy (C), diabetes mellitus, hypothyroidism, lactation, child

<2 yr, increased intracranial pressure, malnutrition, scoliosis, sleep apnea

PHARMACOKINETICS

Bioavailability almost 100%, metabolized in liver/kidney, half-life 5.8 hr

INTERACTIONS

Increase: hypoglycemia—antidiabetics, corticosteroids

NURSING CONSIDERATIONS

Assess:
• Monitor preprandial glucose at beginning of treatment and until well tolerated
• By funduscopic exam at beginning and periodically during treatment
• For allergic reactions; if present, interrupt treatment and notify prescriber
• Growth rate of child at intervals during treatment

Administer:

SUBCUT route
• Rotate inj site; use sterile, disposable syringe/needles; use small-volume syringe for accurate measurement
• Shortly before or after a meal or snack to lessen hypoglycemia

Perform/provide:
• Storage in refrigerator before opening, avoid freezing; after opening, stable for 30 days after initial vial entry, store in refrigerator, do not use if particulate matter is present, avoid direct light, do not use after expiration date

Evaluate:
• Therapeutic response: growth in children

Teach patient/family:
• That treatment may continue for years; regular assessments are required
• To avoid hazardous activities, driving within 2-3 hr of dosing
• Correct administration and needle disposal

---

mechlorethamine (℞)
(me-klor-eth′a-meen)
Mustargen, nitrogen mustard
Func. class.: Antineoplastic alkylating agent
Chem. class.: Nitrogen mustard

Action: Responsible for cross-linking DNA strands leading to cell death; rapidly degraded, a vesicant; activity is not cell cycle phase-specific
Uses: Hodgkin's disease, leukemias, lymphomas, lymphosarcoma; ovarian, breast, lung carcinoma; neoplastic effusions

DOSAGE AND ROUTES
• *Adult:* **IV** 0.4 mg/kg or 10 mg/m^2 as 1 dose or 2-4 divided doses over 2-4 days; second course after 3 wk depending on blood cell count
Neoplastic effusions
• *Adult:* **INTRACAVITARY** 0.4 mg/kg, may be 200-400 mcg/kg
Available forms: Inj 10 mg

SIDE EFFECTS
CNS: Headache, dizziness, drowsiness, paresthesia, peripheral neuropathy, **coma**
EENT: Tinnitus, hearing loss
GI: Nausea, vomiting, diarrhea, stomatitis, weight loss, colitis, **hepatotoxicity**
HEMA: **Thrombocytopenia, leukopenia, agranulocytosis,** anemia
INTEG: Alopecia, pruritus, herpes zoster, extravasation
Contraindications: Pregnancy (D), lactation, myelosuppression, acute herpes zoster
Precautions: Radiation therapy, chronic lymphocytic leukopenia

PHARMACOKINETICS
Metabolized in liver, excreted in urine

INTERACTIONS
Increase: blood dyscrasias—amphotericin B

Increase: bleeding—aspirin, anticoagulants

Increase: toxicity—antineoplastics, radiation

Decrease: antibody reaction—live virus vaccines

NURSING CONSIDERATIONS
Assess:
• CBC, differential, platelet count qwk; withhold drug if WBC is <1000/mm³ or platelet count is <75,000/mm³; notify prescriber, recovery of WBCs, platelets within 20 days
• Renal function tests: BUN, serum uric acid, urine CCr before, during therapy
• I&O ratio; report fall in urine output of 30 ml/hr
• Monitor temp q4h (may indicate beginning infection); no rectal temps
• Hepatic studies before, during therapy (bilirubin, AST, ALT, LDH) as needed or monthly
• Bleeding: hematuria, guaiac, bruising or petechiae, mucosa or orifices q8h
• Jaundiced skin and sclera, dark urine, clay-colored stools, itchy skin, abdominal pain, fever, diarrhea
• Effects of alopecia on body image; discuss feelings about body changes
• Buccal cavity q8h for dryness, sores, ulceration, white patches, oral pain, bleeding, dysphagia
• Local irritation, pain, burning, discoloration at inj site
⚠ Symptoms indicating severe allergic reaction: rash, pruritus, urticaria, purpuric skin lesions, itching, flushing

Administer:
• After using guidelines for preparation of cytotoxic drugs
• Antiemetic 30-60 min before giving drug and prn
• IV after diluting 10 mg/10 ml sterile H₂O or NaCl; leave needle in vial, shake, withdraw dose, give through Y-tube or 3-way stopcock or directly over 3-5 min
• Watch for infiltration; infiltrate area with isotonic sodium thiosulfate or 1% lidocaine; apply ice for 6-12 hr

• Topical or systemic analgesics for pain
• Local or systemic drugs for infection

Y-site compatibilities:
Amifostine, aztreonam, filgrastim, fludarabine, granisetron, melphalan, ondansetron, sargramostim, teniposide, vinorelbine

Perform/provide:
• Storage at room temperature in dry form
• Increase fluid intake to 2-3 L/day to prevent urate deposits, calculi formation
• Diet low in purines: organ meats (kidney, liver), dried beans, peas to maintain alkaline urine
• Preparation under hood using gloves and mask
• Rinsing of mouth tid-qid with water, club soda; brushing of teeth bid-tid with soft brush or cotton-tipped applicators for stomatitis; use unwaxed dental floss
• Warm compresses at inj site for inflammation

Evaluate:
• Therapeutic response: decreased tumor size, spread of malignancy

Teach patient/family:
• The rationale for and techniques of protective isolation
• That sterility, amenorrhea can occur; reversible after discontinuing treatment
• That hair may be lost during treatment; a wig or hairpiece may make patient feel better; new hair may be different in color, texture
• To avoid foods with citric acid, hot or rough texture
• To report any bleeding, white spots, or ulcerations in mouth to prescriber; tell patient to examine mouth daily
• To report signs of infection: fever, sore throat, flulike symptoms
• To report signs of anemia: fatigue, headache, faintness, shortness of breath, irritability
• To avoid use of razors, commercial mouthwash
• To avoid use of aspirin products, NSAIDs
• To notify prescriber if pregnancy is suspected; to use contraception during treatment

M

meclizine (oтc, ℞)

(mek'li-zeen)

Antivert, Antrizine, Bonamine ✦, Bonine, Dramamine Less Drowsy Formula, meclizine HCl, Meni-D, Vergon

Func. class.: Antiemetic, antihistamine, anticholinergic

Chem. class.: H_1-Receptor antagonist, piperazine derivative

Action: Acts centrally by blocking chemoreceptor trigger zone, which in turn acts on vomiting center

Uses: Vertigo, motion sickness

DOSAGE AND ROUTES

Vertigo

• *Adult:* PO 25-100 mg daily in divided doses

Motion sickness

• *Adult:* PO 12.5-25 mg 1 hr before traveling, repeat dose q12-24h prn

Available forms: Tabs 12.5, 25, 50 mg; chew tabs 25 mg; caps 25, 30 mg

SIDE EFFECTS

CNS: Drowsiness, fatigue, restlessness, headache, insomnia

CV: Hypotension

EENT: Dry mouth, blurred vision

GI: Nausea, anorexia, constipation, increased appetite

GU: Urinary retention

Contraindications: Hypersensitivity to cyclizines, shock

Precautions: Pregnancy (B), children, narrow-angle glaucoma, glaucoma, urinary retention, lactation, prostatic hypertrophy, geriatric, CV disease, hypertension, seizure disorder

PHARMACOKINETICS

PO: Onset 1 hr, duration 8-24 hr, half-life 6 hr

INTERACTIONS

Increase: effect of alcohol, opioids, other CNS depressants

Drug/Herb

Increase: anticholinergic effect—corkwood, henbane leaf

Increase: sedative effect—hops, Jamaican dogwood, khat, senega

Drug/Lab Test

False negative: Allergy skin testing

NURSING CONSIDERATIONS

Assess:

• VS, B/P

⚠ Signs of toxicity of other drugs or masking of symptoms of disease: brain tumor, intestinal obstruction

• Observe for drowsiness, dizziness, level of consciousness

• For nausea/vomiting after 1 hr

Administer:

PO route

• Tablets may be swallowed whole, chewed, or allowed to dissolve; give with food to decrease GI upset

• Lowest possible dose in geriatric, anticholinergic effects

Evaluate:

• Therapeutic response: absence of dizziness, vomiting

Teach patient/family:

• That a false-negative result may occur with skin testing for allergies; these procedures should not be scheduled for 4 days after discontinuing use

• To avoid hazardous activities, activities requiring alertness; dizziness may occur; instruct patient to request assistance with ambulation

• To avoid alcohol, other depressants

⚠ Safety alert   ✦ "Tall Man" lettering

*medroxyPROGES-TERone (℞)

(me-drox'ee-proe-jess'te-rone)
Amen, Curretab, Cycrin, Depo-Provera, medroxyPRO-GESTERone, Provera
Func. class.: Antineoplastic, hormone, contraceptive
Chem. class.: Progesterone derivative

Do not confuse:
medroxyPROGESTERone/
methylPREDNISolone
Amen/Ambien
Provera/Premarin/Covera

Action: Inhibits secretion of pituitary gonadotropins, which prevents follicular maturation and ovulation; stimulates growth of mammary tissue; antineoplastic action against endometrial cancer

Uses: Uterine bleeding (abnormal), secondary amenorrhea, prevent endometrial changes associated with estrogen replacement therapy (ERT)

Unlabeled uses: Pickwickian syndrome, sleep apnea

DOSAGE AND ROUTES
Secondary amenorrhea
• *Adult:* **PO** 5-10 mg daily × 5-10 days
Uterine bleeding
• *Adult:* **PO** 5-10 mg daily × 5-10 days starting on 16th or 21st day of menstrual cycle
With ERT
• *Adult:* **PO** monophasic 2.5 mg daily; biphasic 5 mg days 15-28 of cycle
Available forms: Tabs 2.5, 5, 10 mg; inj susp 50, 100, 150, 400 mg/ml

SIDE EFFECTS
CNS: Dizziness, headache, migraines, depression, fatigue
CV: Hypotension, thrombophlebitis, edema, **thromboembolism, stroke, pulmonary embolism, MI**
EENT: Diplopia

GI: Nausea, vomiting, anorexia, cramps, increased weight, **cholestatic jaundice**
GU: Amenorrhea, cervical erosion, breakthrough bleeding, dysmenorrhea, vaginal candidiasis, breast changes, *gynecomastia, testicular atrophy, impotence,* endometriosis, **spontaneous abortion**
INTEG: Rash, urticaria, acne, hirsutism, alopecia, oily skin, seborrhea, purpura, melasma, photosensitivity
META: Hyperglycemia
SYST: **Angioedema, anaphylaxis**

Contraindications: Pregnancy (X), breast cancer, hypersensitivity, thromboembolic disorders, reproductive cancer, genital bleeding (abnormal, undiagnosed)

Precautions: Lactation, hypertension, asthma, blood dyscrasias, gallbladder disease, CHF, diabetes mellitus, bone disease, depression, migraine headache, convulsive disorders, renal/hepatic disease, family history of cancer of breast or reproductive tract

PHARMACOKINETICS
PO: Duration 24 hr, excreted in urine and feces, metabolized in liver

INTERACTIONS
Decrease: medroxyPROGESTERone action—aminoglutethimide
Drug/Lab Test
Increase: Alk phos, sodium (urine), pregnanediol, amino acids
Decrease: GTT, HDL

NURSING CONSIDERATIONS
Assess:
⚠ Symptoms indicating severe allergic reaction, angioedema, have epINEPHrine and rescusitative equipment available
• Weight daily; notify prescriber of weekly weight gain >5 lb
• B/P at beginning of treatment and periodically
• I&O ratio; be alert for decreasing urinary output, increasing edema

• Hepatic studies: ALT, AST, bilirubin, periodically during long-term therapy
• Edema, hypertension, cardiac symptoms, jaundice
• Mental status: affect, mood, behavioral changes, depression

Administer:
• Titrated dose; use lowest effective dose
• Oil solution deep in large muscle mass (IM); rotate sites
• With food or milk to decrease GI symptoms (PO)

Perform/provide:
• Storage in dark area

Evaluate:
• Therapeutic response: decreased abnormal uterine bleeding, absence of amenorrhea

Teach patient/family:
• To avoid sunlight or use sunscreen; photosensitivity can occur
• Cushingoid symptoms: weight gain, moon face, buffalo hump, acne
⚠ To report breast lumps, vaginal bleeding, edema, jaundice, dark urine, clay-colored stools, dyspnea, headache, blurred vision, abdominal pain, numbness or stiffness in legs, chest pain; male to report impotence or gynecomastia
• To report suspected pregnancy

medrysone ophthalmic
See Appendix C

megestrol (℞)
(me-jess'trole)
Megace, Megace ES, megestrol
Func. class.: Antineoplastic hormone
Chem. class.: Progestin

Do not confuse:
Megace/Reglan
Action: Affects endometrium by antiluteinizing effect; this is thought to bring about cell death

Uses: Breast, endometrial cancer, renal cell cancer; cachexia anorexia weight loss in AIDs
Unlabeled uses: Hot flashes

DOSAGE AND ROUTES
Endometrial/ovarian carcinoma
• *Adult:* **PO** 40-320 mg/day in divided doses
Breast carcinoma
• *Adult:* **PO** 40 mg qid or 160 mg daily
Anorexia (AIDS)
• *Adult:* **PO** 800 mg daily (oral susp) or 625 mg/day (ES)
Hot flashes (unlabeled)
• *Adult:* **PO** 20 mg daily
Available forms: Tabs 20, 40 mg; oral susp 40, 125 mg/ml

SIDE EFFECTS
CNS: Mood swings
CV: **Thrombophlebitis, thromboembolism**
GI: Nausea, vomiting, diarrhea, abdominal cramps, weight gain
GU: Gynecomastia, fluid retention, hypercalcemia, vaginal bleeding, discharge, impotence, decreased libido
INTEG: Alopecia, rash, pruritus, purpura, itching
Contraindications: Pregnancy (D) (tabs); (X) (susp), hypersensitivity

PHARMACOKINETICS
PO: Duration 1-3 days, half-life 60 min; metabolized in liver; excreted in feces, breast milk

INTERACTIONS
Drug/Lab Test
Increase: Alk phos, urinary sodium, urinary pregnanediol, plasma amino acids
Decrease: HDL, glucose tolerance test
False positive: Urine glucose

NURSING CONSIDERATIONS
Assess:
• I&O ratio; weights
• Effects of alopecia on body image; discuss feelings about body changes

⚠ Symptoms indicating severe allergic reaction: rash, pruritus, urticaria, purpuric skin lesions, itching, flushing
• Frequency of stools, characteristics: cramping, acidosis, signs of dehydration (rapid respirations, poor skin turgor, decreased urine output, dry skin, restlessness, weakness)
• Anorexia, nausea, vomiting, constipation, weakness, loss of muscle tone
⚠ Thrombophlebitis: Homans' sign, edema, pain in calf, thigh, notify prescriber immediately
Administer:
• Oral susp for AIDS patients; shake well
• Tablets for carcinoma
Perform/provide:
• Nutritious diet with iron, vitamin supplements as ordered
• Storage in tight container at room temperature
Evaluate:
• Therapeutic response: decreased tumor size, spread of malignancy; weight gain in AIDS patients
Teach patient/family:
• To report vaginal bleeding
• That nonhormonal contraception should be used during and 4 mo after treatment
• That gynecomastia can occur; reversible after discontinuing treatment
⚠ To recognize signs of fluid retention, thromboemboli and to report immediately

---

meloxicam (℞)
(mel-ox′i-kam)
Mobic
Func. class.: Nonsteroidal antiinflammatory drugs/nonopioid analgesic (NSAIDs)
Chem. class.: Oxicam

Action: Inhibits prostaglandin synthesis by decreasing an enzyme needed for biosynthesis; analgesic, antiinflammatory, antipyretic effects
Uses: Osteoarthritis, rheumatoid arthritis, juvenile arthritis

DOSAGE AND ROUTES
• *Adult:* **PO** 7.5 mg daily, may increase to 15 mg daily
Available forms: Tabs 7.5 mg; susp 7.5 mg/ml

SIDE EFFECTS
CNS: Dizziness, drowsiness, tremors, headache, nervousness, malaise, fatigue, insomnia, depression, **seizures**
CV: Hypertension, angina, **cardiac failure, MI,** hypotension, palpitations, **dysrhythmias,** tachycardia
EENT: Tinnitus, hearing loss
GI: Pancreatitis, nausea, colitis, GERD, vomiting, diarrhea, constipation, flatulence, cramps, dry mouth, peptic ulcer, **GI bleeding, perforation**
GU: **Nephrotoxicity: dysuria, hematuria, oliguria, azotemia**
HEMA: **Blood dyscrasias,** anemia, prolonged bleeding
INTEG: Rash, urticaria, photosensitivity
SYST: **Angioedema, anaphylaxis, Stevens-Johnson syndrome, toxic epidermal necrolysis**
Contraindications: Pregnancy (D) 2nd/3rd trimester; hypersensitivity, asthma, severe renal/hepatic disease, peptic ulcer disease, L&D, lactation, CV bleeding
Precautions: Pregnancy (C), children, bleeding disorders, GI disorders, cardiac disorders, hypersensitivity to other antiinflammatory agents, geriatric, CCr <25 ml/min

PHARMACOKINETICS
PO: Peak 4-5 hr
IM: Peak 50 min, half-life 6 hr, enters breast milk, <50% metabolized by liver, excreted by kidneys

INTERACTIONS
Increase: nephrotoxicity—cycloSPORINE
Increase: meloxicam action—phenytoin, sulfonamides, salicylates
Increase: action of aminoglycosides, hydantoins, diuretics, anticoagulants

---

Side effects: *italics* = common; **bold** = life-threatening

Decrease: meloxicam action—cholestyramine
Decrease: action of β-blockers
Drug/Herb
Increase: gastric irritation—arginine, gossypol
Increase: NSAIDs effect—bearberry, bilberry
Increase: bleeding risk—bogbean, chondroitin

NURSING CONSIDERATIONS
Assess:
• Renal, hepatic, blood studies: BUN, creatinine, AST, ALT, Hgb before treatment, periodically thereafter
• Bleeding times; check for bruising, bleeding; test for occult blood in urine
⚠ For anaphylaxis and angioedema; emergency equipment should be nearby
⚠ Hepatic dysfunction: jaundice, yellow sclera and skin, clay-colored stools
• Audiometric, ophthalmic exam before, during, after treatment
• GI condition, hypertension, cardiac conditions
Administer:
• May take without regard to meals, to take with food for GI upset
• Take with full glass of water and sit upright for ½ hr
Perform/provide:
• Storage at room temperature
Evaluate:
• Therapeutic response: decreased pain, stiffness, swelling in joints, ability to move more easily
Teach patient/family:
• To report blurred vision or ringing, roaring in ears (may indicate toxicity)
• To avoid driving, other hazardous activities if dizziness or drowsiness occurs
• To report change in urine pattern, weight increase, edema, pain increase in joints, fever, blood in urine (indicates nephrotoxicity); to report rash, black stools, or continuing headache
• To avoid alcohol, aspirin, acetaminophen without consulting prescriber

⚠ High Alert
melphalan (℞)
(mel′fa-lan)
Alkeran, L-PAM, phenylalanine mustard
Func. class.: Antineoplastic, alkylating agent
Chem. class.: Nitrogen mustard

Do not confuse:
melphalan/Myleran
Action: Responsible for cross-linking DNA strands leading to cell death; activity is not cell cycle phase specific
Uses: Multiple myeloma, malignant melanoma, advanced ovarian cancer
Unlabeled uses: Breast, testicular, prostate carcinoma; osteogenic sarcoma, chronic myelogenous leukemia

DOSAGE AND ROUTES
Multiple myeloma
• *Adult:* **PO** 150 mcg/kg/day × 1 wk, then 21 days after, then 50 mcg/kg/day or 100-150 mcg/kg/day or 250 mcg/kg/day × 4 days for 2-3 wk after, then 2-4 mg/day or 7 mg/m^2 × 5 day q5-6wk
• *Adult:* **IV INF** 16 mg/m^2, reduce in renal insufficiency, give over 15-20 min, give at 2-wk intervals × 4 doses, then at 4-wk intervals
Ovarian carcinoma
• *Adult:* **PO** 200 mcg/kg/day for 5 days q4-5wk
Available forms: Tabs 2 mg, powder for inj 50 mg

SIDE EFFECTS
GI: Nausea, vomiting, stomatitis, diarrhea
GU: Amenorrhea, hyperuricemia, gonadal suppression
HEMA: **Thrombocytopenia, neutropenia, leukopenia,** anemia
INTEG: Rash, urticaria, alopecia, pruritus
RESP: **Fibrosis, dysplasia**
SYST: **Anaphylaxis,** allergic reactions

⚠ Safety alert   *"Tall Man" lettering

Contraindications: Pregnancy (D), lactation, hypersensitivity to this drug or other nitrogen mustards

Precautions: Radiation therapy, bone marrow depression, infections, renal disease, children

PHARMACOKINETICS

Metabolized in liver, excreted in urine, half-life 1½ hr

INTERACTIONS

Increase: toxicity—antineoplastics, radiation

Increase: pulmonary toxicity—carmustine

Increase: renal failure risk—cycloSPORINE

Increase: enterocolitis risk—nalidixic acid

Decrease: antibody response—live virus vaccines

NURSING CONSIDERATIONS

Assess:

• CBC, differential, platelet count qwk; withhold drug if WBC is <3000/mm³ or platelet count is <100,000/mm³; notify prescriber; recovery usually occurs in 6 wk

• Renal studies: BUN, serum uric acid, urine CCr before, during therapy

• I&O ratio; report fall in urine output to 30 ml/hr

• For infection: fever, cough, temp, sore throat, notify prescriber

• For bleeding: bruising, blood in urine, stools, emesis

• Hepatic studies before, during therapy (bilirubin, AST, ALT, LDH) as needed or monthly

• Bleeding: hematuria, guaiac, bruising or petechiae, mucosa or orifices q8h

• Jaundiced skin and sclera, dark urine, clay-colored stools, itchy skin, abdominal pain, fever, diarrhea

• Buccal cavity q8h for dryness, sores, ulceration, white patches, oral pain, bleeding, dysphagia

• Local irritation, pain, burning, discoloration at inj site

⚠ Symptoms indicating severe allergic reaction: rash, pruritus, urticaria, purpuric skin lesions, itching, flushing; assess allergy to chlorambucil, cross-sensitivity may occur

Administer:

• Antiemetic 30-60 min before giving drug to prevent vomiting

IV route

• Give by intermittent inf after reconstituting with 10 ml diluent provided (5 mg/ml), shake, dilute dose with 0.9% NaCl (≤0.45 mg/ml), give within 1 hr, run over ≥15 min

Y-site compatibilities: Acyclovir, amikacin, aminophylline, ampicillin, aztreonam, bleomycin, bumetanide, buprenorphine, butorphanol, calcium gluconate, carboplatin, carmustine, cefazolin, cefepime, cefoperazone, cefotaxime, cefotetan, ceftazidime, ceftizoxime, ceftriaxone, cefuroxime, cimetidine, cisplatin, clindamycin, cyclophosphamide, cytarabine, dacarbazine, dactinomycin, DAUNOrubicin, dexamethasone, diphenhydrAMINE, DOXOrubicin, doxycycline, droperidol, enalaprilat, etoposide, famotidine, floxuridine, fluconazole, fludarabine, fluorouracil, furosemide, gallium, ganciclovir, gentamicin, granisetron, haloperidol, heparin, hydrocortisone, hydrocortisone sodium phosphate, hydromorphone, hydrOXYzine, idarubicin, ifosfamide, imipenem-cilastatin, lorazepam, mannitol, mechlorethamine, meperidine, mesna, methotrexate, methylPREDNISolone, metoclopramide, metronidazole, miconazole, minocycline, mitomycin, mitoxantrone, morphine, nalbuphine, netilmicin, ondansetron, pentostatin, piperacillin, plicamycin, potassium chloride, prochlorperazine, promethazine, ranitidine, sodium bicarbonate, streptozocin, teniposide, thiotepa, ticarcillin, ticarcillin/clavulanate, tobramycin, trimethoprim-sulfamethoxazole, vancomycin, vinBLAStine, vinCRIStine, vinorelbine, zidovudine

M

Side effects: *italics* = common; **bold** = life-threatening

Perform/provide:
- Storage in airtight, light-resistant container
- Strict medical asepsis, protective isolation if WBC levels are low
- Increase fluid intake to 2-3 L/day to prevent urate deposits, calculi formation
- Diet low in purines: organ meats (kidney, liver), dried beans, peas to maintain alkaline urine
- Rinsing of mouth tid-qid with water, club soda; brushing of teeth bid-tid with soft brush or cotton-tipped applicators for stomatitis; use unwaxed dental floss
- Warm compresses at inj site for inflammation

Evaluate:
- Therapeutic response: decreased tumor size, spread of malignancy

Teach patient/family:
- That sterility, amenorrhea can occur; reversible after discontinuing treatment
- To avoid foods with citric acid, hot or rough texture
- To report any bleeding, white spots, or ulcerations in mouth to prescriber; tell patient to examine mouth daily
- To report signs of infection: fever, sore throat, flulike symptoms
- To report suspected pregnancy; to use contraception during treatment
- To report signs of anemia: fatigue, headache, faintness, shortness of breath, irritability
- To avoid use of razors, commercial mouthwash
- To avoid use of aspirin products, NSAIDs, alcohol

memantine (R̶)
(me-man′teen)
Namenda
Func. class.: Anti-Alzheimer agent
Chem. class.: NMDA receptor antagonist

Action: Antagonist action of CNS NMDA receptors that may contribute to the symptoms of Alzheimer's disease

Uses: Treatment of moderate to severe dementia in Alzheimer's disease
Unlabeled uses: Vascular dementia

DOSAGE AND ROUTES
- *Adult:* **PO** 5 mg daily, may increase dose in 5 mg increments ≥1 wk intervals; recommended target dose 20 mg/day
Available forms: Tabs 5, 10 mg; oral sol 2 mg/ml

SIDE EFFECTS
CNS: Dizziness, confusion, somnolence, headache, hallucinations
CV: Hypertension
GI: Vomiting, constipation
INTEG: Rash
MISC: Back pain, fatigue, pain
RESP: Coughing, dyspnea
Contraindications: Hypersensitivity
Precautions: Pregnancy (B), renal disease, GU conditions that raise urine pH, lactation, children, seizures

PHARMACOKINETICS
Rapidly absorbed PO, 44% protein binding, very little metabolism, 57%-82% excreted unchanged in urine, terminal elimination half-life 60-80 hr

INTERACTIONS
- May alter levels of both drugs: hydrochlorothiazide, triamterene, cimetidine, quinidine, ranitidine, nicotine
Decrease: clearance of memantine—drugs which makes the urine alkaline (sodium bicarbonate, carbonic anhydrase inhibitors)

NURSING CONSIDERATIONS
Assess:
- B/P: hypertension
- Mental status: affect, mood, behavioral changes; hallucinations, confusion
- GI status: vomiting, constipation, add bulk, increase fluids for constipation
- GU status: urinary frequency

Administer:
- Can be taken without regard to meals
- Twice a day if dose >5 mg

A Safety alert   *"Tall Man" lettering

• Dosage adjusted to response no more than q1wk

• Oral sol using device provided; remove dosing syringe, green cap, and plastic tube from plastic; attach tube to green cap; open cap by pushing down on cap and turning counterclockwise; remove unscrewed cap; carefully remove seal from bottle and discard; insert plastic tube fully into bottle and screw green cap tightly onto bottle by turning cap clockwise; keeping bottle upright on table, remove the lid; with plunger fully depressed, insert tip of syringe into cap; while holding syringe, gently pull up on plunger; remove syringe; invert syringe and slowly press plunger to a level that removes large air bubbles; keep plunger in inverted position; a few small air bubbles may be present

Perform/provide:

• Assistance with ambulation during beginning therapy; dizziness may occur

Evaluate:

• Therapeutic response: decrease in confusion, improved mood

Teach patient/family:

• To report side effects: restlessness, psychosis, visual hallucinations, stupor, loss of consciousness; indicate overdose

• To use drug exactly as prescribed; drug is not a cure

• To use oral solution dispenser

---

menotropins (℞)
(men-oh-troe′pins)
Humegon, Pergonal,
Repronex
Func. class.: Gonadotropin
Chem. class.: Exogenous gonadotropin

Action: In women, increases follicular growth, maturation; in men, when given with hCG, stimulates spermatogenesis
Uses: Infertility, anovulation in women, stimulates spermatogenesis in men

DOSAGE AND ROUTES
Infertility
• *Men:* **IM** 1 ampule 3 × wk with hCG 2000 units 2 × wk × 4 mo
• *Women:* **IM** 75 international units FSH, LH daily × 9-12 days, then 10,000 units hCG 1 day after these drugs; repeat × 2 menstrual cycles, then increase to 150 international units FSH, LH daily × 9-12 days, then 10,000 units hCG 1 day after these drugs × 2 menstrual cycles
Anovulation
• *Women:* **IM** 75 international units FSH, LH daily × 9-12 days, then 10,000 units hCG 1 day after last dose of these drugs; repeat × 1-3 menstrual cycles
Available forms: Powder for inj lyophilized 75 international units FSH, LH activity 150 international units FSH, LH activity

SIDE EFFECTS
CNS: Fever
CV: **Hypovolemia**
GI: Nausea, vomiting, diarrhea, anorexia
GU: Ovarian enlargement, abdominal distention/pain, multiple births, ovarian hyperstimulation: sudden ovarian enlargement, ascites with or without pain; gynecomastia in men
HEMA: **Hemoperitoneum, arterial thromboembolism**
RESP: **ARDS, pulmonary embolism, pulmonary infarction, pleural effusion**
SYST: **Anaphylaxis**
Contraindications: Pregnancy (X), primary ovarian failure, abnormal bleeding, thyroid/adrenal dysfunction, organic intracranial lesion, ovarian cysts, primary testicular failure

NURSING CONSIDERATIONS
Assess:
• Weight daily; notify prescriber if weight increases rapidly
• Estrogen excretion level; if >100 mcg/24 hr, drug is withheld; hyperstimulation syndrome may occur

M

- I&O ratio; be alert for decreasing urinary output
- Ovarian enlargement, abdominal distention/pain; report symptoms immediately

Administer:

IM route

- After reconstituting with 1-2 ml sterile saline inj; use immediately

Evaluate:

- Therapeutic response: ovulation, pregnancy

Teach patient/family:

- That multiple births are possible; if pregnancy occurs, usually 4-6 wk after start of treatment
- To keep appointment during treatment daily × 2 wk

⚠ High Alert

meperidine (℞)

(me-per′i-deen)

Demerol, meperidine, Pethidine

Func. class.: Opioid analgesic

Chem. class.: Phenylpiperidine derivative

Controlled Substance Schedule II

Do not confuse:

meperidine/hydromorphone/meprobamate/morphine

Demerol/Dilaudid

Action: Depresses pain impulse transmission at the spinal cord level by interacting with opioid receptors

Uses: Moderate to severe pain, preoperatively, postoperatively

Unlabeled uses: Rigors

DOSAGE AND ROUTES

Pain

- *Adult:* **PO/SUBCUT/IM** 50-150 mg q3-4h prn; **IV** 15-35 mg/hr as a **CONT INF**; PCA 10 mg, then 1-5 mg incremental dose; lockout interval 6-10 min
- *Child:* **PO/SUBCUT/IM** 1 mg/kg q3-4h prn, not to exceed 100 mg q4h

Labor analgesia

- *Adult:* **SUBCUT/IM** 50-100 mg given when contractions are regularly spaced, repeat q1-3h prn

Preoperatively

- *Adult:* **IM/SUBCUT** 50-100 mg q30-90 min before surgery; dose should be reduced if given **IV**
- *Child:* **IM/SUBCUT** 1-2.2 mg/kg 30-90 min before surgery

Renal disease

- CCr 10-50 ml/min 75% of dose; CCr <10 ml/min 50% of dose

Available forms: Inj 10, 25, 50, 75, 100 mg/ml; tabs 50, 100 mg; syr 50 mg/5 ml

SIDE EFFECTS

CNS: Drowsiness, dizziness, confusion, headache, sedation, euphoria, **increased intracranial pressure, seizures**

CV: Palpitations, bradycardia, change in B/P, tachycardia (IV)

EENT: Tinnitus, blurred vision, miosis, diplopia, depressed corneal reflex

GI: Nausea, vomiting, anorexia, constipation, cramps

GU: Urinary retention, dysuria

INTEG: Rash, urticaria, bruising, flushing, diaphoresis, pruritus

RESP: **Respiratory depression**

Contraindications: Hypersensitivity, addiction (opioid)

Precautions: Pregnancy (B), addictive personality, lactation, increased intracranial pressure, MI (acute), severe heart disease, respiratory depression, renal/hepatic disease, child <18 yr, geriatric

PHARMACOKINETICS

Absorption 50% (PO), well absorbed IM, SUBCUT

PO: Onset 15 min, peak ½-1 hr, duration 2-4 hr

SUBCUT/IM: Onset 10 min, peak ½-1 hr, duration 2-4 hr

IV: Onset 5 min, duration 2 hr

Metabolized by liver (to active/inactive

⚠ Safety alert   *"Tall Man" lettering

metabolites), excreted by kidneys; crosses placenta, excreted in breast milk; half-life 3-4 hr; toxic by-product can result from regular use

INTERACTIONS

⚠ May cause fatal reaction: MAOIs, procarbazine

Increase: effects with other CNS depressants, alcohol, opioids, sedative/hypnotics, antipsychotics, skeletal muscle relaxants

Increase: adverse reactions—protease inhibitor antiretrovirals

Decrease: meperidine effect—phenytoin

Drug/Herb

Increase: CNS depression—chamomile, hops, Jamaican dogwood, kava, lavender, mistletoe, nettle, pokeweed, poppy, senega, skullcap, valerian

Increase: Parsley may promote serotonin syndrome; avoid concurrent medicinal use

Drug/Lab Test

Increase: Amylase, lipase

NURSING CONSIDERATIONS

Assess:

• Pain: location, type, character; give before pain becomes extreme; reassess after 60 min (IM, SUBCUT, PO) and 5-10 min (IV)

• Renal function prior to initiating therapy; poor renal function can lead to accumulation of toxic metabolite and seizures

• I&O ratio; check for decreasing output; may indicate urinary retention

• For constipation; increase fluids, bulk in diet; give laxatives if needed

• CNS changes: dizziness, drowsiness, hallucinations, euphoria, LOC, pupil reactions; at chronic or high-dose use

• Allergic reactions: rash, urticaria

• Respiratory dysfunction: depression, character, rate, rhythm; notify prescriber if respirations are <12/min

• CNS stimulation: occurs with chronic or high doses

Administer:

• Patient should remain recumbent for 1 hr after IM/SUBCUT route

• With antiemetic for nausea, vomiting

• When pain is beginning to return; determine dosage interval by patient response

• In gradually decreasing dose after long-term use; withdrawal symptoms may occur

IV route

• After diluting with 5 ml or more sterile H_2O or NS; give directly over 4-5 min; may be further diluted in sol to 1 mg/ml during anesthesia in D_5W or NS; if diluted in NS, may be given through patient-controlled inf device

Additive compatibilities: Cefazolin, DOBUTamine, ondansetron, scopolamine, succinylcholine, triflupromazine, verapamil

Syringe compatibilities: Atropine, benzquinamide, butorphanol, chlorproMAZINE, cimetidine, dimenhyDRINATE, diphenhydrAMINE, droperidol, fentanyl, glycopyrrolate, hydrOXYzine, ketamine, metoclopramide, midazolam, pentazocine, perphenazine, prochlorperazine, promazine, promethazine, ranitidine, scopolamine

Y-site compatibilities: Amifostine, amikacin, ampicillin, atenolol, aztreonam, bumetanide, cefazolin, cefotaxime, cefotetan, cefoxitin, ceftazidime, ceftizoxime, ceftriaxone, cefuroxime, cephalothin, cephapirin, chloramphenicol, cisatracurium, cladribine, clindamycin, dexamethasone, diltiazem, diphenhydrAMINE, DOBUTamine, DOPamine, DOXOrubicin liposome, doxycycline, droperidol, erythromycin, famotidine, filgrastim, fluconazole, fludarabine, gallium, gentamicin, granisetron, heparin, hydrocortisone, insulin (regular), kanamycin, labetalol, lidocaine, methyldopate, magnesium sulfate, melphalan, methylPREDNISolone, metoclopramide, metoprolol, metronidazole, moxalactam, ondansetron, oxacillin, oxytocin, paclitaxel, penicillin G potassium, piperacillin, potassium chloride, propofol, propranolol, ranitidine,

remifentanil, sargramostim, teniposide, thiotepa, ticarcillin, ticarcillin/
clavulanate, tobramycin, trimethoprim-
sulfamethoxazole, vancomycin, verapamil, vinorelbine

Perform/provide:
• Storage in light-resistant container at
room temperature
• Assistance with ambulation
• Safety measures: night-light, call bell
within easy reach

Evaluate:
• Therapeutic response: decrease in pain

Teach patient/family:
• To report any symptoms of CNS
changes, allergic reactions
• That physical dependency may result
from extended use
• That drowsiness, dizziness may occur;
to call for assistance
• That withdrawal symptoms may occur:
nausea, vomiting, cramps, fever, faintness,
anorexia
• To make position changes slowly; orthostatic hypotension can occur
• To avoid OTC medications, alcohol unless directed by prescriber

Treatment of overdose: Naloxone
(Narcan) 0.2-0.8 mg IV, O$_2$, IV fluids, vasopressors

---

mercaptopurine (℞)
(mer-kap-toe-pyoor'een)
Purinethol, 6-MP
Func. class.: Antineoplastic-anti-
metabolite
Chem. class.: Purine analog

Action: Inhibits purine metabolism at
multiple sites, which inhibits DNA and
RNA synthesis, S phase of cell cycle specific

Uses: Chronic myelocytic or acute lymphoblastic leukemia in children, acute
myelogenous leukemia

Unlabeled uses: Polycythemia vera,
psoriatic arthritis, colitis, lymphoma

DOSAGE AND ROUTES
• *Adult:* **PO** 80-100 mg/m^2 daily max 5
mg/kg/day; maintenance 1.5-2.5 mg/kg/
day
• *Child:* **PO** 75 mg/m^2/day; maintenance
1.5-2.5 mg/kg/day

Available forms: Tabs 50 mg

SIDE EFFECTS
CNS: Fever, headache, weakness
*GI: Nausea, vomiting, anorexia, diar-
rhea, stomatitis,* **hepatotoxicity** (high
doses), jaundice, gastritis
GU: **Renal failure,** hyperuricemia, **oliguria,** crystalluria, **hematuria**
HEMA: **Thrombocytopenia, leukopenia, myelosuppression, anemia**
INTEG: Rash, dry skin, urticaria
Contraindications: Pregnancy (D),
patients with prior drug resistance, leukopenia (<2500/mm^3), thrombocytopenia
(<100,000/mm^3), anemia, lactation
Precautions: Renal disease

PHARMACOKINETICS
Incompletely absorbed when taken
orally; metabolized in liver, excreted in
urine

INTERACTIONS
• Reversal of neuromuscular blockade:
nondepolarizing muscle relaxants
Increase: toxicity—radiation or other
antineoplastics
Increase: bone marrow depression—
allopurinol, co-trimoxazole
Increase or decrease: anticoagulant
action—warfarin
Decrease: antibodies—live virus vaccines

NURSING CONSIDERATIONS
Assess:
• CBC, differential, platelet count qwk;
withhold drug if WBC is <3500 or platelet count is <100,000; notify prescriber;
drug should be discontinued
• Renal studies: BUN, serum uric acid,
urine CCr, electrolytes before, during therapy

⚠ Safety alert   *"Tall Man" lettering

- I&O ratio; report fall in urine output to <30 ml/hr
- Monitor temp q4h; fever may indicate beginning infection; no rectal temps
- Hepatic studies before, during therapy: bilirubin, alk phos, AST, ALT, qwk during beginning therapy
- Bleeding: hematuria, guaiac, bruising, petechiae; mucosa or orifices q8h
- Buccal cavity q8h for dryness, sores, ulceration, white patches, oral pain, bleeding, dysphagia

⚠ Symptoms indicating severe allergic reaction: rash, urticaria, itching, flushing

Administer:
- Antacid before oral agent; give drug after evening meal before bedtime
- Allopurinol or sodium bicarbonate to maintain uric acid levels, alkalinization of urine

Perform/provide:
- Strict medical asepsis, protective isolation if WBC levels are low
- Increase fluid intake to 2-3 L/day to prevent urate deposits, calculi formation, unless contraindicated
- Diet low in purines: absence of organ meats (kidney, liver), dried beans, peas to maintain alkaline urine
- Rinsing of mouth tid-qid with water, club soda; brushing of teeth bid-tid with soft brush or cotton-tipped applicators for stomatitis; use unwaxed dental floss
- Nutritious diet with iron, vitamin supplements as ordered
- Storage in tightly closed container in cool environment

Evaluate:
- Therapeutic response: decreased size of tumor, spread of malignancy

Teach patient/family:
- To avoid foods with citric acid, hot or rough texture for stomatitis
- To report stomatitis: any bleeding, white spots, ulcerations in mouth; tell patient to examine mouth daily, report symptoms
- That contraceptive measures are recommended during therapy; to avoid breastfeeding
- To drink 10-12 (8 oz) glasses of fluid/day

- To notify prescriber of fever, chills, sore throat, nausea, vomiting, anorexia, diarrhea, bleeding, bruising, which may indicate blood dyscrasias
- To report signs of infection: fever, sore throat, flulike symptoms
- To report signs of anemia: fatigue, headache, faintness, shortness of breath, irritability
- To report bleeding: avoid use of razors, commercial mouthwash
- To avoid use of aspirin products, NSAIDs
- To take entire dose at one time

meropenem (℞)
(mer-oh-pen'em)
Merrem IV
Func. class.: Antiinfective—miscellaneous
Chem. class.: Carbapenem

Action: Bactericidal, interferes with cell wall replication of susceptible organisms; osmotically unstable cell wall swells, bursts from osmotic pressure

Uses: Serious infections caused by gram-positive bacteria: *Streptococcus pneumoniae,* group A β-hemolytic streptococci, enterococcus; gram-negative: *Klebsiella, Proteus, Escherichia coli, Pseudomonas aeruginosa;* appendicitis, peritonitis caused by *viridans* group streptococci; *Bacteroides fragilis, Bacteroides thetaiotaomicron,* bacterial meningitis (≥3 mo)

Unlabeled uses: Febrile neutropenic, community-acquired pneumonia

DOSAGE AND ROUTES
- *Adult:* **IV** 1 g q8h, given over 15-30 min or as an **IV BOL** 5-20 ml given over 3-5 min
- *Child ≥3 mo:* **IV** 20-40 mg/kg q8h (max 2g q8h meningitis)
- *Child >50 kg:* **IV** 1 g q8h (intraabdominal infection) or 2 g q8h (meningitis) given over 15-30 min or as an **IV BOL** 5-20 ml over 3-5 min; max 2 g q8h

Renal disease
• *Adult:* IV CCr 26-50 ml/min 1 g q12h; CCr 10-25 ml/min 500 mg q12h; CCr <10 ml/min 500 mg q24h
Available forms: Powder for inj 500 mg, 1 g

SIDE EFFECTS

CNS: Fever, somnolence, **seizures,** dizziness, weakness, myoclonia, *headache,* confusion
CV: Hypotension, palpitations, tachycardia
GI: Diarrhea, nausea, vomiting, **pseudomembranous colitis, hepatitis,** glossitis
HEMA: **Eosinophilia, neutropenia,** decreased Hgb, Hct, **agranulocytosis**
INTEG: *Rash,* urticaria, *pruritus,* pain at inj site, phlebitis, erythema at inj site
RESP: Chest discomfort, dyspnea, hyperventilation, **pulmonary embolism**
SYST: **Anaphylaxis, Stevens-Johnson syndrome, angioedema**
Contraindications: Hypersensitivity to meropenem or imipenem
Precautions: Pregnancy (B), lactation, geriatric, renal disease, seizure disorder

PHARMACOKINETICS

IV: Onset immediate, peak dose dependent, half-life 1 hr, excreted unchanged in urine (70%)

INTERACTIONS

Increase: meropenem plasma levels—probenecid
Decrease: effect of valproic acid
Drug/Herb
• Do not use acidophilus with antiinfectives; separate by several hours
Drug/Lab Test
Increase: AST, ALT, LDH, BUN, alk phos, bilirubin, creatinine
False positive: Direct Coombs' test

NURSING CONSIDERATIONS
Assess:
• Sensitivity to carbapenem antibiotics, penicillins

• Renal disease: lower dose may be required
• Bowel pattern daily; if severe diarrhea occurs, drug should be discontinued; may indicate pseudomembranous colitis
• For infection: temp, sputum, characteristics of wound, before, during, and after treatment
⚠ Allergic reactions, anaphylaxis: rash, urticaria, pruritus; may occur few days after therapy begins
• Overgrowth of infection: perineal itching, fever, malaise, redness, pain, swelling, drainage, rash, diarrhea, change in cough, sputum
Administer:
• By IV inf or IV bol
• After C&S is taken
• Reconstitute with 0.9% NaCl, D₅W, LR; dilute in 5-20 ml comp sol; give by direct IV over 3-5 min; give by intermittent inf, dilute in 5-20 ml of comp sol; give over 15-30 min
Additive compatibilities: Aminophylline, atropine, cimetidine, dexamethasone, DOBUTamine, DOPamine, enalaprilat, fluconazole, furosemide, gentamicin, heparin, insulin (regular), magnesium sulfate, metoclopramide, morphine, norepinephrine, phenobarbital, ranitidine, vancomycin
Y-site compatibilities: Aminophylline, atenolol, atropine, cimetidine, dexamethasone, digoxin, diphenhydrAMINE, enalaprilat, fluconazole, furosemide, gentamicin, heparin, insulin (regular), metoclopramide, morphine, norepinephrine, phenobarbital, vancomycin
Evaluate:
• Therapeutic response: negative C&S; absence of symptoms and signs of infection
Teach patient/family:
• To report severe diarrhea; may indicate pseudomembranous colitis
• To report sore throat, bruising, bleeding, joint pain; may indicate blood dyscrasias (rare)
• To report overgrowth of infection: black, furry tongue; vaginal itching; foul-smelling stools

⚠ Safety alert   *"Tall Man" lettering

- To avoid breastfeeding; drug is excreted in breast milk

Treatment of overdose: EpINEPHrine, antihistamines; resuscitate if needed (anaphylaxis)

---

mesalamine (℞)
(mez-al'a-meen)
Asacol, Canasa, Pentasa,
Rowasa Salofalk ✦
Func. class.: GI antiinflammatory
Chem. class.: 5-Aminosalicylic acid

Do not confuse:
Asacol/Ansaid/Os-Cal

Action: May diminish inflammation by blocking cyclooxygenase, inhibiting prostaglandin production in colon; local action only

Uses: Mild to moderate active distal ulcerative colitis, proctosigmoiditis, proctitis

Unlabeled uses: Crohn's disease

DOSAGE AND ROUTES

- *Adult:* **RECT** 60 ml (4 g) at bedtime, retained for 8 hr × 3-6 wk; **PO** 1000 mg qid for up to 8 wk; **SUPP** 500 mg bid × 3-6 wk, retain 1-3 hr

Available forms: Rect susp 4 g/60 ml; supp 500 mg; ext rel tab 250, 500 mg ✦; ext rel cap 250 mg, 1 g; del rel tab 250 ✦, 400, 500 ✦

SIDE EFFECTS

CNS: Headache, fever, dizziness, insomnia, asthenia, weakness, fatigue
CV: Pericarditis, myocarditis, chest pain, palpitations
EENT: Sore throat, cough, pharyngitis, rhinitis
GI: Cramps, gas, nausea, diarrhea, rectal pain, constipation
INTEG: Rash, itching, acne
SYST: Flulike symptoms, malaise, back pain, peripheral edema, leg and joint pain, arthralgia, dysmenorrhea, **anaphylaxis,** acute intolerance syndrome

Contraindications: Hypersensitivity to this drug or salicylates

Precautions: Pregnancy (B), renal disease, lactation, children, sulfite sensitivity, geriatric, pyloric stenosis

PHARMACOKINETICS

RECT: Primarily excreted in feces but some in urine as metabolite; half-life 1 hr, metabolite half-life 5-10 hr

INTERACTIONS

Increase: mesalamine absorption—omeprazole
Increase: action of azathioprine
Decrease: digoxin level—digoxin
Decrease: mesalamine absorption—lactulose

Drug/Lab Test
Increase: AST, ALT, alk phos, LDH, GGTP, amylase, lipase

NURSING CONSIDERATIONS
Assess:
- For allergy to salicylates, sulfonamides, if allergic reactions occur, discontinue product
- Renal studies: BUN, creatinine before and during treatment; renal toxicity may occur
- GI symptoms: cramps, gas, nausea, diarrhea, rectal pain; if severe, drug should be discontinued
- I&O ratios, increase fluids to 1500 ml daily to prevent crystalluria

Administer:
PO route
- Swallow tabs whole; do not break, crush, or chew tabs
Rectal route
- Drug should be given at bedtime, retained until morning; empty bowel before insertion

Perform/provide:
- Storage at room temperature

Evaluate:
- Therapeutic response: absence of pain, bleeding from GI tract, decrease in number of diarrhea stools

Teach patient/family:
- That usual course of therapy is 3-6 wk
- To shake bottle well (rectal susp)

M

Side effects: *italics* = common; **bold** = life-threatening

- Method of rectal administration
- To inform prescriber of GI symptoms
- To report abdominal cramping, pain, diarrhea with blood, headache, fever, rash, chest pain; drug should be discontinued

---

metaproterenol (℞)
(met-a-proe-ter′e-nole)
Alupent, Arm-a-Med,
Dey-Lute
Func. class.: Bronchodilator-
selective β$_2$-agonist

Do not confuse:
Alupent/Atrovent

Action: Relaxes bronchial smooth muscle by direct action on β$_2$-adrenergic receptors with increased levels of cAMP with increased bronchodilation, diuresis, cardiac CNS stimulation

Uses: Bronchial asthma, bronchospasm

DOSAGE AND ROUTES

- *Adult and child >12 yr:* **INH** 2-3 inhalations; may repeat q3-4h, not to exceed 12 inhalations/day; **IPPB** or **NEB** 0.2-0.3 ml of 5% sol diluted in 2.5 ml of ½ NS or NS; or 2.5 ml of 0.4, 0.6% sol q4h prn
- *Adult:* **PO** 20 mg q6-8h
- *Geriatric:* **PO** 10 mg tid-qid, initially
- *Child 6-12 yr:* **IPPB/NEB** 0.1-0.2 ml of a 5% sol diluted in NS to a final volume of 3 ml q4h prn
- *Child >9 yr or >27 kg:* **PO** 20 mg q6-8h or 0.4-0.9 mg/kg tid
- *Child 6-9 yr or <27 kg:* **PO** 10 mg q6-8h or 0.4-0.9 mg/kg tid
- *Child 2-6 yr:* **PO** 1.3-2.6 mg/kg divided q6-8h
- *Child 1-2 yr:* **PO** 0.4 mg/kg q6-8h

Available forms: Tabs 10, 20 mg; aerosol inhaler 0.65 mg/dose; syr 10 mg/5 ml; neb inhaler 0.4%, 0.6%, 5%

SIDE EFFECTS

CNS: Tremors, anxiety, insomnia, headache, dizziness, stimulation
CV: Palpitations, tachycardia, hypertension, dysrhythmias, **cardiac arrest** (high dose)
GI: Nausea, vomiting, dry mouth
MISC: Hypokalemia, pyrosis
RESP: **Paradoxical bronchospasm**

Contraindications: Hypersensitivity to sympathomimetics, narrow-angle glaucoma, cardiac dysrhythmias with tachycardia

Precautions: Pregnancy (C), cardiac disorders, hyperthyroidism, diabetes mellitus, prostatic hypertrophy, seizure disorder, geriatric, child <6 yr (NEB), child <12 yr (INH)

PHARMACOKINETICS

PO: Onset 15-30 min, peak 1 hr, duration 1-4 hr, excreted in urine as metabolites
INH: Onset 1 min, peak 1 hr, duration 1-2½ hr
NEB: Onset 5-30 min, peak 1 hr, duration 1-2½ hr

INTERACTIONS

⚠ Hypertensive crisis: MAOIs, tricyclics
Increase: effects of both drugs—other sympathomimetics, bronchodilators
Decrease: β-blockers action
Drug/Herb
Increase: effect—black/green tea, coffee, cola nut, guarana, yerba maté
Drug/Lab Test
Decrease: Potassium

NURSING CONSIDERATIONS

Assess:
- Respiratory function: vital capacity, forced expiratory volume, ABGs; also B/P; lung sounds, secretions before and after treatment
- Tolerance over long-term therapy; dose may have to be changed; check for rebound bronchospasm

Administer:
- 2 hr before bedtime to avoid sleeplessness
- PO with food for GI upset

⚠ Safety alert   *"Tall Man" lettering

Perform/provide:
• Storage at room temperature; do not use discolored sol
• Spacer device for geriatric
Evaluate:
• Therapeutic response: absence of dyspnea, wheezing; improved ABGs
Teach patient/family:
• To increase fluid intake (2-3 L/day) to liquefy secretions unless contraindicated
• Not to use OTC medications; excess stimulation may occur
• To notify prescriber of headaches, chest pain, weakness, dizziness, anxiety
• Use of inhaler; review package insert with patient
• To avoid getting aerosol in eyes
• To wash inhaler in warm water and dry daily
• All aspects of drug; avoid smoking, smoke-filled rooms, persons with respiratory infections

metformin (℞)
(met-for′min)
Fortamet, Glucophage, Glucophage XR, Novo-Metformin ✚, Riomet
Func. class.: Antidiabetic, oral
Chem. class.: Biguanide

Action: Inhibits hepatic glucose production and increases sensitivity of peripheral tissue to insulin
Uses: Type 2 diabetes mellitus

DOSAGE AND ROUTES
• *Adult:* **PO** 500 mg bid initially, then increase to desired response 1-2 g; dosage adjustment q2-3wk or 850 mg daily with morning meal with dosage increased every other wk, max 2500 mg/day, **EXT REL** max 2000 mg/day
• *Geriatric:* **PO** use lowest effective dose
Available forms: Tabs 500, 850, 1000 mg; ext rel tab 500 mg; oral sol (Riomet) 500 mg/5 ml

SIDE EFFECTS
CNS: Headache, weakness, dizziness, drowsiness, tinnitus, fatigue, vertigo, *agitation*
ENDO: **Lactic acidosis,** hypoglycemia
GI: Nausea, vomiting, diarrhea, heartburn, anorexia, metallic taste
HEMA: **Thrombocytopenia,** decreased vit B_{12} levels
INTEG: Rash
Contraindications: Hypersensitivity, hepatic, creatinine >1.5 mg/ml (males) ≥1.4 (females), CHF, alcoholism, cardiopulmonary disease, history of lactic acidosis
Precautions: Pregnancy (B), previous hypersensitivity, geriatric, thyroid disease

PHARMACOKINETICS
Excreted by the kidneys unchanged 35%-50%, half-life 1½-5 hr, terminal 6-20 hr, peak 1-3 hr

INTERACTIONS
• Do not give with radiologic contrast media; may cause renal failure
Increase: metformin level—cimetidine, digoxin, morphine, procainamide, quinidine, ranitidine, triamterene, vancomycin
Increase: hypoglycemia—cimetidine, calcium channel blockers, corticosteroids, estrogens, oral contraceptives, phenothiazines, sympathomimetics, diuretics, phenytoin
Drug/Herb
Increase: hyperglycemia—glucosamine
Increase: hypoglycemia—chromium, coenzyme Q-10, fenugreek
Increase: metformin level—quinine
Increase: antidiabetic effect—alfalfa, aloe, basil, bay, bilberry, bitter melon, black catechu, buchu, burdock, coriander, dandelion, eyebright (po), fenugreek, garlic, ginseng, glucomannan, glucosamine, goat's rue, gymnema, horehound, horse chestnut, jambul, myrrh, myrtle
Decrease: antidiabetic effect—bee pollen, blue cohosh, broom, chromium, elecampane, eucalyptus, gotu kola

Side effects: *italics* = common; **bold** = life-threatening

NURSING CONSIDERATIONS

Assess:
• For hypoglycemic reactions (sweating, weakness, dizziness, anxiety, tremors, hunger), hyperglycemic reactions soon after meals
• CBC (baseline, q3mo) during treatment; check LFTs periodically AST, LDH, renal studies: BUN, creatinine during treatment; glucose, A1c
⚠ For lactic acidosis: malaise, myalgia, abdominal distress; risk increases with age, poor renal function; monitor electrolytes, lactate, pyruvate, blood pH, ketones, glucose

Administer:
PO route
• Do not break, crush, chew ext rel tab
• Twice a day given with meals to decrease GI upset and provide best absorption; may also be taken as a single dose
• Tabs crushed and mixed with meal or fluids for patients with difficulty swallowing

Perform/provide:
• Conversion from other oral hypoglycemic agents; change may be made without gradual dosage change; monitor serum or urine glucose and ketones tid during conversion
• Storage in tight container in cool environment

Evaluate:
• Therapeutic response: decrease in polyuria, polydipsia, polyphagia; clear sensorium; absence of dizziness; stable gait, blood glucose at normal level

Teach patient/family:
⚠ Lactic acidosis symptoms: hyperventilation, fatigue, malaise, chills, myalgia, somnolence; to notify prescriber immediately
• To use regular self-monitoring of blood glucose using blood glucose meter
• The symptoms of hypo/hyperglycemia, what to do about each
• That drug must be continued on daily basis; explain consequence of discontinuing drug abruptly

• To avoid OTC medications unless approved by prescriber
• That diabetes is a lifelong illness; that this drug is not a cure; only controls symptoms
• That all food included in diet plan must be eaten to prevent hypoglycemia
• To carry emergency ID and glucagon emergency kit for emergencies
• That Glucophage XR tab may appear in stool

Treatment of overdose: Glucose 25 g IV via dextrose 50% sol, 50 ml or 1 mg glucagon

---

⚠ High Alert

methadone (℞)
(meth'a-done)
Dolophine, methadone, Methadose
Func. class.: Opioid analgesic
Chem. class.: Synthetic diphenylheptane derivative

Controlled Substance Schedule II
Do not confuse:
methadone/methylphenidate
Action: Depresses pain impulse transmission at the spinal cord level by interacting with opioid receptors, produce CNS depression
Uses: Severe pain, opioid withdrawal

DOSAGE AND ROUTES

Severe pain
• *Adult:* **PO/SUBCUT/IM** 2.5-10 mg q3-4h prn
Opioid withdrawal
• *Adult:* **PO** 15-40 mg/day individualized initially, then 20-120 mg/day titrated to patient response
• *Child:* 0.05-0.1 mg/kg/dose q6-12h
Renal disease
• *Adult:* CCr 10-50 ml/min dose q8h; CCr <10 ml/min dose q8-12h
Available forms: Inj 10 mg/ml; tabs 5, 10 mg; oral sol 5, 10 mg/5 ml; dispersible tabs 40 mg; oral conc 10 mg/ml; oral sol 5 mg/5 ml, 10 mg/5 ml, 10 mg/10 ml

---

⚠ Safety alert   *"Tall Man" lettering

SIDE EFFECTS

CNS: Drowsiness, dizziness, confusion, headache, sedation, euphoria, **seizures**
CV: Palpitations, bradycardia, change in B/P, **cardiac arrest, shock**
EENT: Tinnitus, blurred vision, miosis, diplopia
GI: Nausea, vomiting, anorexia, constipation, cramps, biliary tract spasm
GU: Increased urinary output, dysuria, urinary retention
INTEG: Rash, urticaria, bruising, flushing, diaphoresis, pruritus
RESP: **Respiratory depression, respiratory arrest**

Contraindications: Hypersensitivity to this drug or chlorobutanol (inj), addiction (opiate)
Precautions: Pregnancy (C), addictive personality, lactation, increased intracranial pressure, MI (acute), severe heart disease, respiratory depression, renal/hepatic disease, children <18 yr, geriatric

PHARMACOKINETICS

PO: Onset 30-60 min, peak 1½-2 hr, duration 6-8 hr, cumulative 22-48; PO half as active as INJ
SUBCUT/IM: Onset 10-20 min, peak 1½-2 hr, duration 4-6 hr, cumulative 22-48 hr
Metabolized by liver; excreted by kidneys; crosses placenta; excreted in breast milk; half-life 15-30 hr, extended interval with continued dosing; 90% bound to plasma proteins

INTERACTIONS

⚠ Unpredictable reactions: MAOIs, do not use together
Increase: effects with other CNS depressants—alcohol, opiates, sedative/hypnotics, antipsychotics, skeletal muscle relaxants
Decrease: analgesia—rifampin, phenytoin, nalbuphine, pentazine
Drug/Herb
Increase: CNS depression—chamomile, hops, Jamaican dogwood, kava, lavender, mistletoe, nettle, pokeweed, poppy, senega, skullcap, valerian
Increase: anticholinergic effect—corkwood
Drug/Lab Test
Increase: Amylase, lipase

NURSING CONSIDERATIONS

Assess:
• For pain: type, location, intensity, grimacing before and 1½-2 hr after administration; use pain scoring
• I&O ratio; check for decreasing output; may indicate urinary retention
• CNS changes: dizziness, drowsiness, hallucinations, euphoria, LOC, pupil reaction
• Allergic reactions: rash, urticaria
• Respiratory dysfunction: respiratory depression, character, rate, rhythm; notify prescriber if respirations are <10/min
• For opioid detoxification: no analgesia occurs, only prevention of withdrawal symptoms
• B/P, pulse
• Bowel changes, bulk, fluids, laxatives should be used for constipation
Administer:
• With antiemetic if nausea/vomiting occurs
• When pain is beginning to return; determine dosage interval by patient response
• Rotating inj sites, give deep in large muscle mass (IM)
Perform/provide:
• Storage in light-resistant container at room temperature
• Assistance with ambulation
• Safety measures: night-light, call bell within easy reach
Evaluate:
• Therapeutic response: decrease in pain, successful opioid withdrawal
Teach patient/family:
• To report any symptoms of CNS changes, allergic reactions
• That physical dependency may result from extended use
⚠ Withdrawal symptoms may occur:

M

nausea, vomiting, cramps, fever, faintness, anorexia

Treatment of overdose: Naloxone (Narcan) 0.2-0.8 mg IV, O_2, IV fluids, vasopressors

---

methimazole (℞)
(meth-im′a-zole)
Tapazole
Func. class.: Thyroid hormone antagonist (antithyroid)
Chem. class.: Thioamide

Action: Inhibits synthesis of thyroid hormones by decreasing iodine use in manufacture of thyroglobin and iodothyronine; does not affect circulatory T_4, T_3

Uses: Hyperthyroidism, preparation for thyroidectomy, thyrotoxic crisis, thyroid storm

DOSAGE AND ROUTES
Hyperthyroidism
• *Adult:* **PO** 15 mg/day (mild hyperthyroidism); 30-40 mg/day (moderate-severe); 60 mg/day (severe); maintenance 5-15 mg/day
• *Child:* **PO** 0.4 mg/kg/day in divided doses q8h; continue until euthyroid; maintenance dose 0.2 mg/kg/day in divided doses q8h, max 30 mg/24 hr
Preparation and thyroidectomy
• *Adult and child:* **PO** same as above; iodine may be added × 10 days before surgery
Thyrotoxic crisis
• *Adult and child:* **PO** same as hyperthyroidism with iodine and propranolol
Available forms: Tabs 5, 10 mg

SIDE EFFECTS
CNS: Drowsiness, headache, vertigo, fever, paresthesias, neuritis
ENDO: Enlarged thyroid
GI: Nausea, diarrhea, vomiting, **jaundice, hepatitis,** loss of taste
GU: **Nephritis**
HEMA: **Agranulocytosis, leukopenia, thrombocytopenia, hypothrombine-**

mia, lymphadenopathy, bleeding, vasculitis
INTEG: Rash, urticaria, pruritus, alopecia, hyperpigmentation, lupus-like syndrome
MS: Myalgia, arthralgia, nocturnal muscle cramps

Contraindications: Pregnancy (D), hypersensitivity, lactation
Precautions: Infection, bone marrow depression, hepatic disease

PHARMACOKINETICS
PO: Onset 12-18 hr, duration 36-72 hr, half-life 4-12 hr; excreted in urine, breast milk; crosses placenta

INTERACTIONS
• Agranulocytosis: phenothiazines
Increase: bone marrow depression—radiation, antineoplastic agents
Increase: response to digoxin, warfarin
Decrease: effectiveness—amiodarone, potassium iodide
Drug/Lab Test
Increase: PT, AST, ALT, alk phos

NURSING CONSIDERATIONS
Assess:
• Pulse, B/P, temp
• I&O ratio; check for edema: puffy hands, feet, periorbits; indicate hypothyroidism
• Weight daily; same clothing, scale, time of day
• T_3, T_4, which are increased; serum TSH, which is decreased; free thyroxine index, which is increased if dosage is too low; discontinue drug 3-4 wk before RAIU
⚠ Blood work: CBC for blood dyscrasias: leukopenia, thrombocytopenia, agranulocytosis; if these occur, drug should be discontinued and other treatment initiated; LFTs
• Hypersensitivity: rash, enlarged cervical lymph nodes; drug may have to be discontinued
• Hypoprothrombinemia: bleeding, petechiae, ecchymosis

⚠ Safety alert   *"Tall Man" lettering

- Clinical response: after 3 wk should include increased weight, pulse; decreased T$_4$

⚠ Bone marrow depression: sore throat, fever, fatigue

Administer:
- With meals to decrease GI upset
- At same time each day to maintain drug level
- Lowest dose that relieves symptoms; discontinue before RAIU

Perform/provide:
- Storage in light-resistant container
- Fluids to 3-4 L/day, unless contraindicated

Evaluate:
- Therapeutic response: weight gain, decreased pulse, decreased T$_4$, B/P

Teach patient/family:
- Not to breastfeed
- To take pulse daily
- To report redness, swelling, sore throat, mouth lesions, fever, which indicate blood dyscrasias
- To keep graph of weight, pulse, mood
- To avoid OTC products that contain iodine
- That seafood, other iodine products may be restricted
- Not to discontinue this medication abruptly; thyroid crisis may occur; stress patient response
- That response may take several mo if thyroid is large
- The symptoms and signs of overdose: periorbital edema, cold intolerance, mental depression
- The symptoms of inadequate dose: tachycardia, diarrhea, fever, irritability
- To take medication as prescribed; do not skip or double dose

methocarbamol (℞)

(meth-oh-kar′ba-mole)
Carbacot, methocarbamol, Robaxin
Func. class.: Skeletal muscle relaxant, central acting
Chem. class.: Carbamate derivative

Action: Depresses multisynaptic pathways in the spinal cord, causing skeletal muscle relaxation

Uses: Adjunct for relief of spasm and pain in musculoskeletal conditions

DOSAGE AND ROUTES

MS pain
- *Adult:* **PO** 1.5 g qid × 2-3 days, then 1 g qid; **IM** 500 mg in each gluteal region, may repeat q8h; **IV BOL** 1-3 g/day at max 3 ml/min; **IV INF** 1 g/250 ml D$_5$W or NS, not to exceed 3 g/day
- *Geriatric:* **PO** 500 mg qid, titrate to needed dose

Tetanus management
- *Adult:* **IV Direct** 1-2 g or **IV INF** 1-3 g q6h
- *Child:* **IV** 15 mg/kg q6h prn

Available forms: Tabs 500, 750 mg; inj 100 mg/ml

SIDE EFFECTS

CNS: Dizziness, weakness, drowsiness, headache, tremor, depression, insomnia; **seizures** (IV, IM use)
CV: Postural hypotension, **bradycardia**
EENT: Diplopia, temporary loss of vision, blurred vision, nystagmus
GI: Nausea, vomiting, hiccups, anorexia, metallic taste
GU: Brown, black, green urine
HEMA: Hemolysis, increased hemoglobin (IV only)
INTEG: Rash, pruritus, fever, facial flushing, urticaria, phlebitis
SYST: **Anaphylaxis** (IM, IV)

Contraindications: Hypersensitivity, child <12 yr, intermittent porphyria

M

Precautions: Pregnancy (C), renal/hepatic disease, addictive personalities, myasthenia gravis, epilepsy

PHARMACOKINETICS

IM/IV: Onset rapid
PO: Onset ½ hr, peak 1-2 hr, half-life 1-2 hr
Metabolized in liver, excreted in urine unchanged, crosses placenta

INTERACTIONS

Increase: CNS depression—alcohol, tricyclics, opioids, barbiturates, sedatives, hypnotics
Drug/Herb
Increase: CNS depression—chamomile, hops, kava, skullcap, valerian
Drug/Lab Test
False increase: VMA, urinary 5-HIAA

NURSING CONSIDERATIONS

Assess:
• Blood studies: CBC, WBC, differential; blood dyscrasias may occur
• During and after inj: CNS effects, rash, conjunctivitis, nasal congestion may occur
• Hepatic studies: AST, ALT, alk phos; hepatitis may occur
• ECG in epileptic patients; poor seizure control has occurred
• Allergic reactions: rash, fever, respiratory distress
• Severe weakness, numbness in extremities
• Tolerance: increased need for medication, more frequent requests for medication, increased pain
• CNS depression: dizziness, drowsiness, psychiatric symptoms
Administer:
PO route
• With meals for GI symptoms
IM route
• IM deep in large muscle mass; rotate sites
• Do not give SUBCUT
• Considered incompatible with any drug in sol or syringe

IV route
• IV undiluted over 1 min or more; give 300 mg or less/1 min or longer; may be diluted in 250 ml or less D_5 or isotonic NaCl sol for slow IV infusion
• By slow IV to prevent phlebitis; keep recumbent for 15 min to prevent orthostatic hypotension; check for extravasation
• Considered incompatible with any drug in sol or syringe
Perform/provide:
• Storage in tight container at room temperature
• Assistance with ambulation if dizziness/drowsiness occurs
• Recumbent position during and 10-15 min after IV administration
Evaluate:
• Therapeutic response: decreased pain, spasticity
Teach patient/family:
• Not to discontinue medication quickly; insomnia, nausea, headache, spasticity, tachycardia will occur; drug should be tapered off over 1-2 wk
• That urine may turn green, black, or brown
• Not to take with alcohol, other CNS depressants
• To avoid altering activities while taking this drug
• To avoid hazardous activities if drowsiness, dizziness occurs
• To avoid using OTC medication: cough preparations, antihistamines, unless directed by prescriber
Treatment of overdose: Induce emesis of conscious patient, lavage, dialysis; have epINEPHrine, antihistamines, and corticosteroids available, enhance elimination with osmotic diuresis, IV fluids for hypotension

---

⚠ Safety alert   *"Tall Man" lettering

⚠ High Alert

methotrexate (amethopterin, MTX) (℞)
(meth-oh-trex′ate)
methotrexate, Rheumatrex Dose Pack, Trexall
Func. class.: Antineoplastic-antimetabolite
Chem. class.: Folic acid antagonist

Do not confuse:
methotrexate/metolazone

Action: Inhibits an enzyme that reduces folic acid, which is needed for nucleic acid synthesis in all cells; S phase of cell cycle specific; immunosuppressive

Uses: Acute lymphocytic leukemia, in combination for breast, lung, head, neck carcinoma; lymphosarcoma, gestational choriocarcinoma, hydatidiform mole, psoriasis, rheumatoid arthritis, mycosis fungoides

Unlabeled uses: Used investigationally to produce abortion

DOSAGE AND ROUTES

Acute lymphocytic leukemia
• *Adult and child:* **PO/IM/IV** 3.3 mg/m^2/day × 4-6 wk until remission, then 20-30 mg/m^2 **PO/IM** qwk in 2 divided doses or 2.5 mg/kg **IV** × 2 wk

Choriocarcinoma
• *Adult and child:* **PO/IM** 15-30 mg/m^2 daily × 5 days, then off 1 wk; may repeat

Meningeal leukemia
• *Adult and child:* 12 mg/m^2 **INTRATHECALLY** q2-5d until CSF is normal, then 1 additional dose, max 15 mg

Burkitt's lymphoma (stages I, II, III)
• *Adult:* **PO** 10-25 mg daily × 4-8 days with 7-day rest period

Lymphosarcoma (stage III)
• *Adult:* **PO/IM/IV** 0.625-2.5 mg/kg/day

Osteosarcoma
• *Adult and child:* **IV** 12 g/m^2 given over 4 hr, then leucovorin rescue

Mycosis fungoides
• *Adult:* **PO** 2.5-10 mg/day until cleared (may be many months); **IM** 50 mg qwk or 25 mg 2 ×/wk

Psoriasis
• *Adult:* **PO/IM/IV** 10-25 mg qwk or 2.5 mg **PO** q12h × 3 doses, may increase to 25 mg qwk

Breast cancer
• *Adult:* **IV** 40 mg/m^2 on days 1 and 8 with other antineoplastics

Rheumatoid arthritis
• *Adult:* **PO** 7.5 mg/wk or divided doses of 2.5 mg q12h × 3 given qwk; max 20 mg/wk

Polyarticular-course juvenile RA
• *Child:* **PO** 10 mg/m^2 qwk

Available forms: Tabs 2.5, 5, 7.5, 10, 15 mg; inj 25 mg/ml; powder for inj 20, mg, 1 g

SIDE EFFECTS

CNS: Dizziness, **seizures, leukoencephalopathy,** headache, confusion, hemiparesis, malaise, fatigue, chills, fever; **arachnoiditis** (intrathecal)

GI: Nausea, vomiting, anorexia, diarrhea, ulcerative stomatitis, **hepatotoxicity,** cramps, ulcer, gastritis, **GI hemorrhage,** abdominal pain, hematemesis, **hepatic fibrosis, acute toxicity**

GU: Urinary retention, **renal failure,** menstrual irregularities, defective spermatogenesis, **hematuria, azotemia, uric acid nephropathy**

HEMA: **Leukopenia, thrombocytopenia, myelosuppression, anemia**

INTEG: Rash, alopecia, dry skin, urticaria, photosensitivity, folliculitis, vasculitis, petechiae, ecchymosis, acne, alopecia, **severe fatal skin reaction**

RESP: **Methotrexate-induced lung disease**

SYST: **Sudden death, Pneumocystis jiroveci**

Contraindications: Pregnancy (X), hypersensitivity, leukopenia (<3500/mm^3), thrombocytopenia (<100,000/mm^3), anemia, psoriatic patients with severe renal/hepatic disease, alcoholism, HIV

M

Side effects: *italics* = common; **bold** = life-threatening

Precautions: Renal disease, lactation, children

PHARMACOKINETICS
PO: Readily absorbed
PO/IM/IV: Onset unknown; duration unknown
IT: Onset, peak, duration unknown
Not metabolized; excreted in urine (unchanged); crosses placenta, blood-brain barrier; 50% plasma protein bound

INTERACTIONS
Increase: toxicity—salicylates, sulfa drugs, other antineoplastics, radiation, alcohol, probenecid, NSAIDs, phenylbutazone, theophylline, penicillins
Increase: hypoprothrombinemia—oral anticoagulants
Decrease: effect of oral digoxin, vaccines, phenytoin, fosphenytoin
Decrease: effect of methotrexate—folic acid supplements

NURSING CONSIDERATIONS
Assess:
• Make sure that drug is taken weekly in RA, JRA
⚠ CBC, differential, platelet count weekly; withhold drug if WBC is <3500/mm^3 or platelet count is <100,000/mm^3; notify prescriber; drug should be discontinued; WBC, platelet nadirs occur on day 7
• Renal studies: BUN, serum uric acid, urine CCr, electrolytes before, during therapy
• I&O ratio; report fall in urine output to <30 ml/hr
• Monitor temp q4h; fever may indicate beginning infection; no rectal temps
• Hepatic studies before and during therapy: bilirubin, alk phos, AST, ALT; liver biopsy should be done before start of therapy (psoriasis patients)
• Bleeding time, coagulation time during treatment; bleeding: hematuria, guaiac, bruising or petechiae, mucosa or orifices q8h

• Effects of alopecia on body image; discuss feelings about body changes
⚠ Hepatotoxicity: jaundiced skin and sclera, dark urine, clay-colored stools, pruritus, abdominal pain, fever, diarrhea
• Monitor methotrexate levels, adjust leucovorin dose based on the level
• Buccal cavity q8h for dryness, sores, ulceration, white patches, oral pain, bleeding, dysphagia
⚠ Symptoms indicating severe allergic reaction: rash, urticaria, itching, flushing
Administer:
• Antacid before oral agent; give drug after evening meal before bedtime
• Antiemetic 30-60 min before giving drug
• Allopurinol or sodium bicarbonate to maintain uric acid levels, alkalinization of urine (pH >6.5), adequate fluids
IV route
• After diluting 5 mg/2 ml of sterile H$_2$O for inj; give through Y-tube or 3-way stopcock at 10 mg or less/min
⚠ Leucovorin calcium within 24 hr of this drug to prevent tissue damage; check agency policy, continue until methotrexate level <10^{-8}m
⚠ Give sodium bicarbonate tabs or IV fluids to prevent precipitation of drug at high doses; urine pH should be >7; may need to reduce dosage if BUN 20-30 mg/dl or creatinine is 1.2-2 mg/dl; stop drug if BUN >30 mg/dl or creatinine is >2 mg/dl
Additive compatibilities: Cephalothin, cyclophosphamide, cytarabine, fluorouracil, hydrOXYzine, mercaptopurine, ondansetron, sodium bicarbonate, vinCRIStine
Solution compatibilities: Amino acids, 4.25%/D$_{25}$, D$_5$W, sodium bicarbonate 0.05 mol/L, sodium chloride 0.9%
Syringe compatibilities: Bleomycin, cisplatin, cyclophosphamide, doxapram, DOXOrubicin, fluorouracil, furosemide, heparin, leucovorin, mitomycin, vinBLAStine, vinCRIStine
Y-site compatibilities: Allopurinol, amifostine, amphotericin B cholesteryl, asparaginase, aztreonam, bleomycin,

---

cefepime, ceftriaxone, cimetidine, cisplatin, cyclophosphamide, cytarabine, DAUNOrubicin, dexchlorpheniramine, diphenhydrAMINE, DOXOrubicin, DOXOrubicin liposome, etoposide, famotidine, filgrastim, fludarabine, fluorouracil, furosemide, gallium, ganciclovir, granisetron, heparin, hydromorphone, imipenem/cilastatin, leucovorin, lorazepam, melphalan, mesna, methylPREDNISolone, metoclopramide, mitomycin, morphine, ondansetron, oxacillin, paclitaxel, piperacillin/tazobactam, prochlorperazine, ranitidine, sargramostim, teniposide, thiotepa, vinBLAStine, vinCRIStine, vinorelbine

Perform/provide:

• Strict medical asepsis and protective isolation if WBC levels are low

• Liquid diet: carbonated beverage, Jell-O; dry toast, crackers may be added when patient is not nauseated or vomiting

• Increased fluid intake to 2-3 L/day to prevent urate deposits, calculi formation, unless contraindicated

• Diet low in purines: absence of organ meats (kidney, liver), dried beans, peas to maintain alkaline urine

• Rinsing of mouth tid-qid with water, club soda; brushing of teeth bid-tid with soft brush or cotton-tipped applicators for stomatitis; use unwaxed dental floss

• Nutritious diet with iron, vitamin supplements

• Storage in tightly closed container in cool environment; store injection, powder for inj in dark, dry area

Evaluate:

• Therapeutic response: decreased tumor size, spread of malignancy

Teach patient/family:

• To report any complaints, side effects to nurse or prescriber: black tarry stools, chills, fever, sore throat, bleeding, bruising, cough, shortness of breath, dark or bloody urine

• That hair may be lost during treatment; wig or hairpiece may make patient feel better; tell patient that new hair may be different in color, texture (alopecia is rare)

• To avoid foods with citric acid, hot or rough texture if stomatitis is present

• To report stomatitis: any bleeding, white spots, ulcerations in mouth to prescriber; tell patient to examine mouth daily, report symptoms to nurse, use good oral hygiene

• That contraceptive measures are recommended during therapy and for at least 8 wk following cessation of therapy, to discontinue breastfeeding; toxicity to infant may occur

• To drink 10-12 glasses of fluid/day

• To avoid alcohol, salicylates, live vaccines

• To avoid use of razors, commercial mouthwash

• To use sunblock to prevent burns

---

methylcellulose (OTC)

(meth-ill-sell′yoo-lose)
Citrucel
Func. class.: Laxative, bulk forming
Chem. class.: Hydrophilic semisynthetic cellulose derivative

Do not confuse:

Citrucel/Citracal

Action: Attracts water, expands in intestine to increase peristalsis; also absorbs excess water in stool; decreases diarrhea

Uses: Chronic constipation

DOSAGE AND ROUTES

• *Adult:* **PO** up to 6 g daily in divided doses

• *Child 6-12 yr:* **PO** 3 g daily in divided doses

Available forms: Powder 105 mg/g, 196 mg/g

SIDE EFFECTS

GI: **Obstruction,** abdominal distention

Contraindications: Hypersensitivity, GI obstruction, hepatitis

PHARMACOKINETICS

PO: Onset 12-24 hr, peak 1-3 days

---

666   methyldopa/methyldopate

INTERACTIONS

Decrease: absorption—antibiotics, digoxin, nitrofurantoin, salicylates, tetracyclines, oral anticoagulants

Drug/Herb
Increase: laxative action—flax senna

NURSING CONSIDERATIONS

Assess:
• Blood, urine electrolytes if used often
• I&O ratio to identify fluid loss
• Cause of constipation; lack of fluids, bulk, exercise, constipating drugs
• Cramping, rectal bleeding, nausea, vomiting; drug should be discontinued

Administer:
PO route
• Alone for better absorption; do not take within 1 hr of other drugs
• In morning or evening (oral dose)

Evaluate:
• Therapeutic response: decrease in constipation

Teach patient/family:
• To mix powder in water
• To increase fluid intake
• That normal bowel movements do not always occur daily
• Not to use in presence of abdominal pain, nausea, vomiting
• To notify prescriber if constipation unrelieved or if symptoms of electrolyte imbalance occur: muscle cramps, pain, weakness, dizziness, excessive thirst

---

methyldopa/methyl-dopate (℞)

(meth-ill-doe′pa)
Aldomet, Apo-Methyldopa ✦, Dopamet ✦, methyldopa/methyldopate, Novomedopa ✦, Nu-Medopa ✦
Func. class.: Antihypertensive
Chem. class.: Centrally acting α-adrenergic inhibitor

Do not confuse:
methyldopa/L-dopa/levodopa
Action: Stimulates central inhibitory α-adrenergic receptors or acts as false transmitter, resulting in reduction of arterial pressure

Uses: Hypertension, hypertensive crisis

DOSAGE AND ROUTES

• **Adult:** PO 250-500 mg bid or tid, then adjusted q2d as needed, 0.5-2 g daily in 2-4 divided doses (maintenance), not to exceed 3 g/day; **IV** 250-500 mg in 100 ml D_5W q6h, run over 30-60 min, not to exceed 1 g q6h, switch to oral as soon as possible
• **Geriatric:** PO 125 mg bid-tid, increase q2d as needed, max 3 g/day
• **Child:** PO 10 mg/kg/day in 2-4 divided doses, not to exceed 65 mg/kg or 3 g/day, whichever is less; **IV** 20-40 mg/kg/day in 4 divided doses, not to exceed 65 mg/kg or 3 g, whichever is less

Available forms: *Methyldopa:* tabs 125, 250, 500 mg; oral susp 50 mg/ml; *methyldopate:* inj 50 mg/ml

SIDE EFFECTS

CNS: Drowsiness, weakness, dizziness, sedation, headache, depression, psychosis paresthesias, parkinsonism, Bell's palsy, nightmares
CV: Bradycardia, **myocarditis,** orthostatic hypotension, angina, edema, weight gain, **CHF,** paradoxical pressor response (IV use)
EENT: Nasal congestion
ENDO: Breast enlargement, gynecomastia, lactation, amenorrhea
GI: Nausea, vomiting, diarrhea, constipation, **hepatic dysfunction,** sore or "black" tongue, **pancreatitis,** colitis, flatulence
GU: Impotence, failure to ejaculate
HEMA: **Leukopenia, thrombocytopenia, hemolytic anemia, granulocytopenia,** positive Coombs' test
INTEG: Rash, **toxic epidermal necrolysis,** lupuslike syndrome

Contraindications: Active hepatic disease, hypersensitivity

Precautions: Pregnancy (B) (PO); (C) (IV), eclampsia, severe cardiac disease, renal/hepatic disease, CHF, edema

---

⚠ Safety alert   *"Tall Man" lettering

PHARMACOKINETICS

PO: Peak 2-4 hr, duration 12-24 hr
IV: Peak 2 hr, duration 10-16 hr
Metabolized by liver, excreted in urine, half-life 2 hr

INTERACTIONS

• Lithium toxicity: lithium
Increase: pressor effect—sympathomimetic amines, MAOIs
Increase: hypotension, CNS toxicity—levodopa
Increase: hypotension—diuretics, other antihypertensives
Increase: psychosis—haloperidol
Increase: CNS depression—alcohol, antihistamines, antidepressants, analgesics, sedative/hypnotics
Increase: B/P—phenothiazines, β-blockers, amphetamines, NSAIDs, tricyclics, barbiturates
Increase: hypoglycemia—TOLBUTamide
Decrease: methyldopa absorption—iron
Drug/Herb
Increase: toxicity, death—aconite
Increase: antihypertensive effect—barberry, betony, black catechu, black cohosh, bloodroot, broom, burdock, cat's claw, dandelion, goldenseal, hawthorn, Irish moss, Jamaican dogwood, kelp, khella, mistletoe, parsley
Increase or decrease: antihypertensive effect—astragalus, cola tree
Decrease: effect—capsicum, Indian snakeroot
Decrease: antihypertensive effect—coltsfoot, guarana, khat, licorice, yohimbine
Drug/Lab Test
Interference: Urinary uric acid, serum creatinine, AST
False increase: Urinary catecholamines

NURSING CONSIDERATIONS

Assess:
• Blood studies: neutrophils, decreased platelets
• Direct Coombs' test before/after 6, 12 mo of therapy
• Baselines in renal, hepatic studies, before therapy begins
• B/P when beginning treatment, periodically thereafter, report significant changes
• Allergic reaction: rash, fever, pruritus, urticaria; drug should be discontinued if antihistamines fail to help
• CNS symptoms, especially in the geriatric, depression, change in mental status
• Symptoms of CHF: edema, dyspnea, wet crackles, B/P
• Renal symptoms: polyuria, oliguria, urinary frequency; I&O ratio, weight, report weight gain >5 lb
Administer:
PO route
• Shake susp before use
IV route
• After diluting with 100 ml D_5W; run over ½-1 hr
Additive compatibilities: Aminophylline, ascorbic acid, chloramphenicol, diphenhydrAMINE, heparin, magnesium sulfate, multivitamins, netilmicin, potassium chloride, promazine, sodium bicarbonate, succinylcholine, verapamil, vit B/C
Solution compatibilities: D_5W, D_5/0.9% NaCl, Ringer's, sodium bicarbonate 5%, 0.9% NaCl, amino acids 4.25%/D_{25}, Dextran$_6$/0.9% NaCl, Normosol R, Normosol M/D_5W
Y-site compatibilities: Esmolol, heparin, meperidine, morphine, theophylline
Perform/provide:
• Storage of tabs in tight container
Evaluate:
• Therapeutic response: decrease in B/P in hypertension
Teach patient/family:
• To avoid hazardous activities
• Not to discontinue drug abruptly, or withdrawal symptoms may occur: anxiety, increased B/P, headache, insomnia, increased pulse, tremors, nausea, sweating
• Not to use OTC (cough, cold, allergy) products unless directed by prescriber
• To comply with dosage schedule even if feeling better

M

- To rise slowly to sitting or standing position to minimize orthostatic hypotension
- To notify prescriber of mouth sores, sore throat, fever, swelling of hands or feet, irregular heartbeat, chest pain, signs of angioedema
- That excessive perspiration, dehydration, vomiting, diarrhea may lead to fall in blood pressure; consult prescriber
- That dizziness, fainting, light-headedness may occur during first few days of therapy
- That compliance is necessary; not to skip or stop drug unless directed by prescriber
- That drug may cause skin rash or impaired perspiration

Treatment of overdose: Gastric evacuation, sympathomimetics may be indicated; if severe, hemodialysis

---

methylergonovine (℞)
(meth-ill-er-goe-noe′veen)
Methergine,
methylergonovine
Func. class.: Oxytocic
Chem. class.: Ergot alkaloid

Action: Stimulates uterine, vascular, smooth muscle, causing contractions; decreases bleeding; arterial vasoconstriction

Uses: Treatment of hemorrhage postpartum or postabortion, uterine contractions

DOSAGE AND ROUTES

- *Adult:* **PO** 200-400 mcg q6-12h × 2-7 days **IM/IV** 200 mcg q2-4h for 1-5 doses
Available forms: Inj 200 mcg/ml; tabs 200 mcg

SIDE EFFECTS

CNS: Headache, dizziness, **seizures**
CV: **Hypotension,** chest pain, palpitation, **hypertension, dysrhythmias, CVA (IV)**
EENT: Tinnitus
GI: Nausea, vomiting
GU: Cramping

INTEG: Sweating, rash, allergic reactions
RESP: Dyspnea

Contraindications: Pregnancy (4th stage of labor), hypersensitivity to ergot preparations, indication of labor, before delivery of placenta, hypertension, pelvic inflammatory disease, respiratory disease, cardiac disease, peripheral vascular disease

Precautions: Pregnancy (C), severe renal/hepatic disease, jaundice, diabetes mellitus, seizure disorders, sepsis, CAD

PHARMACOKINETICS

PO: Onset 5-25 min, duration 3 hr
IM: Onset 2-5 min, duration 3 hr
IV: Onset immediate, duration 45 min
Metabolized in liver, excreted in urine

INTERACTIONS

Increase: vasoconstriction—vasopressors, nicotine

NURSING CONSIDERATIONS

Assess:
- B/P, pulse, character and amount of vaginal bleeding; watch for indications of hemorrhage
- Respiratory rate, rhythm, depth; notify prescriber of abnormalities
- For uterine relaxation; observe for severe cramping
- ⚠ Ergot toxicity: tinnitus, hypertension, palpitations, chest pain, nausea, vomiting, weakness; cold, numb extremities

Administer:
- Only during fourth stage of labor; not to be used to augment labor
- IM in deep muscle mass; rotate inj sites of additional doses

IV route
- Undiluted through Y-tube or 3-way stopcock; give 0.2 mg or less/min or diluted in 5 ml 0.9% NaCl given through Y-site
- With crash cart available on unit; IV route used only in emergencies

Y-site compatibilities: Heparin, hydrocortisone sodium succinate, potassium chloride, vit B/C

⚠ Safety alert   *"Tall Man" lettering

Evaluate:
• Therapeutic response: absence of hemorrhage

Teach patient/family:
• To report increased blood loss, severe abdominal cramps, fever or foul-smelling lochia
• To avoid smoking
• Not to breastfeed while taking this drug

---

methylphenidate (℞)
(meth-ill-fen'i-date)
Concerta, Daytrana,
Metadate CD, Methylin,
Methylin ER, Methidate,
PMS-Methylphenidate ✤
Riphenidate ✤, Ritalin, Ritalin
LA, Ritalin SR
Func. class.: Cerebral stimulant
Chem. class.: Piperidine derivative

Controlled Substance Schedule II
Do not confuse:
methylphenidate/methadone

Action: Increases release of norepinephrine, dopamine in cerebral cortex to reticular activating system; exact action not known

Uses: Attention deficit disorder (ADD), attention deficit hyperactivity disorder (ADHD); narcolepsy (except Concerta, Metadate CD, Ritalin LA)

Unlabeled uses: Depression in the geriatric, cancer, post-stroke patients, HIV, brain injury, improvement in pain control, sedation in patients receiving opiates

DOSAGE AND ROUTES

Attention deficit hyperactivity disorder
• *Child >6 yr:* **PO** (immediate release tabs, chew tabs, oral sol) 5 mg before breakfast and lunch, increasing by 5-10 mg/wk, not to exceed 60 mg/day; **EXT REL** 20 mg daily-tid

Attention deficit hyperactivity disorder, conversion from PO to transdermal
• *Child 6-12 yr:* Week 1, 12.5 cm^2 (10 mg); week 2, 18.75 cm^2 (15 mg); week 3, 25 cm^2 (20 mg); week 4, 37.5 cm^2 (30 mg)

Narcolepsy
• *Adult:* **PO** 10 mg bid-tid, 30-45 min before meals, may increase up to 40-60 mg/day

Depression (geriatric)
• *Geriatric:* **PO** 2.5 mg q$_{AM}$, increase q3d by 2.5 mg to desired dose, max 20 mg/day

Available forms: Tabs 5, 10, 20 mg; ext rel tabs 10, 20, mg; ext rel tabs (Concerta) 18, 27, 36, 54 mg; ext rel caps 10, 20, 30, 40 mg; oral sol 5 mg, 10 mg/ml; chew tabs (Methylin) 2.5, 5, 10 mg; transdermal patch 12.5 cm^2 (10 mg), 18.75 cm^2 (15 mg), 25 cm^2 (20 mg), 37.5 cm^2 (30 mg)

SIDE EFFECTS

CNS: Hyperactivity, insomnia, restlessness, talkativeness, dizziness, drowsiness, toxic psychosis, headache, akathisia, dyskinesia, masking or worsening of Gilles de la Tourette's syndrome, **seizures**

CV: Palpitations, tachycardia, B/P changes, angina, **dysrhythmias**

ENDO: Growth retardation

GI: Nausea, anorexia, dry mouth, weight loss, abdominal pain

HEMA: **Leukopenia, anemia, thrombocytopenic purpura**

INTEG: **Exfoliative dermatitis,** urticaria, rash, erythema multiforme

MISC: Fever, arthralgia, scalp hair loss

Contraindications: Hypersensitivity, anxiety, history of Gilles de la Tourette's syndrome; children <6 yr, glaucoma, anorexia nervosa, tartrazine dye hypersensitivity

Precautions: Pregnancy (C), hypertension, depression, seizures, lactation, drug abuse

M

Side effects: *italics* = common; **bold** = life-threatening

PHARMACOKINETICS

PO: Onset ½-1 hr, duration 4-6 hr, metabolized by liver, excreted by kidneys

INTERACTIONS

• Hypertensive crisis: MAOIs or within 14 days of MAOIs, vasopressors
Increase: effects of tricyclics, SSRIs, anticonvulsants
Decrease: effect of guanethidine
Drug/Herb
• Synergistic effect: melatonin
Increase: CNS stimulation—cola nut, guarana, horsetail, yerba maté, yohimbe
Drug/Food
Increase: stimulation—caffeine

NURSING CONSIDERATIONS
Assess:
• VS, B/P; may reverse antihypertensives; check patients with cardiac disease more often for increased B/P
• CBC, urinalysis, in diabetes: blood glucose, urine glucose; insulin changes may have to be made, since eating will decrease
• Height, growth rate q3mo in children; growth rate may be decreased
• Mental status: mood, sensorium, affect, stimulation, insomnia, aggressiveness
⚠ Withdrawal symptoms: headache, nausea, vomiting, muscle pain, weakness
• Appetite, sleep, speech patterns
• For attention span, decreased hyperactivity in ADHD persons
Administer:
• Do not crush or chew ext rel medication; caps may be opened and beads sprinkled over spoonful of applesauce
• Gum, hard candy, frequent sips of water for dry mouth
• Chew tab with adequate water to prevent choking; contains phenylalanine
Transdermal route
• Place on clean, dry area of the hip; avoid waist; removal is 9 hr after application; fold after removal and flush down toilet

Evaluate:
• Therapeutic response: decreased hyperactivity (ADHD) or ability to stay awake (narcolepsy)
Teach patient/family:
• To decrease caffeine consumption (coffee, tea, cola, chocolate); may increase irritability, stimulation; not to use guarana, yerba maté, cola nut
• To avoid OTC preparations unless approved by prescriber
• To taper off drug over several weeks, or depression, increased sleeping, lethargy will occur
• To avoid driving, hazardous activities if dizziness, blurred vision occur
• To avoid alcohol ingestion
• To avoid hazardous activities until stabilized on medication
• To get needed rest; patients will feel more tired at end of day
• That shell of Concerta tab may appear in stools
• To take regular tab at least 6 hr prior to sleep; 10 hr for ext rel
• That for transdermal patch, once tray is opened, use within 2 mo; do not store patches without protective patch
Treatment of overdose: Administer fluids; hemodialysis or peritoneal dialysis; antihypertensive for increased B/P; administer short-acting barbiturate before lavage

*methylPRED-NISolone (R)

(meth-il-pred-niss'oh-lone)
A-Methapred, depMedalone, Depoject, Depo-Medrol, Depopred, Depo-Predate, Medrol, Duralone, Medralone, Rep-Pred, Solu-Medrol
Func. class.: Corticosteroid, synthetic
Chem. class.: Glucocorticoid, immediate acting

Do not confuse:
methylPREDNISolone/predniSONE/medroxyPROGESTERone/methylTESTOSTERone

Action: Decreases inflammation by suppression of migration of polymorphonuclear leukocytes, fibroblasts; reversal of increased capillary permeability and lysosomal stabilization

Uses: Severe inflammation, shock, adrenal insufficiency, collagen disorders, management of acute spinal cord injury, multiple sclerosis

DOSAGE AND ROUTES

Adrenal insufficiency/inflammation
• *Adult:* **PO** 2-60 mg in 4 divided doses; **IM** 10-80 mg (acetate); **IM/IV** 10-250 mg (succinate); intraarticular 4-30 mg (acetate); **RECT** 40 mg 3-7 × wk for ≥2 wk
• *Child:* **IV** 117 mcg-1.66 mg/kg in 3-4 divided doses (succinate); **RECT** 0.5-1 mg/kg (15-30 mg/m^2) daily or every other day × 1 wk or more
Shock
• *Adult:* **IV** 100-250 mg q2-6h or 30 mg/kg, then q4-6h prn, for 2-3 days (succinate)
Multiple sclerosis
• *Adult:* **PO** 160 mg/day × 1 wk, then 64 mg every other day × 30 days
Available forms: Tabs 2, 4, 6, 8, 16, 24, 32 mg; inj 20, 40, 80 mg/ml acetate; inj 40, 125, 500, 1000, 2000 mg/vial succinate; susp for inj 20, 40, 80 mg/ml; dose pack 4 mg tabs; enema 40 mg

SIDE EFFECTS

CNS: Depression, flushing, sweating, headache, mood changes
CV: Hypertension, **circulatory collapse, thrombophlebitis, embolism,** tachycardia
EENT: Fungal infections, increased intraocular pressure, blurred vision, cataracts
GI: Diarrhea, nausea, abdominal distention, **GI hemorrhage,** increased appetite, pancreatitis
HEMA: **Thrombocytopenia**
INTEG: Acne, poor wound healing, ecchymosis, petechiae
MS: Fractures, osteoporosis, weakness
Contraindications: Psychosis, hypersensitivity, idiopathic thrombocytopenia, acute glomerulonephritis, amebiasis, fungal infections, nonasthmatic bronchial disease, child <2 yr, AIDS, TB
Precautions: Pregnancy (C), lactation, diabetes mellitus, glaucoma, osteoporosis, seizure disorders, ulcerative colitis, CHF, myasthenia gravis, renal disease, esophagitis, peptic ulcer

PHARMACOKINETICS

Well absorbed PO, IM
PO: Peak 1-2 hr, duration 1½ days
IM: Peak 4-8 days, duration 1-4 wk
Intraarticular: Peak 1 wk
Half-life >3½ hr (plasma), 18-36 hr (tissue); crosses placenta, enters breast milk in small amounts; metabolized in liver, excreted by kidneys (unchanged)

INTERACTIONS

Increase: side effects—amphotericin B, diuretics
Increase: methylPREDNISolone action—oral contraceptives
Decrease: methylPREDNISolone action—rifampin, phenytoin, theophylline

M

Decrease: effects of antidiabetics, vaccines, somatrem

Drug/Herb

Increase: hypokalemia—aloe, buckthorn, cascara sagrada, Chinese rhubarb, senna

Increase: corticosteroid effect—aloe, licorice, perilla

Drug/Food

• Do not use with grapefruit juice; level of methylPREDNISolone will be increased

Drug/Lab Test

Increase: Cholesterol, sodium, blood glucose, uric acid, calcium, urine glucose

Decrease: Ca, K, T_4, T_3, thyroid ^{131}I uptake test, urine 17-OHCS, 17-KS

False negative: Skin allergy tests

NURSING CONSIDERATIONS

Assess:

• Potassium depletion: parethesias, fatigue, nausea, vomiting, depression, polyuria, dysrhythmias, weakness

• Edema, hypertension, cardiac symptoms

• Mental status: affect, mood, behavioral changes, aggression

• Potassium, blood glucose, urine glucose while on long-term therapy; hypokalemia and hyperglycemia

• Joint mobility, pain, edema if given intraarticularly

• B/P q4h, pulse; notify prescriber of chest pain, crackles

• I&O ratio; be alert for decreasing urinary output, increasing edema; weight daily; notify prescriber of weekly gain >5 lb

• Adrenal insufficiency: weight loss, nausea, vomiting, confusion, anxiety, hypotension, weakness

• Plasma cortisol levels during long-term therapy (normal level: 138-635 nmol/L SI units when drawn at 8 AM)

• Growth in children on long-term treatment

Administer:

• Titrated dose; use lowest effective dose

• IM inj deep in large muscle mass; rotate sites; avoid deltoid; use 21G needle; after shaking suspension (parenteral)

• In one dose in AM to prevent adrenal suppression; avoid SUBCUT administration; may damage tissue

• With food or milk to decrease GI symptoms (PO)

⚠ Do not give Solu-Medrol intrathecally

IV route

• After diluting with diluent provided; agitate slowly; give 500 mg or less/1 min or longer; may be given as IV infusion in its own diluent over 10-20 min

Additive compatibilities: Chloramphenicol, cimetidine, clindamycin, DOPamine, granisetron, heparin, norepinephrine, penicillin G potassium, ranitidine, theophylline, verapamil

Syringe compatibilities: Granisetron, metoclopramide

Y-site compatibilities: Acyclovir, amifostine, amphotericin B cholesteryl, amrinone, aztreonam, cefepime, cisplatin, cladribine, cyclophosphamide, cytarabine, DOPamine, DOXOrubicin, enalaprilat, famotidine, fludarabine, granisetron, heparin, melphalan, meperidine, methotrexate, metronidazole, midazolam, morphine, piperacillin/tazobactam, remifentanil, sodium bicarbonate, tacrolimus, teniposide, theophylline, thiotepa

Perform/provide:

• Assistance with ambulation in patient with bone tissue disease to prevent fractures

Evaluate:

• Therapeutic response: ease of respirations, decreased inflammation; decreased symptoms of adrenal insufficiency

• Infection: increased temp, WBC, even after withdrawal of medication; drug masks infection

Teach patient/family:

• To increase intake of potassium, calcium, protein

• To carry emergency ID (steroid user)

- To notify prescriber if therapeutic response decreases; dosage adjustment may be needed
- Not to discontinue abruptly, or adrenal crisis can result
- To avoid OTC products: salicylates, alcohol in cough products, cold preparations unless directed by prescriber; to avoid vaccinations, since immunosuppression occurs
- About cushingoid symptoms
- To recognize the symptoms of adrenal insufficiency: nausea, anorexia, fatigue, dizziness, dyspnea, weakness, joint pain

metipranolol ophthalmic
See Appendix C

metoclopramide (℞)
(met-oh-kloe-pra′mide)
Apo-Metoclop ✦, Emex ✦, Maxeran ✦, metoclopramide, Octamide, Reglan, Sensamide IV
Func. class.: Cholinergic, antiemetic
Chem. class.: Central dopamine receptor antagonist

Do not confuse:
metoclopramide/metolazone
Reglan/Megace/Renagel

Action: Enhances response to acetylcholine of tissue in upper GI tract, which causes contraction of gastric muscle; relaxes pyloric, duodenal segments; increases peristalsis without stimulating secretions, blocks dopamine in chemoreceptor trigger zone of CNS

Uses: Prevention of nausea, vomiting induced by chemotherapy, radiation, delayed gastric emptying, gastroesophageal reflux

Unlabeled uses: Hiccups, migraines, lactation induction, lung cancer

DOSAGE AND ROUTES
Renal dose
- *Adult:* CCr <40 ml/min 50% of dose

Nausea/vomiting
- *Adult:* IV 1-2 mg/kg 30 min before administration of chemotherapy, then q2h × 2 doses, then q3h × 3 doses
- *Child:* IV 0.1-0.2 mg/kg/dose

Facilitate small bowel intubation, in radiologic exams
- *Adult and child >14 yr:* IV 10 mg over 1-2 min
- *Child <6 yr:* IV 0.1 mg/kg
- *Child 6-14 yr:* IV 2.5-5 mg

Diabetic gastroparesis
- *Adult:* PO 10 mg 30 min before meals, at bedtime × 2-8 wk
- *Geriatric:* PO 5 mg ½ hr before meals, at bedtime, increase to 10 mg if needed

Hiccups (unlabeled)
- *Adult:* PO/IM/IV 10 mg q6h

Gastroesophageal reflux
- *Adult:* PO 10-15 mg qid 30 min before meals
- *Child:* PO 0.4-0.8 mg/kg/day in 4 divided doses

Lactation induction (unlabeled)
- *Adult:* PO 10 mg bid-tid, may increase to 20-45 mg/day in divided doses

Non–small cell lung cancer (NSCLC) radiation sensitizer (unlabeled) (Sensamide IV)
- *Adult:* IV 2 mg/kg given 1 hr prior to radiation therapy 3 ×/wk

Available forms: Tabs 5, 10 mg; syr 5 mg/5 ml; inj 5 mg/ml; conc sol 10 mg/ml

SIDE EFFECTS
CNS: Sedation, fatigue, restlessness, headache, sleeplessness, dystonia, dizziness, drowsiness, **suicide ideation, seizures,** EPS
CV: Hypotension, supraventricular tachycardia
GI: Dry mouth, constipation, nausea, anorexia, vomiting, diarrhea

GU: Decreased libido, prolactin secretion, amenorrhea, galactorrhea

HEMA: **Neutropenia, leukopenia, agranulocytosis**

INTEG: Urticaria, rash

Contraindications: Hypersensitivity to this drug or procaine or procainamide, seizure disorder, pheochromocytoma, breast cancer (prolactin dependent), GI obstruction

Precautions: Pregnancy (B), lactation, GI hemorrhage, CHF, Parkinson's disease, tardive dyskinesia

PHARMACOKINETICS

IV: Onset 1-3 min, duration 1-2 hr
PO: Onset ½-1 hr, duration 1-2 hr
IM: Onset 10-15 min, duration 1-2 hr
Metabolized by liver, excreted in urine, half-life 4 hr

INTERACTIONS

• Avoid use with MAOIs
Increase: sedation—alcohol, other CNS depressants
Increase: risk of EPS—haloperidol, phenothiazines
Decrease: action of metoclopramide—anticholinergics, opiates
Drug/Lab Test
Increase: Prolactin, aldosterone, thyrotropin

NURSING CONSIDERATIONS

Assess:
• For EPS and tardive dyskinesia, more likely to occur in geriatric patient
• Mental status: depression, anxiety, irritability
• GI complaints: nausea, vomiting, anorexia, constipation
Administer:
PO route
• ½-1 hr before meals for better absorption
• Gum, hard candy, frequent rinsing of mouth for dry oral cavity

IV route
• DiphenhydrAMINE IV for EPS
• Undiluted if dose is ≤10 mg; give over 2 min; more than 10 mg may be diluted in 50 ml or more D$_5$W, NaCl, Ringer's, LR and given over 15 min or more
Syringe compatibilities: Aminophylline, ascorbic acid, atropine, benztropine, bleomycin, butorphanol, chlorproMAZINE, cisplatin, cyclophosphamide, cytarabine, dexamethasone, dimenhyDRINATE, diphenhydrAMINE, DOXOrubicin, droperidol, fentanyl, fluorouracil, heparin, hydrocortisone, hydrOXYzine, insulin (regular), leucovorin, lidocaine, magnesium sulfate, meperidine, methotrimeprazine, methylPREDNISolone, midazolam, mitomycin, morphine, pentazocine, perphenazine, prochlorperazine, promazine, promethazine, ranitidine, scopolamine, sufentanil, vinBLAStine, vinCRIStine, vit B/C
Y-site compatibilities: Acyclovir, aldesleukin, amifostine, aztreonam, bleomycin, ciprofloxacin, cisatracurium, cisplatin, cladribine, cyclophosphamide, cytarabine, diltiazem, DOXOrubicin, droperidol, famotidine, filgrastim, fluconazole, fludarabine, fluorouracil, foscarnet, gallium, granisetron, heparin, idarubicin, leucovorin, melphalan, meperidine, meropenem, methotrexate, mitomycin, morphine, ondansetron, paclitaxel, piperacillin/tazobactam, propofol, remifentanil, sargramostim, sufentanil, tacrolimus, teniposide, thiotepa, vinBLAStine, vinCRIStine, vinorelbine, zidovudine
Perform/provide:
• Protect from light with aluminum foil during infusion
• Discard open ampules
Evaluate:
• Therapeutic response: absence of nausea, vomiting, anorexia, fullness
Teach patient/family:
• To avoid driving, other hazardous activities until patient is stabilized on this medication
• To avoid alcohol, other CNS depressants that will enhance sedating properties of this drug

---

⚠ Safety alert   *"Tall Man" lettering

metolazone (℞)

(me-tole′a-zone)
Zaroxolyn
Func. class.: Diuretic, antihypertensive
Chem. class.: Thiazide-like quinazoline derivative

Do not confuse:
metolazone/methotrexate/
metoclopramide
methimazole/metoprolol/minoxidil
Action: Acts on distal tubule by increasing excretion of water, sodium, chloride, potassium, magnesium, bicarbonate
Uses: Edema, hypertension, CHF, nephrotic syndrome

DOSAGE AND ROUTES

Edema
• *Adult:* **PO** 2.5-20 mg/day
Hypertension
• *Adult:* **PO** 2.5-5 mg/day (Zaroxolyn)
Available forms: Tabs 2.5, 5, 10 mg

SIDE EFFECTS

CNS: Anxiety, depression, headache, *dizziness, fatigue, weakness*
CV: Orthostatic hypotension, palpitations, volume depletion, hypotension, chest pain
EENT: Blurred vision
ELECT: Hypokalemia, hypercalcemia, hyponatremia
GI: Nausea, vomiting, anorexia, constipation, diarrhea, cramps, pancreatitis, GI irritation, dry mouth, jaundice
GU: Urinary frequency, polyuria, **uremia, glucosuria,** nocturia, impotence
HEMA: **Aplastic anemia, hemolytic anemia, leukopenia, agranulocytosis, neutropenia**
INTEG: Rash, urticaria, purpura, photosensitivity, fever, dry skin
META: Hyperglycemia, increased creatinine, BUN
Contraindications: Hypersensitivity to thiazides or sulfonamides, anuria, hepatic coma

Precautions: Pregnancy (B), hypokalemia, renal/hepatic disease, gout, COPD, lupus erythematosus, diabetes mellitus, geriatric, lactation, hypotension

PHARMACOKINETICS

PO: Onset 1 hr, peak 2 hr, duration 12-24 hr; excreted unchanged by kidneys; crosses placenta; enters breast milk; half-life 8-14 hr

INTERACTIONS

Increase: hypokalemia—mezlocillin, piperacillin, amphotericin B, glucocorticoids, digoxin, stimulant laxatives
Increase: hypotension—alcohol (large amounts), nitrates, antihypertensives, barbiturates, opioids
Increase: toxicity—lithium
Increase: metolazone effects—loop diuretics
Decrease: action of metolazone—NSAIDs, salicylates
Drug/Herb
Increase: hypokalemia—aloe, buckthorn, cascara sagrada, rhubarb, senna
Increase: toxicity, death—aconite
Increase: antihypertensive effect—barberry, betony, black catechu, black cohosh, bloodroot, broom, burdock, cat's claw, dandelion, goldenseal, Irish moss, Jamaican dogwood, kelp, khella, mistletoe, parsley
Increase or decrease: antihypertensive effect—astragalus, cola tree
Decrease: antihypertensive effect—coltsfoot, guarana, khat, licorice

NURSING CONSIDERATIONS
Assess:
• Weight, I&O daily to determine fluid loss; effect of drug may be decreased if used daily
• Rate, depth, rhythm of respiration, effect of exertion
• B/P lying, standing; postural hypotension may occur
• Electrolytes: K, Mg, Na, Cl; include BUN, blood glucose, CBC, serum creatinine, blood pH, ABGs, uric acid, calcium

M

- Improvement in edema of feet, legs, sacral area daily if medication is being used in CHF
- Improvement in CVP q8h
- Signs of metabolic alkalosis: drowsiness, restlessness
- Signs of hypokalemia: postural hypotension, malaise, fatigue, tachycardia, leg cramps, weakness
- Rashes, fever daily
- Confusion, especially in geriatric; take safety precautions if needed

Administer:

- In AM to avoid interference with sleep if using drug as a diuretic
- Potassium replacement if potassium <3 mg/dl
- With food, if nausea occurs; absorption may be decreased slightly
- Extended product is Zaroxolyn, prompt product is Mykrox; they are not interchangeable

Evaluate:

- Therapeutic response: decreased edema, B/P

Teach patient/family:

- To increase fluid intake to 2-3 L/day unless contraindicated, to rise slowly from lying or sitting position
- To notify prescriber of muscle weakness, cramps, nausea, dizziness
- That drug may be taken with food or milk
- To use sunscreen for photosensitivity
- That blood glucose may be increased in diabetics
- To take early in day to avoid nocturia
- To avoid alcohol
- To avoid sodium food, increase potassium foods in diet

Treatment of overdose: Lavage if taken orally; monitor electrolytes; administer dextrose in saline; monitor hydration, CV, renal status

metoprolol (R̶)
(meh-toe′proe-lole)
Betaloc ✦, Betaloc Durules ✦,
Lopresor ✦, Lopressor,
Lopressor SR ✦, Nu-Metop ✦,
Novometoprol ✦, Toprol-XL
Func. class.: Antihypertensive, antianginal
Chem. class.: β_1-Blocker

Do not confuse:
metoprolol/misoprostol

Action: Lowers B/P by β-blocking effects; reduces elevated renin plasma levels; blocks β_2-adrenergic receptors in bronchial, vascular smooth muscle only at high doses

Uses: Mild to moderate hypertension, acute MI to reduce cardiovascular mortality, angina pectoris, NYHA class II, III heart failure

Unlabeled uses: Atrial ectopy, antipsychotic-induced akathisia, rapid heart rate control, unstable angina, variceal bleeding in portal hypotension, migraine prevention

DOSAGE AND ROUTES

Hypertension

- *Adult:* PO 50 mg bid, or 100 mg daily; may give up to 200-450 mg in divided doses; EXT REL give daily
- *Geriatric:* PO 25 mg/day initially, increase weekly as needed

Myocardial infarction

- *Adult:* (early treatment) IV BOL 5 mg q2min × 3, then 50 mg PO 15 min after last dose and q6h × 48 hr; (late treatment) PO maintenance 100 mg bid for 3 mo

Angina

- *Adult:* PO 100 mg daily as a single dose or in two divided doses, increase qwk prn or 100 mg EXT REL daily

Migraine prevention (unlabeled)

- *Adult:* PO 50-100 mg bid-qid

Available forms: Tabs 50, 100 mg; inj 1 mg/ml; ext rel tab (succinate) (XL) 25,

50, 100, 200 mg; ext rel tabs, tartrate: 100 mg

SIDE EFFECTS

CNS: Insomnia, dizziness, mental changes, hallucinations, **depression,** anxiety, headaches, nightmares, confusion, fatigue

CV: Hypotension, **bradycardia, CHF,** *palpitations,* dysrhythmias, **cardiac arrest, AV block, pulmonary edema, chest pain**

EENT: Sore throat; dry, burning eyes

GI: Nausea, vomiting, colitis, cramps, *diarrhea,* constipation, flatulence, dry mouth, *hiccups*

GU: Impotence

HEMA: **Agranulocytosis, eosinophilia, thrombocytopenia, purpura**

INTEG: Rash, purpura, alopecia, dry skin, urticaria, pruritus

RESP: **Bronchospasm,** dyspnea, wheezing

Contraindications: Hypersensitivity to β-blockers, cardiogenic shock, heart block (2nd, 3rd degree), sinus bradycardia, bronchial asthma

Precautions: Pregnancy (C), major surgery, lactation, diabetes mellitus, renal/hepatic disease, thyroid disease, COPD, CAD, nonallergic bronchospasm, CHF, geriatric

PHARMACOKINETICS

PO: Peak 2-4 hr, duration 13-19 hr
PO-ER: Peak 6-12 hr, duration 24 hr
IV: Onset immediate, peak 20 min, duration 6-8 hr
Half-life 3-4 hr; metabolized in liver (metabolites); excreted in urine; crosses placenta; enters breast milk

INTERACTIONS

• Do not use with MAOIs
Increase: hypotension, bradycardia—reserpine, hydrALAZINE, methyldopa, prazosin, amphetamines, epINEPHrine, H_2-antagonists, calcium channel blockers
Increase: hypoglycemic effects—insulin, oral antidiabetics

Increase: metoprolol effect—cimetidine
Increase: effects of benzodiazepines
Decrease: antihypertensive effect—salicylates, NSAIDs
Decrease: metoprolol level—barbiturates
Decrease: effects of DOPamine, DOBUTamine, xanthines

Drug/Herb
Increase: toxicity, death—aconite
Increase: antihypertensive effect—barberry, betony, black catechu, black cohosh, bloodroot, broom, burdock, cat's claw, dandelion, goldenseal, Irish moss, Jamaican dogwood, kelp, khella, mistletoe, parsley
Increase or decrease: antihypertensive effect—astragalus, cola tree
Decrease: antihypertensive effect—coltsfoot, guarana, khat, licorice

Drug/Food
Increase: absorption with food

Drug/Lab Test
Increase: BUN, potassium, ANA titer, serum lipoprotein, triglycerides, uric acid, alk phos, LDH, AST, ALT

NURSING CONSIDERATIONS
Assess:
• ECG directly when giving IV during initial treatment
• I&O, weight daily
• B/P during initial treatment, periodically thereafter; pulse q4h; note rate, rhythm, quality
• Apical/radial pulse before administration; notify prescriber of any significant changes or pulse <50 bpm
• Baselines in renal, hepatic studies before therapy begins
• Edema in feet, legs daily
• Skin turgor, dryness of mucous membranes for hydration status

Administer:
PO route
• Do not break, crush, or chew ext rel tabs
• After meals, at bedtime; tab may be crushed or swallowed whole; take at same time each day

M

IV route
• IV, undiluted, give over 1 min, × 3 doses at 2-5 min intervals; start **PO** 15 min after last IV dose

Y-site compatibilities: Alteplase, meperidine, morphine

Perform/provide:
• Storage in dry area at room temperature, do not freeze

Evaluate:
• Therapeutic response: decreased B/P after 1-2 wk

Teach patient/family:
• To take immediately after meals
• Not to discontinue drug abruptly; taper over 2 wk; may cause precipitate angina
• Not to use OTC products containing α-adrenergic stimulants (nasal decongestants, OTC cold preparations) unless directed by prescriber
• To report bradycardia, dizziness, confusion, depression, fever, sore throat, shortness of breath to prescriber
• To take pulse at home; advise when to notify prescriber
• To avoid alcohol, smoking, sodium intake
• To comply with weight control, dietary adjustments, modified exercise program
• To carry emergency ID to identify drug, allergies
• To avoid hazardous activities if dizziness is present
• To report symptoms of CHF: difficult breathing, especially on exertion or when lying down, night cough, swelling of extremities
• To take medication at bedtime to prevent effect of orthostatic hypotension
• To wear support hose to minimize effects of orthostatic hypotension

Treatment of overdose: Lavage, IV atropine for bradycardia, IV theophylline for bronchospasm, digoxin, O_2, diuretic for cardiac failure, hemodialysis, hypotension administer vasopressor (norepinephrine)

---

metronidazole (R)
(me-troe-ni′da-zole)
Apo-Metronidazole ✚, Flagyl, Flagyl ER, Flagyl IV, Flagyl IV RTU, metronidazole, Novonidazole ✚, Protostat, Trikacide ✚
Func. class.: Antiinfective—miscellaneous
Chem. class.: Nitroimidazole derivative

Action: Direct-acting amebicide/trichomonacide binds, disrupts DNA structure inhibiting bacterial nucleic acid synthesis

Uses: Intestinal amebiasis, amebic abscess, trichomoniasis, refractory trichomoniasis, bacterial anaerobic infections, giardiasis, septicemia, endocarditis, bone, joint infections, lower respiratory tract infections

Unlabeled uses: Crohn's disease, antibiotic-associated diarrhea, rosacea

DOSAGE AND ROUTES

Trichomoniasis
• *Adult:* **PO** 250 mg tid × 7 days or 2 g in single dose; do not repeat treatment for 4-6 wk
• *Child:* **PO** 5 mg/kg tid × 7 days

Refractory trichomoniasis
• *Adult:* **PO** 250 mg bid × 10 days

Amebic hepatic abscess
• *Adult:* **PO** 500-750 mg tid × 5-10 days
• *Child:* **PO** 35-50 mg/kg/day in 3 divided doses × 10 days

Intestinal amebiasis
• *Adult:* **PO** 750 mg tid × 5-10 days
• *Child:* **PO** 35-50 mg/kg/day in 3 divided doses × 10 days; then oral iodoquinol

Anaerobic bacterial infections
• *Adult:* **IV INF** 15 mg/kg over 1 hr, then 7.5 mg/kg **IV** or **PO** q6h, not to exceed 4 g/day; first maintenance dose should be administered 6 hr following loading dose

---

Giardiasis
- *Adult:* **PO** 250 mg tid × 5 days
- *Child:* **PO** 5 mg/kg tid × 5 days

Antibiotic-associated pseudomembranous colitis
- *Adult:* **PO** 250-500 mg 3-4 ×/day × 10-14 days
- *Child:* **PO** 20 mg/kg/day (max 2 g) divided q6h

Bacterial vaginosis
- *Adult:* **PO** ext rel 750 mg daily × 7 days

Available forms: Tabs 250, 500 mg; ext rel tab (ER) 750 mg; caps 375, 500 mg; inj 500 mg/100 ml; powder for inj 500 mg single dose

SIDE EFFECTS

CNS: Headache, dizziness, confusion, irritability, restlessness, ataxia, depression, fatigue, drowsiness, insomnia, paresthesia, peripheral neuropathy, **seizures,** incoordination, depression, encephalopathy

CV: Flattening of T waves

EENT: Blurred vision, sore throat, retinal edema, dry mouth, metallic taste, furry tongue, glossitis, stomatitis, photophobia

GI: Nausea, vomiting, diarrhea, epigastric distress, *anorexia,* constipation, *abdominal cramps,* metallic taste, **pseudomembranous colitis**

GU: Darkened urine, vaginal dryness, polyuria, **albuminuria,** dysuria, cystitis, decreased libido, **neurotoxicity,** incontinence, dyspareunia, candidiasis

HEMA: **Leukopenia, bone marrow, depression, aplasia**

INTEG: Rash, pruritus, urticaria, flushing

Contraindications: Pregnancy 1st trimester, hypersensitivity to this drug, renal/hepatic/GI disease, contracted visual or color fields, blood dyscrasias, lactation, CNS disorders

Precautions: Pregnancy (B) 2nd/3rd trimesters, *Candida* infections, heart failure, fungal infection, geriatric, dental disease

PHARMACOKINETICS

IV: Onset immediate, peak end of inf
PO: Peak 1-2 hr, half-life 6-11 hr, crosses placenta, enters breast milk, excreted in urine (60%-80%), absorbed PO (80%-85%)

INTERACTIONS

- Disulfiram reaction: alcohol
Increase: action of warfarin
Increase: leukopenia—azathioprine, fluorouracil
Decrease: metronidazole action—phenobarbital, phenytoin, cimetidine
Drug/Herb
- Do not use acidphilus with antiinfectives; separate by several hours
Drug/Lab Test
Altered: AST, ALT, LDH

NURSING CONSIDERATIONS
Assess:
- For infection: WBC, wound symptoms, fever, skin or vaginal secretions; start treatment after C&S
- For opportunistic fungal infections
- Stools during entire treatment; should be clear at end of therapy; stools should be free of parasites for 1 yr before patient is considered cured (amebiasis)
- Vision by ophthalmic exam during, after therapy; vision problems often occur
- I&O; weight daily; stools for number, frequency, character

⚠ Neurotoxicity: peripheral neuropathy, seizures, dizziness, uncoordination, pruritus, joint pains; drug may be discontinued
- Allergic reaction: fever, rash, itching, chills; drug should be discontinued if these symptoms occur
- Superinfection: fever, monilial growth, fatigue, malaise
- Renal and reproductive dysfunction: dysuria, polyuria, impotence, dyspareunia, decreased libido
Administer:
PO route
- Do not break, crush, or chew ER products

Side effects: *italics* = common; **bold** = life-threatening

- PO with or after meals to avoid GI symptoms, metallic taste; crush tabs if needed

IV route
- Prediluted; metronidazole IV, dilute with 4.4 ml sterile H_2O or 0.9% NaCl; must be diluted further with 8 mg/ml or more 0.9% NaCl, D_5W, or LR; must neutralize with 5 mEq $NaCO_3$/500 mg; CO_2 gas will be generated and may require venting; run over 1 hr or more; primary IV must be discontinued; may be given as continuous infusion; do not use aluminum products; IV may require venting

Additive compatibilities: Amikacin, aminophylline, cefazolin, cefotaxime, ceftazidime, ceftizoxime, ceftriaxone, cefuroxime, chloramphenicol, ciprofloxacin, clindamycin, disopyramide, floxacillin, fluconazole, gentamicin, heparin, moxalactam, multielectrolyte concentrate, multivitamins, netilmicin, penicillin G potassium, tobramycin

Y-site compatibilities: Acyclovir, allopurinol, amifostine, amiodarone, cefepime, cisatracurium, cyclophosphamide, diltiazem, DOPamine, DOXOrubicin liposome, enalaprilat, esmolol, fluconazole, foscarnet, granisetron, heparin, hydromorphone, labetalol, lorazepam, magnesium sulfate, melphalan, meperidine, methylPREDNISolone, midazolam, morphine, perphenazine, piperacillin/tazobactam, remifentanil, sargramostim, tacrolimus, teniposide, theophylline, thiotepa, vinorelbine

Perform/provide:
- Storage in light-resistant container; do not refrigerate

Evaluate:
- Therapeutic response: decreased symptoms of infection

Teach patient/family:
- That urine may turn dark-reddish brown, drug may cause metallic taste
- Proper hygiene after BM; hand-washing technique
- To notify physician for numbness or tingling of extremities
- To avoid hazardous activities, since dizziness can occur

- Need for compliance with dosage schedule, duration of treatment
- To use condoms if treatment for trichomoniasis, or cross-contamination may occur
- To use frequent sips of water, sugarless gum, candy for dry mouth
- That treatment of both partners is necessary in trichomoniasis
- Not to drink alcohol or use preparations containing alcohol during use or for 48 hr after use of drug; disulfiram-like reaction can occur

metronidazole topical
See Appendix C

mexiletine (Ʀ)
(mex-il'e-teen)
Mexitil
Func. class.: Antidysrhythmic (Class IB)
Chem. class.: Lidocaine analog

Action: Increases electrical stimulation threshold of ventricle, His-Purkinje system, which stabilizes cardiac membrane
Uses: Life-threatening ventricular tachycardia; because of proarrhythmic effects, use with lesser dysrhythmias not recommended
Unlabeled uses: Diabetic neuropathy, ventricular tachycardia, other ventricular dysrhythmias in acute phase of MI

DOSAGE AND ROUTES
- *Adult:* **PO** 200-400 mg (loading dose), then 200 mg q8h, then 200-400 mg q8h
Diabetic neuropathy (unlabeled)
- *Adult:* **PO** 150 mg/day for 3 days, then 300 mg/day for 3 days, followed by 10 mg/kg/day
Available forms: Caps 150, 200, 250 mg

SIDE EFFECTS
CNS: Headache, dizziness, confusion, **seizures,** tremors, psychosis, nervousness,

paresthesias, weakness, fatigue, coordination difficulties, change in sleep habits

CV: Hypotension, bradycardia, angina, PVCs, **heart block, cardiovascular collapse or arrest,** sinus node slowing, **left ventricular failure,** syncope, **cardiogenic shock, AV conduction disturbances, CHF, atrial dysrhythmias, palpitations, ventricular dysrhythmias, ventricular tachycardia, other ventricular arrhythmias in acute phase of MI**

EENT: Blurred vision, tinnitus

GI: Nausea, vomiting, anorexia, diarrhea, abdominal pain, **hepatitis,** dry mouth, peptic ulcer, altered taste, **GI bleeding,** constipation

GU: Urinary hesitancy, decreased libido

HEMA: **Thrombocytopenia, leukopenia, agranulocytosis**

INTEG: Rash, alopecia, dry skin

MISC: Edema, arthralgia, fever, systemic lupus erythematosus syndrome

RESP: Dyspnea

Contraindications: Hypersensitivity, cardiogenic shock, severe heart block (if no pacemaker)

Precautions: Pregnancy (C), lactation, children, hepatic disease, CHF, seizure disorder, hypotension

PHARMACOKINETICS

PO: Peak 2-3 hr; half-life 12 hr, metabolized by liver, excreted unchanged by kidneys (10%), excreted in breast milk

INTERACTIONS

Increase: mexiletine effects—metoclopramide, urinary alkalinizers

Increase: levels of caffeine, theophylline

Decrease or increase: mexiletine effects—cimetidine

Decrease: mexiletine levels—phenytoin, phenobarbital, rifampin, urinary acidifiers, aluminum/magnesium hydroxide, atropine, opiates

Decrease: drug effect—smoking

Drug/Herb

Increase: hypokalemia, increase antidysrhythmic action—aloe, buckthorn, cascara sagrada, rhubarb, senna

Increase: toxicity, death—aconite

Increase: effect—aloe, broom, chronic buckthorn use, cascara sagrada (chronic use), Chinese rhubarb, figwort, fumitory, goldenseal, kudzu, licorice

Increase: serotonin effect—horehound

Decrease: effect—coltsfoot

Drug/Lab Test

Increase: CPK

NURSING CONSIDERATIONS

Assess:

• ECG continuously for increased PR or QRS segments; discontinue or reduce rate; watch for increased ventricular ectopic beats; may have to rebolus

• Blood levels (therapeutic level 0.5-2 mcg/ml)

• B/P continuously for fluctuations in cardiac rate

• I&O ratio, electrolytes (K, Na, Cl), liver enzymes

⚠ Malignant hyperthermia: tachypnea, tachycardia, changes in B/P, fever

• Respiratory status: rate, rhythm, lung fields for crackles, watch for respiratory depression

• CNS effects: dizziness, confusion, psychosis, paresthesias, seizures; drug should be discontinued

• Lung fields, bilateral crackles may occur in CHF patient

• Increased respiration, increased pulse; drug should be discontinued

Administer:

• With food for GI upset

Evaluate:

• Therapeutic response: decreased dysrhythmias

Teach patient/family:

• To take with food or antacid

• Avoid changes in diet that could drastically acidify or alkalinize urine

• Notify prescriber of side effects

Treatment of overdose: O₂, artificial ventilation, ECG; administer DOPamine for circulatory depression, diazepam or thiopental for convulsions, to acidify urine

M

micafungin (℞)
(my-ca-fun′gin)
Mycamine
Func. class.: Antifungal, systemic
Chem. class.: Echinocandin

Action: Inhibits an essential component in fungal cell walls; causes direct damage to fungal cell wall

Uses: Treatment of esophageal candidiasis; prophylaxis of candida infections in patients undergoing hepatopoietic stem cell transplantation (HSCT); susceptible candida species: *C. albicans, C. glabrata, C. krusei, C. parapsilosis, C. tropicalis*

DOSAGE AND ROUTES
Esophageal candidiasis
• *Adult:* IV 150 mg/day, given over 1 hr
Prophylaxis of candida infections
• *Adult:* IV 50 mg/day, given over 1 hr
Available forms: Powder for injection 50 mg, in single dose vials

SIDE EFFECTS
CNS: **Seizures,** dizziness, *headache, somnolence*
CV: Flushing, hypertension, phlebitis
GI: Abdominal pain, *nausea, anorexia, vomiting, diarrhea, increased AST, ALT, alk phos, blood dehydrogenase, hyperbilirubinemia*
HEMA: **Neutropenia, thrombocytopenia, leukopenia, coagulopathy, anemia, hemolytic anemia**
INTEG: *Rash, pruritus, inj site pain*
META: Hypokalemia, hypocalcemia, hypomagnesemia
MS: Rigors
Contraindications: Hypersensitivity to this product or other echinocandins
Precautions: Pregnancy (C), severe hepatic, lactation, children, geriatric

PHARMACOKINETICS
Metabolized liver; excretion feces, urine; terminal half-life 14-20 hr; protein binding 99%

INTERACTIONS
Increase: plasma concentrations—sirolimus, nifedipine; may need dosage reduction

NURSING CONSIDERATIONS
Assess:
• For signs and symptoms of infection, clearing of cultures during treatment; obtain culture baseline and throughout drug may be started as soon as culture is taken (esophageal candidiasis); monitor cultures during HSCT, for prevention of candida infections
• CBC (RBC, Hct, Hgb), differential, platelet count periodically; notify prescriber of results
• Renal studies: BUN, urine CCr, electrolytes before and during therapy
• Hepatic studies before and during treatment: bilirubin, AST, ALT, alk phos, as needed
• Bleeding: hematuria, heme-positive stools, bruising or petechiae, mucosa or orifices; blood dyscrasias can occur
• For hypersensitivity: rash, pruritus, facial swelling; also for phelibits
• For hemolytic anemia
• GI symptoms: frequency of stools, cramping, if severe diarrhea occurs, electrolytes may need to be given
Administer:
• Do not use if cloudy or precipitated; do not admix
• Flush line before and after administration with 0.9% NaCl
IV route
• For candida prevention, reconstitute with provided diluent 0.9% NaCl without bacteriostatic product; 50 mg vial/5 ml (10 mg/ml), swirl to dissolve, do not shake; further dilute with 100 ml 0.9% NaCl, only; run over 1 hr
• For candida infection, reconstitute with provided diluent 50 mg/5 ml (10 mg/ml); further dilute 3 reconstituted vials in 100 ml of 0.9% NaCl, run over 1 hr

Perform/provide:

• Storage at room temperature, away from light, do not freeze; discard unused solution

Evaluate:

• Therapeutic response: prevention of candida infection in HSCT; or decreased symptoms of candida infection, negative culture

Teach patient/family:

• To notify prescriber if pregnancy is suspected or planned; use nonhormonal form of contraception while taking this product

• To avoid breastfeeding while taking this product

• To inform prescriber of kidney or liver disease

• To report bleeding, facial swelling, wheezing, difficulty breathing, itching, rash, hives, increasing warmth, flushing

• To report signs of infection: increased temp, sore throat, flulike symptoms

• To notify prescriber of nausea, vomiting, diarrhea, jaundice, anorexia, clay-colored stools, dark urine; hepatotoxicity may occur

---

miconazole topical
See Appendix C

---

miconazole vaginal antifungal
See Appendix C

---

midazolam (Rx)
(mid'ay-zoe-lam)
Versed
Func. class.: Sedative, hypnotic, antianxiety
Chem. class.: Benzodiazepine, short-acting

Controlled Substance Schedule IV
Do not confuse:
Versed/Vepesid/Vistaril
Action: Depresses subcortical levels in CNS; may act on limbic system, reticular formation; may potentiate γ-aminobutyric acid (GABA) by binding to specific benzodiazepine receptors

Uses: Preoperative sedation, general anesthesia induction, sedation for diagnostic endoscopic procedures, intubation

Unlabeled uses: Epileptic seizures, refractory status epilepticus

DOSAGE AND ROUTES

Preoperative sedation

• *Adult and child ≥12 yr:* **IM** 0.07-0.08 mg/kg ½-1 hr before general anesthesia

• *Child 1-6 mo:* **IM** 0.1-0.15 mg/kg, may give up to 0.5 mg/kg if needed

• *Child 6 mo-5 yr:* **PO** 0.25-1 mg/kg, max 20 mg as a single dose

• *Child 6 yr-11 yr:* **PO/IM** 0.25-0.5 mg/kg, max 20 mg as a single dose

Induction of general anesthesia

• *Adult and child 12-16 yr:* **IV** (unpremedicated patients) 0.3-0.35 mg/kg over 30 sec, wait 2 min, follow with 25% of initial dose if needed; (premedicated patients) 0.15-0.35 mg/kg over 20-30 sec, allow 2 min for effect

• *Child 6-12 yr:* **IV** 0.025-0.05 mg/kg, total dose up to 0.4 mg/kg may be needed

• *Child 6 mo-5 yr:* **IV** 0.05-0.1 mg/kg, total dose up to 0.6 mg/kg may be needed

• *Child <6 mo:* Titrate with small increments, adjust as needed

Continuous infusion for intubation (critical care)

• *Adult:* **IV** 0.01-0.05 mg/kg over several min; repeat at 10-15 min intervals, until adequate sedation; then 0.02-0.10 mg/kg/hr maintenance, adjust as needed

• *Child:* **IV** 0.05-0.2 mg/kg over 2-3 min, then 0.06-0.12 mg/kg/hr by cont inf; adjust as needed

• *Neonates:* **IV** 0.03-0.06 mg/kg/hr, titrate using lowest dose

Available forms: Inj 1, 5 mg/ml, syr 2 mg/ml

SIDE EFFECTS

CNS: Retrograde amnesia, euphoria, confusion, headache, anxiety, insomnia,

slurred speech, paresthesia, tremors, weakness, chills
CV: Hypotension, PVCs, tachycardia, bigeminy, nodal rhythm, **cardiac arrest**
EENT: Blurred vision, nystagmus, diplopia, loss of balance
GI: Nausea, vomiting, increased salivation, hiccups
INTEG: Urticaria, pain at injection site, swelling at inj site, rash, pruritus at injection site
RESP: Coughing, **apnea, bronchospasm, laryngospasm,** dyspnea, **respiratory depression**
Contraindications: Pregnancy (D), hypersensitivity to benzodiazepines, shock, coma, alcohol intoxication, acute narrow-angle glaucoma
Precautions: COPD, CHF, chronic renal failure, chills, geriatric, debilitated, children, lactation, neonates (contains benzyl alcohol)

PHARMACOKINETICS

IM: Onset 15 min, peak ½-1 hr, duration 2-3 hr
IV: Onset 3-5 min, onset of anesthesia 1½-2½ min, duration 2 hr
Protein binding 97%; half-life 1.2-12.3 hr, metabolized in liver; metabolites excreted in urine; crosses placenta, blood-brain barrier

INTERACTIONS

Increase: extended half-life—oral contraceptives
Increase: respiratory depression—other CNS depressants, alcohol, barbiturates, opiate analgesics, verapamil, ritonavir, indinavir, fluvoxamine
Decrease: midazolam metabolism—azole antifungals, cimetidine, erythromycin, ranitidine, theophylline
Drug/Herb
Increase: hypotension—black cohosh
Increase: CNS depression—catnip, chamomile, clary, cowslip, hops, kava, lavender, mistletoe, nettle, pokeweed, poppy, Queen Anne's lace, senega, skullcap, valerian

Drug/Food
Increase: (PO) midazolam effect—grapefruit juice

NURSING CONSIDERATIONS
Assess:
• Inj site for redness, pain, swelling
• Degree of amnesia in geriatric; may be increased
• Anterograde amnesia
• Vital signs for recovery period in obese patient, since half-life may be extended
• Apnea, respiratory depression that may be increased in the geriatric
Administer:
PO route
• Remove cap of press-in bottle adaptor and push adaptor into neck of bottle; close with cap; remove cap and insert tip of dispenser and insert into adaptor; turn upside-down and withdraw correct dose; place in mouth
IM route
• IM deep into large muscle mass
IV route
• May be given diluted or undiluted
• After diluting with D₅W or 0.9% NaCl to 0.25 mg/ml; give over 2 min (conscious sedation) or over 30 sec (anesthesia induction)
Additive compatibility: Hydromorphone
Syringe compatibilities: Alfentanil, atracurium, atropine, benzquinamide, buprenorphine, butorphanol, chlorproMAZINE, cimetidine, cisatracurium, diphenhydrAMINE, droperidol, fentanyl, glycopyrrolate, hydromorphone, hydrOXYzine, ketamine, meperidine, metoclopramide, morphine, nalbuphine, promazine, promethazine, remifentanil, scopolamine, sufentanil, thiethylperazine, trimethobenzamide
Y-site compatibilities: Abciximab, alfentamil, amikacin, amiodarone, argatroban, atracurium, atropine, aztreonam, benzotropine, calcium gluconate, cefazolin, cefotaxime, cefoxitine, ceftriaxone, cimetidine, ciprofloxacin, cisplatin, clinda-

mycin, clonidine, cyanocobalamin, cyclosporine, dactinomycin, digoxin, diltiazem, diphenhydramine, docetaxal, DOPamine, doxycyclin, enalaprilat, epINEPHrine, erythromycin, esmolol, etomidate, etoposide, famotidine, fentanyl, fluconazole, folic acid, gatifloxacin, gemcitabine, gentamicin, glycopyrrolate, granisetron, heparin, hetastarch, hydromorphone, hydroxyzine, inamrinone, isoproterenol, labetalol, lactated Ringer's, levofloxacin, lidocaine, linezolid, lorazepam, magnesium, mannitol, meperdine, methadone, methyldopa, methylPREDNISolone, metoclopramide, metomolol, metronidazole, milrinone, morphine, nalbuphine, naloxone, niCARdipine, nitroglycerin, nitroprusside, norepinephrine, ondansetron, oxacillin, oxytocin, paclitaxel, palonasetron, pancuronium, papaverin, phentolamine, phytonadione, piperacillin, potassium chloride, propanolol, protamine, pyridoxine, ranitidine, remifentanil, sodium nitroprusside, streptokinase, succinylcholine, sufentanil, teniposide, theophylline, thiotepa, ticarcillin, tobramycin, vancomycin, vasopressin, vecuronium, verapamil, voriconazole

Perform/provide:

• Assistance with ambulation until drowsy period relieved

• Storage at room temperature, protect from light

• Immediate availability of resuscitation equipment, O_2 to support airway; do not give by rapid bolus

Evaluate:

• Therapeutic response: induction of sedation, general anesthesia

Teach patient/family:

• That amnesia occurs; events may not be remembered

Treatment of overdose: Flumazenil, O_2

Increase: supine hypertension—fludrocortisone

Increase: lactic acidosis—metformin

NURSING CONSIDERATIONS

Assess:

• VS, B/P (standing, supine); notify prescriber if B/P supine is increased

• Observe for drowsiness, dizziness, LOC

Administer:

• Tablets may be swallowed whole, chewed, or allowed to dissolve

• Upon arising, midday, and late afternoon (no later than 6 PM)

• Avoid administering if patient is to be supine during day

Evaluate:

• Therapeutic response: decreased orthostatic hypotension

Teach patient/family:

• To avoid hazardous activities, activities requiring alertness; dizziness may occur; instruct patient to request assistance with ambulation

• To avoid alcohol, other depressants

---

mifepristone (℞)

(mif-ee-press'tone)

Mifeprex

Func. class.: Abortifacient

Chem. class.: Antiprogestational

Action: Stimulates uterine contractions, causing complete abortion

Uses: Abortion through 49 days' gestation

Unlabeled uses: Postcoital contraception/contragestation, intrauterine fetal death, endometriosis, Cushing's syndrome, unresectable meningioma

DOSAGE AND ROUTES

• *Adult:* **PO** 600 mg day 1, 400 mcg misoprostol day 3

Available forms: Tabs 200 mg

SIDE EFFECTS

CNS: Dizziness, insomnia, anxiety, syncope, fainting, headache

GI: Nausea, vomiting, diarrhea, dyspepsia

GU: Uterine cramping, uterine hemorrhage, vaginitis, pelvic pain

MISC: Fatigue, back pain, fever, viral infections, chills, sinusitis

Contraindications: Hypersensitivity, severe hepatic disease, severe renal disease, IUD, ectopic pregnancy, chronic adrenal failure, bleeding disorder, inherited porphyrias, PID, respiratory disease, cardiac disease

Precautions: Pregnancy (C), asthma, anemia, jaundice, diabetes mellitus, convulsive disorders, women >35 yr/smoke ≥10 cigarettes/day, past uterine surgery

PHARMACOKINETICS

Rapidly absorbed, peak 90 min, 98% bound to plasma proteins, albumin, glycoprotein, excretion via feces, urine

INTERACTIONS

Decrease: metabolism of erythromycin, ketoconazole, itraconazole

Drug/Herb

Decrease: by St. John's wort

Drug/Food

Decrease: metabolism of mifepristone—grapefruit juice

NURSING CONSIDERATIONS

Assess:

• B/P, pulse; watch for change that may indicate hemorrhage

• Respiratory rate, rhythm, depth; notify prescriber of abnormalities

• For length, duration of contraction; notify prescriber of contractions lasting over 1 min or absence of contractions

• For incomplete abortion, pregnancy must be terminated by another method; drug is teratogenic

Perform/provide:

• Emotional support before and after abortion

Evaluate:

• Therapeutic response: expulsion of fetus

Teach patient/family:
• To report increased blood loss, abdominal cramps, increased temp, foul-smelling lochia
• Some methods of comfort control and pain control
• Must continue with follow-up
• That cramping and vaginal bleeding will occur

miglitol (R)
(mig′lih-tol)
Glyset
Func. class.: Oral hypoglycemic
Chem. class.: α-Glucosidase inhibitor

Action: Delays digestion of ingested carbohydrates, results in smaller rise in blood glucose after meals; does not increase insulin production
Uses: Type 2 diabetes mellitus

DOSAGE AND ROUTES
• *Adult:* **PO** 25 mg tid initially, with first bite of meal; maintenance dose may be increased to 50 mg tid; may be increased to 100 mg tid if needed (only in patients >60 kg) with dosage adjustment at 4-8 wk intervals
Available forms: Tabs 25, 50, 100 mg

SIDE EFFECTS
GI: Abdominal pain, diarrhea, flatulence, **hepatotoxicity**
HEMA: Low iron
INTEG: Rash
Contraindications: Hypersensitivity, diabetic ketoacidosis, cirrhosis, inflammatory bowel disease, colonic ulceration, partial intestinal obstruction, chronic intestinal disease
Precautions: Pregnancy (B), lactation, children, renal/hepatic disease

PHARMACOKINETICS
Peak 2-3 hr, not metabolized, excreted in urine as unchanged drug, half-life 2 hr

INTERACTIONS
Decrease: levels of digoxin, propranolol, ranitidine
Decrease: miglitol levels—digestive enzymes, intestinal adsorbents; do not use together
Drug/Herb
• Improved glucose tolerance: karela
Decrease: hypoglycemic effect—broom, buchu, dandelion, juniper
Increase or decrease: hypoglycemic effect—chromium, fenugreek, ginseng
Drug/Food
Increase: diarrhea—carbohydrates

NURSING CONSIDERATIONS
Assess:
• Hypoglycemia, hyperglycemia; even though drug does not cause hypoglycemia, if patient is on sulfonylureas or insulin, hypoglycemia may be additive
• Blood glucose levels, hemoglobin, A1c LFTs; if hypoglycemia occurs with monotherapy, treat with glucose
Administer:
• Tid with first bite of each meal
Perform/provide:
• Storage in tight container in cool environment
Evaluate:
• Therapeutic response: decreased signs/symptoms of diabetes mellitus (polyuria, polydipsia, polyphagia, clear sensorium, absence of dizziness, stable gait)
Teach patient/family:
• The symptoms of hypo/hyperglycemia, what to do about each, that during periods of stress, infection, surgery, insulin may be required
• That medication must be taken as prescribed; explain consequences of discontinuing medication abruptly
• To avoid OTC medications unless approved by health care provider
• That diabetes is lifelong illness; that this drug is not a cure
• To carry ID for emergency purposes
• That diet and exercise regimen must be followed

Rarely Used

miglustat (℞)
(mih'glue-stat)
Zavesca
Func. class.: Miscellaneous agent

Uses: Adults with mild to moderate type 1 Gaucher disease

DOSAGE AND ROUTES

• *Adult:* **PO** 100 mg tid, without regard to food

Contraindications: Pregnancy (X), hypersensitivity

⚠ High Alert

milrinone (℞)
(mill'rih-nohn)
Primacor
Func. class.: Inotropic/vasodilator agent with phosphodiesterase activity
Chem. class.: Bipyridine derivative

Action: Positive inotropic agent, increases contractility of cardiac muscle with vasodilator properties; reduces preload and afterload by direct relaxation on vascular smooth muscle

Uses: Short-term management of advanced HF that has not responded to other medication; can be used with digoxin

DOSAGE AND ROUTES

• *Adult:* **IV BOL** 50 mcg/kg given over 10 min; start inf of 0.375-0.75 mcg/kg/min; reduce dose in renal impairment

Available forms: Inj 1 mg/ml; pre-mixed inj 200 mcg/ml in D_5W

SIDE EFFECTS

CV: **Dysrhythmias,** hypotension, chest pain
GI: Nausea, vomiting, anorexia, abdominal pain, **hepatotoxicity, jaundice**
HEMA: **Thrombocytopenia**
MISC: Headache, hypokalemia, tremor

Contraindications: Hypersensitivity to this drug, severe aortic disease, severe pulmonic valvular disease, acute myocardial infarction

Precautions: Pregnancy (C), lactation, children, renal/hepatic disease, atrial flutter/fibrillation, geriatric

PHARMACOKINETICS

IV: Onset 2-5 min, peak 10 min, duration variable; half-life 2.4 hr; metabolized in liver; excreted in urine as drug (83%) and metabolites (12%)

NURSING CONSIDERATIONS

Assess:

⚠ ECG continuously during IV, ventricular dysrhythmia can occur

• B/P and pulse q5min during infusion; if B/P drops 30 mm Hg, stop infusion and call prescriber

• Electrolytes: K, Na, Cl, Ca; renal studies: BUN, creatinine; blood studies: platelet count

• ALT, AST, bilirubin daily

• I&O ratio and weight daily; diuresis should increase with continuing therapy

• If platelets are <150,000/mm³, drug is usually discontinued and another drug started

• Extravasation; change site q48h

Administer:

• Potassium supplements if ordered for potassium levels <3 mg/dl

IV route

• Give IV loading dose undiluted over 10 min

• Into running dextrose infusion through Y-connector or directly into tubing; dilute with 0.9% NaCl to 1-3 mg/ml; do not mix with glucose for long-term infusion

• By inf pump for doses other than bolus

Additive compatibilities: Quinidine

Syringe compatibilities: Atropine, calcium chloride, digoxin, epINEPHrine, lidocaine, morphine, propranolol, sodium bicarbonate, verapamil

Y-site compatibilities: Digoxin, diltiazem, DOBUTamine, DOPamine, epINEPHrine, fentanyl, heparin, hydromor-

---

⚠ Safety alert   *"Tall Man" lettering

phone, labetalol, lorazepam, midazolam, morphine, niCARdipine, nitroglycerin, norepinephrine, propranolol, quinidine, ranitidine, thiopental, vecuronium

Evaluate:
• Therapeutic response: increased cardiac output, decreased PCWP, adequate CVP, decreased dyspnea, fatigue, edema, ECG

Teach patient/family:
• To report angina immediately during infusion
• To report headache, which can be treated with analgesics

Treatment of overdose: Discontinue drug, support circulation

---

minocycline (Ⓡ)
(min-oh-sye′kleen)
Arestin, Dynacin, Minocin, Myrac, Vectrin
Func. class.: Broad-spectrum antiinfective
Chem. class.: Tetracycline

Action: Inhibits protein synthesis, phosphorylation in microorganisms by binding to 30S ribosomal subunits, reversibly binding to 50S ribosomal subunits; bacteriostatic

Uses: Syphilis, *Chlamydia trachomatis*, gonorrhea, lymphogranuloma venereum, rickettsial infections, inflammatory acne, *Neisseria meningitidis, Neisseria gonorrhoeae, Treponema pallidum, Chlamydia trachomatis, Ureaplasma urealyticum, Mycoplasma pneumoniae, Nocardia,* periodontitis

Unlabeled uses: Rheumatoid arthritis

DOSAGE AND ROUTES

• *Adult:* **PO/IV** 200 mg, then 100 mg q12h or 50 mg q6h, not to exceed 400 mg/24 hr **IV; SUBGINGIVAL** inserted into periodontal pocket
• *Child >8 yr:* **PO/IV** 4 mg/kg then 4 mg/kg/day **PO** in divided doses q12h

Gonorrhea
• *Adult:* **PO** 200 mg, then 100 mg q12h × 4 days or more

Chlamydia trachomatis
• *Adult:* **PO** 100 mg bid × 7 days
Syphilis
• *Adult:* **PO** 200 mg, then 100 mg q12h × 10-15 days
Uncomplicated gonococcal urethritis in men
• *Adult:* **PO** 100 mg q12h × 5 days
Rheumatoid arthritis (unlabeled)
• *Adult:* **PO** 100 mg bid for ≤48 wk

Available forms: Caps 50, 75, 100 mg; oral susp 50 mg/5 ml; powder for inj 100 mg; caps, pellet filled 50, 100 mg; tabs 50, 75, 100 mg; ext rel tabs 45, 90, 135 mg

SIDE EFFECTS

CNS: Dizziness, fever, light-headedness, vertigo, **seizures, increased intracranial pressure**
CV: Pericarditis
EENT: Dysphagia, glossitis, decreased calcification of deciduous teeth, permanent discoloration of teeth, oral candidiasis
GI: Nausea, abdominal pain, *vomiting, diarrhea,* anorexia, enterocolitis, **hepatotoxicity,** flatulence, abdominal cramps, epigastric burning, stomatitis
GU: Increased BUN, polyuria, polydipsia, **renal failure, nephrotoxicity**
HEMA: **Eosinophilia, neutropenia, thrombocytopenia, hemolytic anemia, pancytopenia**
INTEG: Rash, urticaria, photosensitivity, increased pigmentation, **exfoliative dermatitis,** pruritus, blue-gray color of skin, mucous membranes
SYST: **Angioedema, Stevens-Johnson syndrome**

Contraindications: Pregnancy (D), hypersensitivity to tetracyclines, children <8 yr
Precautions: Hepatic disease, lactation

PHARMACOKINETICS

PO: Peak 2-3 hr, half-life 11-17 hr; excreted in urine, feces, breast milk; crosses placenta; 70%-75% protein bound

INTERACTIONS

Increase: effect of warfarin, digoxin, insulin, oral anticoagulants, theophylline
Decrease: effect of minocycline—antacids, sodium bicarbonate, alkali products, iron, kaolin/pectin, cimetidine
Decrease: effect of barbiturates, carbamazepine, phenytoin, penicillins, oral contraceptives, calcium

Drug/Herb
• Do not use acidophilus with antiinfectives; separate by several hours

Drug/Lab Test
False negative: Urine glucose with Clinistix or Tes-Tape

NURSING CONSIDERATIONS

Assess:
• I&O ratio
• Blood tests: PT, CBC, AST, ALT, BUN, creatinine
• Signs of anemia: Hct, Hgb, fatigue
• Allergic reactions: rash, itching, pruritus, angioedema
• Nausea, vomiting, diarrhea; administer antiemetic, antacids as ordered
• Overgrowth of infection: fever, malaise, redness, pain, swelling, drainage, perineal itching, diarrhea, changes in cough or sputum, black, furry tongue

Administer:
• After C&S obtained
• With a full glass of water; with food for GI symptoms

PO route
• 2 hr before or after laxative or ferrous products; 3 hr after antacid

IV route
• After diluting 100 mg/5 ml sterile H₂O for inj; further dilute in 500-1000 ml of NaCl, dextrose sol, LR, Ringer's sol; run 100 mg/6 hr

Y-site compatibilities: Aztreonam, cisatracurium, cyclophosphamide, filgrastim, fludarabine, granisetron, heparin, hydrocortisone, magnesium sulfate, melphalan, perphenazine, potassium chloride, remifentanil, sargramostim, teniposide, vinorelbine, vit B/C

Perform/provide:
• Storage in airtight, light-resistant container at room temperature

Evaluate:
• Therapeutic response: decreased temp, absence of lesions, negative C&S

Teach patient/family:
• To avoid sunlight; sunscreen does not seem to decrease photosensitivity
• That all prescribed medication must be taken to prevent superinfection; not to use outdated product, Fanconi's syndrome may occur
• To avoid taking with antacids, iron, cimetidine; absorption may be decreased

---

minoxidil (℞, OTC)
(mi-nox′i-dill)
Loniten, minoxidil, Rogaine (top)
Func. class.: Antihypertensive
Chem. class.: Vasodilator, peripheral

Do not confuse:
minoxidil/Monopril
Loniten/Lotensin
Action: Directly relaxes arteriolar smooth muscle, causing vasodilation
Uses: Severe hypertension unresponsive to other therapy (use with diuretic); topically to treat alopecia

DOSAGE AND ROUTES
Severe hypertension
• *Adult:* **PO** 2.5-5 mg/day in 1-2 divided doses; max 100 mg daily; usual range 10-40 mg/day in single doses
• *Geriatric:* **PO** 2.5 mg daily, may be increased gradually
• *Child <12 yr:* **PO** (initial) 0.1-0.2 mg/kg/day; (effective range) 0.25-1 mg/kg/day; (max) 50 mg/day
Alopecia
• *Adult:* **TOP** 1 ml bid, rub into scalp daily, max 2 ml/day
Available forms: Tabs 2.5, 10 mg; top 2% sol

⚠ Safety alert   *"Tall Man" lettering

SIDE EFFECTS

Systemic

CNS: Headache, fatigue

CV: Severe rebound hypertension on withdrawal in children, tachycardia, angina, increased T wave, **CHF, pulmonary edema, pericardial effusion,** edema, sodium, water retention

GI: Nausea, vomiting

GU: Breast tenderness

HEMA: Hct, Hgb, erythrocyte count may decrease initially

INTEG: Pruritus, **Stevens-Johnson syndrome,** rash, hirsutism

Contraindications: Acute MI, dissecting aortic aneurysm, hypersensitivity, pheochromocytoma

Precautions: Pregnancy (C), lactation, children, renal disease, CAD, CHF, geriatric, CVD

PHARMACOKINETICS

PO: Onset 30 min, peak 2-3 hr, duration 48-120 hr; half-life 4.2 hr; metabolized in liver; metabolites excreted in urine, feces

INTERACTIONS

Increase: orthostatic hypotension—antihypertensives

Decrease: antihypertensive effect—NSAIDs, salicylates

Drug/Herb

Increase: antihypertensive effect—hawthorn

Decrease: antihypertensive effect—yohimbine

Drug/Lab Test

Increase: Renal studies

Decrease: Hgb/Hct/RBC

NURSING CONSIDERATIONS

Assess:

⚠ Monitor closely, usually given with β-blocker to prevent tachycardia and increased myocardial workload, usually given with diuretic to prevent serious fluid accumulation, patient should be hospitalized during beginning treatment

• Nausea, edema in feet, legs daily

• Skin turgor, dryness of mucous membranes for hydration status

• Crackles, dyspnea, orthopnea

• Electrolytes: K, Na, Cl, CO_2

• Renal studies: catecholamines, BUN, creatinine

• Hepatic studies: AST, ALT, alk phos

• B/P, pulse

• Weight daily, I&O

Administer:

PO route

• With meals for better absorption, to decrease GI symptoms

• With β-blocker and/or diuretic for hypertension

Topical route

• 1 ml no matter how much balding has occurred; increasing dosage does not speed growth

Perform/provide:

• Storage protected from light and heat

Evaluate:

• Therapeutic response: decreased B/P or increased hair growth

Teach patient/family:

• That body hair will increase but is reversible after discontinuing treatment

• Not to discontinue drug abruptly

• To report pitting edema, dizziness, weight gain >5 lb, shortness of breath, bruising or bleeding, heart rate >20 beats/min over normal, severe indigestion, dizziness, light-headedness, panting, new or aggravated symptoms of angina

• To take drug exactly as prescribed, or serious side effects may occur

Topical

• That for topical use, treatment must continue long-term or new hair will be lost

• Not to use except on scalp

Treatment of overdose: Administer normal saline IV, vasopressors

M

mirtazapine (Ŗ)
(mer-ta′za-peen)
Remeron, Remeron Soltab
Func. class.: Antidepressant
Chem. class.: Tetracyclic

Action: Blocks reuptake of norepinephrine, serotonin into nerve endings, increasing action of norepinephrine, serotonin in nerve cells
Uses: Depression, dysthymic disorder, bipolar disorder—depressed, agitated depression

DOSAGE AND ROUTES
• *Adult:* **PO** 15 mg/day at bedtime, maintenance to continue for 6 mo, titrate up to 45 mg/day; orally disintegrating tabs: open blister pack, place tab on tongue, allow to disintegrate, swallow
• *Geriatric:* **PO** 7.5 mg at bedtime, increase by 7.5 mg q1-2wk to desired dose, max 45 mg/day
Available forms: Tabs 15, 30 mg; orally disintegrating tab (soltab) 15, 30, 45 mg

SIDE EFFECTS
CNS: Dizziness, drowsiness, confusion, headache, anxiety, tremors, stimulation, weakness, insomnia, nightmares, EPS (geriatric), increased psychiatric symptoms, **seizures**
CV: Orthostatic hypotension, ECG changes, tachycardia, **hypertension,** palpitations
EENT: Blurred vision, tinnitus, mydriasis
GI: Diarrhea, dry mouth, nausea, vomiting, **paralytic ileus,** increased appetite, cramps, epigastric distress, constipation, **jaundice, hepatitis,** stomatitis
GU: Urinary retention, **acute renal failure**
HEMA: **Agranulocytosis, thrombocytopenia, eosinophilia, leukopenia**
INTEG: Rash, urticaria, sweating, pruritus, photosensitivity
SYST: Flulike symptoms

Contraindications: Hypersensitivity to tricyclics, recovery phase of MI, convulsive disorders, prostatic hypertrophy
Precautions: Pregnancy (C), suicidal patients, severe depression, increased intraocular pressure, narrow-angle glaucoma, urinary retention, renal/hepatic/cardiac disease, hypothyroidism, hyperthyroidism, electroshock therapy, elective surgery, geriatric

PHARMACOKINETICS
PO: Peak 12 hr, metabolized by liver; excreted in urine, feces; crosses placenta; half-life 20-40 hr

INTERACTIONS
⚠ Hyperpyretic crisis, seizures, hypertensive episode: MAOIs
Increase: CNS depression, alcohol, barbiturates, benzodiazepines, other CNS depressants
Decrease: effects of clonidine, indirect-acting sympathomimetics (epHEDrine)
Drug/Herb
• Serotonin syndrome: SAM-e, St. John's wort
Increase: anticholinergic effect—belladonna, henbane
Increase: antidepressant action—scopolia
Increase: CNS depression—chamomile, hops, kava, skullcap, valerian
Drug/Lab Test
Increase: Serum bilirubin, blood glucose, alk phos
Decrease: VMA, 5-HIAA
False increase: Urinary catecholamines

NURSING CONSIDERATIONS
Assess:
• B/P (lying, standing), pulse q4h; if systolic B/P drops 20 mm Hg, hold drug, notify prescriber; take vital signs q4h in patients with CV disease
• Blood studies: CBC, leukocytes, differential, cardiac enzymes if patient is receiving long-term therapy
• Hepatic studies: AST, ALT, bilirubin, creatinine

⚠ Safety alert   *"Tall Man" lettering

• Weight qwk; appetite may increase with drug
• ECG for flattening of T wave, bundle branch block, AV block, dysrhythmias in cardiac patients
• EPS primarily in geriatric: rigidity, dystonia, akathisia
• Mental status: mood, sensorium, affect, suicidal tendencies, increase in psychiatric symptoms: depression, panic
• Alcohol consumption; if alcohol is consumed, hold dose until morning

Administer:
• Increased fluids, bulk in diet for constipation, especially geriatric
• With food, milk for GI symptoms
• Dosage at bedtime if oversedation occurs during day; may take entire dose at bedtime; geriatric may not tolerate once/day dosing
• Gum, hard candy, or frequent sips of water for dry mouth
• Orally disintegrating tab: no water needed; allow to dissolve on tongue

Perform/provide:
• Storage in tight container at room temperature; do not freeze
• Assistance with ambulation during beginning therapy, since drowsiness/dizziness occurs
• Safety measures, including side rails, primarily in geriatric
• Checking to see PO medication swallowed

Evaluate:
• Therapeutic response: decreased depression

Teach patient/family:
• That therapeutic effects may take 2-3 wk
• To use caution in driving, other activities requiring alertness, because of drowsiness, dizziness, blurred vision
• To report immediately urinary retention
• To avoid alcohol ingestion, other CNS depressants

Treatment of overdose: ECG monitoring, induce emesis; lavage, activated charcoal; administer anticonvulsant

---

misoprostol (℞)
(mye-soe-prost'ole)
Cytotec
Func. class.: Gastric mucosa protectant, antiulcer
Chem. class.: Prostaglandin E_1-analog

Do not confuse:
misoprostol/metoprolol
cytotec/Cytoxan

Action: Inhibits gastric acid secretion; may protect gastric mucosa; can increase bicarbonate, mucus production

Uses: Prevention of nonsteroidal antiinflammatory drug-induced gastric ulcers

Unlabeled uses: Used investigationally with methotrexate to produce abortion, chronic idiopathic constipation, postpartum hemorrhage; cervical ripening/labor induction (vaginal)

DOSAGE AND ROUTES
• *Adult:* **PO** 200 mcg qid with food for duration of nonsteroidal antiinflammatory therapy with last dose at bedtime; if 200 mcg is not tolerated, 100 mcg may be given

Available forms: Tabs 100, 200 mcg

SIDE EFFECTS
GI: Diarrhea, nausea, vomiting, flatulence, constipation, dyspepsia, abdominal pain
GU: Spotting, cramps, hypermenorrhea, menstrual disorders

Contraindications: Pregnancy (X), hypersensitivity to this drug or prostaglandins

Precautions: Lactation, children, geriatric, renal disease, CV disease

PHARMACOKINETICS
PO: Peak 12 min, plasma steady state achieved within 2 days, excreted in urine

---

Side effects: *italics* = common; **bold** = life-threatening

INTERACTIONS
Drug/Food
Decrease: maximum concentrations when taken with food

NURSING CONSIDERATIONS
Assess:
- GI symptoms: hematemesis, occult or frank blood in stools, gastric aspirate, cramping, severe diarrhea
- Obtain a negative pregnancy test; miscarriages are common
- Gastric pH (>5 should be maintained)

Administer:
- PO with meals for prolonged drug effect; avoid use of magnesium antacids

Perform/provide:
- Storage at room temperature

Evaluate:
- Therapeutic response: absence of pain or GI complaints; prevention of ulcers

Teach patient/family:
- To take only as directed, read patient information leaflet
- Not to take if pregnant (can cause miscarriage) and not to become pregnant while taking this medication; if pregnancy occurs during therapy, discontinue drug, notify prescriber; not to administer to nursing mothers
- Not to give drug to anyone else or take for more than 4 wk unless directed by prescriber
- To avoid OTC preparations: aspirin, cough, cold products; condition may worsen

---

⚠ High Alert

mitomycin (℞)
(mye-toe-mye'sin)
mitomycin, Mutamycin
Func. class.: Antineoplastic, antibiotic

Action: Inhibits DNA synthesis, primarily; derived from *Streptomyces caespitosus;* appears to cause cross-linking of DNA, a vesicant

Uses: Pancreas, stomach cancer, head and neck or breast cancer
Unlabeled uses: Palliative treatment of head, neck, colon, breast, biliary, cervical, lung malignancies

DOSAGE AND ROUTES
- *Adult:* IV 10-20 mg/m^2 q6-8wk
Available forms: Inj 5, 20, 40 mg/vial

SIDE EFFECTS
CNS: Fever, headache, confusion, drowsiness, syncope, fatigue
EENT: Blurred vision
GI: Nausea, vomiting, anorexia, stomatitis, **hepatotoxicity,** diarrhea
GU: Urinary retention, **renal failure,** edema
HEMA: **Thrombocytopenia, leukopenia, anemia**
INTEG: Rash, alopecia, **extravasation**
MISC: **Hemolytic uremic syndrome**
RESP: **Fibrosis, pulmonary infiltrate,** dyspnea
Contraindications: Pregnancy (D) 1st trimester, hypersensitivity, as a single agent, thrombocytopenia, coagulation disorders, lactation
Precautions: Renal disease, bone marrow depression

PHARMACOKINETICS
Half-life 1 hr, metabolized in liver, 10% excreted in urine (unchanged)

INTERACTIONS
Increase: toxicity—other antineoplastics, radiation

NURSING CONSIDERATIONS
Assess:
- CBC, differential, platelet count weekly; withhold drug if WBC is <2000/mm^3, granulocyte count <1000/mm^3, or platelet count is <100,000/mm^3; notify prescriber
- Pulmonary function tests, chest x-ray before, during therapy; chest x-ray should be obtained q2wk during treatment
⚠ Fatal hemolytic uremic syndrome: hy-

pertension, thrombocytopenia, microangiopathic hemolytic anemia, occurs in those on long-term therapy

• Renal studies: BUN, serum uric acid, urine CCr, electrolytes before, during therapy

• I&O ratio; report fall in urine output to <30 ml/hr

• Monitor temp q4h; fever may indicate beginning infection

• Hepatic studies before, during therapy: bilirubin, AST, ALT, alk phos as needed or monthly; check for jaundiced skin and sclera, dark urine, clay-colored stools, itchy skin, abdominal pain, fever, diarrhea

• Bleeding: hematuria, guaiac, bruising, petechiae, mucosa or orifices q8h

⚠ Pulmonary fibrosis: bronchospasm

• Dyspnea, crackles, unproductive cough; chest pain, tachypnea, fatigue, increased pulse, pallor, lethargy

• Effects of alopecia on body image; discuss feelings about body changes

• Inflammation of mucosa, breaks in skin

• Buccal cavity q8h for dryness, sores, ulceration, white patches, oral pain, bleeding, dysphagia

• Local irritation, pain, burning at inj site

• GI symptoms: frequency of stools, cramping

• Acidosis, signs of dehydration: rapid respirations, poor skin turgor, decreased urine output, dry skin, restlessness, weakness

Administer:

IV route

• Apply ice compress for extravasation; stop infusion

• Antiemetic 30-60 min before giving drug to prevent vomiting

• IV after diluting 5 mg/10 ml or 10 mg/40 ml sterile H_2O for inj; shake, allow to stand, give through Y-tube or 3-way stopcock; give over 5-10 min, color of reconstituted sol is gray

Additive compatibilities: Dexamethasone, hydrocortisone

Solution compatibilities: LR, 0.3% NaCl, 0.5% NaCl

Syringe compatibilities: Bleomycin, cisplatin, cyclophosphamide, DOXOrubi-

cin, droperidol, fluorouracil, furosemide, heparin, leucovorin, methotrexate, metoclopramide, vinBLAStine, vinCRIStine

Y-site compatibilities: Allopurinol, amifostine, bleomycin, cisplatin, cyclophosphamide, DOXOrubicin, droperidol, fluorouracil, furosemide, granisetron, heparin, leucovorin, melphalan, methotrexate, metoclopramide, ondansetron, teniposide, thiotepa, vinBLAStine, vinCRIStine

Perform/provide:

• Rinsing of mouth tid-qid with water; brushing of teeth with baking soda bid-tid with soft brush or cotton-tipped applicators for stomatitis; use unwaxed dental floss

• Storage at room temperature 1 wk after reconstituting or 2 wk refrigerated

Evaluate:

• Therapeutic response: decreased tumor size, spread of malignancy

Teach patient/family:

• To report any complaints, side effects to nurse or prescriber

• That hair may be lost during treatment and wig or hairpiece may make the patient feel better; tell patient that new hair may be different in color, texture

• To avoid foods with citric acid, hot or rough texture

• To report any bleeding, white spots, ulcerations in mouth; tell patient to examine mouth daily

• To avoid crowds, persons with infections if granulocyte count is low

M

Rarely Used

mitotane (Ᵽ)
(mye'toe-tane)
Lysodren, p'-DDD
Func. class.: Antineoplastic

Uses: Adrenocortical carcinoma

DOSAGE AND ROUTES

• *Adult:* **PO** 9-10 g/day in divided doses tid or qid; may have to decrease dose for severe reaction

Contraindications: Hypersensitivity

⚠ High Alert

mitoxantrone (℞)
(mye-toe-zan'trone)
Novantrone
Func. class.: Antineoplastic, antiinfective, immunomodulator
Chem. class.: Synthetic anthraquinone

Action: DNA reactive agent, cytocidal effect on both proliferating and nonproliferating cells, suggesting lack of cell cycle phase specificity (vesicant)
Uses: Acute nonlymphocytic leukemia (adult), relapsed leukemia, breast cancer; used with steroids to treat bone pain (advanced prostate cancer), multiple sclerosis (MS)
Unlabeled uses: Liver malignancies, non-Hodgkin's lymphoma

DOSAGE AND ROUTES
Induction
• *Adult:* IV INF 12 mg/m^2/day on days 1-3, and 100 mg/m^2 cytosine arabinoside × 7 days as a continuous 24-hr inf
Consolidation
• *Adult:* IV 12 mg/m^2 given as a short 5-15 min inf
Multiple sclerosis
• *Adult:* IV INF 12 mg/m^2 as a 5-15 min inf q3mo
Available forms: Inj 2 mg/ml

SIDE EFFECTS
CNS: Headache, **seizures**
CV: **CHF, cardiopathy, dysrhythmias**
EENT: Conjunctivitis, blue/green sclera
GI: Nausea, vomiting, diarrhea, anorexia, mucositis, **hepatotoxicity**
HEMA: **Thrombocytopenia, leukopenia, myelosuppression, anemia**
INTEG: Rash, necrosis at inj site, dermatitis, thrombophlebitis at inj site, alopecia
MISC: Fever
RESP: Cough, dyspnea
Contraindications: Pregnancy (D), hypersensitivity

Precautions: Myelosuppression, lactation, children; renal/hepatic/cardiac disease; gout

PHARMACOKINETICS
Highly bound to plasma proteins, metabolized in liver, excreted via renal, hepatobiliary systems; half-life 24-72 hr

INTERACTIONS
• Do not mix with heparin; precipitate will form
• Do not mix with any other drug
Increase: bone marrow depression toxicity—radiation, other antineoplastics
Increase: adverse reactions—live virus vaccines

NURSING CONSIDERATIONS
Assess:
• CBC, differential, platelet count qwk; withhold drug if WBC is <4000/mm^3 or platelet count is <75,000/mm^3; notify prescriber of these results
• Hepatic studies before, during therapy: bilirubin, AST, ALT, alk phos prn or qmo
• Renal studies: BUN, serum uric acid, urine CCr, electrolytes before, during therapy
• Bleeding, hematuria, guaiac, bruising or petechiae, mucosa or orifices q8h
• Jaundiced skin and sclera, dark urine, clay-colored stools, itchy skin, abdominal pain, fever, diarrhea
⚠ ECG, ECHO, chest x-ray RAI angiography to assess ejection fraction before and during treatment, cardiotoxic, may develop during treatment or months to years after treatment
• Acidosis, signs of dehydration: rapid respirations, poor skin turgor, decreased urine output, dry skin, restlessness, weakness
⚠ For secondary acute myelogenous leukemia (AML) that can develop after taking this drug
⚠ For MS: obtain MUGA, LVEF baselines; repeat LVEF if symptoms of CHF occur or

---

⚠ Safety alert   *"Tall Man" lettering

if cumulative dose is >100 mg/m^2; do not administer to patients who have received a lifetime dose of ≥140 mg/m^2 or if LVEF <50% or significant LVEF
• Do not administer to patients with MS if neutrophils <1500 cells/mm^3
• Obtain pregnancy test in all women of childbearing age, even if birth control is used

Administer:
• Medications by oral route if possible; avoid IM, SUBCUT, IV routes to prevent infections
• Antiemetic 30-60 min before giving drug to prevent vomiting

IV route
• IV after diluting with 50 ml or more NS or D$_5$W; give over 3-5 min, running IV of D$_5$W or NS; may be diluted further in D$_5$W, NS and run over 15-30 min; check for extravasation; give into freely flowing IV infusion; do not give IM, SUBCUT, or intraarterially

Additive compatibilities: Cyclophosphamide, cytarabine, fluorouracil, hydrocortisone, potassium chloride

Solution compatibilities: D$_5$/0.9 NaCl, D$_5$W, 0.9% NaCl

Y-site compatibilities: Allopurinol, amifostine, cladribine, filgrastim, fludarabine, granisetron, melphalan, ondansetron, sargramostim, teniposide, thiotepa, vinorelbine

Perform/provide:
• Liquid diet: carbonated beverages, Jell-O; dry toast, crackers may be added if patient is not nauseated or vomiting
• Rinsing of mouth tid-qid with water, club soda; brushing of teeth bid-qid with soft brush or cotton-tipped applicators for stomatitis; use unwaxed dental floss
• Increase fluids to 2-3 L/day unless contraindicated

Evaluate:
• Therapeutic response: decreased tumor size, spread of malignancy

Teach patient/family:
• To report side effects to nurse or physician
• To avoid foods with citric acid, rough texture, or hot

• To report any bleeding, white spots, ulcerations in mouth; tell patient to examine mouth daily
• To avoid crowds, persons with infections
• That sclera, urine may turn blue or green, hair loss may occur
• To notify prescriber if pregnancy is suspected or planned, use effective contraception

---

⚠ High Alert

mivacurium (℞)
(miv-a-kure′ee-um)
Mivacron
Func. class.: Neuromuscular blocker—nondepolarizing

Action: Inhibits transmission of nerve impulses by binding competitively with cholinergic receptor sites, antagonizing action of acetylcholine

Uses: Facilitation of endotracheal intubation, skeletal muscle relaxation during mechanical ventilation, surgery, or general anesthesia

DOSAGE AND ROUTES
• *Adult:* **IV** 0.15 mg/kg; maintenance 0.10/mg/kg q15min
• *Child 2-12 yr:* **IV** 0.2 mg/kg for a 10 min block

Available forms: 5-, 10-ml single-use vial (2 mg/ml); premixed infusion in D$_5$W 50-ml flex container

SIDE EFFECTS
CV: Decreased B/P, bradycardia, tachycardia
EENT: Diplopia
INTEG: Rash, urticaria
MS: Weakness, prolonged skeletal muscle relaxation, **paralysis**
RESP: **Prolonged apnea, bronchospasm, wheezing, respiratory depression**

Contraindications: Hypersensitivity
Precautions: Pregnancy (C), renal/hepatic disease, lactation, children <3

mo, fluid and electrolyte imbalances, neuromuscular disease, respiratory disease, obesity, geriatric

PHARMACOKINETICS

Rapidly hydrolyzed by plasma cholinesterases, peak 2-3 min, reversal within 15-30 min

INTERACTIONS

Increase: neuromuscular blockade—aminoglycosides, amphotericin B, bacitracin, carbamazepine, clindamycin, colistin, diuretics, enflurane, halothane, isoflurane, lincomycin, lithium, local anesthetics, magnesium, phenytoin, polymyxin antibiotics, procainamide, quinidine, tetracyclines

NURSING CONSIDERATIONS

Assess:
• For electrolyte imbalances (K, Mg); may lead to increased action of this drug
• VS (B/P, pulse, respirations, airway) until fully recovered; rate, depth, pattern of respirations, strength of hand grip
• I&O ratio; check for urinary retention, frequency, hesitancy
• Recovery: decreased paralysis of face, diaphragm, leg, arm, rest of body
• Allergic reactions: rash, fever, respiratory distress, pruritus; drug should be discontinued

Administer:
• Using nerve stimulator by anesthesiologist to determine neuromuscular blockade
• Anticholinesterase to reverse neuromuscular blockade
• By slow IV over 1-2 min (only by qualified persons, usually an anesthesiologist)
• Only fresh sol

Y-site compatibilities: Etomidate, thiopental

Perform/provide:
• Storage at room temperature; do not freeze
• Reassurance if communication is diffi-

cult during recovery from neuromuscular blockade
• Frequent (q2h) instillation of artificial tears and covering eyes to prevent drying of cornea

Evaluate:
• Therapeutic response: paralysis of jaw, eyelid, head, neck, rest of body

Treatment of overdose: Neostigmine, monitor VS; may require mechanical ventilation

---

Rarely Used

modafinil (℞)

(moh-daf′ih-nil)
Provigil
Func. class.: Cerebral stimulant

Controlled Substance Schedule IV
Uses: Narcolepsy, sleep apnea
Unlabeled uses: Fatigue

DOSAGE AND ROUTES

• *Adult:* **PO** 200 mg daily in the AM, may increase to 400 mg daily if needed

Hepatic dose
• Reduce dose by 50%

Contraindications: Hypersensitivity, hyperthyroidism, hypertension, glaucoma, severe arteriosclerosis, drug abuse, cardiovascular disease, anxiety

---

moexipril (℞)

(moe-ex′ih-prill)
Univasc
Func. class.: Antihypertensive
Chem. class.: Angiotensin-converting enzyme inhibitor

Action: Selectively suppresses renin-angiotensin-aldosterone system; inhibits ACE; prevents conversion of angiotensin I to angiotensin II; results in dilation of arterial, venous vessels

Uses: Hypertension, alone or in combination with thiazide diuretics

---

⚠ Safety alert   *"Tall Man" lettering

DOSAGE AND ROUTES

• *Adult:* **PO** 7.5 mg 1 hr before meals initially, may be increased or divided depending on B/P response; maintenance dosage 7.5-30 mg daily in 1-2 divided doses 1 hr before meals

Renal dose

• *Adult:* **PO** CCr <40 ml/min 3.75 mg/day titrate to desired dose; max 15 mg/day

Available forms: Tabs 7.5, 15 mg

SIDE EFFECTS

CNS: Fever, chills

CV: Hypotension, postural hypotension

GI: Loss of taste

GU: Impotence, dysuria, nocturia, proteinuria, nephrotic syndrome, acute reversible renal failure, polyuria, oliguria, frequency

HEMA: **Neutropenia**

INTEG: Rash

META: Hypokalemia

RESP: **Bronchospasm,** dyspnea, dry cough

SYST: **Angioedema, anaphylaxis**

Contraindications: Pregnancy (D) 2nd/3rd trimesters, hypersensitivity, children, lactation, heart block, bilateral renal stenosis, history of angioedema

Precautions: Pregnancy (C) 1st trimester, dialysis patients, hypovolemia, leukemia, scleroderma, lupus erythematosus, blood dyscrasias, CHF, diabetes mellitus, renal disease, thyroid disease, COPD, asthma, potassium-sparing diuretics

PHARMACOKINETICS

Peak 1.5 hr; metabolized by liver (metabolites); excreted in urine, breast milk; crosses placenta; protein binding 50%-70%, half-life 2-10 hr

INTERACTIONS

• Do not use with potassium-sparing diuretics, sympathomimetics, potassium supplements

Increase: hypotension—diuretics, other antihypertensives, ganglionic blockers, adrenergic blockers, phenothiazines

Increase: toxicity—digoxin, lithium

Increase: hyperkalemia—cycloSPORINE, potassium-sparing diuretics

Increase: myelosuppression—azathioprine

Decrease: antihypertensive effect—NSAIDs

Drug/Herb

Increase: antihypertensive effect—hawthorn

Decrease: antihypertensive effect—yohimbine

Drug/Lab Test

False positive: Urine acetone

NURSING CONSIDERATIONS

Assess:

• Blood tests: neutrophils, decreased platelets

• B/P

• Renal studies: protein, BUN, creatinine; watch for increased levels that may indicate nephrotic syndrome

• Baselines in renal, hepatic studies before therapy begins

• Potassium levels, although hyperkalemia rarely occurs

• Edema in feet, legs daily

• Allergic reaction: rash, fever, pruritus, urticaria; drug should be discontinued if antihistamines fail to help

• Symptoms of CHF; edema, dyspnea, wet crackles, B/P

• Renal symptoms: polyuria, oliguria, frequency

Administer:

• PO 1 hr before meals

• Do not use with potassium-sparing diuretics, sympathomimetics, potassium supplements

Perform/provide:

• Storage in tight container at 86° F (30° C) or less

Evaluate:

• Therapeutic response: decrease in B/P in hypertension

Teach patient/family:

• To take 1 hr before meals

• Not to discontinue drug abruptly

• Not to use OTC (cough, cold, or al-

M

lergy) products unless directed by prescriber
• To comply with dosage schedule, even if feeling better
• To rise slowly to sitting or standing position to minimize orthostatic hypotension
• To notify prescriber of mouth sores, sore throat, fever, swelling of hands or feet, irregular heartbeat, chest pain, signs of angioedema
• That excessive perspiration, dehydration, vomiting, diarrhea may lead to fall in blood pressure; consult prescriber if these occur
• That dizziness, fainting, lightheadedness may occur during first few days of therapy
• That skin rash or impaired perspiration may occur
• How to take B/P
Treatment of overdose: 0.9% NaCl IV inf, hemodialysis

---

montelukast (℞)
(mon-teh-loo'kast)
Singulair
Func. class.: Bronchodilator
Chem. class.: Leukotriene antagonist, cysteinyl

Action: Inhibits leukotriene (LTD$_4$) formation; leukotrienes exert their effects by increasing neutrophil, eosinophil migration; aggregation of neutrophils, monocytes; smooth muscle contraction, capillary permeability; these actions further lead to bronchoconstriction, inflammation, edema
Uses: Chronic asthma in adults and children, seasonal allergic rhinitis
Unlabeled uses: Chronic urticaria

DOSAGE AND ROUTES
• *Adult and child ≥15 yr:* **PO** 10 mg daily PM
• *Child 6-14 yr:* **PO** 5 mg chew tab daily PM
• *Child 2-5 yr:* **PO** chew tab 4 mg daily

Asthma
• *Child 12-23 mo:* **PO** 1 packet (4 mg) of granules taken PM
Available forms: Tabs 10 mg; chew tabs 4, 5 mg; oral granules 4 mg/packet

SIDE EFFECTS
CNS: Dizziness, fatigue, headache
GI: Abdominal pain, dyspepsia, nausea, vomiting, diarrhea
INTEG: Rash
MS: Asthenia
RESP: Influenza, cough, nasal congestion
Contraindications: Hypersensitivity
Precautions: Pregnancy (B), acute attacks of asthma, alcohol consumption, lactation, child <6 yr, aspirin sensitivity, severe hepatic disease

PHARMACOKINETICS
Rapidly absorbed, peak 3-4 hr, half-life 2.7-5.5 hr; protein binding 99%; metabolized by liver, excreted via bile

INTERACTIONS
Decrease: montelukast levels—phenobarbital, rifampin
Drug/Herb
Increase: stimulation—black, green tea, guarana
Drug/Lab Test
Increase: ALT, AST

NURSING CONSIDERATIONS
Assess:
⚠ Adult patients carefully for symptoms of Churg-Strauss syndrome (rare), including eosinophilia, vasculitic rash, worsening pulmonary symptoms, cardiac complications, and/or neuropathy
• CBC, blood chemistry, during treatment
• Respiratory rate, rhythm, depth; auscultate lung fields bilaterally; notify prescriber of abnormalities
• Allergic reactions: rash, urticaria; drug should be discontinued
Administer:
PO route
• In PM daily

• Granules directly in the mouth or mixed with a spoonful of soft food (carrots, applesauce, ice cream, rice)

• Do not open granules packet until ready to use; mix whole dose; give within 15 min

Evaluate:

• Therapeutic response: ability to breathe more easily

Teach patient/family:

• To check OTC medications, current prescription medications for epHEDrine, which will increase stimulation; to avoid alcohol

• To avoid hazardous activities; dizziness may occur

• That drug is not to be used for acute asthma attacks

• If aspirin sensitivity is known, do not take NSAIDs while taking this product

• To continue to use inhaled beta-agonists if exercise-induced asthma occurs

---

moricizine (Ŗ)

(more-i′siz-een)

Ethmozine

Func. class.: Antidysrhythmic, group 1A

Chem. class.: Phenothiazine

Action: Decreased rate of rise of action potential, prolonging refractory period and shortening the action potential duration; depression of inward influx if sodium mediates the effects; drug may slow atrial and AV nodal conduction

Uses: Life-threatening ventricular dysrhythmias

DOSAGE AND ROUTES

Hospitalization is required when initiating therapy

• *Adult:* PO 10-15 mg/kg/day or 600-900 mg/day in 2-3 divided doses

Hepatic dose

• *Adult:* PO 600 mg or less daily

Available forms: Film-coated tabs 200, 250, 300 mg

SIDE EFFECTS

CNS: Dizziness, headache, fatigue, perioral numbness, euphoria, nervousness, sleep disorders, depression, tinnitus, fatigue, anxiety

CV: Palpitations, chest pain, **CHF,** hypertension, syncope, dysrhythmias, bradycardia, **MI, thrombophlebitis,** ECG abnormalities, **cardiac arrest**

GI: Nausea, abdominal pain, vomiting, diarrhea

GU: Sexual dysfunction, difficult urination, dysuria, incontinence, urinary retention

MISC: Sweating, musculoskeletal pain, drug fever, blurred vision, dry mouth

RESP: Dyspnea, hyperventilation, **apnea,** asthma, pharyngitis, cough

Contraindications: 2nd-/3rd-degree AV block, right bundle branch block, cardiogenic shock, hypersensitivity

Precautions: Pregnancy (B), CHF, hypokalemia, hyperkalemia, sick sinus syndrome, lactation, children, impaired hepatic and renal function, cardiac dysfunction

PHARMACOKINETICS

Half-life 1.5-3.5 hr; peak 0.5-2.2 hr; metabolized by the liver; metabolites excreted in feces and urine, protein binding >90%

INTERACTIONS

• Digoxin or propranolol may enhance some cardiac effects of moricizine; moricizine may decrease effects of theophylline

Increase: plasma levels of moricizine—cimetidine

Decrease: effects of theophylline

Drug/Herb

Increase: anticholinergic effect—henbane

Increase: hypokalemia, increase antidysrhythmic action—aloe, buckthorn, cascara sagrada, rhubarb, senna

Increase: toxicity, death—aconite
Increase: effect—aloe, broom, chronic buckthorn use, cascara sagrada (chronic use), Chinese rhubarb, figwort, fumitory, goldenseal, kudzu, licorice
Increase: serotonin effect—horehound
Decrease: effect—coltsfoot
Drug/Lab Test
Increase: CPK

NURSING CONSIDERATIONS
Assess:
• GI status: bowel pattern, number of stools
• Cardiac status: rate, rhythm, quality
• Chest x-ray, pulmonary function test during treatment
• I&O ratio; check for decreasing output
• B/P for fluctuations
• Lung fields: bilateral crackles may occur in CHF patient
• Increased respirations, increased pulse; drug should be discontinued
⚠ Toxicity: fine tremors, dizziness, emesis, lethargy, coma, syncope, hypotension, conduction disturbances
• Cardiac status: respiration, rate, rhythm, character continuously
Administer:
• Initiate therapy in hospital
• Dosage adjustment should be ≥3 days
Evaluate:
• Therapeutic response: absence of dysrhythmias
Teach patient/family:
• To report side effects to prescriber
• To take exactly as prescribed, take consistently with respect to meals
Treatment of overdose: O₂ artificial ventilation, ECG; administer DOPamine for circulatory depression, diazepam or thiopental for seizures

⚠ High Alert

morphine (℞)
(mor′feen)
Astramorph, Astramorph PF, Avinza, Duramorph, Epimorph ♣, Infumorph, Kadian, morphine sulfate, Morphitec ♣, M.O.S. ♣, M.O.S.-S.R. ♣, MS Contin, MSIR, OMS Concentrate, Oramorph SR, RMS, Roxanol, Roxanol Rescudose, Roxanol-T, Statex
Func. class.: Opioid analgesic

Controlled Substance Schedule II
Do not confuse:
morphine/hydromorphone
Roxanol/Roxicet
Action: Depresses pain impulse transmission at the spinal cord level by interacting with opioid receptors
Uses: Severe pain

DOSAGE AND ROUTES
• *Adult:* **SUBCUT/IM** 5-20 mg q4h prn; **PO** 10-30 mg q4h prn; **EXT REL** 70-kg patient q8-12h; **RECT** 10-30 mg q4h prn; **IV** 4-10 mg diluted in 4-5 ml H₂O for inj, over 5 min; **SUS REL** caps (Kadian), **EXT REL** caps (Avinza) give total daily dose q24h; for those with no tolerance to opioids, 30 mg daily; may adjust by no more than 30 mg q4d.
• *Child:* **SUBCUT/IV** 0.1-0.2 mg/kg, not to exceed 15 mg; **PO** 0.2-0.5 mg/kg q4-6h (reg rel), q12h (sus rel)
Available forms: Inj 0.5, 1, 2, 3, 4, 5, 8, 10, 15, 25, 50 mg/ml; sol tabs 10, 15, 30 mg; oral sol 10, 20 mg/5 ml, 20 mg/10 ml, 20 mg/ml; oral tabs 15, 30 mg; rect supp 5, 10, 20, 30 mg; ext rel tabs 15, 30, 60, 100, 200 mg; caps 15, 30 mg; syr 1, 5 mg/ml; cont rel cap pellets (Kadian) 20, 30, 50, 60, 100 mg; ext rel caps (Avinza) 30, 60, 90, 120 mg

SIDE EFFECTS

CNS: Drowsiness, dizziness, confusion, headache, sedation, euphoria

CV: Palpitations, **bradycardia**, change in B/P, **shock, cardiac arrest**

EENT: Tinnitus, blurred vision, miosis, diplopia

GI: Nausea, vomiting, anorexia, constipation, cramps, biliary tract pressure

GU: Urinary retention

HEMA: **Thrombocytopenia**

INTEG: Rash, urticaria, bruising, flushing, diaphoresis, pruritus

RESP: **Respiratory depression, respiratory arrest, apnea**

Contraindications: Hypersensitivity, addiction (opioid), hemorrhage, bronchial asthma, increased intracranial pressure

Precautions: Pregnancy (C), addictive personality, lactation, acute MI, severe heart disease, geriatric, respiratory depression, renal/hepatic disease, child <18 yr

PHARMACOKINETICS

PO: Onset variable, peak variable, duration variable

IM: Onset ½ hr, peak ½-1 hr, duration 3-7 hr

SUBCUT: Onset 15-20 min, peak 50-90 min, duration 3-5 hr

IV: Peak 20 min

RECT: Peak ½-1 hr, duration 4-5 hr

Intrathecal: Onset rapid, duration up to 24 hr

Metabolized by liver, crosses placenta; excreted in urine, breast milk; half-life 1½-2 hr

INTERACTIONS

• Unpredictable reaction, avoid use: MAOIs

Increase: effects with other CNS depressants—alcohol, opiates, sedative/hypnotics, antipsychotics, skeletal muscle relaxants

Decrease: morphine action—rifampin

Drug/Herb

Increase: anticholinergic effect—corkwood

Increase: CNS depression—chamomile, hops, Jamaican dogwood, kava, lavender, mistletoe, nettle, pokeweed, poppy, senega, skullcap, valerian

Decrease: morphine effect—cranberry juice (excessive amounts), oats

Drug/Lab Test

Increase: Amylase

NURSING CONSIDERATIONS

Assess:

• Pain: location, type, character; give dose before pain becomes severe

• Bowel status; constipation common

• I&O ratio; check for decreasing output; may indicate urinary retention

• B/P, pulse, respirations (character, depth, rate)

• CNS changes: dizziness, drowsiness, hallucinations, euphoria, LOC, pupil reaction

• Allergic reactions: rash, urticaria

• Respiratory dysfunction: depression, character, rate, rhythm; notify prescriber if respirations are <12/min

Administer:

• May be given by patient: controlled analgesia

• Epidural cautiously in the geriatric

• Kadian is not bioequivalent to other controlled release forms

• Kadian caps may be opened and sprinkled on applesauce immediately before use; pellets in the cap should not be chewed, crushed, or dissolved, which may lead to overdose; adjustments may need to be made when converting from another form of morphine

PO route

• Do not break, crush, or chew controlled or sus rel products

• With antiemetic for nausea, vomiting

• When pain is beginning to return; determine dosage interval by response; continuous dosing is more effective than prn

IV route

• After diluting with 5 ml or more sterile H_2O or NS; give 15 mg or less over 4-5 min; give through Y-tube or 3-way stopcock; may be added to IV sol, each 0.1-1 mg diluted in 1 ml D_5W, $D_{10}W$, 0.9% NaCl, 0.45% NaCl, Ringer's sol, LR, given with inf pump titrated to patient response

M

Side effects: *italics* = common; **bold** = life-threatening

Additive compatibilities: Alteplase, atracurium, baclofen, bupivacaine, DOBUTamine, fluconazole, furosemide, meropenem, metoclopramide, ondansetron, succinylcholine, verapamil

Syringe compatibilities: Atropine, benzquinamide, bupivacaine, butorphanol, cimetidine, dimenhyDRINATE, diphenhydrAMINE, droperidol, fentanyl, glycopyrrolate, hydrOXYzine, ketamine, metoclopramide, midazolam, milrinone, pentazocine, perphenazine, promazine, ranitidine, scopolamine

Y-site compatibilities: Allopurinol, amifostine, amikacin, aminophylline, amiodarone, ampicillin, ampicillin/sulbactam, amsacrine, atenolol, atracurium, aztreonam, bumetanide, calcium chloride, cefamandole, cefazolin, cefmetazole, cefo perazone, cefotaxime, cefotetan, cefoxitin, ceftazidime, ceftizoxime, ceftriaxone, cefuroxime, cephalothin, cephapirin, chloramphenicol, cisatracurium, cisplatin, cladribine, clindamycin, cyclophosphamide, cytarabine, dexamethasone, digoxin, diltiazem, DOBUTamine, DOPamine, doxycycline, enalaprilat, epiNEPHrine, erythromycin, esmolol, etomidate, famotidine, fentanyl, filgrastim, fluconazole, fludarabine, foscarnet, gentamicin, granisetron, heparin, hydrocortisone, hydromorphone, IL-2, insulin (regular), kanamycin, labetalol, lidocaine, lorazepam, magnesium sulfate, melphalan, meropenem, methotrexate, methyldopate, methylPREDNISolone, metoclopramide, metoprolol, metronidazole, mezlocillin, midazolam, milrinone, moxalactam, nafcillin, niCARdipine, nitroglycerin, norepinephrine, ondansetron, oxacillin, oxytocin, paclitaxel, pancuronium, penicillin G potassium, piperacillin, piperacillin/tazobactam, potassium chloride, propofol, propranolol, ranitidine, remifentanil, sodium bicarbonate, sodium nitroprusside, teniposide, thiotepa, ticarcillin, ticarcillin/clavulanate, tobramycin, trimethoprim-sulfamethoxazole, vancomycin, vecuronium, vinorelbine, vit B/C, warfarin, zidovudine

Perform/provide:
• Storage in light-resistant container at room temperature
• Assistance with ambulation
• Safety measures: side rails, night-light, call bell within easy reach
• Gradual withdrawal after long-term use

Evaluate:
• Therapeutic response; decrease in pain intensity

Teach patient/family:
• To change position slowly; orthostatic hypotension may occur
• To report any symptoms of CNS changes, allergic reactions
• That physical dependency may result from long-term use
• To avoid use of alcohol, CNS depressants
• That withdrawal symptoms may occur: nausea, vomiting, cramps, fever, faintness, anorexia

Treatment of overdose: Naloxone (Narcan) 0.2-0.8 mg IV, O_2, IV fluids, vasopressors

moxifloxacin
Avelox, Avelox IV
Func. class.: Antiinfective
Chem. class.: Fluoroquinolone

Action: Interferes with conversion of intermediate DNA fragments into high-molecular-weight DNA in bacteria; DNA gyrase inhibitor

Uses: Acute bacterial sinusitis: *Streptococcus pneumoniae, Haemophilus influenzae, Moraxella catarrhalis;* acute bacterial exacerbation of chronic bronchitis: *S. pneumoniae, H. influenzae, Haemophilus parainfluenzae, Klebsiella pneumoniae, Staphylococcus aureus, M. catarrhalis;* community-acquired pneumonia: *S. pneumoniae, H. influenzae, Mycoplasma pneumoniae, Chlamydia pneumoniae, M. catarrhalis;* uncomplicated skin/skin structure infections: *S. aureus, Streptococcus pyogenes;* complicated intraabdominal infections including polymicrobial infections: *E. coli,*

A Safety alert   *"Tall Man" lettering

Bacterioides fragilis, S. anginosus, S. constellatus, Enterococcus faecalis, Proteus mirabilis, Clostridium perfringens, Bacteroides thetaiotaomicron, Peptostreptococcus, sp; complicated skin, skin structure infections caused by methicillin-susceptible: *S. aureus, E. coli, K. pneumoniae, Enterobacter cloacae*

DOSAGE AND ROUTES
Acute bacterial sinusitis
• *Adult:* **PO/IV** 400 mg q24h × 10 days
Acute bacterial exacerbation of chronic bronchitis
• *Adult:* **PO/IV** 400 mg q24h × 5 days
Community-acquired pneumonia
• *Adult:* **PO/IV** 400 mg q24h × 7-14 days
Uncomplicated skin/skin structure infections
• *Adult:* **PO/IV** 400 mg q24h × 7 days
Complicated intraabdominal infections
• *Adult:* **IV** 400 mg daily × 5-14 days
Complicated skin, skin structure infections
• *Adult:* **PO/IV** 400 mg daily × 7-21 days
Available forms: Tabs 400 mg; inj premix 400 mg

SIDE EFFECTS
CNS: Headache, dizziness, fatigue, insomnia, depression, *restlessness,* **seizures,** confusion, **increased intracranial pressure**
CV: Prolonged QT interval, **dysrhythmias,** torsade de pointes, tachycardia
EENT: Blurred vision, tinnitus
GI: Nausea, diarrhea, increased ALT, AST, flatulence, heartburn, *vomiting,* oral candidiasis, dysphagia, **pseudomembranous colitis**
INTEG: Rash, pruritus, urticaria, photosensitivity, flushing, fever, chills
MS: Tremor, arthralgia, tendon rupture
SYST: **Anaphylaxis, Stevens-Johnson syndrome**
Contraindications: Hypersensitivity to quinolones
Precautions: Pregnancy (C), lactation, children, renal/GI disease, epilepsy, uncorrected hypokalemia, prolonged QT interval, patients receiving class IA, III antidysrhythmics, tendon pain, seizure disorder

PHARMACOKINETICS
Excreted in urine as active drug, metabolites; parent drug excreted in urine and feces

INTERACTIONS
• Prolonged QT: antidysrhythmics class IA, III
Increase: moxifloxacin serum levels—probenecid
Increase: warfarin, cycloSPORINE effect
Decrease: moxifloxacin absorption—magnesium antacids, aluminum hydroxide, zinc, iron, sucralfate, calcium, enteral feeding, didanosine
Drug/Herb
• Do not use acidophilus with antiinfectives; separate by several hours
Increase: antiinfective effect—cola tree

NURSING CONSIDERATIONS
Assess:
• CNS symptoms: headache, dizziness, fatigue, insomnia, depression, seizures
• Renal, hepatic studies: BUN, creatinine, AST, ALT
• I&O ratio, urine pH <5.5 is ideal
⚠ Allergic reactions and anaphylaxis: fever, flushing, rash, urticaria, pruritus; keep epINEPHrine, emergency equipment nearby for anaphylaxis
Administer:
PO route
• 4 hr before or 8 hr after antacids, zinc, iron, calcium
IV route
• Discontinue primary IV while administering moxifloxacin
• Do not give SUBCUT, IM
Solution compatibilities: 0.9% NaCl, D_5, D_{10}, LR, sterile water for inj
Perform/provide:
• Limited intake of alkaline foods, drugs: milk, dairy products, alkaline antacids, sodium bicarbonate

• That fluids must be increased to 3 L/day to avoid crystallization in kidneys

Evaluate:

• Therapeutic response: decreased pain, C&S; absence of infection

Teach patient/family:

• Not to take any products containing magnesium or calcium (such as antacids), iron, or aluminum with this drug or within 8 hr of drug

• That photosensitivity may occur; patient should avoid sunlight or use sunscreen to prevent burns

• To use frequent rinsing of mouth, sugarless candy or gum for dry mouth

• To take as prescribed, not to double or miss doses

• If dizziness occurs, to ambulate, perform activities with assistance

• To complete full course of drug therapy

• To contact prescriber if adverse reaction occurs or if inflammation or pain in tendon occurs

---

moxifloxacin ophthalmic
See Appendix C

---

multivitamins (otc, ℞)

Adavite, Dayalets, LKV Drops, Multi-75, Multiday, One-A-Day, Optilets, Poly-Vi-sol, Quin tabs, Ru-Lets, Sesame Street Vitamins, Tab-A-Vite, Therabid, Theragran, Unicaps, Vita-Bob, Vita-Kid, many other brands

Func. class.: Vitamins, multiple

Do not confuse:

Theragran/Phenergan

Action: Needed for adequate metabolism

Uses: Prevention and treatment of vitamin deficiencies

DOSAGE AND ROUTES

• *Adult and child:* **PO/IV**—depends on brand

Available forms: Many

SIDE EFFECTS

None known at recommended dosage

Precautions: Pregnancy (A)

NURSING CONSIDERATIONS

Assess:

• Vitamin deficiency: usually more than one vitamin is deficient

Administer:

• Liquid multivitamins diluted or dropped into patient's mouth using dropper provided with some brands

• Chew tabs should be chewed, not swallowed whole

• Give by cont IV inf only after diluting 5-10 ml multivitamins/500-1000 ml of D_5W, $D_{10}W$, $D_{20}W$, LR, D_5/LR, D_5/0.9% NaCl, 0.9% NaCl, 3% NaCl

• Do not use sol with crystals, precipitate, or color other than bright yellow

Additive compatibilities: Cefoxitin, isoproterenol, methyldopa, metoclopramide, metronidazole, netilmicin, norepinephrine, sodium bicarbonate, verapamil

Y-site compatibilities: Acyclovir, ampicillin, cefazolin, cephalothin, cephapirin, diltiazem, erythromycin, fludarabine, gentamicin, tacrolimus

Evaluate:

• Therapeutic response: check each individual vitamin for guidelines

Teach patient/family:

• That adequate nutrition must be maintained to prevent further deficiencies

• To comply with regimen

• To avoid presenting flavored multivitamins as candy; child may overdose

• To store out of children's reach

---

mupirocin topical
See Appendix C

---

muromonab-CD3 (℞)
(mur-oo-mone′ab)
Orthoclone OKT3
Func. class.: Immunosuppressant
Chem. class.: Murine monoclonal antibody

Action: Reverses graft rejection by blocking T-cell function
Uses: Acute allograft rejection in renal, cardiac/hepatic transplant patients

DOSAGE AND ROUTES
• *Adult:* **IV BOL** 5 mg/day × 10-14 days
• *Child:* **IV** 100 mcg/kg/day × 10-14 days

Cardiac/hepatic allograft rejection, steroid resistant
• *Adult:* **IV BOL** 5 mg/day × 10-14 days; begin when it is known that rejection has not been reversed by steroids
Available forms: Inj 5 mg/5 ml

SIDE EFFECTS
CNS: Pyrexia, chills, tremors, **aseptic meningitis,** *fever*
CV: Chest pain
GI: Vomiting, nausea, diarrhea
MISC: **Infection, cytokine release syndrome, anaphylaxis**
RESP: Dyspnea, wheezing, **pulmonary edema**

Contraindications: Hypersensitivity to murine origin, fluid overload
Precautions: Pregnancy (C), child <2 yr, fever

PHARMACOKINETICS
Trough level steady state 3-14 days

INTERACTIONS
Increase: immunosuppression—immunosuppressants
Increase: infection risk—cycloSPORINE, corticosteroids, azathioprine
Increase: CNS symptoms—indomethacin
Decrease: immune response—vaccines

Drug/Herb
• Interference with immunosuppression: astragalus, echinacea, melatonin
Decrease: effect—ginseng, maitake, mistletoe, schisandra, St. John's wort, turmeric

NURSING CONSIDERATIONS
Assess:
⚠ For cytokine release syndrome (CRS): nausea, vomiting, chills, fever, joint pain, weakness, dizziness, diarrhea, tremors, abdominal pain; usually occurs within 30-48 hr and may last 6 hr; treat with antihistamines, acetaminophen
⚠ For hypersensitivity, anaphylaxis: dyspnea, bronchospasm, urticaria, tachycardia, angioedema; emergency equipment must be available
• Blood studies: Hgb, WBC, platelets during treatment qmo; if leukocytes are <3000/mm³, drug should be discontinued; CD3, CD4, CD8, CD3 ≤25 cells/mm³
• Hepatic studies: alk phos, AST, ALT, bilirubin
⚠ Hepatotoxicity: dark urine, jaundice, itching, light-colored stools; drug should be discontinued
• For infection: sore throat, fever, chills, temp, notify prescriber immediately
⚠ For aseptic meningitis: fever, headache, photophobia
⚠ For fluid overload: increased weight, I&O, edema, crackles
Administer:
• Pretreat with corticosteroids, acetaminophen, or antihistamines
• For several days before transplant surgery
• All medications PO if possible; avoid IM injection, since infection may occur
IV route
• IV undiluted; withdraw with a 0.2-0.22 low protein-binding μm filter, discard and use new needle for administration; give over 1 min
• Incompatible with any drug in syringe or sol; do not admix
Evaluate:
• Therapeutic response: absence of graft rejection

Teach patient/family:
• To report fever, chills, sore throat, fatigue, since serious infection may occur; rash, dyspnea, fast heartbeat
• To use contraceptive measures during treatment
• To report cytokine release syndrome, give symptoms
• To avoid vaccinations during treatment
• To avoid persons with infections, crowds; infections may occur

mycophenolate (Ṝ)
(mye-koe-phen′oh-late)
CellCept, Myfortic
Func. class.: Immunosuppressant

Action: Inhibits inflammatory responses that are mediated by the immune system; prolongs the survival of allogenic transplants
Uses: Organ transplants (to prevent rejection); prophylaxis of organ rejection in allogenic cardiac, hepatic, renal transplants
Unlabeled uses: Refractory uveitis, second-line therapy for Churg-Strauss syndrome, diffuse proliferative lupus nephritis (in combination), rheumatoid arthritis, psoriasis

DOSAGE AND ROUTES
Renal transplant
• *Adult:* **PO/IV** give initial dose 72 hr prior to transplantation; 1 g bid given to renal transplant patients in combination with corticosteroids, cycloSPORINE; **TAB ER** 720 mg bid on empty stomach
• *Child:* **PO-ER** 400 mg/m² bid, max 720 mg bid
Renal dose
• *Adult:* **PO/IV** GFR <25 ml/min, max 2 g/day
Cardiac transplant
• *Adult:* **PO/IV** 1.5 g bid, IV can be started ≤24 hr after transplant, switch to **PO** when able
Hepatic transplant
• *Adult:* **PO/IV** 1.5 g bid; give IV over ≥2 hr

Available forms: Caps 250 mg; tabs 500 mg; inj (powder) 500 mg/20-ml vial; powder for oral susp 200 mg/ml; ext rel tab (Myfortic) 180, 360 mg

SIDE EFFECTS
CNS: Tremor, dizziness, insomnia, headache, fever
CV: Hypertension, chest pain
GI: Diarrhea, constipation, nausea, vomiting, stomatitis, **GI bleeding**
GU: UTI, hematuria, **renal tubular necrosis**
HEMA: **Leukopenia, thrombocytopenia, anemia, pancytopenia**
INTEG: Rash
META: Peripheral edema, hypercholesterolemia, hypophosphatemia, edema, hyperkalemia, hypokalemia, hyperglycemia
MS: Arthralgia, muscle wasting
RESP: Dyspnea, respiratory infection, increased cough, pharyngitis, bronchitis, pneumonia
SYST: **Lymphoma,** *nonmelanoma skin carcinoma,* **sepsis**
Contraindications: Hypersensitivity to this drug or mycophenolic acid
Precautions: Pregnancy (C), lymphomas, malignancies, neutropenia, renal disease, lactation

PHARMACOKINETICS
Rapidly and completely absorbed, metabolized to active metabolite (MPA), excreted in urine, feces, protein binding (MPA) 97%, half-life (MPA) 17.9 hr

INTERACTIONS
• Avoid administration with azathioprine
Increase: effects of phenytoin, theophylline
Increase: concentration of both drugs—acyclovir, ganciclovir
Increase: mycophenolate levels—probenecid, salicylates
Decrease: mycophenolate levels—antacids, cholestyramine

Decrease: protein binding of phenytoin, theophylline
Decrease: effect of live attenuated vaccines, oral contraceptives
Drug/Herb
Interference with immunosuppressant astragalus, echinacea, melatonin
Drug/Food
Decrease: absorption if taken with food

NURSING CONSIDERATIONS

Assess:
• Blood studies: CBC during treatment monthly
• Hepatic studies: alk phos, AST, ALT, bilirubin
• Renal studies and electrolytes
Administer:
• 72 hr prior to transplantation; may be given in combination with corticosteroids, cycloSPORINE
PO route
• Do not break, crush, or chew tabs; do not open caps
• At same time each day
• Avoid inhalation or direct contact with skin, mucous membranes, teratogenic in animals
• Oral susp: tap the closed bottle several times to loosen powder, use 94 ml of water in graduated cylinder, add ½ the total amount of water for constitution and shake the closed bottle, add remaining water and shake, again remove child resistant cap and push adapter into neck of the bottle, close tightly
• Give alone for better absorption
IV route
• Do not give by rapid or bolus inj; reconstitute and dilute to 6 mg/ml with D₅W, give over ≥2 hr
• Do not admix with mycophenolate IV in infusion catheter or with other IV drugs or infusion admixtures
Evaluate:
• Therapeutic response: absence of graft rejection
Teach patient/family:
• To report fever, rash, severe diarrhea, chills, sore throat, fatigue, since serious infections may occur

• To reduce risk of infection by avoiding crowds
• The need for repeated lab tests
• To limit exposure to sunlight/UV light
• To use contraception before, during, and 6 wk after therapy
• To take at same time each day

---

nabilone (℞)
(nab'ih-lohn)
Cesamet
Func. class.: Antiemetic
Chem. class.: Cannabinoid—miscellaneous

Action: Orally, active cannabinoid, chemically related to marijuana; may decrease nausea by action on cannabinoid receptors in the CNS
Uses: Prevention of nausea, vomiting associated with cancer chemotherapy, in those who have not responded to other treatment; not to be used on an as needed basis

DOSAGE AND ROUTES

• *Adult:* **PO** 1-2 mg bid; give initial dose 1-3 hr prior to chemotherapy; start with lower dose and increase as needed; may give dose of 1-2 mg the night before chemotherapy; may give 2-3 times daily during chemotherapy cycle
Available forms: Caps 1 mg

SIDE EFFECTS

CNS: Headache, ataxia, drowsiness, dysphoria, euphoria, sleep disturbance, vertigo, asthenia, concentration difficulties, depression, syncope, hallucinations
CV: Chest discomfort, **tachycardia,** orthostatic hypotension
GI: Dry mouth, nausea, *anorexia,* increased appetite
INTEG: Allergic reactions, rash, photosensitivity, pruritus
MS: Back, joint, muscle, neck pain
Contraindications: Hypersensitivity to this product or cannabinoids

---

Precautions: Pregnancy (C), lactation, depression, mental disorders, severe renal/hepatic disease, hypertension, tachycardia, CV disorders

PHARMACOKINETICS

Absorption rapid, 10%-20% absorbed, duration is unpredictable, psychiatric symptoms may occur for up to 72 hr after treatment is concluded, terminal half-life 2 hr, metabolized by the liver, excreted via biliary system in feces

INTERACTIONS

• Hypomanic reaction: disulfiram and possibly fluoxetine
Increase: hypertension, tachycardia, and possibly cardiotoxicity—sympathomimetics (amphetamines, cocaine)
Increase: tachycardia, drowsiness—anticholinergics (antihistamines, atropine, scopolamine)
Increase: drowsiness, CNS depression—CNS depressants (alcohol, barbiturates, benzodiazepines, busPIRone, lithium, muscle relaxants, opioids)
Increase: action or nabilone—naltrexone
Increase: action of both—opioids
Increase: tachycardia, hypertension, drowsiness—tricyclics
Decrease: metabolism of theophylline

NURSING CONSIDERATIONS

Assess:
• For absence of nausea and vomiting during chemotherapy
• CNS symptoms: headache, depression, ataxia, drowsiness, dysphoria, euphoria, sleep disturbances, concentration difficulties
• CV symptoms, cardiac status: tachycardia, orthostatic hypotension, hypertension
• Psychiatric symptoms: euphoria, depression, sleep disturbance
Administer:
• PO, not to be used on an as-needed basis

Perform/provide:
• Storage of capsules at room temperature, away from light and moisture
Evaluate:
• Therapeutic response: decreased nausea and vomiting associated with chemotherapy
Teach patient/family:
• That mood, behavioral changes may occur while taking this product
• To notify prescriber if pregnancy is suspected
• To avoid breastfeeding while taking this product
• Not to use alcohol or other CNS depressants unless approved by prescriber
• Not to operate machinery or perform other hazardous activities while taking this product

nabumetone (℞)
(na-byoo'me-tone)
Relafen
Func. class.: Nonsteroidal antiinflammatory
Chem. class.: Acetic acid derivative

Action: Inhibits prostaglandin synthesis by decreasing enzyme needed for biosynthesis; analgesic, antiinflammatory
Uses: Osteoarthritis, rheumatoid arthritis, acute or chronic treatment

DOSAGE AND ROUTES

• *Adult:* **PO** 1 g as a single dose; may increase to 2 g/day if needed; may give daily or bid as a divided dose
Available forms: Tabs 500, 750 mg

SIDE EFFECTS

CNS: Dizziness, headache, drowsiness, fatigue, tremors, confusion, insomnia, anxiety, depression, nervousness
CV: Tachycardia, peripheral edema, palpitations, dysrhythmias, **CHF, MI, stroke**
GI: Nausea, anorexia, vomiting, diarrhea, jaundice, **cholestatic hepatitis**, constipation, flatulence, cramps, dry mouth, peptic ulcer, gastritis, **ulceration, perforation, bleeding**

GU: **Nephrotoxicity, dysuria, hematuria, oliguria, azotemia,** cystitis
HEMA: **Blood dyscrasias**
INTEG: Purpura, rash, pruritus, sweating, photosensitivity
RESP: Dyspnea, pharyngitis, **bronchospasm**
SYST: **Anaphylaxis, angioneurotic edema**

Contraindications: Hypersensitivity to this drug or aspirin, iodides, NSAIDs, asthma, severe renal/hepatic disease, avoid in late pregnancy, perioperative pain
Precautions: Pregnancy (C); lactation, children, bleeding disorders, GI disorders, cardiac disorders, renal disorders, hepatic dysfunction, geriatric

PHARMACOKINETICS

PO: Peak 2½-4 hr, plasma protein binding >90%, half-life 22-30 hr; metabolized in liver to active metabolite; excreted in urine (metabolites), breast milk

INTERACTIONS

Increase: bleeding risk—anticoagulants, thrombolytics, valproic acid, cefamandole, cefotetan, cefoperazone, plicamycin, clopidogrel, eptifibatide, ticlopidine
Increase: hematologic reactions risk—antineoplastics, radiation
Increase: GI reactions—salicylates, NSAIDs, alcohol, potassium, corticosteroids
Decrease: effect of diuretics, antihypertensives

Drug/Herb
Increase: gastric irritation—arginine, gossypol
Increase: NSAIDs effect—bearberry, bilberry
Increase: bleeding risk—bogbean, chondroitin

Drug/Lab Test
Increase: Bleeding time, K, BUN, AST, ALT, LDH, alk phos, creatinine
Decrease: CCr, blood glucose, Hct, Hgb

NURSING CONSIDERATIONS

Assess:
⚠ Cardiac status: CV thrombotic events, MI, stroke; may be fatal
⚠ GI status: ulceration, bleeding, perforation; may be fatal
• Pain: frequency, intensity, characteristics; relief of pain after med
• Asthma, aspirin sensitivity or nasal polyps; increased hypersensitivity reactions
• Renal, hepatic studies: BUN, creatinine, AST, ALT, Hgb, LDH, blood glucose, WBC, platelets, CCr before treatment, periodically thereafter
• Audiometric, ophthalmic exam before, during, after treatment
• For eye, ear problems: blurred vision, tinnitus; may indicate toxicity

Administer:
• With food for GI symptoms

Perform/provide:
• Storage at room temperature

Evaluate:
• Therapeutic response: decreased pain and stiffness in joints

Teach patient/family:
• To avoid alcoholic beverages and aspirin
• To report blurred vision, ringing, roaring in ears; may indicate toxicity
• To avoid driving, other hazardous activities if dizziness, drowsiness occur
• To report change in urine pattern, increased weight, edema, increased pain in joints, fever, blood in urine; indicates nephrotoxicity
• That therapeutic effects may take up to 1 mo
• To take with a full glass of water to enhance absorption and sit upright for 30 min
• To report dark stools; may indicate GI bleeding
• To use sunscreen, protective clothing if in the sun

nadolol (℞)

(nay-doe'lole)
Corgard, Syn-Nadolol ♣
Func. class.: Antihypertensive, anti-anginal
Chem. class.: β-Adrenergic receptor blocker

Do not confuse:

Corgard/Cognex

Action: Long-acting, nonselective β-adrenergic receptor blocking agent, blocks β_1 in the heart and β_2 in the lungs, uterus, and circulatory system; mechanism is similar to that of propranolol

Uses: Chronic stable angina pectoris, mild to moderate hypertension

Unlabeled uses: Tachydysrhythmias, aggression, anxiety, tremors, esophageal varices (rebleeding only), hyperthyroidism adjunctive therapy, prophylaxis of migraine headaches

DOSAGE AND ROUTES

• *Adult:* **PO** 40 mg daily, increase by 40-80 mg q3-7d; maintenance 40-240 mg/day for angina, 40-320 mg/day for hypertension
• *Geriatric:* **PO** 20 mg/day, may increase by 20 mg until desired dose
Renal dose
• *Adult:* **PO** CCr 31-50 ml/min give q24-36h; CCr 10-30 ml/min give q24-48h; CCr <10 ml/min give q40-60h

Available forms: Tabs 20, 40, 80, 120, 160 mg

SIDE EFFECTS

CNS: Depression, dizziness, *fatigue,* lethargy, paresthesias, headache, *weakness,* insomnia, memory loss, nightmares
CV: **Bradycardia,** *hypotension,* **CHF,** palpitations, **AV block,** chest pain, peripheral ischemia, flushing, edema, vasodilation, conduction disturbances
EENT: Blurred vision, dry eyes, nasal congestion

ENDO: Hyperglycemia, hypoglycemia
GI: Nausea, vomiting, diarrhea, colitis, constipation, cramps, dry mouth, flatulence, hepatomegaly, **pancreatitis,** taste distortion
GU: Impotence, decreased libido
HEMA: **Agranulocytosis, thrombocytopenia**
INTEG: Rash, pruritus, fever, alopecia
RESP: Dyspnea, respiratory dysfunction, **bronchospasm,** cough, wheezing, **pulmonary edema,** pharyngitis, **laryngospasm**

Contraindications: Hypersensitivity to this drug, cardiac failure, cardiogenic shock, 2nd, 3rd degree heart block, bronchospastic disease, sinus bradycardia, CHF, COPD

Precautions: Pregnancy (C), diabetes mellitus, renal disease, lactation, hyperthyroidism, peripheral vascular disease, myasthenia gravis, major surgery, nonallergic bronchospasm

PHARMACOKINETICS

PO: Onset variable, peak 3-4 hr, duration 17-24 hr; half-life 20-24 hr; not metabolized; excreted in urine (unchanged), bile, breast milk; protein binding 30%

INTERACTIONS

• Do not use with MAOIs; bradycardia may occur
• Peripheral ischemia: ergots
Increase: bradycardia—digoxin
Increase: hypotension, bradycardia—clonidine, epINEPHrine
Increase: hypotensive effects—other hypotensive agents, phenothiazines
Decrease: β-blocking effect—thyroid hormones
Decrease: antihypertensive effect—NSAIDs
Drug/Herb
Increase: toxicity, death—aconite
Increase: antihypertensive effect—barberry, betony, black catechu, black cohosh, bloodroot, broom, burdock, cat's claw, dandelion, goldenseal, Irish moss,

Jamaican dogwood, kelp, khella, mistletoe, parsley

Increase or decrease: antihypertensive effect—astragalus, cola tree

Decrease: antihypertensive effect—coltsfoot, guarana, khat, licorice

Drug/Lab Test

Increase: Serum potassium, serum uric acid, ALT, AST, alk phos, LDH, blood glucose, cholesterol, ANA, triglycerides

NURSING CONSIDERATIONS

Assess:

• B/P, pulse, respirations during beginning therapy, orthostatic hypotension may occur

• Weight daily; report gain of 5 lb

• I&O ratio, CCr if kidney damage is diagnosed; crackles, jugular vein distention, fatigue, dyspnea

• Pain: duration, time started, activity being performed, character

• Headache, light-headedness, decreased B/P; may indicate a need for decreased dosage

Administer:

• With 8 oz water

Evaluate:

• Therapeutic response: decreased B/P, heart rate, symptoms of angina

Teach patient/family:

• That drug may mask signs of hypoglycemia or alter blood glucose in diabetics

⚠ Not to discontinue abruptly, serious dysrhythmias may occur

• To avoid OTC drugs unless prescriber approves

• To avoid hazardous activities if dizziness occurs

• To comply with complete medical regimen

• To rise slowly to prevent orthostatic hypotension

• How and when to check B/P and pulse; to hold dose if pulse ≤50 bpm and contact prescriber

nafarelin (Ƀ)
(naf-ah-rell′in)
Synarel
Func. class.: Gonadotropin
Chem. class.: Analog of gonadotropin-releasing hormone

Action: Stimulates the release of LH and FSH, which increases ovarian steroid production; repeated dosing prevents stimulation of the pituitary gland

Uses: Endometriosis, gonadotropin-dependent precocious puberty

DOSAGE AND ROUTES

• *Adult:* **NASAL** 400 mcg/day as one spray (200 mcg) into one nostril in morning and one spray into other nostril in evening; start treatment between days 2 and 4 of menstrual cycle; may increase to 800 mcg/day (one spray into each nostril twice a day); recommended duration of treatment is 6 mo

• *Child:* **NASAL** 2 sprays in each nostril AM and PM, may increase to 3 sprays alternating nostril tid

Available forms: Nasal spray 2 mg/ml (200 mcg/spray)

SIDE EFFECTS

CNS: Headache, flushing, depression, insomnia, *emotional lability,* hot flashes

GU: Decreased libido, vaginal dryness, breast tenderness, increased pubic hair, *impaired fertility, reduction in breast size, absence of menses, hot flashes*

INTEG: Nasal irritation, *acne*

MISC: Body odor, seborrhea, rhinitis, *nasal irritation*

SENSITIVITY: Shortness of breath, chest pain, urticaria, pruritus

Contraindications: Pregnancy (X), hypersensitivity to this product, GnRH, sorbitol; lactation, undiagnosed abnormal vaginal bleeding

Precautions: Children

N

PHARMACOKINETICS

Rapidly absorbed, peak 10-40 min, half-life 3 hr; 80% bound to plasma proteins

INTERACTIONS

Decrease: nafarelin absorption—nasal decongestants (nasal sprays)

NURSING CONSIDERATIONS

Assess:

• Pain in endometriosis during treatment
• Central precocious puberty: endocrine studies, bone age, sex steroids, RHCG, GnRH, baseline q8wk
• For precocious puberty including secondary sex characteristics
• Test results: pituitary/hypothalamus dysfunction (decreased LH); postmenopausal (increased LH)

Administer:

• Repeated doses may be necessary to elevate pituitary gonadotropin reserve; in endometriosis treatment continues for up to 6 mo

Perform/provide:

• Storage at room temp; protect from light

Evaluate:

• Therapeutic response: decreased symptoms of endometriosis; adequate resolution of central precocious puberty

Teach patient/family:

• To use nonhormonal contraception
• About correct nasal use; one spray in right nostril AM, one in left nostril PM for endometriosis; 2 sprays in each nostril in AM and PM for central precocious puberty
• That medication may cause hot flashes, decreased libido, vaginal dryness

---

nafcillin (Ŗ)
(naf-sill'in)
nafcillin sodium
Func. class.: Antiinfective, broad-spectrum
Chem. class.: Penicillinase-resistant penicillin

Action: Interferes with cell wall replication of susceptible organisms; cell lysis mediated by cell wall autolytic enzymes
Uses: Effective for gram-positive cocci *(Staphylococcus aureus, Streptococcus viridans, Streptococcus pneumoniae)*, infections caused by penicillinase-producing *Staphylococcus*

DOSAGE AND ROUTES

• *Adult:* **IV** 500-2000 mg q4h
• *Child and infant >1 mo:* **IV** 50-200 mg/kg/day in divided doses q4-6h
• *Neonates >7 days (weight >2 kg):* **IV** 25 mg/kg q8h
• *Neonates ≤7 days (weight <2 kg):* **IV** 25 mg/kg q12h
Meningitis
• *Adult:* **IV** 100-200 mg/kg/day divided q4-6h, max 12 g/day
• *Neonates >7 days (weight >2 kg):* **IV** 50 mg/kg q6h
• *Neonates ≤7 days (weight <2 kg):* **IV** 50 mg/kg q12h
Available forms: Powder for inj 1, 2, 10 g

SIDE EFFECTS

CNS: Lethargy, hallucinations, anxiety, depression, twitching, **coma, seizures**
GI: Nausea, vomiting, diarrhea, increased AST, ALT, abdominal pain, glossitis, **pseudomembranous colitis**
GU: Oliguria, **proteinuria, hematuria,** vaginitis, moniliasis, **glomerulonephritis,** interstitial nephritis
HEMA: Anemia, increased bleeding time, **bone marrow depression, granulocytopenia**
SYST: **Anaphylaxis, serum sickness, Stevens-Johnson syndrome**

Contraindications: Hypersensitivity to penicillins

Precautions: Pregnancy (B), hypersensitivity to cephalosporins, neonates, GI disease, asthma, lactation

PHARMACOKINETICS

Half-life 1 hr, metabolized by liver, excreted in bile, urine

INTERACTIONS

Increase: nafcillin concentrations—probenecid

Decrease: effect—oral contraceptives, heparin

Drug/Herb
• Do not use acidophilus with antiinfectives; separate by several hours
Decrease: absorption—khat

Drug/Food
Decrease: absorption—food, carbonated drinks, citrus fruit juices

Drug/Lab Test
False-positive: Urine glucose, urine protein

NURSING CONSIDERATIONS

Assess:
• I&O ratio; report hematuria, oliguria, since penicillin in high doses is nephrotoxic

⚠ Any patient with compromised renal system, since drug is excreted slowly in poor renal system function; toxicity may occur rapidly
• Hepatic studies: AST, ALT
• Blood studies: WBC, RBC, H&H, bleeding time
• Renal studies: urinalysis, protein, blood, BUN, creatinine
• C&S before drug therapy; drug may be given as soon as culture is taken
• Bowel pattern before and during treatment
• Respiratory status: rate, character, wheezing, and tightness in chest

⚠ Allergies before initiation of treatment; monitor for anaphylaxis, dyspnea, rash, laryngeal edema; stop drug; keep emergency equipment nearby; skin eruptions after administration of penicillin to 1 wk after discontinuing drug
• Differential WBC in patients on long-term therapy

Administer:
• Drug after C&S has been completed

IV route
• After diluting 1 g/3.4 ml or 2 g/6.8 ml to 250 mg/ml sterile H_2O for inj; further dilute 15-30 ml sterile H_2O or NS sol; give through Y-tube or 3-way stopcock; 500 mg or less/5-10 min; may be further diluted and run over 24 hr

Additive compatibilities: Chloramphenicol, chlorothiazide, dexamethasone, diphenhydrAMINE, epHEDrine, heparin, hydrOXYzine, lidocaine, potassium chloride, prochlorperazine, sodium bicarbonate, sodium lactate

Syringe compatibilities: Cimetidine, heparin

Y-site compatibilities: Acyclovir, atropine, cyclophosphamide, diazepam, enalaprilat, esmolol, famotidine, fentanyl, fluconazole, foscarnet, hydromorphone, magnesium sulfate, morphine, perphenazine, propofol, theophylline, zidovudine

Perform/provide:
• Adrenalin, suction, tracheostomy set, endotracheal intubation equipment
• Adequate fluid intake (2 L) during diarrhea episodes
• Scratch test to assess allergy after securing order from prescriber; usually done when penicillin is only drug of choice
• Storage in tight container; refrigerate reconstituted sol

Evaluate:
• Therapeutic response: absence of fever, draining wounds

Teach patient/family:
• To report sore throat, fever, fatigue (may indicate superinfection)
• To wear or carry emergency ID if allergic to penicillins
• To notify nurse of diarrhea

Treatment of anaphylaxis: Withdraw drug; maintain airway; administer epINEPHrine, aminophylline, O_2, IV corticosteroids

N

⚠ High Alert

nalbuphine (℞)
(nal′byoo-feen)
Nubain, nalbuphine HCl
Func. class.: Opioid analgesic
Chem. class.: Synthetic opioid agonist, antagonist

Action: Depresses pain impulse transmission at the spinal cord level by interacting with opioid receptors
Uses: Moderate to severe pain

DOSAGE AND ROUTES
Analgesic
• *Adult:* SUBCUT/IM/IV 10-20 mg q3-6h prn, not to exceed 160 mg/day
Balanced anesthesia supplement
• *Adult:* IV 0.3-3 mg/kg given over 10-15 min, may give 0.25-0.5 mg/kg as needed for maintenance
Available forms: Inj 10, 20 mg/ml

SIDE EFFECTS

CNS: Drowsiness, dizziness, confusion, headache, sedation, euphoria, dysphoria (high doses), hallucinations, dreaming, tolerance, physical, psychological dependency
CV: Palpitations, bradycardia, change in B/P, orthostatic hypotension
EENT: Tinnitus, blurred vision, miosis, diplopia
GI: Nausea, vomiting, anorexia, constipation, cramps
GU: Increased urinary output, dysuria, urinary retention, urgency
INTEG: Rash, urticaria, bruising, flushing, diaphoresis, pruritus
RESP: **Respiratory depression,** pulmonary edema
Contraindications: Hypersensitivity, addiction (opiate)
Precautions: Pregnancy (C), addictive personality, lactation, increased intracranial pressure, MI (acute), severe heart disease, respiratory depression, renal/hepatic disease

PHARMACOKINETICS
SUBCUT/IM/IV: Duration 3-6 hr; metabolized by liver, excreted by kidneys, half-life 5 hr

INTERACTIONS
⚠ Avoid use with MAOIs, unpredictable reactions may occur
Increase: effects with other CNS depressants—alcohol, opiates, sedative/hypnotics, antipsychotics, skeletal muscle relaxants
Drug/Herb
Increase: CNS depression—chamomile, hops, Jamaican dogwood, kava, lavender, mistletoe, nettle, pokeweed, poppy, senega, skullcap, valerian
Increase: anticholinergic effect—corkwood
Drug/Lab Test
Increase: Amylase, lipase

NURSING CONSIDERATIONS
Assess:
• I&O ratio; check for decreasing output; may indicate urinary retention
⚠ For withdrawal reactions in opiate-dependent individuals: PE, vascular occlusion; abscesses, ulcerations, nausea, vomiting, seizures; however, there is a low potential for dependence
• CNS changes: dizziness, drowsiness, hallucinations, euphoria, LOC, pupil reaction
• Allergic reactions: rash, urticaria
• Respiratory dysfunction: respiratory depression, character, rate, rhythm; notify prescriber if respirations are <10/min
• Need for pain medication by pain sedation scoring, physical dependency
Administer:
• With antiemetic if nausea, vomiting occur
• When pain is beginning to return; determine dosage interval by response

IM route

• IM deep in large muscle mass, rotate inj sites

IV route

• Undiluted 10 mg or less over 3-5 min

Syringe compatibilities: Atropine, cimetidine, diphenhydrAMINE, droperidol, glycopyrrolate, hydrOXYzine, lidocaine, midazolam, prochlorperazine, ranitidine, scopolamine, trimethobenzamide

Y-site compatibilities: Amifostine, aztreonam, cefmetazole, cisatracurium, cladribine, filgrastim, fludarabine, granisetron, melphalan, paclitaxel, propofol, remifentanil, teniposide, thiotepa, vinorelbine

Perform/provide:

• Storage in light-resistant area at room temperature

• Assistance with ambulation

• Safety measures: night-light, call bell within easy reach

Evaluate:

• Therapeutic response: decrease in pain

Teach patient/family:

• To report any symptoms of CNS changes, allergic reactions

• That physical dependency may result from long-term use

• That withdrawal symptoms may occur: nausea, vomiting, cramps, fever, faintness, anorexia

Treatment of overdose: Naloxone (Narcan) 0.2-0.8 mg IV, O_2, IV fluids, vasopressors

---

naloxone (℞)

(nal-oks′one)

naloxone HCl, Narcan

Func. class.: Opioid antagonist, antidote

Chem. class.: Thebaine derivative

Do not confuse:

Narcan/Norcuron

Action: Competes with opioids at opiate receptor sites

Uses: Respiratory depression induced by opioids, pentazocine, propoxyphene; refractory circulatory shock, asphyxia neonatorum, coma, hypotension

Unlabeled uses: IBS, opiate agonist dependence, opiate agonist-induced constipation, pruritus

DOSAGE AND ROUTES

Opioid-induced respiratory depression

• *Adult:* **IV/SUBCUT/IM** 0.4-2 mg; repeat q2-3min if needed

• *Child:* **IV/SUBCUT/IM** 0.01 mg/kg slowly or as **INF** titrated to response

Postoperative opioid-induced respiratory depression

• *Adult:* **IV** 0.1-0.2 mg q2-3min prn

• *Child:* **IV/SUBCUT/IM** 0.01 mg/kg q2-3min prn

Opioid overdose

• *Adult:* **IV/SUBCUT/IM** 0.4 mg (10 mcg/kg) (not opioid dependent) may repeat q2-3min; 0.1-0.2 mg q2-3min (opioid dependent)

• *Child:* **IV/SUBCUT/IM** 10 mcg (0.01 mg/kg) q2-3min

Available forms: Inj 0.02, 0.4 mg/ml

SIDE EFFECTS

CNS: Drowsiness, nervousness

CV: Rapid pulse, increased systolic B/P (high doses), **ventricular tachycardia, fibrillation**

GI: Nausea, vomiting

RESP: Hyperpnea

Contraindications: Hypersensitivity

Precautions: Pregnancy (B), children, cardiovascular disease, opioid dependency, lactation, seizure disorder

PHARMACOKINETICS

Well absorbed IM, SUBCUT; metabolized by liver, crosses placenta; excreted in urine, breast milk; half-life 1 hr

IV: Onset 1 min, duration 45 min

IM/SUBCUT: Onset 2-5 min, duration 45-60 min

N

Side effects: *italics* = common; **bold** = life-threatening

INTERACTIONS

Decrease: effect of opioid analgesics
Drug/Lab Test
Interference: Urine VMA, 5-HIAA, urine glucose

NURSING CONSIDERATIONS

Assess:

• Withdrawal: cramping, hypertension, anxiety, vomiting, signs of withdrawal in drug-dependent individuals may occur up to 2 hr after administration
• VS q3-5min
• ABGs including Po_2, Pco_2
• Cardiac status: tachycardia, hypertension; monitor ECG
• Respiratory dysfunction: respiratory depression, character, rate, rhythm; if respirations are <10/min, administer naloxone; probably due to opioid overdose; monitor LOC
• For pain: duration, intensity, location, before and after administration; may be used for respiratory depression
Administer:

• Only with resuscitative equipment, O_2 nearby
• Only sol prepared within 24 hr
IV route
• Undiluted with sterile H_2O for inj; may be further diluted with NS or D_5 and given as an inf; give 0.4 mg or less over 15 sec or titrate inf to response
Additive compatibilities: Verapamil
Syringe compatibilities: Benzquinamide, heparin, ondansetron
Y-site compatibilities: Gatifloxacin, linezolid, propofol
Perform/provide:

• Dark storage at room temperature
Evaluate:

• Therapeutic response: reversal of respiratory depression; LOC—alert

---

naltrexone (R)

(nal-trex′one)
Depade, ReVia, Vivitrol
Func. class.: Opioid antagonist
Chem. class.: Thebaine derivative

Action: Competes with opioids at opioid receptor sites
Uses: Blockage of opioid analgesics, used in treatment of opiate addiction, alcoholism
Unlabeled uses: Nicotine withdrawal

DOSAGE AND ROUTES

Adjunct in opiate agonist dependence
• *Adult:* **PO** 25 mg; if no withdrawal symptoms in 1 hr, then 25 mg additionally; if no withdrawal symptoms, then 50-150 mg/day or in divided doses
Adjunct in alcoholism treatment
• *Adult:* **PO** 50 mg daily with food × 12 wk; **IM** (Vivitrol) 380 mg q4wk
Pruritus (unlabeled)
• *Adult:* **PO** 50 mg daily × 7 day to 4 wks
Available forms: Tabs 25, 50, 100 mg; susp for inj 380 mg

SIDE EFFECTS

CNS: Stimulation, drowsiness, dizziness, confusion, **seizures,** headache, flushing, hallucinations, nervousness, irritability, **suicidal ideation**
CV: Rapid pulse, **pulmonary edema,** hypertension
EENT: Tinnitus, hearing loss, blurred vision
GI: Nausea, vomiting, diarrhea, heartburn, anorexia, **hepatitis,** constipation
GU: Delayed ejaculation, decreased potency
INTEG: Rash, urticaria, bruising, oily skin, acne, pruritus
MISC: Increased thirst, chills, fever
MS: Joint and muscle pain
RESP: Wheezing, hyperpnea, nasal congestion, rhinorrhea, sneezing, sore throat
Contraindications: Hypersensitivity,

⚠ Safety alert   *"Tall Man" lettering

opioid dependence, hepatic failure, hepatitis
Precautions: Pregnancy (C), hepatic disease, lactation, children

PHARMACOKINETICS

PO: Onset 15-30 min, peak 1-2 hr, duration is dose dependent
IM: Peak 2 hr
Metabolized by liver, excreted by kidneys; crosses placenta, excreted in breast milk; half-life 4 hr; extensive first-pass metabolism; protein binding 21%-28%

INTERACTIONS

Increase: lethargy—phenothiazines
Increase: hepatotoxicity—disulfiram
Decrease: effect of analgesics, antidiarrheals, cough preparations

NURSING CONSIDERATIONS

Assess:
• VS q3-5min
• ABGs including Po_2, Pco_2
• Signs of withdrawal in drug-dependent individuals
• Cardiac status: tachycardia, hypertension
• Respiratory dysfunction: respiratory depression, character, rate, rhythm; if respirations are <10/min, respiratory stimulant should be administered
Administer:
• Only if resuscitative equipment is nearby
Perform/provide:
• Storage in tight container
Evaluate:
• Therapeutic response: blocking opiate ingestion
Teach patient/family:
• That they must be drug-free to start treatment
• That using opioid while taking this drug could prove fatal because high dose is needed to overcome this antagonist
• To carry emergency ID stating med used
• If surgery is needed, all involved should be aware of this drug

nandrolone (℞)

(nan′droe-lone)
Deca-Durabolin, Hybolin Decanoate, Kabolin
Func. class.: Androgenic anabolic steroid, antianemic
Chem. class.: Halogenated testosterone derivative

Controlled Substance Schedule III
Action: May stimulate bone marrow development, stimulates erythropoietin production
Uses: Anemia associated with renal disease

DOSAGE AND ROUTES

• *Adult and child ≥14 yr:* **IM** women 50-100 mg qwk; men 100-200 mg qwk
• *Child 2-13 yr:* **IM** 25-50 mg q3-4wk
Available forms: Inj 100, 200 mg/ml

SIDE EFFECTS

CNS: Dizziness, headache, fatigue, tremors, paresthesias, flushing, sweating, anxiety, lability, insomnia, carpal tunnel syndrome, chills
CV: Increased B/P
EENT: Conjunctival edema, nasal congestion
ENDO: Abnormal GTT, *virilism (women, prepubescent boys)*
GI: Nausea, vomiting, constipation, weight gain, **cholestatic jaundice**
GU: **Hematuria,** amenorrhea, vaginitis, decreased libido, decreased breast size, clitoral hypertrophy, testicular atrophy, priapism
INTEG: Rash, acneiform lesions, oily hair/skin, flushing, sweating, acne vulgaris, alopecia, hirsutism
MISC: Hypercalcemia, chills
MS: Cramps, spasms
Contraindications: Pregnancy (X), severe renal/hepatic/cardiac disease, hypersensitivity, lactation, abnormal genital bleeding, males with cancer of breast, prostate
Precautions: Diabetes mellitus, CV disease, MI

N

Side effects: *italics* = common; **bold** = life-threatening

PHARMACOKINETICS
Well absorbed, peak up to 6 days

INTERACTIONS

Increase: bleeding—anticoagulants, NSAIDs, salicylates
Increase: hepatotoxicity—hepatotoxics

Drug/Lab Test

Increase: Serum cholesterol, blood glucose, urine glucose
Decrease: Serum calcium, serum potassium, T_4, T_3, thyroid ^{131}I uptake test, urine 17-OHCS, 17-KS, PBI, BSP

NURSING CONSIDERATIONS

Assess:
• Anemia symptoms: dyspnea, fatigue, weakness, pallor
• Weight daily; notify prescriber if weekly weight gain is >5 lb
• B/P q4h
• I&O ratio; be alert for decreasing urinary output, increasing edema
• Growth rate in children, since growth rate may be uneven (linear/bone growth) with extended use
• Electrolytes: K, Na, Cl, Ca; cholesterol
• Hepatic studies: ALT, AST, bilirubin
• Edema, hypertension, cardiac symptoms, jaundice
• Mental status: affect, mood, behavioral changes, aggression
• Signs of masculinization in female: increased libido, deepening of voice, decreased breast tissue, enlarged clitoris, menstrual irregularities; male: gynecomastia, impotence, testicular atrophy
• Hypercalcemia: lethargy, polyuria, polydipsia, nausea, vomiting, constipation, drug may have to be decreased
• Hypoglycemia in diabetics, since oral antidiabetic action is increased

Administer:
• Titrated dose; use lowest effective dose
• Inject deeply, use large muscle mass

Perform/provide:
• Diet with increased calories, protein; decrease sodium if edema occurs

Evaluate:
• Therapeutic response: increased appetite, increased stamina

Teach patient/family:
• That drug must be combined with complete health plan: diet, rest, exercise
• To notify prescriber if therapeutic response decreases
• Not to discontinue abruptly
• About changes in sex characteristics
• That females should report menstrual irregularities

---

naphazoline nasal agent
See Appendix C

---

naphazoline ophthalmic
See Appendix C

---

naproxen (OTC, ℞)
(na-prox′en)
Apo-Naproxen ✦, EC-Naprosyn, Naprosyn-E ✦, Naprosyn-SR ✦, Naxen ✦, Novo-Naprox ✦, Nu-Naprox ✦

naproxen sodium
Aleve, Anaprox, Anaprox DS, Apo-Napro-Na ✦, Midol Extended Relief, Naprelan, Novo-Naprox Sodium ✦, Novo-Naprox Sodium DS ✦, Synflex ✦, Synflex DS ✦
Func. class.: Nonsteroidal antiinflammatory, nonopioid analgesic
Chem. class.: Propionic acid derivative

Action: Inhibits prostaglandin synthesis by decreasing an enzyme needed for biosynthesis; analgesic, antiinflammatory, antipyretic

Uses: Mild to moderate pain, osteoarthritis, rheumatoid, gouty arthritis, juvenile arthritis, primary dysmenorrhea

---

⚠ Safety alert   ✦"Tall Man" lettering

DOSAGE AND ROUTES
*Antiinflammatory/analgesic/
antidysmenorrheal*
- *Adult:* **PO** 250-500 mg bid, max 1.5
g/day; **DEL REL** 375-500 mg bid
- *Child ≥2 yr:* **PO** 5 mg/kg/day bid

Antigout
- *Adult:* **PO** 750 mg, then 250 mg q8h

OTC use
- *Adult:* **PO** 200 mg q8-12h or 400 mg,
then 200 mg q12h, max 600 mg/24hr
- *Geriatric >65 yr:* **PO** max 200 mg
q12h

Available forms: *Naproxen:* tabs 250,
375, 500 mg; cont rel tabs (Naprelan)
375, 500 mg; del rel tabs (EC-Naprosyn,
Naprosyn-E) 250 ✤, 375, 500 mg; oral
susp 125 mg/5 ml; ext rel tabs (SR) 750
mg ✤; *naproxen sodium:* tabs 250, 375,
500 mg; supp (Naprosyn, Naxen) 500 mg

✤

SIDE EFFECTS
CNS: Dizziness, drowsiness, fatigue, tremors, confusion, insomnia, anxiety, depression
CV: Tachycardia, peripheral edema, palpitations, dysrhythmias, **MI, stroke**
EENT: Tinnitus, hearing loss, blurred vision
GI: Nausea, anorexia, vomiting, diarrhea, jaundice, **cholestatic hepatitis**, constipation, flatulence, cramps, dry mouth, peptic ulcer, **GI ulceration, bleeding, perforation**
GU: **Nephrotoxicity: dysuria, hematuria, oliguria, azotemia**
HEMA: **Blood dyscrasias**
INTEG: Purpura, rash, pruritus, sweating
SYST: **Anaphylaxis**
Contraindications: Pregnancy (D)
2nd/3rd trimester, hypersensitivity, asthma, severe renal/hepatic disease, ulcer disease, perioperative pain
Precautions: Pregnancy (B) 1st trimester, lactation, children <2 yr, bleeding disorders, GI disorders, cardiac disorders, hypersensitivity to other antiinflammatory agents, geriatric, CCr <25 ml/min

PHARMACOKINETICS
PO: Peak 2-4 hr, half-life 3-3½ hr; metabolized in liver; excreted in urine (metabolites), breast milk; 99% protein binding

INTERACTIONS
- Possible renal impairment: ACE inhibitors
- Toxicity risk: methotrexate, lithium, antineoplastics, radiation treatment
Increase: bleeding risk—oral anticoagulants, thrombolytic agents, eptifibatide, tirofiban, cefamandole, cefotetan, cefoperazone, clopidogrel, ticlopidine, plicamycin, valproic acid
Increase: GI side effects risk—aspirin, corticosteroids, alcohol, NSAIDs
Decrease: effect of antihypertensives, diuretics

Drug/Herb
- Bleeding risk: anise, arnica, bogbean, chamomile, chondroitin, clove, dong quai, fenugreek, feverfew, garlic, ginger, ginkgo, ginseng *(Panax),* licorice

Increase: gastric irritation—arginine, gossypol
Increase: NSAIDs effect—bearberry, bilberry

Drug/Lab Test
Increase: BUN, alk phos
False increase: 5-HIAA, 17KS

NURSING CONSIDERATIONS
Assess:
⚠ Cardiac status: CV thrombotic events, MI, stroke; may be fatal
⚠ GI status: ulceration, bleeding, perforation; may be fatal
- Pain: frequency, characteristics, intensity; relief prior to and 1-2 hr after med
⚠ Asthma, aspirin hypersensitivity or nasal polyps, increased risk of hypersensitivity
- Renal, hepatic, blood studies: BUN, creatinine, AST, ALT, Hgb, LDH, blood glu-

cose, Hct, WBC, platelets CCr before treatment, periodically thereafter
• Audiometric, ophthalmic exam before, during, after treatment
• For eye, ear problems: blurred vision, tinnitus (may indicate toxicity)
Administer:
• With food to decrease GI symptoms; take on empty stomach to facilitate absorption
Perform/provide:
• Storage at room temperature
Evaluate:
• Therapeutic response: decreased pain, stiffness, swelling in joints, ability to move more easily
Teach patient/family:
• To use sunscreen to prevent photosensitivity
• To report blurred vision, ringing, roaring in ears (may indicate toxicity)
• To avoid driving, other hazardous activities if dizziness or drowsiness occurs
• To report change in urine pattern, weight increase, edema (face, lower extremities), pain increase in joints, fever, blood in urine (indicates nephrotoxicity); black stools, flulike symptoms
• That therapeutic effects may take up to 1 mo
• To avoid ASA, alcohol, steroids or other OTC medications without prescriber approval

---

naratriptan (Rx)
(nair'ah-trip-tan)
Amerge
Func. class.: Antimigraine agent, abortive
Chem. class.: 5-HT$_1$ receptor agonist, triptan

Action: Binds selectively to the vascular 5-HT$_1$ receptor subtype, exerts antimigraine effect; causes vasoconstriction in cranial arteries
Uses: Acute treatment of migraine with or without aura

DOSAGE AND ROUTES
• *Adult:* PO 1 or 2.5 mg with fluids, if headache returns, repeat once after 4 hr, max 5 mg/24 hr
Hepatic/renal dose
• Max 2.5 mg/24 hr
Available forms: Tabs 1, 2.5 mg

SIDE EFFECTS
CNS: Dizziness, sedation, fatigue
CV: Increased B/P, palpitations, **tachydysrhythmias, PR, QTc prolongation, ST/T wave changes, PVCs, atrial flutter/fibrillation, coronary vasospasm**
EENT: EENT infections, photophobia
GI: Nausea, vomiting
MISC: Temperature change sensations; tightness, pressure sensations
MS: Weakness, neck stiffness, myalgia
Contraindications: Hypersensitivity, angina pectoris, history of MI, documented silent ischemia, ischemic heart disease, concurrent ergotamine-containing preparations, uncontrolled hypertension, CV syndromes, hemiplegic or basilar migraines, severe renal disease (CCr <15 ml/min); severe hepatic disease (Child-Pugh grade C)
Precautions: Pregnancy (C), postmenopausal women, men >40 yr, risk factors for CAD, hypercholesterolemia, obesity, diabetes, impaired hepatic or renal function, lactation, children, geriatric, peripheral vascular disease

PHARMACOKINETICS
Onset 2-3 hr; peak 2-3 hr; 28%-31% protein binding; half-life 6 hr; metabolized in the liver (metabolite); excreted in urine, feces; may be excreted in breast milk

INTERACTIONS
Increase: weakness, hyperreflexia, incoordination—SSRIs (fluoxetine, fluvoxamine, paroxetine, sertraline)

⚠ Safety alert   *"Tall Man" lettering

Increase: vasospastic effects—ergot, ergot derivatives, other 5-HT$_1$ agonists

Increase: adverse reactions risk—MAOIs, do not use together

Increase: naratriptan effect—sibutramine

Drug/Herb

• Serotonin syndrome: SAM-e, St. John's wort

Increase: effect—butterbur

NURSING CONSIDERATIONS

Assess:

• Migraine symptoms: aura, duration, effect on lifestyle, aggravating/alleviating factors

• For stress level, activity, recreation, coping mechanisms

• Neurologic status: LOC blurred vision, nausea, vomiting, tingling in extremities preceding headache

Administer:

• With fluids as soon as symptoms appear, may take another dose after 4 hr; do not take >5 mg in any 24-hr period

Perform/provide:

• Quiet, calm environment with decreased stimulation for noise, bright light, excessive talking

Evaluate:

• Therapeutic response: decrease in frequency, severity of headache

Teach patient/family:

• To report pain, tightness in chest, neck, throat, or jaw; notify prescriber immediately if sudden, severe abdominal pain occurs

• Not to use if another 5-HT$_1$ agonist or an ergot preparation has been used in the past 24 hr; avoid using >2 days/wk, rebound headache may occur

• Advise patient to notify prescriber if pregnancy is planned or suspected, avoid breastfeeding

---

natalizumab (℞)

(na-ta-liz´-u-mab)

Tysabri

Func. class.: Multiple sclerosis agent, monoclonal antibody

Action: Action not clearly understood; biologic response modifying properties mediated through specific receptors on cells, may be secondary of blockade of the interaction by inflammatory cells on vascular endothelial cells

Uses: Ambulatory patients with relapsing-remitting multiple sclerosis who have not responded to other treatment

Unlabeled uses: Crohn's disease

DOSAGE AND ROUTES

• *Adult:* **IV INF** 300 mg q4wk, give over 1 hr, observe during and for 1 hr after infusion

Available forms: Single-use vial, 300 mg/100 ml 0.9% NaCl

SIDE EFFECTS

CNS: Headache, fatigue, rigors, syncope, tremors, *depression,* **progressive multifocal leukoencephalopathy (PML), suicidal ideation**

CV: Chest discomfort, hyper/hypotension

GI: Abdominal discomfort, abnormal LFT, gastroentritis

GU: Amenorrhea, *UTI, irregular menses,* vaginitis, urinary frequency

INTEG: Rash, dermatitis, pruritus

MS: Arthralgia

RESP: Lower respiratory tract infection

SYST: **Anaphylaxis, angioedema**

Contraindications: Hypersensitivity, immunocompromised individuals (HIV, AIDS, leukemia, lymphoma, transplants), PML, murine (mouse) protein allergy

Precautions: Pregnancy (C), lactation, chronic progressive MS, depression, mental disorders, diabetes, TB, geriatric, active infections

PHARMACOKINETICS

Half-life approximately 11 days

N

INTERACTIONS
• Do not use with vaccines
Increase: infection—immunosuppressants, antineoplastics, immunomodulators

NURSING CONSIDERATIONS
Assess:
• Blood, renal, hepatic studies: CBC, differential, platelet counts, BUN, creatinine, ALT, urinalysis, for hypersensitivity reactions
• CNS symptoms: headache, fatigue, depression, rigors, tremors
• GI status: abdominal discomfort
• Mental status: depression, depersonalization, suicidal thoughts, insomnia
• For MS symptoms; this product should only be used in patients who have not responded to other treatments
⚠ Anaphylaxis: shortness of breath, hives; swelling, tightness in throat, chest pain; usually within 2 hr of infusion
• PML using gadolinium-enhanced MRI scan of the brain, possibly cerebrospinal fluid for JC viral DNA
Administer:
• Acetaminophen for fever, headache
• Only after being enrolled in the TOUCH Prescribing Program
IV infusion
• Use only clear, colorless solution, without particulates
• Withdraw 15 ml from the vial using aseptic technique: inj concentration into 100 ml 0.9% NaCl; do not use other diluents; mix completely; do not shake; infuse immediately or refrigerate for up to 8 hr; warm to room temp before using; flush with 0.9% NaCl before and after infusion; do not admix or use in same line with other agents
• Withhold product at first sign of PML
Perform/provide:
• Storage of solution in refrigerator; do not freeze or shake; protect from light; use within 8 hr of preparation
Evaluate:
• Therapeutic response: decreased symptoms of MS

Teach patient/family:
• To provide patient or family member with written, detailed information about the drug
• That female patients may experience irregular menses, amenorrhea
• To use sunscreen to prevent photosensitivity
• To notify prescriber if pregnancy is suspected
• To avoid breastfeeding while taking this product
• To notify prescriber of possible infection: sore throat, cough, increased temp

natamycin ophthalmic
See Appendix C

nedocromil (℞)
(ned-o-kroe'mill)
Tilade
Func. class.: Antiasthmatic
Chem. class.: Mast cell stabilizer

Action: Stabilizes the membrane of the sensitized mast cell, preventing release of chemical mediators after an antigen-IgE interaction
Uses: Severe perennial bronchial asthma, exercise-induced bronchospasm (prevention), prevention of acute bronchospasm induced by environmental pollutants; *not* for treatment of acute asthma attacks

DOSAGE AND ROUTES
• *Adult and child >12 yr:* **INH** 2 inhalations 2-4 ×/day at regular intervals to provide 14 g/day
Available forms: Inh cap 20 mg; inh aerosol spray 800 mcg/spray, 14.2 g container; neb sol 10 mg/ml; nasal sol 40 mg/ml; nasal insufflation 10 mg/cartridge ✦

SIDE EFFECTS
CNS: Headache, dizziness, neuritis, dysphonia

EENT: Throat irritation, cough, nasal congestion, burning eyes, rhinitis
GI: Nausea, vomiting, anorexia, dry mouth, *bitter taste*
MISC: **Anaphylaxis**

Contraindications: Hypersensitivity to this drug or lactose, status asthmaticus
Precautions: Pregnancy (B), lactation, children

PHARMACOKINETICS

INH: Peak 15 min, duration 4-6 hr; excreted unchanged in urine; half-life 80 min

NURSING CONSIDERATIONS
Assess:
• Pulmonary function testing baseline (asthma)
• Respiratory status: rate, rhythm, characteristics, lung sounds, cough, wheezing, dyspnea
• For rhinitis if using intranasal
Administer:
• By inhalation only, with spacer device if needed
• Gargle, sip of water to decrease irritation in throat
Evaluate:
• Therapeutic response: decrease in asthmatic symptoms, congested, runny nose
Teach patient/family:
• To clear mucus before using
• The proper technique: exhale; using inhaler, inhale deeply with head tipped back to open airway; remove, hold breath, exhale; use Halermatic or Spinhaler with Intal caps
• That therapeutic effect may take up to 4 wk
• That drug is preventive only, not restorative

---

nelarabine (R)
(nella-ra′ben)
Arranon
Func. class.: Antineoplastic
Chem. class.: Purine analog

Action: Leukemic blasts allow for incorporation into DNA, thus interfering with cell replication lending to cell death
Uses: T-cell lymphoblastic leukemia, T-cell lymphoblastic lymphoma post relapse or treatment failure with at least two chemotherapeutic agents

DOSAGE AND ROUTES
• *Adult:* **IV** 1500 mg/m² over 2 hr on days 1, 3, 5, repeated q21d
• *Child:* **IV** 650 mg/m² over 1 hr daily × 5 days, repeated q21d
Available forms: Sol for inj 5 mg/ml

SIDE EFFECTS
CNS: Dizziness, *fatigue,* insomnia, rigors, **seizures,** peripheral neuropathy, **paralysis,** confusion, headache
CV: Edema
GI: Nausea, vomiting, anorexia, diarrhea, stomatitis, constipation
HEMA: **Neutropenia,** leukopenia, **thrombocytopenia,** anemia
META: Decreased potassium, calcium, magnesium, albumin, bilirubin, AST, ALT, hyperuricemia; increased glucose
MS: Myalgia, arthralgia, back pain, weakness
RESP: **Pleural effusion,** cough, dyspnea, wheezing, epistaxis
Contraindications: Pregnancy (D), hypersensitivity, severe neurotoxicity
Precautions: Renal/hepatic disease, lactation, children, geriatric

PHARMACOKINETICS
Metabolized in the liver, excreted kidneys, half-life 30 min-3 hr

INTERACTIONS
• Do not use with live virus vaccinations

NURSING CONSIDERATIONS
Assess:
• CBC (RBC, Hct, Hgb), differential platelet count weekly; withhold drugs if WBC is <4000/mm³, platelet count is <75,000/mm³, or RBC, Hct, Hgb low; notify prescriber of these results
• Renal studies: BUN, serum uric acid, urine CCr, electrolytes before and during therapy
• Monitor temp q4h; fever may indicate beginning infection; no rectal temps
• Hepatic studies before and during therapy: bilirubin, ALT, AST, alk phos as needed or monthly
• Bleeding: hematuria, heme-positive stools, bruising or petechiae, mucosa or orifices q8h
• Neurotoxicity: somnolence, confusion, seizures, ataxia, paresthesias, hypoesthesia, coma, status epilepticus, craniospinal demyelination; contact prescriber immediately
• Dyspnea, crackles, unproductive cough, chest pain, tachypnea, fatigue, increased pulse, pallor, lethargy, personality changes
• Buccal cavity q8h for dryness, sores or ulceration, white patches, oral pain, bleeding, dysphagia
• GI symptoms: frequency of stools, cramping; if severe diarrhea occurs, fluid and electrolytes may need to be given
Administer:
• IV hydration, and allopurinol in risk of hyperuricemia
• Use procedures for proper handling/disposal of anticancer drugs
Perform/provide:
• Rinsing of mouth tid-qid with water, club soda; brushing of teeth bid-tid with soft brush or cotton-tipped applicators for stomatitis; use unwaxed dental floss
• Storage at room temp
Evaluate:
• Therapeutic response: decreased spread of malignancy
Teach patient/family:
• To avoid foods with citric acid, hot or rough texture if stomatitis is present
• Use contraception while taking this product
• To avoid using while lactating
• To report signs of infection: increased temp, sore throat, flulike symptoms
• To report signs of anemia: fatigue, headache, faintness, shortness of breath, irritability
• To report bleeding; to avoid use of razors, commercial mouthwash
• That seizures may occur, do not operate machinery or drive until effects are known
• Not to receive vaccinations while taking this product

nelfinavir (℞)
(nell-fin'a-ver)
Viracept
Func. class.: Antiretroviral
Chem. class.: HIV protease inhibitor

Action: Inhibits human immunodeficiency virus (HIV-1) protease, which prevents maturation of the infectious virus
Uses: HIV-1 in combination with other antiretrovirals

DOSAGE AND ROUTES
HIV infection
• *Adult and child >13 yr:* **PO** 750 mg tid or 1250 mg bid
• *Child 2-13 yr:* **PO** 20-30 mg/kg tid, max 750 mg tid
Prevention of HIV infection after exposure
• *Adult:* **PO** 750 mg tid with two other antiretroviral agents × 4 wks
Available forms: Tabs 250, 625 mg; powder, oral 50 mg/g/scoop

SIDE EFFECTS
CNS: Headache, asthenia, poor concentration, **seizures, suicidal ideation**
CV: Bleeding
ENDO: Hypoglycemia, hyperlipidemia
GI: *Diarrhea,* anorexia, dyspepsia, *nausea, flatulence,* **hepatitis, pancreatitis**

⚠ Safety alert *"Tall Man" lettering

HEMA: Anemia, leukopenia, thrombocytopenia, Hgb abnormalities
INTEG: **Rash,** dermatitis
MS: Pain, arthralgia, myalgia, myopathy
OTHER: **Hypoglycemia,** redistribution/accumulation of body fat

Contraindications: Hypersensitivity to protease inhibitors

Precautions: Pregnancy (B), renal/hepatic disease, lactation, hemophilia, PKU, pancreatitis

PHARMACOKINETICS

Half-life 3½-5 hr, excreted urine/feces, peak 2-4 hr, 98% protein binding, metabolized by CYP3A4 enzyme system

INTERACTIONS

Drug/Herb

⚠ Serious dysrhythmias: amiodarone, ergots, lovastatin, midazolam, pimozide, quinidine, simvastatin, triazolam

Increase: effect—atorvastatin, azithromycin, rifabutin, indinavir, saquinavir, cycloSPORINE, tacrolimus, sirolimus, sildenafil

Increase: nelfinavir levels—ketoconazole, indinavir, ritonavir

Increase: protease inhibitor levels—delavirdine, HIV protease inhibitors

Decrease: nelfinavir levels—rifamycins, nevirapine, phenobarbital, phenytoin, carbamazepine

Decrease: effect of didanosine, methadone, oral contraceptives, phenytoin

Drug/Herb

Decrease: antiretroviral effect—St. John's wort

Drug/Food

Increase: absorption with food

Drug/Lab Test

Increase: AST, ALT, alk phos, total bilirubin, CPK, LDH

NURSING CONSIDERATIONS

Assess:

• Signs of infection, anemia
• Hepatic studies: ALT, AST

• C&S before drug therapy; drug may be taken as soon as culture is taken; repeat C&S after treatment; determine the presence of other sexually transmitted diseases
• Bowel pattern before, during treatment; if severe abdominal pain with bleeding occurs, drug should be discontinued; monitor hydration
• Skin eruptions, rash, urticaria, itching
• Allergies before treatment, reaction of each medication; place allergies on chart
• Viral load, CD4 cell counts baseline and throughout treatment

Administer:

• With food
• Oral powder mixed with fluids if desired; do not mix with juice or acidic fluids; stable mixed for 6 hr

Teach patient/family:

• To avoid taking with other medications unless directed by prescriber
• That drug does not cure, but does manage symptoms; does not prevent transmission of HIV to others
• To use a nonhormonal form of birth control while taking this drug
• If dose is missed, to take as soon as remembered up to 1 hr before next dose; do not double dose
• To take with food

Rarely Used

neomycin (℞)
(nee-oh-mye'sin)
Mycifradin, Myciguent
Func. class.: Antiinfective

Uses: Severe systemic infections of CNS, respiratory, GI, urinary tract, eye, bone, skin, soft tissues caused by *Pseudomonas aeruginosa, Escherichia coli, Enterobacter, Klebsiella pneumoniae, Proteus vulgaris;* also used for hepatic coma, preoperatively to sterilize bowel, infectious diarrhea caused by enteropathogenic *E. coli*

N

DOSAGE AND ROUTES
Hepatic encephalopathy
• *Adult:* **PO** 4-12 g/day in divided doses × 5-6 days
• *Child:* **PO** 50-100 mg/kg/day in divided doses q6h × 5-6 days
Preoperative intestinal antisepsis
• *Adult:* **PO** 1 g qhr × 4hr, then 1 g q4h for remaining 24 hr
Contraindications: Bowel obstruction (oral use), severe renal disease, hypersensitivity, infants, children, GI disease

---

neomycin topical
See Appendix C

---

neostigmine (℞)
(nee-oh-stig'meen)
neostigmine, Prostigmin
Func. class.: Cholinergic stimulant; anticholinesterase
Chem. class.: Quaternary compound

Action: Inhibits destruction of acetylcholine, which increases concentration at sites where acetylcholine is released; this facilitates transmission of impulses across myoneural junction
Uses: Diagnosis/treatment of myasthenia gravis, nondepolarizing neuromuscular blocker antagonist, postoperative ileus, urinary retention

DOSAGE AND ROUTES
Myasthenia gravis diagnosis
• *Adult:* **IM** 0.02 mg/kg as a single dose
• *Child:* **IM** 0.04 mg/kg as a single dose
Myasthenia gravis treatment
• *Adult:* **PO** 15 mg q3-4h, may increase to 375 mg/day; **IM/IV** 0.5-2 mg q1-3h up to 10 mg/day
• *Child:* **PO** 2 mg/kg/day q3-4h; **IM/IV/SUBCUT** 0.01-0.04 mg/kg q2-4h
Nondepolarizing neuromuscular blocker antagonist
• *Adult:* **IV** 0.5-2 mg slowly, may repeat if needed, max 5 mg (give 0.6-1.2 mg atropine several min before this product)
• *Infant and child:* **IV** 0.025-0.1 mg/kg/dose (give atropine several min before this product)
Postoperative abdominal distention/ileus
• *Adult:* **IM/SUBCUT** 0.25-1 mg (1:4000) q4-6h depending on condition × 2-3 days
Urinary retention treatment
• *Adult:* **IM/SUBCUT** 0.5-1 mg q3h × 5 doses after bladder is emptied
Renal dose
• CCr 10-50 ml/min 50% of dose; CCr <10 ml/min 25% of dose
Available forms: Tabs 15 mg; inj 1:1000, 1:2000, 1:4000

SIDE EFFECTS
CNS: Dizziness, headache, sweating, weakness, **seizures**, incoordination, **paralysis**, drowsiness, loss of consciousness
CV: Tachycardia, dysrhythmias, bradycardia, hypotension, AV block, ECG changes, **cardiac arrest,** syncope
EENT: Miosis, blurred vision, lacrimation, visual changes
GI: Nausea, diarrhea, vomiting, cramps, increased peristalsis, salivary and gastric secretions
GU: Urinary frequency, incontinence, urgency
INTEG: Rash, urticaria, flushing
RESP: **Respiratory depression, bronchospasm, constriction, laryngospasm, respiratory arrest,** dyspnea
Contraindications: Obstruction of intestine, renal system, bromide sensitivity, peritonitis, urinary tract obstruction, ileus
Precautions: Pregnancy (C), bradycardia, hypotension, seizure disorders, bronchial asthma, coronary occlusion, hyperthyroidism, dysrhythmias, peptic ulcer, megacolon, poor GI motility, lactation, children

---

⚠ Safety alert   *"Tall Man" lettering

PHARMACOKINETICS

PO: Onset 45-75 min, duration 2½-4 hr

IM/SUBCUT: Onset 20-30 min, duration 2½-4 hr

IV: Onset 1-2 min, duration 1-2 hr, metabolized in liver, excreted in urine

INTERACTIONS

Increase: action of decamethonium, succinylcholine

Increase: bradycardia—β-blockers, calcium channel blockers, digoxin

Decrease: neostigmine action—aminoglycosides, antihistamines, antidepressants, atropine, anticholinergics, local/general anesthetics, corticosteroids, haloperidol, phenothiazines, quinidine, disopyramide

Drug/Herb
Increase: effect: pill-bearing spurge

NURSING CONSIDERATIONS

Assess:
• VS, respiration q8h
• I&O ratio; check for urinary retention or incontinence
⚠ For bradycardia, hypotension, bronchospasm, headache, dizziness, seizures, respiratory depression; drug should be discontinued if toxicity occurs

Administer:
• Only with atropine sulfate available for cholinergic crisis
• Only after all other cholinergics have been discontinued
• Increased doses, as ordered if tolerance occurs
• Larger doses after exercise or fatigue, as ordered

PO route
• On empty stomach for better absorption

IV route
• Undiluted, give through Y-tube or 3-way stopcock; give 0.5 mg or less over 1 min

Additive compatibilities: Netilmicin

Syringe compatibilities: Glycopyrrolate, heparin, ondansetron, pentobarbital, thiopental

Y-site compatibilities: Heparin, hydrocortisone, potassium chloride, vit B/C

Perform/provide:
• Storage at room temperature

Evaluate:
• Therapeutic response: increased muscle strength, hand grasp, improved gait, absence of labored breathing (if severe)

Teach patient/family:
• That drug is not a cure; it only relieves symptoms
• To wear emergency ID specifying myasthenia gravis, drugs taken

Treatment of overdose: Respiratory support, atropine 1-4 mg (IV)

---

nepafenac ophthalmic
See Appendix C

⚠ High Alert

nesiritide (℞)
(neh-seer′ih-tide)
Natrecor
Func. class.: Vasodilator
Chem. class.: Human B-type natriuretic peptide

Action: Uses DNA technology; human B-type natriuretic peptide binds to the receptor in vascular smooth muscle and endothelial cells, leading to smooth muscle relaxation

Uses: Acutely decompensated CHF

DOSAGE AND ROUTES
• *Adult:* **IV BOL** 2 mcg/kg, then **CONT IV INF** 0.01 mcg/kg/min

Available forms: Powder for inj, 1.5 mg single-use vial

SIDE EFFECTS

CNS: Headache, insomnia, dizziness, anxiety, confusion, paresthesia, tremor

CV: *Hypotension,* **tachycardia,** dysrhythmias, bradycardia, ventricular tachycardia, ventricular extrasystoles, atrial fibrillation

GI: Vomiting, nausea

INTEG: Rash, sweating, pruritus, inj site reaction

MISC: Abdominal pain, back pain

RESP: Increased cough, hemoptysis, **apnea**

Contraindications: Hypersensitivity, cardiogenic shock or B/P <90 mm Hg as primary therapy

Precautions: Pregnancy (C); mitral stenosis; significant valvular stenosis, restriction, or obstructive cardiomyopathy, or any condition that is dependent upon venous return; renal disease, lactation, children, constrictive pericarditis

PHARMACOKINETICS

Half-life 18 min

INTERACTIONS

Increase: symptomatic hypotension with ACE inhibitors

NURSING CONSIDERATIONS

Assess:

• PCWP, RAP, cardiac index, MPAP
• B/P, pulse during treatment until stable
• I&O, daily weight
• For CHF: weight gain, dyspnea, crackles, edema

Administer:

IV route

• Do not administer nesiritide through a central catheter containing other drugs; administer other drugs through a separate catheter or a central line heparin-coated catheter as nesiritide binds to heparin
• Prime IV fluid with infusion of 25 ml before connecting to patient's vascular access port and before bolus dose or IV infusion
• Reconstitute one 1.5 mg vial/5 ml of diluent from prefilled 250-ml plastic IV bag with diluent of choice (D$_5$, 0.9% NaCl, D$_5$/½ NaCl, D$_5$/0.2% NaCl); do not shake vial, roll gently; use only clear sol
• Withdraw all contents of reconstituted vial and add to the 250-ml plastic IV bag (6 mcg/ml), invert bag several times
• Use within 24 hr of reconstituting

IV BOLUS route

• Withdraw prescribed bolus dose (volume) from prepared infusion bag; give over 1 min through IV port

Intermittent IV route

• After bolus dose, use infusion, give at 0.1 ml/kg/hr (0.01 mcg/kg/min)

Y-site compatibilities: Bumetanide, enalaprilat, furosemide, heparin, hydrALAZINE, regular insulin

Evaluate:

• Therapeutic response: improvement in CHF with improved PCWP, RAP, MPAP

Teach patient/family:

• To explain purpose of medication and expected results
• To report dizziness, blurred vision, light-headedness, sweating

---

nevirapine

(ne-veer′a-peen)
Viramune

Func. class.: Antiretroviral
Chem. class.: Nonnucleoside reverse transcriptase inhibitor (NNRTI)

Do not confuse

nevirapine/nelfinavir
Viramune/Viracept

Action: Binds directly to reverse transcriptase and blocks RNA, DNA, causing a disruption of the enzyme's site

Uses: HIV-1 in combination with other highly active antiretroviral therapy (HAART)

DOSAGE AND ROUTES

• *Adult:* **PO** 200 mg daily × 2 wk, then 200 mg bid in combination
• *Child ≥8 yr:* **PO** 4 mg/kg/daily × 2 wk, then 4 mg/kg/bid, max 200 mg bid
• *Child 2 mo-8 yr:* **PO** 4 mg/kg daily × 2 wk, then 7 mg/kg bid

Available forms: Tabs 200 mg; oral susp 50 mg/5 ml

SIDE EFFECTS

CNS: Paresthesia, headache, fever, peripheral neuropathy

▲ Safety alert   *"Tall Man" lettering

GI: Diarrhea, abdominal pain, *nausea, stomatitis,* **hepatotoxicity**
HEMA: **Neutropenia, anemia, thrombocytopenia**
INTEG: Rash, **toxic epidermal necrolysis**
MISC: **Stevens-Johnson syndrome**
MS: Pain, myalgia
Contraindications: Hypersensitivity
Precautions: Pregnancy (C), renal/hepatic disease, lactation, children

PHARMACOKINETICS

Rapidly absorbed, peak 4 hr, 60% bound to plasma proteins, metabolized by liver; metabolized by hepatic P450 enzyme system, excreted 91% in urine, terminal half-life 2.5-3 hr

INTERACTIONS

Increase: nevirapine levels—cimetidine, macrolide antiinfectives
Decrease: effects of protease inhibitors, oral contraceptives, ketoconazole, methadone
Decrease: nevirapine levels—rifamycins, anticonvulsants, clonazepam, diazepam, warfarin
Drug/Herb
Decrease: action of antiretroviral—St. John's wort, do not use concurrently
Drug/Lab Test
Increase: ALT, AST, GGT, bilirubin, Hgb
Decrease: Neutrophil count

NURSING CONSIDERATIONS

Assess:
• Signs of infection, anemia
• Hepatic, blood studies during treatment: ALT, AST, viral load, CD4; renal studies; if LFTs are elevated significantly, drug should be withheld
• C&S before drug therapy; drug may be taken as soon as culture is taken; repeat C&S after treatment; determine the presence of other sexually transmitted disease
• Bowel pattern before, during treatment; if severe abdominal pain with bleeding oc-

curs, drug should be discontinued; monitor hydration
⚠ Allergies before treatment, reaction to each medication; skin eruptions; rash, urticaria, itching; if rash is severe or systemic symptoms occur, discontinue immediately
Administer:
• Without regard to meals
• Oral susp should be shaken prior to giving
Teach patient/family:
⚠ To report any right quadrant pain, jaundice, rash immediately
• That drug may be taken with food, antacids, didanosine
• To take as prescribed; if dose is missed, take as soon as remembered up to 1 hr before next dose; do not double dose
• That drug is not a cure, controls symptoms of HIV
• To avoid OTC agents unless approved by prescriber
• To use a nonhormonal form of contraception during treatment
• That drug must be taken in equal intervals around the clock to maintain blood levels for duration of therapy

N

niacin (otc, ℞)
(nye′a-sin)
Edur-Acin, Nia-Bid, Niac, Niacels, Niacor, Niaspan, Nicobid, Nico-400, Nicolar, Nicotinex
nicotinic acid (otc, ℞)
Novo-Niacin ✦, Slo-Niacin, vitamin B
niacinamide (otc, ℞)
nicotinamide (otc, ℞)
Func. class.: Vit B₃, antihyperlipidemic
Chem. class.: Water-soluble vitamin

Do not confuse:
Nicobid/Nitro-Bid
Action: Needed for conversion of fats, protein, carbohydrates, by oxidation reduction; acts directly on vascular smooth

muscle, causing vasodilation, reduces LDL, HDL, triglycerides, and lipoprotein A

Uses: Pellagra, hyperlipidemias (types 4, 5), peripheral vascular disease that presents a risk for pancreatitis

DOSAGE AND ROUTES

Niacin deficiency

• *Adult:* **PO** 100-500 mg/day in divided doses; **IM/SUBCUT** 5-100 mg 5 or more ×/day; **IV** 25-100 mg bid or tid
• *Child*: **PO** up to 300 mg/day in divided doses

Adjunct in hyperlipidemia

• *Adult:* **PO** 250 mg after evening meal; may increase dose at 1-4 wk intervals to 1-2 g tid, max 6 g/day; ext rel 500 mg at bedtime, × 4 wk, then 1000 mg at bedtime for wk 5-8, do not increase by more than 500 mg q4wk, max 2000 mg/day

Pellagra

• *Adult:* **PO** 300-500 mg daily in divided doses
• *Child:* **PO** 100-300 mg daily in divided doses

Peripheral vascular disease

• *Adult:* **PO** 250-800 mg daily in divided doses

Available forms: *Niacin:* tabs 25, 50, 100, 250, 500, 1000 mg; time rel caps 250, 500 mg; timed rel tabs 250, 500 mg; ext rel caps 250, 400 mg; sus rel tabs 500 mg; cont rel tabs 250, 500, 750 mg; sus rel cap 125, 500 mg; elix 50 mg/5 ml; *nicotinamide:* tabs 100, 250, 500 mg

SIDE EFFECTS

CNS: Paresthesias, headache, dizziness, anxiety
CV: Postural hypotension, vasovagal attacks, dysrhythmias, vasodilation
EENT: Blurred vision, ptosis
GI: Nausea, vomiting, anorexia, **jaundice, hepatotoxicity,** diarrhea, peptic ulcer, dyspepsia
GU: Hyperuricemia, **glycosuria, hypoalbuminemia**
INTEG: Flushing, dry skin, rash, pruritus, itching, tingling

Contraindications: Hypersensitivity, peptic ulcer, hepatic disease, lactation, hemorrhage, severe hypotension

Precautions: Pregnancy (C), glaucoma, cardiovascular disease, CAD, diabetes mellitus, gout, schizophrenia, lactation

PHARMACOKINETICS

PO: Peak 30-70 min (depends on formulation) half-life 45 min; metabolized in liver; 30% excreted unchanged in urine

INTERACTIONS

• Postural hypotension: ganglionic blockers
Increase: myopathy, rhabdomyolysis—HMG-CoA reductase inhibitors
Increase: flushing, pruritus—alcohol, avoid use

Drug/Lab Test
Increase: Bilirubin, alk phos, hepatic enzymes, LDH, uric acid, glucose
Decrease: Cholesterol
False increase: Urinary catecholamines
False positive: Urine glucose

NURSING CONSIDERATIONS

Assess:
• Hepatic studies: AST, ALT, bilirubin, uric acid, alk phos; blood glucose before and during treatment
• Cardiac status: rate, rhythm, quality; postural hypotension, dysrhythmias
• Nutritional status: liver, yeast, legumes, organ meat, lean poultry; fat in diet
• Hepatic dysfunction: clay-colored stools, itching, dark urine, jaundice
• CNS symptoms: headache, paresthesias, blurred vision
• For symptoms of niacin deficiency: nausea, vomiting, anemia, poor memory, confusion, dermatitis
• For lipid, triglyceride, cholesterol level, if using for hyperlipidemia

Administer:
• Do not break, crush, or chew ext rel tabs, caps
• With meals for GI symptoms, and 81-

▲ Safety alert   *"Tall Man" lettering

325 mg aspirin or NSAIDs ½ hr before dose to decrease flushing

Evaluate:

• Therapeutic response: decreased lipids, warm extremities, absence of numbness in extremities

Teach patient/family:

• That flushing and increase in feelings of warmth will occur several hr after taking drug (PO); after 2 wk of therapy, these side effects diminish

• To remain recumbent if postural hypotension occurs; to rise slowly to prevent orthostatic hypotension

• To abstain from alcohol if drug is prescribed for hyperlipidemia

• To avoid sunlight if skin lesions are present

⚠ To report clay-colored stools, anorexia, jaundiced sclera, skin; dark urine, hepatotoxicity may occur

---

* **niCARdipine** (R)

(nye-card′i-peen)
Cardene, Cardene IV,
Cardene SR

Func. class.: Calcium channel blocker, antianginal, antihypertensive

Chem. class.: Dihydropyridine

Do not confuse:
niCARdipine/NIFEdipine
Cardene/Cardizem
Cardene SR/Cardizem SR

Action: Inhibits calcium ion influx across cell membrane during cardiac depolarization; produces relaxation of coronary vascular smooth muscle, peripheral vascular smooth muscle; dilates coronary vascular arteries; increases myocardial oxygen delivery in patients with vasospastic angina

Uses: Chronic stable angina pectoris, hypertension

DOSAGE AND ROUTES

Hypertension

• *Adult:* **PO** 20 mg tid initially, may increase after 3 days (range 20-40 mg tid)

or 30 mg bid sus rel, may increase to 60 mg bid or **IV** 5 mg/hr, may increase by 2.5 mg/hr q15min, max 15 mg/hr

Angina

• *Adult:* **PO** 20 mg tid, may be adjusted q3d, may use 20-40 mg tid

Renal dose

• *Adult:* **PO** 20 mg tid; or 30 mg bid (sus rel)

Hepatic dose

• *Adult:* **PO** 20 mg bid

Available forms: Caps 20, 30 mg; sus rel caps 30, 45, 60 mg; inj 2.5 mg/ml

SIDE EFFECTS

CNS: Headache, dizziness, anxiety, depression, confusion, paresthesia, somnolence
CV: Edema, bradycardia, hypotension, palpitations, **pulmonary edema,** chest pain, tachycardia, increased angina, **arrhythmias, CHF**
GI: Nausea, vomiting, gastric upset, constipation, **hepatitis,** abdominal cramps, dry mouth, sore throat
GU: Nocturia, polyuria, **acute renal failure**
INTEG: Rash, infusion site discomfort **Stevens-Johnson syndrome**
OTHER: Blurred vision, flushing, sweating, shortness of breath, impotence

Contraindications: Sick sinus syndrome, 2nd-/3rd-degree heart block, hypersensitivity

Precautions: Pregnancy (C), CHF, hypotension, hepatic injury, lactation, children, renal disease, geriatric

PHARMACOKINETICS

PO: Onset 30 min, peak 1-2 hr, duration 8 hr
PO-SR: Onset unknown, peak 2-6 hr, duration 10-12 hr, half-life 2-5 hr
Metabolized by liver, excreted in urine 60%, 35% feces

INTERACTIONS

Increase: effects of digoxin, neuromuscular blocking agents, theophylline, other antihypertensives, nitrates, alcohol, quinidine

Increase: niCARdipine effects—cimetidine

Increase: toxicity risk—cycloSPORINE, prazosin, carbamazepine, quinidine, propranolol

Decrease: antihypertensive effect—NSAIDs, rifampin

Drug/Herb

Increase: effect—barberry, betel palm, burdock, goldenseal, khat, khella, lily of the valley, plantain

Decrease: effect—yohimbe

Drug/Food

Increase: hypotensive effect—grapefruit juice

NURSING CONSIDERATIONS

Assess:

⚠ Cardiac status: B/P, pulse, respiration, ECG during long-term treatment

• Anginal pain: intensity, location, duration, alleviating factors

• Potassium, renal, hepatic studies, periodically

⚠ CHF: weight gain, crackles, jugular venous distention, dyspnea, I&O

Administer:

PO route

• Do not break, crush, chew, or open sus rel cap

• Without regard to meals

IV route

• Dilute each 25 mg/240 ml of compatible sol (0.1 mg/ml), give slowly

• Stable at room temperature 24 hr

Solution compatibilities: D₅W, D₅/0.45% NaCl, D₅/0.9% NaCl

Y-site compatibilities: Diltiazem, DOBUTamine, DOPamine, epINEPHrine, fentanyl, hydromorphone, labetalol, lorazepam, midazolam, milrinone, morphine, nitroglycerin, norepinephrine, ranitidine, vecuronium

Evaluate:

• Therapeutic response: decreased anginal pain, decreased B/P

Teach patient/family:

• To avoid hazardous activities until stabilized on drug, dizziness is no longer a problem

• To limit caffeine consumption, take no alcohol products

• To avoid OTC drugs unless directed by prescriber

• To comply in all areas of medical regimen: diet, exercise, stress reduction, drug therapy

⚠ To notify prescriber of irregular heartbeat, shortness of breath, swelling of feet and hands, pronounced dizziness, constipation, nausea, hypotension

Treatment of overdose: Defibrillation, β-agonists, IV calcium, diuretics, atropine for AV block, vasopressor for hypotension

nicotine (otc, ℞)
(nik′o-teen)

nicotine chewing gum (otc, ℞)
Nicorette

nicotine inhaler (otc, ℞)
Nicotrol Inhaler

nicotine lozenge (otc)
Commit

nicotine nasal spray (℞)
Nicotrol NS

nicotine transdermal (otc, ℞)
Clear Nicoderm CQ, Habitrol, Nicoderm CQ, Nicotrol, Nicotrol TD

Func. class.: Smoking deterrent
Chem. class.: Ganglionic cholinergic agonist

Action: Agonist at nicotinic receptors in peripheral, central nervous systems; acts at sympathetic ganglia, on chemoreceptors of aorta, carotid bodies; also affects adrenalin-releasing catecholamines

Uses: Deter cigarette smoking

Unlabeled uses: Gilles de la Tourette's syndrome

DOSAGE AND ROUTES

Nicotine chewing gum

• *Adult:* If patient smokes <25 cigarettes/day, start with 2 mg gum; if >25 cigarettes/day, start with 4 mg gum; then 1 piece of gum q1-2h × 6 wk; then 1 piece of gum q2-4h × 2 wk, then 1 piece of gum q4-8h × 2 wk, then discontinue; not to exceed 24/day

Nicotine inhaler

• *Adult:* **INH** 6 cartridges/day for first 3-6 wk, max 16/day × 12 wk

Nicotine lozenge

• *Adult:* If cigarette is desired >30 min after awakening, start with 1 2-mg lozenge; if <30 min after awakening, start with 4-mg lozenge; then 1 q1-2h, max 20 lozenges/day or 5 lozenges/6 hr × 6 wk, then 1 lozenge q2-4h × 2 wk, then 1 lozenge q4-8h × 2 wk, then discontinue

Nicotine nasal spray

• *Adult:* 1 spray in each nostril 1-2 ×/hr, max 5 ×/hr or 40 ×/day, max 3 mo

Nicotine transdermal/inhaler system

• *Habitrol, Nicoderm:* 21 mg/day × 4-8 wk; 14 mg/day × 2-4 wk; 7 mg/day × 2-4 wk

• *Nicotrol:* 15 mg/day × 12 wk; 10 mg/day × 2 wk; 5 mg/day × 2 wk

• *Nicotrol Inhaler:* delivers 30% of what a smoker receives from an actual cigarette

Gilles de la Tourette's syndrome (unlabeled)

• *Adult and child:* Chewing gum: 2 mg chewed × ½ hr bid for 1-6 mo; TD: 7- or 10-mg patch daily × 2 days

Available forms: Transdermal patch (Habitrol, Nicoderm, nicotine transdermal system) delivering 7, 14, 21 mg/day; (Nicoderm) 5, 10, 15 mg/day; nicotine inhaler 4 mg delivered; nasal spray 0.5 mg nicotine/actuation; gum 2 mg/piece; lozenge 2 mg, 4 mg

SIDE EFFECTS

CNS: Dizziness, vertigo, insomnia, headache, confusion, seizures, depression, euphoria, numbness, tinnitus, strange dreams

CV: Dysrhythmias, tachycardia, palpitations, edema, flushing, hypertension

EENT: Jaw ache, irritation in buccal cavity

GI: Nausea, vomiting, anorexia, indigestion, diarrhea, abdominal pain, constipation, eructation

RESP: Breathing difficulty, cough, hoarseness, sneezing, wheezing, bronchial spasm

Contraindications: Pregnancy (X), gum; (D), transdermal; hypersensitivity, immediate post MI recovery period, severe angina pectoris

Precautions: Vasospastic disease, dysrhythmias, diabetes mellitus, hyperthyroidism, pheochromocytoma, coronary disease, esophagitis, peptic ulcer, lactation, renal/hepatic disease

PHARMACOKINETICS

Onset 15-30 min, metabolized in liver, excreted in urine, half-life 2-3 hr, 30-120 hr (terminal)

INTERACTIONS

• Smoking cessation increases diuretic effects of furosemide

Increase: absorption—SUBCUT insulin

Increase: blood levels with cessation of smoking—caffeine, theophylline, pentazocine, imipramine, oxazepam, propranolol, acetaminophen

Decrease: absorption—glutethimide

Decrease: metabolism of propoxyphene

Drug/Herb

Increase: effect—blue cohosh, lobelia

Decrease: effect—oats

NURSING CONSIDERATIONS

Assess:

• Adverse reaction: irritation of buccal cavity, dislike of taste, jaw ache

Administer:

Gum

• Chew gum slowly for 30 min to promote buccal absorption of the drug; do not chew over 45 min

• Begin drug withdrawal after 3 mo use; do not exceed 6 mo

Transdermal patch

• Once a day to a nonhairy, clean, dry area of skin on upper body or upper outer arm; rotate sites to prevent skin irritation

Inhaler

• Puffing on mouthpiece delivers nicotine through the mouth

Evaluate:

• Therapeutic response: decrease in urge to smoke, decreased need for gum after 3-6 mo

Teach patient/family:

Gum

• All aspects of drug use; give package insert to patient and explain

• That gum will not stick to dentures, dental appliances

• That gum is as toxic as cigarettes; to be used only to deter smoking

• Not to use during pregnancy; birth defects may occur

Transdermal patch

• That patch is as toxic as cigarettes; to be used only to deter smoking

• Not to use during pregnancy; birth defects may occur

• To keep used and unused system out of reach of children and pets

• To stop smoking immediately when beginning patch treatment

• To apply promptly after removing from protective patch; system may lose strength

---

*NIFEdipine (R)

(nye-fed'i-peen)

Adalat, Adalat CC, Apo-Nifed ✱, Nifedical XL, Novo-Nifedin ✱, Nu-Nifedin ✱, Procardia, Procardia XL

Func. class.: Calcium-channel blocker, antianginal, antihypertensive

Chem. class.: Dihydropyridine

Do not confuse:

NIFEdipine/niCARdipine

Action: Inhibits calcium ion influx across cell membrane during cardiac depolarization; relaxes coronary vascular smooth muscle; dilates coronary arteries; increases myocardial oxygen delivery in patients with vasospastic angina; dilates peripheral arteries

Uses: Chronic stable angina pectoris, vasospastic angina, hypertension

Unlabeled uses: Migraines, CHF, Raynaud's disease, anal fissures, preterm labor

DOSAGE AND ROUTES

• *Adult:* **PO** immediate release 10 mg tid, increase in 10-mg increments q7-14d, not to exceed 180 mg/24 hr or single dose of 30 mg; **SUS REL** 30-60 mg daily, may increase q7-14d, doses >120 mg not recommended

• *Child:* **PO** 0.25-0.5 mg/kg/dose q4-6h, max 1-2 mg/kg/day

Available forms: Caps 5 ✱, 10, 20 mg; ext rel tabs (CC, XL) 10 ✱, 20 ✱, 30, 60, 90 mg; tabs 10 mg ✱

SIDE EFFECTS

CNS: Headache, fatigue, drowsiness, dizziness, anxiety, depression, weakness, insomnia, light-headedness, paresthesia, tinnitus, blurred vision, nervousness, tremor

CV: **Dysrhythmias,** edema, hypotension, palpitations, tachycardia

GI: Nausea, vomiting, diarrhea, gastric upset, constipation, increased LFTs, dry mouth, flatulence, gingival hyperplasia, **hepatotoxicity**

GU: Nocturia, polyuria

INTEG: Rash, pruritus, flushing, hair loss

MISC: Sexual difficulties, cough, fever, chills

SYST: **Stevens-Johnson syndrome**

Contraindications: Hypersensitivity

Precautions: Pregnancy (C), CHF, hypotension, sick sinus syndrome, 2nd-, 3rd-degree heart block, hypotension less than 90 mm Hg systolic, hepatic injury, lactation, children, renal disease

---

⚠ Safety alert   *"Tall Man" lettering

PHARMACOKINETICS

Well-absorbed PO

PO-ER: Duration 24 hr

PO: Onset 20 min, peak 0.5-6 hr, duration 6-8 hr, half-life 2-5 hr

Metabolized by liver; excreted in urine 60-80% (metabolites), feces 15%; protein binding 90%-98%

INTERACTIONS

Increase: level of digoxin, phenytoin, cycloSPORINE, prazosin, carbamazepine

Increase: NIFEdipine, toxicity—cimetidine, ranitidine

Increase: effects of β-blockers, antihypertensives

Decrease: antihypertensive effect—NSAIDs

Decrease: effects of quinidine

Decrease: NIFEdipine level—smoking

Drug/Herb

Increase: effect—barberry, betel palm, burdock, goldenseal, khat, khella, lily of the valley, plantain

Decrease: effect—yohimbe

Food/Drug

Increase: NIFEdipine level—grapefruit juice

Drug/Lab Test

Increase: CPK, LDH, AST

Positive: ANA, direct Coombs' test

NURSING CONSIDERATIONS

Assess:

• Anginal pain: location, intensity, duration, character, alleviating, aggravating factors

• Cardiac status: B/P, pulse, respiration, ECG

• Potassium, renal, hepatic studies periodically during treatment

Administer:

• Do not break, crush, or chew ext rel tabs

• Without regard to meals

• SL: may puncture liquid-filled cap and squeeze drug into buccal pouch

Evaluate:

• Therapeutic response: decreased anginal pain, B/P, activity tolerance

Teach patient/family:

• To avoid hazardous activities until stabilized on drug, dizziness is no longer a problem

• To limit caffeine consumption; take no alcohol products

• To avoid OTC drugs unless directed by a prescriber

• That ext rel nonabsorbable shell may appear in stools

• To comply with all areas of medical regimen: diet, exercise, stress reduction, drug therapy

• To change position slowly; orthostatic hypotension is common

⚠ To notify prescriber of dyspnea, edema of extremities, nausea, vomiting, severe ataxia, severe rash

• To increase fluid intake to prevent constipation

• To check for gingival hyperplasia and report promptly

Treatment of overdose: Defibrillation, atropine for AV block, vasopressor for hypotension

N

---

nilutamide

(nye-loo'ta-mide)

Anandron ✦, Nilandron

Func. class.: Antineoplastic-hormone

Chem. class.: Antiandrogen

Action: Interferes with testosterone uptake in the nucleus or testosterone activity in target tissues; arrests tumor growth in androgen-sensitive tissue (e.g., prostate gland); prostatic carcinoma is androgen-sensitive, so tumor growth is arrested

Uses: Metastatic prostatic carcinoma, stage D2 in combination with surgical castration

DOSAGE AND ROUTES

• *Adult:* **PO** 300 mg daily × 30 days, then 150 mg daily

Available forms: Tabs 100 ✦, 150 mg

SIDE EFFECTS

CNS: Hot flashes, drowsiness, insomnia, dizziness, hyperthesia, depression
EENT: Delay in adaptation to dark
GI: Diarrhea, nausea, vomiting, increased LFTs, constipation, dyspepsia, **hepatotoxicity**
GU: Decreased libido, impotence, testicular atrophy, UTI, hematuria, nocturia, gynecomastia
HEMA: Anemia
INTEG: Rash, sweating, alopecia, dry skin
MISC: Edema
RESP: Dyspnea, URI, pneumonia, **interstitial pneumonitis**
Contraindications: Hypersensitivity, severe hepatic impairment, severe respiratory disease, women
Precautions: Pregnancy (C)

PHARMACOKINETICS

Rapidly and completely absorbed; excreted in urine and feces as metabolites

INTERACTIONS

Increase: toxicity of vit K, phenytoin, theophylline

NURSING CONSIDERATIONS

Assess:
⚠ Hepatic studies: AST, ALT, alk phos, which may be elevated; if elevated 3× normal, discontinue drug
• For CNS symptoms: drowsiness, insomnia, dizziness
• Chest x-rays, routinely, baseline pulmonary function studies; dyspnea, cough, which may indicate interstitial pneumonitis; discontinue treatment if this condition is suspected
• For hyperglycemia, increased BUN, creatinine, alk phos, leukopenia
Administer:
• Without regard to meals
Perform/provide:
• Storage at room temperature

Evaluate:
• Therapeutic response: decrease in prostatic tumor size, decrease in spread of cancer
Teach patient/family:
⚠ To report side effects: decreased libido, impotence, breast enlargement, hot flashes, diarrhea, dyspnea, cough, shortness of breath; if SOB occurs notify prescriber immediately
⚠ To report signs of hepatotoxicity: dark urine, abdominal pain, clay-colored stools, jaundice eyes, skin
• To wear tinted lens to alleviate delay in adapting to the dark
• That drug is started on day of or day after surgical castration
• To avoid alcohol consumption
Treatment of overdose: Induce vomiting, provide supportive care

nisoldipine
(nye-sole′dih-peen)
Sular
Func. class.: Calcium channel blocker, antihypertensive
Chem. class.: Dihydropyridine

Action: Inhibits calcium ion influx across cell membrane, resulting in dilation of peripheral arteries
Uses: Essential hypertension, alone or with other antihypertensives

DOSAGE AND ROUTES

• *Adult:* **PO** 20 mg daily initially, may increase by 10 mg/wk, usual dose 20-40 mg daily, max 60 mg/day
• *Geriatric/hepatic dose:* **PO** 10 mg/day, increase by 10 mg/wk
Available forms: Ext rel tabs 10, 20, 30, 40 mg

SIDE EFFECTS

CNS: Headache, fatigue, drowsiness, dizziness, anxiety, depression, nervousness, insomnia, light-headedness, paresthesia, tinnitus, psychosis, somnolence, ataxia, confusion, malaise, migraine

CV: Dysrhythmia, edema, CHF, hypotension, palpitations, **MI, pulmonary edema,** tachycardia, syncope, AV block, angina, chest pain, ECG abnormalities

GI: Nausea, vomiting, diarrhea, gastric upset, constipation, increased LFTs, dry mouth, dyspepsia, dysphagia, flatulence

GU: Nocturia, hematuria, dysuria

HEMA: Anemia, leukopenia, petechia

INTEG: Rash, pruritus

MISC: Sexual difficulties, cough, nasal congestion, SOB, wheezing, epistaxis, dyspnea, gingival hyperplasia, chills, fever, gout, sweating

Contraindications: Hypersensitivity; sick sinus syndrome; 2nd-, 3rd-degree heart block; aortic stenosis

Precautions: Pregnancy (C), CHF, hypotension <90 mm Hg systolic, hepatic injury, lactation, children, renal disease, geriatric, acute MI, unstable angina, CAD

PHARMACOKINETICS

Metabolized by liver, excreted in urine, peak 6-12 hr, protein binding 99%, half-life 7-12 hr

INTERACTIONS

Increase: effects of β-blockers, antihypertensives, digoxin

Increase: nisoldipine level—CYP3A4 inhibitors, cimetidine, ranitidine, azole antifungals

Decrease: nisoldipine effect—CYP3A4 inducers, hydantoins

Drug/Herb

Increase: effect—barberry, betel palm, burdock, goldenseal, hawthorn, khat, khella, lily of the valley, plantain

Decrease: effect—St. John's wort, yohimbe

Drug/Food

Increase: nisoldipine level—high-fat foods

Increase: hypotensive effect—grapefruit juice

NURSING CONSIDERATIONS

Assess:
• Cardiac status: B/P, pulse, respiration, ECG
• I&O ratios, weight daily
• For CHF: weight gain, jugular vein distention, edema, crackles

Administer:
• Swallow whole; do not break, crush, or chew
• Once daily as whole tablet; avoid high-fat foods, grapefruit juice

Evaluate:
• Therapeutic response: decreased B/P

Teach patient/family:
• To avoid hazardous activities until stabilized on drug, dizziness is no longer a problem
• To report nausea, dizziness, edema, shortness of breath, palpitations
• To limit caffeine consumption
• To avoid OTC drugs unless directed by a prescriber
• The importance of complying with all areas of medical regimen: diet, exercise, stress reduction, drug therapy
• To rise slowly to prevent orthostatic hypotension

Treatment of overdose: Defibrillation, atropine for AV block, vasopressor for hypotension

nitazoxanide (℞)
(nye-taz-ox'a-nide)
Alinia
Func. class.: Antiprotozoal

Action: Interferes with DNA/RNA synthesis in protozoa
Uses: Diarrhea caused by *Cryptosporidium parvum* or *Giardia lamblia*

DOSAGE AND ROUTES

• *Child 4-11 yr:* **PO** 10 ml (200 mg) q12h × 3 days
• *Child 12-47 mo:* **PO** 5 ml (100 mg) q12h × 3 days
Available forms: Powder for oral susp 100 mg/5 ml

SIDE EFFECTS

CNS: Dizziness, fever, headache
CV: Hypotension
GI: Nausea, anorexia, flatulence, increased appetite, enlarged salivary glands, abdominal pain, diarrhea, vomiting
HEMA: Anemia, **leukopenia,** neutropenia
INTEG: Pruritus, sweating
MISC: Increased creatinine, pale yellow eye discoloration, rhinitis, discolored urine, infection, malaise
Contraindications: Hypersensitivity
Precautions: Pregnancy (B), renal/hepatic disease, lactation, child <1 yr or >11 yr, diabetes mellitus (contains sucrose)

PHARMACOKINETICS

Excreted in urine, bile, feces; hydrolyzed to active metabolite, which undergoes conjugation; metabolite protein binding >99%

INTERACTIONS

• Competes for binding sites: other highly protein-bound drugs

NURSING CONSIDERATIONS

Assess:
• Signs of infection
• Bowel pattern before, during treatment
Administer:
PO route
• With food
Evaluate:
• Therapeutic response: C&S negative for organism
Teach patient/family:
• To take with food; shake susp well before each dose

nitrofurantoin (R)
(nye-troe-fyoor'an-toyn)
Apo-Nitrofurantoin ✦,
Furadantin, Macrobid,
Macrodantin, nitrofurantoin
Func. class.: Urinary tract antiinfective
Chem. class.: Synthetic nitrofuran derivative

Action: Inhibits bacterial acetyl-CoA intefering with carbohydrate metabolism
Uses: Urinary tract infections caused by *Escherichia coli, Klebsiella, Pseudomonas, Proteus vulgaris, Proteus morganii, Serratia, Citrobacter, Staphylococcus aureus, Staphylococcus epidermidis, Enterococcus, Salmonella, Shigella*

DOSAGE AND ROUTES
Active infections
• *Adult:* **PO** 50-100 mg qid pc or 50-100 mg at bedtime for long-term treatment
• *Child 1 mo:* **PO** 5-7 mg/kg/day in 4 divided doses; 1-3 mg/kg/day for long-term treatment, max 7 mg/kg/day
Chronic suppression
• *Adult:* **PO** 50-100 mg qPM
• *Child:* **PO** 1 mg/kg/day qPM or 0.5-1 mg/kg q12h if dose is not well tolerated
Available forms: Caps 25, 50, 100 mg; tabs 50, 100 mg; susp 25 mg/5 ml; macrocrystal caps (Macrodantin) 25, 50, 100 mg; Macrobid cap 100 mg (25 macrocrystals, 75 monohydrate)

SIDE EFFECTS
CNS: Dizziness, headache, drowsiness, peripheral neuropathy, chills, confusion
CV: **Bundle branch block**
GI: Nausea, vomiting, abdominal pain, diarrhea, **cholestatic jaundice,** loss of appetite, **pseudomembranous colitis, hepatitis**
HEMA: **Anemia, agranulocytosis**
INTEG: Pruritus, rash, urticaria, angioedema, alopecia, tooth staining, **exfoliative dermatitis**

SYST: **Stevens-Johnson syndrome, superinfection**
Contraindications: Hypersensitivity, anuria, severe renal disease, infants <1 mo
Precautions: Pregnancy (B), lactation, G6PD deficiency, geriatric, CCr <60, GI disease, diabetes

PHARMACOKINETICS

PO: Half-life 20-60 min; crosses blood-brain barrier, placenta; enters breast milk; excreted as inactive metabolites in liver, unchanged in urine

INTERACTIONS

Increase: antagonistic effect—norfloxacin
Increase: levels of nitrofurantoin—probenecid
Decrease: absorption of magnesium trisilicate antacid
Drug/Herb
• Do not use acidophilus with antiinfectives; separate by several hours
Drug/Lab Test
Increase: BUN, alk phos, bilirubin, creatinine, blood glucose

NURSING CONSIDERATIONS

Assess:
• Blood count during chronic therapy
• Urinary tract infection: burning, pain on urination, fever, cloudy, foul-smelling urine; I&O ratio: C&S before treatment, after completion
• CNS symptoms: insomnia, vertigo, headache, drowsiness, convulsions
• Allergy: fever, flushing, rash, urticaria, pruritus
Administer:
PO route
• Do not break, crush, chew, or open tabs, caps
• Two daily doses if urine output is high or if patient has diabetes
• Use calibrated device to measure liquid product; may mix water, fruit juice; rinse mouth after liquid product; staining of teeth may occur

Evaluate:
• Therapeutic response: decreased dysuria, fever; neg C&S
Teach patient/family:
• To notify prescriber of diarrhea containing mucus or if pus occurs; pseudomembranous colitis may occur
• To take with food or milk; avoid alcohol
• To protect susp from freezing and shake well before taking
• That drug may cause drowsiness; instruct client to seek aid in walking and other activities; advise client not to drive or operate machinery while on medication
• That diabetics should monitor blood glucose level
• That drug may turn urine rust-yellow to brown
⚠ To notify prescriber of symptoms of pseudomembranous colitis: fever, diarrhea with mucus, pus, or blood

---

nitrofurazone topical
See Appendix C

N

nitroglycerin (℞)

(nye-troe-gli'ser-in)

transmucosal tablets (℞)

Nitrogard, Nitrogard SR

extended release caps (℞)

Nitrocot, Nitroglyn E-R, Nitro-par, Nitro-Time, Nitrong

extended release buccal tabs (℞)

Nitrogard, Nitrogard SR ✚

IV (℞)

Nitro-Bid I.V., Tridil

ointment (℞)

Nitro-Bid, Nitrol

SL (℞)

Nitrostat, NitroQuick

translingual spray (℞)

Nitrolingual Translingual Spray

transdermal (℞)

Deponit, Minitran, Nitrek, Nitrocine, Nitrodisc, Nitro-Dur, Transderm-Nitro

Func. class.: Coronary vasodilator, antianginal

Chem. class.: Nitrate

Do not confuse:

Nitro-Bid/Nicobid

Action: Decreases preload, afterload, which is responsible for decreasing left ventricular end-diastolic pressure, systemic vascular resistance; dilates coronary arteries, improves blood flow through coronary vasculature, dilates arterial, venous beds systemically

Uses: Chronic stable angina pectoris, prophylaxis of angina pain, CHF associated with acute MI, controlled hypotension in surgical procedures

DOSAGE AND ROUTES

• *Adult:* **SL** dissolve tab under tongue when pain begins; may repeat q5min until relief occurs; take no more than 3 tabs/15 min; use 1 tab prophylactically 5-10 min before activities; **SUS CAP** q6-12h on empty stomach; **TOP** 1-2 in q8h, increase to 4 in q4h as needed; **IV** 5 mcg/min, then increase by 5 mcg/min q3-5min; if no response after 20 mcg/min, increase by 10-20 mcg/min until desired response; **TRANS PATCH** apply a pad daily to a site free of hair; remove patch at bedtime to provide 10-12h nitrate-free interval to avoid tolerance; **BUCCAL** 1 mg q5h

• *Child:* **IV** initial: 0.25-0.5 mcg/kg/min, titrate to patient response, usual dose 1-3 mcg/kg/min transmucosal

Available forms: Buccal tabs 1, 2, 3 mg; translingual aero 0.4 mg/metered spray; sus rel caps 2.5, 6.5, 9, 13 mg; sus rel tabs 2.6, 6.5, 9 mg; SL tabs 0.3, 0.4, 0.6 mg; oint 2%; trans syst 0.1, 0.2, 0.3, 0.4, 0.6, 0.8 mg/hr; inj sol 25 mg/250 ml, 50 mg/250 ml, 50 mg/500 ml, 100 mg/250 ml, 200 mg/500 ml

SIDE EFFECTS

CNS: Headache, flushing, dizziness

CV: Postural hypotension, tachycardia, **collapse,** syncope, palpitations

GI: Nausea, vomiting

INTEG: Pallor, sweating, rash

Contraindications: Hypersensitivity to this drug or nitrites, severe anemia, increased intracranial pressure, cerebral hemorrhage, closed-angle glaucoma

Precautions: Pregnancy (C), postural hypotension, lactation, children, severe renal/hepatic disease

PHARMACOKINETICS

SUS REL: Onset 20-45 min, duration 3-8 hr

SL: Onset 1-3 min, duration 30 min

TRANSDERMAL: Onset ½-1 hr, duration 12-24 hr

IV: Onset 1-2 min, duration 3-5 min

TRANSMUC: Onset 1-2 min, duration 3-5 hr

AEROSOL: Onset 2 min, duration 30-60 min

TOP OINT: Onset 30-60 min, duration 2-12 hr

Metabolized by liver, excreted in urine, half-life 1-4 min

INTERACTIONS

• Severe hypotension, CV collapse: alcohol

Increase: effects of β-blockers, diuretics, antihypertensives, calcium channel blockers

Increase: hypotension—sildenafil, tadalafil, vardenafil

Increase: nitrate level—aspirin

Decrease: heparin—IV nitroglycerin

Drug/Lab Test

Increase: Urine catecholamine, urine VMA

False increase: Cholesterol

NURSING CONSIDERATIONS

Assess:

• Pain: duration, time started, activity being performed, character

• Orthostatic B/P, pulse prior to and after administration

• Tolerance if taken over long period

• Headache, light-headedness, decreased B/P; may indicate a need for decreased dosage

Administer:

PO route

• Swallow sus rel products whole; do not break, crush, or chew

• With 8 oz H_2O on empty stomach (oral tablet) 1 hr before or

• 2 hr after meals

• SL should be dissolved under tongue, not swallowed

• Aerosol sprayed under tongue, not inhaled

Transdermal route

• Transmucosal tab should be placed between cheek and gum line

• Topical ointment should be measured on papers supplied

• Apply a new TD patch daily and remove after 12-14 hr to prevent tolerance

IV route

• Diluted in amount specified D_5, D_5W, 0.9% NaCl for infusion; use glass infusion bottles, non–polyvinyl chloride infusion tubing; titrate to patient response; do not use filters

Y-site compatibilities: Amiodarone, amphotericin B cholesteryl, amrinone, atracurium, cefmetazole, cisatracurium, diltiazem, DOBUTamine, DOPamine, epiNEPHrine, esmolol, famotidine, fentanyl, fluconazole, furosemide, haloperidol, heparin, hydromorphone, insulin (regular), labetalol, lidocaine, lorazepam, midazolam, milrinone, morphine, niCARdipine, norepinephrine, pancuronium, propofol, ranitidine, remifentanil, sodium nitroprusside, streptokinase, tacrolimus, theophylline, thiopental, vecuronium, warfarin

Evaluate:

• Therapeutic response: decrease, prevention of anginal pain

Teach patient/family:

• To place buccal tab between lip and gum above incisors or between cheek and gum

• To keep tabs in original container; to replace q6mo, as effectiveness is lost; keep away from heat, moisture, light

• If 3 SL tabs in 15 min do not relieve pain, to seek immediate medical attention

• To avoid alcohol

• That drug may cause headache; tolerance usually develops; use nonopioid analgesic

• That drug may be taken before stressful activity: exercise, sexual activity

• That SL may sting when drug comes in contact with mucous membranes

• To avoid hazardous activities if dizziness occurs

• To comply with complete medical regimen

• To make position changes slowly to prevent fainting

⚠ To never use erectile dysfunction products (sildenafil, tadalafil, vardenafil); may cause severe hypotension, death

⚠ High Alert

nitroprusside (℞)
(nye-troe-pruss'ide)
Nitropress, sodium nitro-
prusside
Func. class.: Antihypertensive, vasodilator

Action: Directly relaxes arteriolar, venous smooth muscle, resulting in reduction in cardiac preload, afterload
Uses: Hypertensive crisis, to decrease
bleeding by creating hypotension during
surgery, acute CHF

DOSAGE AND ROUTES

• *Adult and child:* **IV INF** 0.3-8 mcg/kg/
min; max 10 mcg/kg/min
Available forms: Inj 50 mg

SIDE EFFECTS

CNS: Dizziness, headache, agitation,
twitching, decreased reflexes, restlessness
CV: Bradycardia, ECG changes, tachycardia, hypotension
GI: Nausea, vomiting, abdominal pain
INTEG: Pain, irritation at inj site, sweating
MISC: **Cyanide, thiocyanate toxicity,**
flushing, hypothyroidism
Contraindications: Hypersensitivity,
hypertension (compensatory) due to aortic coarctation or AV shunting, acute CHF
associated with reduced peripheral vascular resistance
Precautions: Pregnancy (C), lactation,
children, fluid, electrolyte imbalances,
renal/hepatic disease, hypothyroidism, geriatric

PHARMACOKINETICS

IV: Onset 1-2 min, duration 1-10 min,
half-life 3 days in patients with abnormal renal function, circulating half-life
2 min; metabolized in liver, excreted in
urine

INTERACTIONS

• Severe hypotension: ganglionic blockers, volatile liquid anesthetics, halothane,
enflurane, circulatory depressants
Drug/Herb
Increase: toxicity, death—aconite
Increase: antihypertensive effect—
barberry, betony, black catechu, black cohosh, bloodroot, broom, burdock, cat's
claw, dandelion, goldenseal, Irish moss,
Jamaican dogwood, kelp, khella, mistletoe, parsley
Increase or decrease: antihypertensive
effect—astragalus, cola tree
Decrease: antihypertensive effect—
coltsfoot, guarana, khat, licorice

NURSING CONSIDERATIONS
Assess:

• Electrolytes: K, Na, Cl, CO_2, CBC, serum glucose, serum methemoglobin if
pulmonary O_2 levels are decreased; use
IV 1-2 mg/kg methylene blue given over
several min for methemoglobinemia
• Renal studies: catecholamines, BUN,
creatinine
• Hepatic studies: AST, ALT, alk phos
• B/P by direct means if possible; check
ECG continuously; pulse, jugular vein distention; PCWP; rebound hypertension may
occur after nitroprusside is discontinued
• Weight daily, I&O
⚠ Thiocyanate, lactate, cyanide levels
daily in infusions >3 mcg/kg/min; thiocyanate level should be ≤1 mmol/L; thiocy-
anate toxicity includes confusion, weakness, seizures, hyperreflexia, psychosis,
tinnitus, coma
• Nausea, vomiting, diarrhea
• Edema in feet, legs daily; skin turgor,
dryness of mucous membranes for hydration status
• Crackles, dyspnea, orthopnea q30min
• For decrease in bicarbonate, P_{CO_2} blood
pH, acidosis
Administer:
• Antidote is sodium thiosulfate

IV route
• Depending on B/P reading q15min
• IV after diluting 50 mg/2-3 ml of D_5W, further dilute in 250 ml of D_5W; use an infusion pump only; wrap bottle with aluminum foil to protect from light; observe for color change in the infusion; discard if highly discolored (blue, green, dark red); titrate to patient response

Syringe compatibilities: Heparin
Y-site compatibilities: Amrinone, atracurium, diltiazem, DOBUTamine, DOPamine, enalaprilat, famotidine, lidocaine, nitroglycerin, pancuronium, tacrolimus, theophylline, vecuronium

Evaluate:
• Therapeutic response: decreased B/P, absence of bleeding

Teach patient/family:
• To report headache, dizziness, loss of hearing, blurred vision, dyspnea, faintness
• The reason for giving product and expected results

---

nizatidine (otc, ℞)
(ni-za'ti-deen)
Axid, Axid AR
Func. class.: H_2-receptor antagonist
Chem. class.: Substituted thiazole

Action: Blocks H_2-receptors, thereby reducing gastric acid output
Uses: Benign gastric and duodenal ulceration, prevention of duodenal ulcer recurrence, symptomatic relief of gastroesophageal reflux, heartburn prevention

DOSAGE AND ROUTES
Gastric and duodenal ulcer
• *Adult:* PO 300 mg at night or 150 mg bid for 4-8 wk; maintenance 150 mg at night
Prophylaxis of duodenal ulcer
• *Adult:* PO 150 mg daily at bedtime
Gastroesophageal reflux
• *Adult:* PO 150 mg bid
Heartburn prevention
• *Adult:* PO 75 mg before eating

Renal dose
• *Adult:* **PO** CCr 20-50 ml/min give 150 mg/day; CCr <20 ml/min give 150 mg every other day
Available forms: Caps 150, 300 mg; tabs 75 mg

SIDE EFFECTS
CNS: Headache, somnolence, confusion, abnormal dreams, dizziness
CV: **Cardiac dysrhythmias, cardiac arrest**
ENDO: Gynecomastia
GI: Elevated hepatic enzymes, **hepatitis,** jaundice, nausea
HEMA: **Thrombocytopenia, agranulocytosis, aplastic anemia**
INTEG: Pruritus, sweating, urticaria, **exfoliative dermatitis**
METAB: Hyperuricemia
MS: Myalgia
RESP: **Bronchospasm, laryngeal edema**
Contraindications: Hypersensitivity
Precautions: Pregnancy (B), renal/hepatic impairment (reduce dose in renal impairment), lactation

PHARMACOKINETICS
Partially metabolized by liver, excreted by kidneys, plasma half-life 1½ hr, 70% absorbed orally, small amount (0.1% of plasma concentration) enters breast milk, 35% bound to plasma proteins

NURSING CONSIDERATIONS
Assess:
⚠ CBC with differential if on long-term therapy, agranulocytosis may occur
• Gastric pH (>5 should be maintained)
• Fluid balance, I&O
Administer:
• With meals for prolonged drug effect; antacids 1 hr before or 1 hr after drug; at bedtime if taken daily
Evaluate:
• Mental status, confusion, dizziness, depression, anxiety, weakness, tremors, psychosis, diarrhea, jaundice, report immediately

---

♣ Canada only

Side effects: *italics* = common; **bold** = life-threatening

- For GI symptoms: nausea, vomiting, diarrhea, cramps

Teach patient/family:
- That gynecomastia, impotence may occur, are reversible
- To avoid driving or other hazardous activities until patient is stabilized on this medication; dizziness may occur
- To avoid black pepper, caffeine, alcohol, harsh spices, extremes in temp of food
- To avoid OTC preparations: aspirin, cough, cold preparations

Treatment of overdose: Symptomatic and supportive therapy is recommended; activated charcoal, emesis, or lavage may reduce absorption

---

⚠ High Alert

norepinephrine (℞)
(nor-ep-i-nef'rin)
Levophed
Func. class.: Adrenergic
Chem. class.: Catecholamine

Do not confuse:
norepinephrine/epINEPHrine

Action: Causes increased contractility and heart rate by acting on β-receptors in heart; also acts on α-receptors, causing vasoconstriction in blood vessels; B/P is elevated, coronary blood flow improves, cardiac output increases

Uses: Acute hypotension, shock

DOSAGE AND ROUTES

- *Adult:* IV INF 2-4 mcg/min titrated to B/P; max 30 mcg/min
- *Child:* IV INF 0.1-0.2 mcg/kg/min titrated to B/P; max 2 mcg/kg/min

Available forms: Inj 1 mg/ml

SIDE EFFECTS

CNS: Headache, anxiety, dizziness, insomnia, restlessness, tremor
CV: Palpitations, tachycardia, hypertension, ectopic beats, angina
GI: Nausea, vomiting
GU: Decreased urine output

INTEG: Necrosis, tissue sloughing with extravasation, **gangrene**
RESP: Dyspnea
SYST: **Anaphylaxis**

Contraindications: Hypersensitivity, ventricular fibrillation, tachydysrhythmias, pheochromocytoma, hypotension, hypovolemia

Precautions: Pregnancy (C), lactation, arterial embolism, peripheral vascular disease, hypertension, hyperthyroidism, geriatric, heart disease

PHARMACOKINETICS

IV: Onset 1-2 min; metabolized in liver; excreted in urine (inactive metabolites); crosses placenta

INTERACTIONS

- Dysrhythmias: general anesthetics, bretylium
- Incompatible with alkaline solutions: sodium, HCO_3^-
- Severe hypertension: guanethidine
⚠ Do not use within 2 wk of MAOIs, antihistamines, ergots, methyldopa, oxytocics, tricyclics, guanethidine, or hypertensive crisis may result

Increase: B/P—oxytocics
Increase: pressor effect—tricyclics, MAOIs
Decrease: norepinephrine action—α-blockers

NURSING CONSIDERATIONS

Assess:
- I&O ratio; notify prescriber if output <30 ml/hr
- ECG during administration continuously; if B/P increases, drug is decreased
- B/P and pulse q2-3min after parenteral route
- CVP or PWP during infusion if possible
- For paresthesias and coldness of extremities; peripheral blood flow may decrease
- Inj site: tissue sloughing; administer phentolamine mixed with 0.9% NaCl
- Sulfite sensitivity, which may be life-threatening

Administer:
- Plasma expanders for hypovolemia
- IV after diluting with 500-1000 ml D$_5$W or D$_5$/0.9% NaCl; average dilution is 4 mg/1000 ml diluent (4 mcg base/ml); give as infusion 2-3 ml/min; titrate to response
- Using 2-bottle setup so drug may be discontinued while IV is still running; use infusion pump

Additive compatibilities: Amikacin, calcium chloride, calcium gluconate, cimetidine, corticotropin, dimenhyDRINATE, DOBUTamine, heparin, hydrocortisone, magnesium sulfate, meropenem, methylPREDNISolone, multivitamins, netilmicin, potassium chloride, succinylcholine, verapamil, vit B/C

Syringe compatibilities: Heparin

Y-site compatibilities: Amiodarone, amrinone, cisatracurium, diltiazem, DOBUTamine, DOPamine, epINEPHrine, esmolol, famotidine, fentanyl, furosemide, haloperidol, heparin, hydrocortisone, hydromorphone, labetalol, lorazepam, meropenem, midazolam, milrinone, morphine, niCARdipine, nitroglycerin, potassium chloride, propofol, ranitidine, remifentanil, vecuronium, vit B/C

Perform/provide:
- Storage of reconstituted sol in refrigerator no longer than 24 hr
- Do not use discolored sol

Evaluate:
- Therapeutic response: increased B/P with stabilization

Teach patient/family:
- The reason for drug administration and to report dyspnea, dizziness, chest pain

Treatment of overdose: Administer fluids, electrolyte replacement

norethindrone (℞)
(nor-eth-in′drone)
Aygestin, Camila, Errin, Micronor, Nora-BE, Nor-QD
Func. class.: Progestogen
Chem. class.: Progesterone derivative

Action: Inhibits secretion of pituitary gonadotropins, which prevents follicular maturation, ovulation; stimulates growth of mammary tissue; antineoplastic action against endometrial cancer

Uses: Uterine bleeding (abnormal), amenorrhea, endometriosis, contraception

DOSAGE AND ROUTES
Amenorrhea, abnormal uterine bleeding (Aygestin)
- *Adult:* PO 2.5-10 mg daily days 5-25 of menstrual cycle

Endometriosis (Aygestin)
- *Adult:* PO 5 mg daily × 2 wk, then increased by 2.5 mg daily × 2 wk, up to 15 mg daily

Contraception
- *Adult:* PO 0.35 mg on 1st day of menses, then 0.35 mg daily

Available forms: Tabs (Aygestin) 5 mg; tabs 0.35 mg

SIDE EFFECTS
CNS: Dizziness, headache, migraines, depression, fatigue
CV: Hypotension, **thrombophlebitis**, edema, **thromboembolism, CVA, stroke, pulmonary embolism, MI**
EENT: Diplopia
GI: Nausea, vomiting, anorexia, cramps, increased weight, **cholestatic jaundice**
GU: Amenorrhea, cervical erosion, breakthrough bleeding, dysmenorrhea, vaginal candidiasis, breast changes, (gynecomastia, testicular atrophy, impotence), endometriosis, **spontaneous abortion**
INTEG: Rash, urticaria, acne, hirsutism, alopecia, oily skin, seborrhea, purpura, melasma
META: Hyperglycemia

Contraindications: Pregnancy (X), breast cancer, hypersensitivity, thromboembolic disorders, reproductive cancer, genital bleeding (abnormal, undiagnosed)

Precautions: Lactation, hypertension, asthma, blood dyscrasias, gallbladder disease, CHF, diabetes mellitus, bone disease, depression, migraine headache, convulsive disorders, renal/hepatic disease, family history of breast or reproductive tract cancer

PHARMACOKINETICS

PO: Duration 24 hr, excreted in urine, feces, metabolized in liver

INTERACTIONS

Decrease: progestin effect—barbiturates, carbamazepine, fosphenytoin, phenytoin, rifampin

Drug/Herb

Increase: stimulation—black/green tea, coffee, cola nut, guarana, yerba maté

Decrease: contraception—St. John's wort

Drug/Food

• Caffeine: increase caffeine level

Drug/Lab Test

Increase: Alk phos, nitrogen (urine), pregnanediol, amino acids, factors VII, VIII, IX, X

Decrease: GTT, HDL

NURSING CONSIDERATIONS

Assess:

• Weight daily: notify prescriber of weekly weight gain >5 lb

• B/P at beginning of treatment and periodically

• I&O ratio; be alert for decreasing urinary output, increasing edema

• Hepatic studies: ALT, AST, bilirubin, periodically during long-term therapy

• Edema, hypertension, cardiac symptoms, jaundice, thromboembolism

• Mental status: affect, mood, behavioral changes, depression

• Hypercalcemia

Administer:

• Titrated dose; use lowest effective dose

• In one dose in AM

• With food or milk to decrease GI symptoms

Perform/provide:

• Storage in dark area

Evaluate:

• Therapeutic response: decreased abnormal uterine bleeding, absence of amenorrhea

Teach patient/family:

• About cushingoid symptoms

• To report breast lumps, vaginal bleeding, amenorrhea, edema, jaundice, dark urine, clay-colored stools, dyspnea, headache, blurred vision, abdominal pain, numbness or stiffness in legs, chest pain; men to report impotence or gynecomastia

• To report suspected pregnancy immediately, to wait ≥3 mo after stopping medication to become pregnant

• To avoid smoking; CV reactions may occur

norfloxacin (℞)
(nor-flox'-a-sin)
Noroxin
Func. class.: Urinary antiinfective
Chem. class.: Fluoroquinolone

Action: Interferes with conversion of intermediate DNA fragments into high-molecular-weight DNA in bacteria, inhibits DNA gyrase

Uses: Adult urinary tract infections (including complicated) caused by *Escherichia coli, Enterobacter cloacae, Proteus mirabilis, Klebsiella pneumoniae,* group D strep, indole-positive *Proteus, Citrobacter freundii, Staphylococcus aureus;* uncomplicated gonorrhea; prostatitis; cystitis

DOSAGE AND ROUTES

Uncomplicated infections

• *Adult:* **PO** 400 mg bid × 3-10 days 1 hr before or 2 hr after meals

---

⚠ Safety alert   *"Tall Man" lettering

Complicated infections
• *Adult:* PO 400 mg bid × 10-21 days; 400 mg daily × 7-10 days in impaired renal function
Uncomplicated gonorrhea
• *Adult:* PO 800 mg as a single dose
Prostatitis
• *Adult:* PO 400 mg bid × 4 wk
Renal dose
• *Adult:* PO CCr ≤30 ml/min 400 mg PO daily
Available forms: Tabs 400 mg

SIDE EFFECTS

CNS: Headache, dizziness, fatigue, somnolence, depression, insomnia
CV: **QT prolongation**
EENT: Visual disturbances
GI: Nausea, constipation, **hepatic necrosis,** increased ALT, AST, flatulence, heartburn, vomiting, diarrhea, dry mouth, **pseudomembranous colitis**
HEMA: **Agranulocytosis**
INTEG: Rash, photosensitivity
SYST: **Stevens-Johnson syndrome, angioedema**
Contraindications: Children, hypersensitivity to quinolones
Precautions: Pregnancy (C), lactation, children, renal disease, seizure disorders

PHARMACOKINETICS

Peak 1 hr, half-life 3-4 hr; steady state 2 days; excreted in urine as active drug, metabolites

INTERACTIONS

Increase: levels, toxicity—theophylline, caffeine; do not use together
Increase: serum concentrations of cycloSPORINE
Increase: norfloxacin level—probenecid
Increase: anticoagulation—warfarin
Decrease: effects of norfloxacin—nitrofurantoin; monitor closely
Decrease: norfloxacin effect—antacids, iron products, sucralfate; give 2 hr apart
Drug/Herb
• Do not use acidophilus with antiinfectives; separate by several hours

Drug/Lab Test
Increase: AST, ALT, BUN, creatinine, alk phos

NURSING CONSIDERATIONS

Assess:
• Renal, hepatic studies: BUN, creatinine, AST, ALT
• I&O ratio
• For tendon pain
• CNS symptoms: insomnia, vertigo, headache, agitation, confusion
• Allergic reactions: fever, flushing, rash, urticaria, pruritus
Administer:
• After clean-catch urine for C&S
• Two daily doses if urine output is high or if patient has diabetes
Evaluate:
• Therapeutic response: decreased pain, frequency, urgency, C&S, absence of infection
Teach patient/family:
• That if dizziness occurs, to walk, perform activities with assistance
• To complete full course of drug therapy, to take at same time of day
• To contact prescriber if adverse reaction occurs
• To take 1 hr before or 2 hr after meals; not to take antacids with or within 2 hr of this drug; to sip water or use hard candy for dry mouth

N

---

norfloxacin ophthalmic
See Appendix C

---

norgestrel (℞)
(nor-jess'trel)
Ovrette
Func. class.: Progestogen
Chem. class.: Progesterone derivative

Action: Inhibits secretion of pituitary gonadotropins, which prevents follicular maturation, ovulation, stimulates growth

---

Side effects: *italics* = common; **bold** = life-threatening

of mammary tissue, antineoplastic action against endometrial cancer

Uses: Female contraception

DOSAGE AND ROUTES

• *Adult:* **PO** 1 tab daily

Available forms: Tabs 0.075 mg

SIDE EFFECTS

CNS: Dizziness, headache, migraines, depression, fatigue

CV: Hypotension, **thrombophlebitis,** edema, **thromboembolism, stroke, pulmonary embolism, myocardial infarction**

EENT: Diplopia

GI: Nausea, vomiting, anorexia, cramps, increased weight, **cholestatic jaundice**

GU: Amenorrhea, cervical erosion, breakthrough bleeding, dysmenorrhea, vaginal candidiasis, breast changes, *gynecomastia, testicular atrophy, impotence,* endometriosis, **spontaneous abortion**

INTEG: Rash, urticaria, acne, hirsutism, alopecia, oily skin, seborrhea, purpura, melasma

META: Hyperglycemia

Contraindications: Pregnancy (X), lactation, breast cancer, hypersensitivity, thromboembolic disorders, reproductive cancer, genital bleeding (abnormal, undiagnosed), cerebral hemorrhage

Precautions: Hypertension, asthma, blood dyscrasias, gallbladder disease, CHF, diabetes mellitus, bone disease, depression, migraine headache, convulsive disorders, renal/hepatic disease, family history of breast or reproductive tract cancer

PHARMACOKINETICS

PO: Duration 24 hr; excreted in urine, feces; metabolized in liver

INTERACTIONS

Drug/Lab Test

Increase: Alk phos, nitrogen (urine), pregnanediol, amino acids, factors VII, VIII, IX, X

Decrease: GTT, HDL

NURSING CONSIDERATIONS

Assess:

• Weight daily; notify prescriber of weekly weight gain >5 lb

• B/P at beginning of treatment and periodically

• I&O ratio; be alert for decreasing urinary output, increasing edema

• Hepatic studies: ALT, AST, bilirubin, periodically during long-term therapy

• Edema, hypertension, cardiac symptoms, jaundice

• Mental status: affect, mood, behavioral changes, depression

• Hypercalcemia

Administer:

• Titrated dose; use lowest effective dose

• In one dose in AM

• With food or milk to decrease GI symptoms

• After warming to dissolve crystals

Perform/provide:

• Storage in dark area

Evaluate:

• Therapeutic response: absence of pregnancy

Teach patient/family:

• About cushingoid symptoms

• To report breast lumps, vaginal bleeding, edema, jaundice, dark urine, clay-colored stools, dyspnea, headache, blurred vision, abdominal pain, numbness or stiffness in legs, chest pain

• To report suspected pregnancy, to wait ≥3 mo after stopping medication to get pregnant

• To monitor blood glucose if diabetic

---

nortriptyline (℞)

(nor-trip'ti-leen)

Aventyl, Pamelor

Func. class.: Antidepressant, tricyclic

Chem. class.: Dibenzocycloheptene—secondary amine

Do not confuse:

nortriptyline/amitriptyline

Action: Blocks reuptake of norepinephrine, serotonin into nerve endings, in-

---

creasing action of norepinephrine, serotonin in nerve cells
Uses: Major depression
Unlabeled uses: Chronic pain management

DOSAGE AND ROUTES

• *Adult:* **PO** 25 mg tid or qid; may increase to 150 mg/day; may give daily dose at bedtime
• *Geriatric:* **PO** 10-25 mg at bedtime, increase by 10-25 mg at weekly intervals to desired dose; usual maintenance 75 mg
Available forms: Caps 10, 25, 50, 75 mg; sol 10 mg/5 ml

SIDE EFFECTS

CNS: Dizziness, drowsiness, confusion, headache, anxiety, tremors, stimulation, weakness, insomnia, nightmares, EPS (geriatric), increased psychiatric symptoms
CV: Orthostatic hypotension, ECG changes, tachycardia, **hypertension,** palpitations, **dysrhythmias**
EENT: Blurred vision, tinnitus, mydriasis
GI: Constipation, dry mouth, nausea, vomiting, **paralytic ileus,** increased appetite, cramps, epigastric distress, jaundice, **hepatitis,** stomatitis
GU: Urinary retention, **acute renal failure**
HEMA: **Agranulocytosis, thrombocytopenia, eosinophilia, leukopenia**
INTEG: Rash, urticaria, sweating, pruritus, photosensitivity
Contraindications: Hypersensitivity to tricyclics, recovery phase of MI, convulsive disorders, prostatic hypertrophy
Precautions: Pregnancy (C), suicidal patients, severe depression, increased intraocular pressure, narrow-angle glaucoma, urinary retention, hepatic/cardiac disease, hyperthyroidism, electroshock therapy, elective surgery, lactation, children

PHARMACOKINETICS

PO: Steady state 4-19 days; metabolized by liver; excreted by kidneys; crosses placenta; excreted in breast milk; half-life 18-28 hr

INTERACTIONS

• Heavy smoking: decreased drug effect
⚠ Hyperpyretic crisis, seizures, hypertensive episode: MAOI
Increase: effects of direct-acting sympathomimetics (epINEPHrine), alcohol, barbiturates, benzodiazepines, CNS depressants
Decrease: effects of guanethidine, clonidine, indirect-acting sympathomimetics (epHEDrine)
Drug/Herb
• Serotonin syndrome: SAM-e, St. John's wort
Increase: anticholinergic effect—belladonna, corkwood, henbane, jimsonweed
Increase: antidepressant action—scopolia
Increase: CNS effect—hops, lavender
Drug/Lab Test
Increase: Serum bilirubin, blood glucose, alk phos
Decrease: VMA, 5-HIAA
False increase: Urinary catecholamines

NURSING CONSIDERATIONS

Assess:
• B/P (lying, standing), pulse q4h; if systolic B/P drops 20 mm Hg, hold drug, notify prescriber; take vital signs q4h in patients with CV disease
• Blood studies: CBC, leukocytes, differential, cardiac enzymes if patient is receiving long-term therapy
• Hepatic studies: AST, ALT, bilirubin
• Weight qwk; appetite may increase with drug
• ECG for flattening of T wave, bundle branch block, AV block, dysrhythmias in cardiac patients
• EPS primarily in geriatric: rigidity, dystonia, akathisia
• Mental status changes: mood, sensorium, affect, suicidal tendencies, increase in psychiatric symptoms, depression, panic

N

• Urinary retention, constipation; constipation is more likely to occur in children
⚠ Withdrawal symptoms: headache, nausea, vomiting, muscle pain, weakness; do not usually occur unless drug was discontinued abruptly
• Alcohol intake; if alcohol is consumed, hold dose until AM

Administer:
• Increased fluids, bulk in diet if constipation occurs
• With food, milk for GI symptoms
• Dosage at bedtime for oversedation during day; may take entire dose at bedtime; geriatric may not tolerate once/day dosing
• Gum, hard candy, frequent sips of water for dry mouth
• Concentrate with fruit juice, water, or milk to disguise taste

Perform/provide:
• Storage in tight, light-resistant container at room temperature
• Assistance with ambulation during beginning therapy, since drowsiness/dizziness occurs
• Safety measures including side rails, primarily for geriatric
• Checking to see if PO medication swallowed

Evaluate:
• Therapeutic response: decreased depression

Teach patient/family:
• That therapeutic effects may take 2-3 wk
• To use caution in driving, other activities requiring alertness because of drowsiness, dizziness, blurred vision
• To avoid alcohol ingestion, other CNS depressants
• Not to discontinue medication quickly after long-term use; may cause nausea, headache, malaise
• To wear sunscreen or large hat, since photosensitivity occurs
• To report immediately urinary retention

Treatment of overdose: ECG monitoring; induce emesis; lavage, activated charcoal; administer anticonvulsant

---

nystatin (R)
(nye-stat′in)
Mycostatin, Nadostine ✦,
Nilstat, Nystex, PMS-Nystatin ✦,
Pastilles, nystatin
Func. class.: Antifungal
Chem. class.: Amphoteric polyene

Action: Interferes with fungal DNA replication; binds sterols in fungal cell membrane, which increases permeability, leaking of cell nutrients
Uses: Lozenges, oral: *Candida* species causing oral, intestinal infections

DOSAGE AND ROUTES
Oral infection
• *Adult:* **SUSP** 400,000-600,000 units qid, use ½ dose in each side of mouth, swish and swallow
• *Infant:* **SUSP** 200,000 units qid (100,000 units in each side of mouth)
• *Newborn and premature infant:* **SUSP** 100,000 units qid
• *Adult and child:* **TROCHES** 200,000-400,000 units qid × up to 2 wk
GI infection
• *Adult:* **PO** 500,000-1,000,000 units tid
Available forms: Tabs 500,000 units; powder for oral susp 50 million, 150 million, 500 million, 1 billion, 2 billion, 5 billion units; susp 100,000 units per ml; troches 200,000 units; oral caps 500,000, 1,000,000 units
Side effects/adverse reactions:
GI: Nausea, vomiting, anorexia, diarrhea, cramps
INTEG: Rash, urticaria (rare)
Contraindications: Hypersensitivity
Precautions: Pregnancy (B)

PHARMACOKINETICS
PO: Little absorption, excreted in feces

NURSING CONSIDERATIONS
Assess:
• For allergic reaction: rash, urticaria; drug may have to be discontinued
• For predisposing factors: antibiotic

⚠ Safety alert   *"Tall Man" lettering

therapy, pregnancy, diabetes mellitus, sexual partner infection (vaginal infections)
Administer:
• Oral susp dose by placing ½ in each cheek, then swallow
• Topical dose after cleansing area; mouth may be swabbed
Perform/provide:
• Storage in refrigerator for oral susp; tabs in tight, light-resistant containers at room temperature
Evaluate:
• Therapeutic response: culture negative for *Candida*
Teach patient/family:
• That long-term therapy may be needed to clear infection; to complete entire course of medication
• Using no commercial mouthwashes for mouth infection
• Shake susp before measuring each dose
• To notify prescriber of irritation; drug may have to be discontinued

nystatin topical
See Appendix C

nystatin vaginal antifungal
See Appendix C

octreotide (℞)
(ok-tree'oh-tide)
Sandostatin, Sandostatin LAR Depot
Func. class.: Hormone, antidiarrheal
Chem. class.: Octapeptide

Action: A potent growth hormone similar to somatostatin
Uses: Sandostatin: acromegaly, improves symptoms in carcinoid tumors, vasoactive intestinal peptide tumors (VIPomas); LAR Depot: long-term maintenance of acromegaly, carcinoid tumors, VIPomas

Unlabeled uses: GI fistula, variceal bleeding, diarrheal conditions, pancreatic fistula, irritable bowel syndrome, dumping syndrome

DOSAGE AND ROUTES
Acromegaly
• *Adult:* **SUBCUT/IV** (Sandostatin) 50-100 mcg bid-tid, adjust q2wk based on growth hormone levels, or **IM** (Sandostatin LAR) 20 mg q4wk × 3 mo, adjust by growth hormone levels
VIPomas
• *Adult:* **SUBCUT/IV** (Sandostatin) 0.2-0.3 mg daily in 2-4 doses for 2 wk, not to exceed 0.45 mg daily, or **IM** (Sandostatin LAR) 20 mg q2wk × 2 mo, adjust dose
Carcinoid tumors
• *Adult:* **SUBCUT/IV** (Sandostatin) 0.1-0.6 mg daily in 2-4 doses for 2 wk, titrated to patient response, or **IM** (Sandostatin LAR) 20 mg q4wk × 2 mo, adjust dose
GI fistula
• *Adult:* **SUBCUT** (Sandostatin) 50-200 mcg q8h
Antidiarrheal in AIDS patients
• *Adult:* **SUBCUT/IV** (Sandostatin) 100-1800 mcg/day
Irritable bowel syndrome
• *Adult:* **SUBCUT** (Sandostatin) 100 mcg single dose to 125 mcg bid
Dumping syndrome
• *Adult:* **SUBCUT** (Sandostatin) 50-150 mcg/day
Variceal bleeding
• *Adult:* **IV** (Sandostatin) 25-50 mcg/hr CONT **IV** INF for 18 hr-5 days
Available forms: Inj (Sandostatin) 0.05, 0.1, 0.2, 0.5, 1 mg/ml; inj (LAR depot) 10, 20, 30 mg/5 ml

SIDE EFFECTS
CNS: Headache, dizziness, fatigue, weakness, depression, anxiety, tremors, **seizure,** paranoia
CV: Sinus bradycardia, conduction abnormalities, **dysrhythmias,** chest pain,

SOB, thrombophlebitis, ischemia, **CHF**, hypertension, palpitations

ENDO: Hyperglycemia, ketosis, hypothyroidism, hypoglycemia, galactorrhea, diabetes insipidus

GI: Diarrhea, nausea, abdominal pain, vomiting, flatulence, distention, constipation, **hepatitis,** increased LFTs, **GI bleeding, pancreatitis**

GU: UTI, pollakiuria

HEMA: Hematoma of inj site, bruise

INTEG: Rash, urticaria, pain; inflammation at inj site

MS: Joint and muscle pain

Contraindications: Hypersensitivity

Precautions: Pregnancy (B), diabetes mellitus, hypothyroidism, geriatric, lactation, children, renal disease

PHARMACOKINETICS

Absorbed rapidly, completely, peak ½ hr, half-life 1.7 hr, duration 12 hr, excreted unchanged in urine

INTERACTIONS

Increase: rejection—cycloSPORINE

Drug/Food

Decrease: absorption of dietary fat, vit B_{12} levels

Drug/Lab Test

Decrease: T_4

NURSING CONSIDERATIONS

Assess:

• Growth hormone antibodies, IGF-1, 1-4 hr intervals for 8-12 hr post dose in acromegaly; 5-HIAA, plasma serotonin, plasma substance P in carcinoid; VIP in VIPomas

• Thyroid function tests: T_3, T_4, T_7, TSH to identify hypothyroidism

• Fecal fat, serum carotene

• Allergic reaction: rash, itching, fever, nausea, wheezing

• For cardiac status: bradycardia, conduction abnormalities, dysrhythmias; monitor ECG for QT prolongation, low voltage, axis shifts, early repolarization, R/S transition, early wave progression

Administer:

IM route

• Reconstitute with diluent provided; give into gluteal

SUBCUT route

• Rotate inj site; use hip, thigh, abdomen

• Avoid using medication that is cold; allow to reach room temperature

IV route

• May use IV bolus if required; give over 3 min

• To use by intermittent infusion, dilute in 50-200 ml D_5W, 0.9% NaCl; give 15-30 min

Perform/provide:

• Storage in refrigerator for unopened amps, vials; or room temperature for 2 wk, protect from light; do not use discolored or cloudy sol

Evaluate:

• Therapeutic response: relief of diarrhea in AIDS, improves symptoms in carcinoid or VIP tumors, data is insufficient if drugs decrease size/rate of tumor growth, decreasing symptoms of acromegaly

Teach patient/family:

• Regular assessments are required

• Regarding SUBCUT inj if patient or other persons will be giving inj

• To change position slowly to prevent orthostatic hypotension

---

ofloxacin (℞)

(o-flox′a-sin)

Floxin

Func. class.: Antiinfective

Chem. class.: Fluoroquinolone

Action: Interferes with conversion of intermediate DNA fragments into high-molecular-weight DNA in bacteria, inhibits DNA gyrase

Uses: Treatment of lower respiratory tract infections (pneumonia, bronchitis), genitourinary infections (prostatitis, UTIs) caused by *Escherichia coli, Klebsiella pneumoniae, Chlamydia trachomatis, Neisseria gonorrhoeae;* skin and skin

---

structure infections; conjunctivitis (oph-thalmic) (refer to Appendix C)

DOSAGE AND ROUTES

Lower respiratory tract infections/ skin and skin structure infections
• *Adult:* **PO, IV** 400 mg q12h × 10 days
Cervicitis, urethritis
• *Adult:* **PO, IV** 300 mg q12h × 7 days
Prostatitis
• *Adult:* **PO, IV** 300 mg q12h × 6 wk
Acute, uncomplicated gonorrhea
• *Adult:* **PO, IV** 400 mg as a single dose
Urinary tract infection
• *Adult:* **PO, IV** 200-400 mg q12h × 3-10 days
Renal dose
• *Adult:* **PO** CCr 20-50 ml/min give q24h; CCr <20 ml/min give ½ of dose q24h
Available forms: Tabs 200, 300, 400 mg; inj 20, 40 mg/ml; 200 mg/50 ml; 400 mg/100 ml

SIDE EFFECTS

CNS: Dizziness, headache, fatigue, som-nolence, depression, insomnia, lethargy, malaise, **seizures**
CV: **QT prolongation, dysrhythmias**
EENT: Visual disturbances
GI: Diarrhea, nausea, vomiting, an-orexia, flatulence, heartburn, dry mouth, increased AST, ALT, abdominal pain, con-stipation, **pseudomembranous colitis**
HEMA: **Blood dyscrasias**
INTEG: Rash, pruritus
SYST: **Anaphylaxis, Stevens-Johnson syndrome, toxic epidermal necroly-sis**

Contraindications: QT prolongation, hypersensitivity to quinolones
Precautions: Pregnancy (C), lactation, children, geriatric, renal disease, seizure disorders, excessive sunlight, hypokale-mia

PHARMACOKINETICS

PO: Peak 1-2 hr, half-life 9 hr, steady state 2 days; excreted in urine as active drug, metabolites; 90%-95% bioavailability

INTERACTIONS

• May alter blood glucose levels: antidia-betics
• Possible theophylline toxicity: theoph-ylline, do not use together
Increase: CNS stimulation, seizures—NSAIDs
Increase: anticoagulation—warfarin
Decrease: absorption—antacids with aluminum, magnesium, iron products, su-cralfate, zinc products; separate by 2 hr
Drug/Herb
• Do not use acidophilus with antiinfec-tives; separate by several hours
Increase: effect—cola nut

NURSING CONSIDERATIONS

Assess:
• Renal, hepatic studies: BUN, creatinine, AST, ALT
• Cardiac status: QT prolongation
• CNS symptoms: insomnia, vertigo, headache, agitation, confusion
• Allergic reactions: rash, flushing, urti-caria, pruritus
Administer:
PO route
• 2 hr before or 2 hr after antacids, cal-cium, iron, zinc products
• After clean-catch urine for C&S
IV route
• Dilute to 4 mg/ml with 0.9% NaCl, D_5W, D_5/LR, $D_5/0.9\%$ NaCl, 5% $NaCO_3$, D_5 plas-malyte 56, sodium lactate; give over 1 hr or more
Y-site compatibilities: Ampicillin, bivalrudin, cefotaxime, ceftazidime, cisa-tracurium, clindamycin, docetaxel, etopo-side, gemcitabine, gentamicin, grani-setron, linezolid, piperacillin, propofol, remifentanil, thiotepa, tobramycin, vanco-mycin
Perform/provide:
• Storage for 2 wk refrigerated or 6 mo frozen after reconstitution
Evaluate:
• Therapeutic response: urine culture, absence of symptoms of infection

Side effects: *italics* = common; **bold** = life-threatening

Teach patient/family:
• That if dizziness or light-headedness occurs, ambulate, perform activities with assistance
• To complete full course of therapy
• To avoid iron- or mineral-containing supplements within 2 hr before or after dose
• To avoid sun exposure, photosensitivity can occur

---

ofloxacin ophthalmic
See Appendix C

---

olanzapine
(oh-lanz'a-peen)
Zyprexa, Zyprexa
IntraMuscular
Func. class.: Antipsychotic, neuroleptic
Chem. class.: Thienbenzodiazepine

Action: Unknown; may mediate antipsychotic activity by both dopamine and serotonin type 2 (5-HT2) antagonist; also, may antagonize muscarinic receptors, histaminic (H_1)- and α-adrenergic receptors

Uses: Schizophrenia, acute manic episodes in bipolar disorder
Unlabeled uses: Dementia related to Alzheimer's disease, OCD

DOSAGE AND ROUTES
Schizophrenia
• *Adult:* **PO** 5-10 mg initially daily, may increase dosage by 5 mg at 1 wk or more intervals; orally disintegrating tabs: open blister pack, place tab on tongue, let disintegrate, swallow
• *Geriatric:* **PO** 5 mg, may increase cautiously at 1-wk intervals
Bipolar mania
• *Adult:* **PO** 10-15 mg daily, may increase dose >24 hr, by 5 mg
Agitation associated with schizophrenia, bipolar I mania
• *Adult:* **IM** 10 mg

Available forms: Tab 2.5, 5, 7.5, 10, 15, 20 mg; orally disintegrating tabs 5, 10, 15, 20 mg; powder for inj 10 mg

SIDE EFFECTS
CNS: EPS: pseudoparkinsonism, akathisia, dystonia, tardive dyskinesia, **seizures**, headache, **neuroleptic malignant syndrome (rare)**, somnolence, agitation, nervousness, hostility, *dizziness,* hypertonia, *tremor,* euphoria, confusion, *drowsiness,* fatigue, *abnormal gait, insomnia, fever*
CV: Hypotension, tachycardia, chest pain, **heart failure, sudden death (geriatric, IM)**
ENDO: Increased prolactin levels
GI: Dry mouth, nausea, vomiting, appetite, dyspepsia, anorexia, *constipation,* abdominal pain, *weight gain*
GU: Urinary retention, urinary frequency, enuresis, impotence, amenorrhea, gynecomastia, breast engorgement, premenstrual syndrome
INTEG: Rash
MISC: Peripheral edema, accidental injury, hypertonia
MS: Joint pain, twitching
RESP: Cough, pharyngitis; **fatal pneumonia (geriatric, IM)**
Contraindications: Hypersensitivity
Precautions: Pregnancy (C), lactation, hypertension, hepatic/cardiac disease, geriatric

PHARMACOKINETICS
Well absorbed (60%), peak 6 hr, metabolized by liver, glucuronidation/oxidation by CYP1A2 and CYP2D6, excreted in urine (57%), feces (30%), 93% bound to plasma proteins, half-life 21-54 hr, extended in geriatric; clearance decreased in women, increased in smokers

INTERACTIONS
Increase: sedation—other CNS depressants, alcohol, barbiturate anesthetics, antihistamines, sedatives/hypnotics, antidepressants

---

⚠ Safety alert   *"Tall Man" lettering

Increase: olanzapine levels—CYP1A2 inhibitors (fluvoxamine)
Increase: hypotension—antihypertensives, alcohol, diazepam
Increase: anticholinergic effects—anticholinergics
Decrease: olanzapine levels—CYP1A2 inducers: carbamazepine, omeprazole, rifampin
Decrease: antiparkinson activity—levodopa, bromocriptine, other DOPamine agonists

Drug/Herb
Increase: EPS—betel palm, kava
Increase: effect—cola tree, hops, nettle, nutmeg

Drug/Lab Test
Increase: LFTs, prolactin, CPK

NURSING CONSIDERATIONS
Assess:
• Mental status: orientation, mood, behavior, presence of hallucinations and type before initial administration and monthly
• Swallowing of PO medication: check for hoarding or giving of medication to other patients
• I&O ratio; palpate bladder if low urinary output occurs, urinary retention may be the cause especially in geriatric
• Bilirubin, CBC
• Urinalysis recommended before, during prolonged therapy
• Affect, orientation, LOC, reflexes, gait, coordination, sleep pattern disturbances
• B/P sitting, standing, lying: take pulse and respirations q4h during initial treatment; establish baseline before starting treatment; report drops of 30 mm Hg; obtain baseline ECG
• Dizziness, faintness, palpitations, tachycardia on rising
⚠ Geriatric for serious reactions: fatal pneumonia, heart failure leading to death (IM)
⚠ For neuroleptic malignant syndrome: hyperpyrexia, muscle rigidity, increased CPK, altered mental status, for acute dystonia (check chewing, swallowing, eyes, pill rolling)

• EPS, including akathisia (inability to sit still, no pattern to movements), tardive dyskinesia (bizarre movements of the jaw, mouth, tongue, extremities), pseudoparkinsonism (rigidity, tremors, pill rolling, shuffling gait)
• Skin turgor daily
• Constipation, urinary retention daily; increase bulk, H_2O in diet

Administer:
• Antiparkinsonian agent for EPS
• Decreased dose in geriatric

PO route
• PO with full glass of water, milk; or with food to decrease GI upset
• Orally disintegrating tabs: open blister pack; place tab on tongue until dissolved; swallow; no water needed

IM route
• Dissolve contents of vials with 2.1 ml sterile water for injection (5 mg/ml), use immediately
• Do not use IV or SUBCUT
• Inject slowly, deep into muscle mass

Perform/provide:
• Decreased stimuli by dimming light, avoiding loud noises
• Supervised ambulation until stabilized on medication; do not involve in strenuous exercise program because fainting is possible; patient should not stand still for long periods
• Increased fluids, bulk in diet to prevent constipation
• Sips of water, candy, gum for dry mouth
• Storage in tight, light-resistant container

Evaluate:
• Therapeutic response: decrease in emotional excitement, hallucinations, delusion, paranoia, reorganization of patterns of thought, speech

Teach patient/family:
• To use good oral hygiene; frequent rinsing of mouth, sugarless gum, candy, ice chips for dry mouth
• To avoid hazardous activities until drug response is determined
• That orthostatic hypotension occurs often and to rise from sitting or lying position gradually

---

• To avoid hot tubs, hot showers, tub baths, since hypotension may occur
• To avoid abrupt withdrawal of this drug, or EPS may result; drug should be withdrawn slowly
• To avoid OTC preparations (cough, hay fever, cold) unless approved by prescriber, since serious drug interactions may occur; avoid use with alcohol, CNS depressants; increased drowsiness may occur
• That in hot weather, heat stroke may occur; take extra precautions to stay cool
Treatment of overdose: Lavage if orally ingested; provide airway; do not induce vomiting or use epINEPHrine

---

olmesartan (℞)
(ol-meh-sar'tan)
Benicar
Func. class.: Antihypertensive
Chem. class.: Angiotensin II receptor (type AT₁) antagonist

Action: Blocks the vasoconstrictor and aldosterone-secreting effects of angiotensin II; selectively blocks the binding of angiotensin II to the AT₁ receptor found in tissues
Uses: Hypertension, alone or in combination with other antihypertensives

DOSAGE AND ROUTES
• *Adult:* **PO,** single agent 20 mg daily initially in patients who are not volume depleted, may be increased to 40 mg daily if needed after 2 wk
Available forms: Tabs 5, 20, 40 mg

SIDE EFFECTS
CNS: Dizziness, fatigue, headache, insomnia
CV: Chest pain, peripheral edema, tachycardia
EENT: Sinusitis, rhinitis, pharyngitis
GI: Diarrhea, abdominal pain
MS: Arthralgia, pain
RESP: Upper respiratory infection, bronchitis
SYST: **Angioedema**

Contraindications: Pregnancy (D) 2nd/3rd trimesters, hypersensitivity
Precautions: Pregnancy (C) 1st trimester, lactation, children, geriatric, hepatic disease, CHF

PHARMACOKINETICS
Peak 12 hr, excreted in urine and feces, half-life 13 hr, protein binding 99%

INTERACTIONS
Increase: antihypertensive effects—other antihypertensives, diuretics
Increase: hyperkalemia—potassium supplements, potassium-sparing diuretics
Increase: effect of lithium
Decrease: antihypertensive effect—NSAIDs, salicylates
Drug/Herb
Increase: toxicity, death—aconite
Increase: antihypertensive effect—barberry, betony, black catechu, black cohosh, bloodroot, broom, burdock, cat's claw, dandelion, goldenseal, hawthorn, Irish moss, Jamaican dogwood, kelp, khella, mistletoe, parsley
Increase or decrease: antihypertensive effect—astragalus, cola tree
Decrease: antihypertensive effect—coltsfoot, guarana, khat, licorice, yohimbine

NURSING CONSIDERATIONS
Assess:
⚠ For pregnancy; this drug can cause fetal death when given in pregnancy
• Response and adverse reactions especially in renal disease
• B/P, pulse q4h; note rate, rhythm, quality; electrolytes: K, Na, Cl; baselines in renal, hepatic studies before therapy begins
• Skin turgor, dryness of mucous membranes for hydration status; for angioedema: facial swelling, dyspnea
Administer:
• Without regard to meals

⚠ Safety alert   *"Tall Man" lettering

Evaluate:
• Therapeutic response: decreased B/P
Teach patient/family:
• To comply with dosage schedule, even if feeling better
• To notify prescriber of mouth sores, fever, swelling of hands or feet, irregular heartbeat, chest pain
• That excessive perspiration, dehydration, vomiting, diarrhea may lead to fall in blood pressure; to consult prescriber if these occur
• That drug may cause dizziness, fainting; light-headedness may occur
• To rise slowly to sitting or standing position to minimize orthostatic hypotension
• To notify prescriber immediately if pregnant; not to use during lactation
• To avoid all OTC medications, unless approved by prescriber
• To inform all health care providers of medication use
• To use proper technique for obtaining B/P and acceptable parameters

olopatadine ophthalmic
See Appendix C

olsalazine (℞)
(ohl-sal'ah-zeen)
Dipentum
Func. class.: Antiinflammatory
Chem. class.: Salicylate derivative

Action: Bioconverted to 5-aminosalicylic acid, which decreases inflammation
Uses: Maintenance of remission of ulcerative colitis in patients intolerant to sulfasalazine

DOSAGE AND ROUTES
• *Adult:* **PO** 500 mg bid
Available forms: Caps 250 mg

SIDE EFFECTS
CNS: Headache, hallucinations, depression, vertigo, fatigue, dizziness
GI: Nausea, vomiting, abdominal pain, **hepatitis,** diarrhea, bloating, pancreatitis
HEMA: **Leukopenia, neutropenia, thrombocytopenia, agranulocytosis, anemia**
INTEG: Rash, dermatitis, urticaria
Contraindications: Hypersensitivity to salicylates
Precautions: Pregnancy (C), child <14 yr, lactation; impaired hepatic/renal function; severe allergy; bronchial asthma

PHARMACOKINETICS
PO: Partially absorbed, peak 1½ hr, half-life 5-10 hr, excreted in urine as 5-aminosalicylic acid and metabolites, crosses placenta

INTERACTIONS
Drug/Lab Test
Increase: AST, ALT

NURSING CONSIDERATIONS
Assess:
⚠ Blood dyscrasias: skin rash, fever, sore throat, bruising, bleeding, fatigue, joint pain (rare)
• Allergic reaction: rash, dermatitis, urticaria, pruritus, dyspnea, bronchospasm
Administer:
• Medication after C&S; repeat C&S after full course of medication
• Total daily dose evenly spaced to minimize GI intolerance, with food
Perform/provide:
• Storage in tight, light-resistant container at room temperature
Evaluate:
• Therapeutic response: absence of fever, mucus in stools

Side effects: *italics* = common; **bold** = life-threatening

omalizumab (℞)
(oh-mah-lye-zoo′mab)
Xolair
Func. class.: Antiasthmatic
Chem. class.: Monoclonal antibody

Action: Recombinant DNA-derived humanized IgG murine monoclonal antibody that selectively binds to IgE to limit the release of mediators in the allergic response

Uses: Moderate to severe persistent asthma

Unlabeled uses: Seasonal allergic rhinitis, food allergy

DOSAGE AND ROUTES
• *Adult:* **SUBCUT** 150-375 mg × 2-4 wk, divide inj into 2 sites, if dose is >150 mg; dose is adjusted based on IgE levels, and significant changes in body weight

Available forms: Powder for inj, lyophilized 202.5 mg (150 mg/1.2 ml after reconstitution)

SIDE EFFECTS
INTEG: Pruritus, dermatitis, inj site reactions, rash
MISC: Earache, dizziness, fatigue, pain, **malignancies**, viral infections, **anaphylaxis**
MS: Arthralgia, fracture, leg, arm pain
RESP: Sinusitis, upper respiratory infections, pharyngitis

Contraindications: Hypersensitivity to this drug or hamster protein

Precautions: Pregnancy (B), acute attacks of asthma, lactation, children <12 yr, lymphoma, nephrotic disease

PHARMACOKINETICS
Slowly absorbed, peak 7-8 days, half-life 26 days, degradation by liver, excretion in bile

INTERACTIONS
• None known

NURSING CONSIDERATIONS
Assess:
• Respiratory rate, rhythm, depth; auscultate lung fields bilaterally; notify prescriber of abnormalities

⚠ Anaphylaxis, allergic reactions: rash, urticaria, inability to breathe, edema of throat; drug should be discontinued; have emergency equipment available

Administer:
SUBCUT route
• Reconstitute using 1.4 ml sterile water for inj; gently swirl to dissolve; invert vial to allow to drain; use large-bore needle to withdraw medication; replace needle with small-bore needle
• Given q2-4 wk, product is viscous; if >150 mg is given divide into two sites; the inj may take 5-10 seconds to administer

Evaluate:
• Therapeutic response: ability to breathe more easily

Teach patient/family:
• That improvement will not be immediate
• Not to stop taking or decrease current asthma medications unless instructed by prescriber
• Avoid live virus vaccines while taking this product

omeprazole (OTC, ℞)
(oh-mep′ray-zole)
Losec ✦, Prilosec, Prilosec OTC, Zegerid
Func. class.: Antiulcer, proton pump inhibitor
Chem. class.: Benzimidazole

Do not confuse:
Prilosec/Prinivil/Prozac/predniSONE

Action: Suppresses gastric secretion by inhibiting hydrogen/potassium ATPase enzyme system in gastric parietal cell; characterized as gastric acid pump inhibitor, since it blocks final step of acid production

---

⚠ Safety alert   *"Tall Man" lettering

Uses: Gastroesophageal reflux disease (GERD), severe erosive esophagitis, poorly responsive systemic GERD, pathologic hypersecretory conditions (Zollinger-Ellison syndrome, systemic mastocytosis, multiple endocrine adenomas); treatment of active duodenal ulcers with or without antiinfectives for *Helicobacter pylori*

Unlabeled uses: GERD-related laryngitis, enhancing pancreatin

DOSAGE AND ROUTES

Active duodenal ulcers
• *Adult:* PO 20 mg daily × 4-8 wk; associated with *H. pylori* 40 mg qAM and clarithromycin 500 mg tid on days 1-14, then 20 mg daily on days 15-28

Severe erosive esophagitis/poorly responsive GERD
• *Adult:* PO 20 mg daily × 4-8 wk

Pathologic hypersecretory conditions
• *Adult:* PO 60 mg/day; may increase to 120 mg tid; daily doses >80 mg should be divided

Gastric ulcer
• *Adult:* PO 40 mg daily 4-8 wk
• *Geriatric:* ≤20 mg/day

Heartburn (OTC)
• *Adult:* PO 1 delayed rel tab (20 mg) daily before AM meal with glass of water

Laryngitis (unlabeled)
• *Adult:* PO 20-40 mg at bedtime × 6-24 wk or 20 mg bid × 4-12 wk

Available forms: Delayed rel caps 10, 20, 40 mg; delayed rel tabs (Prilosec OTC) 20 mg

SIDE EFFECTS

CNS: Headache, dizziness, asthenia
CV: Chest pain, angina, tachycardia, bradycardia, palpitations, peripheral edema
EENT: Tinnitus, taste perversion
GI: Diarrhea, abdominal pain, vomiting, nausea, constipation, flatulence, acid regurgitation, abdominal swelling, anorexia, irritable colon, esophageal candidiasis, dry mouth
GU: UTI, urinary frequency, increased creatinine, **proteinuria, hematuria,** testicular pain, glycosuria

HEMA: **Pancytopenia, thrombocytopenia, neutropenia, leukocytosis,** anemia
INTEG: Rash, dry skin, urticaria, pruritus, alopecia
META: Hypoglycemia, increased hepatic enzymes, weight gain
MISC: Back pain, fever, fatigue, malaise
RESP: Upper respiratory infections, cough, epistaxis

Contraindications: Hypersensitivity
Precautions: Pregnancy (C), lactation, children

PHARMACOKINETICS

Bioavailabity 30%-40%; peak ½-3½ hr; half-life ½-1 hr; protein binding 95%; eliminated in urine as metabolites and in feces; in geriatric elimination rate decreased, bioavailability increased; metabolized by CYP450 enzyme system

INTERACTIONS

Increase: bleeding—warfarin
Increase: serum levels of diazepam, phenytoin, flurazepam, triazolam, cycloSPORINE, disulfiram, digoxin
Decrease: absorption of iron salts, ketoconazole, cyanocobalamin, calcium carbonate

Drug/Lab Test
Increase: Alk phos, AST, ALT, bilirubin, gastrin

NURSING CONSIDERATIONS
Assess:
• GI system: bowel sounds q8h, abdomen for pain, swelling, anorexia
• Hepatic enzymes: AST, ALT, alk phos during treatment; blood studies: CBC, differential during treatment

Administer:
• Swallow caps whole; do not crush or chew
• Caps may be opened and sprinkled over applesauce
• Before eating, usually in the AM

Evaluate:
• Therapeutic response: absence of epigastric pain, swelling, fullness

Teach patient/family:

• To report severe diarrhea; drug may have to be discontinued

• That diabetic patient should know hypoglycemia may occur

• To avoid hazardous activities; dizziness may occur

• To avoid alcohol, salicylates, ibuprofen; may cause GI irritation

---

ondansetron (R̶)
(on-dan-seh'tron)
Zofran, Zofran ODT
Func. class.: Antiemetic
Chem. class.: 5-HT₃ receptor antagonist

Chem. class.: 5-HT$_3$ receptor antagonist

Do not confuse:
Zofran/Zantac

Action: Prevents nausea, vomiting by blocking serotonin peripherally, centrally, and in the small intestine

Uses: Prevention of nausea, vomiting associated with cancer chemotherapy, radiotherapy, and prevention of postoperative nausea, vomiting

Unlabeled uses: Bulimia; pruritus (rectal use), alcoholism, hyperemesis gravidarum

DOSAGE AND ROUTES

Prevention of nausea/vomiting of cancer chemotherapy

• *Adult and child 4-18 yr:* **IV** 0.15 mg/kg infused over 15 min, 30 min before start of cancer chemotherapy; 0.15 mg/kg given 4 hr and 8 hr after first dose or 32 mg as a single dose; dilute in 50 ml of D$_5$ or 0.9% NaCl before giving; rectal use (unlabeled) 16 mg daily 2 hr prior to chemotherapy; **PO** 8 mg ½ hr prior to chemotherapy, repeat 8 hr later

• *Child ≥4 yr:* **PO** 4 mg ½ hr prior to chemotherapy

Prevention of nausea/vomiting of radiotherapy

• *Adult:* **PO** 8 mg tid, may repeat q8hr

Prevention of postoperative nausea/vomiting

• *Adult:* **IV/IM** 4 mg undiluted over >30 sec prior to induction of anesthesia

• *Child 2-12 yr:* **IV** 0.1 mg/kg (≤40 kg); **IV** 4 mg (≥40 kg) give ≥30 sec

Hyperemesis gravidarum (unlabeled)

• *Adult:* **PO/IV** 4-8 mg bid-tid

Hepatic dose

• *Adult:* **PO/IM/IV** Max dose 8 mg daily

Bulimia (unlabeled)

• *Adult:* **PO** 4 mg tid (base dose); prn during bingeing/purging

Pruritus (unlabeled)

• *Adult:* **PO** 4 mg bid

Alcoholism (unlabeled)

• *Adult:* **PO** 4 mcg/kg bid

Available forms: Inj 2 mg/ml, 32 mg/50 ml (premixed); tabs 4, 8 mg; oral sol 4 mg/5 ml; oral disintegrating tabs 4, 8 mg

SIDE EFFECTS

CNS: Headache, dizziness, drowsiness, fatigue, EPS

GI: Diarrhea, constipation, abdominal pain, dry mouth

MISC: Rash, **bronchospasm** (rare), *musculoskeletal pain, wound problems, shivering, fever, hypoxia, urinary retention*

Contraindications: Hypersensitivity

Precautions: Pregnancy (B), lactation, children, geriatric, granisetron hypersensitivity

PHARMACOKINETICS

IV: Mean elimination half-life 3.5-4.7 hr, plasma protein binding 70%-76%, extensively metabolized in the liver, excreted 45%-60% in urine

INTERACTIONS

Decrease: ondansetron effect—rifampin

NURSING CONSIDERATIONS
Assess:
• For absence of nausea, vomiting during chemotherapy
• Hypersensitivity reaction: rash, bronchospasm
• For EPS: shuffling gait, tremors, grimacing, rigidity
Administer:
IV route
• After diluting a single dose in 50 ml NS or D₅W, 0.45% NaCl or NS; give over 15 min
Additive compatibilities: Cisplatin, cyclophosphamide, cytarabine, dacarbazine, dexamethasone, DOXOrubicin, etoposide, fluconazole, hydromorphone, meperidine, methotrexate, morphine
Solution compatibilities: May also be diluted with D₅W, lactated Ringer's, D₅/0.9% NaCl, D₅/0.45% NaCl
Y-site compatibilities: Aldesleukin, amifostine, amikacin, aztreonam, bleomycin, carboplatin, carmustine, cefazolin, cefmetazole, cefotaxime, cefoxitin, ceftazidime, ceftizoxime, cefuroxime, chlorproMAZINE, cimetidine, cisatracurium, cisplatin, cladribine, clindamycin, cyclophosphamide, cytarabine, dacarbazine, dactinomycin, DAUNOrubicin, dexamethasone, diphenhydrAMINE, DOPamine, DOXOrubicin, DOXOrubicin liposome, doxycycline, droperidol, etoposide, famotidine, filgrastim, floxuridine, fluconazole, fludarabine, gallium, gentamicin, haloperidol, heparin, hydrocortisone, hydromorphone, hydrOXYzine, ifosfamide, imipenem/cilastatin, magnesium sulfate, mannitol, mechlorethamine, melphalan, meperidine, mesna, methotrexate, metoclopramide, miconazole, mitomycin, mitoxantrone, morphine, paclitaxel, pentostatin, piperacillin/tazobactam, potassium chloride, prochlorperazine, promethazine, ranitidine, remifentanil, streptozocin, teniposide, thiotepa, ticarcillin, ticarcillin/clavulanate, vancomycin, vinBLAStine, vinCRIStine, vinorelbine, zidovudine

Perform/provide:
• Storage at room temperature 48 hr after dilution
Evaluate:
• Therapeutic response: absence of nausea, vomiting during cancer chemotherapy
Teach patient/family:
• To report diarrhea, constipation, rash, or changes in respirations or discomfort at insertion site
• Headache requiring analgesic is common

---

orlistat (℞)
(or'lih-stat)
Xenical
Func. class.: Weight control agent
Chem. class.: Lipase inhibitor

Action: Inhibits the absorption of dietary fats
Uses: Obesity management

DOSAGE AND ROUTES
• *Adult:* **PO** 120 mg tid with each main meal containing fat
Available forms: Caps 120 mg

SIDE EFFECTS
CNS: Insomnia, depression, anxiety, dizziness, headache, fatigue
GI: Oily spotting, flatus with discharge, fecal urgency, fatty/oily stool, oily evacuation, fecal incontinence, frequent defecation, nausea, vomiting, abdominal pain, infectious diarrhea, rectal pain, tooth disorder, hypovitaminosis
GU: UTI, vaginitis, menstrual irregularity
INTEG: Dry skin, rash
MS: Back pain, arthritis, myalgia, tendinitis
RESP: Influenza, URI, LRI, EENT symptoms
Contraindications: Hypersensitivity, chronic malabsorption syndrome, cholestasis, lactation
Precautions: Pregnancy (B), hypothyroidism, other organic causes of obesity, children, anorexia nervosa, bulimia,

---

Side effects: *italics* = common; **bold** = life-threatening

nephrolithiasis, GI disease, diabetes, fat-soluble vitamin deficiency

PHARMACOKINETICS

Minimal absorption, peak 8 hr, 99% protein binding, excretion in feces, half-life 1-2 hr

INTERACTIONS

Increase: lipid-lowering effect—pravastatin

Increase: effects of warfarin

Decrease: absorption—fat-soluble vitamins (A, D, E, K), cycloSPORINE

NURSING CONSIDERATIONS

Assess:

• Weight weekly, diabetic patients may need reduction in oral hypoglycemics

• For misuse in certain populations (anorexia nervosa, bulimia)

Administer:

• For obesity only if patient is on weight-reduction program that includes dietary changes, exercise; patient should be on a diet with 30% of calories from fat, omit dose of orlistat if a meal contains no fat

Evaluate:

• Therapeutic response: decrease in weight

Teach patient/family:

• Safety and effectiveness beyond 2 yr have not been determined

• By instructing patient to read patient's information sheet, discuss unpleasant GI side effects

• To take a multivitamin containing fat-soluble vitamins 2 hr before or after orlistat; phyllium taken with each dose or at bedtime may decrease GI symptoms

• To avoid hazardous activities until stabilized on medication, discuss unpleasant side effects

• To notify prescriber if pregnancy is planned or suspected

---

oseltamivir (℞)

(oss-el-tam′ih-veer)

Tamiflu

Func. class.: Antiviral

Chem. class.: Neuramidase inhibitor

Action: Inhibits influenza virus neuraminidase with possible alteration of virus particle aggregation and release

Uses: Prevention/treatment of influenza type A or B

Unlabeled uses: Possibly effective for Arian flu (H5N1)

DOSAGE AND ROUTES

Treatment of influenza

• *Adult and child >40 kg:* **PO** 75 mg bid × 5 days, begin treatment within 2 days of onset of symptoms

• *Child 23-40 kg and ≥1 yr:* **PO** 60 mg bid

• *Child 15-23 kg and ≥1 yr:* **PO** 45 mg bid

• *Child ≤15 kg and ≥1 yr:* **PO** 30 mg bid

Prevention of influenza

• *Adult and child ≥13 yr:* **PO** 75 mg daily × ≥7 days; begin treatment within 2 days of contact, max use 6 wk

Renal dose

• *Adult:* **PO** CCr 10-30 ml/min 75 mg daily × 5 days

Available forms: Caps 75 mg; powder for oral susp 12 mg/ml after reconstitution

SIDE EFFECTS

CNS: Headache, dizziness, fatigue, *insomnia,* delirium, **self-injury (children)**

GI: Nausea, vomiting, diarrhea, abdominal pain

INTEG: **Toxic epidermal necrolysis, Stevens-Johnson syndrome, erythema multiforme**

RESP: Cough

Contraindications: Hypersensitivity

Precautions: Pregnancy (C), renal/hepatic disease, geriatric

PHARMACOKINETICS

Rapidly absorbed, protein binding 40%-45%, converted to oseltamivir carboxylate, half-life 1-3 hr, metabolite 6-10 hr, excreted in urine

NURSING CONSIDERATIONS

Assess:
• Bowel pattern before, during treatment
• Signs of infection: fever, fatigue, sore throat, headache, muscle soreness, aches

Administer:
• Within 2 days of symptoms of influenza; continue for 5 days
• At least 4 hr before bedtime to prevent insomnia

Perform/provide:
• Storage in tight, dry container

Evaluate:
• Therapeutic response: absence of fever, malaise, cough, dyspnea in infection

Teach patient/family:
• About aspects of drug therapy
• To avoid hazardous activities if dizziness occurs
• To take missed dose as soon as remembered within 2 hr of next dose
⚠ To stop immediately; report to prescriber skin rash, delirium (child)

---

oxacillin (℞)

(ox-a-sill'in)
Bactocill, oxacillin sodium
Func. class.: Broad-spectrum antiinfective
Chem. class.: Penicillinase-resistant penicillin

Do not confuse:
Bactocill/Pathocil

Action: Interferes with cell wall replication of susceptible organisms; osmotically unstable cell wall swells, bursts from osmotic pressure

Uses: Effective for gram-positive cocci *(Staphylococcus aureus, Streptococcus pneumoniae)*, infections caused by penicillinase-producing *Staphylococcus*

DOSAGE AND ROUTES

• *Adult:* **IM/IV** 2-12 g/day in divided doses q4-6h
• *Child:* **IM/IV** 50-100 mg/kg/day in divided doses q4-6h

Available forms: Powder for inj 250, 500 mg, 1, 2, 4, 10 g

SIDE EFFECTS

CNS: Lethargy, hallucinations, anxiety, depression, twitching, **coma, seizures**

GI: Nausea, vomiting, diarrhea, increased AST, ALT, abdominal pain, glossitis, colitis, **pseudomembranous colitis**

GU: **Oliguria, proteinuria, hematuria,** *vaginitis, moniliasis,* **glomerulonephritis**

HEMA: Anemia, increased bleeding time, **bone marrow depression, granulocytopenia**

INTEG: **Exfoliative dermatitis, Stevens-Johnson syndrome**

SYST: **Anaphylaxis, serum sickness**

Contraindications: Hypersensitivity to penicillins

Precautions: Pregnancy (B), hypersensitivity to cephalosporins, neonates, renal/hepatic/GI disease, lactation

PHARMACOKINETICS

IM: Peak 30-60 min, duration 4-6 hr
IV: Peak 5 min, duration 4-6 hr, half-life 30-60 min
Metabolized in the liver; excreted in urine, bile, breast milk; crosses placenta

INTERACTIONS

Increase: oxacillin concentrations—probenecid

Decrease: oxacillin antimicrobial effectiveness—tetracyclines, rifampin, erythromycins, chloramphenicol, cholestyramine, colestipol

Decrease: oral contraceptives effect

Drug/Herb

Decrease: absorption—khat, separate by ≥2 hr

Drug/Lab Test
False positive: Urine glucose, urine protein

NURSING CONSIDERATIONS
Assess:
• I&O ratio; report hematuria, oliguria, since penicillin in high doses is nephrotoxic

⚠ Any patient with compromised renal system, since drug is excreted slowly in poor renal system function; toxicity may occur rapidly
• Hepatic studies: AST, ALT
• Blood studies: WBC, RBC, Hct/Hgb, bleeding time
• Renal studies: urinalysis, protein
• C&S before therapy; drug may be given as soon as culture is taken
• Bowel pattern before and during treatment
• Skin eruptions after administration of penicillin to 1 wk after discontinuing drug
• Respiratory status: rate, character, wheezing, tightness in chest
• Allergies before initiation of treatment, and reaction of each medication

Administer:
• Drug after C&S completed
• IM inj deep in gluteal muscle

IV route
• After diluting 500 mg or less/5 ml sterile H$_2$O or NaCl for inj; may dilute further in D$_5$W, NS, LR and give 1 g over 10 min; may be given as infusion over 6 hr

Additive compatibilities: Cephapirin, chloramphenicol, DOPamine, potassium chloride, sodium bicarbonate

Y-site compatibilities: Acyclovir, cyclophosphamide, diltiazem, famotidine, fluconazole, foscarnet, heparin, hydrocortisone, hydromorphone, labetalol, magnesium sulfate, meperidine, methotrexate, morphine, perphenazine, potassium chloride, tacrolimus, vit B/C, zidovudine

Perform/provide:
• Adrenalin, suction, tracheostomy set, endotracheal intubation equipment
• Scratch test to assess allergy, after securing order from prescriber; usually done when penicillin is only drug of choice

Evaluate:
• Therapeutic response: absence of fever, draining wounds

Teach patient/family:
• All aspects of drug therapy, including need to complete course of medication to ensure organism death (10-14 days); culture may be taken after completed course
• To report sore throat, fever, fatigue (may indicate superinfection); persistent diarrhea
• To wear or carry emergency ID if allergic to penicillins

Treatment of anaphylaxis: Withdraw drug, maintain airway, administer epiNEPHrine, aminophylline, O$_2$, IV corticosteroids

---

oxaliplatin (℞)
(ox-al-i′plat-in)
Eloxatin
Func. class.: Antineoplastic
Chem. class.: Platinum coordination complex

Action: Forms crosslinks, inhibiting DNA replication and transcription, cell-cycle nonspecific

Uses: Metastatic carcinoma of the colon or rectum in combination with 5-FU/leucovorin

Unlabeled uses: Relapsed or refractory non-Hodgkin lymphoma, advanced ovarian cancer

DOSAGE AND ROUTES
Dosage protocols may vary
• *Adult:* **IV INF** *Day 1:* oxaliplatin 85 mg/m^2 in 250-500 ml D$_5$W and leucovorin 200 mg/m^2 in D$_5$W, give both over 2 hr at the same time in separate bags using a Y-line, followed by 5-FU 400 mg/m^2 **IV BOL** over 2-4 min, then 5-FU 600 mg/m^2 **IV INF** in 500 ml D$_5$W as a 22-hr **CONT INF;** *Day 2:* leucovorin 200 mg/m^2 **IV INF** over 2 hr, then 5-FU 400 mg/m^2

⚠ Safety alert   *"Tall Man" lettering

IV BOL over 2-4 min, then 5-FU 600 mg/m^2 **IV INF** in 500 D$_5$W as a 22-hr **CONT INF**; repeat cycle q2wk

Available forms: Powder for inj 50, 100 mg single-use vials

SIDE EFFECTS

CNS: Peripheral neuropathy, fatigue, headache, dizziness, insomnia

CV: Cardiac abnormalities

EENT: Decreased visual acuity, tinnitus, hearing loss

GI: Severe nausea, vomiting, diarrhea, weight loss, stomatitis, anorexia, gastroesophageal reflux, constipation, dyspepsia, mucositis, flatulence

GU: Hematuria, dysuria, creatinine

HEMA: **Thrombocytopenia, leukopenia, pancytopenia, neutropenia, anemia, hemolytic uremic syndrome**

INTEG: Alopecia, rash, flushing, extravasation, redness, swelling, pain at inj site

META: Hypokalemia

RESP: Fibrosis, dyspnea, cough, rhinitis, URI, pharyngitis

SYST: **Anaphylaxis, angioedema**

Contraindications: Pregnancy (D), lactation, hypersensitivity to this drug or other platinum products, radiation therapy or chemotherapy within 1 mo, thrombocytopenia, smallpox vaccination

Precautions: Pneumococcus vaccination, children, geriatric

PHARMACOKINETICS

Metabolized in liver, excreted in urine; after administration, 15% of platinum is in systemic circulation, 85% is either in tissues or being eliminated in urine; half-life 390 h; protein binding >90%

INTERACTIONS

Increase: risk of bleeding—aspirin, NSAIDs, alcohol, anticoagulants

Increase: myelosuppression—myelosuppressive agents, radiation

Increase: nephrotoxicity—aminoglycosides, loop diuretics

Decrease: antibody response—live virus vaccines

NURSING CONSIDERATIONS

Assess:

For bone marrow depression

• CBC, differential, platelet count each cycle; withhold drug if WBC is <4000 or platelet count is <100,000; notify prescriber of results

• Renal studies: BUN, creatinine, serum uric acid, urine CCr before, electrolytes during therapy; dose should not be given if BUN <25 mg/dl; creatinine <1.5 mg/dl; I&O ratio; report fall in urine output of <30 ml/hr

A For anaphylaxis: wheezing, tachycardia, facial swelling, fainting; discontinue drug and report to prescriber; resuscitation equipment should be nearby

A For pulmonary fibrosis: cough, crackles, dyspnea, pulmonary infiltrate; discontinue immediately, death may occur

• Monitor temp q4h (may indicate beginning infection)

• Hepatic studies before each cycle (bilirubin, AST, ALT, LDH) as needed or monthly

• Bleeding: hematuria, guaiac, bruising or petechiae, mucosa or orifices q8h; obtain prescription for viscous lidocaine (Xylocaine)

• Effects of alopecia on body image; discuss feelings about body changes

• Jaundice of skin, sclera; dark urine; clay-colored stools; itchy skin; abdominal pain; fever; diarrhea

• Edema in feet, joint pain, stomach pain, shaking

Administer:

IV route

• Do not reconstitute or dilute with sodium chloride or any chloride-containing solutions

• Do not use aluminum equipment during any preparation or administration, will degrade platinum; do not refrigerate unopened powder or solution; do not freeze; protect from light

• Use cytotoxic handling procedures; prepare in biologic cabinet using gown, gloves, mask; do not allow drug to come

in contact with skin; use soap and water if contact occurs
• Hydrate patient with 0.9% NaCl over 8-12 hr before treatment
• EpINEPHrine, antihistamines, corticosteroids for hypersensitivity reaction
• Antiemetic 30-60 min before giving drug and prn
• Allopurinol to maintain uric acid levels, alkalinization of urine
• Diuretic (furosemide 40 mg IV) or mannitol after infusion

Perform/provide:
• Comprehensive oral hygiene
• All medications PO, if possible, avoid IM inj when platelets <100,000/mm^3
• Increase fluid intake to 2-3 L/day to prevent urate deposits, calculi formation; elimination of drug

Evaluate:
• Therapeutic response: decreased tumor size, spread of malignancy

Teach patient/family:
• To report signs of infection: increased temp, sore throat, flulike symptoms
• To report signs of anemia: fatigue, headache, faintness, shortness of breath, irritability
• To report bleeding: avoid use of razors, commercial mouthwash
• To avoid aspirin, ibuprofen, NSAIDs, alcohol; may cause GI bleeding
• To report any complaints or side effects to nurse or prescriber
• To report any changes in breathing, coughing
• That hair may be lost during treatment; a wig or hairpiece may make patient feel better; new hair may be different in color, texture
• To report numbness, tingling in face or extremities, poor hearing or joint pain, swelling
• Not to receive vaccines during treatment
• To use contraception during treatment and 4 mo after; this drug may cause infertility

oxaprozin (℞)

(ox-a-proe′zin)
Daypro, Daypro ALTA
Func. class.: Nonsteroidal antiinflammatory, antirheumatics
Chem. class.: Propionic acid derivative

Do not confuse:
Daypro/Diupres

Action: May inhibit prostaglandin synthesis by decreasing enzyme needed for biosynthesis; analgesic, antiinflammatory

Uses: Acute and long-term management of osteoarthritis, rheumatoid arthritis, juvenile rheumatoid arthritis

DOSAGE AND ROUTES

• *Adult:* **PO** 600-1200 mg daily; maximum dose 1800 mg/day or 26 mg/kg, whichever is lower
• *Adult <50 kg:* **PO** 600 mg daily

Available forms: Tabs 600 mg; tabs oxaprozin potassium 678 mg (equal to 600 mg oxaprozin); caps 600 mg

SIDE EFFECTS

CNS: Dizziness, headache, drowsiness, fatigue, tremors, confusion, insomnia, anxiety, depression
CV: Tachycardia, peripheral edema, palpitations, dysrhythmias, **MI, stroke**
EENT: Tinnitus, hearing loss, blurred vision
GI: Nausea, anorexia, vomiting, diarrhea, jaundice, **cholestatic hepatitis**, constipation, flatulence, cramps, dry mouth, peptic ulcer, **GI bleeding, perforation, ulceration**
GU: **Nephrotoxicity: dysuria, hematuria, oliguria, azotemia**
HEMA: **Increased bleeding time**
INTEG: Purpura, rash, pruritus, sweating
MISC: **Anaphylaxis, angioneurotic edema, toxic epidermal necrolysis, Stevens-Johnson syndrome**
Contraindications: Hypersensitivity, asthma, patients in whom aspirin and io-

---

dides have induced symptoms of allergic reactions or asthma, perioperative pain
Precautions: Pregnancy (C), avoid in late pregnancy, lactation, children, bleeding disorders, GI disorders, cardiac disorders, hypersensitivity to other antiinflammatory agents, severe renal/hepatic disease, geriatric, CHF

PHARMACOKINETICS

PO: Onset 1 wk, peak unknown, duration unknown, half-life 40-50 hr; metabolized in liver; excreted in urine (metabolites), breast milk; 99% plasma protein binding

INTERACTIONS

Increase: toxicity—aspirin, cycloSPORINE, methotrexate
Increase: bleeding risk—oral anticoagulants, thrombolytics, cefamandole, cefotetan, cefoperazone, clopidogrel, eptifibatide, plicamycin, ticlopidine, tirofiban
Increase: levels of phenytoin, lithium, avoid concomitant use
Increase: GI side effects—aspirin, corticosteroids, NSAIDs, alcohol, potassium supplements
Decrease: effect—antihypertensives, diuretics

Drug/Herb
• NSAIDs effect: bearberry, bilberry
Increase: bleeding risk—anise, arnica, chamomile, clove, dong quai, fenugreek, feverfew, garlic, ginger, ginkgo, ginseng *(Panax)*, licorice, bogbean, chondroitin
Increase: gastric irritation—arginine, gossypol

NURSING CONSIDERATIONS

Assess:
• Pain: frequency, intensity, characteristics; relief of pain after med
⚠ Cardiac status: CV thrombotic events, MI, stroke; may be fatal
⚠ GI status: ulceration, bleeding, perforation; may be fatal
⚠ For Stevens-Johnson syndrome, anaphylaxis, toxic epidermal necrolysis, angioneurotic edema

⚠ Asthma, aspirin hypersensitivity, oronasal polyps; increased hypersensitivity reactions
• Renal, hepatic, blood studies: BUN, creatinine, AST, ALT, Hgb, before treatment, periodically thereafter
• Audiometric, ophthalmic exam before, during, after treatment
• For eye, ear problems: blurred vision, tinnitus; may indicate toxicity

Administer:
• With food, antacids to decrease GI symptoms

Perform/provide:
• Storage at room temperature

Evaluate:
• Therapeutic response: decreased pain, stiffness in joints, decreased swelling in joints, ability to move more easily

Teach patient/family:
⚠ To report blurred vision, ringing, roaring in ears; may indicate toxicity
• To avoid driving, other hazardous activities if dizziness/drowsiness occurs
⚠ To report change in urine pattern, increased weight, edema, increased pain in joints, fever, blood in urine; indicates nephrotoxicity
• That therapeutic effects may take up to 1 mo
• To take with a full glass of water to enhance absorption, sit upright for ½ hr after dose

oxazepam (℞)
(ox-ay′ze-pam)
Apo-Oxazepam ✦, Novoxapam ✦, oxazepam
Func. class.: Sedative/hypnotic; antianxiety
Chem. class.: Benzodiazepine

Controlled Substance Schedule IV
Action: Potentiates the actions of GABA, especially in limbic system and reticular formation
Uses: Anxiety, alcohol withdrawal

Side effects: *italics* = common; **bold** = life-threatening

DOSAGE AND ROUTES
Anxiety
• *Adult:* **PO** 10-30 mg tid-qid
• *Geriatric:* **PO** 5 mg daily-bid initially, may increase
Alcohol withdrawal
• *Adult:* **PO** 15-30 mg tid-qid
Available forms: Caps 10, 15, 30 mg

SIDE EFFECTS

CNS: Dizziness, drowsiness, confusion, headache, anxiety, tremors, fatigue, depression, insomnia, hallucinations, paradoxical excitement, transient amnesia
CV: Orthostatic hypotension, **ECG changes, tachycardia,** hypotension
EENT: Blurred vision, tinnitus, mydriasis
GI: Nausea, vomiting, anorexia
HEMA: Leukopenia
INTEG: Rash, dermatitis, itching
Contraindications: Pregnancy (D), hypersensitivity to benzodiazepines, narrow-angle glaucoma, psychosis, lactation, child <12 yr
Precautions: Geriatric, debilitated, renal/hepatic disease

PHARMACOKINETICS

PO: Peak 2-4 hr; metabolized by liver; excreted by kidneys; half-life 5-15 hr; crosses placenta, breast milk; protein binding 97%

INTERACTIONS

Increase: oxazepam effects—CNS depressants, alcohol, disulfiram, oral contraceptives
Decrease: oxazepam effects—oral contraceptives, phenytoin, theophylline, valproic acid
Decrease: effects of levodopa
Drug/Herb
Increase: CNS depression—catnip, chamomile, clary, cowslip, hops, kava, lavender, mistletoe, nettle, pokeweed, poppy, Queen Anne's lace, senega, skullcap, valerian
Increase: hypotension—black cohosh

Drug/Lab Test
Increase: AST, ALT, serum bilirubin
Decrease: RAIU
False increase: 17-OHCS

NURSING CONSIDERATIONS
Assess:
• B/P (lying, standing), pulse; if systolic B/P drops 20 mm Hg, hold drug, notify prescriber
• Blood studies: CBC during long-term therapy; blood dyscrasias have occurred rarely
• Hepatic studies: AST, ALT, bilirubin, creatinine, LDH, alk phos if taking long term
• Mental status: mood, sensorium, affect, sleeping pattern, drowsiness, dizziness
⚠ Physical dependency, withdrawal symptoms: headache, nausea, vomiting, muscle pain, weakness, tremors, seizures (long-term use)
• Suicidal tendencies
Administer:
• With food, milk for GI symptoms
• Sugarless gum, hard candy, frequent sips of water for dry mouth
Perform/provide:
• Assistance with ambulation during beginning therapy; drowsiness/dizziness occurs
• Safety measures, including side rails
• Check to see if PO medication has been swallowed
Evaluate:
• Therapeutic response: decreased anxiety, restlessness, insomnia
Teach patient/family:
• That drug may be taken with food
• That medication is not to be used for everyday stress or used longer than 4 mo unless directed by prescriber; not to take more than prescribed dose; may be habit forming
• To avoid OTC preparations (cough, cold, hay fever) unless approved by prescriber
• To avoid driving, activities that require alertness, since drowsiness may occur

- To avoid alcohol ingestion, other psychotropic medications unless directed by prescriber
- Not to discontinue medication abruptly after long-term use
- To rise slowly, or fainting may occur, especially geriatric
- That drowsiness may worsen at beginning of treatment

Treatment of overdose: Lavage, VS, supportive care, flumazenil

---

oxcarbazepine (℞)
(ox′kar-baz′uh-peen)
Trileptal
Func. class.: Anticonvulsant
Chem. class.: Carbamazepine analog

Action: May inhibit nerve impulses by limiting influx of sodium ions across cell membrane in motor cortex

Uses: Partial seizures

Unlabeled uses: Trigeminal neuralgia, atypical panic disorder, bipolar disorder

DOSAGE AND ROUTES

Seizures, adjunctive therapy
- *Adult:* **PO** 300 mg bid, may be increased to 600 mg/day in divided doses bid; maintenance 1200 mg/day
- *Child 4-16 yr:* **PO** 8-10 mg/kg/day divided bid, max 600 mg/day; dose is determined by weight

Conversion to monotherapy in partial seizures
- *Adult:* **PO** 300 mg bid with reduction in other anticonvulsants, increase oxcarbazepine to max 600 mg/day q1wk over 2-4 wk; withdraw other anticonvulsants over 3-6 wk

Initiation of monotherapy in partial seizures
- *Adult:* **PO** 300 mg bid, increase by 300 mg/day q3d to 1200 mg divided bid

Renal dose
- *Adult:* **PO** CCr <30 ml/min 150 mg bid and increase slowly

Available forms: Tabs, film-coated, 150, 300, 600 mg; oral susp 300 mg/5 ml

SIDE EFFECTS

CNS: Headache, dizziness, confusion, fatigue, feeling abnormal, ataxia, abnormal gait, tremors, anxiety, agitation, **worsening of seizures**

CV: Hypotension, chest pain, edema

EENT: Blurred vision, diplopia, nystagmus, rhinitis, sinusitis

GI: Nausea, constipation, diarrhea, anorexia, vomiting, abdominal pain, gastritis, dry mouth, thirst, **rectal hemorrhage**

GU: Frequency, UTI, vaginitis

INTEG: Purpura, rash, acne

Contraindications: Hypersensitivity

Precautions: Pregnancy (C), hypersensitivity to carbamazepine, lactation, child <4 yr, renal disease, fluid restriction

PHARMACOKINETICS

PO: Onset unknown; peak unknown; metabolized by liver to active metabolite; terminal half-life 7-9 hr metabolite; inhibits P450 CYP2C19, induces CYP3A4/5

INTERACTIONS

Increase: CNS depression—alcohol

Decrease: effects—felodipine, oral contraceptive, carbamazepine

Decrease: oxcarbazepine levels—phenobarbital, phenytoin, valproic acid, verapamil

Drug/Herb

Increase: anticonvulsant effect—ginkgo

Decrease: anticonvulsant effect—ginseng, santonica

NURSING CONSIDERATIONS

Assess:
- Description of seizures: frequency, duration, aura
- For hyponatremia: headache, nausea, confusion
- Electrolyte: sodium; T_4; phenytoin (when given together)

Side effects: *italics* = common; **bold** = life-threatening

• CNS/mental status: mood, sensorium, affect, behavioral changes, confusion; if mental status changes, notify prescriber
• Eye problems: need for ophthalmic exams before, during, after treatment (slit lamp, funduscopy, tonometry)

Administer:

PO route

• With food, milk to decrease GI symptoms

Perform/provide:

• Storage at room temperature
• Hard candy, gum, frequent rinsing for dry mouth
• Assistance with ambulation during early part of treatment; dizziness occurs

Evaluate:

• Therapeutic response: decreased seizure activity

Teach patient/family:

• To carry emergency ID stating patient's name, drugs taken, condition, prescriber's name and phone number
• To avoid driving, other activities that require alertness
• Not to discontinue medication quickly after long-term use
• To inform prescriber if hypersensitive to carbamazepine
• To avoid use of alcohol while taking this medication
• To use alternative contraception if using hormonal method

---

oxybutynin (R)
(ox-i-byoo'ti-nin)
Ditropan, Ditropan XL, oxybutynin, Oxytrol Transdermal
Func. class.: Anticholinergic
Chem. class.: Synthetic tertiary amine

Do not confuse:
Ditropan/diazepam
Action: Relaxes smooth muscles in urinary tract by inhibiting acetylcholine at postganglionic sites
Uses: Antispasmodic for neurogenic bladder, overactive bladder

DOSAGE AND ROUTES

• *Adult:* **PO** 5 mg bid-tid, not to exceed 5 mg qid; **ER** 5-10 mg daily, may increase by 5 mg, max 30 mg/day; **TD** apply one patch to abdomen, hip, buttock 2 ×/wk (q3-4 days)
• *Geriatric:* **PO** 2.5-5 mg bid-tid, increase by 2.5 mg q several days
• *Child >6 yr:* **PO** 5 mg bid, max 5 mg tid; **ER** 5 mg daily, max 20 mg/day
• *Child 1-5 yr:* **PO** 0.2 mg/kg/dose 2-4 ×/day

Available forms: Syr 5 mg/5 ml; tabs 5 mg; ext rel tabs 5, 10, 15 mg; TD 3.9 mg/day

SIDE EFFECTS

CNS: Anxiety, restlessness, dizziness, somnolence, insomnia, nervousness, **seizures,** headache, drowsiness, confusion
CV: Palpitations, sinus tachycardia, hypertension, peripheral edema
EENT: Blurred vision, dry eyes, increased intraocular tension, *dry mouth,* throat
GI: Nausea, vomiting, anorexia, abdominal pain, *constipation, dyspepsia,* diarrhea, taste perversion, GERD
GU: Dysuria, impotence, urinary retention, hesitancy

Contraindications: Hypersensitivity, GI obstruction, GU obstruction, glaucoma, severe colitis, myasthenia gravis, unstable CV

Precautions: Pregnancy (B), lactation, suspected glaucoma, children <12 yr, geriatric

PHARMACOKINETICS

Onset ½-1 hr, peak 3-6 hr, duration 6-10 hr; metabolized by liver, excreted in urine

INTERACTIONS

Increase: levels of atenolol, digoxin, nitrofurantoin

Increase: anticholinergic effects—antihistamines, amantidine, other anticholinergics
Increase or decrease: levels of phenothiazines
Decrease: levels of acetaminophen, haloperidol, levodopa
Drug/Herb
Increase: constipation—black catechu
Increase: anticholinergic action—butterbur, jimsonweed, scopolia
Decrease: anticholinergic effect—jaborandi tree, pill-bearing spurge

NURSING CONSIDERATIONS
Assess:
• Urinary patterns: distention, nocturia, frequency, urgency, incontinence
• Allergic reactions: rash, urticaria; if these occur, drug should be discontinued
• CNS effects: confusion, anxiety; anticholinergic effects in the geriatric
Administer:
• Without regard to meals
Evaluate:
• Urinary status: dysuria, frequency, nocturia, incontinence
Teach patient/family:
• To avoid hazardous activities; dizziness, blurred vision may occur
• To avoid OTC medications with alcohol, other CNS depressants
• To prevent photophobia by wearing sunglasses
• Avoid hot weather, strenuous activity, drug decreases perspiration

⚠ High Alert
oxycodone (℞)
(ox-i-koe′done)
Endocodone, M-Oxy, Oxy-Contin, OxyFAST, OxyLR, Roxicodone, Roxicodone SR, Supeudol ✣
oxycodone/aspirin
Endodan ✣, Oxycodan ✣, Percodan, Percodan-Demi, Roxiprin
oxycodone/ acetaminophen
Endocet ✣, Oxycocet ✣, Percocet, Roxicet, Roxilox, Tylox
Func. class.: Opiate analgesic
Chem. class.: Semisynthetic derivative

Controlled Substance Schedule II
Do not confuse:
Percodan/Decadron
Roxicet/Roxanol
Tylox/Xanax/Trimox/Wymox
Action: Inhibits ascending pain pathways in CNS, increases pain threshold, alters pain perception
Uses: Moderate to severe pain
Unlabeled uses: Postherpetic neuralgic (cont rel)

DOSAGE AND ROUTES
• *Adult:* **PO** 10-30 mg q4hr (5 mg q6h for OxyLR, OxyFAST) **OxyFAST Conc Sol is extremely concentrated; do not use interchangeably**
• *Child:* **PO** 0.05-0.15 mg/kg/dose up to 5 mg/dose q4-6h; not recommended in children
Available forms: *Oxycodone:* cont rel tabs (Oxy Contin) 10, 20, 40, 80, 160 mg; immediate rel tabs 15, 30 mg; tabs 5 mg; immediate rel caps 5 mg; oral sol 5 mg/5 ml, 20 mg/ml; *oxycodone with acetaminophen:* tabs 5 mg/325 mg; caps 5 mg/500 mg; oral sol 5 mg/325 mg/5 ml; *oxycodone with aspirin:* 2.44 mg/325 mg, 4.88/325 mg

SIDE EFFECTS

CNS: Drowsiness, dizziness, confusion, headache, sedation, euphoria
CV: Palpitations, bradycardia, change in B/P
EENT: Tinnitus, blurred vision, miosis, diplopia
GI: Nausea, vomiting, anorexia, constipation, cramps
GU: Increased urinary output, dysuria, urinary retention
INTEG: Rash, urticaria, bruising, flushing, diaphoresis, pruritus
RESP: **Respiratory depression**
Contraindications: Hypersensitivity, addiction (opiate)
Precautions: Pregnancy (B), addictive personality, lactation, increased intracranial pressure, MI (acute), severe heart disease, respiratory depression, renal/hepatic disease, child <18 yr

PHARMACOKINETICS

PO: Onset 15-30 min, peak 1 hr, duration 4-6 hr, metabolized by liver, excreted in urine, crosses placenta, excreted in breast milk, half-life 2-3 hr

INTERACTIONS

Increase: effects with other CNS depressants—alcohol, opioids, sedative/hypnotics, antipsychotics, skeletal muscle relaxants
Drug/Herb
Increase: anticholinergic effect—corkwood
Increase: sedative effect—Jamaican dogwood, lavender, mistletoe, nettle, pokeweed, poppy, senega, valerian
Drug/Lab Test
Increase: Amylase, lipase

NURSING CONSIDERATIONS

Assess:
• I&O ratio; check for decreasing output; may indicate urinary retention
• CNS changes: dizziness, drowsiness, hallucinations, euphoria, LOC, pupil reaction
• Allergic reactions: rash, urticaria

• Respiratory dysfunction: respiratory depression, character, rate, rhythm; notify prescriber if respirations are <10/min; also B/P, pulse
• For pain: intensity, location, type, characteristics; need for pain medication by pain/sedation scoring; physical dependence

Administer:
• Do not break, crush, or chew controlled rel tabs
• 80, 160 mg cont rel tabs (OxyContin) only in opioid-tolerant patients
• With antiemetic if nausea, vomiting occur
• When pain is beginning to return; determine dosage interval by response

Perform/provide:
• Storage in light-resistant area at room temperature
• Assistance with ambulation
• Safety measures: night-light, call bell within easy reach

Evaluate:
• Therapeutic response: decrease in pain

Teach patient/family:
• To report any symptoms of CNS changes, allergic reactions
• That physical dependency may result from extended use
• That withdrawal symptoms may occur: nausea, vomiting, cramps, fever, faintness, anorexia

Treatment of overdose: Naloxone (Narcan) 0.2-0.8 mg IV, O_2, IV fluids, vasopressors

oxymetazoline nasal agent
See Appendix C

oxymetazoline ophthalmic
See Appendix C

⚠ High Alert

oxymorphone (℞)
(ox-i-mor′fone)
Numorphan
Func. class.: Opiate analgesic
Chem. class.: Semisynthetic phenanthrene derivative

Controlled Substance Schedule II
Action: Inhibits ascending pain pathways in CNS, increases pain threshold, alters pain perception
Uses: Moderate to severe pain

DOSAGE AND ROUTES
• *Adult:* **IM/SUBCUT** 1-1.5 mg q4-6h prn; **IV** 0.5 mg q4-6h prn; **RECT** 5 mg q4-6h prn
Labor analgesia
• *Adult:* **IM:** 0.5-1 mg
Available forms: Inj 1, 1.5 mg/ml; supp 5 mg

SIDE EFFECTS
CNS: Drowsiness, dizziness, confusion, headache, sedation, **seizures,** *euphoria (geriatric)*
CV: Palpitations, **bradycardia,** change in B/P
EENT: Tinnitus, blurred vision, miosis, diplopia
GI: Nausea, vomiting, anorexia, constipation, cramps
GU: Increased urinary output, dysuria, urinary retention
INTEG: Rash, urticaria, bruising, flushing, diaphoresis, pruritus
RESP: **Respiratory depression**
Contraindications: Hypersensitivity, addiction (opiate)
Precautions: Pregnancy (B) (short-term), addictive personality, lactation, increased intracranial pressure, MI (acute), severe heart disease, respiratory depression, renal/hepatic disease, child <18 yr

PHARMACOKINETICS
SUBCUT/IM: Onset 10-15 min, peak 1½ hr, duration, 3-6 hr
IV: Onset 5-10 min, peak 15-30 min, duration 3-6 hr
RECT: Onset 15-30 min, duration 3-6 hr
Metabolized by liver, excreted in urine, crosses placenta, half-life 2.5-4 hr

INTERACTIONS
Increase: effects with other CNS depressants—alcohol, opiates, sedative/hypnotics, antipsychotics, skeletal muscle relaxants
⚠ *Increase:* unpredictable effects/reactions—MAOIs
Drug/Herb
Increase: anticholinergic effect—corkwood
Increase: sedative effect—Jamaican dogwood, lavender, mistletoe, nettle, pokeweed, poppy, senega, valerian
Drug/Lab Test
Increase: Amylase

NURSING CONSIDERATIONS
Assess:
• For pain: location, intensity, type, other characteristics, before and 1 hr after (IM) IV 30 min; need for pain medication, physical dependence
• I&O ratio for decreasing output; may indicate urinary retention
• CNS changes: dizziness, drowsiness, hallucinations, euphoria, LOC, pupil reaction
• Allergic reactions: rash, urticaria
• Respiratory dysfunction: respiratory depression, character, rate, rhythm; notify prescriber if respirations are <10/min
Administer:
• With antiemetic for nausea, vomiting
• When pain is beginning to return; determine interval by response
IV route
• After diluting with 5 ml sterile H_2O or NS for inj; give over 2-5 min through Y-tube or 3-way stopcock

Syringe compatibilities: Glycopyrrolate, hydrOXYzine, ranitidine
Perform/provide:
• Storage in light-resistant area at room temperature
• Assistance with ambulation
• Safety measures: night-light, call bell within easy reach
Evaluate:
• Therapeutic response: decrease in pain
Teach patient/family:
• To report any symptoms of CNS changes, allergic reactions
• That physical dependency may result from extended use
• That withdrawal symptoms may occur: nausea, vomiting, cramps, fever, faintness, anorexia
Treatment of overdose: Naloxone (Narcan) 0.2-0.8 mg IV, O_2, IV fluids, vasopressors

⚠ High Alert

oxytocin (℞)
(ox-i-toe'sin)
Pitocin
Func. class.: Hormone
Chem. class.: Oxytocic, uterine-active agent

Action: Acts directly on myofibrils, producing uterine contraction; stimulates milk ejection by the breast; vasoactive antidiuretic effect
Uses: Stimulation, induction of labor; missed or incomplete abortion; postpartum bleeding

DOSAGE AND ROUTES
Postpartum hemorrhage
• *Adult:* IV 10-40 units in 1000 ml non-hydrating diluent infused at 20-40 mU/min
• *Adult:* IM 10 units after delivery of placenta
Contraction stress test (CST)
• *Adult:* IV 0.5 mU/min, increase q20min until 3 contractions within 10 min

Stimulation of labor
• *Adult:* IV 1-2 mU/min, increase by 1-2 mU q15-60min until contractions occur; then decrease dose
Incomplete abortion
• *Adult:* IV INF 10 units/500 ml D_5W or 0.9% NaCl at 10-20 mU/min, max 30 units/12 hr
Available forms: Inj 10 units/ml

SIDE EFFECTS
CNS: **Seizures, tetanic contractions**
CV: Hypotension, hypertension, dysrhythmias, increased pulse, bradycardia, tachycardia, PVC
FETUS: Dysrhythmias, jaundice, hypoxia, **intracranial hemorrhage**
GI: Anorexia, nausea, vomiting, constipation
GU: **Abruptio placentae, decreased uterine blood flow**
HEMA: Increased hyperbilirubinemia
INTEG: Rash
RESP: **Asphyxia**
SYST: Water intoxication of mother
Contraindications: Hypersensitivity, serum toxemia, cephalopelvic disproportion, fetal distress, hypertonic uterus, prolapsed umbilical cord, active genital herpes
Precautions: Cervical/uterine surgery, uterine sepsis, primipara >35 yr, 1st, 2nd stage of labor

PHARMACOKINETICS
IM: Onset 3-7 min, duration 1 hr, half-life 12-17 min
IV: Onset 1 min, duration 30 min, half-life 12-17 min

INTERACTIONS
• Hypertension: vasopressors
Drug/Herb
• Hypertension: ephedra

NURSING CONSIDERATIONS
Assess:
• I&O ratio
• Respiration
• B/P, pulse; watch for changes that may indicate hemorrhage

- Respiratory rate, rhythm, depth; notify prescriber of abnormalities
- Length, intensity, duration of contraction; notify prescriber of contractions lasting over 1 min or absence of contractions; turn patient on her side; discontinue oxytocin
- FHTs, fetal distress; watch for acceleration, deceleration; notify prescriber if problems occur; fetal presentation, pelvic dimensions; turn patient on left side if FHT change in rate, give O_2

⚠ For signs and symptoms of water intoxication; confusion, anuria, drowsiness, headache

Administer:
Labor induction
- After diluting 10 units/L of 0.9% NS or D_5 NS run at 1-2 mU/min at 15-30 min intervals to begin normal labor; dilute 10-40 mU/min; titrate to control postpartum bleeding; dilute 10 units/500 ml sol; run 10 units-20 mU/ml; administer by only 1 route at a time; use inf pump; rotate inf to provide mixing; do not shake

Control of postpartum bleeding
- Dilute 10-40 units/1 L of sol; run at 10-20 mU/min; adjust rate as needed
- With crash cart available on unit (magnesium sulfate at bedside)

Additive compatibilities: Chloramphenicol, metaraminol, netilmicin, sodium bicarbonate, thiopental, verapamil

Y-site compatibilities: Heparin, hydrocortisone, insulin (regular), meperidine, morphine, potassium chloride, vit B/C, warfarin

Evaluate:
- Therapeutic response: stimulation of labor, control of postpartum bleeding

Teach patient/family:
- To report increased blood loss, abdominal cramps, fever, foul-smelling lochia
- That contractions will be similar to menstrual cramps, gradually increasing in intensity

paclitaxel (℞)
(pa-kli-tax'el)
Onxol, Taxol
paclitaxel protein bound particles (℞)
Abraxane
Func. class.: Antineoplastic—miscellaneous
Chem. class.: Toxoid

Do not confuse:
paclitaxel/paroxetine/Paxil
Taxol/Paxil/Taxotere

Action: Inhibits reorganization of microtubule network needed for interphase and mitotic cellular functions; also causes abnormal bundles of microtubules during cell cycle and multiple esters of microtubules during mitosis

Uses: Taxol: metastatic carcinoma of the ovary, breast; AIDS-related Kaposi's sarcoma (2nd-line), non–small cell lung cancer (1st-line), adjuvant treatment for node-positive breast cancer; Onxol: failure of other treatment in breast cancer, advanced carcinoma in ovarian cancer

Unlabeled uses: Advanced head, neck, small cell lung cancer; non-Hodgkin's lymphoma, adenocarcinoma of the upper GI tract, hormone-refractory prostate cancer

DOSAGE AND ROUTES
Paclitaxel
Ovarian carcinoma
- *Adult:* **IV INF** 135 mg/m² given over 24 hr q3wk then cisplatin 75 mg/m²; or 175 mg/m² over 3 hr q3wk; or 175 mg/m² over 3 hr

Advanced ovarian carcinoma
- *Adult:* **IV/INF** 175 mg/m² with cisplatin 75 mg/m² using a 3-hr regimen q3wk

Breast carcinoma
- *Adult:* **IV INF** 175 mg/m² over 3 hr q3wk × 4 courses

AIDS-related Kaposi's sarcoma
- *Adult:* **IV INF** 135 mg/m² over 3 hr q3wk or 100 mg/m² over 3 hr q2wk

1st-line non–small cell lung cancer
• *Adult:* IV INF 135 mg/m²/24 hr inf with cisplatin 75 mg/m² × 3 wk
Paclitaxel protein-bound particles
• *Adult:* IV 260 mg/m² q3wk
Available forms: Inj 30 mg/5 ml vial (6 mg/ml); powder for inj, lyophilized 100 mg in single-use vials

SIDE EFFECTS

CV: Bradycardia, *hypotension,* abnormal ECG
GI: Nausea, vomiting, diarrhea, mucositis, increased bilirubin, alk phos, AST
HEMA: **Neutropenia, leukopenia, thrombocytopenia, anemia,** bleeding, infections
INTEG: Alopecia
MS: Arthralgia, myalgia
NEURO: Peripheral neuropathy
SYST: Hypersensitivity reactions, **anaphylaxis, Stevens-Johnson syndrome, toxic epidermal necrolysis**
Contraindications: Pregnancy (D), hypersensitivity to paclitaxel or other drugs with polyoxyethylated castor oil, neutropenia of <1500/mm³
Precautions: Children, lactation; hepatic, cardiovascular disease; CNS disorder

PHARMACOKINETICS

89%-98% of drug is serum protein bound, metabolized in liver, excreted in bile and urine; terminal half-life 5.3-17.4 hr

INTERACTIONS

Increase: myelosuppression—other antineoplastics, radiation
Increase: DOXOrubicin levels—DOXOrubicin
⚠ *Increase:* toxicity, decrease metabolism—ketoconazole; avoid concurrent use
Decrease: paclitaxel metabolism—verapamil, diazepam, cycloSPORINE, teniposide, etoposide, quinidine, dexamethasone, vinCRIStine, testosterone

Decrease: immune response—live virus vaccines

NURSING CONSIDERATIONS
Assess:
• CBC, differential, platelet count prior to and qwk; withhold drug if WBC is <1500/mm³ or platelet count is <100,000/mm³, notify prescriber
• Monitor temp q4h (may indicate beginning infection)
• Hepatic studies before, during therapy (bilirubin, AST, ALT, LDH) prn or qmo, check for jaundiced skin and sclera, dark urine, clay-colored stool, itchy skin, abdominal pain, fever, diarrhea
• VS during 1st hr of infusion, check IV site for signs of infiltration
⚠ Hypersensitive reactions, anaphylaxis including hypotension, dyspnea, angioedema, generalized urticaria; discontinue infusion immediately; keep emergency equipment available
• Bleeding: hematuria, guaiac, bruising or petechiae, mucosa or orifices q8h; obtain prescription for viscous lidocaine (Xylocaine)
• Effects of alopecia on body image; discuss feelings about body changes
Administer:
• Antiemetic 30-60 min before giving drug and prn
IV route
• After diluting in 0.9% NaCl, D₅, D₅ and 0.9% NaCl, D₅LR to a concentration of 0.3-1.2 mg/ml
• Using an in-line filter ≤0.22 μm
• After premedicating with dexamethasone 20 mg PO 12 hr and 6 hr before paclitaxel, diphenhydrAMINE 50 mg IV ½-1 hr before paclitaxel and cimetidine 300 mg or ranitidine 50 mg IV ½-1 hr before paclitaxel
• Using only glass bottles, polypropylene, polyolefin bags and administration sets; do not use PVC infusion bags or sets
• Using gloves and cytotoxic handling precautions
Abraxane
• Reconstitute vial by injecting 20 ml of 0.9% NaCl

• Slowly inject the 20 ml of 0.9% NaCl over at least 1 min to direct the sol flow on wall of vial
• Do not inject 0.9% NaCl directly onto lyophilized cake (foaming will occur)
• Allow vial to sit for at least 5 min to ensure proper wetting of lyophilized cake
• Gently swirl or invert vial slowly for at least 2 min until completely dissolved
• Calculate dosing by dosing vol/ml = total dose (mg) ÷ 5 (mg/ml)

Y-site compatibilities: Acyclovir, amikacin, aminophylline, ampicillin/sulbactam, bleomycin, butorphanol, calcium chloride, carboplatin, cefepime, cefotetan, ceftazidime, ceftriaxone, cimetidine, cisplatin, cladribine, cyclophosphamide, cytarabine, dacarbazine, dexamethasone, diphenhydrAMINE, DOXOrubicin, droperidol, etoposide, famotidine, floxuridine, fluconazole, fluorouracil, furosemide, ganciclovir, gentamicin, granisetron, haloperidol, heparin, hydrocortisone, hydromorphone, ifosfamide, lorazepam, magnesium sulfate, mannitol, meperidine, mesna, methotrexate, metoclopramide, morphine, nalbuphine, ondansetron, pentostatin, potassium chloride, prochlorperazine, propofol, ranitidine, sodium bicarbonate, thiotepa, vancomycin, vinBLAStine, vinCRIStine, zidovudine

Perform/provide:
• Confirmation that dexamethasone was given 12 hr and 6 hr before infusion begins
• Storage of prepared sol up to 27 hr in refrigerator

Evaluate:
• Therapeutic response: decreased tumor size, spread of malignancy

Teach patient/family:
• To report signs of infection: fever, sore throat, flulike symptoms
• To report signs of anemia: fatigue, headache, faintness, shortness of breath, irritability
• To report bleeding; avoid use of razors, commercial mouthwash
• To avoid use of aspirin, ibuprofen

• To report any complaints or side effects to nurse or prescriber
• That hair may be lost during treatment; a wig or hairpiece may make patient feel better; new hair may be different in color, texture
• That pain in muscles and joints 2-5 days after infusion is common
• To use nonhormonal type of contraception
• To avoid receiving vaccinations while on this drug

---

palivizumab (℞)
(pal-ih-viz′uh-mab)
Synagis
Func. class.: Monoclonal antibody

Action: A humanized monoclonal antibody that exhibits neutralizing and fusion-inhibitory activity against respiratory syncytial virus (RSV)

Uses: Prevention of serious lower respiratory tract disease caused by RSV in pediatric patients

DOSAGE AND ROUTES
• *Child:* IM 15 mg/kg, those patients who develop RSV should receive monthly doses during RSV season (November-April)

Available forms: Powder for reconstitution 50, 100 mg; solution 50 mg/0.5 ml, 100 mg/1 ml

SIDE EFFECTS
CNS: Fever
EENT: Otitis media, rhinitis, pharyngitis
GI: Nausea, vomiting, diarrhea, increased AST
INTEG: Rash, inj site reaction
RESP: URI, **apnea,** cough
SYST: **Anaphylaxis**

Contraindications: Hypersensitivity, adults, cyanotic congenital heart disease
Precautions: Pregnancy (C), thrombocytopenia, coagulation disorders, established RSV, congenital heart disease, chronic lung disease, systemic allergic reactions

---

Side effects: *italics* = common; **bold** = life-threatening

PHARMACOKINETICS

Mean half-life 20 days

NURSING CONSIDERATIONS

Assess:

• For presence of RSV infection, drug is given to prevent infection. For side effects; report if allergic reaction is evident

⚠ For anaphylaxis: difficulty breathing; drug should be discontinued and have emergency equipment nearby

Administer:

• IM only

• After adding 1 ml of sterile water for inj per 100-mg vial, add 0.6 ml sterile water for inj for 50-mg vial; gently swirl for 30 sec to avoid foaming; do not shake; let stand at room temperature for 20 min until sol clarifies; given within 6 hr of reconstitution

Teach patient/family:

• To report upper respiratory infections, earaches, rash, sore throat

---

palonosetron (℞)

(pa-lone-o′se-tron)

Aloxi

Func. class.: Antiemetic

Chem. class.: 5-HT₃ receptor antagonist

Action: Prevents nausea, vomiting by blocking serotonin peripherally, centrally, and in the small intestine at the 5-HT₃ receptor

Uses: Prevention of nausea, vomiting associated with cancer chemotherapy

DOSAGE AND ROUTES

• *Adult:* **IV** 0.25 mg as a single dose over 30 secs, ½ hr prior to chemotherapy, max 25 mg IV over q7d

Available forms: Inj 0.25 mg/5 ml

SIDE EFFECTS

CNS: Headache, dizziness, drowsiness, fatigue, insomnia

GI: Diarrhea, constipation, abdominal pain

MISC: Weakness, hyperkalemia, anxiety, rash, **bronchospasm** (rare), arthralgia, *fever, urinary retention*

Contraindications: Hypersensitivity

Precautions: Pregnancy (B), lactation, children, geriatric, prolongation of QT interval or other cardiac conduction intervals (patients with hypokalemia, hypomagnesium, taking diuretics, congenital QT syndrome, those taking antidysrhythmics or other drugs that may prolong QT interval and cumulative high-dose antithramycline therapy)

PHARMACOKINETICS

62% protein bound; metabolized by liver; unchanged drug and metabolites excreted by kidney; terminal elimination half-life: 40 hr

NURSING CONSIDERATIONS

Assess:

• For absence of nausea, vomiting during chemotherapy

• Hypersensitivity reaction: rash, bronchospasm

Administer:

IV route

• Give as a single dose over 30 sec

• Do not mix with other drugs, flush IV line before and after administration with 0.9% NaCl

Perform/provide:

• Storage at room temperature

Evaluate:

• Therapeutic response: absence of nausea, vomiting during cancer chemotherapy

Teach patient/family:

• To report diarrhea, constipation, rash, or changes in respirations or discomfort at insertion site

• To avoid alcohol, barbiturates

---

pamidronate (℞)

(pam-i-drone'ate)

Aredia

Func. class.: Bone-resorption inhibitor, electrolyte modifier

Chem. class.: Bisphosphonate

Do not confuse:

Aredia/Adriamycin

Action: Inhibits bone resorption, apparently without inhibiting bone formation and mineralization; absorbs calcium phosphate crystals in bone and may directly block dissolution of hydroxyapatite crystals of bone

Uses: Moderate to severe Paget's disease, mild to moderate hypercalcemia associated with malignancy with or without bone metastases, osteolytic bone metastases in breast cancer, multiple myeloma patients

Unlabeled uses: Postmenopausal osteoporosis, hyperparathyroidism, reduction of bone pain in prostatic carcinoma, immobilization-related hypercalcemia

DOSAGE AND ROUTES

Hypercalcemia of malignancy

• *Adult:* **IV INF** 60-90 mg as a single dose in moderate hypercalcemia, 90 mg in severe hypercalcemia over 24 hr; dose should be diluted in 1000 ml 0.45% NaCl, 0.9% NaCl or D_5W, wait 7 days before 2nd course

Osteolytic lesions from multiple myeloma

• *Adult:* **IV** 90 mg/500 ml of D_5W, 0.45% NaCl, or 0.9% NaCl given over 4 hr on a monthly basis

Paget's disease

• *Adult:* **IV** 90-180 mg/treatment, may use 30 mg daily × 3 days

Available forms: Powder for inj 30, 60, 90 mg/vial; inj 3, 6, 9 mg/ml

SIDE EFFECTS

CNS: Fever, fatigue, psychosis

CV: Hypertension

GI: Abdominal pain, anorexia, constipation, nausea, vomiting, diarrhea, dyspepsia

GU: UTI, fluid overload

INTEG: Redness, swelling, induration, pain on palpation at site of catheter insertion

META: Anemia, *hypokalemia, hypomagnesemia, hypophosphatemia, hypocalcemia,* hypothyroidism

MS: Bone pain, myalgia

RESP: Coughing, dyspnea, URI

Contraindications: Pregnancy (D), hypersensitivity to bisphosphonates

Precautions: Children, nursing mothers, renal dysfunction

PHARMACOKINETICS

Rapidly cleared from circulation and taken up mainly by bones, primarily in areas of high bone turnover, eliminated primarily by kidneys

INTERACTIONS

• Hypomagnesemia, hypokalemia: digoxin

Decrease: pamidronate effect—calcium, vit D

NURSING CONSIDERATIONS

Assess:

• Electrolytes, Ca, P, Mg, K

• For hypercalcemia: nausea, vomiting, constipation, thirst, dysrhythmias; hypocalcemia, paresthesia, twitching, laryngospasm, Chvostek's, Trousseau's signs

• For bone pain; use analgesics

• I&O, check for fluid overload edema, crackles, increased B/P

Administer:

IV route

• After reconstituting by adding 10 ml of sterile water for inj to each vial (30 mg/10 ml, or 60 mg/10 ml, or 90 mg/10 ml depending on vial used), then add to 1000 ml of sterile 0.45%, 0.9% NaCl, D_5W, run over 24 hr for hypercalcemia or 60 mg ≥4 hr, 90 mg over 24 hr; dilute reconstituted sol in 500 ml of 0.9% NaCl, 0.45% NaCl, or D_5W, give over 4 hr (multiple myeloma, Paget's disease)

• Do not mix with calcium-containing infusion sol such as Ringer's sol

Side effects: *italics* = common; **bold** = life-threatening

Perform/provide:
• Storage of infusion sol up to 24 hr at room temperature
• Reconstituted sol with sterile water may be stored under refrigeration for up to 24 hr

Evaluate:
• Therapeutic response: decreased calcium levels

Teach patient/family
• To report hypercalcemic relapse: nausea, vomiting, bone pain, thirst; unusual muscle twitching, muscle spasms, severe diarrhea, constipation
• To continue with dietary recommendations including calcium and vit D
• To obtain an analgesic from provider for bone pain
• That if nausea/vomiting occur, small, frequent meals may help
• To report vision symptoms: blurred vision, edema, inflammation; report to prescriber

---

pancreatin (℞)

(pan′kree-a-tin)

Creon, Donnazyme, Hi-Vegi-Lip, 4× Pancreatin 600 mg, 8× Pancreatin 900 mg, Pancrezyme 4×

Func. class.: Digestant

Chem. class.: Pancreatic enzyme concentrate—bovine/porcine

Action: Pancreatic enzyme needed for breakdown of substances released from the pancreas

Uses: Exocrine pancreatic secretion insufficiency, cystic fibrosis (digestive aid)

Dosage and routes:
• *Adult:* **PO** 8000-24,000 USP units with meals

Available forms: Tabs 650, 2000, 12,000 units, others in combination

SIDE EFFECTS

EENT: Buccal soreness

GI: Anorexia, nausea, vomiting, diarrhea, glossitis, anal soreness

GU: Hyperuricuria, hyperuricemia

INTEG: Rash, hypersensitivity

Contraindications: Hypersensitivity to pork, chronic pancreatic disease

Precautions: Pregnancy (C), lactation, ileus, esophageal stricture, Crohn's disease

INTERACTIONS

Decrease: absorption—cimetidine, antacids, oral iron

Decrease: effect of acarbose, miglitol

NURSING CONSIDERATIONS

Assess:
• I&O ratio; watch for increasing urinary output
• Fecal fat, nitrogen, PT, calcium during treatment
• For polyuria, polydipsia, polyphagia (may indicate diabetes mellitus)
• For allergy to pork

Administer:

PO route
• Swallow tabs whole; do not break, crush, or chew enteric-coated tabs
• After antacid or H₂-blockers; decreased pH inactivates drug
• Low-fat diet for GI symptoms

Perform/provide:
• Storage in tight container at room temperature

Evaluate:
• Therapeutic response: relief of GI symptoms

⚠ Safety alert   *"Tall Man" lettering

pancrelipase (R̥)
(pan-kre-li′pase)
Cotazym, Cotazym-65B ✦,
Cotazym E.C.S. 8, Cotazym
E.C.S. 20, Cotazym Capsules,
Cotazym-S, Creon, Ilozyme,
Ku-Zyme HP, Lipram-PN16,
Lipram-CR20, Lipram-UL12,
Lipram-PN10, Pancrease
Capsules, Pancrease MT 4,
Pancrease MT 10, Pancrease
MT 16, Protilase, Ultrase MT
12, Ultrase MT 20, Viokase,
Zymase
Func. class.: Digestant
Chem. class.: Pancreatic enzyme—
bovine/porcine

Action: Pancreatic enzyme needed for breakdown of substances released from the pancreas
Uses: Exocrine pancreatic secretion insufficiency, cystic fibrosis (digestive aid), steatorrhea, pancreatic enzyme deficiency

DOSAGE AND ROUTES
Many products listed above are not interchangeable
• *Adult and child:* **PO** 1-3 caps/tabs before meals or with meals, or 1 cap/tab with snack or 1-2 powder pkt before meals
Available forms: Powder 16,800 units lipase/70,000 units protease and amylase; caps 8000 units lipase/30,000 units protease and amylase; delayed rel cap 4000 units lipase/12,000 units protease and amylase, 4000 units lipase/25,000 units protease/20,000 units amylase, 5000 units lipase/20,000 units protease and amylase, 10,000 units lipase/30,000 units protease and amylase, 12,000 units lipase/24,000 units protease and amylase, 12,000 units lipase/39,000 units protease and amylase, 16,000 units lipase/48,000 units protease and amylase, 20,000 units lipase/65,000 units protease and amylase, 24,000 units lipase/78,000 units protease and amylase

SIDE EFFECTS
GI: Anorexia, nausea, vomiting, diarrhea
GU: Hyperuricuria, hyperuricemia
Contraindications: Allergy to pork
Precautions: Pregnancy (C), ileus, pancreatitis, Crohn's disease

INTERACTIONS
Decrease: absorption—cimetidine, antacids, oral iron
Decrease: effect of acarbose, miglitol

NURSING CONSIDERATIONS
Assess:
• For appropriate height, weight development; may be delayed
• I&O ratio; watch for increasing urinary output
• Fecal fat, nitrogen, PT during treatment
• For polyuria, polydipsia, polyphagia (may indicate diabetes mellitus)
• For pork sensitivity, cross-sensitivity may occur
Administer:
• After antacid or cimetidine; decreased pH inactivates drug
• Powder mixed in prepared fruit juice for infants, children
• Low-fat diet for GI symptoms
• With 8 oz water or more; do not allow to sit in mouth; have patient sit up during administration
Perform/provide:
• Storage in tight container at room temperature
Evaluate:
• Therapeutic response: improved digestion of carbohydrates, protein, fat; absence of steatorrhea
Teach patient/family:
• Not to inhale powder; may be very irritating to mucous membranes; some powder may irritate skin
• To notify prescriber of allergic reactions, abdominal pain, cramping, or blood in the urine

Side effects: *italics* = common; **bold** = life-threatening

⚠ High Alert

pancuronium (℞)
(pan-kyoo-roe'nee-um)
pancuronium bromide,
Pavulon
Func. class.: Neuromuscular
blocker (nondepolarizing)
Chem. class.: Synthetic curariform

Action: Inhibits transmission of nerve impulses by binding with cholinergic receptor sites, antagonizing action of acetylcholine

Uses: Facilitation of endotracheal intubation, skeletal muscle relaxation during mechanical ventilation, surgery, or general anesthesia

DOSAGE AND ROUTES
• *Adult and child >1 mo:* **IV** 0.04-0.1 mg/kg, then 0.01 mg/kg q½-1h
Available forms: Inj 1, 2 mg/ml

SIDE EFFECTS

CV: Bradycardia; tachycardia; increased, decreased B/P; ventricular extrasystoles, edema
EENT: Increased secretions
INTEG: Rash, flushing, pruritus, urticaria, sweating, salivation
MS: Weakness to prolonged skeletal muscle relaxation
RESP: **Prolonged apnea, bronchospasm, cyanosis, respiratory depression, wheezing**
SYST: **Anaphylaxis**
Contraindications: Hypersensitivity to bromide ion
Precautions: Pregnancy (C), renal/hepatic/cardiac disease, lactation, children <2 yr, electrolyte imbalances, dehydration, neuromuscular disease, respiratory disease

PHARMACOKINETICS

IV: Onset 3-5 min, dose dependent, peak 3-5 min; metabolized (small amounts), excreted in urine (unchanged), crosses placenta

INTERACTIONS
• Dysrhythmias: theophylline
Increase: neuromuscular blockade—aminoglycosides, clindamycin, enflurane, isoflurane, lincomycin, lithium, local anesthetics, opioid analgesics, polymyxin antiinfectives, quinidine, thiazides
Drug/Lab Test
Decrease: Cholinesterase

NURSING CONSIDERATIONS
Assess:
• For electrolyte imbalances (K, Mg); may lead to increased action of this drug
• VS (B/P, pulse, respirations, airway) until fully recovered; rate, depth, pattern of respirations, strength of hand grip
• I&O ratio; check for urinary retention, frequency, hesitancy
• Recovery: decreased paralysis of face, diaphragm, leg, arm, rest of body; allow to recover fully before neuro assessment
⚠ Allergic reactions, anaphylaxis: rash, fever, respiratory distress, pruritus; drug should be discontinued

Administer:
IV, direct route
• With diazepam or morphine when used for therapeutic paralysis; this drug provides no sedation
• Using nerve stimulator by anesthesiologist to determine neuromuscular blockade
• Atropine to counteract muscarinic effects
• After succinylcholine effects subside
• Anticholinesterase to reverse neuromuscular blockade
• IV undiluted, give over 1-2 min (only by qualified persons)
Additive compatibilities: Verapamil
Syringe compatibilities: Heparin
Y-site compatibilities: Aminophylline, cefazolin, cefuroxime, cimetidine, DOBUTamine, DOPamine, epINEPHrine, esmolol, fentanyl, fluconazole, gentamicin, heparin, hydrocortisone, isoproterenol,

---

⚠ Safety alert   *"Tall Man" lettering

lorazepam, midazolam, morphine, nitroglycerin, nitroprusside, ranitidine, trimethoprim-sulfamethoxazole, vancomycin

Perform/provide:
• Storage in refrigerator; do not store in plastic; use only fresh sol
• Reassurance if communication is difficult during recovery from neuromuscular blockade
• Frequent (q2h) instillation of artificial tears and covering eyes to prevent drying of cornea

Evaluate:
• Therapeutic response: paralysis of jaw, eyelid, head, neck, rest of body

Treatment of overdose: Edrophonium or neostigmine, atropine, monitor VS; may require mechanical ventilation

panitumumab (Rx)
(pan-i-tue′moo-mab)
Vectibix
Func. class.: Antineoplastic—miscellaneous
Chem. class.: Multikinase inhibitor, signal transduction inhibitor

Action: Decreases growth and survival of cancer cells by competitive inhibition of EGF receptor
Uses: EGFR expressing metastatic colorectal cancer

DOSAGE AND ROUTES
• *Adult:* IV INF 6 mg/kg over 60 min every 2 wk
Available forms: Sol for inj 20 mg/ml

SIDE EFFECTS
CNS: Fatigue, ocular toxicity
CV: Peripheral edema
GI: Nausea, diarrhea, vomiting, anorexia, mouth ulceration, abdominal pain, constipation
HEMA: Thrombophlebitis
INTEG: Rash, pruritus, **exfoliative dermatitis,** skin fissure

META: Hypocalcemia, hypomagnesemia, antibody formation
RESP: **Bronchospasm, cough,** dyspnea, **hypoxia, pulmonary fibrosis,** pneumonitis, wheezing
Contraindications: Hypersensitivity
Precautions: Pregnancy (C), lactation, children, hepatic disease, acute bronchospasm, diarrhea, exfoliative dermatitis, hamster protein allergy, hypomagnesemia, hypotension, pulmonary fibrosis, sepsis

PHARMACOKINETICS
Bioavailability 38%-49%; elimination half-life 7.5 days; peak 3 hr; high-fat meal decreases bioavailability; plasma protein binding 99.5%; metabolized in the liver; oxidative metabolism by CYP3A4, glucuronidation by UGT1A9; 77% excreted in feces

NURSING CONSIDERATIONS
Assess:
• Serum electrolytes periodically
• Signs of infection: increased temperature
• Signs of infusion reactions: bronchospasm, fever, chills, hypotension
• Signs of ocular toxicity
Administer:
• Give in hospital or clinic setting with full resuscitation equipment
• Only as IV infusion using controlled IV infusion pump; do not give IV push or bolus; use low-protein binding 0.2 or 0.22 micron in-line filter; flush line with 0.9% NaCl before and after administration
• Give over 60 min through a peripheral line or indwelling catheter; infuse doses of >1000 mg over 90 min
• Dilute in 100 ml of 0.9% NaCl; dilute doses >1000 mg in 150 ml of 0.9% NaCl; mix by inverting; do not exceed 10 mg/ml; use within 6 hr if stored at room temp; can be stored between 2° and 8° C for up to 24 hr

Side effects: *italics* = common; **bold** = life-threatening

Perform/provide:
- Storage of unopened vials in refrigerator; do not shake; protect from direct sunlight; do not freeze

Evaluate:
- Therapeutic response: decrease in colon carcinoma progression

Teach patient/family:
⚠ To report adverse reactions immediately: difficulty breathing, mouth sores, skin rash, ocular toxicity
- Reason for treatment, expected results, adverse reactions

---

pantoprazole (℞)
(pan-toe-pray′zole)
Protonix, Prontonix IV
Func. class.: Proton pump inhibitor
Chem. class.: Benzimidazole

Action: Suppresses gastric secretion by inhibiting hydrogen/potassium ATPase enzyme system in gastric parietal cell; characterized as gastric acid pump inhibitor, since it blocks final step of acid production

Uses: Gastroesophageal reflux disease (GERD), severe erosive esophagitis, maintenance, long-term pathologic hypersecretory conditions including Zollinger-Ellison syndrome

DOSAGE AND ROUTES
GERD
- *Adult:* **PO** 40 mg daily × 8 wk, may repeat course

Erosive esophagitis
- *Adult:* **IV** 40 mg daily × 7-10 day **PO** 40 mg daily × 8 wk; may repeat **PO** course

Pathologic hypersecretory conditions
- *Adult:* **IV** 80 mg q12h; max 240 mg/day

Available forms: Delayed rel tabs 20, 40 mg; powder for inj, freeze-dried 40 mg/vial

SIDE EFFECTS
CNS: Headache, insomnia
GI: Diarrhea, abdominal pain, flatulence
INTEG: Rash
META: Hyperglycemia
Contraindications: Hypersensitivity
Precautions: Pregnancy (C), lactation, children

PHARMACOKINETICS
Peak 2.4 hr, duration >24 hr, half-life 1.5 hr, protein binding 97%, eliminated in urine as metabolites and in feces; in geriatric elimination rate decreased

INTERACTIONS
Increase: pantoprazole serum levels—diazepam, phenytoin, flurazepam, triazolam, clarithromycin
Increase: bleeding—warfarin
Decrease: absorption—sucralfate, calcium carbonate, vit B_{12}

NURSING CONSIDERATIONS
Assess:
- GI system: bowel sounds q8h, abdomen for pain, swelling, anorexia
- Hepatic studies: AST, ALT, alk phos during treatment

Administer:
PO route
- Swallow del rel tabs whole; do not break, crush, or chew
- Take del rel tabs at same time of day
- May take with or without food

IV route
- Reconstitute with 10 ml 0.9% NaCl, further dilute with 80 ml LR, D_5, 0.9% NaCl (0.8 mg/ml), give over 15 min (≤6 mg/min) using in-line filter provided

Evaluate:
- Therapeutic response: absence of epigastric pain, swelling, fullness

Teach patient/family:
- To report severe diarrhea; drug may have to be discontinued
- That diabetic patient should know hypoglycemia may occur
- To avoid hazardous activities; dizziness may occur

• To avoid alcohol, salicylates, ibuprofen; may cause GI irritation
• To notify prescriber if pregnant or plan to become pregnant, do not breastfeed

Rarely Used

papaverine (℞)
(pa-pav′er-een)
Func. class.: Peripheral vasodilator

Uses: Arterial spasm resulting in cerebral and peripheral ischemia; myocardial ischemia associated with vascular spasm or dysrhythmias; angina pectoris; peripheral pulmonary embolism; visceral spasm as in ureteral, biliary, GI colic, peripheral vascular disease

DOSAGE AND ROUTES
• *Adult:* **SUS REL** 150-300 mg q8-12h; **IM/IV** 30-120 mg
Contraindications: Hypersensitivity, complete AV heart block

Rarely Used

paraldehyde (℞)
(par-al′de-hyde)
Func. class.: Anticonvulsant

Uses: Refractory seizures, status epilepticus, sedation, insomnia, alcohol withdrawal, tetanus, eclampsia

DOSAGE AND ROUTES
Seizures
• *Adult:* **IM** 5-10 ml; divide 10 ml into 2 inj; **IV** 0.2-0.4 ml/kg in **NS** inj
• *Child:* **IM** 0.15 ml/kg; **RECT** 0.3 ml/kg q4-6h or 1 ml/yr of age, not to exceed 5 ml; may repeat in 1 hr prn; **IV** 5 ml/90 ml **NS** inj; begin infusion at 5 ml/hr; titrate to patient response
Alcohol withdrawal
• *Adult:* **PO/RECT** 5-10 ml, not to exceed 60 ml; **IM** 5 ml q4-6h × 24 hr, then q6h on following days, not to exceed 30 ml

Sedation
• *Adult:* **PO/REC** 4-10 ml; **IM** 5 ml; **IV** 3-5 ml in emergency only
• *Child:* **PO/RECT/IM** 0.15 ml/kg
Tetanus
• *Adult:* **IV** 4-5 ml or 12 ml by gastric tube q4h diluted with water; **IM** 5-10 ml prn
Contraindications: Hypersensitivity, gastroenteritis with ulceration

paricalcitol (℞)
(par-ih-cal′sih-tol)
Zemplar
Func. class.: Vit D analog
Chem. class.: Fat-soluble vitamin

Action: Reduces parathyroid hormone (PTH) levels; suppresses PTH levels in patients with chronic renal failure with absence of hypercalcemia/hyperphosphatemia; serum PO_4, calcium, CaXP may increase
Uses: Hyperparathyroidism in chronic renal failure

DOSAGE AND ROUTES
• *Adult:* **IV BOL** 0.04-0.1 mcg/kg (2.8-7 mcg) no more than every other day during dialysis; may increase by 2-4 mcg q2-4wk until target serum intact PTH (1.5 − 3 × nonuremic upper limit of normal) is achieved
Available forms: Inj 5 mcg/ml

SIDE EFFECTS
CNS: Lightheadedness
CV: Palpitations
GI: Nausea, vomiting, anorexia, dry mouth
OTHER: Pneumonia, edema, chills, fever, flu, **sepsis**
Contraindications: Hypersensitivity, hypercalcemia
Precautions: Pregnancy (C), cardiovascular disease, renal calculi, geriatric, lactation, children

INTERACTIONS
• Digoxin toxicity: digoxin

NURSING CONSIDERATIONS

Assess:
• Ca, PO_4 2 ×/wk during initial therapy; after dose is established take calcium and phosphorus qmo

Administer:
IV route
• By IV bolus only

Evaluate:
• Decreased hypoparathyroidism in chronic renal disease

Teach patient/family:
• To report weakness, lethargy, headache, anorexia, loss of weight
• To report nausea, vomiting, palpitations

Rarely Used

paromomycin (℞)
(par-oh-moe-mye'sin)
Humatin
Func. class.: Amebicide, aminoglycoside

Uses: Intestinal amebiasis, adjunct in hepatic coma

DOSAGE AND ROUTES
Intestinal amebiasis
• *Adult and child:* **PO** 25-35 mg/kg/day in 3 divided doses × 5-10 day with meals
Hepatic coma
• *Adult:* **PO** 4 g daily in divided doses × 5-6 day

Contraindications: Hypersensitivity, renal disease, GI obstruction

---

paroxetine (℞)
(par-ox'e-teen)
Paxil, Paxil CR
Func. class.: Antidepressant, SSRI
Chem. class.: Phenylpiperidine derivative

Do not confuse:
paroxetine/paclitaxel
Paxil/paclitaxel/Taxol

Action: Inhibits CNS neuron uptake of serotonin but not of norepinephrine or DOPamine

Uses: Major depressive disorder, obsessive-compulsive disorder, panic disorder, generalized anxiety disorder, posttraumatic stress disorder, premenstrual disorders, social anxiety disorder

Unlabeled uses: Diabetic neuropathy, headaches, premature ejaculation, bipolar depression with lithium, fibromyalgia

DOSAGE AND ROUTES
Generalized anxiety disorder
• *Adult:* **PO** 20 mg/day AM range 20-50 mg/day
Posttraumatic stress disorder
• *Adult:* **PO** 20 mg/day range 20-50 mg/day
Depression
• *Adult:* **PO** 20 mg daily in AM; after 4 wk if no clinical improvement is noted, dose may be increased by 10 mg/day qwk to desired response, not to exceed 60 mg/day or **CONTROLLED REL** 25 mg/day, may increase by 12.5 mg/day weekly up to 62.5 mg/day
• *Geriatric:* **PO** 10 mg daily, increase by 10 mg to desired dose, max 40 mg/day
Obsessive-compulsive disorder
• *Adult:* **PO** 20 mg/day in AM, start with 20 mg/day, increase 10 mg/day increments, max 60 mg/day
Panic disorder
• *Adult:* **PO** 40 mg/day, start with 10 mg/day and increase in 10 mg/day increments, max 60 mg/day or **CONTROLLED REL** 12.5 mg/day, max 75 mg/day
Premenstrual disorders
• *Adult:* **CONTROLLED REL** 12.5 mg/day in AM
Renal dose
• *Adult:* **PO** 10 mg daily in AM, may increase by 10 mg/day qwk, max 50 mg daily or **CONTROLLED REL** 12.5 mg/day, max 50 mg/day

Available forms: Tabs 10, 20, 30, 40 mg; oral susp 10 mg/5 ml; controlled rel tab 12.5, 25, 37.5 mg

---

⚠ Safety alert   *"Tall Man" lettering

SIDE EFFECTS

CNS: Headache, nervousness, insomnia, *drowsiness, anxiety, tremor, dizziness,* fatigue, sedation, abnormal dreams, agitation, apathy, euphoria, hallucinations, delusions, psychosis

CV: Vasodilation, postural hypotension, palpitations

EENT: Visual changes

GI: Nausea, diarrhea, dry mouth, anorexia, dyspepsia, *constipation,* cramps, vomiting, taste changes, flatulence, decreased appetite

GU: Dysmenorrhea, decreased libido, urinary frequency, UTI, amenorrhea, cystitis, impotence, *abnormal ejaculation (male)*

INTEG: Sweating, rash

MS: Pain, arthritis, myalgia, myopathy, myosthenia

RESP: Infection, pharyngitis, nasal congestion, sinus headache, sinusitis, cough, dyspnea

SYST: Asthenia, fever

Contraindications: Hypersensitivity, patients taking MAOIs, alcohol use

Precautions: Pregnancy (D), lactation, children, geriatric, seizure history, patients with history of mania, renal/hepatic disease

PHARMACOKINETICS

PO: Peak 5.2 hr; metabolized in liver by CPY50 enzyme system, unchanged drugs and metabolites excreted in feces and urine; half-life 21 hr; protein binding 95%

INTERACTIONS

• Paroxetine may decrease digoxin levels

⚠ Do not use with MAOIs, thioridazine; potentially fatal reactions can occur

Increase: bleeding—warfarin

Increase: paroxetine plasma levels—cimetidine

Increase: agitation—L-tryptophan

Increase: side effects—highly protein-bound drugs

Increase: theophylline levels—theophylline

Decrease: paroxetine levels—phenobarbital and phenytoin

Drug/Herb

• Possible serotonin syndrome: SAM-e, St. John's wort

• Hypertensive crisis: ephedra

Increase: anticholinergic effect—corkwood, jimsonweed

Increase: sedative—hops, lavender

Increase: CNS stimulation—yohimbe

Drug/Lab Test

Increase: Serum bilirubin, blood glucose, alk phos

Decrease: VMA, 5-HIAA

False increase: Urinary catecholamines

NURSING CONSIDERATIONS

Assess:

• Mental status: mood, sensorium, affect, suicidal tendencies, increase in psychiatric symptoms, depression, panic; OCD: decreasing obsessive thoughts, compulsive behaviors

• B/P (lying/standing), pulse q4h; if systolic B/P drops 20 mm Hg, hold drug, notify prescriber; take vital signs q4h in patients with CV disease

• Blood studies: CBC, leukocytes, differential, cardiac enzymes if patient is receiving long-term therapy

• Hepatic studies: AST, ALT, bilirubin, creatinine

• Weight qwk; appetite may decrease with drug

• ECG for flattening of T wave, bundle branch, AV block, dysrhythmias in cardiac patients

• EPS primarily in geriatric: rigidity, dystonia, akathisia

• Urinary retention, constipation

• Withdrawal symptoms: headache, nausea, vomiting, muscle pain, weakness; not usual unless drug discontinued abruptly

• Alcohol intake; if alcohol is consumed, hold dose until morning

Administer:

• Increased fluids, bulk in diet for constipation, urinary retention

• With food, milk for GI symptoms

- Crushed if patient is unable to swallow medication whole
- Dosage at bedtime for oversedation during day; may take entire dose at bedtime; geriatric may not tolerate once/day dosing
- Gum, hard candy, frequent sips of water for dry mouth
- Avoid use with other CNS depressants

Perform/provide:
- Storage at room temperature; do not freeze
- Assistance with ambulation during therapy, since drowsiness, dizziness occur
- Safety measures primarily in geriatric
- Checking to see if PO medication swallowed

Evaluate:
- Therapeutic response: decreased depression

Teach patient/family:
- That therapeutic effect may take 1-4 wk
- To use caution in driving, other activities requiring alertness because of drowsiness, dizziness, blurred vision
- Not to discontinue medication quickly after long-term use; may cause nausea, headache, malaise
- To avoid alcohol ingestion

Treatment of overdose: Airway, for seizures give diazepam, symptomatic treatment

---

pegaptanib (℞)
(peg-ap'ta-nib)
Macugen
Func. class.: Ophthalmic agent—miscellaneous

Action: Binds to vascular endothelial growth factor (VEGF), thereby inhibiting angiogenesis

Uses: Treatment of neovascular (wet) age-related macular degeneration; may be used alone or with photodynamic therapy

DOSAGE AND ROUTES

- *Adult:* **INTRAVITREAL INJ** 0.3 mg injected q6wk

Available forms: Inj 0.3 mg, single glass syringes

SIDE EFFECTS

EENT: Anterior chamber inflammation, blurred vision, conjunctival hemorrhage, corneal edema, cataract, eye discharge, eye pain, increased intraocular pressure, punctuate keratitis, reduced visual acuity, vitreous floaters, vitreous opacities, blepharitis, conjunctivitis, photophobia, retinal detachment, iatrogenic traumatic cataract

Contraindications: Hypersensitivity, ocular or periocular infections

Precautions: Pregnancy (B), inflammatory eye disease, ocular hypertension

PHARMACOKINETICS:

Half-life 87-100 hr in vitreous humor of the monkey, may remain fully active in the eye for 7-28 days

INTERACTIONS

- None known

NURSING CONSIDERATIONS

Assess:
- Visual acuity periodically
- Treated eye for increased intraocular pressure, infection, endophthalmitis
- Perfusion of the optic nerve head immediately after inj, tonometry ½ hr after inj, biomicroscopy 2-7 days after inj

Administer:
- Anesthesia and a broad-spectrum anti-infective agent before injection
- The inj should be done under aseptic conditions

Perform/provide:
- Storage at 36°-46° F, do not freeze or shake vigorously

Evaluate:
- Therapeutic response: macular degeneration stabilized

Teach patient/family:
- To report any inflammation, bleeding, eye discharge, opacities to prescriber
- To continue with follow-up care during treatment

⚠ Safety alert   *"Tall Man" lettering

⚠ High Alert

pegaspargase (℞)
(peg-as'per-gase)
Oncaspar, PEG-L-
asparaginase
Func. class.: Antineoplastic
Chem. class.: Escherichia coli enzyme

Action: Indirectly inhibits protein synthesis in tumor cells; without amino acid, DNA, RNA synthesis is halted; asparagine, protein synthesis is halted; G_1 phase; cell-cycle specific; a nonvesicant; a modified version of L-asparaginase

Uses: Acute lymphocytic leukemia in combination with other antineoplastics

DOSAGE AND ROUTES

In combination
• *Adult and child with BSA ≥0.6 m²:*
IV/IM 2500 international units/m² q14d, run **IV** over 1-2 hr in 100 ml of NaCl or D₅ through a running **IV**; **IM** should be no more than 2 ml in one inj site
• *Child with BSA <0.6 m²:* **IV/IM** 82.5 international units/kg q14d

Sole induction
• *Adult:* **IV** 2500 international units/m² q14d

Available forms: Inj 750 international units/ml in a phosphate buffered saline sol

SIDE EFFECTS

CNS: Neuritis, dizziness, headache, **coma, depression**, fatigue, confusion, hallucinations, **seizures**
CV: Chest pain, **hypertension**
ENDO: Hyperglycemia
GI: Nausea, vomiting, anorexia, cramps, stomatitis, **hepatotoxicity, pancreatitis,** *diarrhea*
GU: Urinary retention, **renal failure,** glycosuria, polyuria, azotemia, uric acid neuropathy
HEMA: **Thrombocytopenia, leukopenia, myelosuppression, anemia,** decreased clotting factors, pancytopenia
INTEG: **Rash,** urticaria, chills, fever
RESP: **Fibrosis, pulmonary infiltrate, severe bronchospasm**
SYST: **Anaphylaxis, hypersensitivity**
Contraindications: Hypersensitivity, infant, lactation, pancreatitis
Precautions: Pregnancy (C), renal/hepatic disease, CNS disease

PHARMACOKINETICS

Half-life 5½ days, onset rapid, duration 2 wk, metabolized in reticuloendothelial system

INTERACTIONS
• Do not use with radiation
• Coagulation factor imbalances: heparin, warfarin, aspirin, NSAIDs
Decrease: action of methotrexate

NURSING CONSIDERATIONS
Assess:
⚠ For signs and symptoms of pancreatitis (nausea, vomiting, severe abdominal pain), anaphylaxis (bronchospasm, dyspnea), cyanosis
• CBC, differential, platelet count qwk; withhold drug if WBC count is <4000 or platelet count is <75,000; notify prescriber of results
• Pulmonary function tests, chest x-ray studies before and during therapy; chest x-ray film should be obtained q2wk during treatment, watch for severe bronchospasm, fibrosis, pulmonary infiltrate
• Renal studies: BUN, serum uric acid, ammonia, urine CCr, electrolytes before and during therapy
• I&O ratio; report fall in urine output to ≤30 ml/hr, may indicate renal failure
• Temp q4h (may indicate beginning infection)
• Hepatic studies before and during therapy (bilirubin, AST, ALT, LDH) as needed or monthly; hepatotoxicity can occur; check for jaundiced skin, sclera; dark urine, clay-colored stools, itchy skin, abdominal pain, fever, diarrhea

- RBC, Hct, Hgb; may be decreased
- Serum, urine glucose levels, glycosuria can occur
- Bleeding: hematuria, stool guaiac, bruising or petechiae, mucosa or orifices q8h
- Dyspnea, crackles, nonproductive cough, chest pain, tachypnea, fatigue, increased pulse, pallor, lethargy, swelling around eyes or lips; anaphylaxis may occur
- B/P, since hypertension can occur
- Local irritation, pain, burning, discoloration at inj site
- ⚠ Symptoms of severe allergic reaction: rash, pruritus, urticaria, purpuric skin lesions, itching, flushing, dyspnea
- Frequency of stools, characteristics; cramping, acidosis; signs of dehydration: rapid respirations, poor skin turgor, decreased urine output, dry skin, restlessness, weakness

Administer:
- Antispasmodic if GI symptoms occur
- Allopurinol or sodium bicarbonate to reduce uric acid levels, alkalinization of urine

IV INF route
- Using 21, 23, 25G needle; administer by slow IV infusion via Y-tube or 3-way stopcock of flowing D$_5$W or NS infusion over 2 hr after diluting
- Considered incompatible with other drugs in syringe or sol

Perform/provide:
- Deep-breathing exercises with patient tid-qid; place in semi-Fowler's position
- Increase fluid intake to 2-3 L/day to prevent urate deposits, calculi formation
- Diet low in purines: no organ meats (kidney, liver); dried beans, peas to maintain alkaline urine
- Rinsing of mouth tid-qid with water, club soda; brushing of teeth bid-tid with soft brush or cotton-tipped applicator for stomatitis; use unwaxed dental floss
- Warm compresses at inj site for inflammation
- Nutritious diet with iron, vitamin supplements
- HOB raised to facilitate breathing

Evaluate:
- Therapeutic response: decreased exacerbations in acute lymphocytic leukemia

Teach patient/family:
- To report nausea, vomiting, bruising, bleeding, stomatitis, severe diarrhea, jaundice, chest pain, abdominal pain, trouble breathing, rash
- To avoid vaccinations without advice of prescriber
- Not to use hard-bristled toothbrush, razors
- To avoid OTC medications, alcohol

Treatment of anaphylaxis: Administer epINEPHrine, diphenhydrAMINE, IV corticosteroids

pegfilgrastim (℞)
(peg-fill-grass′stim)
Neulasta
Func. class.: Hematopoietic agent
Chem. class.: Granulocyte colony-stimulating factor

Action: Stimulates proliferation and differentiation of neutrophils

Uses: To decrease infection in patients receiving antineoplastics that are myelosuppressive; to increase WBC in patients with drug-induced neutropenia

DOSAGE AND ROUTES
- *Adult:* **SUBCUT** 6 mg give once per chemotherapy cycle

Available forms: Sol for inj 6 mg/0.6 ml

SIDE EFFECTS
CNS: Fever, fatigue, headache, dizziness, insomnia, peripheral edema
GI: Nausea, vomiting, diarrhea, mucositis, anorexia, constipation, dyspepsia, abdominal pain, stomatitis, **splenic rupture**
HEMA: **Leukocytosis, granulocytopenia, sickle cell crisis, hemoglobin S disease with crisis**
INTEG: Alopecia
MISC: Chest pain, hyperuricemia, **anaphylaxis, influenza-like illness**

MS: Skeletal pain

RESP: **Respiratory distress syndrome**

Contraindications: Hypersensitivity to proteins of *Escherichia coli,* filgrastim; ARDS

Precautions: Pregnancy (C), lactation, myeloid malignancies, sickle cell disease, adolescents, child <45 kg, leukocytosis, splenic rupture, ARDs, allergic-type reactions

PHARMACOKINETICS

Half-life: 15-80 hr

INTERACTIONS

• Do not use this drug concomitantly or 2 wk before or 24 hr after administration of cytotoxic chemotherapy

Increase: release of neutrophils—lithium

Drug/Lab Test

Increase: Uric acid, LDH, alk phos

NURSING CONSIDERATIONS

Assess:

⚠ Allergic reactions, anaphylaxis: rash, urticaria; discontinue this drug, have emergency equipment nearby

• Blood studies: CBC, platelet count before treatment and twice weekly; neutrophil counts may be increased for 2 days after therapy

• B/P, respirations, pulse before and during therapy

• Bone pain, give mild analgesics

Administer:

• Using single-use vials; after dose is withdrawn, do not reenter vial

• Do not use 6 mg fixed dose in infants, children, or others <45 kg

• Inspect sol for discoloration, particulates; if present, do not use

• Do not administer in the period 14 days before and 24 hr after cytotoxic chemotherapy

Perform/provide:

• Storage in refrigerator; do not freeze; may store at room temperature up to 6 hr, avoid shaking, protect from light

Evaluate:

• Therapeutic response: absence of infection

Teach patient/family:

• The technique for self-administration: dose, side effects, disposal of containers and needles; provide instruction sheet

---

peginterferon alfa-2a (℞)

(peg-in-ter-feer′on)

Pegasys

Func. class.: Immunomodulator

Action: Stimulates genes to modulate many biologic effects, including inhibition of viral replication; inhibits ion cell proliferation, immunomodulation, stimulates effector proteins, decreases leukocyte, platelet counts

Uses: Chronic hepatitis C infections in adults with compensated liver disease; chronic hepatitis B in adults with HBe AG-positive, HBe AG-negative

Unlabeled uses: Renal cell carcinoma, chronic myelogenous leukemia

DOSAGE AND ROUTES

• *Adult:* SUBCUT 180 mcg qwk × 48 wk; if poorly tolerated, reduce dose to 135 mcg qwk; in some cases reduction to 90 mcg may be needed

Available forms: Inj 180 mcg/0.5 ml

SIDE EFFECTS

CNS: Headache, insomnia, dizziness, anxiety, hostility, lability, nervousness, depression, fatigue, poor concentration, pyrexia, **suicidal ideation, homicidal ideation,** relapse of drug addiction

ENDO: Hypothyroidism

GI: Abdominal pain, nausea, diarrhea, anorexia, vomiting, dry mouth, **fatal colitis, fatal pancreatitis**

HEMA: **Thrombocytopenia,** neutropenia, anemia, lymphopenia

INTEG: Alopecia, pruritus, rash, dermatitis

MISC: Blurred vision, inj site reaction, rigors

Side effects: *italics* = common; **bold** = life-threatening

MS: Back pain, myalgia, arthralgia
RESP: Cough, dyspnea
Contraindications: Hypersensitivity to interferons, neonates, infants, autoimmune hepatitis, decompensated hepatic disease prior to use of this drug
Precautions: Pregnancy (C), thyroid disorders, myelosuppression, renal/hepatic/cardiac disease, lactation, children <18 yr, depression, suicidal/homicidal ideation, preexisting ophthalmologic disorders, pancreatitis, geriatric

PHARMACOKINETICS

Half-life 15-80 hr, large variability in other pharmacokinetics

INTERACTIONS

• Use caution when giving with theophylline, myelosuppressive agents
Drug/Lab Test
Increase: Triglycerides, ALT, neutrophils, platelets
Abnormal: Thyroid function test

NURSING CONSIDERATIONS

Assess:
• ALT, HCV viral load; patients who show no reduction in ALT, HCV are unlikely to show benefit of treatment after 6 mo
• Platelet counts, heme concentration, ANC, serum creatinine concentration, albumin, bilirubin, TSH, T_4, AFP
• For myelosuppression, hold dose if neutrophil count is <500 × 10⁶/L or if platelets are <50 × 10⁹/L
• For hypersensitivity: discontinue immediately if hypersensitivity occurs
Administer:
• In evening to reduce discomfort, sleep through some side effects
Evaluate:
• Therapeutic response: decreased chronic hepatitis C signs/symptoms, undetectable viral load
Teach patient/family:
• Provide patient or family member with written, detailed information about drug
• Instructions for home use if appropriate

• Use 2 forms of effective contraception throughout treatment and for 6 mo after treatment (men and women) (combination therapy with ribavirin)
• To avoid driving or other hazardous activity if dizziness, confusion, fatigue, somnolence occur
• To use puncture-resistant container for disposal of needles/syringes if using at home
• To report suicidal/homicidal ideation

Rarely Used

pegvisomant (℞)
(peg-vi'soe-mant)
Somavert
Func. class.: Miscellaneous agent

Uses: Acromegaly, in those patients who have an inadequate response to other treatment

DOSAGE AND ROUTES

• *Adult:* **SUBCUT** Loading dose of 40 mg, under supervision of prescriber, then **SUBCUT** 10 mg daily, measure IGF-I levels q4-6wk
Contraindications: Hypersensitivity, latex allergy

⚠ High Alert

pemetrexed (℞)
(pem-ah-trex'ed)
Alimta
Func. class.: Antineoplastic-antimetabolite
Chem. class.: Folic acid antagonist

Action: Inhibits an enzyme that reduces folic acid, which is needed for cell replication
Uses: Malignant pleural mesothelioma in combination with cisplatin; non–small cell lung cancer as a single agent

DOSAGE AND ROUTES

• *Adult:* **IV INF** 500 mg/m² given over 10 min on day 1 of a 21-day cycle with

⚠ Safety alert   *"Tall Man" lettering

cisplatin 75 mg/m^2 infused over 2 hr, beginning ½ hr after end of pemetrexed infusion

• Nadir ANC <500/mm^3 and platelets ≥50,000/mm^3, 75% of previous dose

Available forms: Inj, single-use vials, 500 mg

SIDE EFFECTS

CNS: Fatigue, fever, mood alteration, neuropathy

CV: **Thrombosis/embolism,** *chest pain*

GI: Nausea, vomiting, anorexia, diarrhea, ulcerative stomatitis, constipation, dysphagia, dehydration

GU: Renal failure, creatinine elevation

HEMA: **Neutropenia, leukopenia, thrombocytopenia, myelosuppression, anemia**

INTEG: Rash, desquamation

RESP: Dyspnea

SYST: **Infection with/without neutropenia**

Contraindications: Pregnancy (D), hypersensitivity, ANC <1500 cells/mm^3, CCr <45 ml/min, thrombocytopenia (<100,000/mm^3), anemia

Precautions: Renal/hepatic disease, lactation, children

PHARMACOKINETICS

Not metabolized; excreted in urine (unchanged 70%-90%); not known if it is excreted in breast milk; half-life 3.5 hr, 81% protein binding

INTERACTIONS

Decrease: pemetrexed's clearance—nephrotoxic drugs (NSAIDs)

NURSING CONSIDERATIONS

Assess:

⚠ CBC, differential, platelet count, monitor for nadir and recovery; a new cycle should not begin if ANC <1500 cells/mm^3, platelets are <100,000 cells/mm^3, creatinine clearance <45 ml/min

• Renal studies: BUN, serum uric acid, urine CCr, electrolytes before, during therapy

• I&O ratio; report fall in urine output to <30 ml/hr

• Monitor temp q4h; fever may indicate beginning infection; no rectal temps

• Bleeding time, coagulation time during treatment; bleeding: hematuria, guaiac, bruising or petechiae, mucosa or orifices q8h

• Buccal cavity q8h for dryness, sores, ulceration, white patches, oral pain, bleeding, dysphagia

⚠ Symptoms indicating severe allergic reaction: rash, urticaria, itching, flushing

Administer:

• Vit B$_{12}$ and low-dose folic acid as a prophylactic measure to treat related hematologic, GI toxicity; at least 5 daily doses of folic acid must be taken in the 7 days preceding first dose

• Premedicate with a corticosteroid (dexamethasone) given PO bid the day before, day of, and day after administration of pemetrexed

IV route

• Use aseptic technique during reconstitution, dilution

• Reconstitute 500 mg vial/20 ml 0.9% NaCl inj (preservative free) = 25 mg/ml, swirl until dissolved, further dilute with 100 ml 0.9% NaCl inj (preservative free), give as IV infusion over 10 mg

• Use only 0.9% NaCl inj (preservative free) for reconstitution, dilution

Perform/provide:

• Strict medical asepsis and protective isolation if WBC levels are low

• Liquid diet: carbonated beverage, Jell-O; dry toast, crackers may be added when patient is not nauseated or vomiting

• Rinsing of mouth tid-qid with water, club soda; brushing of teeth bid-tid with soft brush or cotton-tipped applicators for stomatitis; use unwaxed dental floss

• Storage at 77° F, excursions permitted 59°-86° F, not light sensitive, discard unused portions

Evaluate:
• Therapeutic response: decreased spread of malignancy

Teach patient/family:
• To report any complaints, side effects to nurse or prescriber: black tarry stools, chills, fever, sore throat, bleeding, bruising, cough, shortness of breath, dark or bloody urine
• To avoid foods with citric acid, hot or rough texture if stomatitis is present
• To report stomatitis: any bleeding, white spots, ulcerations in mouth to prescriber; tell patient to examine mouth daily, report symptoms to nurse, use good oral hygiene
• That contraceptive measures are recommended during therapy and for at least 8 wk after cessation of therapy, to discontinue breastfeeding; toxicity to infant may occur
• To avoid alcohol, salicylates, live vaccines
• To avoid use of razors, commercial mouthwash

penciclovir topical
See Appendix C

PENICILLINS

penicillin G benzathine (℞)
(pen-i-sill'in)
Bicillin L-A, Megacillin ✹, Permapen
penicillin G (℞)
Pfizerpen
penicillin G procaine (℞)
Ayercillin ✹, Wycillin
penicillin V (℞)
Apo-Pen-VK ✹, Beepen-VK, Nadopen-V ✹, Novopen-VK ✹, Pen-Vee K ✹, PVF K ✹, Veetids
Func. class.: Broad-spectrum antiinfective
Chem. class.: Natural penicillin

Action: Interferes with cell wall replication of susceptible organisms; lysis is mediated by cell wall autolytic enzymes, results in cell death
Uses: Respiratory infections, scarlet fever, erysipelas, otitis media, pneumonia, skin and soft tissue infections, gonorrhea; effective for gram-positive cocci *(Staphylococcus, Streptococcus pyogenes, S. viridans, S. faecalis, S. bovis, S. pneumoniae)*, gram-negative cocci *(Neisseria gonorrhoeae)*, gram-positive bacilli *(Actinomyces, Bacillus anthracis, Clostridium perfringens, C. tetani, Corynebacterium diphtheriae, Listeria monocytogenes)*, gram-negative bacilli *(Escherichia coli, Proteus mirabilis, Salmonella, Shigella, Enterobacter, Streptobacillus moniliformis)*, spirochetes *(Treponema pallidum)*

DOSAGE AND ROUTES
Penicillin G benzathine
Early syphilis
• *Adult:* **IM** 2.4 million units in single dose
Congenital syphilis
• *Child <2 yr:* **IM** 50,000 units/kg in single dose

Prophylaxis of rheumatic fever, glomerulonephritis
• *Adult and child:* **IM** 1.2 million units in single dose qmo or 600,000 units q2wk
Upper respiratory infections (group A streptococcal)
• *Adult:* **IM** 1.2 million units in single dose
• *Child >27 kg:* **IM** 900,000 units in single dose
• *Child <27 kg:* **IM** 300,000-600,000 units in single dose
Available forms: Inj 300,000, 600,000 units/ml

Penicillin G
• CCr <10 ml/min, give full loading dose, then ½ of loading dose q8-10h
Pneumococcal/streptococcal infections (serious)
• *Adult:* **IM/IV** 5-24 million units in divided doses q4-6h
• *Child <12 yr:* **IV** 150,000 units/kg/day in 4-6 divided doses
Available forms: Powder for inj 1, 5, 20 million units/vial; inj 1, 2, 3 million units/50 ml

Penicillin G procaine
Moderate to severe pneumococcal infections
• *Adult and child:* **IM** 600,000-1.2 million units in 1 or 2 doses/day for 10 days to 2 wk
• *Newborn:* Avoid use in newborns
Pneumococcal pneumonia
• *Adult and child >12 yr:* **IM** 600,000-1.2 million units/day × 7-10 days
Available forms: Inj 600,000, 1,200,000 units/unit dose

Penicillin V
• Dosage reduction indicated in renal impairment (CCr <50 ml/min) based on clinial response, degree of impairment
Pneumococcal/staphylococcal infections
• *Adult:* **PO** 250-500 mg q6h
• *Child <12 yr:* **PO** 25-50 mg/kg/day in divided doses q6-8h; max 3 g/day
Streptococcal infections
• *Adult:* **PO** 125-250 mg q6-8h × 10 days

Prevention of recurrence of rheumatic fever/chorea
• *Adult:* **PO** 125-250 mg bid continuously
Vincent's gingivitis/pharyngitis
• *Adult:* **PO** 250-500 mg q6-8h
Available forms: Tabs 250, 500 mg; powder for oral sol 125, 250 mg/5 ml

SIDE EFFECTS

CNS: Lethargy, hallucinations, anxiety, depression, twitching, **coma, seizures**
GI: Nausea, vomiting, diarrhea, increased AST, ALT, abdominal pain, glossitis, colitis, **pseudomembranous colitis**
GU: **Oliguria, proteinuria, hematuria,** *vaginitis, moniliasis,* **glomerulonephritis**
HEMA: Anemia; increased bleeding time; **bone marrow depression, granulocytopenia**
META: Hyperkalemia, hypokalemia, alkalosis, hypernatremia
MISC: **Anaphylaxis, serum sickness, Stevens-Johnson syndrome,** *local pain,* tenderness and fever with IM inj
Contraindications: Hypersensitivity to penicillins; neonates
Precautions: Pregnancy (B), hypersensitivity to cephalosporins, lactation, severe renal disease, GI disease, asthma

PHARMACOKINETICS

Penicillin G benzathine
IM: Very slow absorption, duration 21-28 days, half-life 30-60 min; excreted in urine, feces, breast milk; crosses placenta
Penicillin G
IV: Peak immediate
IM: Peak ¼-½ hr
PO: Peak 1 hr, duration 6 hr
Excreted in urine unchanged, excreted in breast milk, crosses placenta, half-life 30-60 min
Penicillin G procaine
IM: Peak 1-4 hr, duration 15 hr, excreted in urine
Penicillin V
PO: Peak 30-60 min, duration 6-8 hr, half-life 30 min, excreted in urine, breast milk

Side effects: *italics* = common; **bold** = life-threatening

INTERACTIONS

Increase: penicillin concentrations—aspirin, probenecid

Increase: effect of heparin, methotrexate

Decrease: effect of oral contraceptives, typhoid vaccine

Decrease: antimicrobial effect of penicillin—tetracyclines

Drug/Herb

• Do not use acidophilus with antiinfectives; separate by several hours

Decrease: absorption of penicillin—khat

Drug/Lab Test

False positive: Urine glucose, urine protein

NURSING CONSIDERATIONS

Assess:

• For infection: temp, characteristics of sputum, wounds, urine, stools before, during, and after treatment

• I&O ratio; report hematuria, oliguria, since penicillin in high doses is nephrotoxic

⚠ Any patient with compromised renal system, since drug is excreted slowly in poor renal system function; toxicity may occur rapidly

• Hepatic studies: AST, ALT

• Blood studies: WBC, RBC, Hct, Hgb, bleeding time

• Renal tests: urinalysis, protein, blood

• C&S before therapy; drug may be given as soon as culture is taken

⚠ For pseudomembranous colitis: diarrhea, mucus, pus; bowel pattern before and during treatment

• Skin eruptions after administration of penicillin to 1 wk after discontinuing drug

• Respiratory status: rate, character, wheezing, tightness in chest

⚠ Allergies before initiation of treatment, reaction of each medication; because of prolonged action, allergic reaction may be prolonged and severe; watch for anaphylaxis: rash, dyspnea, pruritus, laryngeal edema

Administer:

Penicillin G benzathine

• Drug after C&S completed

• After shaking well, deep IM inj in large muscle mass; avoid intravascular inj; aspirate; do not give IV

Penicillin G

• Drug after C&S

Y-site compatibilities: Acyclovir, amiodarone, cyclophosphamide, diltiazem, enalaprilat, esmolol, fluconazole, foscarnet, heparin, hydromorphone, labetalol, magnesium sulfate, meperidine, morphine, perphenazine, potassium chloride, tacrolimus, theophylline, verapamil, vit B/C

Penicillin G procaine

• Drug after C&S

• Deep IM inj; avoid intravascular inj

• Aspirate; do not give IV

Penicillin V

• Orally on empty stomach for best absorption

• Drug after C&S

Perform/provide:

• EpINEPHrine, suction, tracheostomy set, endotracheal intubation equipment

• Adequate fluid intake (2 L) during diarrhea episodes

• Scratch test to assess allergy after securing order from prescriber; usually done when penicillin is only drug of choice

• Storage in dry, tight container; oral susp refrigerated 2 wk

Evaluate:

• Therapeutic response: absence of fever, draining wounds

• Allergies before initiation of treatment, reaction of each medication; highlight allergies on chart; hypersensitivity reaction may be delayed

Teach patient/family:

• To report sore throat, fever, fatigue; may indicate superinfection

• To wear or carry emergency ID if allergic to penicillins

• To report diarrhea, prevent dehydration

• To shake susp well before each dose; store in refrigerator for up to 2 wk

• To use all medication prescribed

⚠ Safety alert   *"Tall Man" lettering

• To use additional contraception if using any of these drugs

Treatment of anaphylaxis: Withdraw drug; maintain airway; administer epINEPHrine, aminophylline, O_2, IV corticosteroids

---

pentamidine (R)
(pen-tam'i-deen)
Nebupent, Pentam 300,
Pentacarinat ✤
Pneumopent ✤
Func. class.: Antiprotozoal
Chem. class.: Aromatic diamide derivative

Action: Interferes with DNA/RNA synthesis in protozoa

Uses: Treatment/prevention of *Pneumocystis jiroveci* infections

Unlabeled uses: *Leishmania* infections, *Trypanosoma* infections

DOSAGE AND ROUTES

• *Adult and child:* **IV/IM** 4 mg/kg/day × 2-3 wk; **NEB** 300 mg via specific nebulizer given q4wk for prevention

Available forms: Inj, aerosol 300 mg/vial; sol for aerosol 60 mg/vial ✤

SIDE EFFECTS

CNS: Disorientation, hallucinations, *dizziness,* confusion

CV: Hypotension, ventricular tachycardia, ECG abnormalities, **dysrhythmias**

GI: Nausea, vomiting, anorexia; increased AST, ALT; **acute pancreatitis,** metallic taste

GU: **Acute renal failure, increased serum creatinine, renal toxicity**

HEMA: Anemia, **leukopenia, thrombocytopenia**

INTEG: Sterile abscess, pain at injection site, pruritus, urticaria, *rash*

META: *Hyperkalemia,* hypocalcemia, hypoglycemia

MISC: Fatigue, chills, night sweats, **anaphylaxis, Stevens-Johnson syndrome**

RESP: Cough, shortness of breath, **bronchospasm** (with aerosol)

Precautions: Pregnancy (C), blood dyscrasias, renal/hepatic/cardiac disease, diabetes mellitus, hypocalcemia, hypertension, hypotension, lactation, children

PHARMACOKINETICS

Excreted unchanged in urine (66%)

INTERACTIONS

• Nephrotoxicity: aminoglycosides, amphotericin B, cisplatin, NSAIDs, vancomycin

⚠ Fatal dysrhythmias: erythromycin IV

Increase: QT prolongation—class IA, class III antidysrhythmics; phenothiazines

Increase: myelosuppression—antineoplastics, radiation

NURSING CONSIDERATIONS

Assess:

• Blood tests, blood glucose, CBC, platelets, calcium, magnesium

• I&O ratio; report hematuria, oliguria

• ECG for cardiac dysrhythmias

• Patient should be lying down when receiving drug; severe hypotension may develop; monitor B/P during administration and until B/P stable

⚠ Any patient with compromised renal system; drug is excreted slowly in poor renal system function; toxicity may occur rapidly

• Hepatic studies: AST, ALT

• Renal studies: urinalysis, BUN, creatinine; nephrotoxicity may occur

• Signs of infection, anemia

• Bowel pattern before, during treatment

• Sterile abscess, pain at inj site

• Respiratory status: rate, character, wheezing, dyspnea

• Dizziness, confusion, hallucination

• Allergies before treatment, reaction of each medication; place allergies on chart in bright red letters; notify all people giving drugs

• Diabetic patients, hypoglycemia may occur, then hyperglycemia with prolonged therapy

P

✤ Canada only   Side effects: *italics* = common; **bold** = life-threatening

Administer:

Inhalation route

• Through nebulizer; mix contents in 6 ml of sterile H_2O; do not use low pressure (<20 psi); flow rate should be 5-7 L/min (40-50 psi) air or O_2 source over 30-45 min until chamber is empty

IM route

• 300 mg diluted in 3 ml sterile H_2O; give deep IM by Z-track; painful by this route

IV route

• Reconstitute 300 mg/3-5 ml of sterile water for inj, D_5W, withdraw dose and further dilute in 50-250 ml D_5W, give over 1-2 hr

Y-site compatibilities: Aldesleukin, cefazolin, cefoperazone, cefotaxime, cefoxitin, ceftazidine, ceftriaxone, diltiazem, fluconazole, foscarnet, gatifloxacin, linezolid, zidovudine

Perform/provide:

• Storage in refrigerator protected from light

Evaluate:

• Therapeutic response: decreased temp, increased ability to breathe

Teach patient/family:

• To report sore throat, fever, fatigue (may indicate superinfection)

• To maintain adequate fluid intake

⚠ High Alert

pentazocine (℞)
(pen-taz′oh-seen)
Talwin, Talwin NX
Func. class.: Opiate analgesic, antagonist
Chem. class.: Synthetic benzomorphan

Controlled Substance Schedule IV
Action: Inhibits ascending pain pathways in CNS, increases pain threshold, alters pain perception
Uses: Moderate to severe pain

DOSAGE AND ROUTES

• *Adult:* **PO** 50-100 mg q3-4h prn, not to exceed 600 mg/day; **IV/IM/SUBCUT** 30 mg q3-4h prn, not to exceed 360 mg/day
Labor
• *Adult:* **IM** 60 mg; **IV** 30 mg q2-3h when contractions are regular
Renal dose
• CCr 10-50 ml/min reduce dose by 25%; CCr <10 ml/min reduce dose by 50%
Available forms: Inj 30 mg/ml; tabs 50 mg

SIDE EFFECTS

CNS: Drowsiness, dizziness, confusion, headache, sedation, euphoria, hallucinations, dreaming
CV: Palpitations, bradycardia, change in B/P, tachycardia, increased B/P (high doses)
EENT: Tinnitus, blurred vision, miosis, diplopia
GI: Nausea, vomiting, anorexia, constipation, *cramps,* dry mouth
GU: Increased urinary output, dysuria, urinary retention
INTEG: Rash, urticaria, bruising, flushing, diaphoresis, pruritus, severe irritation at inj sites
RESP: **Respiratory depression**
Contraindications: Hypersensitivity, addiction (opiate)
Precautions: Pregnancy (C), addictive personality, lactation, increased intracranial pressure, MI (acute), severe heart disease, respiratory depression, renal/hepatic disease, seizure disorder, child <18 yr, head trauma

PHARMACOKINETICS

SUBCUT/IM: Onset 15-30 min, peak 1-2 hr, duration 2-4 hr
IV: Onset 2-3 min, duration 4-6 hr; metabolized by liver, excreted by kidneys, crosses placenta, half-life 2-3 hr, extensive first-pass metabolism with less than 20% entering circulation

---

⚠ Safety alert   *"Tall Man" lettering

INTERACTIONS

⚠ Unpredictable reactions: MAOIs
Increase: effects—CNS depressants; alcohol, sedative/hypnotics, antipsychotics, skeletal muscle relaxants
Decrease: effects—opiates
Drug/Lab Test
Increase: Amylase

NURSING CONSIDERATIONS

Assess:
• For pain: intensity, duration, location prior to and 1 hr after dose
• I&O ratio; check for decreasing output; may indicate urinary retention
• For withdrawal symptoms in opiate-dependent patients
• Pulmonary embolism, abscesses, ulcerations, vascular occlusion, WBC
• CNS changes: dizziness, drowsiness, hallucinations, euphoria, LOC, pupil reaction
• Allergic reactions: rash, urticaria
• Respiratory dysfunction: respiratory depression, character, rate, rhythm; notify prescriber if respirations are <10/min
• Need for pain medication, physical dependence

Administer:
• With antiemetic if nausea, vomiting occur
• When pain is beginning to return; determine dosage interval by patient response

IM/SUBCUT route
• Give IM deeply into large muscle mass, rotate sites; SUBCUT may cause necrosis with repeated inj

IV route
• Undiluted or diluted 5 mg/ml of sterile H₂O for inj; give 5 mg or less over 1 min

Syringe compatibilities: Atropine, benzquinamide, butorphanol, chlorproMAZINE, cimetidine, dimenhyDRINATE, diphenhydrAMINE, droperidol, fentanyl, hydromorphone, hydrOXYzine, meperidine, metoclopramide, morphine, perphenazine, prochlorperazine, promazine, promethazine, ranitidine, scopolamine
Y-site compatibilities: Heparin, hydrocortisone, potassium chloride, vit B/C

Perform/provide:
• Storage in light-resistant area at room temperature
• Assistance with ambulation
• Safety measures: night-light, call bell within easy reach
Evaluate:
• Therapeutic response: decrease in pain
Teach patient/family:
• To report any symptoms of CNS changes, allergic reactions
• That physical dependency may result from extended use
• That withdrawal symptoms may occur: nausea, vomiting, cramps, fever, faintness, anorexia
Treatment of overdose: Naloxone (Narcan) 0.2-0.8 mg IV, O₂, IV fluids, vasopressors

---

⚠ High Alert

pentobarbital (℞)
(pen-toe-bar′bi-tal)
Nembutal, Novopentobarb ✿
Nova-Rectal ✿, pentobarbital sodium
Func. class.: Sedative/hypnotic barbiturate; anticonvulsant
Chem. class.: Barbitone, short acting

Controlled Substance Schedule II (USA), Schedule G (CDSA IV) (Canada)
Do not confuse:
pentobarbital/phenobarbital
Action: Depresses activity in brain cells, primarily in reticular activating system in brain stem; selectively depresses neurons in posterior hypothalamus, limbic structures
Uses: Insomnia, sedation, preoperative medication, increased intracranial pressure, dental anesthetic

DOSAGE AND ROUTES

Insomnia
• *Adult:* **PO** 100-200 mg at bedtime; **IM** 150-200 mg at bedtime; **IV** 100 mg ini-

P

tially, then up to 500 mg; **RECT** 120-200 mg at bedtime
• *Child:* **IM** 2-6 mg/kg, not to exceed 100 mg; **PO** 2-6 mg/kg/day in divided doses; **PO** preoperatively 2-6 mg/kg, max 100 mg/dose; **IV** 100 mg (hypnotic/anticonvulsant)

Available forms: Caps 50, 100 mg; elix 20 mg/5 ml; rect supp 25, 30, 50, 60, 120, 200 mg; inj 50 mg/ml

SIDE EFFECTS

CNS: Lethargy, drowsiness, hangover, dizziness, paradoxical stimulation in geriatric and children, light-headedness, dependence, **CNS depression**, mental depression, slurred speech
CV: Hypotension, bradycardia
GI: Nausea, vomiting, diarrhea, constipation
HEMA: **Agranulocytosis, thrombocytopenia, megaloblastic anemia** (long-term treatment)
INTEG: Rash, urticaria, pain, abscesses at inj site, angioedema, thrombophlebitis, **Stevens-Johnson syndrome**
RESP: **Respiratory depression, apnea, laryngospasm, bronchospasm**
Contraindications: Pregnancy (D), hypersensitivity to barbiturates, respiratory depression, addiction to barbiturates; severe renal/hepatic impairment; porphyria, uncontrolled pain
Precautions: Anemia, lactation, renal/hepatic disease, hypertension, geriatric, acute/chronic pain

PHARMACOKINETICS

PO: Onset 15-30 min, duration 4-6 hr
RECT: Onset slow, duration 4-6 hr
Metabolized by liver, excreted by kidneys (metabolites); half-life 15-48 hr

INTERACTIONS

Increase: CNS depression—alcohol, MAOIs, sedatives, other CNS depressants, antihistamines, opiates
Increase: half-life of doxycycline
Decrease: effect of oral anticoagulants, corticosteroids, griseofulvin, quinidine

Drug/Herb
Increase: pentobarbital levels—eucalyptus, Jamaican dogwood, kava, lemon balm nettle, pill-bearing spurge, poppy, quinine, senega, valerian
Drug/Lab Test
False increase: Sulfobromophthalein

NURSING CONSIDERATIONS
Assess:
• VS q30min after parenteral route for 2 hr
• Blood studies: Hct, Hgb, RBCs, serum folate, vit D (long-term therapy); PT in patients receiving anticoagulants
• Hepatic studies: AST, ALT, bilirubin; if increased, drug is usually discontinued
• Mental status: mood, sensorium, affect, memory (long, short)
• Physical dependency: more frequent requests for medication, shakes, anxiety
⚠ Barbiturate toxicity: hypotension; pupillary constriction; cold, clammy skin; cyanosis of lips; insomnia; nausea; vomiting; hallucinations; delirium; weakness; coma; mild symptoms may occur in 8-12 hr without drug
• Respiratory changes: respiratory depression, character, rate, rhythm; hold drug if respirations are <10/min or if pupils are dilated
• Blood dyscrasias: fever, sore throat, bruising, rash, jaundice, epistaxis
Administer:
• For <14 days, since not effective after that; tolerance develops
• After removal of cigarettes to prevent fires
• After trying conservative measures for insomnia
• Avoid use with CNS depressants; serious CNS depression may result
PO route
• Use elixir alone or diluted in fluids
• ½-1 hr before bedtime for sleeplessness
• On empty stomach for best absorption
• Crushed or whole
• Alone; do not mix with other drugs or inject if there is precipitate

IM route
• Inj deep in large muscle mass to prevent tissue sloughing and abscesses; do not inject more than 5 ml in one site

IV route
• IV undiluted or dilute in sterile H_2O, LR, NaCl, give 50 mg or less/min; titrate to patient response; use only clear sol; avoid extravasation
• IV only with resuscitative equipment available; administer at <100 mg/min (only by qualified personnel)

Additive compatibilities: Amikacin, aminophylline, calcium chloride, cephapirin, chloramphenicol, dimenhyDRINATE, erythromycin lactobionate, lidocaine, thiopental, verapamil

Syringe compatibilities: Aminophylline, epHEDrine, hydromorphone, neostigmine, scopolamine, sodium bicarbonate, thiopental

Y-site compatibilities: Acyclovir, insulin (regular), propofol

Perform/provide:
• Assistance with ambulation after receiving dose
• Safety measures: night-light, call bell within easy reach
• Checking to see if PO medication has been swallowed
• Storage of suppositories in refrigerator; do not use aqueous solutions that contain precipitate

Evaluate:
• Therapeutic response: ability to sleep at night, less early morning awakening if taking drug for insomnia, or decrease in number, severity of seizures if taking drug for seizure disorder

Teach patient/family:
• That hangover is common
• That drug is indicated only for short-term treatment of insomnia; probably ineffective after 2 wk
• That physical dependency may result from extended use (45-90 days depending on dose)
• To avoid driving, other activities requiring alertness
• To avoid alcohol ingestion
• Not to discontinue medication quickly

after long-term use; drug should be tapered over 1-2 wk
• To tell all prescribers that a barbiturate is being taken
• That withdrawal insomnia may occur after short-term use; not to start using drug again; insomnia will improve in 1-3 nights
• That effects may take 2 nights for benefits to be noticed
• Alternative measures to improve sleep (reading, exercise several hr before bedtime, warm bath, warm milk, TV, self-hypnosis, deep breathing)

Treatment of overdose: Lavage, activated charcoal, warming blanket, vital signs, hemodialysis, I&O ratio

> ### ⚠ High Alert
>
> ### pentostatin (℞)
> (pen-toh-stat'in)
> Nipent
> *Func. class.:* Antineoplastic, enzyme inhibitor
> *Chem. class.: Streptomyces antibioticus derivative*

Action: Inhibits the enzyme adenosine deaminase (ADA), which is able to block DNA synthesis and some RNA synthesis

Uses: α-Interferon-refractory hairy cell leukemia

Unlabeled uses: Chronic lymphocytic leukemia

DOSAGE AND ROUTES
• *Adult:* **IV** 4 mg/m^2 every other wk; may be given **IV BOL,** or diluted in a larger volume and given over 20-30 min

Available forms: Powder for inj 10 mg/vial

SIDE EFFECTS
CNS: Headache, anxiety, confusion, depression, dizziness, insomnia, nervousness, paresthesia
GI: Nausea, vomiting, anorexia, diarrhea, constipation, flatulence, stomatitis, elevated LFTs

---

GU: **Hematuria,** dysuria, increased BUN/creatinine

HEMA: **Leukopenia, anemia, thrombocytopenia,** *ecchymosis,* **lymphadenopathy,** petechiae

INTEG: Rash, eczema, dry skin, pruritus, sweating, herpes simplex/zoster

RESP: Cough, upper respiratory infection, bronchitis, dyspnea, epistaxis, pneumonia, pharyngitis, rhinitis, sinusitis

SYST: Fever, infection, fatigue, pain, allergic reaction, chills, **death, sepsis,** chest pain, flulike symptoms

Contraindications: Pregnancy (D), hypersensitivity to this drug or mannitol

Precautions: Renal disease, lactation, children, bone marrow depression

PHARMACOKINETICS

IV: Elimination half-life 5.7 hr, low protein binding, 90% excreted in urine unchanged or as metabolites

INTERACTIONS

⚠ Fatal pulmonary toxicity: fludarabine

Increase: adverse reactions—vidarabine

Drug/Lab Test

Increase: Uric acid

NURSING CONSIDERATIONS

Assess:

• CBC, differential, platelet count qwk; withhold drug if WBC is <2000/mm^3 or platelet count is <75,000/mm^3; notify prescriber

• Renal studies; BUN, serum uric acid, urine CCr, electrolytes before, during therapy

• I&O ratio; report fall in urine output to <30 ml/hr

• Monitor temp q4h; fever may indicate beginning infection

• Hepatic studies before, during therapy: bilirubin, AST, ALT, alk phos, prn or qmo; check for jaundiced skin and sclera, dark urine, clay-colored stools, itchy skin, abdominal pain, fever, diarrhea

• Bleeding: hematuria, guaiac stools, bruising, petechiae, mucosa or orifices q8h

• Effects of alopecia on body image; discuss feelings about body changes

• Inflammation of mucosa, breaks in skin

• Buccal cavity q8h for dryness, sores, ulceration, white patches, oral pain, bleeding, dysphagia

• Local irritation, pain, burning at inj site

• Symptoms of severe allergic reaction: rash, pruritus, urticaria, purpuric skin lesions, itching, flushing

• GI symptoms: frequency of stools, cramping

• Acidosis, signs of dehydration; rapid respiration, poor skin turgor, decreased urine output, dry skin, restlessness, weakness

Administer:

• Antiemetic 30-60 min before giving drug to prevent vomiting

• Antibiotics as ordered for prophylaxis of infection

IV route

• Hydrate with 500-1000 ml D$_5$½ NS or equivalent before administration; administer another 500 ml D$_5$ or equivalent after pentostatin

• After diluting, use with 5 ml sterile H$_2$O for injection and mix thoroughly (2 mg/ml); may be given by bolus or diluted in 25-50 ml 5% dextrose, or 0.9% NaCl (0.33 or 0.18 mg/ml)

Solution compatibilities: D$_5$W, 0.9% NaCl, LR

Y-site compatibilities: Fludarabine, melphalan, ondansetron, paclitaxel, sargramostim

Perform/provide:

• Hydrocortisone, sodium thiosulfate to infiltration area, and ice compress after stopping infusion

• Strict hand-washing technique, gloves, protective covering

• Liquid diet: carbonated beverages; gelatin may be added if patient is not nauseated or vomiting

• Rinsing of mouth tid-qid with water, club soda; brushing of teeth bid-qid with soft brush or cotton-tipped applicators for stomatitis; use unwaxed dental floss

• Storage in refrigerator; reconstituted or

diluted sol may be stored at room temperature up to 8 hr

Evaluate:
• Therapeutic response: decrease in tumor size, spread of malignancy

Teach patient/family:
• To report any complaints, side effects to nurse or prescriber
• That hair may be lost during treatment and wig or hairpiece may make patient feel better; tell patient that new hair may be different in color, texture
• To avoid foods with citric acid, hot or rough texture
• To report any bleeding, white spots, ulcerations in mouth to prescriber; tell patient to examine mouth daily
• To avoid crowds and sources of infection when granulocyte count is low

---

pentoxifylline (℞)
(pen-tox′ih-fill-in)
Trental
Func. class.: Hemorheologic agent
Chem. class.: Dimethylxanthine derivative

Action: Decreases blood viscosity, stimulates prostacyclin formation, increases blood flow by increasing flexibility of RBCs; decreases RBC hyperaggregation; reduces platelet aggregation, decreases fibrinogen concentration

Uses: Intermittent claudication related to chronic occlusive vascular disease

Unlabeled uses: Cerebrovascular insufficiency, diabetic neuropathies, TIAs, leg ulcers, strokes, aphthous stomatitis, sickle cell anemia

DOSAGE AND ROUTES
• *Adult:* **PO** 400 mg tid with meals, may decrease to bid if side effects occur; must be taken for ≥8 wk for maximal effect

Stomatitis (unlabeled)
• *Adult:* **PO** 400 mg tid × 1-6 mo

Available forms: Cont release tabs 400 mg; ext rel tabs 400 mg

SIDE EFFECTS

CNS: Headache, anxiety, *tremors,* confusion, *dizziness*
CV: Angina, dysrhythmias, palpitation, hypotension, chest pain, dyspnea, edema
EENT: Blurred vision, earache, increased salivation, sore throat, conjunctivitis
GI: Dyspepsia, nausea, vomiting, anorexia, bloating, belching, constipation, cholecystitis, dry mouth, thirst, bad taste
INTEG: Rash, pruritus, urticaria, brittle fingernails
MISC: Epistaxis, flulike symptoms, laryngitis, nasal congestion, **leukopenia,** malaise, weight changes

Contraindications: Hypersensitivity to this drug or xanthines, retinal/cerebral hemorrhage

Precautions: Pregnancy (C), angina pectoris, lactation, children, impaired renal function, recent surgery, peptic ulceration, hepatic/cardiac disease

PHARMACOKINETICS
PO: Peak 8 wk, half-life ½-1 hr, degradation in liver, excreted in urine

INTERACTIONS
Increase: risk of bleeding—warfarin, salicylates, NSAIDs, thrombolytics, abciximab, eptifibatide, tirofiban, ticlopidine
Increase: theophylline level—theophylline
Increase: hypotension—antihypertensives, nitrates
Increase: pentoxifylline—cimetidine

Drug/Herb
Increase: bleeding potential—anise, arnica, chamomile, clove, dong quai, fenugreek, feverfew, garlic, ginger, ginkgo, ginseng *(Panax),* licorice

NURSING CONSIDERATIONS
Assess:
• B/P, respirations of patient also taking antihypertensives; intermittent claudication baseline and throughout

Administer:
- Do not break, crush, or chew ext rel tabs
- With meals to prevent GI upset

Evaluate:
- Therapeutic response: decreased pain, cramping, increased ambulation

Teach patient/family:
- That therapeutic response may take 2-4 wk, 8-12 wk to reach full benefit
- To observe feet for arterial insufficiency
- To use cotton socks, well-fitted shoes; not to go barefoot
- To watch for bleeding, bruises, petechiae, epistaxis
- To avoid smoking, to prevent blood vessel constriction

perindopril (℞)
(per-in′doe-pril)
Aceon
Func. class.: Antihypertensive
Chem. class.: Angiotensin-converting enzyme inhibitor

Action: Selectively suppresses renin-angiotensin-aldosterone system; inhibits ACE; prevents conversion of angiotensin I to angiotensin II, dilation of arterial, venous vessels

Uses: Hypertension, stable artery disease

DOSAGE AND ROUTES

Hypertension
- *Adult:* **PO** 4 mg/day, may increase or decrease to desired response range 4-8 mg/day; may give in 2 divided doses or as a single dose, max 16 mg/day

Patients on diuretics
- Discontinue diuretic 2-3 days prior to perindopril then resume diuretic if needed

Renal dose
- *Adult:* **PO** CCr 16-29 ml/min, 2 mg every other day; CCr 30-59 2 mg daily

Stable CAD
- *Adult:* **PO** 4 mg/day × 2 wk then increase as tolerated to 8 mg/day

Available forms: Tabs scored 2, 4, 8 mg

SIDE EFFECTS

CNS: Insomnia, dizziness, paresthesias, headache, fatigue, anxiety, depression
CV: Hypotension, chest pain, tachycardia, dysrhythmias, syncope
EENT: Tinnitus, visual changes, sore throat, double vision, dry burning eyes
GI: Nausea, vomiting, colitis, cramps, diarrhea, constipation, flatulence, dry mouth, loss of taste
GU: **Proteinuria, renal failure,** increased frequency of polyuria or oliguria
HEMA: **Agranulocytosis, neutropenia**
INTEG: Rash, purpura, alopecia, hyperhidrosis
META: Hyperkalemia
RESP: Dyspnea, *dry cough,* crackles
SYST: **Angioedema**

Contraindications: Pregnancy (D) 2nd/3rd trimester, hypersensitivity, history of angioedema

Precautions: Pregnancy (C) 1st trimester, renal disease, hyperkalemia, lactation, hepatic failure, dehydration, bilateral renal artery stenosis, cough, angioedema, severe CHF

PHARMACOKINETICS

Bioavailability 75%; peak 1 hr parent drug, 3-7 hr prodrug; protein binding 68%; metabolized by liver (active metabolite perindoprilat); half-life 0.8-10 hr; excreted in urine

INTERACTIONS

Increase: effects of neuromuscular blocking agents, antihypertensives, lithium
Increase: diuretics
Increase: hypersensitivity—allopurinol
Increase: severe hypotension—diuretics, other antihypertensives
Increase: hyperkalemia—salt substitutes, potassium-sparing diuretics, potassium supplements
Decrease: effects of NSAIDs
Decrease: antihypertensive effect—NSAIDs, salicylates

Drug/Herb
Increase: toxicity, death—aconite
Increase: antihypertensive effect—barberry, betony, black catechu, black cohosh, bloodroot, broom, burdock, cat's claw, dandelion, goldenseal, hawthorn, Irish moss, Jamaican dogwood, kelp, khella, mistletoe, parsley
Increase or decrease: antihypertensive effect—astragalus, cola tree
Decrease: antihypertensive effect—coltsfoot, guarana, khat, licorice, yohimbine
Drug/Lab Test
Interference: Glucose/insulin tolerance tests

NURSING CONSIDERATIONS
Assess:
• B/P, pulse q4h; note rate, rhythm, quality
• Electrolytes: K, Na, Cl during 1st 2 wk of therapy
• Baselines in renal, hepatic studies before therapy begins and 1 wk into therapy
• Edema in feet, legs daily
• Skin turgor, dryness of mucous membranes for hydration status, dry mouth
• Symptoms of CHF: edema, dyspnea, wet crackles
Administer:
• As a single dose or in 2 divided doses
Evaluate:
• Therapeutic response: decreased B/P
Teach patient/family:
• Not to use OTC (cough, cold, or allergy) products unless directed by prescriber; to avoid salt substitutes
• To avoid sunlight or wear sunscreen for photosensitivity
• To comply with dosage schedule, even if feeling better
• To notify prescriber of mouth sores, sore throat, fever, swelling of hands or feet, irregular heartbeat, chest pains, signs of angioedema
• That excessive perspiration, dehydration, vomiting, diarrhea may lead to fall in blood pressure; consult prescriber if these occur

• That drug may cause dizziness, fainting; light-headedness may occur during 1st few days of therapy
• That drug may cause skin rash or impaired perspiration; angioedema may occur and to discontinue if it occurs
• Not to discontinue drug abruptly
• To rise slowly to sitting or standing position to minimize orthostatic hypotension
Treatment of overdose: Lavage, IV atropine for bradycardia, IV theophylline for bronchospasm, digoxin, O_2, diuretic for cardiac failure

Rarely Used
permethrin (OTC, ℞)
(per-meth'rin)
Acticin, Elimite, Nix
Func. class.: Pediculicide

Uses: Lice, nits, ticks, flea nits

DOSAGE AND ROUTES
Lice (head)
• *Adult and child:* Wash hair, towel dry; apply liberally to hair; leave on 10 min; rinse with water; repeat in 7-10 days
Scabies
• *Adult and child:* **TOP** 5% cream applied and massaged into all skin surfaces; leave cream on 8-14 hr, then wash; repeat in 7-10 days
Contraindications: Hypersensitivity

perphenazine (℞)
(per-fen'a-zeen)
Apo-Perphenazine ♣, perphenazine, PMS Perphenazine ♣
Func. class.: Antipsychotic, neuroleptic
Chem. class.: Phenothiazine piperidine

Action: Depresses cerebral cortex, hypothalamus, limbic system, which control activity, aggression; blocks neurotransmission produced by dopamine at synapse; exhibits strong α-adrenergic, anticholinergic blocking action; as antiemetic inhibits medullary chemoreceptor trigger zone; receptor affinity dopamine D_2, histamine H_1, α-adrenergic

Uses: Psychotic disorders, schizophrenia, nausea, vomiting

DOSAGE AND ROUTES

• *Geriatric:* PO 2-4 mg daily-bid, increase by 2-4 mg/wk to desired dose

Nausea/vomiting

• *Adult and child >12 yr:* IM 5-10 mg prn, max 15 mg in ambulatory patients, 30 mg in hospitalized patients; PO 8-16 mg/day in divided doses, up to 24 mg; **IV** not to exceed 5 mg, give diluted or slow **IV** drip

Psychiatric use in hospitalized patients

• *Adult:* PO 8-16 mg bid-qid, gradually increased to desired dose, not to exceed 64 mg/day; **IM** 5 mg q6h, not to exceed 30 mg/day

• *Child >12 yr:* PO 6-12 mg in divided doses

Nonhospitalized patients

• *Adult:* PO 4-8 mg tid

Available forms: Tabs 2, 4, 8, 16 mg; oral conc 16 mg/5 ml; syr 2 mg/5 ml ✿

SIDE EFFECTS

CNS: EPS: pseudoparkinsonism, akathisia, dystonia, tardive dyskinesia, **seizures,** *headache,* **neuroleptic malignant syndrome,** dizziness

CV: Orthostatic hypotension (geriatric), **cardiac arrest,** ECG changes, **tachycardia**

EENT: Blurred vision, glaucoma

GI: Dry mouth, nausea, vomiting, anorexia, constipation, diarrhea, jaundice, weight gain

GU: Urinary retention, urinary frequency, enuresis, impotence, amenorrhea, gynecomastia

HEMA: Anemia, **leukopenia, leukocytosis, agranulocytosis**

INTEG: Rash, photosensitivity, dermatitis

RESP: **Laryngospasm,** dyspnea, **respiratory depression**

Contraindications: Hypersensitivity, blood dyscrasias, coma, child <12 yr, brain damage, bone marrow depression

Precautions: Pregnancy (C), lactation, seizure disorders, hypertension, hepatic/cardiac disease, geriatric, narrow-angle glaucoma

PHARMACOKINETICS

Bioavailability 20%; metabolized by liver (sulfoxidation, hydroxylation, dealkylation; glucuronidation by CYP2D6); excreted in urine, breast milk; crosses placenta, half-life 9-12 hr

PO: Onset erratic, peak 2-4 hr

IM: Onset 10 min, peak 1-2 hr; duration 6 hr, occasionally 12-24 hr

INTERACTIONS

• Oversedation: other CNS depressants, alcohol, barbiturate anesthetics

• Toxicity: epINEPHrine

Increase: risk of EPS—lithium

Increase: effects of both drugs—β-adrenergic blockers, alcohol

Increase: anticholinergic effects—anticholinergics

Increase: perphenazine effect—ritonavir

Increase: hypotension—thiazide diuretics, meperidine

Decrease: absorption—aluminum hydroxide or magnesium hydroxide antacids

Decrease: antiparkinson effect—levodopa

Decrease: oral anticoagulant effect—oral anticoagulants

Drug/Herb

Increase: anticholinergic effect—henbane leaf

Increase: EPS—betel palm, kava

Increase: action—cola tree, hops, nettle, nutmeg

Drug/Lab Test

Increase: LFTs, cardiac enzymes, cholesterol, blood glucose, prolactin, bilirubin, PBI, cholinesterase, ^{131}I

Decrease: Hormones (blood, urine)

False positive: Pregnancy tests, PKU
False negative: Urinary steroids, 17-OHCS

NURSING CONSIDERATIONS
Assess:
• Mental status before initial administration
• Swallowing of PO medication; check for hoarding or giving of medication to other patients
• I&O ratio; palpate bladder if urinary output is low, urinary retention may be the cause
• Bilirubin, CBC, LFTs qmo
• Urinalysis is recommended before and during prolonged therapy
• Affect, orientation, LOC, reflexes, gait, coordination, sleep pattern disturbances
• B/P standing and lying; also include pulse, respirations q4h during initial treatment; establish baseline before starting treatment; report drops of 30 mm Hg
• Dizziness, faintness, palpitations, tachycardia on rising
• EPS including akathisia (inability to sit still, no pattern to movements), tardive dyskinesia (bizarre movements of jaw, mouth, tongue, extremities), pseudoparkinsonism (rigidity, tremors, pill rolling, shuffling gait)
• Skin turgor daily
A For neuroleptic malignant syndrome: hyperthermia, altered mental status, increased CPK, muscle rigidity
• Constipation, urinary retention daily; increase bulk, water in diet
Administer:
• Antiparkinsonian agent on order from prescriber for EPS
• Avoid use with CNS depressants
PO route
• Concentrate mixed in water, orange, pineapple, apricot, prune, tomato, grapefruit juice; do not mix with caffeine beverages (coffee, cola), tannics (tea), or pectinates (apple juice), since incompatibility may result; use 60 ml diluent for each 5 ml of concentrate
IM route
• IM inj into large muscle mass

• Remain lying down after IM inj for at least 30 min
IV route
• After diluting each 5 mg/9 ml of NaCl, shake, give 0.5 mg or less (1 ml = 0.5 mg) over 1 min; may be further diluted and infused
Additive compatibilities: Ascorbic acid, ethacrynate, netilmicin
Syringe compatibilities: Atropine, benztropine, butorphanol, chlorproMAZINE, cimetidine, dimenhyDRINATE, diphenhydrAMINE, droperidol, fentanyl, hydrOXYzine, meperidine, methotrimeprazine, metoclopramide, morphine, pentazocine, prochlorperazine, promethazine, ranitidine, scopolamine
Y-site compatibilities: Acyclovir, amikacin, ampicillin, azlocillin, cefazolin, cefotaxime, cefoxitin, cefuroxime, cephalothin, cephapirin, chloramphenicol, clindamycin, doxycycline, erythromycin, famotidine, gentamicin, kanamycin, metronidazole, mezlocillin, minocycline, moxalactam, nafcillin, oxacillin, penicillin G potassium, piperacillin, tacrolimus, ticarcillin, ticarcillin/clavulanate, tobramycin, trimethoprim-sulfamethoxazole, vancomycin
Perform/provide:
• Supervised ambulation until stabilized on medication; do not involve in strenuous exercise program because fainting is possible; patient should not stand still for long periods
• Increased fluids, bulk in diet to prevent constipation
• Sips of water, sugarless candy, gum, ice chips for dry mouth
• Storage in tight, light-resistant container
Evaluate:
• Therapeutic response: decrease in emotional excitement, hallucinations, delusions, paranoia, reorganization of patterns of thought, speech
Teach patient/family:
• That orthostatic hypotension occurs frequently and to rise from sitting or lying position gradually; to avoid hazardous activities until stabilized on medication

• To avoid hot tubs, hot showers, tub baths, since hypotension may occur; that in hot weather, heat stroke may occur; take extra precautions to stay cool
• To avoid abrupt withdrawal of this drug, or EPS may result; drug should be withdrawn slowly
• To avoid OTC preparations (cough, hay fever, cold) unless approved by prescriber, since serious drug interactions may occur; avoid use with alcohol; increased drowsiness may occur
• To use a sunscreen to prevent burns
• About compliance with drug regimen
• About necessity for meticulous oral hygiene, since oral candidiasis may occur
• To report sore throat, malaise, fever, bleeding, mouth sores; if these occur, CBC should be drawn and drug discontinued
• That urine may turn reddish-brown

Treatment of overdose: Lavage if orally ingested; provide an airway; *do not induce vomiting*

---

phenazopyridine
(R̶, OTC)
(fen-az-oh-peer'i-deen)
Azo-Standard, Baridium, Eridium, Geridium, Phenazo ✦, phenazopyridine, Phenazodine, Prodium, Pyridiate, Pyridium, Urodine, Urogesic
Func. class.: Interstitial cystitis agent
Chem. class.: Azodye

Action: Exerts analgesic, anesthetic action on the urinary tract mucosa
Uses: Urinary tract irritation, infection used with a urinary antiinfective

DOSAGE AND ROUTES

• *Adult:* **PO** 200 mg tid × 2 days or less when used with antibacterial for UTI
• *Child 6-12 yr:* **PO** 4 mg/kg tid × 2 days
Renal dose
• Do not use in CCr <50 ml/min

Available forms: Tabs 95, 97.2, 100, 200 mg

SIDE EFFECTS

CNS: Headache
GI: Nausea, vomiting, diarrhea, heartburn, anorexia, **hepatic toxicity**
GU: **Renal toxicity,** *orange-red urine*
HEMA: **Thrombocytopenia, agranulocytosis, leukopenia, neutropenia, hemolytic anemia, methemoglobinemia**
INTEG: Rash, skin pigmentation, pruritus
Contraindications: Hypersensitivity, renal insufficiency
Precautions: Pregnancy (B), lactation, children <12 yr

PHARMACOKINETICS

Metabolized by liver, excreted by kidneys, crosses placenta, duration 6-8 hr

INTERACTIONS

Drug/Lab Test
Interference: Urinalysis

NURSING CONSIDERATIONS

Assess:
• Urinary status: burning, pain, itching, urgency, frequency, hematuria, before/after treatment completed
• Hepatic studies: AST, ALT, bilirubin if patient is on long-term therapy
⚠ Hepatotoxicity: dark urine, clay-colored stools, jaundiced skin and sclera, itching, abdominal pain, fever, diarrhea if patient is on long-term therapy
• Allergic reactions: rash, urticaria; drug may have to be discontinued

Administer:
• To patient crushed or whole; chewable tablets may be chewed
• With food or milk to decrease gastric symptoms

Evaluate:
• Therapeutic response: decrease in urinary pain

Teach patient/family:
• Not to exceed recommended dosage and to take with meals
• To discontinue after pain is relieved but

⚠ Safety alert *"Tall Man" lettering

continue to take concurrent prescribed antiinfective until finished

• That urine may turn red-orange; may stain clothing or contact lenses

Treatment of overdose: Methylene blue 1-2 mg/kg IV or 100-200 mg vit C PO

phenelzine (℞)
(fen'el-zeen)
Nardil
Func. class.: Antidepressant, MAOI
Chem. class.: Hydrazine

Action: Increases concentrations of endogenous epinephrine, norepinephrine, serotonin, dopamine in storage sites in CNS by inhibition of MAO; increased concentration reduces depression

Uses: Depression, when uncontrolled by other means

DOSAGE AND ROUTES

• *Adult:* PO 45 mg/day in divided doses; may increase to 60 mg/day; dose should be reduced to 15 mg/day, not to exceed 90 mg/day

• *Geriatric:* PO 7.5 mg daily, increase by 7.5-15 mg q3-4d; usual dose 15-60 mg/day in divided doses

Available forms: Tabs 15 mg

SIDE EFFECTS

CNS: Dizziness, drowsiness, confusion, headache, anxiety, tremors, stimulation, weakness, hyperreflexia, mania, insomnia, fatigue, weight gain

CV: Orthostatic hypotension, hypertension, dysrhythmias, **hypertensive crisis,** tachycardia, peripheral edema

EENT: Blurred vision

ENDO: **SIADH-like syndrome**

GI: Constipation, dry mouth, nausea, vomiting, *anorexia,* diarrhea, weight gain

GU: Change in libido, urinary frequency

HEMA: **Anemia**

INTEG: Rash, flushing, increased perspiration

Contraindications: Hypersensitivity to MAOIs, hypertension, CHF, severe renal/

hepatic disease, pheochromocytoma, severe cardiac disease, active alcoholism

Precautions: Pregnancy (C), seizure disorders, severe depression, schizophrenia, hyperactivity, diabetes mellitus, child <16 yr, suicidal ideation in children/adolescents

PHARMACOKINETICS

Metabolized by liver, excreted by kidneys

INTERACTIONS

• Toxicity: sumatriptan, sulfonamides
• Confusion, shivering, hyperreflexia: L-tryptophan

⚠ Hyperpyretic crisis, convulsions, hypertensive episode: tricyclics, SSRIs, meperidine, methylphenidate, amphetamines, nasal decongestants, sinus medications, appetite suppressants, asthma inhalants

Increase: hypotension—thiazide diuretics

Increase: hypoglycemic effect—antidiabetics

Increase: pressor effects—guanethidine, clonidine, indirect-acting or mixed sympathomimetics (epHEDrine)

Increase: effects of direct-acting sympathomimetics (epINEPHrine)—alcohol, barbiturates, benzodiazepines, CNS depressants, levodopa

Decrease: serotonin, norepinephrine—rauwolfia alkaloids

Drug/Herb

• Serotonin syndrome: parsley, St. John's wort
• Hypertension: brewer's yeast
• Tension headaches, irritability, visual hallucinations, mania: ginseng

Increase: sympathomimetic action—betel palm, butcher's broom, capsicum peppers, galanthamine, green tea (large amounts), guarana (large amounts), night-blooming cereus

Increase: effect—ginkgo, nutmeg, yohimbe

P

Increase: anticholinergic effect—jimsonweed
Decrease: effect—valerian
Drug/Food
• Avoid tyramine foods, caffeine

NURSING CONSIDERATIONS
Assess:
• B/P (lying, standing), pulse; if systolic B/P drops 20 mm Hg, hold drug, notify prescriber
• Blood studies: CBC, leukocytes, cardiac enzymes (long-term therapy)
• Hepatic studies: ALT, AST, bilirubin; hepatotoxicity may occur
⚠ Toxicity: increased headache, palpitation; discontinue drug immediately; prodromal signs of hypertensive crisis
⚠ Mental status changes: mood, sensorium, affect, memory (long, short); increase in psychiatric symptoms; suicidal ideation in children/adolescents
• Urinary retention, constipation, edema; take weight qwk
• Withdrawal symptoms: headache, nausea, vomiting, muscle pain, weakness
Administer:
• Increased fluids, bulk in diet for constipation
• With food, milk for GI symptoms
• Crushed if patient cannot swallow medication whole
• Dosage at bedtime for oversedation during day
• Gum, hard candy, or frequent sips of water for dry mouth
• Phentolamine for severe hypertension
• Avoid use with CNS depressants
Perform/provide:
• Storage in tight container in cool environment
• Ambulation assistance at start of therapy, since drowsiness/dizziness occurs, especially geriatric
• Safety measures including side rails
• Checking to see if PO medication swallowed
Evalute:
• Therapeutic response: decreased depression

Teach patient/family:
• That therapeutic effects may take 1-4 wk
• To avoid driving, other activities requiring alertness
• To avoid alcohol ingestion, OTC medications: cold, weight loss, hay fever, cough syrup
• To rise slowly to prevent orthostatic hypotension
• Not to discontinue medication quickly after long-term use
• To avoid high-tyramine foods: cheese (aged), sour cream, beer, wine, pickled products, liver, raisins, bananas, figs, avocados, meat tenderizers, chocolate, yogurt; provide complete list of tyramine-containing foods; increased caffeine, may cause hypertensive reactions
• To report headache, palpitation, neck stiffness, dizziness, constriction in chest, throat, rash, insomnia, change in strength, changes in urinary patterns, color of urine
Treatment of overdose: Lavage, activated charcoal, monitor electrolytes, vital signs, diazepam IV, $NaHCO_3$

⚠ High Alert

phenobarbital (℞)
(fee-noe-bar′bi-tal)
Ancalixir ♣, Barbita, Luminal, phenobarbital sodium, Solfoton
Func. class.: Anticonvulsant
Chem. class.: Barbiturate

Controlled Substance Schedule IV
Do not confuse:
phenobarbital/pentobarbital
Action: Decreases impulse transmission; increases seizure threshold at cerebral cortex level
Uses: All forms of epilepsy, status epilepticus, febrile seizures in children, sedation, insomnia
Unlabeled uses: Hyperbilirubinemia, chronic cholestasis

⚠ Safety alert   *"Tall Man" lettering

DOSAGE AND ROUTES

Seizures

- *Adult:* **PO** 60-200 mg/day in divided doses tid or total dose at bedtime
- *Child:* **PO** 4-6 mg/kg/day in divided doses q12h; may be given as single dose

Status epilepticus

- *Adult:* **IV INF** 10 mg/kg; run no faster than 50 mg/min; may give up to 20 mg/kg
- *Child:* **IV INF** 5-10 mg/kg; may repeat q10-15min up to 20 mg/kg; run no faster than 50 mg/min

Insomnia

- *Adult:* **PO/IM** 100-320 mg
- *Child:* **PO/IM** 3-5 mg/kg

Sedation

- *Adult:* **PO** 30-120 mg/day in 2-3 divided doses
- *Child:* **PO** 3-5 mg/kg/day in 3 divided doses

Preoperative sedation

- *Adult:* **IM** 100-200 mg 1-1½ hr before surgery
- *Child:* **IM** 16-100 mg or **PO/IM/IV** 1-3 mg/kg 1-1½ hr before surgery

Available forms: Caps 15 mg; elix 20 mg/5 ml; tabs 8, 15, 30, 60, 100 mg; inj 30, 60, 65, 130 mg/ml

SIDE EFFECTS

CNS: Paradoxic excitement (geriatric), drowsiness, lethargy, hangover headache, flushing, hallucinations, **coma**
GI: Nausea, vomiting, diarrhea, constipation
INTEG: Rash, urticaria, **Stevens-Johnson syndrome, angioedema,** local pain, swelling, necrosis, **thrombophlebitis**
Contraindications: Pregnancy (D), hypersensitivity to barbiturates, porphyria, hepatic disease, respiratory disease, nephritis, hyperthyroidism, diabetes mellitus, geriatric, lactation
Precautions: Anemia

PHARMACOKINETICS

IV: Onset 5 min, peak 30 min, duration 4-6 hr
IM/SUBCUT: Onset 10-30 min, duration 4-6 hr

PO: Onset 20-60 min, peak 8-12 hr, duration 6-10 hr
Metabolized by liver; crosses placenta; excreted in urine, breast milk; half-life 53-118 hr

INTERACTIONS

Increase: effects—CNS depressants, alcohol, chloramphenicol, valproic acid, disulfiram, nondepolarizing skeletal muscle relaxants, sulfonamides
Increase: orthostatic hypotension—furosemide
Decrease: effects—theophylline, oral anticoagulants, corticosteroids, metronidazole, doxycycline, quinidine
Drug/Herb
Increase: phenobarbital levels—quinine
Increase: CNS depression—chamomile, eucalyptus, hops, Jamaican dogwood, kava, lemon balm, nettle, pill-bearing spurge, poppy, senega, skullcap, valerian
Decrease: barbiturate effect—St. John's wort

NURSING CONSIDERATIONS

Assess:
- Mental status: mood, sensorium, affect, memory (long, short)
- For respiratory depression
- Blood dyscrasias: fever, sore throat, bruising, rash, jaundice
- Convulsion activity: type, duration, precipitating factors
- Blood studies, LFTs during long-term treatment
- Therapeutic blood level periodically: 15-40 mcg/ml
- Respiratory status: rate, rhythm, depth

Administer:
- Avoid use with other CNS depressants

IM route
- IM inj deep in large muscle mass to prevent tissue sloughing; use <5 ml in each site

IV route
- Slow IV after dilution with at least 10 ml sterile H_2O for inj regardless of dose; give 65 mg or less/min; titrate to patient response

P

Additive compatibilities: Amikacin, aminophylline, calcium chloride, calcium gluconate, cephapirin, colistimethate, dimenhyDRINATE, meropenem, polymyxin B, sodium bicarbonate, thiopental, verapamil

Solution compatibilities: D_5W, $D_{10}W$, 0.45% NaCl, 0.9% NaCl, Ringer's, dextrose/saline combinations, dextrose/Ringer's, dextrose/LR combinations, sodium lactate

Syringe compatibilities: Heparin

Y-site compatibilities: Enalaprilat, meropenem, propofol, sufentanil

Perform/provide:
• Supervision of ambulation for dizziness, drowsiness

Evaluate:
• Therapeutic response: decreased seizures, increased sedation

Teach patient/family:
• To use exactly as ordered
• To avoid alcohol use
• To avoid hazardous activities until stabilized on drug; drowsiness may occur
• Never to withdraw drug abruptly; withdrawal symptoms may occur
• That therapeutic effects (PO) may not be seen for 2-3 wk

Treatment of overdose: Lavage, activated charcoal, warming blanket, vital signs, hemodialysis, I&O ratio

---

phentolamine (℞)
(fen-tole′a-meen)
Regitine, Rogitine ✤
Func. class.: Antihypertensive
Chem. class.: α-Adrenergic blocker

Do not confuse:
phentolamine/phentermine
Action: α-Adrenergic blocker, binds to α-adrenergic receptors, dilating peripheral blood vessels, lowering peripheral resistances, lowering blood pressure
Uses: Hypertension, pheochromocytoma, prevention, treatment of dermal necrosis following extravasation of norepinephrine or DOPamine

Unlabeled uses: Impotence, hypertensive crisis due to MAOIs

DOSAGE AND ROUTES

Treatment of hypertensive episodes in pheochromocytoma
• *Adult:* **IV/IM,** 5 mg, repeat if necessary
• *Child:* **IV/IM,** 0.5-1 mg/kg, repeat if necessary; max 5 mg

Diagnosis of pheochromocytoma
• *Adult:* **IV** 2.5 mg; if negative, repeat with 5 mg IV
• *Child:* **IV** 0.05 mg/kg; if negative, repeat with 0.1 mg/kg IV

Treatment of necrosis
• *Adult:* 5-10 mg/10 ml **NS** injected into area of norepinephrine extravasation within 12 hr
• *Child:* 0.1-0.2 mg/kg, max 5 mg

Prevention of necrosis
• *Adult:* 10 mg/L of norepinephrine-containing sol
• *Child:* **IV** 0.1-0.2 mg/kg, max 5 mg

Available forms: Inj 5 mg/ml

SIDE EFFECTS

CNS: Dizziness, flushing, weakness, **cerebrovascular spasm**
CV: Hypotension, tachycardia, angina, dysrhythmias, **MI**
EENT: Nasal congestion
GI: Dry mouth, nausea, vomiting, diarrhea, abdominal pain
Contraindications: Hypersensitivity, MI, coronary insufficiency, angina
Precautions: Pregnancy (C), lactation, dysrhythmia

PHARMACOKINETICS

IV: Peak 2 min, duration 10-15 min
IM: Peak 15-20 min, duration 3-4 hr
Metabolized in liver, excreted in urine

INTERACTIONS

Increase: effects of epINEPHrine, antihypertensives
Drug/Herb
Increase: toxicity, death—aconite
Increase: antihypertensive effect—

⚠ Safety alert   *"Tall Man" lettering

barberry, betony, black catechu, black cohosh, bloodroot, broom, burdock, cat's claw, dandelion, goldenseal, hawthorn, Irish moss, Jamaican dogwood, kelp, khella, mistletoe, parsley

Increase or decrease: antihypertensive effect—astragalus, cola tree

Decrease: antihypertensive effect—coltsfoot, guarana, khat, licorice, yohimbine

NURSING CONSIDERATIONS

Assess:
• Weight daily, I&O
• B/P lying, standing before starting treatment, q4h after
• Nausea, vomiting, diarrhea, edema in feet, legs daily; skin turgor, dryness of mucous membranes for hydration status, postural hypotension, cardiac system: pulse, ECG

Administer:
• Gum, frequent rinsing of mouth, or hard candy for dry mouth
• With vasopressor available
• After discontinuing all medication for 24 hr
• Treatment during required bed rest, 1 hr after

IV route
• After diluting 5 mg/1 ml sterile H₂O for inj; give 5 mg or less/min; patient to remain recumbent during administration

CONT INF route
• Dilute 5-10 mg/500 ml D₅W, titrate to patient response
• 10 mg/L may be added to norepinephrine in IV sol for prevention of dermal necrosis

Additive compatibilities: DOBUTamine, verapamil
Syringe compatibilities: Papaverine
Y-site compatibilities: Amiodarone
Evaluate:
• Therapeutic response: decreased B/P
Teach patient/family:
• That bed rest is required during treatment, 1 hr after
Treatment of overdose: Administer norepinephrine; discontinue drug

phenylephrine (Rx)
(fen-ill-ef'rin)
Neo-Synephrine
Func. class.: Adrenergic, direct-acting
Chem. class.: Substituted phenylethylamine

Action: Powerful and selective (α₁) receptor agonist causing contraction of blood vessels
Uses: Hypotension, paroxysmal supraventricular tachycardia, shock, maintain B/P for spinal anesthesia

DOSAGE AND ROUTES

Hypotension
• *Adult:* **SUBCUT/IM** 2-5 mg; may repeat q10-15min if needed; do not exceed initial dose; **IV** 0.1-0.5 mg; may repeat q10-15min if needed; do not exceed initial dose
• *Child:* **IM/SUBCUT** 0.1 mg/kg/dose q1-2h prn
Supraventricular tachycardia
• *Adult:* **IV BOL** 0.5-1 mg given rapidly, not to exceed prior dose by >0.1 mg, total dose ≤1 mg
Shock
• *Adult:* **IV INF** 10 mg/500 ml D₅W given 100-180 mcg/min (if 20 gtt/ml inf device), then maintenance of 40-60 mcg/min; use infusion device
• *Child:* **IV BOL** 5-20 mcg/kg/dose q10-15min; **IV INF** 0.1-0.5 mcg/kg/min
Available forms: Inj 1% (10 mg/ml)

SIDE EFFECTS

CNS: Headache, anxiety, tremor, insomnia, dizziness
CV: Palpitations, tachycardia, hypertension, ectopic beats, angina, reflex bradycardia, **dysrhythmias**
GI: Nausea, vomiting
INTEG: Necrosis, tissue sloughing with extravasation, **gangrene**
SYST: **Anaphylaxis**
Contraindications: Hypersensitivity, ventricular fibrillation, tachydysrhythmias,

pheochromocytoma, narrow-angle glaucoma, severe hypertension

Precautions: Pregnancy (C), lactation, arterial embolism, peripheral vascular disease, geriatric, hyperthyroidism, bradycardia, myocardial disease, severe arteriosclerosis, partial heart block

PHARMACOKINETICS

IV: Onset immediate, duration 20-30 min

IM/SUBCUT: Onset 10-15 min, duration 45-60 min

INTERACTIONS

• Dysrhythmias: general anesthetics, digoxin, bretylium

⚠ Do not use within 2 wk of MAOIs, or hypertensive crisis may result

Increase: in B/P—oxytocics

Increase: pressor effect—tricyclics, β-blockers, H₁ antihistamines

Decrease: phenylephrine action—α-blockers

NURSING CONSIDERATIONS

Assess:

• I&O ratio; notify prescriber if output <30 ml/hr

• ECG during administration continuously; if B/P increases, drug is decreased

• B/P and pulse q5min after parenteral route

• CVP or PWP during inf if possible

• For paresthesias and coldness of extremities; peripheral blood flow may decrease

Administer:

IV route

• Plasma expanders for hypovolemia

• IV after diluting 1 mg/9 ml sterile H_2O for inj; give dose over ½-1 min; may be diluted 10 mg/500 ml of D_5W or NS; titrate to response (normal B/P); check for extravasation, check site for infiltration, use infusion pump

Additive compatibilities: Chloramphenicol, DOBUTamine, lidocaine, potassium chloride, sodium bicarbonate

Y-site compatibilities: Amiodarone, amrinone, cisatracurium, famotidine, haloperidol, remifentanil, zidovudine

Perform/provide:

• Storage of reconstituted sol if refrigerated for no longer than 24 hr

• Discard discolored sol

Evaluate:

• Therapeutic response: increased B/P with stabilization

Teach patient/family:

• The reason for administration

• To report pain at infusion site or other adverse reactions immediately

Treatment of overdose: Administer an α-blocker

phenylephrine nasal agent
See Appendix C

phenylephrine ophthalmic
See Appendix C

phenytoin (℞)
(fen'i-toh-in)
Dilantin, Dilantin Infatab, Phenytex
Func. class.: Anticonvulsant; antidysrhythmic (IB)
Chem. class.: Hydantoin

Action: Inhibits spread of seizure activity in motor cortex by altering ion transport; increases AV conduction

Uses: Generalized tonic-clonic seizures; status epilepticus; nonepileptic seizures associated with Reye's syndrome or after head trauma; migraines, trigeminal neuralgia, Bell's palsy, ventricular dysrhythmias uncontrolled by antidysrhythmics

⚠ Safety alert   *"Tall Man" lettering

DOSAGE AND ROUTES

Seizures

• *Adult:* **PO** 1 g or 20 mg/kg (ext rel) in 3-4 divided doses given q2h, or 400 mg, then 300 mg q2h × 2 doses, maintenance 300-400 mg/day, max 600 mg/day; **IV** 15-20 mg/kg, max 25-50 mg/min, then 100 mg q6-8h

• *Child:* **PO** 5 mg/kg/day in 2-3 divided doses, maintenance 4-8 mg/kg/day in 2-3 divided doses, max 300 mg/day; **IV** 15-20 mg/kg at 1-3 mg/kg/min

Status epilepticus

• *Adult:* **IV** 10-15 mg/kg, max 25-50 mg/min, may give 100 mg q6-8h thereafter

• *Child:* **IV** 15-20 mg/kg, max in divided doses 1-3 mg/kg/min

Neuritic pain

• *Adult:* **PO** 200-600 mg/day in divided doses

Ventricular dysrhythmias

• *Adult:* **PO** loading dose 1 g divided over 24 hr, then 500 mg/day × 2 days; **IV** 250 mg over 5 min until dysrhythmias subside or until 1 g is given, or 100 mg q15min until dysrhythmias subside or until 1 g is given

• *Child:* **PO** 3-8 mg/kg or 250 mg/m^2/day as single dose or 2 divided doses; **IV** 3-8 mg/kg over several min, or 250 mg/m^2/day as single dose or 2 divided doses

Renal dose

• Do not use loading dose CCr <10 ml/min or hepatic failure

Available forms: Susp 30, 125 mg/5 ml; chewable tabs 50 mg; inj 50 mg/ml; ext rel caps 30, 100 mg; prompt rel caps 30, 100 mg

SIDE EFFECTS

CNS: Drowsiness, dizziness, insomnia, paresthesias, depression, suicidal tendencies, aggression, headache, confusion, slurred speech

CV: Hypotension, **ventricular fibrillation**

EENT: Nystagmus, diplopia, blurred vision

ENDO: Diabetes insipidus

GI: Nausea, vomiting, constipation, anorexia, weight loss, **hepatitis,** jaundice, gingival hyperplasia

GU: **Nephritis,** urine discoloration

HEMA: **Agranulocytosis, leukopenia, aplastic anemia, thrombocytopenia, megaloblastic anemia**

INTEG: Rash, **lupus erythematosus, Stevens-Johnson syndrome,** hirsutism

SYST: Hypocalcemia

Contraindications: Hypersensitivity, psychiatric condition, bradycardia, SA and AV block, Stokes-Adams syndrome, hepatic failure, acute intermittent porphyria

Precautions: Pregnancy (C), allergies, renal/hepatic disease, geriatric, petit mal seizures, hypotension, myocardial insufficiency

PHARMACOKINETICS

PO-ER: Onset 2-24 hr, peak 4-12 hr, duration 12-36 hr

IV: Onset 1-2 hr, duration 12-24 hr

PO: Onset 2-24 hr, peak 1½-2½ hr, duration 6-12 hr

Metabolized by liver, excreted by kidneys; highly protein-bound, half-life 22 hr, dose dependent

INTERACTIONS

Increase: phenytoin effect—benzodiazepines, cimetidine, tricyclics, salicylates, valproate, cycloSERINE, diazepam, chloramphenicol

Decrease: phenytoin effects—alcohol (chronic use), antacids, barbiturates, carbamazepine, diazoxide, rifampin, folic acid

Drug/Herb

Increase: potassium loss, increase antidysrhythmic action—aloe, buckthorn, cascara sagrada, senna

Increase: action—ginkgo

Decrease: anticonvulsant effect—ginseng, santonica, valerian

Drug/Lab Test

Increase: Glucose, alk phos, BSP

Decrease: Dexamethasone, metyrapone test serum, PBI, urinary steroids

NURSING CONSIDERATIONS

Assess:

⚠ For phenytoin hypersensitivity syndrome 3-12 wk after start of treatment: rash, temp, lymphadenopathy; may cause hepatotoxicity, renal failure, rhabdomyolysis

⚠ For beginning rash that may lead to Stevens-Johnson syndrome or toxic epidermal necrolysis; phenytoin should not be used again

• Drug level: toxic level 30-50 mcg/ml, ther level: 7.5-20 mcg/ml, wait ≥1 wk to draw levels

• For seizures: duration, type, intensity precipitating factors

• Blood studies: CBC, platelets q2wk until stabilized, then qmo × 12, then q3mo; discontinue drug if neutrophils <1600/mm³; renal function: albumin conc

• Mental status: mood, sensorium, affect, memory (long, short)

• Respiratory depression; rate, depth, character

• Blood dyscrasias: fever, sore throat, bruising, rash, jaundice

Administer:

• Do not interchange chewable product with caps, not equivalent; only ext rel caps are to be used for once-a-day dosing

• Shake susp well before each dose G tube/NG tube; dilute susp prior to administration; flush tube with 20 ml H_2O after dose

• Allow 7-10 days between dosage changes

• Divided PO doses with or after meals to decrease adverse effects

• 2 hr before or after antacid or antidiarrheal use

IV route

• After diluting with diluent provided (2.2 ml/100 mg, 5.2 ml/250 mg, 1 ml/50 mg); shake; give through Y-tube or 3-way stopcock; inject slowly <50 mg/min; clear IV tubing first with NS sol; use in-line filter; discard 4 hr after preparation; inject into large veins to prevent purple glove syndrome

Additive compatibilities: Bleomycin, sodium bicarbonate, verapamil

Y-site compatibilities: Esmolol, famotidine, fluconazole, foscarnet, tacrolimus

Evaluate:

• Therapeutic response; decrease in severity of seizures, ventricular dysrhythmias

Teach patient/family:

• That if diabetic, urine glucose should be monitored

• That urine may turn pink

• Not to discontinue drug abruptly; seizures may occur

• Proper brushing of teeth using a soft toothbrush, flossing to prevent gingival hyperplasia; need to see dentist frequently

• To avoid hazardous activities until stabilized on drug

• To carry emergency ID stating drug use

• That heavy use of alcohol may diminish effect of drug; to avoid OTC medications

• Not to change brands or forms once stabilized on therapy; brands may vary

---

Rarely Used

physostigmine (℞)
(fi-zoe-stig′meen)
Antilirium
Func. class.: Antidote, reversible anticholinesterase

Uses: To reverse CNS effects of anticholinergic

DOSAGE AND ROUTES

Overdose of anticholinergics

• *Adult:* **IM/IV/SUBCUT** 0.5-2 mg; give no more than 1 mg/min; may repeat q20 min until response or adverse reactions; repeat 1-4 mg q30-60 min as life-threatening signs reoccur

• *Child:* **IM/IV** inj 0.02 mg/kg, not more than 0.5 mg/min; may repeat at 5-10 min intervals until max dose of 2 mg, response or adverse reactions

Contraindications: Hypotension, obstruction of intestine or renal system, asthma, gangrene, CV disease, choline esters, depolarizing neuromuscular blocking agents, diabetes

physostigmine ophthalmic
See Appendix C

phytonadione (vit K₁) (℞)
(fye-toe-na-dye'one)
AquaMEPHYTON, Mephyton
Func. class.: Vit K₁, fat-soluble vitamin

Action: Needed for adequate blood clotting (factors II, VII, IX, X)

Uses: Vit K malabsorption, hypoprothrombinemia, prevention of hypoprothrombinemia caused by oral anticoagulants, prevention of hemorrhagic disease of the newborn

DOSAGE AND ROUTES
Hypoprothrombinemia caused by vit K malabsorption
- *Adult:* **PO/IM** 2.5-25 mg, may repeat or increase to 50 mg
- *Child:* **PO/IM** 5-10 mg
- *Infant:* **PO/IM** 2 mg

Prevention of hemorrhagic disease of the newborn
- *Neonate:* **IM** 0.5-1 mg within 1 hr after birth, repeat in 2-3 wk if required

Hypoprothrombinemia caused by oral anticoagulants
- *Adult and child:* **PO/SUBCUT/IM** 1-10 mg, may repeat 12-48 hr after **PO** dose or 6-8 hr after **SUBCUT/IM** dose, based on PT

Available forms: Tabs 5 mg; inj 2 m/10 ml aqueous colloidal; inj aqueous dispersion 10 mg/ml (IM)

SIDE EFFECTS
CNS: Headache, **brain damage** (large doses)
GI: Nausea, decreased LFTs

HEMA: **Hemolytic anemia, hemoglobinuria, hyperbilirubinemia**
INTEG: Rash, urticaria

Contraindications: Hypersensitivity, severe hepatic disease, last few weeks of pregnancy
Precautions: Pregnancy (C), neonates

PHARMACOKINETICS
PO/INJ: Metabolized, crosses placenta

INTERACTIONS
Decrease: action of phytonadione—cholestyramine, mineral oil
Decrease: action of oral anticoagulants
Drug/Food
- Olestra, decreased vit K levels

NURSING CONSIDERATIONS
Assess:
- For bleeding: emesis, stools, urine
- PT during treatment (2-sec deviation from control time, bleeding time, and clotting time); monitor for bleeding, pulse, and B/P
- Nutritional status: liver (beef), spinach, tomatoes, coffee, asparagus, broccoli, cabbage, lettuce, greens

Administer:
IV route
- After diluting with D₅NS 10 ml or more; give 1 mg/min or more
⚠ IV only when other routes not possible (deaths have occurred)

Additive compatibilities: Amikacin, calcium gluceptate, cephapirin, chloramphenicol, cimetidine, netilmicin, sodium bicarbonate
Syringe compatibilities: Doxapram
Y-site compatibilities: Ampicillin, epINEPHrine, famotidine, heparin, hydrocortisone, potassium chloride, tolazoline, vit B/C

Perform/provide:
- Storage in tight, light-resistant container

Evaluate:
- Therapeutic response: decreased bleeding tendencies, decreased PT, decreased clotting time

P

Teach patient/family:
- Not to take other supplements unless directed by prescriber
- The necessary foods for diet
- To avoid IM inj site, use soft toothbrush, do not floss, use electric razor until coagulation defect corrected
- To report symptoms of bleeding
- Not to use OTC medications unless approved by prescriber
- The importance of frequent lab tests to monitor coagulation factors

pilocarpine ophthalmic
See Appendix C

pimecrolimus topical
See Appendix C

pindolol (℞)
(pin´doe-lole)
Novo-Pindol ✹, Syn-Pindolol ✹, Visken
Func. class.: Antihypertensive
Chem. class.: Nonselective β-blocker

Do not confuse:
pindolol/Parlodel/Plendil

Action: Competitively blocks stimulation of β-adrenergic receptor within vascular smooth muscle; decreases rate of SA node discharge, increases recovery time, slows conduction of AV node, decreases heart rate, which decreases O_2 consumption in myocardium; also decreases renin-aldosterone-angiotensin system, at high doses inhibits $β_2$ receptors in bronchial system

Uses: Mild to moderate hypertension

DOSAGE AND ROUTES
- *Adult:* **PO** 5 mg bid, usual dose 15 mg/day (5 mg tid), may increase by 10 mg/day q3-4wk to a max of 60 mg/day
- *Geriatric:* **PO** 5 mg daily, increase by 5 mg q3-4wk

Available forms: Tabs 5, 10 mg

SIDE EFFECTS
CNS: Insomnia, dizziness, hallucinations, anxiety, fatigue, headache, depression
CV: Hypotension, bradycardia, **CHF,** edema, chest pain, palpitation, claudication, tachycardia, **AV block, pulmonary edema, bradycardia, dysrhythmias**
EENT: Visual changes, sore throat, *double vision;* dry, burning eyes, nasal stuffiness
GI: Nausea, vomiting, **ischemic colitis,** diarrhea, *abdominal pain,* **mesenteric arterial thrombosis,** flatulence, constipation
GU: Impotence, urinary frequency
HEMA: **Agranulocytosis, thrombocytopenia, purpura**
INTEG: Rash, alopecia, pruritus, fever
MISC: Joint pain, muscle pain
RESP: **Bronchospasm,** *dyspnea,* cough, crackles

Contraindications: Hypersensitivity to β-blockers, cardiogenic shock; 2nd-, 3rd-degree heart block; sinus bradycardia, CHF, cardiac failure, bronchial asthma, severe COPD

Precautions: Pregnancy (B), major surgery, lactation, diabetes mellitus, thyroid disease, COPD, well-compensated heart failure, CAD, nonallergic bronchospasm, peripheral vascular disease, renal/hepatic disease

PHARMACOKINETICS
PO: Peak 1-3 hr; half-life 3-4 hr, excreted 30%-50% unchanged; 60%-65% metabolized by liver; excreted in breast milk; protein binding 40%-60%

INTERACTIONS
- May alter hypoglycemic effect: insulin, oral hypoglycemics
Increase: hypotension, bradycardia—reserpine, hydrALAZINE, methyldopa, prazosin, anticholinergics, other antihypertensives

Increase: effects of β-blockers, calcium channel blockers

Decrease: antihypertensive effects—NSAIDs, salicylates, sympathomimetics, thyroid

Decrease: bronchodilation—theophyllines, β$_2$-agonists

Drug/Herb

Increase: toxicity, death—aconite

Increase: antihypertensive effect—barberry, betony, black catechu, black cohosh, bloodroot, broom, burdock, cat's claw, dandelion, goldenseal, hawthorn, Irish moss, Jamaican dogwood, kelp, khella, mistletoe, parsley

Increase or decrease: antihypertensive effect—astragalus, cola tree

Decrease: antihypertensive effect—coltsfoot, guarana, khat, licorice, St. John's wort, yohimbine

Drug/Lab Test

Increase: Renal, hepatic studies

Interference: Glucose, insulin tolerance test

NURSING CONSIDERATIONS

Assess:
- I&O, weight daily
- B/P during initial treatment, periodically thereafter; pulse q4h, note rate, rhythm, quality; apical, radial pulse before administration; notify prescriber of any significant changes
- Baselines in renal, hepatic studies before therapy begins
- Skin turgor, dryness of mucous membranes for hydration status; edema in feet, legs daily

Administer:
- PO before meals, at bedtime; tablet may be crushed or swallowed whole

Perform/provide:
- Storage in dry area at room temperature; do not freeze

Evaluate:
- Therapeutic response: decreased B/P after 1-2 wk

Teach patient/family:
- To take with or immediately after meals if GI symptoms occur

⚠ Not to discontinue drug abruptly; ta-per over 2 wk; may cause precipitate angina

- Not to use OTC products containing α-adrenergic stimulants (nasal decongestants, OTC cold preparations) unless directed by prescriber
- To report bradycardia, dizziness, confusion, depression, fever, sore throat, shortness of breath to prescriber
- To take pulse at home; to notify prescriber if pulse <60 bpm
- To avoid alcohol, smoking, sodium
- To comply with weight control, dietary adjustments, modified exercise program
- To carry emergency ID to identify drug, allergies
- To avoid hazardous activities if dizziness is present
- To report symptoms of CHF: difficult breathing, especially on exertion or when lying down, night cough, swelling of extremities
- To take medication at bedtime to prevent orthostatic hypotension
- To wear support hose to minimize effects of orthostatic hypotension

Treatment of overdose: Lavage, IV atropine for bradycardia, IV theophylline for bronchospasm, digitalis, O$_2$, diuretic for cardiac failure, hemodialysis, hypotension; give vasopressor (norepinephrine)

pioglitazone (℞)
(pie-oh-glye'ta-zone)
Actos
Func. class.: Antidiabetic, oral
Chem. class.: Thiazolidinedione

Action: Specifically targets insulin resistance, an insulin sensitizer; regulates the transcription of a number of insulin responsive genes

Uses: Type 2 diabetes mellitus

DOSAGE AND ROUTES

Monotherapy
- *Adult:* PO 15-30 daily, may increase to 45 mg/day

Combination therapy
- *Adult:* PO 15-30 mg daily with a sulfo-

nylurea, metformin, or insulin; decrease sulfonylurea dose if hypoglycemia occurs; decrease insulin dose by 10%-25% if hypoglycemia occurs or if plasma glucose is <100 mg/dl, max 45 mg/day

Hepatic dose
• Do not use in active hepatic disease or if ALT >2.5 times ULN

Available forms: Tabs 15, 30, 45 mg

SIDE EFFECTS

CNS: Headache
ENDO: Aggravated diabetes mellitus
MISC: Myalgia, sinusitis, URI, pharyngitis
MS: Fractures (females)

Contraindications: Hypersensitivity to thiazolidinedione, lactation, children, diabetic ketoacidosis

Precautions: Pregnancy (C), geriatric, renal/hepatic/thyroid disease, edema, CHF

PHARMACOKINETICS

Maximal reduction in FBS after 12 wk; half-life 3-7 hr, terminal 16-24 hr

INTERACTIONS

Decrease: effect of oral contraceptives, use an alternative contraceptive method
Decrease: pioglitazone effect—ketoconazole

Drug/Herb
• Poor blood glucose control: glucosamine

Increase: hypoglycemia—chromium, coenzyme Q10, fenugreek
Increase: antidiabetic effect—alfalfa, aloe, basil, bay, bilberry, bitter melon, black catechu, buchu, burdock, coriander, dandelion, eyebright (po), fenugreek, garlic, ginseng, glucomannan, glucosamine, goat's rue, gymnema, horehound, horse chestnut, jambul, myrrh, myrtle
Decrease: antidiabetic effect—bee pollen, blue cohosh, broom, chromium, elecampane, eucalyptus, gotu kola

NURSING CONSIDERATIONS

Assess:
• For hypoglycemic reactions (sweating, weakness, dizziness, anxiety, tremors, hunger), hyperglycemic reactions soon after meals
• Check LFTs periodically AST, LDH
• FBS, glycosylated Hgb, fasting plasma insulin, plasma lipids/lipoproteins, B/P, body weight during treatment

Administer:
• Once a day; give with meals to decrease GI upset and provide best absorption
• Tabs crushed and mixed with food or fluids for patients with difficulty swallowing

Perform/provide:
• Conversion from other oral hypoglycemic agents; change may be made with gradual dosage change; monitor serum glucose during conversion
• Storage in tight container in cool environment

Evaluate:
• Therapeutic response: Decrease in polyuria, polydipsia, polyphagia; clear sensorium; absence of dizziness; stable gait, blood glucose at normal level

Teach patient/family:
• To self-monitor using a blood glucose meter
• The symptoms of hypo/hyperglycemia, what to do about each
• That the drug must be continued on daily basis; explain consequence of discontinuing drug abruptly
• To avoid OTC medications or herbal preparations unless approved by prescriber
• That diabetes is lifelong illness; that this drug is not a cure; only controls symptoms
• That all food included in diet plan must be eaten to prevent hypoglycemia
• To carry emergency ID and glucagon emergency kit for emergencies
• To notify prescriber if oral contraceptives are used
• Not to use if breastfeeding
• To report symptoms of hepatic dysfunction (nausea, vomiting, abdominal pain, fatigue, anorexia, dark urine, jaundice)

piperacillin (℞)

(pip′er-ah-sill′in)

Pipracil

Func. class.: Broad-spectrum antiinfective

Chem. class.: Extended-spectrum penicillin

Action: Lysis mediated by cell wall autolytic enzymes

Uses: Respiratory, skin, urinary tract, bone infections; gonorrhea; pneumonia; effective for gram-positive cocci *(Staphylococcus aureus, Streptococcus pyogenes, Streptococcus viridans, Streptococcus faecalis, Streptococcus bovis, Streptococcus pneumoniae)*, gram-negative cocci *(Neisseria gonorrhoeae, Neisseria meningitidis)*, gram-positive bacilli *(Acinetobacter, Clostridium perfringens, Clostridium tetani)*, gram-negative bacilli *(Bacteroides, Citrobacter, Enterobacter, Escherichia coli, Eubacterium, Fusobacterium nucleatum, Klebsiella, Morganella morganii, Peptococcus, Peptostreptococcus, Proteus mirabilis, Proteus vulgaris, Providencia rettgeri, Pseudomonas aeruginosa, Serratia)*

DOSAGE AND ROUTES

Urinary tract infections
• *Adult:* **IV** 8-16 g/day (125-200 mg/kg/day) in divided doses q6-8h

Serious systemic infections
• *Adult and child >12 yr:* **IM/IV** 2-4 g q4-6h (2 g/site **IM**)
• *Child <12 yr:* **IM/IV** 200-300 mg/kg/day in divided doses q4-6h
• *Neonate <36 wk:* **IV** 75 mg/kg q12h in the 1st wk of life, then q8h in 2nd wk
• *Full-term infant:* **IV** 75 mg/kg q8h in 1st wk of life; q6h thereafter

Prophylaxis of surgical infections
• *Adult:* **IV** 2 g ½-1 hr before procedure; may be repeated during surgery or after surgery

Renal dose
• *Adult:* **IV** CCr 20-40 ml/min give q8h; CCr <20 ml/min give q12h

Available forms: Powder for inj 2, 3, 4, 40 g

SIDE EFFECTS

CNS: Lethargy, hallucinations, anxiety, depression, twitching, **coma, seizures**
GI: Nausea, vomiting, diarrhea; increased AST, ALT; abdominal pain; glossitis; **pseudomembranous colitis;** hepatitis
GU: **Oliguria, proteinuria, hematuria,** *vaginitis, moniliasis,* **glomerulonephritis**
HEMA: Anemia, increased bleeding time, **bone marrow depression,** thrombocytopenia
META: Hypokalemia, hypernatremia
SYST: **Serum sickness, anaphylaxis, Stevens-Johnson syndrome, exfoliative dermatitis**

Contraindications: Hypersensitivity to penicillins, neonates
Precautions: Pregnancy (B), lactation, hypersensitivity to cephalosporins; CHF, renal/GI disease, seizures, children

PHARMACOKINETICS

IM: Peak 30-50 min
IV: Peak 20-30 min
Half-life 0.7-1.33 hr; excreted in urine, bile, breast milk; crosses placenta

INTERACTIONS

Increase: piperacillin concentrations—aspirin, probenecid
Increase: levels of methotrexate, neuromuscular blockers
Decrease: antimicrobial effect of piperacillin—tetracyclines (with high concentrations of piperacillin), aminoglycosides
Decrease: effect of oral contraceptives
Drug/Herb
• Do not use acidophilus with antiinfectives; separate by several hours
Decrease: Absorption—khat

Drug/Lab Test
False positive: Urine glucose, urine protein, Coombs' test

NURSING CONSIDERATIONS
Assess:
• For infection: temp, WBC, sputum, stools, urine, wounds
• I&O ratio; report hematuria, oliguria, since penicillin in high doses is nephrotoxic

⚠ Any patient with compromised renal system, since drug is excreted slowly in poor renal system function; toxicity may occur rapidly
• Hepatic studies: AST, ALT
• Blood studies: WBC, RBC, Hgb, Hct, bleeding time prior to and periodically during treatment
• Renal studies: urinalysis, protein, blood, BUN, creatinine prior to and periodically during treatment
• C&S before drug therapy; drug may be taken as soon as culture is taken
• Bowel pattern before and during treatment
• Skin eruptions after administration of penicillin to 1 wk after discontinuing drug
• Respiratory status: rate, character, wheezing, tightness in chest
• Allergies before initiation of treatment, reaction of each medication
Administer:
• Drug after C&S completed
IM route
• 2 g/4 ml, 3 g/6 ml, 4 g/8 ml of sterile water, 0.9% NaCl max 2 g/site
IV route
• After diluting 1 g or less/5 ml or more sterile H₂O or 0.9% NaCl; shake; give dose over 3-5 min; may further dilute to 50-100 ml with D₅W, 0.9% NS, and give over ½ hr; discontinue primary IV
Additive compatibilities: Ciprofloxacin, clindamycin, fluconazole, hydrocortisone, ofloxacin, potassium chloride, verapamil
Syringe compatibilities: Heparin
Y-site compatibilities: Acyclovir, allopurinol, amifostine, aztreonam, ciprofloxacin, cyclophosphamide, diltiazem, DOXOrubicin liposome, enalaprilat, esmolol, famotidine, fludarabine, foscarnet, gallium, granisetron, heparin, hydromorphone, IL-2, labetalol, lorazepam, magnesium sulfate, melphalan, meperidine, midazolam, morphine, perphenazine, propofol, ranitidine, remifentanil, tacrolimus, teniposide, theophylline, thiotepa, verapamil, zidovudine
Perform/provide:
• EpINEPHrine, suction, tracheostomy set, endotracheal intubation equipment on unit
• Adequate intake of fluids (2 L) during diarrhea episodes
• Scratch test to assess allergy after securing order from prescriber; usually done when penicillin is only drug of choice
• Storage of reconstituted sol 24 hr at room temperature or 7 days refrigerated
Evaluate:
• Therapeutic response: absence of fever, purulent drainage, redness, inflammation
Teach patient/family:
• That culture may be taken after completed course of medication
• To report sore throat, fever, fatigue; may indicate superinfection
• To wear or carry emergency ID if allergic to penicillins
• To notify nurse of diarrhea
Treatment of anaphylaxis: Withdraw drug, maintain airway, administer epINEPHrine, aminophylline, O₂, IV corticosteroids

---

**piperacillin/
tazobactam (℞)**
(pip′er-ah-sill′in &
ta-zoe-bak′tam)
Zosyn
Func. class.: Antiinfective, broad-spectrum
Chem. class.: Extended-spectrum penicillin, β-lactamase inhibitor

Action: Interferes with cell wall replication of susceptible organisms; osmotically unstable cell wall swells and bursts from osmotic pressure; tazobactam is a β-lactamase inhibitor, protects piperacillin from enzymatic degradation

Uses: Moderate to severe infections: piperacillin-resistant, β-lactamase-producing strains causing infections in respiratory, skin, urinary tract, bone, gonorrhea, pneumonia; effective for resistant *Staphylococcus aureus,* resistant *Escherichia coli, Bacteroides fragilis, Bacteroides ovatus, Bacteroides thetaiotaomicron, Bacteroides vulgatus, Haemophilus influenzae*

DOSAGE AND ROUTES
Nosocomial pneumonia
• *Adult:* IV 3.375 g q6-8h with an aminoglycoside × 1-2 wk; continue aminoglycoside only if *Pseudomonas aeruginosa* is isolated
Other infections
• *Adult:* IV INF 6-12 g/day given 2.25 g q8h to 3.375 g q6h over 30 min × 7-10 days
Renal dose
• *Adult:* IV CCr 20-40 ml/min give 2.25 g q6h; CCr <20 ml/min give 2.25 g q8h

Available forms: Powder for inj 2 g piperacillin/0.25 g tazobactam, 3 g piperacillin/0.375 g tazobactam, 4 g piperacillin/0.5 g tazobactam, 36 g piperacillin/4.5 g tazobactam

SIDE EFFECTS
CNS: Lethargy, hallucinations, anxiety, depression, twitching, insomnia, headache, fever, dizziness, **seizures**

GI: Nausea, vomiting, diarrhea; increased AST, ALT; abdominal pain, glossitis, **pseudomembranous colitis,** constipation

GU: **Oliguria, proteinuria, hematuria,** *vaginitis, moniliasis,* **glomerulonephritis, renal failure**

HEMA: Anemia, increased bleeding time, **bone marrow depression, agranulocytosis**

INTEG: Rash, pruritus, **exfoliative dermatitis**

META: Hypokalemia, hypernatremia

SYST: **Serum sickness, anaphylaxis**

Contraindications: Hypersensitivity to penicillins; neonates; carbapenem allergy

Precautions: Pregnancy (B), lactation, hypersensitivity to cephalosporins, CHF, renal insufficiency in children, seizures, GI disease, electrolyte imbalances

PHARMACOKINETICS
IV: Peak completion of IV, duration 6 hr
Half-life 0.7-1.2 hr; excreted in urine, bile, breast milk; crosses placenta; 33% bound to plasma proteins

INTERACTIONS
Increase: effect of neuromuscular blockers, oral anticoagulants, methotrexate
Increase: piperacillin concentrations—aspirin, probenecid
Decrease: antimicrobial effect of piperacillin—tetracyclines, aminoglycosides IV
Decrease: effect of oral contraceptives
Drug/Herb
• Do not use acidophilus with antiinfectives; separate by several hours
Decrease: absorption—khat
Drug/Lab Test
Increase: Platelet count, eosinophilia, neutropenia, leukopenia, serum creatinine, PTT, AST, ALT, alk phos, bilirubin, BUN, electrolytes
Decrease: Hct, Hgb, electrolytes
False positive: Urine glucose, urine protein, Coombs' test

NURSING CONSIDERATIONS
Assess:
• For infection: temp, stools, urine, sputum, wounds
• I&O ratio; report hematuria, oliguria, since penicillin in high doses is nephrotoxic
⚠ Any patient with compromised renal system, since drug is excreted slowly in poor renal system function; toxicity may occur rapidly
• Hepatic studies: AST, ALT prior to and periodically thereafter

P

- Blood studies: WBC, RBC, Hct, Hgb, bleeding time prior to and periodically thereafter
- Renal studies: urinalysis, protein, blood, BUN, creatinine prior to and periodically thereafter
- C&S before drug therapy; drug may be given as soon as culture is taken
- Bowel pattern before and during treatment
- Skin eruptions after administration of penicillin to 1 wk after discontinuing drug
- Respiratory status: rate, character, wheezing, tightness in chest
- Allergies before initiation of treatment, reaction of each medication

Administer:
- Separate aminoglycoside from piperacillin to avoid inactivation
- Drug after C&S is complete

IV route
- After diluting 5 ml 0.9% NaCl for injection or sterile H_2O for inj, dextran 6% in NS, dextrose 5%, KCl 40 mEq, bacteriostatic saline/parabens, bacteriostatic saline/benzyl alcohol, bacteriostatic H_2O/benzyl alcohol per 1 g piperacillin; shake well; further dilute in at least 50 ml compatible IV sol and run as int inf over at least 30 min

Y-site compatibilities: Aminophylline, aztreonam, bleomycin, bumetanide, buprenorphine, butorphanol, calcium gluconate, carboplatin, carmustine, cefepime, cimetidine, clindamycin, cyclophosphamide, cytarabine, dexamethasone, diphenhydrAMINE, DOPamine, enalaprilat, etoposide, floxuridine, fluconazole, fludarabine, fluorouracil, furosemide, gallium, granisetron, heparin, hydrocortisone, hydromorphone, ifosfamide, leucovorin, lorazepam, magnesium sulfate, mannitol, meperidine, mesna, methotrexate, methylPREDNISolone, metoclopramide, metronidazole, morphine, ondansetron, plicamycin, potassium chloride, ranitidine, remifentanil, sargramostim, sodium bicarbonate, thiotepa, trimethoprim-sulfamethoxazole, vinBLAStine, vinCRIStine, zidovudine

Perform/provide:
- EpINEPHrine, suction, tracheostomy set, endotracheal intubation equipment on unit
- Adequate intake of fluids (2 L) during diarrhea episodes
- Scratch test to assess allergy on order from prescriber; usually when penicillin is only drug of choice
- Discard after 24 hr if stored at room temperature or after 48 hr if refrigerated; use single-dose vials immediately after reconstitution; stable in ambulatory IV pump for 12 hr

Evaluate:
- Therapeutic response: absence of fever, purulent drainage, redness, inflammation; culture shows decreased organisms

Teach patient/family:
- That culture may be taken after completed course of medication
- To report sore throat, fever, fatigue (may indicate superinfection)
- To wear or carry emergency ID if allergic to penicillins
- To notify nurse of diarrhea

Treatment of overdose: Withdraw drug, maintain airway, administer epINEPHrine, aminophylline, O_2, IV corticosteroids for anaphylaxis

pirbuterol (R)
(peer-byoo'ter-ole)
Maxair
Func. class.: Bronchodilator
Chem. class.: β-Adrenergic agonist

Action: Causes bronchodilation with little effect on heart rate by action on β-receptors, causing increased cAMP and relaxation of smooth muscle
Uses: Reversible bronchospasm (prevention, treatment) including asthma; may be given with theophylline or steroids

DOSAGE AND ROUTES
- *Adult and child >12 yr:* **INH** 1-2 puffs (0.4 mg) q4-6h; max 12 **INH**/day

Available forms: Aerosol delivery 0.2 mg pirbuterol/actuation

SIDE EFFECTS

CNS: Tremors, anxiety, insomnia, headache, dizziness, stimulation, restlessness, hallucinations, drowsiness, irritability
CV: Palpitations, tachycardia, hypertension, angina, hypotension, dysrhythmias
EENT: Dry nose and mouth, irritation of nose, throat
GI: Gastritis, nausea, vomiting, anorexia
MS: Muscle cramps
RESP: **Paradoxical bronchospasm,** dyspnea, coughing

Contraindications: Hypersensitivity to sympathomimetics, tachycardia
Precautions: Pregnancy (C), lactation, cardiac disorders, hyperthyroidism, hypertension, diabetes mellitus, prostatic hypertrophy

PHARMACOKINETICS

INH: Onset 3 min, peak ½-1 hr, duration 5 hr, terminal half-life 2 hr

INTERACTIONS

⚠ Hypertensive crisis: MAOIs
Increase: action of other aerosol bronchodilators
Increase: pirbuterol action—tricyclics, antihistamines, levothyroxine
Decrease: pirbuterol action—β-blockers
Drug/Herb
Increase: action of both—cola nut, guarana, yerba maté
Increase: effect—green tea (large amounts), guarana

NURSING CONSIDERATIONS

Assess:
• Respiratory function: vital capacity, forced expiratory volume, ABGs, B/P, lung sounds, pulse, characteristics of sputum
⚠ Paradoxical bronchospasm, that can occur rapidly, hold drug, notify prescriber

Administer:
• After shaking; exhale; place mouthpiece in mouth; inhale slowly; hold breath; remove; exhale slowly
• Gum, sips of water for dry mouth
Perform/provide:
• Storage in light-resistant container; do not expose to temperatures over 86° F (30° C)
• Fluid intake >2 L/day to liquefy thick secretions
Evaluate:
• Therapeutic response: absence of dyspnea, wheezing over 1 hr
Teach patient/family:
• Not to use OTC medications; extra stimulation may occur
• Use of inhaler; review package insert with patient
• To avoid getting aerosol in eyes
• Actuator is for Maxair autoinhaler; do not use with other inhaler canister
• About all aspects of drug; avoid smoking, smoke-filled rooms, persons with respiratory infections
• To keep fluid intake >2 L/day to liquefy thick secretions
Treatment of overdose: Administer a β-adrenergic blocker

piroxicam (Rx)
(peer-ox'i-kam)
Apo-Piroxicam ✦, Feldene, Novopirocam ✦, PMS-Piroxicam ✦
Func. class.: Nonsteroidal antiinflammatory
Chem. class.: Oxicam derivative

Action: Inhibits prostaglandin synthesis by decreasing an enzyme needed for biosynthesis; has analgesic, antiinflammatory, antipyretic properties
Uses: Mild to moderate pain, osteoarthritis, rheumatoid arthritis

DOSAGE AND ROUTES

• *Adult:* **PO** 20 mg daily or 10 mg bid
Available forms: Caps 10, 20 mg

SIDE EFFECTS

CNS: Dizziness, *drowsiness,* fatigue, tremors, confusion, insomnia, anxiety, depression, *headache*

CV: Tachycardia, peripheral edema, palpitations, dysrhythmias, hypertension, **MI, stroke**

EENT: Tinnitus, hearing loss, blurred vision

GI: Nausea, anorexia, vomiting, diarrhea, jaundice, **cholestatic hepatitis,** constipation, flatulence, cramps, dry mouth, peptic ulcer, **bleeding, ulceration, perforation**

GU: **Nephrotoxicity: dysuria, hematuria, oliguria, azotemia**

HEMA: **Blood dyscrasias**

INTEG: Purpura, rash, pruritus, sweating, photosensitivity

SYST: **Anaphylaxis**

Contraindications: Hypersensitivity, asthma, severe renal/hepatic disease, ulcer/cardiac disease, perioperative pain

Precautions: Pregnancy (B), avoid in late pregnancy, lactation, children, bleeding disorders, GI disorders, cardiac disorders, hypersensitivity to other antiinflammatory agents, CHF

PHARMACOKINETICS

PO: Peak 2 hr; duration 48-72 hr, half-life 30-80 hr; metabolized in liver; excreted in urine (metabolites), breast milk; 99% protein binding

INTERACTIONS

• Hypoglycemia: oral antidiabetics

Increase: toxicity—cycloSPORINE, methotrexate, lithium, alcohol, oral anticoagulants, aspirin, corticosteroids

Decrease: effects of antihypertensives, diuretics

Drug/Herb

Increase: gastric irritation—arginine, gossypol

Increase: NSAIDs effect—bearberry, bilberry

Increase: bleeding risk—bogbean, chondroitin

NURSING CONSIDERATIONS

Assess:

⚠ Cardiac status: CV thrombotic events, MI, stroke; may be fatal

⚠ GI status: ulceration, bleeding, perforation; may be fatal

• For pain: location, duration, type, ROM before and 1-2 hr after administration

• Renal, hepatic, blood studies: BUN, creatinine, AST, ALT, Hgb, before treatment, periodically thereafter

• Audiometric, ophthalmic exam before, during, after treatment

• For eye, ear problems: blurred vision, tinnitus (may indicate toxicity)

⚠ Those with aspirin sensitivity, asthma, nasal polyps may develop allergic reactions

Administer:

• Do not break, crush, or chew caps

• With food to decrease GI symptoms; take on empty stomach to facilitate absorption; take drug same time daily

Perform/provide:

• Storage at room temperature

• At least 6-8 glasses of water/day

Evaluate:

• Therapeutic response: decreased pain, stiffness, swelling in joints; ability to move more easily

Teach patient/family:

• To report blurred vision or ringing, roaring in ears (may indicate toxicity)

• To avoid driving, other hazardous activities if dizzy or drowsy

• That patient should drink at least 6-8 glasses of water/day

• To report change in urine pattern, weight increase, edema, pain increase in joints, fever, blood in urine (indicates nephrotoxicity)

• That therapeutic effects may take up to 1 mo

• To avoid ASA, other OTC meds, alcohol; advise patient to use sunscreen

---

⚠ Safety alert   *"Tall Man" lettering

plasma protein fraction (℞)
Plasmanate, Plasma Plex, Plasmatein, Protenate
Func. class.: Blood derivative
Chem. class.: Human plasma in NaCl

Action: Exerts similar oncotic pressure as human plasma, expands blood volume
Uses: Hypovolemic shock, hypoproteinemia, ARDS, preoperative cardiopulmonary bypass, acute hepatic failure, nephrotic syndrome, cardiogenic shock

DOSAGE AND ROUTES
Hypovolemia
• *Adult:* IV INF 250-500 ml (12.5-25 g protein), not to exceed 10 ml/min
• *Child:* IV INF 22-33 ml/kg at 5-10 ml/min
Hypoproteinemia
• *Adult:* IV INF 1000-1500 ml daily, not to exceed 8 ml/min
Available forms: Inj 5%

SIDE EFFECTS
CNS: Fever, chills, headache, paresthesias, flushing
CV: **Fluid overload,** hypotension, erratic pulse
GI: Nausea, vomiting, increased salivation
INTEG: Rash, urticaria, cyanosis
RESP: Altered respirations, dyspnea, **pulmonary edema**
Contraindications: Hypersensitivity, CHF, severe anemia, renal insufficiency
Precautions: Pregnancy (C), decreased salt intake, decreased cardiac reserve, lack of albumin deficiency, hepatic disease

PHARMACOKINETICS
Metabolized as a protein/energy source

INTERACTIONS
Drug/Lab Test
False increase: Alk phos

NURSING CONSIDERATIONS
Assess:
• Blood studies: Hct, Hgb, electrolytes, serum protein; if serum protein declines, dyspnea, hypoxemia can result
• B/P (decreased), pulse (erratic), respiration during infusion
• I&O ratio; urinary output may decrease
• CVP, pulmonary wedge pressure (increases if overload occurs), jugular vein distention
• Allergy: fever, rash, itching, chills, flushing, urticaria, nausea, vomiting, or hypotension requires discontinuation of infusion; use new lot if therapy reinstituted, premedicate with diphenhydrAMINE
⚠ Increased CVP reading: distended neck veins indicate circulatory overload; SOB, anxiety, insomnia, expiratory crackles, frothy blood-tinged cough, cyanosis indicate pulmonary overload
Administer:
IV route
• IV access at distant site from infection or trauma; no dilution required; use infusion pump, use large-gauge needle (≥20G); discard unused portion; infuse slowly
• Within 4 hr of opening, discard partially used vials
Additive compatibilities: Carbohydrate and electrolyte sol, whole blood, packed red blood cells, chloramphenicol, tetracycline
Perform/provide:
• Adequate hydration before administration
• Storage—check type of albumin, date; may have to refrigerate
Evaluate:
• Therapeutic response: increased B/P, decreased edema, increased serum albumin

⚠ High Alert

plicamycin (℞)
(ply-ka-my'sin)
Mithramycin, Mithracin
Func. class.: Antineoplastic,
antibiotic; hypocalcemic
Chem. class.: Crystalline aglycone

Action: Inhibits DNA, RNA, protein synthesis; derived from *Streptomyces plicatus;* replication is decreased by binding to DNA; demonstrates calcium-lowering effect not related to its tumoricidal activity; also acts on osteoclasts and blocks action of parathyroid hormone; a vesicant

Uses: Testicular cancer, hypercalcemia, hypercalciuria, symptomatic treatment of advanced neoplasms

DOSAGE AND ROUTES

Testicular tumors
• *Adult:* IV 25-30 mcg/kg/day × 8-10 days, not to exceed 30 mcg/kg/day
Hypercalcemia/hypercalciuria
• *Adult:* IV 25 mcg/kg/day × 3-4 days, repeat at intervals of 1 wk
Available forms: Inj 2500 mcg/vial powder

SIDE EFFECTS

CNS: Drowsiness, weakness, lethargy, headache, flushing, fever, depression
GI: Nausea, vomiting, anorexia, diarrhea, stomatitis, increased liver enzymes
GU: Increased BUN, creatinine; **proteinuria**
HEMA: **Hemorrhage, thrombocytopenia,** decreased PT, WBC count
INTEG: Rash, cellulitis, **extravasation,** facial flushing
META: Decreased serum Ca, P, K
Contraindications: Pregnancy (X), hypersensitivity, thrombocytopenia, bone marrow depression, bleeding disorders, lactation, child <15 yr

Precautions: Renal/hepatic disease, electrolyte imbalances

PHARMACOKINETICS

Crosses blood-brain barrier, excreted in urine; little known about pharmacokinetics

INTERACTIONS

Increase: toxicity—other antineoplastics or radiation
Drug/Herb
Increase: bleeding risk—anise, arnica, chamomile, clove, dong quai, fenugreek, garlic, ginger, ginkgo, ginseng *(Panax),* licorice

NURSING CONSIDERATIONS
Assess:
• CBC, differential, platelet count qwk; withhold drug if WBC is <4000/mm³ or platelet count is <50,000/mm³; notify prescriber
• Renal studies: BUN, serum uric acid, urine CCr, electrolytes before, during therapy
• I&O ratio; report urine output <30 ml/hr
• Monitor temp q4h; fever may indicate beginning infection
• Hepatic studies before, during therapy: bilirubin, AST, ALT, alk phos prn or qmo; jaundiced skin, sclera; dark urine, clay-colored stools, itchy skin, abdominal pain, fever, diarrhea
• Alkalosis if severe vomiting is present
⚠ Toxicity: facial flushing, epistaxis, increased PT, thrombocytopenia; drug should be discontinued
⚠ Bleeding: hematuria, guaiac stools, bruising or petechiae, mucosa or orifices q8h; may progress to severe bleeding
• Inflammation of mucosa, breaks in skin
• Buccal cavity q8h for dryness, sores, ulceration, white patches, oral pain, bleeding, dysphagia
• Local irritation, pain, burning at inj site
• Frequency of stools, characteristics, cramping

• Acidosis, signs of dehydration: rapid respirations, poor skin turgor, decreased urine output, dry skin, restlessness, weakness

Administer:

• Antiemetic 30-60 min before giving drug and 4-10 hr after treatment to prevent vomiting

• Transfusion for anemia

• Antispasmodic for diarrhea, phenothiazine for nausea and vomiting

IV route

• Dilute 2.5 mg/4.9 ml of sterile H_2O; (500 mcg/ml) dilute single dose in 1000 ml of D_5W run over 4-6 hr

• EDTA for extravasation, apply ice compress

• Slow IV infusion using 20G, 21G needle

Y-site compatibilities: Allopurinol, amifostine, aztreonam, filgrastim, granisetron, melphalan, piperacillin/tazobactam, teniposide, thiotepa, vinorelbine

Perform/provide:

• Liquid diet: carbonated beverages; gelatin may be added if patient is not nauseated or vomiting

• Rinsing of mouth tid-qid with water; brushing of teeth with baking soda bid-tid with soft brush or cotton-tipped applicator for stomatitis; unwaxed dental floss

• Usage immediately after mixing

Evaluate:

• Therapeutic response: decreased tumor size, spread of malignancy

Teach patient/family:

• To report any complaints or side effects to nurse or prescriber

• To avoid foods with citric acid, hot or rough texture

• To use effective contraception, avoid breastfeeding

• To report to prescriber any bleeding, white spots, ulcerations in the mouth; tell patient to examine mouth daily

• To avoid driving, activities requiring alertness; drowsiness may occur

• To report leg cramps, tingling of fingertips, weakness; may indicate hypocalcemia

• To avoid crowds, persons with infections when granulocyte count is low

---

Rarely Used

poly-L-lactic acid (℞)
(pol'i-el-lak'tik-as'id)
Sculptra
Func. class.: Physical adjuncts

Uses: Facial fat loss (lipoatrophy) in those with HIV

DOSAGE AND ROUTES

• *Adult:* **INJ** injected deep into dermic or subcut layer to avoid superficial inj using a 26G sterile needle; the number of inj depends on quantity of fat loss

Contraindications: Hypersensitivity

Rarely Used ⚠ High Alert

poractant alfa (℞)
Curosurf
Func. class.: Lung surfactant extract

Uses: Treatment (rescue) of respiratory distress syndrome in premature infants

DOSAGE AND ROUTES

• *Premature infant:* **INTRATRACHEAL INSTILL** 2.5 ml/kg birth weight up to 2 subsequent doses of 1.25 ml/kg birth weight can be administered at 12-hr intervals, max 5 ml/kg

Contraindications: Full-term infant, hypersensitivity

P

---

porfimer (Ꭱ)

(pour′fih-mur)

Photofrin

Func. class.: Antineoplastic—miscellaneous

Action: Used in photodynamic treatment of tumors (PDT); antitumor and cytotoxic actions are light and O_2 dependent; used with 630-nm laser light

Uses: Esophageal cancer (completely obstructing), endobronchial non–small cell lung cancer, Barrett's esophagus

Unlabeled uses: AIDS-related cutaneous Kaposi's sarcoma; basal cell, squamous cell carcinoma

DOSAGE AND ROUTES

Refer to Optiguide for complete instructions

• *Adult:* IV 2 mg/kg, then illumination with laser light 40-50 hr after inj; a second laser light application may be given 96-120 hr after inj; may repeat q30 days × 3

Endobronchial cancer

• *Adult:* 200 joules/cm of tumor length

Available forms: Cake/powder for inj 75 mg

SIDE EFFECTS

CNS: Anxiety, confusion, insomnia

CV: Hypotension, hypertension, atrial fibrillation, **cardiac failure,** *tachycardia*

GI: Abdominal pain, constipation, diarrhea, dyspepsia, dysphagia, eructation, esophageal edema/bleeding, hematemesis, melena, nausea, vomiting, anorexia

MISC: Dehydration, weight decrease, anemia, photosensitivity reaction, UTI, moniliasis

RESP: **Pleural effusion,** pneumonia, dyspnea, respiratory insufficiency, **tracheoesophageal fistula**

Contraindications: Porphyria, porphyrin allergy (porfimer); tracheoesophageal, bronchoesophageal fistula; major blood vessels with eroding tumors (PDT)

Precautions: Pregnancy (C), geriatric, lactation, children

PHARMACOKINETICS

Half-life 250 hr, 90% protein bound

INTERACTIONS

Increase: photosensitivity—tetracyclines, sulfonamides, phenothiazines, sulfonylureas, thiazides

NURSING CONSIDERATIONS

Assess:

• Ocular sensitivity: sensitivity to sun, bright lights, car headlights, patients should wear dark sunglasses with an average light transmittance of <4%

• Chest pain: may be so severe as to necessitate opiate analgesics

• For extravasation at inj site: take care to protect from light

Administer:

• As a single slow IV inj over 3-5 min at 2 mg/kg; reconstitute each vial with 31.8 ml D_5 or 0.9% NaCl (2.5 mg/ml), shake well; do not mix with other drugs or sol; protect from light and use immediately

• Laser light is initiated 630-nm wave length laser light

Perform/provide:

• Wiping of spills with damp cloth, avoid skin/eye contact, use rubber gloves, eye protection, dispose of material in polyethylene bag according to policy

Teach patient/family:

• To report chest pain, eye sensitivity

• To wear sunglasses; avoid exposure to sunlight or bright light for 30 days

posaconazole

See Appendix A—Selected New Drugs

potassium acetate
potassium bicarbonate
(otc, ℞)
K+ Care ET, K-Electrolyte, K-Ide, Klor-Con EF, K-Lyte, K-Vescent

potassium bicarbonate and potassium chloride (otc, ℞)
Klorvess, Klorvess Effervescent Granules, K-Lyte/Cl, Neo-K ♣

potassium bicarbonate and potassium citrate (otc, ℞)
Effer-K, K-Lyte DS

potassium chloride (otc, ℞)
Apo-K ♣, Cena-K, Gen-K, K+ Care, K+ 10, Kalium Durules ♣, Kaochlor, Kaochlor S-F, Kaon-Cl, Kay Ciel, KCl, K-Dur, K-Lease, K-Long ♣, K-Lor, Klor-Con, Klorvess, Klotrix, K-Lyte/C1 powder, K-med, K-Norm, K-Sol, K-tab, Micro-K, Micro-LS, Potasalan, Roychlor, Rum-K, Slow-K, Ten-K

potassium chloride/ potassium bicarbonate/ potassium citrate (otc, ℞)
Kaochlor Eff

potassium gluconate (otc, ℞)
Kaon, Kaylixir, K-G Elixir, Potassium-Rougier ♣

potassium gluconate/ potassium chloride (otc, ℞)
Kolyum

potassium gluconate/ potassium citrate (otc, ℞)
Twin-K

Func. class.: Electrolyte, mineral replacement
Chem. class.: Potassium

Action: Needed for adequate transmission of nerve impulses and cardiac contraction, renal function, intracellular ion maintenance

Uses: Prevention and treatment of hypokalemia

DOSAGE AND ROUTES
Potassium acetate—hypokalemia
• *Adult and child:* PO 40-100 mEq/day in divided doses 2-4 days
Potassium bicarbonate
• *Adult:* PO dissolve 25-50 mEq in water daily-qid
Hypokalemia (prevention)
• *Adult and child:* PO 20 mEq/day in 2-4 divided doses
Potassium chloride
• *Adult:* PO 40-100 mEq in divided doses tid-qid; IV 20 mEq/hr when diluted as 40 mEq/1000 ml, not to exceed 150 mEq/day
• *Child:* PO 2-4 mEq/kg/day
Potassium gluconate
• *Adult:* PO 40-100 mEq in divided doses tid-qid
Potassium phosphate
• *Adult:* IV 1 mEq/hr in sol of 60 mEq/L, not to exceed 150 mEq/day; PO 40-100 mEq/day in divided doses
• *Child:* IV max rate of inf 1 mEq/kg/hr
Available forms: Tabs for sol 6.5, 25 mEq; ext rel caps 8, 10 mEq; powder for sol 3.3, 5, 6.7, 10, 13.3 mEq/5 ml; tabs 2, 4, 5, 13.4 mEq; ext rel tabs 6.7, 8, 10 mEq; elix 6.7 mEq/5 ml; oral sol 2.375 mEq/5 ml; inj for prep of IV 1.5, 2, 2.4, 3, 3.2, 4.4, 4.7 mEq/ml

SIDE EFFECTS
CNS: Confusion
CV: Bradycardia, **cardiac depression, dysrhythmias, arrest, peaking T waves, lowered R and depressed RST, prolonged P-R interval, widened QRS complex**
GI: Nausea, vomiting, cramps, pain, *diarrhea,* ulceration of small bowel
GU: Oliguria
INTEG: Cold extremities, rash
Contraindications: Renal disease (severe), severe hemolytic disease, Addison's

disease, hyperkalemia, acute dehydration, extensive tissue breakdown

Precautions: Pregnancy (C), cardiac disease, potassium-sparing diuretic therapy, systemic acidosis

PHARMACOKINETICS

PO: Excreted by kidneys and in feces; onset of action ≈30 min
IV: Immediate onset of action

INTERACTIONS

• Hyperkalemia: potassium phosphate IV and products containing calcium or magnesium; potassium-sparing diuretic, or other potassium products, ACE inhibitors

NURSING CONSIDERATIONS

Assess:
• ECG for peaking T waves, lowered R, depressed RST, prolonged P-R interval, widening QRS complex, hyperkalemia; drug should be reduced or discontinued
• Potassium level during treatment (3.5-5 mg/dl is normal level)
• I&O ratio; watch for decreased urinary output; notify prescriber immediately
• Cardiac status: rate, rhythm, CVP, PWP, PAWP, if being monitored directly

Administer:
PO route
• Do not break, crush, or chew ext rel tabs/caps or enteric products
• With or after meals; dissolve effervescent tabs, powder in 8 oz cold water or juice; do not give IM, SUBCUT
• Caps with full glass of liquid

IV route
• Through large-bore needle to decrease vein inflammation; check for extravasation
• In large vein, avoiding scalp vein in child (IV)
• IV after diluting in large volume of IV sol and give as an inf, slowly by IV inf to prevent toxicity; never give IV bolus or IM

Potassium acetate
Additive compatibilities: Metoclopramide

Y-site compatibilities: Ciprofloxacin
Potassium chloride
Additive compatibilities: Aminophylline, amiodarone, atracurium, bretylium, calcium gluconate, cefepime, cephalothin, cephapirin, chloramphenicol, cimetidine, ciprofloxacin, cisatracurium, clindamycin, cloxacillin, corticotropin, cytarabine, dimenhyDRINATE, DOPamine, DOXOrubicin liposome, enalaprilat, erythromycin, floxacillin, fluconazole, fosphenytoin, furosemide, heparin, hydrocortisone, isoproterenol, lidocaine, metaraminol, methicillin, methyldopa, metoclopramide, mitoxantrone, nafcillin, netilmicin, norepinephrine, oxacillin, penicillin G potassium, phenylephrine, piperacillin, ranitidine, sodium bicarbonate, thiopental, vancomycin, verapamil, vit B/C

Y-site compatibilities: Acyclovir, aldesleukin, allopurinol, amifostine, aminophylline, amiodarone, ampicillin, amrinone, atropine, aztreonam, betamethasone, calcium gluconate, cephalothin, cephapirin, chlordiazepoxide, chlorproMAZINE, ciprofloxacin, cladribine, cyanocobalamin, dexamethasone, digoxin, diltiazem, diphenhydrAMINE, DOBUTamine, DOPamine, droperidol, edrophonium, enalaprilat, epINEPHrine, esmolol, estrogens, ethacrynate, famotidine, fentanyl, filgrastim, fludarabine, fluorouracil, furosemide, gallium, granisetron, heparin, hydrALAZINE, idarubicin, indomethacin, insulin (regular), isoproterenol, kanamycin, labetalol, lidocaine, lorazepam, magnesium sulfate, melphalan, meperidine, methicillin, methoxamine, methylergonovine, midazolam, minocycline, morphine, neostigmine, norepinephrine, ondansetron, oxacillin, oxytocin, paclitaxel, penicillin G potassium, pentazocine, phytonadione, piperacillin/tazobactam, prednisoLONE, procainamide, prochlorperazine, propofol, propranolol, pyridostigmine, remifentanil, sargramostim, scopolamine, sodium bicarbonate, succinylcholine, tacrolimus, teniposide, theophylline, thiotepa, trimethaphan, trimethonzamide, vinorelbine, warfarin, zidovudine

Perform/provide:
• Storage at room temperature
Evaluate:
• Therapeutic response: absence of fatigue, muscle weakness; decreased thirst and urinary output; cardiac changes
Teach patient/family:
• To add potassium-rich foods to diet: bananas, orange juice, avocados; whole grains, broccoli, carrots, prunes, cocoa after this medication is discontinued
• To avoid OTC products: antacids, salt substitutes, analgesics, vitamin preparations, unless specifically directed by prescriber
• To report hyperkalemia symptoms (lethargy, confusion, diarrhea, nausea, vomiting, fainting, decreased output) or continued hypokalemia symptoms (fatigue, weakness, polyuria, polydipsia, cardiac changes)
• To dissolve powder or tablet completely in at least 120 ml water or juice
• Importance of regular follow-up visits

potassium iodide (℞)
Pima, saturated solution (SSKI), strong iodine solution (Lugol's solution), Thyro-Block
Func. class.: Thyroid hormone antagonist
Chem. class.: Iodine product

Action: Inhibits secretion of thyroid hormone, fosters colloid accumulation in thyroid follicles, decreases vascularity of gland
Uses: Preparation for thyroidectomy, thyrotoxic crisis, neonatal thyrotoxicosis, radiation protectant, thyroid storm

DOSAGE AND ROUTES
Thyrotoxic crisis
• *Adult and child:* **PO** 500 mg q4h (10 gtt SSKI), or 1 ml of strong iodine sol tid; give ≥1 hr after 1st dose of propylthiouracil, or methimazole

Preparation for thyroidectomy
• *Adult and child:* **PO** 3-5 gtt strong iodine sol tid, or 1-5 drops SSKI in water tid after meals for 10 days prior to surgery
Available forms: Oral sol (Lugol's solution) iodine 5%/potassium iodide 10%; oral sol (SSKI) 1 g/ml; syrup 325 mg/5 ml; tabs 130 mg

SIDE EFFECTS
CNS: Headache, confusion, paresthesias
EENT: Metallic taste, stomatitis, salivation, periorbital edema, sore teeth and gums, cold symptoms
ENDO: Hypothyroidism, hyperthyroid adenoma
GI: Nausea, diarrhea, vomiting, small-bowel lesions, upper gastric pain
INTEG: Rash, urticaria, **angioneurotic edema,** acne, mucosal hemorrhage, fever
MS: Myalgia, arthralgia, weakness
Contraindications: Pregnancy (D), hypersensitivity to iodine, pulmonary edema, pulmonary TB
Precautions: Lactation, children

PHARMACOKINETICS
PO: Onset 24-48 hr, peak 10-15 days after continuous therapy, uptake by thyroid gland or excreted in urine; crosses placenta

INTERACTIONS
• Hypothyroidism: lithium, other antithyroid agents
Drug/Lab Test
Interference: Urinary 17-OHCS

NURSING CONSIDERATIONS
Assess:
• Pulse, B/P, temp
• I&O ratio; check for edema: puffy hands, feet, periorbit; indicate hypothyroidism
• Weight daily; same clothing, scale, time of day
• T_3, T_4, which is increased; serum TSH, which is decreased; free thyroxine index,

836 pralidoxime

which is increased if dosage is too low; discontinue drug 3-4 wk before RAIU

⚠ Overdose: peripheral edema, heat intolerance, diaphoresis, palpitations, dysrhythmias, severe tachycardia, fever, delirium, CNS irritability

• Hypersensitivity: rash; enlarged cervical lymph nodes may indicate drug should be discontinued

• Hypoprothrombinemia: bleeding, petechiae, ecchymosis

• Clinical response: after 3 wk should include increased weight, pulse; decreased T_4

Administer:

• Strong iodine solution after diluting with water or juice to improve taste

• Through straw to prevent tooth discoloration

• With meals to decrease GI upset

• At same time each day to maintain drug level

• Lowest dose that relieves symptoms, discontinue before RAIU

Perform/provide:

• Fluids to 3-4 L/day, unless contraindicated

Evaluate:

• Therapeutic response: weight gain, decreased pulse, T_4, size of thyroid gland

Teach patient/family:

• To abstain from breastfeeding after delivery

• To keep graph of weight, pulse, mood

• To avoid OTC products that contain iodine

• That seafood, other iodine products may be restricted

• Not to discontinue this medication abruptly; thyroid crisis may occur; stress response

• That response may take several mo if thyroid is large

• To discontinue drug, notify prescriber of fever, rash, metallic taste, swelling of throat; burning of mouth, throat; sore gums, teeth; severe GI distress, enlargement of thyroid, cold symptoms

Rarely Used

pralidoxime (℞)
(pra-li-dox'eem)
Protopam Chloride
Func. class.: Cholinesterase reactivator, nerve gas antidote

Uses: Cholinergic crisis in myasthenia gravis, organophosphate poisoning antidote (early), relief of paralysis of respiratory muscles; used as an adjunct to systemic atropine administration

DOSAGE AND ROUTES
Anticholinesterase overdose
• *Adult:* **IV** 1-2 g, then 250 mg q5min until desired response
Organophosphate poisoning
• *Adult:* **IV INF** 1-2 g/100 ml 0.9% NaCl over 15-30 min; may repeat in 1 hr; **PO** 1-3 g q5h
• *Child:* **IV INF** 20-40 mg/kg/dose diluted in 100 ml 0.9% NaCl over 15-30 min
Contraindications: Hypersensitivity, carbamate insecticide poisoning

pramipexole (℞)
(pra-mi-pex'ol)
Mirapex
Func. class.: Antiparkinson agent
Chem. class.: Dopamine-receptor agonist, non-ergot

Action: Selective agonist for D_2 receptors (presynaptic/postsynaptic sites); binding at D_3 receptor contributes to antiparkinson effects
Uses: Parkinson's disease
Unlabeled uses: Restless leg syndrome

DOSAGE AND ROUTES
Initial treatment
• *Adult:* **PO** from a starting dose of 0.375 mg/day given in 3 divided doses; increase gradually by 0.125 mg/dose at 5-7 day intervals until total daily dose of 4.5 mg is reached

⚠ Safety alert   *"Tall Man" lettering

Maintenance treatment
• *Adult:* **PO** 1.5-4.5 mg daily in 3 divided doses
Restless leg syndrome (unlabeled)
• *Adult:* **PO** 0.125-0.375 mg 1-2 hr prior to bedtime, increase gradually
Renal dose
• *Adult:* **PO** CCr 35-59 ml/min-0.125 mg bid, may increase q5-7 days to 1.5 mg bid; CCr 15-34 ml/min 0.125 mg daily, increase q5-7 days to 1.5 mg daily
Available forms: Tabs 0.125, 0.25, 0.5, 1, 1.5 mg

SIDE EFFECTS

CNS: Agitation, insomnia, psychosis, hallucination, depression, dizziness, headache, confusion, amnesia, dream disorder, asthenia
CV: Orthostatic hypotension, edema, syncope, tachycardia
EENT: Blurred vision
GI: Nausea, anorexia, constipation, dysphagia, dry mouth
GU: Impotence, urinary frequency
HEMA: **Hemolytic anemia, leukopenia, agranulocytosis**
Contraindications: Hypersensitivity
Precautions: Pregnancy (C), renal/cardiac disease, MI with dysrhythmias, affective disorders, psychosis, preexisting dyskinesias

PHARMACOKINETICS

Minimally metabolized, peak 2 hr, half-life 8 hr, 8.5-12 hr in geriatric

INTERACTIONS

Increase: pramipexole levels—levodopa, cimetidine, ranitidine, diltiazem, triamterene, verapamil, quinidine
Decrease: pramipexole levels—DOPamine antagonists, phenothiazines, metoclopramide, butyrophenones
Drug/Herb
Decrease: effect of pramipexole—chaste tree fruit, kava

NURSING CONSIDERATIONS

Assess:
• Renal studies
• Involuntary movements in parkinsonism: bradykinesia, tremors, staggering gait, muscle rigidity, drooling
• B/P, ECG, respiration during initial treatment; hypo/hypertension should be reported
• Mental status: affect, mood, behavioral changes, depression; complete suicide assessment
⚠ For sleep attacks: may fall asleep during activities without warning; may need to discontinue medication
Administer:
• Adjust dosage to patient response, titrate slowly
• With meals to minimize GI symptoms
Perform/provide:
• Assistance with ambulation during beginning therapy
• Testing for diabetes mellitus, acromegaly if on long-term therapy
Evaluate:
• Therapeutic response: movement disorder improves
Teach patient/family:
• That therapeutic effects may take several weeks to a few months
• To change positions slowly to prevent orthostatic hypotension
• To use drug exactly as prescribed: if drug is discontinued abruptly, parkinsonian crisis may occur, avoid alcohol, OTC sleeping products
• To notify prescriber if pregnancy is planned or suspected

P

---

pramlintide (℞)
(pram′lin-tide)
Symlin
Func. class.: Antidiabetic
Chem. class.: Synthetic human amylin analog

Action: Modulates and slows stomach emptying, prevents postprandial rise in plasma glucagon, decreases appetite, leads to decreased caloric intake and weight loss

Uses: Type 1 diabetes mellitus, type 2 diabetes mellitus as an adjunct to insulin therapy with uncontrolled type 1 or type 2 diabetes

DOSAGE AND ROUTES

• *Adult:* **SUBCUT** 15 mcg, may increase by 15 mcg to 30-60 mcg, max 120 mcg/dose

Available forms: Inj 5-ml vials (0.6 mg/ml)

SIDE EFFECTS

CNS: Headache, fatigue, dizziness
GI: Nausea, vomiting, anorexia, abdominal pain
INTEG: Inj site reactions
META: Hypoglycemia (while used with insulin)
MS: Arthralgia
RESP: Cough, pharyngitis
SYST: Systemic allergy

Contraindications: Hypersensitivity to this product or metacresol, gastroparesis
Precautions: Pregnancy (C), lactation

PHARMACOKINETICS

Absorption 30%-40%, extensively bound to blood cells or albumin, half-life 48 min, metabolized by kidneys

INTERACTIONS

• Do not use with erythromycin, metoclopramide
Increase: effect of acetaminophen
Increase: pramlintide action—antimuscarinics, α-glucosidase inhibitors, diphenoxylate, loperamide, octreotide, opiate agonist, tricyclic antidepressants
Increase: hypoglycemia—ACE inhibitors, disopyramide, anabolic steroids, androgens, fibric acid derivatives, alcohol, corticosteroids, insulin
Increase: hyperglycemia—phenothiazines
Decrease: hypoglycemia—niacin, dextrothyroxine, thiazide diuretics, triam-

terene, estrogens, progestins, oral contraceptives, MAOIs

NURSING CONSIDERATIONS

Assess:
• Fasting blood glucose, 2 hr PP (80-150 mg/dl, normal fasting level; 70-130 mg/dl, normal 2 hr level); A1c may also be drawn to identify treatment effectiveness; also monitor weight, appetite
• For hypoglycemic reaction (sweating, weakness, dizziness, chills, confusion, headache, nausea, rapid weak pulse, fatigue, tachycardia, memory lapses, slurred speech, staggering gait, anxiety, tremors, hunger)
• For hyperglycemia: acetone breath, polyuria, fatigue, polydipsia, flushed, dry skin, lethargy
Administer:
SUBCUT route
• Take prior to mealtime, or if 30 g of carbohydrates will be consumed
• Do not use if a meal is skipped
• Do not use if discolored
Syringe compatibilities: Do not mix with insulin, give separately
Perform/provide:
• Storage at room temperature, keep away from heat and sunlight; refrigerate all other supply
Evaluate:
• Therapeutic response: decrease in polyuria, polydipsia, polyphagia, clear sensorium, absence of dizziness, stable gait; improving A1c
Teach patient/family:
• That drug does not cure diabetes but controls symptoms
• To carry emergency ID as diabetic
• To recognize hypoglycemia reaction: headache, fatigue, weakness
• The dosage, route, mixing instructions, if any diet restrictions, disease process
• To carry a glucose source (candy or lump sugar) to treat hypoglycemia
• The symptoms of ketoacidosis: nausea, thirst, polyuria, dry mouth, decreased B/P, dry, flushed skin, acetone breath, drowsiness, Kussmaul respirations
• That a plan is necessary for diet, exer-

cise; all food on diet should be eaten; exercise routine should not vary
• About blood glucose testing; make sure patient is able to determine glucose level
• To avoid OTC drugs unless directed by prescriber, alcohol
• Not to operate machinery or drive until effect is known

Treatment of overdose: Glucose 25 g IV, via dextrose 50% sol, 50 ml or glucagon 1 mg SUBCUT

---

pramoxine topical
See Appendix C

---

pravastatin (Ŗ)
(pra'va-sta-tin)
Pravachol
Func. class.: Antilipidemic
Chem. class.: HMG-CoA reductase enzyme

Do not confuse:
Pravachol/Prevacid
Action: Inhibits HMG-CoA reductase enzyme, which reduces cholesterol synthesis
Uses: As an adjunct in primary hypercholesterolemia (types IIa, IIb, III, IV), to reduce the risk of recurrent MI, atherosclerosis, primary/secondary CV events, reduce stroke, TIAs

DOSAGE AND ROUTES
• *Adult:* **PO** 40-80 mg daily at bedtime (range 20-80 mg daily)
• *Adolescent 14-18 yr:* **PO** 40 mg daily
• *Child 8-13 yr:* **PO** 20 mg daily
• *Geriatric/renal/hepatic disease:* **PO** 10 mg/day initially
Available forms: Tabs 10, 20, 40, 80 mg

SIDE EFFECTS
CNS: Headache, dizziness, fatigue
EENT: Lens opacities
GI: Nausea, constipation, diarrhea, flatus, abdominal pain, heartburn, **hepatic dysfunction,** pancreatitis, **hepatitis**
INTEG: Rash, pruritus, photosensitivity
MISC: Chest pain, rash, pruritus, photosensitivity
MS: Muscle cramps, myalgia, **myositis, rhabdomyolysis**
RESP: Common cold, rhinitis, cough
Contraindications: Pregnancy (X), hypersensitivity, lactation, active hepatic disease
Precautions: Past hepatic disease, alcoholism, severe acute infections, trauma, severe metabolic disorders, electrolyte imbalances

PHARMACOKINETICS
Peak 1-1½ hr; metabolized by the liver, protein binding 80%; excreted in urine 20%, feces 70%, breast milk; crosses placenta

INTERACTIONS
Increase: myopathy risk—erythromycin, niacin, cycloSPORINE, gemfibrozil, clofibrate, clarithromycin, itraconazole, protease inhibitors
Increase: effects of warfarin, digoxin
Decrease: bioavailability of pravastatin—bile acid sequestrants
Drug/Herb
Increase: effect—glucomannan
Decrease: effect—gotu kola, oat bran, St. John's wort
Drug/Lab Test
Increase: CPK, LFTs
Altered: Thyroid function tests

NURSING CONSIDERATIONS
Assess:
• Fasting lipid profile: LDL, HDL, triglycerides, cholesterol q8wk, then q3-6mo when stable; obtain diet history
• Hepatic studies: baseline, q6wk during the first 3 mo, q8wk for remainder of yr, then q6mo; AST, ALT, LFTs may increase
• Renal studies in patients with compromised renal system: BUN, I&O ratio, creatinine

⚠ For muscle tenderness, pain, obtain CPK baseline and if these occur; rhabdomyolysis may occur, therapy should be discontinued

Administer:
• Without regard to meals, at bedtime
• Give 1 hr before or 4 hr after bile acid sequestrants

Perform/provide:
• Storage in cool environment in tight container protected from light

Evaluate:
• Therapeutic response: decrease in cholesterol to desired level after 8 wk

Teach patient/family:
• That blood work will be necessary during treatment
⚠ To report blurred vision, severe GI symptoms, dizziness, headache, muscle pain, weakness, fever
• That regimen will continue: low-cholesterol diet, exercise program
• To report suspected, planned pregnancy, not to use during pregnancy
• To use sunscreen, protective clothing to prevent burns

---

prazosin (℞)
(pray′zoe-sin)
Minipress, prazosin
Func. class.: Antihypertensive
Chem. class.: α_1-Adrenergic blocker

Action: Blocks α-mediated vasoconstriction of adrenergic receptors, inducing peripheral vasodilation

Uses: Hypertension, refractory CHF, Raynaud's vasospasm

Unlabeled uses: Benign prostatic hypertrophy to decrease urine outflow obstruction

DOSAGE AND ROUTES

Hypertension
• *Adult:* PO 1 mg bid or tid, increasing to 20 mg daily in divided doses if required; usual range 6-15 mg/day, not to exceed 1 mg initially; max 20-40 mg/day
• *Child:* PO 5 mcg/kg q6h; max 400 mcg/kg/day

Benign prostatic hyperplasia
• *Adult:* PO 1-9 mg daily
Available forms: Caps 1, 2, 5 mg

SIDE EFFECTS

CNS: Dizziness, headache, drowsiness, anxiety, depression, vertigo, weakness, fatigue
CV: Palpitations, orthostatic hypotension, tachycardia, edema, rebound hypertension
EENT: Blurred vision, epistaxis, tinnitus, dry mouth, red sclera
GI: Nausea, vomiting, diarrhea, constipation, abdominal pain
GU: Urinary frequency, incontinence, impotence, priapism, H_2O, sodium retention

Contraindications: Hypersensitivity
Precautions: Pregnancy (C), children, lactation, hepatic disease, prostate cancer

PHARMACOKINETICS

PO: Onset 2 hr, peak 2-4 hr, duration 6-12 hr; half-life 2 hr, metabolized in liver, excreted via bile, feces (>90%), in urine (<10%), protein binding 97%

INTERACTIONS

Increase: hypotensive effects—β-blockers, nitroglycerin, alcohol, verapamil
Decrease: antihypertensive effect—NSAIDs, clonidine, salicylates

Drug/Herb
Increase: toxicity, death—aconite
Increase: antihypertensive effect—barberry, betony, black catechu, black cohosh, bloodroot, broom, burdock, cat's claw, dandelion, goldenseal, hawthorn, Irish moss, Jamaican dogwood, kelp, khella, mistletoe, parsley
Increase or decrease: antihypertensive effect—astragalus, cola tree
Decrease: antihypertensive effect—coltsfoot, guarana, khat, licorice, yohimbine

Drug/Lab Test
Increase: Urinary norepinephrine, VMA

NURSING CONSIDERATIONS

Assess:

• B/P (sitting, standing) during initial treatment, periodically thereafter; pulse, jugular venous distention q4h

• BUN, uric acid if on long-term therapy

• Weight daily, I&O; edema in feet, legs daily

• Skin turgor, dryness of mucous membranes for hydration status

• Crackles, dyspnea, orthopnea q30min

Administer:

• 1st dose at bedtime to avoid fainting

Perform/provide:

• Storage in tight container in cool environment

Evaluate:

• Therapeutic response: decreased B/P

Teach patient/family:

• That fainting occasionally occurs after 1st dose; take 1st dose at bedtime or do not drive or operate machinery for 4 hr after 1st dose

• To change positions slowly, to prevent orthostatic hypotension

• To avoid OTC medications unless approved by prescriber

Treatment of overdose: Administer volume expanders or vasopressors, discontinue drug, place in supine position

*prednisoLONE (℞)

(pred-niss'oh-lone)
Articulose-50, Delta-Cortef, Hydeltrasol, Hydeltra-T.B.A., Key-Pred 25, Key-Pred 50, Key-Pred-SP, Orapred, Pediapred, Predaject-50, Predalone 50, Predalone-T.B.A., Predcor-25, Predcor-50, prednisoLONE, PrednisoLONE Acetate, Prednisol TBA, Prelone

Func. class.: Corticosteroid, synthetic

Chem. class.: Glucocorticoid, immediate acting

Do not confuse:
prednisoLONE/predniSONE

Action: Decreases inflammation by suppression of migration of polymorphonuclear leukocytes, fibroblasts; reversal to increase capillary permeability and lysosomal stabilization

Uses: Severe inflammation, immunosuppression, neoplasms

DOSAGE AND ROUTES

• *Adult:* **PO** 2.5-15 mg bid-qid; **IM** 2-30 mg (acetate, phosphate) q12h; **IV** 2-30 mg (phosphate) q12h; 2-30 mg in joint or soft tissue (phosphate), 4-40 mg in joint of lesion (tebutate)

Asthma/antiinflammatory

• *Child:* **PO/IV** 1 mg/kg q6h × 2 days, then 1-2 mg/kg; max 60 mg/day

Available forms: Tabs 5 mg; syr 5 mg/5 ml, 15 mg/15 ml; acetate: inj 25, 50 mg/ml; tebutate: inj 20 mg/ml; phosphate: inj 20 mg/ml, oral liquid 5 mg/ml, tabs 1, 2.5, 5, 10, 20, 50 mg, oral sol 5 mg/ml, 5 mg/5 ml, syr 5 mg/5 ml

SIDE EFFECTS

CNS: Depression, flushing, sweating, headache, mood changes

CV: Hypertension, **circulatory collapse, thrombophlebitis, embolism,** tachycardia

EENT: Fungal infections, increased intra-ocular pressure, blurred vision

GI: Diarrhea, nausea, abdominal distention, **GI hemorrhage,** increased appetite, **pancreatitis**

HEMA: **Thrombocytopenia**

INTEG: Acne, poor wound healing, ecchymosis, petechiae

MS: Fractures, osteoporosis, weakness

Contraindications: Psychosis, hypersensitivity, idiopathic thrombocytopenia, acute glomerulonephritis, amebiasis, fungal infections, nonasthmatic bronchial disease, child <2 yr

Precautions: Pregnancy (C), diabetes mellitus, glaucoma, osteoporosis, seizure disorders, ulcerative colitis, CHF, myasthenia gravis

PHARMACOKINETICS

PO: Peak 1-2 hr, duration 2 days
IM: Peak 3-45 hr

INTERACTIONS

Increase: side effects—alcohol, salicylates, indomethacin, amphotericin B, digitalis, cycloSPORINE, diuretics

Increase: prednisoLONE action—salicylates, estrogens, indomethacin, oral contraceptives, ketoconazole, macrolide antibiotics

Decrease: prednisoLONE action—cholestyramine, colestipol, barbiturates, rifampin, epHEDrine, phenytoin, theophylline

Decrease: effects of anticoagulants, anticonvulsants, antidiabetics, ambenonium, neostigmine, isoniazid, toxoids, vaccines, anticholinesterases, salicylates, somatrem

Drug/Herb

• Hypokalemia: aloe, buckthorn, cascara sagrada, Chinese rhubarb, senna

Increase: effect—aloe, licorice, perilla

Drug/Lab Test

Increase: Cholesterol, sodium, blood glucose, uric acid, calcium, urine glucose

Decrease: Calcium, potassium, T_4, T_3, thyroid ^{131}I uptake test, urine 17-OHCS, 17-KS, PBI

False negative: Skin allergy tests

NURSING CONSIDERATIONS

Assess:

• Potassium, blood glucose, urine glucose while on long-term therapy; hypokalemia and hyperglycemia

• Weight daily; notify prescriber if weekly gain >5 lb

• B/P q4h, pulse; notify prescriber if chest pain occurs

• I&O ratio; be alert for decreasing urinary output, increasing edema

• Plasma cortisol levels (long-term therapy) (normal level: 138-635 nmol/L SI units when drawn at 8 AM)

• Infection: increased temp, WBC, even after withdrawal of medication; drug masks infection

• Potassium depletion: paresthesias, fatigue, nausea, vomiting, depression, polyuria, dysrhythmias, weakness

• Edema, hypertension, cardiac symptoms

• Mental status: affect, mood, behavioral changes, aggression

Administer:

IM route

• After shaking suspension (parenteral)

• Titrated dose; use lowest effective dose

• IM inj deep in large muscle mass; rotate sites; avoid deltoid; use 21G needle

• In 1 dose in AM to prevent adrenal suppression; avoid SUBCUT administration; may damage tissue

• With food or milk to decrease GI symptoms

IV route

• Undiluted or added to NaCl or D_5 and given by IV inf; give 10 mg or less/1 min; decrease rate if burning occurs

Additive compatibilities: Ascorbic acid, cephalothin, cytarabine, erythromycin, fluorouracil, heparin, methicillin, penicillin G potassium, penicillin G sodium, vit B/C

Y-site compatibilities: Ciprofloxacin, heparin/hydrocortisone, potassium chloride, vit B/C

⚠ Safety alert   *"Tall Man" lettering

Perform/provide:

• Assistance with ambulation to patient with bone tissue disease to prevent fractures

Evaluate:

• Therapeutic response: ease of respirations, decreased inflammation

Teach patient/family:

• That emergency ID as steroid user should be carried

• To notify prescriber if therapeutic response decreases; dosage adjustment may be needed

• Not to discontinue abruptly; adrenal crisis can result; take exactly as prescribed

• To avoid OTC products: salicylates, cough products with alcohol, cold preparations unless directed by prescriber

• About cushingoid symptoms

• The symptoms of adrenal insufficiency: nausea, anorexia, fatigue, dizziness, dyspnea, weakness, joint pain

**prednisoLONE
ophthalmic**
See Appendix C

*predniSONE (℞)
(pred′ni-sone)
Apo-Prednisone ✤,
Deltasone ✤, Liquid Pred,
Meticorten, Orasone,
Panasol-S, Prednicen-M,
PredniSONE, Sterapred,
Winpred
Func. class.: Corticosteroid
Chem. class.: Intermediate-acting glucocorticoid

Do not confuse:
predniSONE/methylPREDNISolone/ prednisoLONE/Prilosec

Action: Decreases inflammation by suppression of migration of polymorphonuclear leukocytes, fibroblasts, reversal to increase capillary permeability, and lysosomal stabilization

Uses: Severe inflammation, immunosuppression, neoplasms, multiple sclerosis, collagen disorders, dermatologic disorders

DOSAGE AND ROUTES

• *Adult:* **PO** 5-60 mg daily or divided bid-qid

• *Child:* **PO** 0.05-2 mg/kg/day divided 1-4 ×/day

Nephrosis

• *Child:* **PO** 2 mg/kg/day in divided doses, max 28 days, then 1-1.5 mg/kg/day every other day × 4 wk

Multiple sclerosis

• *Adult:* **PO** 200 mg/day × 1 wk, then 80 mg every other day × 1 mo

Available forms: Tabs 1, 2.5, 5, 10, 20, 50 mg; oral sol 5 mg/5 ml; syr 5 mg/5 ml

SIDE EFFECTS

CNS: Depression, flushing, sweating, headache, mood changes

CV: Hypertension, **circulatory collapse, thrombophlebitis, embolism,** tachycardia

EENT: Fungal infections, increased intraocular pressure, blurred vision

GI: Diarrhea, nausea, abdominal distention, **GI hemorrhage,** increased appetite, pancreatitis

HEMA: **Thrombocytopenia**

INTEG: Acne, poor wound healing, ecchymosis, petechiae

META: Hyperglycemia

MS: Fractures, osteoporosis, weakness

Contraindications: Psychosis, hypersensitivity, idiopathic thrombocytopenia, acute glomerulonephritis, amebiasis, fungal infections, nonasthmatic bronchial disease, child <2 yr, AIDS, TB

Precautions: Pregnancy (C), diabetes mellitus, glaucoma, osteoporosis, seizure disorders, ulcerative colitis, CHF, myasthenia gravis, renal disease, esophagitis, peptic ulcer, cataracts, coagulopathy

PHARMACOKINETICS

PO: Well absorbed PO, peak 1-2 hr, duration 1-1½ days, half-life 3½-4 hr
Crosses placenta, enters breast milk, metabolized by liver after conversion, excreted in urine

INTERACTIONS

Increase: side effects—alcohol, salicylates, indomethacin, amphotericin B, digitalis, cycloSPORINE, diuretics
Increase: predniSONE action—salicylates, estrogens, indomethacin, oral contraceptives, ketoconazole, macrolide antiinfectives
Decrease: predniSONE action—cholestyramine, colestipol, barbiturates, rifampin, epHEDrine, phenytoin, theophylline
Decrease: effects of anticoagulants, anticonvulsants, antidiabetics, ambenonium, neostigmine, isoniazid, toxoids, vaccines, anticholinesterases, salicylates, somatrem

Drug/Herb
• Hypokalemia: aloe, buckthorn, Chinese rhubarb, senna
Increase: effect—aloe, licorice, perilla

Drug/Lab Test
Increase: Cholesterol, sodium, blood glucose, uric acid, calcium, urine glucose
Decrease: Calcium, potassium, T_4, T_3, thyroid ^{131}I uptake test, urine 17-OHCS, 17-KS, PBI
False negative: Skin allergy tests

NURSING CONSIDERATIONS

Assess:
• Adrenal insufficiency: nausea, vomiting, anorexia, confusion, hypotension
• Potassium, blood glucose, urine glucose while on long-term therapy; hypokalemia and hyperglycemia
• Weight daily; notify prescriber of weekly gain >5 lb
• B/P q4h, pulse; notify prescriber of chest pain; monitor for crackles, dyspnea if edema is present
• I&O ratio; be alert for decreasing urinary output, increasing edema

• Plasma cortisol (long-term therapy) (normal: 138-635 nmol/L SI units drawn at 8 AM)
• Infection: increased temp, WBC, even after withdrawal of medication; drug masks infection
• Potassium depletion: paresthesias, fatigue, nausea, vomiting, depression, polyuria, dysrhythmias, weakness
• Edema, hypertension, cardiac symptoms
• Mental status: affect, mood, behavioral changes, aggression

Administer:
• For long-term use, alternate-day therapy is recommended to decrease adverse reactions
• Titrated dose; use lowest effective dose
• With food or milk to decrease GI symptoms

Perform/provide:
• Assistance with ambulation to patient with bone tissue disease to prevent fractures

Evaluate:
• Therapeutic response: ease of respirations, decreased inflammation

Teach patient/family:
• That emergency ID as steroid user should be carried; information on drug being taken and condition
• To notify prescriber if therapeutic response decreases; dosage adjustment may be needed
• To avoid vaccinations
• Not to discontinue abruptly, or adrenal crisis can result
• To avoid OTC products: salicylates, cough products with alcohol, cold preparations unless directed by prescriber
• About cushingoid symptoms: moon face, weight gain
• That drug causes immunosuppression; to report any symptoms of infection (fever, sore throat, cough)
• The symptoms of adrenal insufficiency: nausea, anorexia, fatigue, dizziness, dyspnea, weakness, joint pain

pregabalin (℞)
(pre-gab′a-lin)
Lyrica
Func. class.: Anticonvulsant
Chem. class.: Gamma aminobutyric acid (GABA) analog

Controlled Substance Schedule V
Action: Binds to high-voltage–gated calcium channels in CNS tissues; this may lead to anticonvulsant action, similar to the inhibitory neurotransmitter GABA, anxiolytic, analgesics, and antiepileptic properties
Uses: Neuropathic pain associated with diabetic peripheral neuropathy, partial-onset seizures, postherpetic neuralgia
Unlabeled uses: Generalized anxiety disorder (GAD), moderate pain, social anxiety disorder

DOSAGE AND ROUTES
Diabetic peripheral neuropathic pain
• *Adult:* **PO** 50 mg tid, may increase to 300 mg/day (max) within 1 wk, adjust in renal disease
Partial-onset seizures
• *Adult:* **PO** 75 mg bid or 50 mg tid; may increase to 600 mg/day (max)
Postherpetic neuralgia
• *Adult:* **PO** 75-150 mg bid or 50-100 mg tid in patient with CCr ≥60 ml/min, initially give 75 mg bid or 50 mg tid and may increase to 600 mg/day (max) within 1 wk
Renal dose
• *Adult:* **PO** CCr 30-60 ml/min 75-300 mg/day in 2-3 divided doses; CCr 15-30 ml/min 25-150 mg/day in 1-2 divided doses; CCr <15 ml/min 25-75 mg/day in a single dose
Available forms: Caps 25, 50, 75, 100, 150, 200, 225, 300 mg

SIDE EFFECTS
CNS: Dizziness, fatigue, confusion, euphoria, incoordination, nervousness, neurop-athy, tremor, vertigo, somnolence, ataxia, amnesia, abnormal thinking
EENT: Dry mouth, blurred vision, nystagmus, amblyopia
GI: Constipation, flatulence, abdominal pain, weight gain
HEMA: Ecchymosis
MS: Back pain
OTHER: Pruritus, impotence
RESP: Dyspnea
Contraindications: Hypersensitivity, abrupt discontinuation
Precautions: Pregnancy (C), renal disease, lactation, children <12 yr, elderly, PR interval prolongation, creatine kinase elevations, CHF (class III, IV), decreased platelets, drug abuse, dependence, glaucoma, myopathy

PHARMACOKINETICS
Well absorbed, absorption decreased with food, 90% recovered in urine unchanged, negligible metabolism, not bound to plasma proteins, half-life 6 hr

INTERACTIONS
Increase: weight gain/fluid retention—thiazolidinedione, avoid use if possible
Increase: CNS depression—anxiolytics, sedatives, hypnotics, barbiturates, general anesthetics, opiate agonists, phenothiazines, sedating H_1 blockers, thiazolidinediones, tricyclic antidepressants
Drug/Lab Test
Increase: Creatine kinase
Decrease: Platelets

NURSING CONSIDERATIONS
Assess:
• Seizures: aura, location, duration, activity at onset
• Pain: location, duration, characteristics if using for diabetic neuropathy
• Renal studies: urinalysis, BUN, urine creatinine q3mo, creatine kinase; if markedly increased, discontinue
• Mental status: mood, sensorium, affect, behavioral changes; if mental status changes, notify prescriber

Side effects: *italics* = common; **bold** = life-threatening

Administer:
- Do not crush or chew caps; caps may be opened and contents put in applesauce or dissolved in juice
- Give without regard to meals
- Gradually withdraw over 7 days; abrupt withdrawal may precipitate seizures

Perform/provide:
- Storage at room temperature away from heat and light
- Hard candy, frequent rinsing of mouth, gum for dry mouth
- Assistance with ambulation during early part of treatment; dizziness occurs
- Seizure precautions: padded side rails; move objects that may harm patient
- Increased fluids, bulk in diet for constipation

Evaluate:
- Therapeutic response: decreased seizure activity; decrease in neuropathic pain

Teach patient/family:
- To carry emergency ID stating patient's name, drugs taken, condition, prescriber's name, and phone number
- To avoid driving, other activities that require alertness: dizziness, drowsiness may occur
- Not to discontinue medication quickly after long-term use, taper over ≥1 wk; withdrawal-precipitated seizures may occur, not to double doses if dose is missed, take if 2 hr or more before next dose
- To notify prescriber if pregnancy planned or suspected; avoid breastfeeding
- To report muscle pain, tenderness, weakness, when accompanied by fever, malaise
- To avoid alcohol

Treatment of overdose: Lavage, VS, hemodialysis

---

primaquine (℞)
(prim′a-kween)
Func. class.: Antimalarial
Chem. class.: Synthetic 8-amino-quinolone

Action: Unknown; thought to destroy exoerythrocytic forms by gametocidal action

Uses: Malaria caused by *Plasmodium vivax,* in combination with clindamycin for *Pneumocystis jiroveci* pneumonia

DOSAGE AND ROUTES
- *Adult:* **PO** 15 mg (base) daily × 2 wk; 26.3-mg tab is 15-mg base
- *Child:* **PO** 0.5 mg/kg (0.3 mg/base/day) daily × 2 wk

Available forms: Tabs 26.3 mg, powder

SIDE EFFECTS
CNS: Headache, dizziness
CV: Hypertension
EENT: Blurred vision, difficulty focusing
GI: Nausea, vomiting, anorexia, cramps
HEMA: **Agranulocytosis, granulocytopenia, leukopenia, hemolytic anemia, leukocytosis,** mild anemia, **methemoglobinemia**
INTEG: Pruritus, skin eruptions, pallor, weakness

Contraindications: Hypersensitivity, anemia, lupus erythematosus, methemoglobinemia, porphyria, rheumatoid arthritis, methemoglobin reductase deficiency, G6PD deficiency, iodine hypersensitivity

Precautions: Pregnancy (C), bone marrow suppression, lactation, children

PHARMACOKINETICS
PO: Metabolized by liver (metabolites), half-life 3.7-9.6 hr

INTERACTIONS
- Toxicity: quinacrine

⚠ Safety alert   *"Tall Man" lettering

NURSING CONSIDERATIONS
Assess:
• Ophthalmic test if long-term treatment or drug dosage >150 mg/day
• Hepatic studies qwk: AST, ALT, bilirubin, if on long-term therapy
• Blood studies: CBC; blood dyscrasias occur
• Allergic reactions: pruritus, rash, urticaria
• Blood dyscrasias: malaise, fever, bruising, bleeding (rare)
• For renal status: dark urine, hematuria, decreased output
⚠ For hemolytic reaction: chills, fever, chest pain, cyanosis; drug should be discontinued immediately
Administer:
PO route
• Before or after meals at same time each day to maintain drug level; take with food to decrease GI upset
Evaluate:
• Therapeutic response: decreased symptoms of malaria
Teach patient/family:
• To report visual problems, fever, fatigue, dark urine, bruising, bleeding; may indicate blood dyscrasias
• To complete full course of therapy

---

primidone (℞)
(pri′mi-done)
Apo-Primidone ♣, Mysoline, PMS-Primidone ♣, primidone, Sertan ♣
Func. class.: Anticonvulsant
Chem. class.: Barbiturate derivative

Action: Raises seizure threshold by conversion of drug to phenobarbital, decreases neuron firing
Uses: Generalized tonic-clonic (grand mal), complex-partial psychomotor seizures, essential tremors

DOSAGE AND ROUTES
• *Adult and child >8 yr:* **PO** 100-125 mg at bedtime on days 1, 2, 3; then 100-125 mg bid on days 4, 5, 6; then 100-125 mg tid on days 7, 8, 9; then maintenance 250 mg tid-qid, max 2 g/day in divided doses
• *Child <8 yr:* **PO** 50 mg at bedtime on days 1, 2, 3; then 50 mg bid on days 4, 5, 6; then 100 mg bid on days 7, 8, 9; maintenance 125-250 mg tid or 10-25 mg/kg/day in divided doses
Available forms: Tabs 50, 250 mg; susp 250 mg/5 ml; chew tabs 125 mg ♣

SIDE EFFECTS
CNS: Stimulation, drowsiness, irritability, psychosis, ataxia, vertigo, fatigue, emotional disturbances, mood changes, paranoia
EENT: Diplopia, nystagmus, edema of eyelids
GI: Nausea, vomiting, anorexia, **hepatitis**
GU: Impotence
HEMA: **Thrombocytopenia, leukopenia, neutropenia, eosinophilia, megaloblastic anemia,** decreased serum folate level, lymphadenopathy
INTEG: Rash, edema, alopecia, lupuslike syndrome
Contraindications: Pregnancy (D), hypersensitivity, porphyria
Precautions: COPD, renal/hepatic disease, hyperactive children

PHARMACOKINETICS
PO: Peak 4 hr; excreted by kidneys, in breast milk; half-life 3-12 hr

INTERACTIONS
• Primidone levels are decreased by acetaZOLAMIDE, succinimides, carbamazepine
• May decrease effect of oral contraceptives, acebutolol, metoprolol, propranolol, tricyclics, phenothiazines
Increase: primidone levels—alcohol, heparin, CNS depressants, hydantoins, isoniazid, nicotinamide, phenytoin, phenobarbital

Side effects: *italics* = common; **bold** = life-threatening

Drug/Herb
Increase: effect—ginkgo
Decrease: effect—ginseng, santonica

NURSING CONSIDERATIONS
Assess:
• For seizures: location, duration, type; folic acid deficiency; fatigue, weakness, neuropathy, depression
• Drug level: therapeutic level 5-15 mcg/ml; CBC should be done q6mo
• Mental status: mood, sensorium, affect, memory (long, short)
• Respiratory depression, wheezing
• Blood dyscrasias: fever, sore throat, bruising, rash, jaundice

Administer:
PO route
• After shaking liquid susp well
• With food for GI upset
• Tablets crushed and mixed with food or fluid for swallowing difficulties
• Avoid use with CNS depressants

Evaluate:
• Therapeutic response: decreased seizures

Teach patient/family:
• Not to withdraw drug quickly; withdrawal symptoms may occur
• To avoid hazardous activities until stabilized on drug; drowsiness, dizziness may occur
• To carry emergency ID with condition and medication
• To recognize the signs of blood dyscrasias; when to notify prescriber
• To avoid alcohol

---

probenecid (℞)
(proe-ben′e-sid)
Benemid, Benuryl ✦, probenecid
Func. class.: Uricosuric, antigout agent
Chem. class.: Sulfonamide derivative

Action: Inhibits tubular reabsorption of urates, with increased excretion of uric acids

Uses: Hyperuricemia in gout, gouty arthritis, adjunct to cephalosporin, cidofovir, or penicillin treatment

DOSAGE AND ROUTES
Gonorrhea
• *Adult:* **PO** 1 g with 3.5 g ampicillin or 1 g ½ hr before 4.8 million units of aqueous penicillin G procaine injected into 2 sites **IM**

Gout/gouty arthritis
• *Adult:* **PO** 250 mg bid for 1 wk, then 500 mg bid, not to exceed 2 g/day; maintenance: 500 mg/day × 6 mo

Adjunct in penicillin/cephalosporin treatment
• *Adult and child >50 kg:* **PO** 500 mg qid
• *Child <50 kg:* **PO** 25 mg/kg, then 40 mg/kg in divided doses qid

Minimize nephrotoxicity in cidofovir therapy
• *Adult:* **PO** 2 g 3 hr prior to cidofovir dose, followed by 1 g at 2 and 8 hr after end of cidofovir infusion

Renal dose
• Avoid use if CCr <50 ml/min

Available forms: Tabs 0.5 g

SIDE EFFECTS
CNS: Drowsiness, headache
CV: Bradycardia
GI: Gastric irritation, nausea, vomiting, anorexia, **hepatic necrosis**
GU: Glycosuria, thirst, frequency, **nephrotic syndrome**
INTEG: Rash, dermatitis, pruritus, fever
META: Acidosis, hypokalemia, hyperchloremia, hyperglycemia
RESP: **Apnea,** irregular respirations

Contraindications: Hypersensitivity, severe renal/hepatic disease, CCr <50 mg/min, history of uric acid calculus

Precautions: Pregnancy (B), child <2 yr

PHARMACOKINETICS
PO: Peak 2-4 hr, duration 8 hr, half-life 5-8 hr; metabolized by liver; excreted in urine

---

⚠ Safety alert   ✦"Tall Man" lettering

INTERACTIONS

Increase: effect of acyclovir, barbiturates, allopurinol, benzodiazepines, dyphylline, zidovudine

Increase: toxicity—sulfa drugs, dapsone, clofibrate, indomethacin, rifampin, naproxen, methotrexate

Decrease: action of probenecid—salicylates

Drug/Lab Test

Increase: BSP/urinary PSP, theophylline levels

False positive: Urine glucose with copper sulfate test (Clinitest)

NURSING CONSIDERATIONS

Assess:
• Uric acid levels (3-7 mg/dl); mobility, joint pain, swelling
• Respiratory rate, rhythm, depth; notify prescriber of abnormalities
• Electrolytes, CO_2 before, during treatment
• Urine pH, output, glucose during beginning treatment

⚠ For CNS symptoms: confusion, twitching, hyperreflexia, stimulation, headache; may indicate overdose

Administer:
• After meals or with milk if GI symptoms occur
• Increase fluid intake to 2-3 L/day to prevent urinary calculi

Evaluate:
• Therapeutic response: absence of pain, stiffness in joints

Teach patient/family:
• To avoid OTC preparations (aspirin) unless directed by prescriber; increase water intake, avoid alcohol, caffeine

---

procainamide (R)
(proe-kane-ah'mide)
procainamide, Procanbid, Promine, Pronestyl, Pronestyl-SR
Func. class.: Antidysrhythmic (Class IA)
Chem. class.: Procaine HCl amide analog

Action: Depresses excitability of cardiac muscle to electrical stimulation and slows conduction in atrium, bundle of His, and ventricle increases refractory period

Uses: Life-threatening ventricular dysrhythmias

DOSAGE AND ROUTES

Atrial fibrillation/PAT
• *Adult:* PO 1-1.25 g; may give another 750 mg if needed; if no response, 500 mg-1 g q2h until desired response; maintenance 50 mg/kg in divided doses q6h

Ventricular tachycardia
• *Adult:* PO 1 g; maintenance 50 mg/kg/day given in 3-hr intervals; SUS REL 500 mg-1.25 g q6h

Other dysrhythmias
• *Adult:* IV BOL 100 mg q5min, given 25-50 mg/min, not to exceed 500 mg; or 17 mg/kg total then IV INF 2-6 mg/min

Renal dose
• *Adult:* IV CCr 10-50 ml/min give q6-12h; CCr <10 ml/min give q8-24h

Available forms: Caps 250, 375, 500 mg; tabs 250, 375, 500 mg; sus rel tabs 500, 750, 1000 mg; inj 100, 500 mg/ml

SIDE EFFECTS

CNS: Headache, dizziness, confusion, psychosis, restlessness, irritability, weakness

CV: Hypotension, **heart block, cardiovascular collapse, arrest**

GI: Nausea, vomiting, anorexia, diarrhea, hepatomegaly, pain, bitter taste

HEMA: SLE syndrome, **agranulocytosis, thrombocytopenia, neutropenia, hemolytic anemia**

P

INTEG: Rash, urticaria, edema, swelling (rare), pruritus, flushing

Contraindications: Hypersensitivity, severe heart block, lupus erythematosus, torsades de pointes

Precautions: Pregnancy (C), lactation, children, renal/hepatic disease, CHF, respiratory depression, cytopenia, bone marrow failure, dysrhythmia associated with digoxin toxicity, myasthenia gravis, digoxin toxicity

PHARMACOKINETICS

PO: Peak 1-2 hr, duration 3 hr (8 hr extended)

IM: Peak 10-60 min, duration 3 hr; half-life 3 hr

Metabolized in liver to active metabolites, excreted unchanged by kidneys (60%)

INTERACTIONS

Increase: effects of neuromuscular blockers

Increase: procainamide effects—cimetidine, quinidine, trimethoprim, β-blockers, ranitidine

Increase: toxicity—other antidysrhythmics, thioridazine, quinolones

Drug/Herb

Increase: anticholinergic effect—henbane

Increase: toxicity, death—aconite

Increase: effect—aloe, broom, chronic buckthorn use, cascara sagrada (chronic use), Chinese rhubarb, figwort, fumitory, goldenseal, kudzu, licorice

Increase: serotonin effect—horehound

Decrease: effect—coltsfoot

Drug/Lab Test

Increase: ALT, AST, alk phos, LDH, bilirubin

NURSING CONSIDERATIONS

Assess:

⚠ ECG continuously if using IV to determine increased PR or QRS segments; discontinue immediately; watch for increased ventricular ectopic beats, maximum need to rebolus

• Blood levels, 3-10 mcg/ml or NAPA levels 10-20 mcg/ml

⚠ CBC q2wk × 3 mo; leukocyte, neutrophil, platelet counts may be decreased, treatment may need to be discontinued

• I&O ratio; electrolytes (K, Na, Cl), weigh weekly, report gain >2 lb

⚠ Toxicity: confusion, drowsiness, nausea, vomiting, tachydysrhythmias, oliguria

• ANA titer, during long-term treatment, watch for lupuslike symptoms

• Cardiac rate, rhythm, character, B/P continuously for fluctuations

• Respiratory status: rate, rhythm, character, lung fields; bilateral crackles may occur in CHF patient; watch for respiratory depression

⚠ CNS effects: dizziness, confusion, psychosis, paresthesias, seizures; drug should be discontinued

Administer:

PO route

• Do not break, crush, or chew sus rel tabs

IM route

• IM inj in deltoid; aspirate to avoid intravascular administration

IV route

• After diluting 100 mg/ml of D_5W or sterile H_2O for inj; give 20 mg or less/1 min; may dilute 1 g/250-500 ml D_5W, run at 2-6 mg/min

• Check IV site q8h for infiltration or extravasation

Additive compatibilities: Amiodarone, atracurium, DOBUTamine, flumazenil, lidocaine, netilmicin, verapamil

Solution compatibilities: D_5W, D_5/0.9% NaCl, 0.45% NaCl, 0.9% NaCl, water for inj

Y-site compatibilities: Amiodarone, cisatracurium, famotidine, heparin, hydrocortisone, potassium chloride, ranitidine, remifentanil, vit B/C

Evaluate:

• Therapeutic response: decreased dysrhythmias

Teach patient/family:

• That wax matrix may appear in stools

• Not to discontinue without health-care provider's advice

⚠ Safety alert   *"Tall Man" lettering

To notify prescriber immediately if lupuslike symptoms appear (joint pain, butterfly rash, fever, chills, dyspnea)

To notify prescriber of leukopenia (sore mouth, gums, throat) or thrombocytopenia (bleeding, bruising)

• How to take pulse and when to report to prescriber

Treatment of overdose: O$_2$, artificial ventilation, ECG, administer DOPamine for circulatory depression, diazepam or thiopental for seizures, isoproterenol

---

procaine (℞)
(proe′kane)
Novocain, Unicaine
Func. class.: Local anesthetic
Chem. class.: Ester

Action: Competes with calcium for sites in nerve membrane that control sodium transport across cell membrane; decreases rise of depolarization phase of action potential

Uses: Spinal anesthesia, epidural, peripheral nerve block, perineum, lower extremities, infiltration

DOSAGE AND ROUTES

Spinal anesthesia
• *Adult:* 100 mg
Perineum anesthesia
• *Adult:* 50 mg
Available forms: Inj 1%, 2%, 10%

SIDE EFFECTS

CNS: Anxiety, restlessness, **seizures, loss of consciousness,** drowsiness, disorientation, tremors, shivering

CV: **Myocardial depression, cardiac arrest, dysrhythmias,** bradycardia, hypotension, hypertension, fetal bradycardia

EENT: Blurred vision, tinnitus, pupil constriction

GI: Nausea, vomiting

INTEG: Rash, urticaria, allergic reactions, edema, burning, skin discoloration at inj site, tissue necrosis

RESP: **Status asthmaticus, respiratory arrest, anaphylaxis**

Contraindications: Hypersensitivity, sulfite allergy, myasthenia gravis, child <12 yr, severe hepatic disease

Precautions: Pregnancy (C), geriatric, severe drug allergies

PHARMACOKINETICS

Onset 2-5 min, duration 1 hr; metabolized by liver, excreted in urine (metabolites)

INTERACTIONS

• Dysrhythmias: epINEPHrine, halothane, enflurane
• Hypertension: MAOIs, tricyclics, phenothiazines

Decrease: action of aminosalicylic acid, sulfonamides

Decrease: action of procaine—chloroprocaine

NURSING CONSIDERATIONS

Assess:
• B/P, pulse, respiration during treatment
• Fetal heart tones if drug is used during labor
• Allergic reactions: rash, urticaria, itching
• Cardiac status: ECG for dysrhythmias, pulse, B/P during anesthesia

Administer:
• Only drugs that are not cloudy, do not contain precipitate
• Only with crash cart, resuscitative equipment nearby
• Only drugs without preservatives for epidural or caudal anesthesia

Additive compatibilities: Ascorbic acid, hydrocortisone, penicillin G, penicillin G sodium, vit B/C

Syringe compatibilities: Ampicillin, cloxacillin, glycopyrrolate, hydroxyzine, gentamicin

Solution compatibilities: D$_5$, D$_{10}$, NS, LR, Y$_2$, NS

Perform/provide:
• Use of new sol; discard unused portions, protect from light

P

Evaluate:
• Therapeutic response: anesthesia necessary for procedure

Treatment of overdose: Airway, O_2, vasopressor, IV fluids, anticonvulsants for seizures

---

procarbazine (Ᵽ)
(proe-kar′ba-zeen)
Matulane, Natulan ✚
Func. class.: Antineoplastic, alkylating agent
Chem. class.: Hydrazine derivative

Action: Inhibits DNA, RNA, protein synthesis; has multiple sites of action; a nonvesicant

Uses: Lymphoma, Hodgkin's disease, cancers resistant to other therapy

Unlabeled uses: Brain, lung malignancies, other lymphomas, multiple myeloma, malignant melanoma, polycythemia vera

DOSAGE AND ROUTES

• *Adult:* PO 2-4 mg/kg/day for first wk; maintain dosage of 4-6 mg/kg/day until platelets and WBC fall; after recovery, 1-2 mg/kg/day

• *Child:* PO 50 mg/m²/day for 7 days, then 100 mg/m² until desired response, leukopenia, or thrombocytopenia occurs; 50 mg/day is maintenance after bone marrow recovery

Available forms: Caps 50 mg

SIDE EFFECTS

CNS: Headache, dizziness, insomnia, hallucinations, confusion, **coma**, pain, chills, fever, sweating, paresthesias, **seizures**
EENT: Retinal hemorrhage, nystagmus, photophobia, diplopia
GI: Nausea, vomiting, anorexia, diarrhea, constipation, dry mouth, stomatitis
GU: Azoospermia, cessation of menses
HEMA: **Thrombocytopenia, anemia, leukopenia, myelosuppression, bleeding tendencies,** purpura, petechiae, epistaxis

INTEG: Rash, pruritus, dermatitis, alopecia, herpes, hyperpigmentation
MS: Arthralgias, myalgias
RESP: Cough, pneumonitis

Contraindications: Pregnancy (D), hypersensitivity, thrombocytopenia, bone marrow depression, lactation

Precautions: Renal/hepatic disease, radiation therapy

PHARMACOKINETICS

Half-life 1 hr; concentrates in liver, kidney, skin; metabolized in liver, excreted in urine

INTERACTIONS

• Hypotension: meperidine, do not use together
• Disulfiram-like reaction: alcohol, MAOIs, tricyclics, tyramine foods, sympathomimetic drugs
• Hypertension: guanethidine, levodopa, methyldopa, reserpine, caffeine
⚠ Life-threatening hypertension: sympathomimetics
Increase: hypoglycemia—insulin, oral hypoglycemics
Increase: CNS depression—barbiturates, antihistamines, opioids, hypotensive agents, phenothiazines
Drug/Food
• Hypertensive crisis: tyramine foods

NURSING CONSIDERATIONS

Assess:
• CBC, differential, platelet count qwk; withhold drug if WBC is <4000/mm³ or platelet count is <100,000/mm³; notify prescriber
• Renal studies: BUN, serum uric acid, urine CCr, electrolytes before, during therapy
• I&O ratio, report fall in urine output to <30 ml/hr
• Monitor temp q4h; fever may indicate beginning infection
• Hepatic studies before, during therapy: bilirubin, AST, ALT, alk phos prn or qmo

---

⚠ Safety alert   *"Tall Man" lettering

- CNS changes: confusion, paresthesias, neuropathies, drug should be discontinued

⚠ For tyramine foods in diet, hypertensive crisis can occur

⚠ Toxicity: facial flushing, epistaxis, increased PT, thrombocytopenia; drug should be discontinued

- Bleeding: hematuria, guaiac stools, bruising or petechiae, mucosa or orifices q8h
- Effects of alopecia on body image; discuss feelings about body changes
- Jaundiced skin, sclera; dark urine, clay-colored stools, itchy skin, abdominal pain, fever, diarrhea
- Buccal cavity q8h for dryness, sores or ulceration, white patches, oral pain, bleeding, dysphagia
- Alkalosis if vomiting is severe
- GI symptoms: frequency of stools, cramping
- Acidosis, signs of dehydration: rapid respirations, poor skin turgor, decreased urine output, dry skin, restlessness, weakness

Administer:
- In divided doses and at bedtime to minimize nausea and vomiting
- Nonphenothiazine antiemetic 30-60 min before giving drug and 4-10 hr after treatment to prevent vomiting
- Transfusion for anemia
- Antispasmodic for GI symptoms

Perform/provide:
- Liquid diet: carbonated beverages; gelatin may be added if patient is not nauseated or vomiting
- Storage in tight, light-resistant container in cool environment

Evaluate:
- Therapeutic response: decreased tumor size, spread of malignancy

Teach patient/family:
- To report any complaints, side effects to nurse or prescriber; cough, shortness of breath, fever, chills, sore throat, bleeding, bruising, vomiting blood; black, tarry stools
- That hair may be lost during treatment and wig or hairpiece may make patient

feel better; tell patient that new hair may be different in color, texture
- To avoid sunlight or UV exposure, wear sunscreen or protective clothing
- To avoid foods with citric acid, hot, or rough texture
- To report any bleeding, white spots, ulcerations in mouth to prescriber; tell patient to examine mouth daily
- To avoid driving, activities requiring alertness; dizziness may occur
- To use effective contraception, avoid breastfeeding
- To avoid ingestion of alcohol, caffeine, tyramine-containing foods; cold, hay fever, weight-reducing products may cause serious drug interactions
- To avoid crowds, persons with infections if granulocytes are low

prochlorperazine (℞)
(proe-klor-pair'a-zeen)
Chlorpazine, Compa-Z, Compazine, Contranzine, Provacin ✦, Stemetil ✦, Ultrazine
Func. class.: Antiemetic, antipsychotic
Chem. class.: Phenothiazine, piperazine derivative

Do not confuse:
prochlorperazine/chlorproMAZINE
Compazine/Coumadin
Action: Acts centrally by blocking chemoreceptor trigger zone, which in turn acts on vomiting center
Uses: Nausea, vomiting, psychotic disorders

DOSAGE AND ROUTES
Postoperative nausea/vomiting
- *Adult:* **IM** 5-10 mg 1-2 hr before anesthesia; may repeat in 30 min; **IV** 5-10 mg 15-30 min before anesthesia; **IV INF** 20 mg/L D₅W or NS 15-30 min before anesthesia, not to exceed 40 mg/day

Severe nausea/vomiting
- *Adult:* PO 5-10 mg tid-qid; **SUS REL** 15 mg daily in AM or 10 mg q12h; **RECT** 25 mg/bid; **IM** 5-10 mg; may repeat q4h, not to exceed 40 mg/day
- *Child 18-39 kg:* PO 2.5 mg tid or 5 mg bid, not to exceed 15 mg/day; **IM** 0.132 mg/kg
- *Child 14-17 kg:* **PO/RECT** 2.5 mg bid-tid, not to exceed 10 mg/day; **IM** 0.132 mg/kg
- *Child 9-13 kg:* **PO/RECT** 2.5 mg daily-bid, not to exceed 7.5 mg/day; **IM** 0.132 mg/kg

Antipsychotic
- *Adult and child ≥12 yr:* PO 5-10 mg tid-qid; may increase q2-3d, max 150 mg/day; **IM** 10-20 mg q2-4h up to 4 doses, then 10-20 mg q4-6h, max 200 mg/day; **RECT** 10 mg tid-qid, may increase by 5-10 mg q2-3d as needed
- *Child 2-12 yr:* PO 2.5 mg bid-tid; **IM** 0.132 mg/kg

Antianxiety
- *Adult and child ≥12 yr:* 5 mg tid-qid, max 20 mg/day or >12 wk; **IM** 5-10 mg q3-4h, max 40 mg/day; **IV** 2.5-10 mg; max 40 mg/day
- *Child 2-12 yr:* **IM** 132 mcg/kg

Available forms: Syr 5 mg/ml; inj 5 mg/ml; tabs 5, 10, 25 mg; sus rel caps 10, 15 mg; supp 2.5, 5, 25 mg

SIDE EFFECTS

CNS: **Neuroleptic malignant syndrome,** *extrapyramidal reactions, tardive dyskinesia, euphoria,* **depression,** drowsiness, restlessness, tremor, dizziness

CV: **Circulatory failure, tachycardia**

EENT: Blurred vision

GI: Nausea, vomiting, anorexia, dry mouth, diarrhea, constipation, weight loss, metallic taste, cramps

HEMA: **Agranulocytosis**

RESP: **Respiratory depression**

Contraindications: Hypersensitivity to phenothiazines, coma, seizure, encephalopathy, bone marrow depression, narrow-angle glaucoma

Precautions: Pregnancy (C), children <2 yr, geriatric, lactation

PHARMACOKINETICS

PO: Onset 30-40 min, duration 3-4 hr
SUS REL: Onset 30-40 min, duration 10-12 hr
RECT: Onset 60 min, duration 3-4 hr
IM: Onset 10-20 min, duration 12 hr
Metabolized by liver; excreted in urine, breast milk; crosses placenta

INTERACTIONS

Increase: anticholinergic action—anticholinergics, antiparkinson drugs, antidepressants

Decrease: prochlorperazine effect—barbiturates, antacids

Drug/Herb

Increase: CNS depression—chamomile, cola nut, hops, kava, nettle, nutmeg, skullcap, valerian

Increase: anticholinergic effect—henbane, jimsonweed, scopolia

Increase: EPS—betel palm, kava

Drug/Lab Test

Increase: LFTs, cardiac enzymes, cholesterol, blood glucose, prolactin, bilirubin, PBI, ^{131}I, alk phos, leukocytes, granulocytes, platelets

Decrease: Hormones (blood and urine)

False-positive: Pregnancy tests, urine bilirubin

False-negative: Urinary steroids, 17-OHCS, pregnancy tests

NURSING CONSIDERATIONS

Assess:
- EPS: abnormal movement, tardive dyskinesia, akathisia
- VS, B/P; check patients with cardiac disease more often
- ⚠ For neuroleptic malignant syndrome: seizures, hyper/hypotension, fever, tachycardia, dyspnea, fatigue, muscle stiffness, loss of bladder control; notify prescriber immediately
- ⚠ CBC, LFTs during course of treatment, blood dyscrasias, hepatotoxicity may occur

---

• Respiratory status before, during, after administration of emetic; check rate, rhythm, character; respiratory depression can occur rapidly with geriatric or debilitated patients

Administer:
• Avoid other CNS depressants

IM route
• IM inj in large muscle mass; aspirate to avoid IV administration
• Keep patient recumbent for ½ hr

IV route
• IV after diluting 5 mg/9 ml of NaCl for inj (0.5 mg/ml); give 5 mg or less/min; may dilute 10-20 mg/L NaCl and give as infusion; can cause contact dermatitis

Additive compatibilities: Amikacin, ascorbic acid, dexamethasone, dimenhyDRINATE, erythromycin, ethacrynate, lidocaine, nafcillin, sodium bicarbonate, vit B/C

Syringe compatibilities: Atropine, butorphanol, chlorproMAZINE, cimetidine, diamorphine, diphenhydrAMINE, droperidol, fentanyl, glycopyrrolate, hydrOXYzine, meperidine, metoclopramide, nalbuphine, pentazocine, perphenazine, promazine, promethazine, ranitidine, scopolamine, sufentanil

Y-site compatibilities: Amsacrine, calcium gluconate, cisatracurium, cisplatin, cladribine, cyclophosphamide, cytarabine, DOXOrubicin, DOXOrubicin liposome, fluconazole, granisetron, heparin, hydrocortisone, melphalan, methotrexate, ondansetron, paclitaxel, potassium chloride, propofol, remifentanil, sargramostim, sufentanil, teniposide, thiotepa, vinorelbine, vit B/C

Evaluate:
• Therapeutic response: absence of nausea, vomiting; reduced anxiety, agitation, excitability

Teach patient/family:
• To avoid hazardous activities, activities requiring alertness; dizziness may occur
• To avoid alcohol
• Not to double or skip doses
• That urine may be pink to reddish brown

• To report dark urine, clay-colored stools, bleeding, bruising, rash, blurred vision
• To avoid sun or wear sunscreen, protective clothing

---

progesterone (℞)
(proe-jess'ter-one)
Crinone, progesterone, Prochieve, Prometrium
Func. class.: Progestogen
Chem. class.: Progesterone derivative

Action: Inhibits secretion of pituitary gonadotropins, which prevents follicular maturation, ovulation; stimulates growth of mammary tissue; antineoplastic action against endometrial cancer

Uses: Contraception, amenorrhea, premenstrual syndrome, abnormal uterine bleeding, endometrial hyperplasia prevention, assisted reproductive technology (ART) gel

DOSAGE AND ROUTES
Infertility
• *Adult:* **VAG** 90 mg daily
Amenorrhea/functional uterine bleeding
• *Adult:* **IM** 5-10 mg daily × 6-8 doses
Endometrial hyperplasia prevention
• *Adult:* **PO** 200 mg/day × 12 days
ART
• *Adult:* **GEL** 90 mg (8%) vaginally daily, for supplementation; 90 mg (8%) vaginally bid for replacement, if pregnancy occurs continue × 10-12 wk

Available forms: Inj 50 mg/ml; vag gel 4%, 8%; caps 100, 200 mg

SIDE EFFECTS
CNS: Dizziness, headache, migraines, depression, fatigue
CV: Hypotension, **thrombophlebitis,** edema, **thromboembolism, stroke, pulmonary embolism, MI**
EENT: Diplopia, retinal thrombosis
GI: Nausea, vomiting, anorexia, cramps, increased weight, **cholestatic jaundice**

Side effects: *italics* = common; **bold** = life-threatening

GU: Amenorrhea, cervical erosion, breakthrough bleeding, dysmenorrhea, vaginal candidiasis, breast changes, *gynecomastia, testicular atrophy, impotence,* endometriosis, **spontaneous abortion**

INTEG: Rash, urticaria, acne, hirsutism, alopecia, oily skin, seborrhea, purpura, melasma

META: Hyperglycemia

SYST: **Angioedema, anaphylaxis**

Contraindications: Pregnancy (D), breast cancer, hypersensitivity, thromboembolic disorders, reproductive cancer, genital bleeding (abnormal, undiagnosed), cerebral hemorrhage

Precautions: Lactation, hypertension, asthma, blood dyscrasias, gallbladder disease, CHF, diabetes mellitus, bone disease, depression, migraine headache, convulsive disorders, renal/hepatic disease, family history of breast or reproductive tract cancer

PHARMACOKINETICS

IM, RECT, VAG: Duration 24 hr
Excreted in urine, feces; metabolized in liver

INTERACTIONS

Decrease: progesterone effect—barbiturates, phenytoin

Drug/Herb
Increase: hormonal effect—alfalfa

Drug/Lab Test
Increase: Alk phos, nitrogen (urine), pregnanediol, amino acids, factors VII, VIII, IX, X
Decrease: GTT, HDL

NURSING CONSIDERATIONS

Assess:
• Weight daily; notify prescriber of weekly weight gain >5 lb
• B/P at beginning of treatment and periodically
• I&O ratio; be alert for decreasing urinary output, increasing edema

• Hepatic studies: ALT, AST, bilirubin periodically during long-term therapy
• Edema, hypertension, cardiac symptoms, jaundice, thromboembolism
• Mental status: affect, mood, behavioral changes, depression
• Hypercalcemia

Administer:
• Do not break, crush, or chew caps
• Titrated dose; use lowest effective dose
• After warming to dissolve crystals
• In one dose in AM
• With food or milk to decrease GI symptoms

Perform/provide:
• Storage in dark area

Evaluate:
• Therapeutic response: decreased abnormal uterine bleeding, absence of amenorrhea

Teach patient/family:
⚠ To report breast lumps, vaginal bleeding, edema, jaundice, dark urine, clay-colored stools, dyspnea, headache, blurred vision, abdominal pain, numbness or stiffness in legs, chest pain
• To report suspected pregnancy
• To monitor blood glucose if diabetic

---

promethazine (℞)
(proe-meth′a-zeen)
Histanil ✦, Phenadoz, Phenergan, promethazine HCl
Func. class.: Antihistamine, H_1-receptor antagonist
Chem. class.: Phenothiazine derivative

Do not confuse:
Phenergan/Theragran

Action: Acts on blood vessels, GI, respiratory system by competing with histamine for H_1-receptor site; decreases allergic response by blocking histamine

Uses: Motion sickness, rhinitis, allergy symptoms, sedation, nausea, preoperative and postoperative sedation

---

⚠ Safety alert   *"Tall Man" lettering

DOSAGE AND ROUTES
Nausea
• *Adult:* **PO/IM/IV/REC** 12.5-25 mg; q4-6h prn
• *Child >2 yr:* **PO/IM/IV/REC** 0.25-0.5 mg/kg q4-6h prn
Motion sickness
• *Adult:* **PO** 25 mg bid, give ½-1 hr before departure and q8-12h prn
• *Child >2 yr:* **PO/IM/RECT** 12.5-25 mg bid, give ½-1 hr before departure and q8-12h prn
Allergy/rhinitis
• *Adult:* **PO** 12.5 mg qid, or 25 mg at bedtime
• *Child >2 yr:* **PO** 6.25-12.5 mg tid or 25 mg at bedtime
Sedation
• *Adult:* **PO/IM** 25-50 mg at bedtime
• *Child >2 yr:* **PO/IM/RECT** 12.5-25 mg at bedtime
Sedation (preoperative/postoperative)
• *Adult:* **PO/IM/IV** 25-50 mg
• *Child >2 yr:* **PO/IM/IV** 0.5-1.1 mg/kg
Available forms: Tabs 12.5, 25, 50 mg; supp 12.5, 25 mg; inj 25, 50 mg/ml, syr 6.25 mg/5 ml

SIDE EFFECTS
CNS: Dizziness, drowsiness, poor coordination, fatigue, anxiety, euphoria, confusion, paresthesia, neuritis, EPS, **neuroleptic malignant syndrome**
CV: Hypotension, palpitations, tachycardia
EENT: Blurred vision, dilated pupils, tinnitus, nasal stuffiness; dry nose, throat, mouth; photosensitivity
GI: Constipation, dry mouth, nausea, vomiting, anorexia, diarrhea
GU: Urinary retention, dysuria, frequency
HEMA: **Thrombocytopenia, agranulocytosis, hemolytic anemia**
INTEG: Rash, urticaria, photosensitivity
RESP: Increased thick secretions, wheezing, chest tightness, **apnea in neonates, infants, young children**

Contraindications: Hypersensitivity to H_1-receptor antagonist, acute asthma attack, lower respiratory tract disease; sulfite allergy, child <2 yr
Precautions: Pregnancy (C), increased intraocular pressure, renal/cardiac disease, hypertension, bronchial asthma, seizure disorder, stenosed peptic ulcers, hyperthyroidism, prostatic hypertrophy, bladder neck obstruction

PHARMACOKINETICS
PO: Onset 20 min, duration 4-12 hr
IV: Onset 3-5 min
Metabolized in liver; excreted by kidneys, GI tract (inactive metabolites)

INTERACTIONS
Increase: CNS depression—barbiturates, opioids, hypnotics, tricyclics, alcohol
Increase: promethazine effect—MAOIs
Decrease: oral anticoagulants effect—heparin
Drug/Herb
Increase: anticholinergic effect—henbane, jimsonweed, scopolia
Drug/Lab Test
False negative: Skin allergy test
False positive: Urine pregnancy test

NURSING CONSIDERATIONS
Assess:
• I&O ratio; be alert for urinary retention, frequency, dysuria; drug should be discontinued
⚠ CBC during long-term therapy; blood dyscrasias may occur
• Respiratory status: rate, rhythm, increase in bronchial secretions, wheezing, chest tightness
• Cardiac status: palpitations, increased pulse, hypotension
Administer:
• Avoid use with other CNS depressants
PO route
• With meals for GI symptoms; absorption may slightly decrease
• When used for motion sickness, 30 min–1 hr before travel

IM route
• IM inj deep in large muscle; rotate site
IV route
• After diluting each 25-50 mg/9 ml of NaCl for inj; give 25 mg or less/2 min

Additive compatibilities: Amikacin, ascorbic acid, chloroquine, hydromorphone, netilmicin, vit B/C

Syringe compatibilities: Atropine, butorphanol, chlorproMAZINE, cimetidine, dimenhyDRAMINE, droperidol, fentanyl, glycopyrrolate, hydromorphone, hydrOXYzine, meperidine, metoclopramide, midazolam, pentazocine, perphenazine, prochlorperazine, promazine, ranitidine, scopolamine

Y-site compatibilities: Amifostine, amsacrine, aztreonam, ciprofloxacin, cisatracurium, cisplatin, cladribine, cyclophosphamide, cytarabine, DOXOrubicin, filgrastim, fluconazole, fludarabine, granisetron, melphalan, ondansetron, remifentanil, sargramostim, teniposide, thiotepa, vinorelbine

Perform/provide:
• Hard candy, gum, frequent rinsing of mouth for dryness
• Storage in tight, light-resistant container
Evaluate:
• Therapeutic response: absence of running, congested nose, rashes, absence of motion sickness, nausea; sedation
Teach patient/family:
• That drug may cause photosensitivity; to avoid prolonged sunlight
• To notify prescriber of confusion, sedation, hypotension
• To avoid driving, other hazardous activity if drowsy
• To avoid concurrent use of alcohol

---

propafenone (℞)
(pro-paff'e-nown)
Rythmol
Func. class.: Antidysrhythmic (Class IC)

Action: Slows conduction velocity; reduces membrane responsiveness; inhibits automaticity; increases ratio of effective refractory period to action potential duration; β-blocking activity

Uses: Life-threatening dysrhythmias, sustained ventricular tachycardia

Unlabeled uses: Atrial fibrillation (single dose)

DOSAGE AND ROUTES
• *Adult:* **PO** 150 mg q8h; allow a 3-4 day interval before increasing dose, max 900 mg/day
Atrial fibrillation (unlabeled)
• *Adult:* **PO** 450 or 600 mg as a single dose

Available forms: Tabs 150, 225, 300 mg

SIDE EFFECTS
CNS: Headache, dizziness, abnormal dreams, syncope, confusion, **seizures**
CV: **Supraventricular dysrhythmia, ventricular dysrhythmia, bradycardia,** prodysrhythmia, palpitations, AV block, intraventricular conduction delay, AV dissociation, hypotension, chest pain
EENT: Blurred vision, altered taste, tinnitus
GI: Nausea, vomiting, constipation, dyspepsia, cholestasis, abnormal hepatic studies, dry mouth
HEMA: **Leukopenia, agranulocytosis, granulocytopenia, thrombocytopenia,** anemia, bruising
INTEG: Rash
RESP: Dyspnea

Contraindications: 2nd/3rd-degree AV block, right bundle branch block, cardiogenic shock, hypersensitivity, bradycardia, uncontrolled CHF, sick-sinus syndrome, marked hypotension, bronchospastic disorders

Precautions: Pregnancy (C), CHF, hypokalemia, hyperkalemia, recent MI, nonallergic bronchospasm, lactation, children, renal/hepatic disease, geriatric

PHARMACOKINETICS
Peak 3-5 hr, half-life 2-10 hr; metabolized in liver; excreted in urine (metabolite)

⚠ Safety alert   *"Tall Man" lettering

INTERACTIONS

Increase: anticoagulation—warfarin
Increase: CNS effects—local anesthetics
Increase: digoxin level—digoxin
Increase: β-blocker effect—propranolol, metoprolol
Increase: cycloSPORINE levels—cycloSPORINE
Decrease: propafenone effect—rifampin, cimetidine, quinidine

Drug/Herb

• Hypokalemia, increased antidysrhythmic action: aloe, buckthorn, cascara sagrada, senna pod/leaf
Increase: toxicity, death—aconite
Increase: effect—aloe, broom, chronic buckthorn use, cascara sagrada (chronic use), Chinese rhubarb, figwort, fumitory, goldenseal, kudzu, licorice
Increase: serotonin effect—horehound
Decrease: effect—coltsfoot

Drug/Lab Test
Increase: CPK

NURSING CONSIDERATIONS

Assess:

• GI status: bowel pattern, number of stools
⚠ Cardiac status: rate, rhythm, quality; ECG or Holter monitor prior to and during therapy; watch for PR, QT prolongation
• Chest x-ray film, pulmonary function test during treatment
• I&O ratio; check for decreasing output; daily weight
• B/P for fluctuations
• Lung fields; bilateral crackles, dyspnea, peripheral edema, weight gain, jugular venous distention may occur in CHF patient
⚠ Toxicity: fine tremors, dizziness, hypotension, drowsiness, abnormal heart rate
• Cardiac function: respiratory rate, rhythm, character continuously

Administer:

• To hospitalized patients, since heart monitoring is required
• After hypo/hyperkalemia is corrected
• Dosage adjustment q3-4 days

Evaluate:
• Therapeutic response: absence of dysrhythmias

Teach patient/family:
• To avoid hazardous activities until response is known
• To report fever, chills, sore throat, bleeding, shortness of breath, chest pain, palpitations, blurred vision
• Take tab with food
• To carry emergency ID identifying medication and prescriber

Treatment of overdose: O_2, artificial ventilation, defibrillation ECG; administer DOPamine for circulatory depression, diazepam or thiopental for convulsions, isoproterenol

---

propantheline (℞)
(proe-pan'the-leen)
Pro-Banthine, Propanthel ✽,
Func. class.: GI anticholinergic, antiulcer agent
Chem. class.: Synthetic quaternary ammonium compound

Action: Inhibits actions of acetylcholine at postganglionic parasympathetic neuroeffector sites
Uses: Treatment of urinary incontinence, peptic ulcer disease, irritable bowel syndrome, duodenography

DOSAGE AND ROUTES

• *Adult:* **PO** 15 mg tid before meals, 30 mg at bedtime
• *Geriatric, small patients:* **PO** 7.5 mg tid before meals
• *Child:* **PO** 0.375 mg/kg (10 mg/m^2) qid
Available forms: Tabs 15 mg

SIDE EFFECTS

CNS: Confusion, stimulation in geriatric, headache, insomnia, dizziness, drowsiness, anxiety, weakness, hallucinations
CV: Palpitations, tachycardia, orthostatic hypotension (geriatric)

EENT: Blurred vision, photophobia, mydriasis, cycloplegia, increased ocular tension
GI: Dry mouth, constipation, **paralytic ileus,** heartburn, nausea, vomiting, dysphagia, absence of taste
GU: Urinary hesitancy, retention, impotence
INTEG: Urticaria, rash, pruritus, anhidrosis, fever, allergic reactions

Contraindications: Hypersensitivity to anticholinergics, narrow-angle glaucoma, GI obstruction, myasthenia gravis, paralytic ileus, GI atony, toxic megacolon, urinary tract obstruction

Precautions: Pregnancy (C), hyperthyroidism, coronary artery disease, dysrhythmias, CHF, ulcerative colitis, hypertension, hiatal hernia, renal/hepatic disease, urinary retention, prostatic hypertrophy, geriatric

PHARMACOKINETICS

PO: Onset 30-45 min, duration 6 hr; metabolized by liver, GI system; excreted in urine, bile

INTERACTIONS

Increase: anticholinergic effect—tricyclics, MAOIs, H₁-antihistamines, belladonna alkaloids, opioids, disopyramide, procainamide, quinidine, phenothiazines

Drug/Herb
Increase: anticholinergic effect—henbane, jimsonweed, scopolia

NURSING CONSIDERATIONS

Assess:
• VS, cardiac status: checking for dysrhythmias, increased rate, palpitations
• I&O ratio; check for urinary retention or hesitancy
• GI complaints: pain, bleeding (frank or occult), nausea, vomiting, anorexia

Administer:
• ½-1 hr before meals for better absorption
• Decreased dose to geriatric patients; metabolism may be slowed
• Gum, hard candy, frequent rinsing for dry mouth

• Avoid use with other CNS depressants

Perform/provide:
• Storage in tight container protected from light
• Increased fluids, bulk, exercise to decrease constipation

Evaluate:
• Therapeutic response: absence of epigastric pain, bleeding, nausea, vomiting

Teach patient/family:
• To avoid driving, other hazardous activities until stabilized on medication; may cause blurred vision; to use caution when standing due to orthostatic hypotension
• To avoid alcohol; will enhance sedating properties of this drug
• To drink plenty of fluids
• To report dysphagia

---

proparacaine ophthalmic
See Appendix C

⚠ High Alert

propofol (℞)
(pro′poh-fole)
Diprivan, Disoprofol
Func. class.: General anesthetic

Action: Produces dose-dependent CNS depression; action is unknown

Uses: Induction or maintenance of anesthesia as part of balanced anesthetic technique; sedation in mechanically ventilated patients

DOSAGE AND ROUTES

Induction
• *Adult:* IV 2-2.5 mg/kg, approximately 40 mg q10sec until induction onset
• *Child 3-16 yr:* IV 2.5-3.5 mg/kg over 20-30 sec
• *Geriatric:* IV 1-1.5 mg/kg, approximately 20 mg q10sec until induction onset

Maintenance
• *Adult:* IV 0.1-0.2 mg/kg/min (6-12 mg/kg/hr)

⚠ Safety alert   *"Tall Man" lettering

• *Child ≥3 yr:* IV 0.125-0.3 mg/kg/min (7.5-18 mg/kg/hr)
• *Geriatric:* IV 0.05-0.1 mg/kg/min (3-6 mg/kg/hr)
ICU sedation
• *Adult:* IV 5 mcg/kg/min over 5 min; may give 5-10 mcg/kg/min over 5-10 min until desired response
Available forms: Inj 10 mg/ml in 20-ml ampule, 50-ml and 100-ml vials

SIDE EFFECTS

CNS: Involuntary movement, headache, jerking, fever, dizziness, shivering, tremor, confusion, somnolence, paresthesia, agitation, abnormal dreams, euphoria, fatigue, **increased ICP, impaired cerebral flow, seizures**

CV: Bradycardia, hypotension, hypertension, PVC, PAC, tachycardia, abnormal ECG, ST segment depression, **asystole**

EENT: Blurred vision, tinnitus, eye pain, strange taste, diplopia

GI: Nausea, vomiting, abdominal cramping, dry mouth, swallowing, hypersalivation, **pancreatitis**

GU: Urine retention, green urine, cloudy urine, oliguria

INTEG: Flushing, phlebitis, hives, burning/stinging at inj site, rash, pain of extremities

MS: Myalgia

RESP: **Apnea,** *cough, hiccups,* dyspnea, hypoventilation, sneezing, wheezing, tachypnea, hypoxia

Contraindications: Hypersensitivity to drug or soybean oil, egg; hyperlipidemia

Precautions: Pregnancy (B), geriatric, respiratory depression, severe respiratory disorders, cardiac dysrhythmias, labor and delivery, lactation, children

PHARMACOKINETICS

Onset 15-30 sec, rapid distribution, half-life 1-8 min, terminal elimination half-life 5-10 hr; 70% excreted in urine; metabolized in liver by conjugation to inactive metabolites

INTERACTIONS

Increase: CNS depression—alcohol, opioids, sedative/hypnotics, antipsychotics, skeletal muscle relaxants, inhalational anesthetics

NURSING CONSIDERATIONS

Assess:
• Inj site: phlebitis, burning, stinging
• ECG for changes: PVC, PAC, ST segment changes; monitor VS
• CNS changes: movement, jerking, tremors, dizziness, LOC, pupil reaction
• Allergic reactions: hives

⚠ Respiratory dysfunction: respiratory depression, character, rate, rhythm; notify prescriber if respirations are <10/min

Administer:
IV route
• Shake well before use; if diluted, use only D_5W to not less than 2 mg/ml; give over 3-5 min, titrate to needed level of sedation; use only glass containers when mixing, not stable in plastic
• May be given by cont inf; give by inf pump
• Only with resuscitative equipment available
• Only by qualified persons trained in anesthesia

Y-site compatibilities: Acyclovir, alfentanil, aminophylline, ampicillin, aztreonam, bumetanide, buprenorphine, butorphanol, calcium gluconate, carboplatin, cefazolin, cefoperazone, cefotaxime, cefotetan, cefoxitin, ceftizoxime, ceftriaxone, cefuroxime, chlorproMAZINE, cimetidine, cisplatin, clindamycin, cyclophosphamide, cycloSPORINE, cytarabine, dexamethasone, diphenhydrAMINE, DOBUTamine, DOPamine, doxycycline, droperidol, enalaprilat, epHEDrine, epINEPHrine, esmolol, famotidine, fentanyl, fluconazole, fluorouracil, furosemide, ganciclovir, glycopyrrolate, granisetron, haloperidol, heparin, hydrocortisone, hydromorphone, hydrOXYzine, ifosfamide,

P

Side effects: *italics* = common; **bold** = life-threatening

imipenem/cilastatin, inamrinone, regular insulin, isoproterenol, ketamine, labetalol, levorphanol, lidocaine, lorazepam, magnesium sulfate, mannitol, meperidine, mezlocillin, miconazole, morphine, nafcillin, nalbuphine, naloxone, nitroglycerin, norepinephrine, ofloxacin, paclitaxel, pentobarbital, phenobarbital, piperacillin, potassium chloride, prochlorperazine, propranolol, ranitidine, scopolamine, sodium bicarbonate, sodium nitroprusside, succinylcholine, sufentanil, thiopental ticarcillin, ticarcillin/clavulanate, vecuronium, verapamil

Solution compatibilities: D_5W, D_5LR, LR, D_5/0.45% NaCl, D_5/0.2% NaCl

Perform/provide:

• Storage in light-resistant area at room temperature, use within 6 hr of opening
• If transferred from original container to another container, complete infusion within 12 hr

Evaluate:

• Therapeutic response: induction of anesthesia

Teach patient/family:

• That this medication will cause dizziness, drowsiness, sedation

Treatment of overdose: Discontinue drug; administer vasopressor agents or anticholinergics, artificial ventilation

---

⚠ High Alert

propoxyphene (℞)

(proe-pox′i-feen)

Darvon, Darvon-N, Dolene, Novopropoxyn ✦

Func. class.: Opiate analgesic

Chem. class.: Synthetic opiate

Controlled Substance Schedule IV

Action: Depresses pain impulse transmission at the spinal cord level by interacting with opioid receptors

Uses: Mild to moderate pain

DOSAGE AND ROUTES

• *Adult:* **PO** 65 mg q4h prn (HCl)
• *Adult:* **PO** 100 mg q4h prn (napsylate)

Available forms: Caps (propoxyphene HCl) 32, 65 mg; tabs (propoxyphene napsylate) 100 mg; oral susp 50 mg/5 ml

SIDE EFFECTS

CNS: Drowsiness, dizziness, confusion, headache, sedation, euphoria, **seizures, hyperthermia** (geriatric)

CV: Palpitations, bradycardia, change in B/P, **dysrhythmias**

EENT: Tinnitus, blurred vision, miosis, diplopia

GI: Nausea, vomiting, anorexia, constipation, cramps

GU: Urinary retention, dysuria

INTEG: Rash, urticaria, bruising, flushing, diaphoresis, pruritus

RESP: **Respiratory depression**

Contraindications: Hypersensitivity to ASA products (some preparations), addiction (opioid)

Precautions: Pregnancy (C), addictive personality, lactation, increased intracranial pressure, MI (acute), severe heart disease, respiratory depression, renal/hepatic disease, child <18 yr, geriatric

PHARMACOKINETICS

PO: Onset ½-1 hr, peak 2-2½ hr, duration 4-6 hr

Metabolized by liver, excreted by kidneys (as metabolites), crosses placenta, excreted in breast milk, half-life 6-12 hr (metabolites)

INTERACTIONS

⚠ Possible fatal reactions: MAOIs, alcohol

Increase: effects with other CNS depressants—opioids, sedative/hypnotics, antipsychotics, skeletal muscle relaxants

Drug/Herb

Increase: CNS depression—chamomile, hops, Jamaican dogwood, kava, lavender, mistletoe, nettle, pokeweed, poppy, senega, skullcap, valerian

---

⚠ Safety alert   *"Tall Man" lettering

Increase: anticholinergic effect—corkwood
Drug/Lab Test
Increase: Amylase

NURSING CONSIDERATIONS

Assess:
• For pain: duration, location, type
• I&O ratio; check for decreasing output; may indicate retention
• CNS changes: dizziness, drowsiness, hallucinations, euphoria, loss of consciousness, pupil reaction
• Allergic reactions: rash, urticaria
• Respiratory dysfunction: respiratory depression, character, rate, rhythm; notify prescriber if respirations are <10/min
• Need for pain medication; physical dependence

Administer:
• With antiemetic for nausea, vomiting
• When pain is beginning to return; determine dosage interval by response

Perform/provide:
• Storage in light-resistant area at room temperature
• Assistance with ambulation

Evaluate:
• Therapeutic response: decrease in pain

Teach patient/family:
• To report any symptoms of CNS changes, allergic reactions
• That physical dependency may result when used for extended periods; not to exceed dose
• That withdrawal symptoms may occur: nausea, vomiting, cramps, fever, faintness, anorexia

Treatment of overdose: Naloxone (Narcan) 0.2-0.8 mg IV, O_2, IV fluids, vasopressors

---

propranolol (℞)
(proe-pran'oh-lole)
Apo-Propranolol ✤
Betaclinron E-R ✤
Detensol ✤, Inderal, Inderal LA, InnoPran XL,
NovoPranol ✤, propranolol HCl, PMS-Propranolol ✤
Func. class.: Antihypertensive, antianginal, antidysrhythmic (class II)
Chem. class.: β-Adrenergic blocker

Do not confuse:
Inderal/Toradol/IMDUR

Action: Nonselective β-blocker with negative inotropic, chronotropic, dromotropic properties

Uses: Chronic stable angina pectoris, hypertension, supraventricular dysrhythmias, migraine, prophylaxis, MI, pheochromocytoma, essential tremor, cyanotic spells related to hypertrophic subaortic stenosis

Unlabeled uses: Anxiety; Parkinson's tremor, prevention of variceal bleeding caused by portal hypertension, akathisia induced by antipsychotics

DOSAGE AND ROUTES

Dysrhythmias
• *Adult:* **PO** 10-30 mg tid-qid; **IV BOL** 0.5-3 mg give 1 mg/min; may repeat in 2 min, may repeat q4h thereafter
• *Child:* **PO** 1 mg/kg/day divided in 2 doses; **IV** 0.01-0.1 mg/kg over 5 min

Hypertension
• *Adult:* **PO** 40 mg bid or 80 mg daily (ext rel) initially; usual dose 120-240 mg/day bid-tid or 120-160 mg daily (ext rel)
• *Child:* **PO** 0.5-1 mg/kg/day divided q6-12h

Angina
• *Adult:* **PO** 80-320 mg in divided doses bid-qid or 80 mg daily (ext rel); usual dose 160 mg daily (ext rel)

MI prophylaxis
• *Adult:* **PO** 180-240 mg/day tid-qid starting 5 days to 2 wk after MI

P

Side effects: *italics* = common; **bold** = life-threatening

Pheochromocytoma
• *Adult:* **PO** 60 mg/day × 3 days preoperatively in divided doses or 30 mg/day in divided doses (inoperable tumor)

Migraine
• *Adult:* **PO** 80 mg/day (ext rel) or in divided doses; may increase to 160-240 mg/day in divided doses
• *Child:* **PO** 0.6-1.5 mg/kg/day divided q8h

Essential tremor
• *Adult:* **PO** 40 mg bid; usual dose 120 mg/day

Available forms: Ext rel caps 60, 80, 120, 160 mg; tabs 10, 20, 40, 60, 80, 90 mg; inj 1 mg/ml; oral sol 4 mg/ml, 8 mg/ml; conc oral sol 80 mg/ml

SIDE EFFECTS

CNS: Depression, hallucinations, dizziness, fatigue, lethargy, paresthesias, bizarre dreams, disorientation
CV: **Bradycardia**, hypotension, **CHF**, palpitations, AV block, peripheral vascular insufficiency, vasodilation, cold extremities, **pulmonary edema, dysrhythmias**
EENT: Sore throat, **laryngospasm**, blurred vision, dry eyes
GI: Nausea, vomiting, diarrhea, colitis, constipation, cramps, dry mouth, hepatomegaly, gastric pain, acute pancreatitis
GU: Impotence, decreased libido, UTIs
HEMA: **Agranulocytosis, thrombocytopenia**
INTEG: Rash, pruritus, fever
META: Hyperglycemia, hypoglycemia
MISC: Facial swelling, weight change, Raynaud's phenomenon
MS: Joint pain, arthralgia, muscle cramps, pain
RESP: Dyspnea, respiratory dysfunction, *bronchospasm,* cough

Contraindications: Hypersensitivity to this drug; cardiac failure; cardiogenic shock, 2nd-, 3rd-degree heart block; bronchospastic disease; sinus bradycardia; CHF, bronchospasm

Precautions: Pregnancy (C), diabetes mellitus, lactation, hyperthyroidism, COPD, renal/hepatic disease, children,

myasthenia gravis, peripheral vascular disease, hypotension, CHF

PHARMACOKINETICS

PO: Onset 30 min, peak 1-1½ hr, duration 12 hr
PO-ER: Peak 6 hr, duration 24 hr, half-life 8-11 hr
IV: Onset 2 min, peak 1 min, duration 5 min
Metabolized by liver; crosses placenta, blood-brain barrier; excreted in breast milk, protein binding 90%

INTERACTIONS

• Smoking decreases propranolol levels
Increase: effect of calcium channel blockers, neuromuscular blocker
Increase: negative inotropic effects—disopyramide
Increase: β-blocking effect—cimetidine
Increase: hypotension—quinidine, haloperidol, prazosin
Decrease: β-blocking effects—barbiturates
Drug/Herb
Increase: toxicity, death—aconite
Increase: antihypertensive effect—barberry, betony, black catechu, black cohosh, bloodroot, broom, burdock, cat's claw, dandelion, goldenseal, Irish moss, Jamaican dogwood, kelp, khella, mistletoe, parsley
Increase or decrease: antihypertensive effect—astragalus, cola tree
Decrease: antihypertensive effect—coltsfoot, guarana, khat, licorice
Drug/Lab Test
Increase: Serum potassium, serum uric acid, ALT, AST, alk phos, LDH
Decrease: Blood glucose
Interference: Glaucoma testing

NURSING CONSIDERATIONS

Assess:
• B/P, pulse, respirations during beginning therapy; notify prescriber if pulse <50 bpm
• Weight daily; report gain of 5 lb
⚠ I&O ratio, CCr if kidney damage is di-

agnosed; watch for fluid overload: fatigue, weight gain, jugular distention, dyspnea, peripheral edema, crackles

⚠ ECG continuously if using as antidysrhythmic, IV, PCWP, CVP

• Hepatic enzymes: AST, ALT, bilirubin
• Angina pain: duration, time started, activity being performed, character
• Tolerance (long-term use)
• Headache, light-headedness, decreased B/P; may indicate a need for decreased dosage

Administer:

PO route

• Do not break, crush, chew, or open ext rel cap
• Do not use ext rel cap for essential tremor, MI, cardiac dysrhythmias; do not use InnoPran XL in hypertropic subaortic stenosis, migraine, angina pectoris
• Ext rel caps should be taken daily; InnoPran XL should be taken at bedtime
• May mix oral sol with liquid or semisolid food; rinse container to get entire dose
• With 8 oz water with food; food enhances bioavailability
• Do not give with aluminum-containing antacid; may decrease GI absorption

IV route

• IV undiluted or diluted 10 ml D₅W for inj; give 1 mg or less/min; may be diluted in 50 ml NaCl and run 1 mg over 10-15 min

Additive compatibilities: DOBUTamine, verapamil

Solution compatibilities: 0.9% NaCl, 0.45 NaCl, Ringer's, D₅W, D₅/0.9% NaCl, D₅/0.45% NaCl

Syringe compatibilities: Inamrinone, milrinone

Y-site compatibilities: Alteplase, amrinone, heparin, hydrocortisone, meperidine, milrinone, morphine, potassium chloride, propofol, tacrolimus, vit B/C

Perform/provide:

• Protection from light

Evaluate:

• Therapeutic response: decreased B/P, dysrhythmias

Teach patient/family:

⚠ Not to discontinue abruptly, may precipitate life-threatening dysrhythmias; to take drug at same time each day; to decrease dosage over 2 wk to prevent cardiac damage
• To avoid OTC drugs unless approved by prescriber; avoid alcohol
• To avoid hazardous activities if dizzy
• The importance of compliance with complete medical regimen; monitor blood glucose, may mask symptoms of hypoglycemia
• To make position changes slowly to prevent fainting
• That sensitivity to cold may occur

---

propylhexadrine nasal agent
See Appendix C

---

propylthiouracil (℞)
(proe-pill-thye-oh-yoor′a-sill)
propylthiouracil, Propyl-Thyracil ✦ PTU
Func. class.: Thyroid hormone antagonist (antithyroid)
Chem. class.: Thioamide

Action: Blocks synthesis peripherally of T₃, T₄ (triiodothyronine, thyroxine), inhibits organification of iodine

Uses: Preparation for thyroidectomy, thyrotoxic crisis, hyperthyroidism, thyroid storm

DOSAGE AND ROUTES

Thyrotoxic crisis
• *Adult and child:* **PO** same as hyperthyroidism with iodine and propranolol
Preparation for thyroidectomy
• *Adult:* 600-1200 mg/day
• *Child:* 10 mg/kg/day in divided doses
Hyperthyroidism
• *Adult:* **PO** 100 mg tid increasing to 300 mg q8h if condition is severe; continue to euthyroid state, then 100 mg daily-tid
• *Child >10 yr:* **PO** 100 mg tid; con-

Side effects: *italics* = common; **bold** = life-threatening

tinue to euthyroid state, then 25 mg tid to 100 mg bid
• *Child 6-10 yr:* **PO** 50-150 mg in divided doses q8h
• *Neonate:* **PO** 10 mg/kg/day in divided doses
Available forms: Tabs 50, 100 mg

SIDE EFFECTS

CNS: Drowsiness, headache, vertigo, fever, paresthesias, neuritis
GI: Nausea, diarrhea, vomiting, **jaundice, hepatitis,** loss of taste
GU: **Nephritis**
HEMA: **Agranulocytosis, leukopenia, thrombocytopenia, hypothrombinemia, lymphadenopathy,** bleeding, vasculitis, periarteritis
INTEG: Rash, urticaria, pruritus, alopecia, hyperpigmentation, lupuslike syndrome
MS: Myalgia, arthralgia, nocturnal muscle cramps, osteoporosis
Contraindications: Pregnancy (D), hypersensitivity, lactation
Precautions: Infection, bone marrow depression, hepatic disease

PHARMACOKINETICS

PO: Onset up to 3 wk, peak 6-10 wk, duration 1 wk to 1 mo, half-life 1-2 hr; excreted in urine, bile, breast milk; crosses placenta; concentration in thyroid gland

INTERACTIONS

• Bone marrow depression: radiation, antineoplastics
• Agranulocytosis: phenothiazines
Increase: anticoagulant effect—heparin, oral anticoagulants
Increase: effects—potassium/sodium iodide, lithium
Drug/Lab Test
Increase: PT, AST, ALT, alk phos

NURSING CONSIDERATIONS

Assess:
• Pulse, B/P, temp
• I&O ratio; check for edema: puffy

hands, feet, periorbits; indicates hypothyroidism
• Weight daily; same clothing, scale, time of day
• T_3, T_4, which are increased; serum TSH, which is decreased; free thyroxine index, which is increased if dosage is too low; discontinue drug 3-4 wk before RAIU
⚠ Blood studies: CBC for blood dyscrasias: leukopenia, thrombocytopenia, agranulocytosis; LFTs
⚠ Overdose: peripheral edema, heat intolerance, diaphoresis, palpitations, dysrhythmias, severe tachycardia, increased temp, delirium, CNS irritability
⚠ Hypersensitivity: rash, enlarged cervical lymph nodes; drug may have to be discontinued
• Hypoprothrombinemia: bleeding, petechiae, ecchymosis
• Clinical response: after 3 wk should include increased weight, pulse; decreased T_4
• Bone marrow depression: sore throat, fever, fatigue
Administer:
• With meals to decrease GI upset
• At same time each day to maintain drug level
• Lowest dose that relieves symptoms
Perform/provide:
• Storage in light-resistant container
• Fluids to 3-4 L/day, unless contraindicated
Evaluate:
• Therapeutic response: weight gain, decreased pulse, decreased T_4, decreased B/P
Teach patient/family:
• To abstain from breastfeeding after delivery
• To take pulse daily
• To report redness, swelling, sore throat, mouth lesions, which indicate blood dyscrasias
• To keep graph of weight, pulse, mood
• To avoid OTC products that contain iodine
• That seafood, other iodine products may be restricted
• Not to discontinue this medication

⚠ Safety alert   *"Tall Man" lettering

abruptly; thyroid crisis may occur; stress response
• That response may take several months if thyroid is large
• The symptoms/signs of overdose: periorbital edema, cold intolerance, mental depression
• The symptoms of inadequate dose: tachycardia, diarrhea, fever, irritability
• To take medication as prescribed; not to skip or double dose; missed doses should be taken when remembered up to 1 hr before next dose
• To carry emergency ID listing condition, medication

---

protamine (℞)
(proe′ta-meen)
Func. class.: Heparin antagonist
Chem. class.: Low-molecular-weight protein

Action: Binds heparin, making it ineffective
Uses: Heparin overdose, hemorrhage

DOSAGE AND ROUTES
• *Adult and child:* **IV** 1 mg of protamine/100 units heparin given or 100 anti-Xa units of LMWH; administer slowly 1-3 min; not to exceed 50 mg/10 min
Available forms: Inj 10 mg/ml

SIDE EFFECTS
CNS: Lassitude
CV: Hypotension, bradycardia, **circulatory collapse**
GI: Nausea, vomiting, anorexia
HEMA: Bleeding
INTEG: *Rash,* dermatitis, urticaria
RESP: Dyspnea, **pulmonary edema, severe respiratory distress**
SYST: **Anaphylaxis, angioedema**
Contraindications: Hypersensitivity
Precautions: Pregnancy (C), lactation, children, allergy to salmon, diabetes mellitus

PHARMACOKINETICS
IV: Onset 5 min, duration 2 hr

NURSING CONSIDERATIONS
Assess:
⚠ Hypersensitivity: urticaria, cough, wheezing, have emergency equipment nearby
• Blood studies (Hct, platelets, occult blood in stools) q3mo
• Coagulation tests (aPTT, ACT) 15 min after dose, then in several hours
• VS, B/P, pulse after 30 min; plus 3 hr after dose
• Skin rash, urticaria, dermatitis
⚠ Allergy to fish; use with caution; men that have had a vasectomy may be more prone to hypersensitivity
Administer:
IV route
• After diluting 50 mg/5 ml sterile bacteriostatic H_2O for inj; shake, give 20 mg or less over 1-3 min; may further dilute with equal volume of NaCl or D_5W and run over 2-3 hr; titrate to aPTT, ACT; use infusion pump
Additive compatibilities: Cimetidine, ranitidine, verapamil
Perform/provide:
• Storage at 36°-46° F (2°-8° C)
Evaluate:
• Therapeutic response: reversal of heparin overdose

P

Side effects: *italics* = common; **bold** = life-threatening

pseudoephedrine
(orc, R)

(soo-doh-eh-fed'rin)
Afrin, Allermed, Cenafed,
Children's Congestion Relief,
Children's Silfedrine,
Congestion Relief, Decofed
Syrup, DeFed-60, Dorcol
Children's Decongestant,
Drixoral Non-Drowsy
Formula, Dynafed,
Efidac/24, Eltor ✦,
Genaphed, Halofed, Mini
Thin Pseudo, PediaCare
Infant's Decongestant,
Pseudo, pseudoephedrine
HCl, Pseudogest, Seudotabs,
Sinustop Pro, Sudafed,
Sudafed 12 Hour, Sudex,
Triaminic AM Decongestant
Formula
Func. class.: Adrenergic
Chem. class.: Substituted phenyl-
ethylamine

Action: Primary activity through α-effects
on respiratory mucosal membranes reducing congestion hyperemia, edema; minimal bronchodilation secondary to β-effects
Uses: Nasal decongestant, adjunct in otitis media; with antihistamines

DOSAGE AND ROUTES

• *Adult and child >12 yr:* **PO** 60 mg q6h;
EXT REL 120 mg q12h or 240 mg q24h
• *Geriatric:* **PO** 30-60 mg q6h prn
• *Child 6-12 yr:* **PO** 30 mg q6h, not to
exceed 120 mg/day
• *Child 2-6 yr:* **PO** 15 mg q6h, not to
exceed 60 mg/day
Available forms: Ext rel caps 120, 240
mg; oral sol 15 mg, 30 mg/5 ml; drops
7.5 mg/0.8 ml; tabs 30, 60 mg; caps 60
mg; ext rel tabs 120, 240 mg

SIDE EFFECTS

CNS: Tremors, anxiety, stimulation, insomnia, headache, dizziness, hallucinations, **seizures** (geriatric)

CV: Palpitations, tachycardia, hypertension,
chest pain, **dysrhythmias, CV collapse**
EENT: Dry nose, irritation of nose and
throat
GI: Anorexia, nausea, vomiting, dry
mouth
GU: Dysuria
Contraindications: Hypersensitivity to
sympathomimetics, narrow-angle glaucoma
Precautions: Pregnancy (C), cardiac
disorders, hyperthyroidism, diabetes mellitus, prostatic hypertrophy, lactation, hypertension

PHARMACOKINETICS

PO: Onset 15-30 min; duration 4-6 hr,
8-12 hr (ext rel); metabolized in liver;
excreted in feces and breast milk; terminal half-life 9-16 hr

INTERACTIONS

⚠ Do not use with MAOIs or tricyclics;
hypertensive crisis may occur
Increase: effect of this drug—urinary alkalizers
Decrease: effect of this drug—
methyldopa, urinary acidifiers, rauwolfia
alkaloids

NURSING CONSIDERATIONS

Assess:
• For nasal congestion; auscultate lung
sounds; check for tenacious bronchial se-
cretions
• B/P, pulse throughout treatment
• For CNS side effects in the geriatric: ex-
citation, seizures, hallucinations
Administer:
• Near bedtime; stimulation can occur
Perform/provide:
• Storage at room temperature
Evaluate:
• Therapeutic response: decreased na-
sal congestion
Teach patient/family:
• The reason for drug administration
• Not to use continuously, or more than
recommended dose; rebound congestion
may occur
⚠ To notify prescriber immediately of

⚠ Safety alert   *"Tall Man" lettering

anxiety; slow, fast heart rate; dyspnea; seizures

• To check with prescriber before using other drugs, as drug interactions may occur

• To avoid taking near bedtime; stimulation can occur

• Not to use if stimulation, restlessness, or tremors occur

• That use in children may cause excessive agitation

---

pseudoephedrine nasal agent
See Appendix C

---

psyllium (OTC, ℞)
(sill′ee-um)
Alramucil, Fiberall, Fiberall Natural Flavor and Orange Flavor, Genfiber, Hydrocil Instant, Karacil ♣, Konsyl, Konsyl Orange, Maalox Daily Fiber Therapy, Metamucil, Metamucil Lemon Lime, Metamucil Orange Flavor, Metamucil Sugar Free, Metamucil Sugar Free Orange Flavor, Modane Bulk, Mylanta Natural Fiber Supplement, Natural Fiber Laxative, Natural Fiber Laxative Sugar Free, Natural Vegetable Reguloid, Perdiem, Prodiem Plain ♣, Reguloid Natural, Reguloid Orange, Reguloid Sugar Free Orange, Reguloid Sugar Free Regular, Restore, Restore Sugar Free, Serutan, Syllact, V-Lax
Func. class.: Bulk laxative
Chem. class.: Psyllium colloid

Action: Bulk-forming laxative
Uses: Chronic constipation, ulcerative colitis, irritable bowel syndrome

DOSAGE AND ROUTES

• *Adult:* **PO** 1-2 tsp in 8 oz H_2O bid or tid, then 8 oz H_2O or 1 premeasured packet in 8 oz H_2O bid or tid, then 8 oz H_2O

• *Child >6 yr:* **PO** 1 tsp in 4 oz H_2O at bedtime

Available forms: Chew pieces 1.7, 3.4 g/piece; effervescent powder 3.4, 3.7 g/packet; powder 3.3, 3.4, 3.5, 4.94 g/tsp; granules 2.5, 4.03 g/tsp; wafers 3.4 g/wafer

SIDE EFFECTS

GI: Nausea, vomiting, anorexia, diarrhea, cramps, intestinal esophageal blockage
Contraindications: Hypersensitivity, intestinal obstruction, abdominal pain, nausea/vomiting, fecal impaction
Precautions: Pregnancy (C)

PHARMACOKINETICS

Onset 12-72 hr, excreted in feces, not absorbed in GI tract

INTERACTIONS

Decrease: absorption of cardiac glycosides, oral anticoagulants, salicylates
Drug/Herb
Increase: laxative effect—flax, senna

NURSING CONSIDERATIONS
Assess:

• Blood, urine electrolytes if used often
• I&O ratio to identify fluid loss
• Cause of constipation; fluids, bulk, exercise missing
• Cramping, rectal bleeding, nausea, vomiting; drug should be discontinued
Administer:
PO route
• Alone for better absorption, separate from other drugs by 1-2 hr
• In morning or evening (oral dose)
• Immediately after mixing with H_2O
• With 8 oz H_2O or juice followed by another 8 oz of fluid

Evaluate:
• Therapeutic response: decrease in constipation or decreased diarrhea in colitis

Teach patient/family:
• To maintain adequate fluid consumption
• That normal bowel movements do not always occur daily
• Not to use in presence of abdominal pain, nausea, vomiting
• To notify prescriber if constipation unrelieved or if symptoms of electrolyte imbalance occur: muscle cramps, pain, weakness, dizziness, excessive thirst

---

pyrantel (OTC)
(pie-ran'tel)
Antiminth, Combantrin ✦
Pin-Rid, Pin-X, Reese's
Pinworm
Func. class.: Anthelmintic
Chem. class.: Pyrimidine derivative

Action: Causes paralysis in worm by neuroblockade via stimulation of ganglionic receptors; worms expelled by normal peristalsis

Uses: Pinworms, roundworms, hookworms

DOSAGE AND ROUTES

• *Adult and child >2 yr:* **PO** 11 mg/kg as single dose, not to exceed 1 g; repeat in 2 wk for pinworms

Available forms: Oral susp 50 mg/ml; liquid 50 mg/ml; soft gel caps 180 mg

SIDE EFFECTS

CNS: Dizziness, headache, drowsiness, insomnia, fever, weakness
GI: Nausea, vomiting, anorexia, diarrhea, distention, abdominal cramps
INTEG: Rash

Contraindications: Hypersensitivity
Precautions: Pregnancy (C), seizure disorders, hepatic disease, dehydration, anemia, child <2 yr, malnutrition

PHARMACOKINETICS

PO: Peak 1-3 hr; metabolized in liver; excreted in feces, urine (unchanged/metabolites)

INTERACTIONS

• Antagonizes effect of pyrantel: piperazine

NURSING CONSIDERATIONS

Assess:
• Stools during entire treatment; specimens must be sent to lab while still warm
• For diarrhea during expulsion of worms
• For allergic reaction: rash

Administer:
• After meals to avoid GI symptoms
• After shaking suspension

Perform/provide:
• Storage in tight, light-resistant container in cool environment

Evaluate:
• Therapeutic response: expulsion of worms, 3 negative stool cultures after completion of treatment

Teach patient/family:
• Proper hygiene after BM, including hand-washing technique; tell patient not to put fingers in mouth
• That infected person should sleep alone; not to shake bed linen; to change bed linen daily, wash in hot water; that all family members should be treated for pinworms; treat dogs/cats; keep children away from animal's feces
• To clean toilet daily with disinfectant (green soap solution)
• The need for compliance with dosage schedule, duration of treatment
• To drink fruit juice to help expel worms
• To wear shoes, wash all fruits, vegetables well before eating

---

⚠ Safety alert   *"Tall Man" lettering

pyrazinamide (℞)
(peer-a-zin′a-mide)
PMS Pyrazinamide ♣,
pyrazinamide, Tebrazid ♣
Func. class.: Antitubercular agent
Chem. class.: Pyrazinoic acid amine,
nicoturimide analog

Action: Bactericidal interference with
lipid, nucleic acid biosynthesis
Uses: Tuberculosis, as an adjunct when
other drugs are not feasible

DOSAGE AND ROUTES
• *Adult and child:* **PO** 15-30 mg/kg/day
not to exceed 2 g/day
Available forms: Tabs 500 mg

SIDE EFFECTS
CNS: Headache
GI: **Hepatotoxicity,** abnormal hepatic
studies, peptic ulcer, nausea, vomiting, an-
orexia, cramps, diarrhea
GU: Urinary difficulty, increased uric acid
HEMA: **Hemolytic anemia**
INTEG: Photosensitivity, urticaria
Contraindications: Hypersensitivity,
severe hepatic damage, acute gout
Precautions: Pregnancy (C), child <13
yr, renal failure, diabetes, porphyria,
chronic gout

PHARMACOKINETICS
PO: Peak 2 hr, half-life 9-10 hr; metabolized in liver, excreted in urine
(metabolites/unchanged drug)

INTERACTIONS
Drug/Lab Test
Increase: PBI
Decrease: 17-KS

NURSING CONSIDERATIONS
Assess:
• Signs of anemia: Hct, Hgb, fatigue
• Temp; if >101° F (38° C), drug should
be reduced
🅐 Hepatic studies qwk: ALT, AST, biliru-
bin

• Renal status before, qmo: BUN, creati-
nine, output, sp gr, urinalysis, uric acid
• Hepatic status: decreased appetite,
jaundice, dark urine, fatigue
Administer:
• With meals for GI symptoms
• After C&S is completed; qmo to detect
resistance
Evaluate:
• Therapeutic response: decreased symp-
toms of TB, culture negative
Teach patient/family:
• That compliance with dosage sched-
ule, length is necessary
• To avoid alcohol
• To report fever, loss of appetite, mal-
aise, nausea, vomiting, darkened urine,
pale stools

pyridostigmine (℞)
(peer-id-oh-stig′meen)
Mestinon, Mestinon SR,
Mestinon Timespan, Regonol
Func. class.: Cholinergic; anticholin-
esterase
Chem. class.: Tertiary amine carba-
mate

Action: Inhibits destruction of acetylcholine, which increases concentration at
sites where acetylcholine is released; this
facilitates transmission of impulses across
myoneural junction
Uses: Nondepolarizing muscle relaxant
antagonist, myasthenia gravis

DOSAGE AND ROUTES
Myasthenia gravis
• *Adult:* **PO** 600 mg/day in 5-6 divided
doses, not to exceed 1.5 g/day; **IM/IV** 2
mg or ⅟₃₀ of **PO** dose; **SUS REL** 180-540
mg daily or bid at intervals of at least 6 hr
• *Child:* **PO** 7 mg/kg/day in 5-6 divided
doses; **IM/IV** 0.05-0.15 mg/kg/dose
*Nondepolarizing neuromuscular
blocker antagonist*
• *Adult:* 0.6-1.2 mg **IV** atropine, then
0.1-0.25 mg/kg/dose
• *Child:* **IV** 0.1-0.25 mg/kg/dose

Available forms: Tabs 60 mg; ext rel tabs 180 mg; syr 60 mg/5 ml; inj 5 mg/ml

SIDE EFFECTS

CNS: Dizziness, headache, sweating, weakness, **seizures**, incoordination, **paralysis**, drowsiness, LOC

CV: Tachycardia, dysrhythmias, bradycardia, AV block, hypotension, ECG changes, **cardiac arrest**, syncope

EENT: Miosis, blurred vision, lacrimation, visual changes

GI: Nausea, diarrhea, vomiting, cramps, increased salivary and gastric secretions, peristalsis

GU: Urinary frequency, incontinence, urgency

INTEG: Rash, urticaria, flushing

RESP: **Respiratory depression, bronchospasm, constriction, laryngospasm, respiratory arrest**

Contraindications: Bradycardia; hypotension; obstruction of intestine, renal system; bromide sensitivity

Precautions: Pregnancy (C), seizure disorders, bronchial asthma, coronary occlusion, hyperthyroidism, dysrhythmias, peptic ulcer, megacolon, poor GI motility

PHARMACOKINETICS

PO: Onset 20-30 min, duration 3-6 hr
PO-EXT REL: Onset 30-60 min, duration 6-12 hr
IM/IV/SUBCUT: Onset 2-15 min, duration 2½-4 hr
Metabolized in liver, excreted in urine

INTERACTIONS

Increase: action—decamethonium, succinylcholine
Decrease: action—gallamine, metocurine, pancuronium, tubocurarine, atropine
Decrease: pyridostigmine action—aminoglycosides, anesthetics, procainamide, quinidine, mecamylamine, polymyxin, magnesium, corticosteroids, antidysrhythmics, quinolones

Drug/Herb
Increase: effect—jaborandi tree, pill-bearing spurge

NURSING CONSIDERATIONS

Assess:
• VS, respiration q8h
• I&O ratio; check for urinary retention or incontinence
• Bradycardia, hypotension, bronchospasm, headache, dizziness, convulsions, respiratory depression; drug should be discontinued if toxicity occurs

Administer:
• Do not break, crush, or chew sus rel tabs
• Only with atropine sulfate available for cholinergic crisis
• Only after all other cholinergics have been discontinued
• Increased doses for tolerance, as ordered
• Larger doses after exercise or fatigue, as ordered
• On empty stomach for better absorption

IV route
• Undiluted, give through Y-tube or 3-way stopcock, give 0.5 mg or less/min
Syringe compatibilities: Glycopyrrolate
Y-site compatibilities: Heparin, hydrocortisone, potassium chloride, vit B/C
Perform/provide:
• Storage at room temperature
Evaluate:
• Therapeutic response: increased muscle strength, hand grasp, improved gait, absence of labored breathing (if severe)
Teach patient/family:
• That drug is not a cure, only relieves symptoms
• To wear emergency ID specifying myasthenia gravis, drugs taken
Treatment of overdose: Discontinue drug, atropine 1-4 mg IV

⚠ Safety alert *"Tall Man" lettering

pyridoxine (vit B$_6$)
(℞, OTC)
(peer-i-dox′een)
Beesix, Doxine, Nestrex,
pyridoxine HCl, Pyri, Rodex,
Vitabee 6, vitamin B$_6$
Func. class.: Vit B$_6$, water soluble

Action: Needed for fat, protein, carbohydrate metabolism; enhances glycogen release from liver and muscle tissue; needed as coenzyme for metabolic transformations of a variety of amino acids

Uses: Vit B$_6$ deficiency of inborn errors of metabolism, seizures, isoniazid therapy, oral contraceptives, alcoholic polyneuritis

Unlabeled uses: Palmar-Plantar erythrodysesthesia syndrome

DOSAGE AND ROUTES
RDA
• *Adult:* **PO** male 1.7-2 mg; female 1.4-1.6 mg
Vit B$_6$ deficiency
• *Adult:* **PO/IM/IV** 5-25 mg daily × 3wk
• *Child:* **PO/IM/IV** 100 mg until desired response
Deficiency caused by isoniazid, cycloSERINE, hydrALAZINE, penicillamine
• *Adult:* **PO** 6-100 mg daily
• *Child:* **PO** 5-25 mg daily
Prevention of deficiency caused by isoniazid, cycloSERINE, hydrALAZINE, penicillamine
• *Adult:* **PO** 6-50 mg daily
• *Child:* **PO** 0.5-1.5 mg daily
• *Infant:* **PO** 0.1-0.5 mg daily
Palmar-Plantar erythrodysesthesia syndrome (unlabeled)
• *Adult:* **PO** 50-150 mg daily
Available forms: Tabs 10, 25, 50, 100 mg; ext rel tabs 100 mg; inj 100 mg/ml; ext rel caps 150 mg

SIDE EFFECTS
CNS: Paresthesia, flushing, warmth, lethargy (rare with normal renal function)
INTEG: Pain at inj site
Contraindications: Hypersensitivity
Precautions: Pregnancy (A), lactation, children, Parkinson's disease, patients taking levodopa should avoid supplemental vitamins with >5 mg pyridoxine

PHARMACOKINETICS
PO/INJ: Half-life 2-3 wk, metabolized in liver, excreted in urine

INTERACTIONS
Decrease: effects of levodopa
Decrease: effects of pyridoxine—oral contraceptives, isoniazid, cycloSERINE, hydrALAZINE, penicillamine, chloramphenicol, immunosuppressants

NURSING CONSIDERATIONS
Assess:
• Pyridoxine levels throughout treatment
• Nutritional status: yeast, liver, legumes, bananas, green vegetables, whole grains
Administer:
PO route
• Do not break, crush, or chew ext rel tabs/caps
IM route
• Rotate sites; burning or stinging at site may occur
• Z-track to minimize pain
IV route
• Undiluted or added to most IV sol; give 50 mg or less/1 min if undiluted
Syringe compatibilities: Doxapram
Perform/provide:
• Storage in tight, light-resistant container
Evaluate:
• Therapeutic response: absence of nausea, vomiting, anorexia, skin lesions, glossitis, stomatitis, edema, seizures, restlessness, paresthesia
Teach patient/family:
• To avoid vitamin supplements unless directed by prescriber
• To keep out of children's reach

• To increase meat, bananas, potatoes, lima beans, whole grain cereals in diet
• To discuss birth control status with prescriber

---

pyrimethamine (℞)
(peer-i-meth′a-meen)
Daraprim, Fansidar (with sulfadoxine)
Func. class.: Antimalarial, antiprotozoal
Chem. class.: Folic acid antagonist

Action: Inhibits folic acid metabolism in parasite, prevents transmission by stopping growth of fertilized gametes
Uses: Malaria prophylaxis, *Plasmodium vivax*
Unlabeled uses: *Pneumocystis jiroveci* pneumonia as an adjunct

DOSAGE AND ROUTES
Prophylaxis of malaria
• *Adult and child >10 yr:* **PO** 25 mg qwk
• *Child 4-10 yr:* **PO** 12.5 mg qwk
• *Child <4 yr:* **PO** 6.25 mg qwk
Toxoplasmosis
• *Adult:* **PO** 100 mg, then 25 mg daily × 4-5 wk, with 1 g sulfadoxine q6h
• *Child:* **PO** 1 mg/kg/day in 2 divided doses or 2 mg/kg/day × 3 days, then 1 mg/kg/day or divided twice daily × 4 wk, max 25 mg/day
Toxoplasmosis in AIDS patients
• *Adult:* **PO** 100-200 mg/day × 1-2 days, then 50-100 mg/day × 3-6 wk, then 25-50 mg/day for life (given with clindamycin or sulfADIAZINE)
Available forms: Tabs 25 mg; combo tabs 500 mg sulfadoxine/25 mg pyrimethamine

SIDE EFFECTS
CNS: Stimulation, irritability, **seizures,** tremors, ataxia, fatigue
CV: **Dysrhythmias**
GI: Nausea, vomiting, cramps, anorexia, diarrhea, atrophic glossitis, gastritis
HEMA: **Thrombocytopenia, leukope-**nia, **pancytopenia, megaloblastic anemia,** decreased folic acid, **agranulocytosis**
INTEG: Skin eruptions, photosensitivity
RESP: **Respiratory failure**
Contraindications: Hypersensitivity, chloroquine-resistant malaria, megaloblastic anemia caused by folate deficiency
Precautions: Pregnancy (C), blood dyscrasias, seizure disorder, lactation, G6PD disease, renal/hepatic disease

PHARMACOKINETICS
PO: Peak 2 hr, half-life 96 hr, metabolized in liver, highly protein bound, excreted in urine (metabolites)

INTERACTIONS
• Synergistic action: folic acid
Increase: bone marrow suppression—bone marrow depressants, radiation therapy

NURSING CONSIDERATIONS
Assess:
• Folic acid level; megaloblastic anemia occurs
⚠ Blood studies, CBC, platelets, since blood dyscrasias occur; twice weekly if dosage is increased
⚠ For toxicity: vomiting, anorexia, seizure, blood dyscrasia, glossitis; drug should be discontinued immediately
Administer:
• Leucovorin IM 3-9 mg/day × 3 days if folic acid deficiency occurs
• Before or after meals at same time each day to maintain drug level, to decrease GI symptoms
Perform/provide:
• Storage in tight, light-resistant container
Evaluate:
• Therapeutic response: decreased symptoms of malaria
Teach patient/family:
• To report visual problems, fever, fatigue, bruising, bleeding; may indicate blood dyscrasias
• To report immediately skin rash; stop use

⚠ Safety alert   *"Tall Man" lettering

Treatment of overdose: Gastric lavage, short-acting barbiturate, leucovorin, respiratory support if needed

quetiapine (℞)
(kwe-tie′a-peen)
Seroquel
Func. class.: Antipsychotic

Action: Functions as an antagonist at multiple neurotransmitter receptors in the brain including $5HT_{1A}$, $5HT_2$, dopamine D_1, D_2, H_1, and adrenergic α_1, α_2 receptors

Uses: Psychotic disorders

DOSAGE AND ROUTES
• *Adult:* **PO** 25 mg bid, with incremental increases of 25 mg bid-tid on days 2 and 3 to a dose of 300-400 mg daily given bid-tid, max 800 mg/day

Available forms: Tabs 25, 100, 200, 300 mg

SIDE EFFECTS
CNS: EPS, pseudoparkinsonism, akathisia, dystonia, tardive dyskinesia; drowsiness, insomnia, agitation, anxiety, *headache,* **seizures, neuroleptic malignant syndrome,** *dizziness*

CV: Orthostatic hypotension, **tachycardia**

GI: Nausea, anorexia, constipation, abdominal pain, dry mouth

INTEG: Rash

MISC: Asthenia, back pain, fever, ear pain

RESP: Rhinitis

Contraindications: Hypersensitivity

Precautions: Pregnancy (C), children, hepatic disease, geriatric, breast cancer, lactation, long-term use, seizures, dementia

PHARMACOKINETICS
PO: Extensively metabolized by liver half-life ≥6 hr; peak 1½ hr; inhibits P450 CYP3A4 enzyme system

INTERACTIONS
Increase: CNS depression—alcohol, opioid analgesics, sedative/hypnotics, antihistamines

Increase: quetiapine clearance—phenytoin, thioridazine, barbiturates, glucocorticoids, carbamazepine, rifampin

Increase: quetiapine action—fluconazole, itraconazole, ketoconazole

Increase: effects of erythromycin

Decrease: quetiapine clearance—cimetidine

Decrease: effects of DOPamine agonists, levodopa, lorazepam

Drug/Herb

Increase: action—cola tree, hops, nettle, nutmeg

Increase: EPS—betel palm, kava

NURSING CONSIDERATIONS
Assess:
• Mental status before initial administration
• Swallowing of PO medication: check for hoarding or giving of medication to other patients
• I&O ratio; palpate bladder if urinary output is low
• Bilirubin, CBC, hepatic studies qmo
• Urinalysis before, during prolonged therapy
• Affect, orientation, LOC, reflexes, gait, coordination, sleep pattern disturbances
• B/P standing and lying; also pulse, respirations; take these q4h during initial treatment; establish baseline before starting treatment; report drops of 30 mm Hg; watch for ECG changes
• Dizziness, faintness, palpitations, tachycardia on rising
• EPS, including akathisia (inability to sit still, no pattern to movements), tardive dyskinesia (bizarre movements of the jaw, mouth, tongue, extremities), pseudoparkinsonism (rigidity, tremors, pill rolling, shuffling gait)

⚠ For neuroleptic malignant syndrome: hyperthermia, increased CPK, altered mental status, muscle rigidity, seizures, tachycardia, diaphoresis, hyper/hypo-

tension, fatigue; notify prescriber immediately if symptoms occur
- Skin turgor daily
- Constipation, urinary retention daily; if these occur, increase bulk and water in the diet

Administer:
- Reduced dose in geriatric
- Antiparkinsonian agent on order from prescriber, to be used for EPS
- Avoid use of CNS depressants

Perform/provide:
- Decreased stimulus by dimming lights, avoiding loud noises
- Supervised ambulation until patient is stabilized on medication; do not involve in strenuous exercise program because fainting is possible; patient should not stand still for a long time
- Sips of water, sugarless candy, gum for dry mouth
- Storage in tight, light-resistant container

Evaluate:
- Therapeutic response: decrease in emotional excitement, hallucinations, delusions, paranoia; reorganization of patterns of thought, speech

Teach patient/family:
- To rise slowly, to prevent orthostatic hypotension
- To take medication only as prescribed
- If drowsiness occurs, avoid hazardous activities such as driving
- To avoid use of OTC meds unless directed by prescriber
- To notify prescriber if pregnancy is planned, suspected
- To notify prescriber immediately of fever, difficulty breathing, fatigue

---

quinapril (℞)
(kwin'a-pril)
Accupril
Func. class.: Antihypertensive
Chem. class.: Angiotensin-converting enzyme (ACE) inhibitor

Action: Selectively suppresses renin-angiotensin-aldosterone system; inhibits ACE, prevents conversion of angiotensin I

to angiotensin II; results in dilation of arterial, venous vessels

Uses: Hypertension, alone or in combination with thiazide diuretics; systolic CHF

DOSAGE AND ROUTES

Hypertension (monotherapy)
- *Adult:* **PO** 10-20 mg daily initially, then 20-80 mg/day divided bid or daily
- *Geriatric:* **PO** 10 mg daily, titrate to desired response

Congestive heart failure
- *Adult:* **PO** 5 mg bid, may increase qwk until 20-40 mg/day in 2 divided doses

Renal dose
Adult: **PO** CCr 30-60 ml/min 5 mg/day initially; CCr <30 ml/min 2.5 mg/day initially

Available forms: Tabs 5, 10, 20, 40 mg

SIDE EFFECTS

CNS: Headache, dizziness, fatigue, somnolence, depression, malaise, nervousness, vertigo

CV: Hypotension, postural hypotension, syncope, palpitations, angina pectoris, **MI, tachycardia,** vasodilation, chest pain

GI: Nausea, diarrhea, constipation, *vomiting,* gastritis, **GI hemorrhage,** dry mouth

GU: Increased BUN, creatinine, decreased libido, impotence

HEMA: **Thrombocytopenia, agranulocytosis**

INTEG: **Angioedema,** rash, sweating, photosensitivity, pruritus

META: Hyperkalemia

MISC: Back pain, amblyopia

MS: Myalgia

RESP: Cough, pharyngitis, dyspnea

Contraindications: Pregnancy (D) 2nd/3rd trimester, hypersensitivity to ACE inhibitors, children, angioedema

Precautions: Pregnancy (C) 1st trimester, impaired renal, hepatic function, dialysis patients, hypovolemia, blood dyscrasias, COPD, bilateral renal stenosis, asthma, geriatric, lactation, cough

---

PHARMACOKINETICS

Bioavailability ≥60%
PO: Onset <1 hr, peak 1-2 hr, duration 24 hr, serum protein binding 97%, half-life 2 hr, metabolized by liver (active metabolites quinaprilat), metabolites excreted in urine (60%)/feces (37%)

INTERACTIONS

• Use caution with vasodilators, hydrALAZINE, prazosin, potassium-sparing diuretics, sympathomimetics, potassium supplements
Increase: hypotension—diuretics, other antihypertensives, ganglionic blockers, adrenergic blockers, phenothiazines, nitrates, acute alcohol ingestion
Increase: toxicity of lithium, digoxin
Decrease: absorption of tetracycline
Decrease: hypotensive effect of quinapril—indomethacin
Drug/Herb
Increase: toxicity, death—aconite
Increase: antihypertensive effect—barberry, betony, black catechu, black cohosh, bloodroot, broom, burdock, cat's claw, dandelion, goldenseal, hawthorn, Irish moss, Jamaican dogwood, kelp, khella, mistletoe, parsley
Increase or decrease: antihypertensive effect—astragalus, cola tree
Decrease: antihypertensive effect—coltsfoot, guarana, khat, licorice, yohimbine
Drug/Lab Test
False positive: Urine acetone, ANA titer

NURSING CONSIDERATIONS

Assess:
⚠ Blood studies: neutrophils, decreased platelets; WBC with differential baseline and periodically q3mo; if neutrophils <1000/mm³, discontinue treatment (recommended in collagen-vascular disease)
• B/P, orthostatic hypotension, syncope
• Renal studies: protein, BUN, creatinine; watch for increased levels; may indicate nephrotic syndrome
• Baselines in renal, hepatic studies before therapy begins and periodically; increased LFTs; uric acid and glucose may be increased
• Potassium levels; hyperkalemia is rare
• Edema in feet, legs daily, weight daily in CHF
⚠ Allergic reactions: rash, fever, pruritus, urticaria; drug should be discontinued if antihistamines fail to help
• Renal symptoms: oliguria, urinary frequency, dysuria
Administer:
• Tabs may be crushed if necessary
Evaluate:
• Therapeutic response: decrease in B/P
Teach patient/family:
• Not to discontinue drug abruptly
• Not to use OTC products (cough, cold, allergy); not to use salt substitutes containing potassium unless directed by prescriber
• To comply with dosage schedule, even if feeling better
• To rise slowly to sitting or standing position to minimize orthostatic hypotension
• To notify prescriber of mouth sores, sore throat, fever, swelling of hands or feet, irregular heartbeat, chest pain, persistent dry cough
• To report excessive perspiration, dehydration, vomiting, diarrhea; may lead to fall in B/P
• That drug may cause dizziness, fainting, light-headedness; may occur during first few days of therapy
• That drug may cause skin rash or impaired taste perception
• How to take B/P, and normal readings for age-group
Treatment of overdose: 0.9% NaCl IV inf

quinidine (℞)
(kwin'i-deen)
quinidine gluconate
Quinaglute Dura-Tabs,
Quinalan, Quinate ✦
quinidine polygalacturonate
Cardioquin
quinidine sulfate
Apo-Quinidine ✦, Cin-Quin,
Novoquinidine ✦, Quinidex
Extentabs, Quinora
Func. class.: Antidysrhythmic (Class IA)
Chem. class.: Quinine dextroisomer

Action: Prolongs duration of action potential and effective refractory period, thus decreasing myocardial excitability; anticholinergic properties

Uses: PVCs, atrial fibrillation, PAT, ventricular tachycardia, atrial flutter, malaria/IV quinidine gluconate

DOSAGE AND ROUTES
Quinidine gluconate
• *Adult:* **PO** 324-660 mg q6-12h (sus rel); **IM** 600 mg, then 400 mg q2h; **IV** give 16 mg/min
Quinidine sulfate
Atrial fibrillation/flutter
• *Adult:* **PO** 200 mg q2-3h × 5-8 doses; may increase daily until sinus rhythm is restored; max 4 g/day given only after digitalization, maintenance 200-300 mg tid-qid or 300-600 mg q8-12h (sus rel)
Paroxysmal supraventricular tachycardia
• *Adult:* **PO** 400-600 mg q2-3h, then 200-300 mg q6-8h or 300-600 mg q8-12h (sus rel)
Premature atrial/ventricular contraction
• *Adult:* **PO** 200-300 mg q6-8h or 300-600 mg (sus rel) q8-12h; max 4 g/day
• *Child:* **PO** 30 mg/kg/day or 900 mg/m^2/day in 5 divided doses
Available forms: *Gluconate:* sus rel tabs 324, 330 mg; inj gluconate 80 mg/ml; *sulfate:* tabs 200, 300 mg; sus rel tabs 300 mg; *polygalacturonate:* tabs 275 mg

SIDE EFFECTS
CNS: Headache, dizziness, involuntary movement, confusion, psychosis, restlessness, irritability, syncope, excitement, depression, ataxia
CV: **Hypotension,** *bradycardia,* PVCs, **heart block, cardiovascular collapse, arrest,** torsades de pointes, widening QRS complex, **ventricular tachycardia**
EENT: Cinchonism: tinnitus, blurred vision, hearing loss, mydriasis, disturbed color vision
GI: Nausea, vomiting, anorexia, abdominal pain, *diarrhea,* **hepatotoxicity**
HEMA: **Thrombocytopenia,** hemolytic anemia, agranulocytosis, hypoprothrombinemia
INTEG: Rash, urticaria, **angioedema,** swelling, photosensitivity, flushing with severe pruritus
RESP: Dyspnea, **respiratory depression**
Contraindications: Hypersensitivity, or idiosyncratic response, digoxin toxicity, history of long QT syndrome, drug-induced torsades de pointe, blood dyscrasias, severe heart block, myasthenia gravis
Precautions: Pregnancy (C), lactation, children, renal disease, potassium imbalance, hepatic disease, CHF, respiratory depression, geriatric

PHARMACOKINETICS
PO: Peak 0.5-6 hr, duration 6-8 hr; half-life 6-7 hr, metabolized in liver, excreted unchanged (10%-50%) by kidneys, protein bound (80%-90%)

INTERACTIONS
• Additive vagolytic effect: anticholinergic blockers
• Additive cardiac depression: other antidysrhythmics, phenothiazines, reserpine
Increase: effects of neuromuscular blockers, digoxin, warfarin, tricyclics, propranolol

---

⚠ Safety alert   *"Tall Man" lettering

Increase: quinidine effects—cimetidine, sodium bicarbonate, carbonic anhydrase inhibitors, antacids, hydroxide suspensions, amiodarone, verapamil, nifedipine
Decrease: quinidine effects—barbiturates, phenytoin, rifampin, sucralfate, cholinergics

Drug/Herb
• Hypokalemia, increased antidysrhythmic action: aloe, buckthorn, cascara sagrada, senna
Increase: toxicity, death—aconite
Increase: effect—aloe, broom, chronic buckthorn use, cascara sagrada (chronic use), Chinese rhubarb, figwort, fumitory, goldenseal, kudzu, licorice
Increase: serotonin effect—horehound
Decrease: effect—coltsfoot

Drug/Food
• Delayed absorption, decreased metabolism: grapefruit juice

Drug/Lab Test
Increase: CPK
Interference: Triamterene therapy interferes with quinidine test levels

NURSING CONSIDERATIONS
Assess:
⚠ ECG continuously to determine increased PR or QRS segments, QT interval; discontinue or reduce dose
• Blood levels (therapeutic level 2-7 mcg/ml)
• B/P continuously for fluctuations
⚠ For cinchonism: tinnitus, headache, nausea, dizziness, fever, vertigo, tremor; may lead to hearing loss
• Cardiac status: rate, rhythm, character, continuously
• Respiratory status: rate, rhythm, lung fields for crackles; increased respiration, increased pulse; drug should be discontinued
• CNS effects: dizziness, confusion, psychosis, paresthesias, convulsions; drug should be discontinued
Administer:
• AV node blocker (digoxin) before starting quinidine to avoid increased ventricular rate

PO route
• Do not break, crush, or chew ext rel products
• With a full glass of water, on empty stomach; if GI upset occurs, may take with food
• Sus rel forms not interchangeable
IM route
• IM inj in deltoid; aspirate to avoid intravascular administration
IV route
• After diluting 800 mg/50 ml or more D_5; give 16 mg or less over 1 min as inf; use infusion pump
Additive compatibilities: Bretylium, cimetidine, milrinone, ranitidine, verapamil
Y-site compatibilities: Diazepam, milrinone
Evaluate:
• Therapeutic response: decreased dysrhythmias
Teach patient/family:
• That if dizziness, drowsiness occur, avoid driving or hazardous activities
• To use sunglasses; may cause sensitivity to light
• To carry emergency ID stating disease and medication use
• How to take pulse and when to notify prescriber
• To avoid OTC meds unless approved by prescriber

quinine (OTC, ℞)
(kwye'nine)
Novoquine ✦ quinine sulfate
Func. class.: Antimalarial
Chem. class.: Cinchona tree alkaloid

Action: Inhibits parasite replications, transcription of DNA to RNA by forming complexes with DNA of parasite
Uses: *Plasmodium falciparum,* malaria, nocturnal leg cramps

DOSAGE AND ROUTES
• *Adult:* **PO** 650 mg q8h × 10 days, given with pyrimethamine 25 mg q12h × 3 days, with sulfADIAZINE 500 mg qid × 5 days

• *Child:* **PO** 25 mg/kg/day divided q8h for 3-7 days in conjunction with another agent

Leg cramps

• *Adult:* **PO** 250-300 mg at bedtime

Available forms: Caps 200, 300, 325 mg; tabs 260, 325 mg

SIDE EFFECTS

CNS: Headache, stimulation, fatigue, irritability, **seizures,** bad dreams, dizziness, fever, confusion, anxiety

CV: Angina, dysrhythmias, tachycardia, hypotension, **acute circulatory failure**

EENT: Blurred vision, corneal changes, retinal changes, difficulty focusing, tinnitus, vertigo, deafness, photophobia, diplopia, night blindness

ENDO: Hypoglycemia

GI: Nausea, vomiting, anorexia, diarrhea, epigastric pain

GU: Renal tubular damage, **anuria**

HEMA: **Thrombocytopenia, purpura, hypothrombinemia, hemolysis**

INTEG: Pruritus, pigmentary changes, skin eruptions, lichen planuslike eruptions, flushing, facial edema, sweating

MISC: **Hemolytic uremic syndrome**

RESP: Dyspnea

Contraindications: Pregnancy (X), hypersensitivity, G6PD deficiency, retinal field changes, lactation, myasthenia gravis

Precautions: Blood dyscrasias, severe GI disease, neurologic disease, severe hepatic disease, psoriasis, cardiac dysrhythmias, tinnitus, hypoglycemia

PHARMACOKINETICS

PO: Peak 1-3 hr, metabolized in liver, excreted in urine, half-life 4-11 hr

INTERACTIONS

Increase: toxicity—$NaHCO_3$, acetaZOLAMIDE

Increase: levels of digoxin, digitoxin, neuromuscular blockers, other anticoagulants

Increase: treatment failure—rifampin

Decrease: absorption—magnesium or aluminum salts (antacids)

Drug/Lab Test

Increase: 17-KS

Interference: 17-OHCS

NURSING CONSIDERATIONS

Assess:

• B/P, pulse, watch for hypotension, tachycardia

• Hepatic studies qwk: ALT, AST, bilirubin

• Blood studies, CBC, since blood dyscrasias occur

• For cinchonism: nausea, blurred vision, tinnitus, headache, difficulty focusing

Administer:

• Take with food to decrease GI upset; if a dose is missed, do not double

• Oral caps are not approved for prevention of malaria, treatment of severe malaria, or treatment/prevention of leg cramps

Perform/provide:

• Storage in tight, light-resistant container

Evaluate:

• Therapeutic response: decreased symptoms of malaria

Teach patient/family:

• Not to breastfeed while taking medication

• To avoid OTC preparations: cold preparations, tonic water

Treatment of overdose: Multiple dosages of activated charcoal

rabeprazole (℞)
(rah-bep′rah-zole)
Aciphex
Func. class.: Antiulcer, proton pump inhibitor
Chem. class.: Benzimidazole

Action: Suppresses gastric secretion by inhibiting hydrogen/potassium ATPase enzyme system in gastric parietal cell; characterized as gastric acid pump inhibitor, since it blocks final step of acid production

Uses: Gastroesophageal reflux disease (GERD), severe erosive esophagitis, poorly responsive systemic GERD, pathologic hypersecretory conditions (Zollinger-Ellison syndrome, systemic mastocytosis, multiple endocrine adenomas); treatment of active duodenal ulcers with or without antiinfectives for *Helicobacter pylori;* daytime, nighttime heartburn

DOSAGE AND ROUTES
Healing of duodenal ulcers
• *Adult:* **PO** 20 mg daily × ≤4 wk to be taken after breakfast
Healing of erosive esophagitis or ulcerative GERD
• *Adult:* **PO** 20 mg daily × 4-8 wk
Pathologic hypersecretory conditions
• *Adult:* **PO** 60 mg/day; may increase to 120 mg in 2 divided doses
Available forms: Del rel tabs 20 mg

SIDE EFFECTS
CNS: Headache, dizziness, asthenia
CV: Chest pain, angina, tachycardia, bradycardia, palpitations, peripheral edema
EENT: Tinnitus, taste perversion
GI: Diarrhea, abdominal pain, vomiting, nausea, constipation, flatulence, acid regurgitation, abdominal swelling, anorexia, irritable colon, esophageal candidiasis, dry mouth
GU: UTI, urinary frequency, increased creatinine, **proteinuria, hematuria,** testicular pain, glycosuria
HEMA: **Pancytopenia, thrombocytopenia, neutropenia, leukocytosis,** anemia
INTEG: Rash, dry skin, urticaria, pruritus, alopecia
META: Hypoglycemia, increased hepatic enzymes, weight gain
MISC: Back pain, fever, fatigue, malaise
RESP: Upper respiratory infections, cough, epistaxis
Contraindications: Hypersensitivity
Precautions: Pregnancy (C), lactation, children

PHARMACOKINETICS
Eliminated in urine as metabolites and in feces, terminal half-life 1-2 hr

INTERACTIONS
Increase: serum levels of rabeprazole—benzodiazepines, phenytoin, clarithromycin
Decrease: levels of rabeprazole—sucralfate, calcium carbonate, vit B_{12}

NURSING CONSIDERATIONS
Assess:
• GI system: bowel sounds q8h, abdomen for pain, swelling, anorexia
• Hepatic studies: AST, ALT, alk phos during treatment
Administer:
• Do not break, crush, or chew del rel tab
• After breakfast daily
Evaluate:
• Therapeutic response: absence of epigastric pain, swelling, fullness
Teach patient/family:
• To report severe diarrhea, drug may have to be discontinued
• That diabetic patient should know hypoglycemia may occur
• To avoid hazardous activities; dizziness may occur
• To avoid alcohol, salicylates, NSAIDs; may cause GI irritation
• To wear sunscreen, protective clothing to prevent burns

R

> ## radioactive iodine (sodium iodide)
> ¹³¹I (℞)
> *Func. class.:* Antithyroid
> *Chem. class.:* Radiopharmaceutical

Action: Converted to protein-bound iodine by thyroid gland for use when needed
Uses:
High dose: Thyroid cancer, hyperthyroidism

Low dose: Visualization to determine thyroid cancer, diagnostic aid in thyroid function studies

DOSAGE AND ROUTES

Thyroid cancer
• *Adult:* **PO** 50-150 mCi, may repeat depending on clinical status

Hyperthyroidism
• *Adult:* **PO** 4-10 mCi, depending on serum thyroxine level

Available forms: Caps 1-50, 0.8-100 mCi; oral sol 7.05 mCi/ml, 3.5-150 mCi/ vial

SIDE EFFECTS

EENT: Sore throat, cough
ENDO: Hypothyroidism, **hyperthyroid adenoma,** transient thyroiditis
GI: Nausea, diarrhea, vomiting
HEMA: **Eosinophilia, lymphedema, leukemia, bone marrow depression, leukopenia,** anemia
INTEG: Alopecia

Contraindications: Pregnancy (X), recent MI, lactation, large nodular goiter, age <30 yr, vomiting/diarrhea, acute hyperthyroidism, use of thyroid drugs, lactation

PHARMACOKINETICS

PO: Onset 3-6 days; excreted in urine, sweat, feces, breast milk; crosses placenta; excreted in 56 days

INTERACTIONS

• Hypothyroidism: lithium
Decrease: uptake if recent intake of stable iodine, thyroid, antithyroid drugs

NURSING CONSIDERATIONS

Assess:
• Weight daily with same clothing, scale, time of day
• Blood work, including CBC for blood dyscrasias (leukopenia, thrombocytopenia, agranulocytosis)
• Overdose: peripheral edema, heat intolerance, diaphoresis, palpitations, dysrhythmias, severe tachycardia, increased temp, delirium, CNS irritability
• Hypersensitivity: rash, enlarged cervical lymph nodes; drug may have to be discontinued
• Hypoprothrombinemia: bleeding, petechiae, ecchymosis
• Clinical response: after 3 wk should include increased weight, pulse; decreased T_4
• Bone marrow depression: sore throat, fever, fatigue

Administer:
• Only after discontinuing all other antithyroid agents × 5-7 days
• After NPO overnight, food delays action
• During or within 10 days after menstruation
• Do not take antithyroid agents except propranolol, which decreases hyperthyroid symptoms, until total effect of taking ^{131}I has occurred (about 6 wk)

Perform/provide:
• Limited contact with patient ½ hr/day for each person
• Adequate rest after treatment
• Fluids to 3-4 L/day for 48 hr to remove agent from body

Evaluate:
• Therapeutic response: weight gain, decreased pulse, decreased T_4, B/P

Teach patient/family:
• To empty bladder often during treatment; avoid irradiation of gonads
• To report redness, swelling, sore throat, mouth lesions; indicate blood dyscrasias
• To avoid extended contact with children, spouse for 1 wk
• That bathroom may be used by entire family
• To avoid coughing, expectorating for 24 hr (saliva and vomitus are highly radioactive for 6-8 hr)

⚠ Safety alert   *"Tall Man" lettering

raloxifene (R)
(ral-ox′ih-feen)
Evista
Func. class.: Bone resorption inhibitor, selective estrogen receptor modulator (SERM)
Chem. class.: Benzothiophene

Action: Reduces resorption of bone and decreases bone turnover; mediated through estrogen receptor binding
Uses: Prevention, treatment of osteoporosis in postmenopausal women

DOSAGE AND ROUTES
• *Adult:* PO 60 mg daily
Available forms: Tabs 60 mg

SIDE EFFECTS
CNS: Insomnia, migraines, depression, fever
CV: Hot flashes, chest pain
EENT: Retinal vein occlusion (rare)
GI: Nausea, vomiting, diarrhea, anorexia, cramps, dyspepsia
GU: Vaginitis, UTI, leukorrhea, cystitis, *hot flashes*
INTEG: Rash, sweating
META: Weight gain, peripheral edema
MS: Arthralgia, myalgia, *leg cramps,* arthritis
RESP: Sinusitis, pharyngitis, increased cough, pneumonia, laryngitis, rhinitis, bronchitis
Contraindications: Pregnancy (X), hypersensitivity, lactation, women with active or history of venous thromboembolic events
Precautions: Venous thromboembolic events, hepatic/CV disease, cervical/uterine cancer, elevated triglycerides, pulmonary embolism

PHARMACOKINETICS
Elimination half-life 28-32 hr; excreted in feces; excreted in breast milk; highly bound to plasma proteins

INTERACTIONS
• Administer cautiously with other highly protein-bound drugs
Decrease: action of anticoagulants
Decrease: action of raloxifene—ampicillin, cholestyramine
Drug/Lab Test
Increase: Apolipoprotein A_1, corticosteroid-binding globulin, thyroxine-binding globulin (TBG)
Decrease: Calcium, total protein, albumin, platelets, apolipoprotein, fibrinogen, LDL cholesterol, total cholesterol

NURSING CONSIDERATIONS
Assess:
• Weight daily, notify prescriber of weekly weight gain >5 lb
• B/P q4h, watch for increase caused by H_2O and sodium retention
• I&O ratio; decreasing urinary output, increasing edema
• Hepatic studies, including AST, ALT, bilirubin, alk phos
• Bone density test baseline and throughout treatment, bone-specific alk phos, osteocalcin, collagen breakdown
Administer:
• Without regard to meals, vit D
• Add calcium supplement if inadequate
Evaluate:
• Therapeutic response: prevention, treatment of osteoporosis
Teach patient/family:
• To weigh weekly, report gain >5 lb
• To discontinue 72 hr before prolonged bedrest; advise to avoid one position for long periods
• To take calcium supplements, vit D if intake is inadequate
• To increase exercise using weights
• To stop smoking and to decrease alcohol consumption
• That this drug does not help control hot flashes
• To report fever, acute migraine, insomnia, emotional distress; urinary tract infection, or vaginal burning/itching; swelling, warmth, or pain in calves

R

ramelteon (Ɍ)
(rah-mel'tee-on)
Rozerem
Func. class.: Sedative/hypnotic,
antianxiety
Chem. class.: Melatonin receptor
agonist

Action: Binds selectively to melatonin receptors (MT_1, MT_2); thought to be involved in circadian rhythm and the normal sleep/wake cycle

Uses: Insomnia

DOSAGE AND ROUTES
• *Adult:* **PO** 8 mg at bedtime
Hepatic dose
• Do not use in severe hepatic disease; use with caution in mild to moderate hepatic disease
Available forms: Tabs 8 mg

SIDE EFFECTS
CNS: Dizziness, somnolence, fatigue, headache, insomnia, depression, complex sleep related reactions: sleep driving, sleep eating
GI: Nausea, diarrhea, dysgeusia, vomiting
MISC: Myalgia, arthralgia, decreased blood cortisol, influenza, upper RI
SYST: **Severe allergic reactions**
Contraindications: Hypersensitivity, children, infants, lactation, alcohol intoxication, hepatic encephalopathy
Precautions: Pregnancy (C), hepatic disease, alcoholism, COPD, seizure disorder, sleep apnea, suicidal ideation

PHARMACOKINETICS
Absorbed rapidly, peak 0.75 hr, protein binding 82%, rapid first pass metabolism via liver, 84% excreted in urine, 4% feces, half-life 2-5 hr

INTERACTIONS
• Possible toxicity: antiretroviral protease inhibitors
Increase: ramelteon effect—alcohol, azole antifungals (ketoconazole, fluconazole), fluvoxamine, anxiolytics, sedatives, hypnotics, barbiturates
Decrease: effect of ramelteon—rifampin
Drug/Herb
• Do not use with melatonin
Increase: CNS depression—catnip, chamomile, clary, cowslip, hops, kava, lavender, mistletoe, nettle, pokeweed, poppy, Queen Anne's lace, senega, skullcap, valerian
Drug/Food
• Food: prolonged absorption, sleep onset reduced—high-fat/heavy meal

NURSING CONSIDERATIONS
Assess:
• Mental status: mood, sensorium, affect, memory (long, short)
• Type of sleep problem: falling asleep, staying asleep
Administer:
• After removal of cigarettes to prevent fires
• After trying conservative measures for insomnia
• Within 30 min of bedtime for sleeplessness
• On empty stomach for fast onset
Perform/provide:
• Assistance with ambulation after receiving dose
• Safety measure: night-light, call bell within easy reach
• Checking to see if PO medication has been swallowed
• Storage in tight container in cool environment
Evaluate:
• Therapeutic response: ability to sleep at night, decreased amount of early morning awakening
Teach patient/family:
• To avoid driving or other activities requiring alertness until drug is stabilized
• To avoid alcohol ingestion or CNS depressants
• Alternative measures to improve sleep: reading, exercise several hr before bedtime, warm bath, warm milk, TV, self-hypnosis, deep breathing
• To take immediately before going to bed

• Not to ingest a high-fat/heavy meal before taking

• To report cessation of menses, galactorrhea (women), decreased libido, infertility; worsening of insomnia, or behavioral changes

---

ramipril (℞)
(ra-mi′pril)
Altace
Func. class.: Antihypertensive
Chem. class.: Angiotensin-converting enzyme inhibitor (ACE)

Do not confuse:
ramipril/enalapril
Altace/alteplase/Artane

Action: Selectively suppresses renin-angiotensin-aldosterone system; inhibits ACE, prevents conversion of angiotensin I to angiotensin II; results in dilation of arterial, venous vessels

Uses: Hypertension, alone or in combination with thiazide diuretics; CHF (post MI), reduction in risk of MI, stroke, death from CV disorders

DOSAGE AND ROUTES

Hypertension
• *Adult:* **PO** 2.5 mg daily initially, then 2.5-20 mg/day divided bid or daily
Renal impairment
• *Adult:* **PO** 1.25 mg daily with CCr <40 ml/min/1.73 m²; increase as needed to max of 5 mg/day
CHF post-MI
• *Adult:* **PO** 1.25-2.5 mg bid; may increase to 5 mg bid
Reduction in risk of MI, stroke, death
• *Adult:* **PO** 2.5 mg daily × 7 days, then 5 mg daily × 21 days; then may increase to 10 mg/day
Renal dose
• *Adult:* **PO** CCr <40 ml/min 50% of dose
Available forms: Caps 1.25, 2.5, 5, 10 mg

SIDE EFFECTS

CNS: Headache, dizziness, anxiety, insomnia, paresthesia, *fatigue,* depression, malaise, vertigo, **seizures**
CV: Hypotension, chest pain, palpitations, angina, syncope, dysrhythmia
EENT: Hearing loss
GI: Nausea, constipation, vomiting, dyspepsia, dysphagia, anorexia, diarrhea, abdominal pain
GU: **Proteinuria,** increased BUN, creatinine, impotence
HEMA: Decreased Hct, Hgb, **eosinophilia, leukopenia**
INTEG: Rash, sweating, photosensitivity, pruritus
META: Hyperkalemia
MISC: **Angioedema**
MS: Arthralgia, arthritis, myalgia
RESP: Cough, dyspnea

Contraindications: Pregnancy (D) 2nd/3rd trimester, hypersensitivity to ACE inhibitors, lactation, children, history of angioedema

Precautions: Pregnancy (C) 1st trimester, impaired renal/hepatic function, dialysis patients, hypovolemia, blood dyscrasias, CHF, COPD, asthma, geriatric, renal artery stenosis, cough

PHARMACOKINETICS

Bioavailability >50%-60%
PO: Onset 1-2 hr, peak 3-6 hr, duration 24 hr, protein binding 73%, half-life 1-2 hr, 9-18 hr for active metabolite, metabolized by liver (metabolites excreted in urine, feces)

INTERACTIONS

Increase: hypotension—diuretics, other antihypertensives, ganglionic blockers, adrenergic blockers, nitrates, acute alcohol ingestion
Increase: toxicity—vasodilators, hydrALAZINE, prazosin, potassium-sparing diuretics, sympathomimetics, potassium supplements
Increase: serum levels of digoxin, lithium
Decrease: absorption—antacids

Decrease: antihypertensive effect—indomethacin, NSAIDs, salicylates
Drug/Herb
Increase: toxicity, death—aconite
Increase: antihypertensive effect—barberry, betony, black catechu, black cohosh, bloodroot, broom, burdock, cat's claw, dandelion, goldenseal, hawthorn, Irish moss, Jamaican dogwood, kelp, khella, mistletoe, parsley
Increase or decreased: antihypertensive effect—astragalus, cola tree
Decrease: antihypertensive effect—coltsfoot, guarana, khat, licorice, yohimbine
Drug/Lab Test
False positive: Urine acetone, ANA titer

NURSING CONSIDERATIONS
Assess:
⚠ Blood studies: neutrophils, decreased platelets; WBC with diff baseline and periodically q3mo, if neutrophils <1000/mm³, discontinue treatment (recommended in collagen-vascular disease)
• B/P, orthostatic hypotension, syncope
• Renal studies: protein, BUN, creatinine; increased levels may indicate nephrotic syndrome
• Baselines in renal, hepatic function tests before therapy begins and periodically; increased LFTs; uric acid and glucose may be increased
• Potassium levels, although hyperkalemia rarely occurs
• Dipstick of urine for protein daily in first morning specimen; if protein is increased, a 24-hr urinary protein should be collected
• Edema in feet, legs daily, weight daily in CHF
⚠ Allergic reactions: rash, fever, pruritus, urticaria; drug should be discontinued if antihistamines fail to help
• Renal symptoms: polyuria, oliguria, urinary frequency, dysuria
Administer:
• Caps can be opened and added to food
Perform/provide:
• Storage in tight container at 86° F (30° C) or less
• Supine position for severe hypotension

Evaluate:
• Therapeutic response: decrease in B/P
Teach patient/family:
• Not to discontinue drug abruptly
• Not to use OTC products (cough, cold, allergy) unless directed by prescriber; not to use salt substitutes containing potassium without consulting prescriber
• To comply with dosage schedule, even if feeling better
• To rise slowly to sitting or standing position to minimize orthostatic hypotension
• To notify prescriber of mouth sores, sore throat, fever, swelling of hands or feet, irregular heartbeat, chest pain
• To report excessive perspiration, dehydration, vomiting, diarrhea; may lead to fall in B/P
• That drug may cause dizziness, fainting, light-headedness; may occur during first few days of therapy
• That drug may cause skin rash or impaired perspiration
• How to take B/P, and normal readings for age group
Treatment of overdose: 0.9% NaCl IV inf, hemodialysis

---

ranibizumab
See Appendix A—Selected New Drugs

---

ranitidine (Rx, OTC)
(ra-nit'i-deen)
Apo-Ranitidine ✦, Zantac, Zantac C ✦, Zantac EFFERdose, Zantac GELdose
ranitidine bismuth citrate
Tritec
Func. class.: H₂-Histamine receptor antagonist

Do not confuse:
ranitidine/amantadine
Zantac/Xanax/Zofran
Action: Inhibits histamine at H₂-receptor site in parietal cells, which inhibits gastric acid secretion

---

⚠ Safety alert   ✦ "Tall Man" lettering

Uses: Duodenal ulcer, Zollinger-Ellison syndrome, gastric ulcers, hypersecretory conditions, gastroesophageal reflux disease, stress ulcers, erosive esophagitis (maintenance), active duodenal ulcers with *Helicobacter pylori* in combination with clarithromycin

Unlabeled uses: Prevention of aspiration pneumonitis, stress ulcers, upper GI bleeding

DOSAGE AND ROUTES

Ranitidine
Duodenal ulcer
• *Adult:* **PO** 150 mg bid, maintenance 150 mg at bedtime
Zollinger-Ellison syndrome
• *Adult:* **PO** 150 mg bid, may increase if needed
Gastric ulcer
• *Adult:* **PO** 150 mg bid × 6 wk, then 150 mg at bedtime
GERD
• *Adult:* **PO** 150 mg bid
Erosive esophagitis
• *Adult:* **PO** 150 mg bid, 300 mg at bedtime; **IM** 50 mg q6-8h; **IV BOL** 50 mg diluted to 20 ml over 5 min q6-8h; **IV INT INF** 50 mg/100 ml D$_5$ over 15-20 min q6-8h
• *Child:* **PO** 4-5 mg/kg/day divided q8-12h, max 6 mg/kg/day or 300 mg; **IV** 2-4 mg/kg/day divided q6-8h
Renal dose
• *Adult:* CCr <50 ml/min give **PO** q24h give **IM/IV** q12-24h
Ranitidine bismuth citrate
• *Adult:* **PO** 400 mg bid × 4 wk with clarithromycin 500 mg tid × 1st 2 wk
Available forms: *Ranitidine:* tabs 75, 150, 300 mg; sol for inj 25 mg/ml; effervescent tabs 75, 150 mg; inj 25 mg/ml; caps 150, 300 mg; syr 15 mg/ml; granules, effervescent 150 mg/packet; *ranitidine bismuth citrate:* tabs 400 mg

SIDE EFFECTS

CNS: Headache, sleeplessness, dizziness, confusion, agitation, depression, hallucination (geriatric)

CV: Tachycardia, bradycardia, PVCs
EENT: Blurred vision, increased ocular pressure
GI: Constipation, abdominal pain, diarrhea, nausea, vomiting, **hepatotoxicity**
GU: Impotence, gynecomastia
INTEG: Urticaria, rash, fever
SYST: **Anaphylaxis (rare)**
Contraindications: Hypersensitivity
Precautions: Pregnancy (B), lactation, child <12 yr, renal/hepatic disease

PHARMACOKINETICS

PO: Peak 2-3 hr; duration 8-12 hr; metabolized by liver; excreted in urine (30% unchanged, PO), breast milk; half-life 2-3 hr; protein binding 15%

INTERACTIONS

Increase: absorption, toxicity—anticoagulants, sulfonylureas, procainamide
Increase: effects of benzodiazepines, calcium channel blockers
Decrease: absorption of ranitidine—antacids, diazepam, anticholinergics, metoclopramide
Decrease: effects of cephalosporins, iron salts, ketoconazole
Drug/Lab Test
Increase: AST, ALT, alk phos, creatinine, LDH, bilirubin
False positive: Urine protein

NURSING CONSIDERATIONS

Assess:
• Gastric pH (>5 should be maintained)
• I&O ratio, BUN, creatinine
• Mental status: confusion, dizziness, depression, anxiety, weakness, tremors, psychosis, diarrhea, abdominal discomfort, jaundice; report immediately
• GI complaints: nausea, vomiting, diarrhea, cramps
Administer:
PO route
• With meals for prolonged effect
• Antacids 1 hr before or 1 hr after ranitidine

Side effects: *italics* = common; **bold** = life-threatening

IV route
• IV after diluting 50 mg/20 ml 0.9% NaCl, D_5W, $D_{10}W$, LR, $NaCO_3$ 5% and give 50 mg or less/5 min or more; may dilute 50 mg/50-100 ml of 0.9% NaCl, D_5W, $D_{10}W$, LR, $NaCO_3$ 5% and give over 15-20 min

Additive compatibilities: AcetaZOLAMIDE, amikacin, aminophylline, chloramphenicol, chlorothiazide, ciprofloxacin, colistimethate, dexamethasone, digoxin, DOBUTamine, DOPamine, doxycycline, epINEPHrine, erythromycin, floxacillin, fluconazole/ondansetron, flumazenil, furosemide, gentamicin, heparin, insulin (regular), isoproterenol, lidocaine, lincomycin, meropenem, methylPREDNISolone, moxalactam, penicillin G potassium, penicillin G sodium, polymyxin B, potassium chloride, protamine, quinidine, sodium nitroprusside, ticarcillin, tobramycin, vancomycin

Syringe compatibilities: Atropine, cyclizine, dexamethasone, dimenhyDRINATE, diphenhydrAMINE, DOBUTamine, DOPamine, fentanyl, glycopyrrolate, hydromorphone, isoproterenol, meperidine, metoclopramide, morphine, nalbuphine, oxymorphone, pentazocine, perphenazine, prochlorperazine, promethazine, scopolamine

Y-site compatibilities: Acyclovir, aldesleukin, allopurinol, amifostine, aminophylline, amsacrine, atracurium, aztreonam, bretylium, cefepime, ceftazidime, ciprofloxacin, cisatracurium, cisplatin, cladribine, cyclophosphamide, cytarabine, diltiazem, DOBUTamine, DOPamine, DOXOrubicin, DOXOrubicin liposome, enalaprilat, epINEPHrine, esmolol, fentanyl, filgrastim, fluconazole, fludarabine, foscarnet, furosemide, gallium, granisetron, heparin, hydromorphone, idarubicin, labetalol, lorazepam, melphalan, meperidine, methotrexate, midazolam, milrinone, morphine, niCARdipine, nitroglycerin, norepinephrine, ondansetron, paclitaxel, pancuronium, piperacillin, piperacillin/tazobactam, procainamide, propofol, remifentanil, sargramostim, tacrolimus, teniposide, theophylline, thiopental, thiotepa, vecuronium, vinorelbine, warfarin, zidovudine

Perform/provide:
• Storage at room temperature
Evaluate:
• Therapeutic response: decreased abdominal pain
Teach patient/family:
• That gynecomastia, impotence may occur but are reversible
• To avoid driving, other hazardous activities until stabilized on this medication
• To avoid black pepper, caffeine, alcohol, harsh spices, extremes in temperature of food
• That drug must be continued for prescribed time to be effective
• To avoid breastfeeding
• Not to take the maximum OTC daily dose for longer than 2 wk

ranolazine
See Appendix A—Selected New Drugs

rasagiline (℞)
(ra-sa′ji-leen)
Azilect
Func. class.: Antiparkinson agent
Chem. class.: MAOI

Action: Inhibits MAOI type B; may increase dopamine levels
Uses: Idiopathic Parkinson's disease monotherapy or with levodopa

DOSAGE AND ROUTES
Monotherapy
• *Adult:* **PO** 1 mg daily
Adjunctive therapy
• *Adult:* **PO** 0.5 mg daily, may be increased to 1 mg daily; change of levodopa dose in adjunct therapy; reduce levodopa dose may be needed
Hepatic dose
• *Adult:* **PO** 0.5 mg in mild hepatic disease
Concomitant ciprofloxacin, other CYP1A2 inhibitors
• *Adult:* **PO** 0.5 mg; plasma concentrations of rasagiline may double

---

⚠ Safety alert   *"Tall Man" lettering

Available forms: Tabs 0.5, 1 mg

SIDE EFFECTS

CNS: Drowsiness, hallucinations, depression, headache, malaise, paresthesia, vertigo, syncope

CV: Angina, **hypertensive crisis** (ingestion of tyramine products), orthostatic hypotension

GI: Nausea, diarrhea, dry mouth, dyspepsia

GU: Impotence, decreased libido

MISC: Conjunctivitis, fever, flu syndrome, neck pain, allergic reaction, alopecia

MS: Arthralgia, arthritis, dyskinesia, fall

RESP: Rhinitis

Contraindications: Hypersensitivity to this drug or MAOIs; lactation, pheochromocytoma

Precautions: Pregnancy (C), psychiatric disorders, children, severe hepatic disorders

PHARMACOKINETICS

Onset, peak, duration is unknown; well-absorbed, protein binding >88%-94%, metabolized by CYP1A2 in the liver, excreted by the kidneys

INTERACTIONS

• Do not give with meperidine, other analgesics, serious reaction including coma and death may occur; do not give with sympathomimetics

Increase: levels of rasagiline up to 2-fold—ciprofloxacin, CYP1A2 inhibitors (atazanavir, mexiletine, taurine)

Increase: severe CNS toxicity with antidepressants (tricyclics, SSRIs, SNRIs, mirtazapine, cyclobenzaprine)

Increase: hypertensive crisis—MAOIs

Drug/Herb

• Do not give with St. John's wort

NURSING CONSIDERATIONS

Assess:

• For Parkinson's symptoms: tremor, ataxia, muscle weakness and rigidity; baseline and periodically

• Mental status: hallucinations, confusion, notify prescriber

• For hypertensive crisis: severe headache, blurred vision, seizures, chest pain, difficulty thinking, nausea/vomiting, signs of stroke; any unexplained severe headache should be considered to be hypertensive crisis

• For increased dyskinesia and postural hypotension if used in combination with levodopa

• For melanomas frequently, perform periodic skin exams by a dermatologist

• Cardiac status: B/P, ECG; periodically during beginning treatment

Administer:

• With meals to prevent nausea; continuing therapy usually reduces or eliminates nausea

• Reduced dose of carbidopa/levodopa, cautiously

Evaluate:

• Therapeutic response: improved symptoms in those with Parkinson's disease

Teach patient/family:

• To change positions slowly to prevent orthostatic hypotension

• To avoid hazardous activities until stabilized; dizziness can occur

• To rinse mouth frequently, use sugarless gum to alleviate dry mouth

• To take as prescribed, not to miss dose or double doses; take missed dose as soon as remembered, if several hours before next dose

• To prevent hypertensive crisis by avoiding tyramine foods

• To report signs of hypertensive crisis

---

rasburicase (℞)
(rass-burr′i-case)
Elitek
Func. class.: Antineoplastic, antimetabolite
Chem. class.: Recombinant urate-oxidase enzyme

Action: Catalyzes enzymatic oxidation of uric acid into an inactive and a soluble metabolite

---

Side effects: *italics* = common; **bold** = life-threatening

Uses: To reduce uric acid levels in children with leukemia, lymphoma, solid tumor malignancies who are receiving chemotherapy

DOSAGE AND ROUTES

• *Adult:* IV INF 0.15 or 0.2 mg/kg as a single daily dose given as **IV INF** over ½ hr

Available forms: Powder for inj 1.5 mg/vial

SIDE EFFECTS

CNS: Headache

GI: Nausea, vomiting, anorexia, diarrhea, abdominal pain, constipation, dyspepsia, mucositis

HEMA: **Neutropenia with fever**

SYST: Anaphylaxis, hemolysis, **methemoglobinemia, sepsis**

Contraindications: Hypersensitivity, G6PD deficiency, hemolytic reactions, or methemoglobinemia reactions to this drug

Precautions: Pregnancy (C), lactation, children <2 yr

PHARMACOKINETICS

Elimination half-life 18 hr

NURSING CONSIDERATIONS

Assess:

• Renal studies: BUN, serum uric acid, urine creatinine clearance, electrolytes before and during therapy

• Monitor temp q4h; fever may indicate beginning infection; no rectal temps

• Anaphylaxis, have emergency equipment nearby

• For G6PD deficiency, hemolytic reactions, methemoglobinemia; these patients should not be given this agent

• For toxicity: severe diarrhea, nausea, vomiting

• GI symptoms: frequency of stools, cramping, if severe diarrhea occurs, fluid and electrolytes may need to be given

Administer:

• Antiemetic 30-60 min before giving drug and prn

Evaluate:

• Therapeutic response: decreased uric acid levels

Teach patient/family:

• Reason for therapy, expected results

⚠ High Alert

remifentanil (℞)

(rem-ih-fin′ta-nill)

Ultiva

Func. class.: Opiate agonist analgesic

Chem. class.: μ-Opioid agonist

Controlled Substance Schedule II

Action: Inhibits ascending pain pathways in limbic system, thalamus, midbrain, hypothalamus

Uses: In combination with other drugs in general anesthesia to provide analgesia

DOSAGE AND ROUTES

• *Adult:* Induction IV 0.5-1 mcg/kg/min with a hypnotic or volative agent; maintenance with isoflurane (0.4-1.5 MAC) or propofol (100-200 mcg/kg/min); CONT INF 0.25-0.4 mcg/kg/min

Available forms: Powder for inj lyophilized 1 mg/ml after reconstitution

SIDE EFFECTS

CNS: Drowsiness, *dizziness,* confusion, *headache,* sedation, euphoria, delirium, agitation, anxiety

CV: Palpitations, *bradycardia,* change in B/P, facial flushing, syncope, **asystole**

EENT: Tinnitus, blurred vision, miosis, diplopia

GI: Nausea, vomiting, anorexia, constipation, cramps, dry mouth

GU: Urinary retention, dysuria

INTEG: Rash, urticaria, bruising, flushing, diaphoresis, pruritus

MS: Rigidity

RESP: **Respiratory depression, apnea**

Contraindications: Child <12 yr, hypersensitivity

Precautions: Pregnancy (C), lactation, increased intracranial pressure, acute MI, severe heart disease, renal/hepatic disease, asthma, respiratory conditions, seizures disorders, geriatric

PHARMACOKINETICS

Unknown

INTERACTIONS

• Respiratory depression, hypotension, profound sedation: alcohol, sedatives, hypnotics, or other CNS depressants; antihistamines, phenothiazines

Drug/Herb

Increase: CNS depression—kava

NURSING CONSIDERATIONS

Assess:

• I&O ratio, check for decreasing output; may indicate urinary retention, especially in geriatric

• CNS changes; dizziness, drowsiness, hallucinations, euphoria, LOC, pupil reaction

• Allergic reactions: rash, urticaria

• Respiratory dysfunction: respiratory depression, character, rate, rhythm; notify prescriber if respirations are <12/min; CV status; bradycardia, syncope

• Use pain scoring to determine pain perception

Administer:

• Add 1 ml diluent per mg remifentanil

• Interruption of infusion results in rapid reversal (no residual opioid effect within 5-10 min)

Y-site compatibilities: Acyclovir, alfentanil, amikacin, aminophylline, ampicillin, ampicillin/sulbactam, aztreonam, bretylium, bumetanide, buprenorphine, butorphanol, calcium gluconate, cefazolin, cefepine, cefotaxime, cefotetan, cefoxitin, ceftazidime, ceftizoxime, ceftriaxone, cefuroxime, cimetidine, ciprofloxacin, cisatracurium, cisplatin, clindamycin, dactinomycin, dexamethasone, digoxin, diltiazem, diphenhydrAMINE, DOBUTamine, docetaxel, DOPamine, doxacurium, doxycycline, droperidol, enalaprilat, epINEPHrine, esmolol, etoposide, famotidine, fentanyl, fluconazole, furosemide, ganciclovir, gatiflexacin, gemcitabine, gentamicin, granisetron, haloperidol, heparin, hetastarch, hydrocortisone sodium succinate, hydromorphone, hydrOXYzine, imipenem/cilastatin, inamrinone, isoproterenol, ketorolac, levofloxacin, lidocaine, lorazepam, magnesium sulfate, mannitol, meperidine, methylPREDNISolone sodium succinate, metoclopramide, metronidazole, midazolam, minocycline, morphine, nalbuphine, netilmicin, nitroglycerin, norepinephrine, ofloxacin, ondansetron, paclitaxel, palonsetron, phenylephrine, piperacillin, potassium chloride, procainamide, prochlorperazine, promethazine, ranitidine, sulfentanil, sulfamethoxazole, teniposide, theophylline, thiopental, thiotepa, ticarcillin, ticarcillin/clavulanale, tobramycin, trimethoprim, vancomycin, voriconazole, zidovudine

Solution compatibilities: D_5, 0.45% NaCl, LR

Perform/provide:

• Storage in light-resistant area at room temperature

Evaluate:

• Therapeutic response: maintenance of anesthesia

Teach patient/family:

• To call for assistance when ambulating or smoking; drowsiness, dizziness may occur

• To make position changes slowly to prevent orthostatic hypotension

R

---

repaglinide (℞)

(re-pag'lih'nide)

Gluco Norm ✤, Prandin

Func. class.: Antidiabetic

Chem. class.: Meglitinide

Action: Causes functioning β-cells in pancreas to release insulin, leading to drop in blood glucose levels; closes ATP-dependent potassium channels in the β-cell membrane; this leads to opening

---

Side effects: *italics* = common; **bold** = life-threatening

of calcium channels; increased calcium influx induces insulin secretion

Uses: Type 2 diabetes mellitus

DOSAGE AND ROUTES

• *Adult:* PO 1-2 mg with each meal, max 16 mg/day, adjust at weekly intervals

Renal dose

• *Adult:* PO 0.5 mg/day; titrate upward cautiously

Available forms: Tabs 0.5, 1, 2 mg

SIDE EFFECTS

CNS: Headache, weakness, paresthesia

ENDO: **Hypoglycemia**

GI: Nausea, vomiting, diarrhea, constipation, dyspepsia

INTEG: Rash, allergic reactions

MISC: Chest pain, UTI, allergy

MS: Back pains, arthralgia

RESP: URI, sinusitis, rhinitis, bronchitis

Contraindications: Hypersensitivity to meglitinides, diabetic ketoacidosis, type 1 diabetes

Precautions: Pregnancy (C), geriatric, cardiac disease, severe renal/hepatic disease, thyroid disease, severe hypoglycemic reactions, lactation, children

PHARMACOKINETICS

PO: Competely absorbed by GI route; onset 30 min, peak 1-1½ hr, duration <4 hr; half-life 1 hr; metabolized in liver; excreted in urine, feces (metabolites); crosses placenta; 98% plasma protein bound

INTERACTIONS

Increase: in both—levonorgestrel/ethinyl estradiol

Increase: repaglinide metabolism—CYP450 inducers: rifampin, barbiturates, carbamazepine

Increase: repaglinide effect—NSAIDs, salicylates, sulfonamides, chloramphenicol, MAOIs, coumarins, β-blockers, probenecid, gemfibrozil, simvastatin

Decrease: repaglinide metabolism—CYP450 inhibitors: antifungals (ketoconazole, miconazole), erythromycin, macrolides

Decrease: repaglinide action—calcium channel blockers, corticosteroids, oral contraceptives, thiazide diuretics, thyroid preparations, estrogens, phenothiazines, phenytoin, rifampin, isoniazid, phenobarbital, sympathomimetics

Drug/Herb

Increase: antidiabetic effect—alfalfa, aloe, basil, bay, bilberry, bitter melon, black catechu, buchu, burdock, coriander, dandelion, eyebright (po), fenugreek, garlic, ginseng, glucomannan, glucosamine, goat's rue, gymnema, horehound, horse chestnut, jambul, myrrh, myrtle

Increase or decrease: hypoglycemic effect—chromium, fenugreek, ginseng

Decrease: hypoglycemic effect—broom, buchu, dandelion, juniper

Decrease: glucose tolerance—karela

Decrease: antidiabetic effect—bee pollen, blue cohosh, broom, chromium, elecampane, eucalyptus, gotu kola

Drug/Food

Decrease: repaglinide level, give before meals

NURSING CONSIDERATIONS

Assess:

⚠ Hypo/hyperglycemic reaction that can occur soon after meals: dizziness, weakness, headache, tremor, anxiety, tachycardia, hunger, sweating, abdominal pain

• A1c, fasting, postprandial glucose during treatment

Administer:

• Up to 15 min before meals; 2, 3, or 4 ×/day preprandially

• Skip dose if meal is skipped; add dose if meal is added

Perform/provide:

• Storage in tight container in cool environment

Evaluate:

• Therapeutic response: decrease in polyuria, polydipsia, polyphagia, clear sensorium, absence of dizziness, stable gait

---

⚠ Safety alert   *"Tall Man" lettering

Teach family/patient:
• Technique of blood glucose monitoring; use blood glucose meter
• The symptoms of hypo/hyperglycemia; what to do about each
• That drug must be continued on daily basis; explain consequences of discontinuing drug abruptly
• To avoid OTC medications unless ordered by prescriber
• That diabetes is a lifelong illness; drug will not cure disease
• That all food included in diet plan must be eaten to prevent hypoglycemia; to have glucagon emergency kit available; take before meals 2, 3, or 4 ×/day
• To carry emergency ID
• To avoid alcohol, explain disulfiram-like reaction

Treatment of overdose: Glucose 25 g IV via dextrose 50% solution, 50 ml or 1 mg glucagon

---

Rarely Used

reserpine (℞)
(re-ser′peen)
Novoreserpine ✽, Reserfia ✽, reserpine
Func. class.: Antihypertensive, antiadrenergic agent, peripheral action

Do not confuse:
reserpine/Risperdal
Uses: Hypertension

DOSAGE AND ROUTES
• *Adult:* **PO** 0.05-0.1 mg daily × 1-2 wk, then 0.1-0.25 mg daily maintenance
• *Geriatric:* **PO** 0.05 mg daily, increase by 0.05 weekly to desired dose
Contraindications: Pregnancy (D), hypersensitivity, depression, suicidal patients, active peptic ulcer disease, ulcerative colitis, Parkinson's disease, renal failure

---

Rh$_o$(D) immune globulin standard dose IM (℞)
BayRho-Full Dose Rho-GAM
Rh$_o$(D) globulin microdose IM (℞)
HypRho-D Mini-Dose, MiCRhoGAM, Mini-Gamulin
Rh$_o$(D) globulin IV (℞)
Rhophylac, WinRho SD, WinRho SDF
Func. class.: Immune globulins

Do not confuse:
Gamulin Rh/MICRh$_o$GAM
Action: Suppresses immune response of nonsensitized Rh$_o$(D or D^u)-negative patients who are exposed to Rh$_o$(D or D^u)-positive blood
Uses: Prevention of isoimmunization in Rh-negative women given Rh-positive blood after abortions, miscarriages, amniocentesis

DOSAGE AND ROUTES
Prior to Rh$_o$(D) immune globulin delivery (IM use only)
• *Adult:* **IM** 1 vial (300 mcg) (standard dose) at 26-28 wk, 1 vial (300 mcg) (standard dose) 72 hr after delivery
Pregnancy termination <13 wk
• *Adult:* **IM** 1 vial (50 mcg) (microdose) within 72 hr
Pregnancy termination >13 wk
• *Adult:* **IM** 1 vial (300 mcg) (standard dose) within 72 hr
Fetal-maternal hemorrhage
• *Adult:* **IM** packed RBCs volume of hemorrhage/15 = needed vials (standard dose)
Following delivery
• *Adult:* **IM** 1 vial (300 mcg) (standard dose) given within 72 hr of delivery or miscarriage
Transfusion error
• *Adult:* **IM** 1 vial (300 mcg) (standard dose) give within 72 hr

R

Side effects: *italics* = common; **bold** = life-threatening

Rh$_o$(D) immune globulin IV (IM or IV use)
Prior to delivery
• *Adult:* **IM/IV** 1500 international units (300 mcg) at 28 wk; if given earlier, repeat q12wk
Following delivery
• *Adult:* **IM/IV** 600 international units (120 mcg) within 72 hr after delivery
Following amniocentesis <34 wk/ chronic villas sample
• *Adult:* **IM/IV** 1500 international units (300 mcg) within 72 hr; repeat q12wk during pregnancy
Transfusion reaction
• *Adult:* **IM** 6000 international units (1200 mcg) q12h until total dose given; **IV** 3000 international units (600 mcg) q8h until total dose given
Immune thrombocytopenic purpura (ITP)
• *Adult and child:* **IV** 250 international units (50 mcg)/kg; frequency of additional doses based on response

Available forms: *Rh$_o$(D) immune globulin (IM use):* inj single-dose vial (50 mcg/vial-microdose; 300 mcg/vial-standard); *Rh$_o$(D) immune globulin IV (IV/IM use):* inj 120, 300, 1000 mcg

SIDE EFFECTS

CNS: Lethargy
INTEG: Irritation at inj site, fever
MS: Myalgia
Contraindications: Previous immunization with this drug, Rh$_o$(O)-positive/D^u-positive patient
Precautions: Pregnancy (C)

INTERACTIONS

Decrease: antibody response—live virus vaccines (measles, mumps, rubella)

NURSING CONSIDERATIONS
Assess:
⚠ Allergies, reactions to immunizations; previous immunization with this drug
⚠ For intravascular hemolysis: back pain, chills, hemoglobinuria, renal insufficiency
• Type, crossmatch mother and newborn's cord blood; if mother is Rh$_o$(D) negative, D^u-negative and newborn Rh$_o$(D) positive, this medication should be given
Administer:
IM route
• Reconstitute Rh$_o$(D) immune globulin IV using 1.25 ml of 0.9% NaCl, swirl
• IM inj in deltoid; aspirate within 3 hr if possible
• Only equal lot numbers of drug, crossmatch
• Only MICRhoGAM for abortions or miscarriages <12 wk unless fetus or father is Rh negative; unless patient is Rh$_o$(D)-positive, D^u-positive, Rh antibodies are present
• Do not use Rh$_o$(D) immune globulin or Rh$_o$(D) immune globulin micro dose by IV
IV, direct route
• Reconstitute Rh$_o$(D) immune globulin IV using 2.5 ml of 0.9% NaCl, swirl, give over 3-5 min
Perform/provide:
• Storage in refrigerator
Evaluate:
• Rh$_o$(D) sensitivity in transfusion error, prevention of erythroblastosis fetalis for normal vision
Teach patient/family:
• How drug works; that drug must be given after subsequent deliveries if subsequent babies are Rh positive

riboflavin (vit B$_2$)
(OTC)
(rye'boh-flay-vin)
Func. class.: Vit B$_2$, water soluble

Action: Needed for respiratory reactions by catalyzing proteins
Uses: Vit B$_2$ deficiency or polyneuritis; cheilosis adjunct with thiamine

DOSAGE AND ROUTES
Deficiency
• *Adult and child >12 yr:* **PO** 5-25 mg daily

- *Child <12 yr:* **PO** 2-10 mg daily, then 0.6 mg/1000 calories ingested
RDA
- *Adult:* **PO** Males 1.4-1.8 mg, females 1.2-1.3 mg
Available forms: Tabs 5, 10, 25, 50, 100, 250 mg

SIDE EFFECTS
GU: Yellow discoloration of urine
Precautions: Pregnancy (A)

PHARMACOKINETICS
PO: Half-life 65-85 min, 60% protein bound, unused amounts excreted in urine (unchanged)

INTERACTIONS
Increase: riboflavin need—alcohol, probenecid, tricyclics, phenothiazines
Decrease: action of tetracyclines
Drug/Lab Test
- May cause false elevations of urinary catecholamines

NURSING CONSIDERATIONS
Assess:
- Nutritional status: liver, eggs, dairy products, yeast, whole grain, green vegetables
Administer:
- With food for better absorption
Perform/provide:
- Storage in airtight, light-resistant container
Evaluate:
- Therapeutic response: absence of headache, GI problems, cheilosis, skin lesions, depression, burning, itchy eyes, anemia
Teach patient/family:
- That urine may turn bright yellow
- About addition of needed foods that are rich in riboflavin
- To avoid alcohol

rifabutin (℞)
(riff′a-byoo-ten)
Mycobutin
Func. class.: Antimycobacterial agent
Chem. class.: Rifamycin S derivative

Do not confuse:
rifabutin/rifampin
Action: Inhibits DNA-dependent RNA polymerase in susceptible strains of *Escherichia coli* and *Bacillus subtilis;* mechanism of action against *Mycobacterium avium* unknown
Uses: Prevention of *M. avium* complex (MAC) in patients with advanced HIV infection
Unlabeled uses: *Helicobacter pylori* that has not responded to other treatment

DOSAGE AND ROUTES
- *Adult:* 300 mg daily (may take as 150 mg bid)
Available forms: Caps 150 mg

SIDE EFFECTS
CNS: Headache, fatigue, anxiety, confusion, insomnia
GI: Nausea, vomiting, anorexia, diarrhea, heartburn, **hepatitis,** discolored saliva
GU: Hematuria, *discolored urine*
HEMA: **Hemolytic anemia, eosinophilia, thrombocytopenia, leukopenia**
INTEG: Rash
MISC: Flulike symptoms, shortness of breath, chest pressure
MS: Asthenia, arthralgia, myalgia
Contraindications: Hypersensitivity, active TB, WBC <1000/mm^3 or platelet count <50,000/mm^3
Precautions: Pregnancy (B), lactation, hepatic disease, blood dyscrasias, children

R

PHARMACOKINETICS

PO: Peak 2-3 hr, duration >24 hr, half-life 3 hr; metabolized in liver (active/inactive metabolites), excreted in urine primarily as metabolites

INTERACTIONS

Increase: levels of rifabutin: ritonavir
Decrease: action of amprenavir, anticoagulants, β-blockers, barbiturates, busPIRone, clofibrate, corticosteroids, cycloSPORINE, dapsone, delavirdine, digoxin, disopyramide, doxycycline, efavirenz, estrogens, fluconazole, indinavir, ketoconazole, losartan, nelfinavir, nevirapine, opioid analgesic, oral contraceptives, phenytoin, quinidine, saquinavir, sulfonylureas, theophylline, tocainide, tricyclics, verapamil, zidovudine, zolpidem

Drug/Food
• High-fat diet decreases absorption
Drug/Lab Test
Interference: Folate level, vit B_{12}, BSP, gallbladder studies

NURSING CONSIDERATIONS

Assess:
• CBC for neutropenia, thrombocytopenia, eosinophilia
• For acute TB: chest x-ray, sputum culture, blood culture, biopsy of lymph nodes, PPD; drug should not be given for active TB
• Signs of anemia: Hct, Hgb, fatigue
• Hepatic studies qwk: ALT, AST, bilirubin
• Renal status before, qmo: BUN, creatinine, output, specific gravity, urinalysis
• Hepatic status: decreased appetite, jaundice, dark urine, fatigue
Administer:
• With food if GI upset occurs; better to take on empty stomach 1 hr before or 2 hr after meals; high-fat foods slow absorption; may take in 2 divided doses
• Antiemetic if vomiting occurs
• After C&S is completed; qmo to detect resistance

Evaluate:
• Therapeutic response: not used for active TB because of risk of development of resistance to rifampin; culture negative
Teach patient/family:
• That patients using oral contraceptives should consider using nonhormonal methods of birth control, since rifabutin may decrease their efficacy
• That compliance with dosage schedule, duration is necessary
• That scheduled appointments must be kept; relapse may occur
• That urine, feces, saliva, sputum, sweat, tears may be colored red-orange; soft contact lenses may be permanently stained
• To report flulike symptoms: excessive fatigue, anorexia, vomiting, sore throat; unusual bleeding, yellowish discoloration of skin, eyes
• To report myositis: muscle or bone pain

rifampin (℞)
(rif'am-pin)
Rifadin, Rimactane, Rofact ✤
Func. class.: Antitubercular
Chem. class.: Rifamycin B derivative

Do not confuse:
rifampin/rifabutin
Action: Inhibits DNA-dependent polymerase, decreases tubercle bacilli replication
Uses: Pulmonary tuberculosis, meningococcal carriers (prevention)

DOSAGE AND ROUTES
Tuberculosis
• *Adult:* **PO/IV** max 600 mg/day as single dose 1 hr before meals or 2 hr after meals or 10 mg/kg/day 2-3 ×/wk
• *Child >5 yr:* **PO/IV** 10-20 mg/kg/day as single dose 1 hr before meals or 2 hr after meals, not to exceed 600 mg/day, with other antituberculars
• 6-mo regimen: 2 mo treatment of isoniazid, rifampin, pyrazinamide and possibly streptomycin or ethambutol; then rifampin and isoniazid × 4 mo

• 9-mo regimen: rifampin and isoniazid supplemented with pyrazinamide, or streptomycin or ethambutol

Meningococcal carriers

• *Adult:* **PO/IV** 600 mg bid × 2 days
• *Child >5 yr:* **PO/IV** 10-20 mg/kg not to exceed 600 mg/dose
• *Infant 3 mo-1 yr:* 5 mg/kg **PO** bid for 2 days

Prevention of H. influenzae *type B* **infection**

• *Adult:* **PO** 600 mg/day × 4 days
• *Child:* **PO** 20 mg/kg/day × 4 days

Available forms: Caps 150, 300 mg; powder for inj 600 mg/vial

SIDE EFFECTS

CNS: Headache, fatigue, anxiety, drowsiness, confusion
EENT: Visual disturbances
GI: Nausea, vomiting, anorexia, diarrhea, **pseudomembranous colitis,** *heartburn,* sore mouth and tongue, **pancreatitis,** increased LFTs
GU: **Hematuria, acute renal failure, hemoglobinuria**
HEMA: **Hemolytic anemia, eosinophilia, thrombocytopenia, leukopenia**
INTEG: Rash, pruritus, urticaria
MISC: Flulike symptoms, menstrual disturbances, edema, shortness of breath
MS: Ataxia, weakness

Contraindications: Hypersensitivity
Precautions: Pregnancy (C), lactation, hepatic disease, blood dyscrasias, child <5 yr

PHARMACOKINETICS

PO: Peak 1-4 hr, duration >24 hr, half-life 3 hr; metabolized in liver (active/inactive metabolites), excreted in urine as free drug (30% crosses placenta) and breast milk

INTERACTIONS

• Lithium toxicity: lithium
• Hepatotoxicity: isoniazid
• Incompatible with sodium lactate
Decrease: action of acetaminophen, alcohol, anticoagulants, antidiabetics, β-blockers, barbiturates, benzodiazepines, chloramphenicol, clofibrate, corticosteroids, cycloSPORINE, dapsone, digoxin, diltiazem, doxycycline, fluoroquinolones, haloperidol, hormones, imidazole antifungals, NIFEdipine, oral contraceptives, phenytoin, protease inhibitors, sulfonamides, theophylline, verapamil, zidovudine

Drug/Lab Test
Interference: Folate level, vit B$_{12}$, gallbladder studies, dexamethasone suppression test
False positive: Direct Coombs' test

NURSING CONSIDERATIONS

Assess:
• For infection: sputum culture, lung sounds
• Signs of anemia: Hct, Hgb, fatigue
• Hepatic studies qmo: ALT, AST, bilirubin
• Renal status before, qmo: BUN, creatinine, output, specific gravity, urinalysis
• Hepatic status: decreased appetite, jaundice, dark urine, fatigue

Administer:
• After C&S is completed; qmo to detect resistance

PO route
• On empty stomach, 1 hr before or 2 hr after meals with a full glass of water
• Antiemetic if vomiting occurs

IV route
• After diluting each 600 mg/10 ml of sterile water for inj (60 mg/ml), agitate, withdraw dose and dilute in 100 ml or 500 ml of D$_5$W or 0.9% NaCl given as an inf over 3 hr, or if diluted in 100 ml, give over ½ hr; do not admix with other sol or medications

Evaluate:
• Therapeutic response: decreased symptoms of TB, culture negative

Teach patient/family:
• That compliance with dosage schedule, duration is necessary
• That scheduled appointments must be kept; relapse may occur

R

- To avoid alcohol, hepatotoxicity may occur
- That urine, feces, saliva, sputum, sweat, tears may be colored red-orange; soft contact lenses may be permanently stained
- To report flulike symptoms: excessive fatigue, anorexia, vomiting, sore throat; unusual bleeding, yellowish discoloration of skin, eyes
- To use nonhormonal form of birth control

rifapentine (℞)
(riff′ah-pen-teen)
Priftin
Func. class.: Antitubercular
Chem. class.: Rifamycin derivative

Action: Inhibits DNA-dependent polymerase, decreases tubercle bacilli replication

Uses: Pulmonary tuberculosis, must be used with at least one other antitubercular agent

DOSAGE AND ROUTES
Intensive phase
- *Adult:* PO 600 mg (four 150-mg tabs 2 ×/wk), with an interval of 72 hr between doses × 2 mo; must be given with at least one other antitubercular agent
Continuation phase
- *Adult:* PO 600 mg qwk × 4 mo in combination with isoniazid or other appropriate antitubercular
Available forms: Tabs 150 mg

SIDE EFFECTS
CNS: Headache, fatigue, anxiety, dizziness
EENT: Visual disturbances
GI: Nausea, vomiting, anorexia, diarrhea, bilirubinemia, hepatitis, increased ALT, AST, *heartburn,* **pancreatitis**
GU: **Hematuria,** pyuria, proteinuria, urinary casts, urine discoloration
HEMA: **Thrombocytopenia, leukopenia, neutropenia, lymphopenia,** anemia, **leukocytosis,** purpura, hematoma
INTEG: Rash, pruritus, urticaria, acne

MISC: Edema, aggressive reaction, increased B/P
MS: Gout, arthrosis
Contraindications: Hypersensitivity to rifamycins, porphyria
Precautions: Pregnancy (C), lactation, hepatic disease, blood dyscrasias, children <12 yr, HIV, geriatric

PHARMACOKINETICS
PO: Peak 5-6 hr, half-life 13 hr; metabolized in liver (active/inactive metabolites), excreted in urine and feces, excreted in breast milk, protein binding 97%, steady state 10 days, CYP450 3A4, 2C8/9 inducer

INTERACTIONS
- Use with extreme caution with protease inhibitors
Decrease: action of amitriptyline, anticoagulants, antidiabetics, barbiturates, β-blockers, chloramphenicol, clarithromycin, clofibrate, corticosteroids, cycloSPORINE, dapsone, delavirdine, diazepam, digoxin, diltiazem, disopyramide, doxycycline, fentanyl, fluconazole, fluoroquinolones, haloperidol, indinavir, itraconazole, ketoconazole, methadone, mexiletine, nelfinavir, NIFEdipine, nortriptyline, oral contraceptives, phenothiazines, phenytoin, progestins, quinidine, quinine, ritonavir, saquinavir, sildenafil, tacrolimus, theophylline, thyroid preparations, tocainide, verapamil, warfarin, zidovudine
Drug/Food
Increase: absorption with food
Drug/Lab Test
Interference: Folate level, vit B_{12}

NURSING CONSIDERATIONS
Assess:
- Baselines in CBC, AST, ALT, bilirubin, platelets
- For infection: sputum culture, lung sounds
- Signs of anemia: Hct, Hgb, fatigue
- Hepatic studies qmo: ALT, AST, bilirubin

A Safety alert   *"Tall Man" lettering

- Renal status qmo: BUN, creatinine, output, specific gravity, urinalysis
- Hepatic status: decreased appetite, jaundice, dark urine, fatigue

Administer:
- May give with food for GI upset
- Antiemetic if vomiting occurs
- After C&S is completed; qmo to detect resistance

Evaluate:
- Therapeutic response: decreased symptoms of TB, culture negative

Teach patient/family:
- That compliance with dosage schedule, duration is necessary
- That scheduled appointments must be kept; relapse may occur
- That urine, feces, saliva, sputum, sweat, tears may be colored red-orange; soft contact lenses, dentures may be permanently stained
- To use alternative method of contraception, oral contraceptive action may be decreased
- To report flulike symptoms: excessive fatigue, anorexia, vomiting, sore throat; unusual bleeding, yellowish discoloration of skin, eyes

---

rifaximin (℞)
(rif-ax′i-min)
Xifaxan
Func. class.: Antiinfective—miscellaneous
Chem. class.: Analog of rifampin

Action: Binds to bacterial DNA–dependent RNA polymerase, thereby inhibiting bacterial RNA synthesis
Uses: Traveler's diarrhea in those ≥12 yr, caused by *E. coli*

DOSAGE AND ROUTES
- *Adult and child ≥12 yr:* **PO** 200 mg tid × 3 days without regard to meals
Available forms: Tabs 200 mg

SIDE EFFECTS
CNS: Abnormal dreams, dizziness, insomnia

GI: Abdominal pain, constipation, defecation urgency, flatulence, nausea, rectal tenesmus, vomiting
MISC: Headache, pyrexia

Contraindications: Hypersensitivity, diarrhea with fever, blood in stool
Precautions: Pregnancy (C), lactation, children

PHARMACOKINETICS
Half-life 6 hr, induces P4503A4 (CYP3A4), excreted in feces

INTERACTIONS
Drug/Herb
- Do not use acidophilus with antiinfectives; separate by several hours

NURSING CONSIDERATIONS
Assess:
- For GI symptoms: amount, character of diarrhea, abdominal pain, nausea, vomiting
- **⚠** For overgrowth of infection and pseudomembranous colitis

Administer:
- Without regard to food

Evaluate:
- Therapeutic response: absence of infection

Teach patient/family:
- To discontinue rifaximin and notify prescriber if diarrhea persists for more than 24-48 hr, if diarrhea worsens, or if blood is in stools and fever is present

---

riluzole (℞)
(rill′you-zole)
Rilutek
Func. class.: ALS agent
Chem. class.: Benzathiazole

Action: May act by modulating the release of glutamate and inactivating voltage-dependent sodium channels
Uses: Amyotropic lateral sclerosis (ALS)

DOSAGE AND ROUTES

• *Adult:* PO 50 mg q12h, take 1 hr before or 2 hr after meals

Available forms: Tabs 50 mg

SIDE EFFECTS

CNS: Hypertonia, depression, dizziness, insomnia, somnolence, vertigo

CV: Hypertension, tachycardia, phlebitis, palpitation, postural hypertension

GI: Nausea, vomiting, dyspepsia, anorexia, diarrhea, flatulence, stomatitis, dry mouth, increased LFTs, jaundice

GU: UTI, dysuria

HEMA: **Neutropenia**

INTEG: Pruritus, eczema, alopecia, **exfoliative dermatitis**

RESP: Decreased lung function, rhinitis, increased cough

Contraindications: Hypersensitivity

Precautions: Pregnancy (C), neutropenia, renal/hepatic disease, geriatric, lactation, children, cigarette smoking

PHARMACOKINETICS

Well absorbed, extensively metabolized by the liver, excretion in urine/feces

INTERACTIONS

Increase: elimination of riluzole—cigarette smoking, rifampin, omeprazole, charcoal-broiled food

Increase: hepatic injury—allopurinol, methyldopa, sulfasalazine, leflunomide, methotrexate, tacrine

Increase: LFTs—barbiturates, carbamazepine

Decrease: elimination of riluzole—caffeine, theophylline, amitriptyline, quinolones

Drug/Food

• High-fat meal: decreased absorption

NURSING CONSIDERATIONS

Assess:

• Hepatic studies: AST, ALT, bilirubin, GGT, baseline and qmo × 3 mo, then q3mo; monitor liver chemistries

• For neutropenia <500/mm

Administer:

• 1 hr before or 2 hr after meals; a high-fat meal decreases absorption

Teach patient/family:

• To report febrile illness, which may indicate neutropenia

• The reason for drug and expected results

---

rimantadine (Rx)

(ri-man'tah-deen)

Flumadine

Func. class.: Synthetic antiviral

Chem. class.: Tricyclic amine

Do not confuse:

rimantadine/amantadine/ranitidine

Action: Prevents uncoating of nucleic acid in viral cell, preventing penetration of virus to host; causes release of dopamine from neurons

Uses: Prophylaxis or treatment of influenza type A

DOSAGE AND ROUTES

Renal/hepatic dose

• Reduce dose as needed

Influenza type A

Prophylaxis

• *Adult and child >10 yr:* PO 100 mg bid; in renal, hepatic disease, lower dose to 100 mg/day

• *Child 1-10 yr:* PO 5 mg/kg/day, not to exceed 150 mg

Treatment

• *Adult:* PO 100 mg bid; in renal, hepatic disease, lower dose to 100 mg/day; start treatment at onset of symptoms, continue for at least 1 wk

• *Geriatric:* PO 100 mg/day × 5-7 days

Available forms: Tabs 100 mg; syr 50 mg/5 ml

SIDE EFFECTS

CNS: *Headache, dizziness,* fatigue, depression, hallucinations, tremors, **seizures,** insomnia, poor concentration, asthenia, gait abnormalities, *anxiety,* confusion

CV: Pallor, palpitations, edema

Safety alert   *"Tall Man" lettering

EENT: Tinnitus, taste abnormality, eye pain
GI: Nausea, vomiting, constipation, *dry mouth, anorexia, abdominal pain,* diarrhea, dyspepsia
INTEG: Rash

Contraindications: Hypersensitivity to drugs of adamantine class (this drug, amantadine)

Precautions: Pregnancy (C), seizure disorders, renal/hepatic disease, lactation, children <1 yr

PHARMACOKINETICS

PO: Peak 6 hr, elimination half-life 25½ hr, plasma protein binding (40%)

INTERACTIONS

Increase: rimantadine concentration—cimetidine
Decrease: peak concentration of rimantadine—acetaminophen, aspirin

NURSING CONSIDERATIONS
Assess:
• Assess for seizures; if seizures occur, drug should be discontinued
• Bowel pattern before, during treatment
• CNS effect in geriatric or patients with severe renal, hepatic disease
• Skin eruptions, photosensitivity after administration of drug
• Respiratory status: rate, character, wheezing, tightness in chest
• Allergies before initiation of treatment, reaction of each medication; list allergies on chart in bright red letters
• Signs of infection
Administer:
• Within 48 hr of exposure to influenza; continue for 10 days after contact
• At least 4 hr before bedtime to prevent insomnia
• After meals for better absorption, to decrease GI symptoms
• In divided doses to prevent CNS disturbances: headache, dizziness, fatigue, drowsiness
Perform/provide:
• Storage in tight, dry container

Evaluate:
• Therapeutic response: absence of fever, malaise, cough, dyspnea in infection
Teach patient/family:
• About aspects of drug therapy: need to report dyspnea, dizziness, poor concentration, behavioral changes
• To avoid hazardous activities if dizziness occurs

rimexolone ophthalmic
See Appendix C

risedronate (℞)
(rih-sed'roh-nate)
Actonel
Func. class.: Bone resorption inhibitor
Chem. class.: Bisphosphonate

Action: Inhibits bone resorption, absorbs calcium phosphate crystal in bone and may directly block dissolution of hydroxyapatite crystals of bone
Uses: Paget's disease, prevention, treatment of osteoporosis in postmenopausal women, glucocorticoid-induced osteoporosis

DOSAGE AND ROUTES
Paget's disease
• *Adult:* **PO** 30 mg daily × 2 mo; patients with Paget's disease should receive calcium and vit D if dietary intake is lacking; if relapse occurs, retreatment is advised
Postmenopausal osteoporosis
• *Adult:* **PO** 5 mg daily or 35 mg qwk
Glucocorticoid osteoporosis
• *Adult:* **PO** 5 mg daily
Available forms: Tabs 5, 30, 35 mg

SIDE EFFECTS
CNS: Dizziness, headache, depression
CV: Chest pain, hypertension
GI: Abdominal pain, anorexia, diarrhea, nausea, constipation

R

MISC: Rash, UTI, pharyngitis

MS: Bone pain, arthralgia

Contraindications: Hypersensitivity to bisphosphonates, inability to stand or sit upright for ≥30 min

Precautions: Pregnancy (C), children, lactation, renal disease, active upper GI disorders

PHARMACOKINETICS

Rapidly cleared from circulation, taken up mainly by bones, eliminated primarily through kidneys

INTERACTIONS

Increase: GI irritation—NSAIDs, salicylates

Decrease: absorption of risedronate—calcium supplements, antacids

Drug/Food

Decrease: bioavailability—take ½ hr before food or drinks other than water

Drug/Lab Test

Interference: Bone-imaging agents

NURSING CONSIDERATIONS

Assess:

• Symptoms of Paget's disease: headache, bone pain, increased head circumference

• Electrolytes: renal function studies; Ca, P, Mg, K

• For hypercalcemia: paresthesia, twitching, laryngospasm, Chvostek's, Trousseau's signs

Administer:

• For 2 months to be effective in Paget's disease

• With a full glass of water, patient should be in upright position for ½ hr

• Supplemental calcium and vit D in Paget's disease

• Give daily ≥30 min before meals

Perform/provide:

• Storage in cool environment, out of direct sunlight

Evaluate:

• Therapeutic response: increased bone mass, absence of fractures

Teach patient/family:

• To sit upright for ½ hr after dose to prevent irritation

• To comply with diet

• To notify prescriber if pregnancy is suspected

---

risperidone (℞)

(ris-pehr′ih-dohn)

Risperdal, Risperdal Consta, Risperdal M-TAB

Func. class.: Antipsychotic

Chem. class.: Benzisoxazole derivative

Do not confuse:

Risperdal/reserpine

Action: Unknown; may be mediated through both dopamine type 2 (D_2) and serotonin type 2 (5-HT_2) antagonism

Uses: Psychotic disorders

DOSAGE AND ROUTES

• *Adult:* **PO** 1 mg bid, with incremental increases of 1 mg bid on days 2 and 3 to a dose of 3 mg bid by day 3; then do not increase dose for at least 1 wk; **IM** 25 mg q2wk; may increase to max 50 mg q2wk

• *Geriatric:* **PO** 0.5 mg daily-bid, increase by 1 mg qwk

Hepatic/renal dose

• *Adult:* **PO** 0.5 mg bid, increase by 0.5 mg bid, increase to 1.5 mg bid

Available forms: Tabs 1, 2, 3, 4 mg; oral sol 1 mg/ml; orally disintegrating tabs 0.5, 1, 2 mg; powder for inj 25, 37.5, 50 mg

SIDE EFFECTS

CNS: EPS, pseudoparkinsonism, akathisia, dystonia, tardive dyskinesia; drowsiness, insomnia, agitation, anxiety, headache, **seizures, neuroleptic malignant syndrome,** dizziness

CV: Orthostatic hypotension, **tachycardia; heart failure, sudden death (geriatric)**

EENT: Blurred vision

GI: Nausea, vomiting, *anorexia, constipation,* jaundice, weight gain

---

⚠ Safety alert   *"Tall Man" lettering

RESP: Rhinitis; **fatal pneumonia (geriatric)**

Contraindications: Hypersensitivity, lactation, seizure disorders

Precautions: Pregnancy (C), children, renal/hepatic disease, geriatric, breast cancer

PHARMACOKINETICS

PO: Extensively metabolized by liver to a major active metabolite, plasma protein binding 90%

INTERACTIONS

Increase: sedation—other CNS depressants, alcohol

Increase: EPS—other antipsychotics

Increase: risperidone excretion—carbamazepine

Decrease: levodopa effect—levodopa

Drug/Herb

Increase: CNS depression—kava

Increase: action—cola tree, hops, nettle, nutmeg

Increase: EPS—betel palm, kava

Drug/Lab Test

Increase: Prolactin levels

NURSING CONSIDERATIONS

Assess:

• Mental status before initial administration

• Swallowing of PO medication; check for hoarding or giving of medication to other patients

• I&O ratio; palpate bladder if urinary output is low

• Bilirubin, CBC, hepatic studies qmo

• Urinalysis before, during prolonged therapy

• Affect, orientation, LOC, reflexes, gait, coordination, sleep pattern disturbances

• B/P standing and lying; also pulse, respirations; take these q4h during initial treatment; establish baseline before starting treatment; report drops of 30 mm Hg; watch for ECG changes

• Dizziness, faintness, palpitations, tachycardia on rising

• EPS, including akathisia, tardive dyskinesia (bizarre movements of the jaw, mouth, tongue, extremities), pseudoparkinsonism (rigidity, tremors, pill rolling, shuffling gait)

⚠ For serious reactions in the geriatric patient: fatal pneumonia, heart failure, sudden death

⚠ For neuroleptic malignant syndrome: hyperthermia, increased CPK, altered mental status, muscle rigidity

• Skin turgor daily

• Constipation, urinary retention daily; if these occur, increase bulk and water in diet

Administer:

• Reduced dose in geriatric

• Antiparkinsonian agent on order from prescriber, to be used for EPS

• Avoid use with CNS depressants

• Oral disintegrating tab: do not open blister pack until ready to use; tear 1 of the 4 units apart at perforation; bend corner where indicated; peel back foil; do not push tab through foil; remove from pack and place on tongue; tab disintegrates in seconds and can be swallowed with or without liquids

• When switching from oral to inj, give oral dose with first inj and continue for 3 wk, then discontinue

Perform/provide:

• Decreased stimulus by dimming lights, avoiding loud noises

• Supervised ambulation until patient is stabilized on medication; do not involve in strenuous exercise program because fainting is possible; patient should not stand still for a long time

• Increased fluids to prevent constipation

• Sips of water, candy, gum for dry mouth

• Storage in tight, light-resistant container

Evaluate:

• Therapeutic response: decrease in emotional excitement, hallucinations, delusions, paranoia; reorganization of patterns of thought, speech

Teach patient/family:

• That orthostatic hypotension may occur and to rise from sitting or lying position gradually

• To avoid hot tubs, hot showers, tub baths; hypotension may occur
• To avoid abrupt withdrawal of this drug; EPS may result; drug should be withdrawn slowly
• To avoid OTC preparations (cough, hay fever, cold) unless approved by prescriber; serious drug interactions may occur; avoid use of alcohol; increased drowsiness may occur
• To avoid hazardous activities if drowsy or dizzy
• Compliance with drug regimen
• To report impaired vision, tremors, muscle twitching
• In hot weather, that heat stroke may occur; take extra precautions to stay cool
• To use contraception, inform prescriber if pregnancy is planned or suspected

Treatment of overdose: Lavage if orally ingested; provide airway; *do not induce vomiting*

ritodrine (℞)
(rih'toh-dreen)
ritodrine, Yutopar
Func. class.: Tocolytic, uterine relaxant
Chem. class.: β_2-Adrenergic agonist

Action: Reduces frequency, intensity of uterine contractions by stimulation of the β_2-receptors in uterine smooth muscle
Uses: Management of preterm labor

DOSAGE AND ROUTES
• *Adult:* **IV INF** 150 mg/500 ml (0.3 mg/ml) given 0.1 mg/min, increased gradually by 0.05 mg/min q10min until desired response, max 0.35 mg/min
Available forms: Inj 10 mg/ml, 15 mg/ml

SIDE EFFECTS
CNS: Headache, restlessness, anxiety, nervousness, sweating, chills, drowsiness, tremor

CV: Altered maternal, fetal heart rate, B/P, dysrhythmias, palpitations, chest pain, maternal pulmonary edema
GI: Nausea, vomiting, anorexia, malaise, bloating, constipation, diarrhea
META: Hyperglycemia, hypokalemia
MISC: Erythema, rash, dyspnea, hyperventilation, glycosuria, **lactic acidosis**

Contraindications: Hypersensitivity, eclampsia, hypertension, dysrhythmias, thyrotoxicosis, before 20th wk of pregnancy, antepartum hemorrhage, intrauterine fetal death, maternal cardiac disease, pulmonary hypertension, uncontrolled diabetes, pheochromocytoma, bronchial asthma

Precautions: Pregnancy (B), migraine, sulfite sensitivity, pregnancy-induced hypertension, diabetes

PHARMACOKINETICS
IV: Immediate, distribution half-life 6 min, 2nd phase 1½-2½ hr, elimination phase >10 hr; metabolized in liver; 90% excreted in urine; crosses placenta

INTERACTIONS
Increase: pulmonary edema—corticosteroids
Increase: systemic hypertension—atropine
Increase: CV effects of ritodrine—magnesium sulfate, diazoxide, meperidine, potent general anesthetics
Increase: effects of sympathomimetic amines
Decrease: action of ritodrine—β-blockers
Drug/Lab Test
Increase: blood glucose, free fatty acids, insulin, GTT
Decrease: potassium

NURSING CONSIDERATIONS
Assess:
• Maternal, fetal heart tones during infusion; maternal ECG to determine CV disease
• Intensity, length of uterine contractions

⚠ Safety alert   *"Tall Man" lettering

• Fluid intake to prevent fluid overload; discontinue if this occurs
• Blood glucose in diabetics
Administer:
• Only clear sol
• After dilution: 150 mg/500 ml D_5W or NS, give at 0.3 mg/ml
• Using infusion pump; product should be continued for 12 hr after contractions stop
• Considered incompatible with any drug in sol or syringe
• In bed during infusion
Perform/provide:
• Positioning of patient in left lateral recumbent position to decrease hypotension, increase renal blood flow
Evaluate:
• Therapeutic response: decreased intensity, length of contraction, absence of preterm labor, decreased B/P

---

ritonavir (℞)
(ri-toe'na-veer)
Norvir
Func. class.: Antiretroviral
Chem. class.: Protease inhibitor

Do not confuse:
ritonavir/Retrovir
Action: Inhibits human immunodeficiency virus (HIV-1) protease and prevents maturation of the infectious virus
Uses: HIV-1 in combination with other antiretrovirals

DOSAGE AND ROUTES

• *Adult:* **PO** 600 mg bid; if nausea occurs begin dose at ½ and gradually increase
• *Child 2-16 yr:* **PO** 400 mg/m² bid up to 1200 mg/day
Available forms: Caps 100 mg; oral sol 80 mg/ml

SIDE EFFECTS

CNS: Paresthesia, *headache*, **seizures,** fever
GI: Diarrhea, buccal mucosa ulceration, abdominal pain, *nausea,* taste perversion,

dry mouth, dizziness, insomnia, vomiting, anorexia
INTEG: Rash
MISC: Asthenia, **angioedema, anaphylaxis, Stevens-Johnson syndrome,** increase lipids, lipodystrophy
MS: Pain
Contraindications: Hypersensitivity
Precautions: Pregnancy (B), hepatic disease, lactation, children, pancreatitis, diabetes

PHARMACOKINETICS

Well absorbed; 98% protein binding, hepatic metabolism, peak 2-4 hr, terminal half-life 3-5 hr

INTERACTIONS

⚠ Toxicity: amiodarone, azole antifungals, benzodiazepines, bepridil, buPROPion, clozapine, desipramine, dihydroergotamine, encainide, ergotamine, flecainide, HMG-CoA reductase inhibitors, interleukins, meperidine, midazolam, pimozide, piroxicam, propafenone, propoxyphene, quinidine, saquinavir, terfenadine, triazolam, zolpidem
Increase: ritonavir levels—fluconazole
Increase: level of both drugs—clarithromycin, ddI
Decrease: ritonavir levels—rifamycins, nevirapine, barbiturates, phenytoin
Decrease: levels of anticoagulants, atovaquone, divalproex, ethinyl estradiol, lamotrigine, phenytoin, sulfamethoxazole, theophylline, zidovudine
Drug/Herb
Decrease: ritonavir levels—St. John's wort; avoid concurrent use
Drug/Lab Test
Increase: AST, ALT, CPK, cholesterol, GGT, triglycerides, uric acid
Decrease: Hct, RBC, Hgb, neutrophils, WBC

NURSING CONSIDERATIONS
Assess:
• Signs of infection, anemia
• Hepatic studies: ALT, AST

R

- Viral load and CD4 baseline and throughout therapy
- C&S before drug therapy; drug may be taken as soon as culture is taken; repeat C&S after treatment; determine the presence of other sexually transmitted diseases
- Bowel pattern before, during treatment; if severe abdominal pain with bleeding occurs, discontinue drug; monitor hydration
- Skin eruptions; rash
- Allergies before treatment, reaction to each medication

Administer:
- With food; mix oral powder with high-calorie drink such as Ensure
- Store caps in refrigerator
- That drug must be taken in equal intervals around the clock to maintain blood levels for duration of therapy
- To take with food; mix liquid formulation with chocolate milk or liquid nutritional supplement

Teach patient/family:
- To take as prescribed; if dose is missed, take as soon as remembered up to 1 hr before next dose; do not double dose
- That drug is not a cure for HIV; opportunistic infections may continue to be acquired
- That redistribution of body fat or accumulation of body fat may occur
- That others may continue to contract HIV from the patient
- Not to use St. John's wort; that it decreases this drug's effect

---

rituximab
(rih-tuks'ih-mab)
Rituxan
Func. class.: Antineoplastic—miscellaneous
Chem. class.: Murine/human monoclonal antibody

Action: Directed against the CD20 antigen that is found on malignant B lymphocytes; CD20 regulates a portion of cell-cycle initiation/differentiation

Uses: Non-Hodgkin's lymphoma (CD20 positive, B-cell), bulky disease (tumors >10 cm)

DOSAGE AND ROUTES
- *Adult:* **IV INF** 375 mg/m² qwk × 4 doses; give at 50 mg/hr for 1st inf; if hypersensitivity does not occur, increase rate by 50 mg/hr q½h, max 400 mg/hr; slow/interrupt inf if hypersensitivity occurs; other inf can be given at 100 mg/hr and increased by 100 mg/hr, max 400 mg/hr
Available forms: Inj 10 mg/ml

SIDE EFFECTS
CNS: **Life-threatening brain infection**
CV: **Cardiac dysrhythmias**
GI: Nausea, vomiting, anorexia
GU: **Renal failure**
HEMA: **Leukopenia, neutropenia, thrombocytopenia**
INTEG: Irritation at site, rash, **fatal mucocutaneous infections (rare)**
OTHER: Fever, chills, asthenia, headache, **angioedema,** hypotension, myalgia, **bronchospasm**
SYST: **Stevens-Johnson syndrome**
Contraindications: Hypersensitivity, murine proteins
Precautions: Pregnancy (C), lactation, children, geriatric, cardiac conditions

PHARMACOKINETICS
Half-life 42-79 min

NURSING CONSIDERATIONS
Assess:
⚠ For signs of fatal infusion reaction: hypoxia, pulmonary infiltrates, acute respiratory distress syndrome, MI, ventricular fibrillation, cardiogenic shock; most fatal infusion reactions occur with first infusion; potentially fatal
⚠ For signs of severe mucocutaneous reactions: Stevens-Johnson syndrome, lichenoid dermatitis, toxic epidermal lysis; occur 1-13 wk after drug is given
⚠ Tumor lysis syndrome: acute renal failure requiring hemodialysis, hyperkale-

---

⚠ Safety alert   *"Tall Man" lettering

mia, hypocalcemia, hyperuricemia, hyperphosphatemia

• CBC, differential, platelet count weekly; withhold drug if WBC is <3500/mm³, or platelet count <100,000/mm³; notify prescriber of these results; drug should be discontinued

• Food preferences: list likes, dislikes

• GI symptoms: frequency of stools

• Signs of dehydration: rapid respirations, poor skin turgor, decreased urine output, dry skin, restlessness, weakness

Administer:

IV INF route

• After diluting to a final conc. of 1-4 mg/ml; use 0.9% NaCl, D₅W, gently invert bag to mix; do not mix with other drugs

Perform/provide:

• Increase fluid intake to 2-3 L/day for dehydration unless contraindicated

• Changing of IV site q48h

• Nutritious diet with iron, vitamin supplement, low fiber, few dairy products

• Storage of vials at 36°-40° F, protect vials from direct sunlight, inf sol is stable at 36°-46° F × 24 hr and room temperature for another 12 hr

Evaluate:

• Therapeutic response: decrease in tumor size, decrease in spread of cancer

Teach patient/family:

• To report adverse reactions

---

rivastigmine (℞)
(riv-as-tig′mine)
Exelon
Func. class.: Anti-Alzheimer agent
Chem. class.: Cholinesterase inhibitor

Action: May enhance cholinergic functioning by increasing acetylcholine
Uses: Mild to moderate Alzheimer's dementia

DOSAGE AND ROUTES

• *Adult:* **PO** 1.5 mg bid with food; after 2 wk or more, may increase to 3 mg bid after 2 wk or more; may increase to 4.5 mg bid and thereafter 6 mg bid, max 12 mg/day

Available forms: Caps 1.5, 3, 4.5, 6 mg; solution 2 mg/ml

SIDE EFFECTS

CNS: Tremors, confusion, insomnia, psychosis, hallucination, depression, dizziness, headache, anxiety, somnolence, fatigue, syncope

GI: Nausea, vomiting, anorexia, abdominal distress, flatulence, diarrhea, constipation, dyspepsia

MISC: Urinary tract infection, asthenia, increased sweating, hypertension, flulike symptoms, weight change

Contraindications: Hypersensitivity to this drug, other carbamates; narrow-angle glaucoma, undiagnosed skin lesions

Precautions: Pregnancy (B), renal/hepatic/cardiac/respiratory disease, seizure disorder, peptic ulcer, cardiac disease, urinary obstruction, asthma, lactation, children

PHARMACOKINETICS

Rapidly and completely absorbed, metabolized to decarbamylated metabolite, half-life is 1.5 hr, excreted via kidneys (metabolites), clearance is lowered in the geriatric, hepatic disease, and increased in nicotine use

INTERACTIONS

• Synergistic effect: cholinomimetics, other cholinesterase inhibitors

Drug/Herb

Increase: effect—pill-bearing spurge

NURSING CONSIDERATIONS

Assess:

• Hepatic studies: AST, ALT, alk phos, LDH, bilirubin, CBC

• For severe GI effects: nausea, vomiting, anorexia, weight loss

• B/P, respiration during initial treatment; hypo/hypertension should be reported

• Mental status: affect, mood, behavioral changes, depression; complete suicide assessment

R

Side effects: *italics* = common; **bold** = life-threatening

Administer:

• With meals; take with morning and evening meal even though absorption may be decreased

• Discontinue treatment for several doses and restart at same or next lower dosage level, if adverse reactions cause intolerance

• If treatment is interrupted for longer than several days, treatment should be initiated with lowest daily dose and titrated as indicated above

Perform/provide:

• Assistance with ambulation during beginning therapy

Evaluate:

• Therapeutic response: decreased dementia

Teach patient/family:

• The procedure for giving oral solution; use instruction sheet provided

• To notify prescriber of severe GI effects

---

rizatriptan (℞)

(rye-zah-trip′tan)
Maxalt, Maxalt-MLT
Func. class.: Migraine agent
Chem. class.: 5-HT$_{1D}$ receptor agonist, abortive agent-triptan

Action: Binds selectively to the vascular 5-HT$_{1D}$ receptor subtype, exerts antimigraine effect; causes vasoconstriction in cranial arteries

Uses: Acute treatment of migraine

DOSAGE AND ROUTES

• *Adult:* **PO** 5-10 mg single dose, redosing separate by 2 hr or more; max 30 mg/24 hr, use 5 mg in patient on propranolol; max 15 mg/24 hr

Available forms: Tabs (Maxalt) 5, 10 mg; orally disintegrating tabs (Maxalt-MLT) 2.5, 5, 10 mg

SIDE EFFECTS

CNS: Dizziness, drowsiness, headache, fatigue, warm/cold sensations, flushing

CV: **MI, ventricular fibrillation, ventricular tachycardia, coronary artery vasospasm**

ENDO: Hot flashes, mild increase in growth hormone

GI: Nausea, dry mouth, diarrhea, abdominal pain

RESP: Chest tightness, pressure, dyspnea

Contraindications: Angina pectoris, history of MI, documented silent ischemia, Prinzmetal's angina, ischemic heart disease, concurrent ergotamine-containing preparations, uncontrolled hypertension, hypersensitivity, basilar or hemiplegic migraine

Precautions: Pregnancy (C), postmenopausal women, men >40 yr, risk factors for CAD, hypercholesterolemia, obesity, diabetes, impaired renal/hepatic function, lactation, children, geriatric

PHARMACOKINETICS

Onset of pain relief 10 min-2 hr, peak 1-1½ hr, duration 14-16 hr, 14% plasma protein binding, metabolized in the liver (metabolite), excreted in urine (82%), feces (12%), half-life 2-3 hr

INTERACTIONS

• Weakness, hyperreflexia, incoordination: SSRIs

Increase: levels of sibutramine

Increase: rizatriptan action—cimetidine, oral contraceptives, MAOIs, nonselective MAOI (type A and B), isocarboxazid, pargyline, phenelzine, propranolol, tranylcypromine

Increase: vasospastic effects—ergot, ergot derivatives, other 5-HT receptor agonists

Drug/Herb

• Serotonin syndrome: SAM-e, St. John's wort

Increase: effect—butterbur, feverfew

NURSING CONSIDERATIONS

Assess:

• For migraine symptoms: visual disturbances, aura

• For stress level, activity, recreation, coping mechanisms

- Neurologic status: LOC, blurring vision, nausea, vomiting, tingling in extremities preceding headache
- Ingestion of tyramine foods (pickled products, beer, wine, aged cheese), food additives, preservatives, colorings, artificial sweeteners, chocolate, caffeine, which may precipitate these types of headaches
- Renal status: urine output

Administer:
- Oral disintegrating tab: do not open blister until use; peel blister open with dry hands; place tab on tongue, where it will dissolve, and swallow with saliva (contains phenylalanine)

Perform/provide:
- Quiet, calm environment with decreased stimulation for noise, bright light, excessive talking

Evaluate:
- Therapeutic response: decrease in frequency, severity of headache

Teach patient/family:
- Use of orally disintegrating tab: instruct patient not to open blister until use, to peel blister open with dry hands, to place tab on tongue, where it will dissolve, and to swallow with saliva (contains phenylalanine)
- To report any side effects to prescriber
- To use alternative contraception while taking drug if oral contraceptives are being used
- That drug does not prevent or reduce number of migraines, main action is abortive

---

⚠ High Alert

rocuronium (℞)
(ro-kyur-oh′nium)
Zemuron
Func. class.: Neuromuscular blocker (nondepolarizing)
Chem. class.: Biquaternary ammonium ester

Action: Inhibits transmission of nerve impulses by binding with cholinergic receptor sites, antagonizing action of acetylcholine

Uses: Facilitation of endotracheal intubation, skeletal muscle relaxation during mechanical ventilation, surgery, or general anesthesia

DOSAGE AND ROUTES
Intubation
- *Adult and child >3 mo:* **IV** 0.6 mg/kg

Available forms: Inj 10 mg/ml

SIDE EFFECTS
CV: Bradycardia, tachycardia, change in B/P, edema
GI: Nausea, vomiting
INTEG: Rash, flushing, pruritus, urticaria
RESP: **Prolonged apnea, bronchospasm, cyanosis, respiratory depression,** wheezing
Contraindications: Hypersensitivity
Precautions: Pregnancy (C), lactation, child <2 yr, electrolyte imbalances, dehydration, renal/hepatic/cardiac/respiratory/neuromuscular disease

PHARMACOKINETICS
Half-life 71-203 min, duration ½ hr, metabolized in liver

INTERACTIONS
- Theophylline increases risk of dysrhythmias

Increase: neuromuscular blockade caused by amphotericin B, verapamil, aminoglycosides, clindamycin, enflurane, isoflurane, lincomycin, lithium, opiates, local anesthetics, polymyxin, antiinfectives, quinidine, thiazides

NURSING CONSIDERATIONS
Assess:
- For electrolyte imbalances (K, Mg), before drug is used; electrolyte imbalances may lead to increased action of this drug
- VS (B/P, pulse, respirations, airway) until fully recovered; rate, depth, pattern of respirations, strength of hand grip; patient should be intubated before use

---

🍁 Canada only   Side effects: *italics* = common; **bold** = life-threatening

- Recovery: decreased paralysis of face, diaphragm, leg, arm, rest of body; residual weakness and respiratory problems may occur during recovery
- Allergic reactions: rash, fever, respiratory distress, pruritus; drug should be discontinued

Administer:
- Using peripheral nerve stimulator by anesthesiologist to determine neuromuscular blockade; deep tendon reflexes should be monitored during extended use
- Undiluted direct IV over 2 min (only by qualified person, usually anesthesiologist); do not administer IM
- Maintenance q20-45min after 1st dose; titrate to response

Perform/provide:
- Storage in light-resistant area
- Reassurance if communication is difficult during recovery from neuromuscular blockade

Evaluate:
- Therapeutic response: paralysis of jaw, eyelid, head, neck, rest of body as evaluated by peripheral nerve stimulator

Teach patient/family:
- About all procedures or treatments; patient will remain conscious if anesthesia is not given also

Treatment of overdose: Edrophonium or neostigmine, atropine, monitor VS; may require mechanical ventilation

ropinirole (Rx)
(roh-pin'ih-role)
Requip
Func. class.: Antiparkinson agent
Chem. class.: Dopamine-receptor agonist, nonergot

Action: Selective agonist for D_2 receptors (presynaptic/postsynaptic sites); binding at D_3 receptor contributes to antiparkinson effects
Uses: Parkinson's disease, restless leg syndrome (RLS)

DOSAGE AND ROUTES
- *Adult:* **PO** 0.25 mg tid, titrate weekly to a max of 24 mg/day
Restless leg syndrome
- *Adult:* **PO** 0.25 mg 1-3 hr before bedtime; may increase until symptom's resolved
Available forms: Tabs 0.25, 0.5, 1, 2, 3, 4, 5 mg

SIDE EFFECTS
CNS: Agitation, insomnia, psychosis, hallucination, dystonia, depression, dizziness, somnolence, **sleep attacks**
CV: Orthostatic hypotension, tachycardia, hypertension, hypotension, syncope, palpitations
EENT: Blurred vision
GI: Nausea, vomiting, anorexia, dry mouth, constipation, dyspepsia, flatulence
GU: Impotence, urinary frequency
HEMA: **Hemolytic anemia, leukopenia, agranulocytosis**
INTEG: Rash, sweating
RESP: Pharyngitis, rhinitis, sinusitis, bronchitis, dyspnea
Contraindications: Hypersensitivity
Precautions: Pregnancy (C), dysrhythmias, affective disorder, psychosis, renal/hepatic/cardiac disease

PHARMACOKINETICS
PO: Peak 1-2 hr; half-life 6 hr; extensively metabolized by the liver by P450 CYP1A2 enzyme system; protein binding 40%

INTERACTIONS
Increase: ropinirole effect—cimetidine, ciprofloxacin, diltiazem, enoxacin, erythromycin, fluvoxamine, mexiletine, norfloxacin, tacrine, digoxin, theophylline, L-dopa
Decrease: ropinirole effects—butyrophenones, metoclopramide, phenothiazines, thioxanthenes
Drug/Herb
Decrease: ropinirole action—chaste tree fruit, kava

⚠ Safety alert   *"Tall Man" lettering

NURSING CONSIDERATIONS

Assess:

• Involuntary movements in parkinsonism: akinesia, tremors, staggering gait, muscle rigidity, drooling

• B/P, respiration during initial treatment; hypo/hypertension should be reported

⚠ For sleep attacks, drowsiness, falling asleep without warning even during hazardous activities

• Mental status: affect, mood, behavioral changes, depression; complete suicide assessment

Administer:

• Drug until NPO before surgery

• Adjust dosage to patient response

• With meals to reduce nausea

Perform/provide:

• Testing for diabetes mellitus, acromegaly if on long-term therapy

Evaluate:

• Therapeutic response: improvement in movement disorder

Teach patient/family:

• That therapeutic effects may take several weeks to a few months

• To change positions slowly to prevent orthostatic hypotension

• To use drug exactly as prescribed; if drug is discontinued abruptly, parkinsonian crisis may occur

---

ropivacaine (℞)

(roe-pi′va-kane)

Naropin

Func. class.: Local anesthetic

Chem. class.: Amide

Action: Competes with calcium for sites in nerve membrane that control sodium transport across cell membrane; decreases rise of depolarization phase of action potential

Uses: Peripheral nerve block, caudal anesthesia, central neural block, vaginal, epidural, spinal block

DOSAGE AND ROUTES

Lumbar epidural block for cesarean section

• *Adult:* 20-30 ml of 0.5% sol

• *Adult:* 15-20 ml of 0.75% sol

Thoracic epidural

• *Adult:* 5-15 ml of 0.5% to 0.75% sol

Major nerve block

• *Adult:* 35-50 ml of 0.5% sol

• *Adult:* 10-40 ml of 0.75% sol

Labor pain (epidural)

• *Adult:* 10-20 ml 0.2% sol then 6-14 ml 1 hr

Postop (lumbar or thoracic epidural)

• *Adult:* 6-14 ml/hr of 0.2% sol

Infiltration/minor nerve block

• *Adult:* 1-100 ml of 0.2% sol

• *Adult:* 1-40 ml of 0.5% sol

Available forms: Inj 2, 5, 7.5 mg/ml

SIDE EFFECTS

CNS: Anxiety, restlessness, **seizures, loss of consciousness,** drowsiness, disorientation, tremors, shivering, paresthesia

CV: **Myocardial depression, cardiac arrest, dysrhythmias,** bradycardia, hypotension, hypertension, **fetal bradycardia**

EENT: Blurred vision, tinnitus, pupil constriction

ENDO: Hypokelamia

GI: Nausea, vomiting

GU: Urinary retention

INTEG: Rash, urticaria, allergic reactions, edema, burning, skin discoloration at inj site, tissue necrosis

RESP: **Status asthmaticus, respiratory arrest, anaphylaxis**

Contraindications: Hypersensitivity to amide local anesthetics, child <12 yr, geriatric, severe hepatic disease, severe hypotension, complete heart block

Precautions: Pregnancy (B), severe drug allergies, hyperthyroidism, CV disease; hepatic/neurologic disease

R

Side effects: *italics* = common; **bold** = life-threatening

PHARMACOKINETICS

Onset varies with inj site, duration varies with inj site; metabolized by liver, excreted in urine (metabolites)

INTERACTIONS

• Dysrhythmias: epINEPHrine, halothane, enflurane
• Hypertension: MAOIs, tricyclics, phenothiazines
Increase: effect—amiodarone, ciprofloxacin, fluvoxamine, azole antifungal
Decrease: action of ropivacaine—chloroprocaine

NURSING CONSIDERATIONS
Assess:
• B/P, pulse, respiration during treatment
• Fetal heart tones during labor
• Allergic reactions: rash, urticaria, itching
• Cardiac status: ECG for dysrhythmias, pulse, B/P during anesthesia
Administer:
• Only with crash cart, resuscitative equipment nearby
• Only drugs without preservatives for epidural or caudal anesthesia
Perform/provide:
• Use of new sol; discard unused portions
Evaluate:
• Therapeutic response: anesthesia necessary for procedure
Treatment of overdose: Airway, O_2, vasopressor, IV fluids, anticonvulsants for seizures

---

rosiglitazone (℞)
(ros-ih-glit'ah-zone)
Avandia
Func. class.: Antidiabetic, oral
Chem. class.: Thiazolidinedione

Action: Improves insulin resistance by hepatic glucose metabolism, insulin receptor kinase activity, insulin receptor phosphorylation

Uses: Type 2 diabetes mellitus, alone or in combination with sulfonylureas, metformin, or insulin
Unlabeled uses: Increased ovulation frequency in those with polycystic ovary syndrome; reduced in-stent restenosis in those with diabetes

DOSAGE AND ROUTES
Monotherapy
• *Adult:* **PO** 4 mg daily or in 2 divided doses, may increase to 8 mg daily or in 2 divided doses after 12 wk
Combination therapy
• *Adult:* **PO** This drug should be added to metformin, sulfonylurea at the adult dose
Available forms: Tabs 2, 4, 8 mg

SIDE EFFECTS
CNS: Fatigue, headache
ENDO: Hyper/hypoglycemia
MISC: Accidental injury, URI, sinusitis, anemia, back pain, diarrhea, edema
Contraindications: Hypersensitivity to thiazolidinediones, children, lactation, diabetic ketoacidosis
Precautions: Pregnancy (C), geriatric, thyroid disease, renal/hepatic disease

PHARMACOKINETICS
Maximal reductions in FBS after 6-12 wk, protein binding 99.8%, excreted in urine, feces, elimination half-life 3-4 hr, may be excreted in breast milk

INTERACTIONS
Decrease: effect of oral contraceptives, alternative method advised
Drug/Herb
• Hypoglycemia: chromium, coenzyme Q10, fenugreek
• Poor glucose control: glucosamine
Increase: antidiabetic effect—alfalfa, aloe, basil, bay, bilberry, bitter melon, black catechu, buchu, burdock, coriander, dandelion, eyebright (po), fenugreek, garlic, ginseng, glucomannan, glucosamine, goat's rue, gymnema, horehound, horse chestnut, jambul, myrrh, myrtle

Decrease: antidiabetic effect—bee pollen, blue cohosh, broom, chromium, elecampane, eucalyptus, gotu kola

NURSING CONSIDERATIONS

Assess:

• For hypoglycemic reactions (sweating, weakness, dizziness, anxiety, tremors, hunger), hyperglycemic reactions soon after meals

• Check LFTs periodically AST, ALT (if ALT >2.5 × ULN, do not use)

• Fast blood sugar, A1c, fasting plasma insulin, plasma lipids/lipoproteins, B/P, body weight during treatment

Administer:

• Once or in 2 divided doses

• Tabs crushed and mixed with food or fluids for patients with difficulty swallowing

Perform/provide:

• Conversion from other oral hypoglycemic agents if needed; change may be made without gradual dosage change; monitor serum or urine glucose and ketones tid during conversion

• Storage in tight container in cool environment

Teach patient/family:

• To monitor blood glucose; that periodic LFTs mandatory

• The symptoms of hypo/hyperglycemia, what to do about each

• That the drug must be continued on daily basis; explain consequences of discontinuing drug abruptly

• To avoid OTC medications or herbal preparations unless approved by prescriber

• That diabetes is lifelong illness; that this drug is not a cure; only controls symptoms

• That all food included in diet plan must be eaten to prevent hypoglycemia

• To carry emergency ID and glucagon emergency kit for emergencies

• To report symptoms of hepatic dysfunction (nausea, vomiting, abdominal pain, fatigue, anorexia, dark urine, jaundice)

• That 2 wk is needed to see a reduction

in blood glucose and 2-3 months to see full effect

• To notify prescriber if oral contraceptives are used

• Not to use if breastfeeding, may be secreted in breast milk

Evaluate:

• Therapeutic response: Decrease in polyuria, polydipsia, polyphagia; clear sensorium; absence of dizziness; stable gait, blood glucose at normal level

---

rosuvastatin (℞)

(roe-soo′va-sta-tin)
Crestor
Func. class.: Antilipemic
Chem. class.: HMG-CoA reductase inhibitor

Action: Inhibits HMG-CoA reductase enzyme, which reduces cholesterol synthesis

Uses: As an adjunct in primary hypercholesterolemia (types IIa, IIb), and mixed dyslipidemia elevated serum triglycerides, homozygous familial hypercholesterolemia (FH)

DOSAGE AND ROUTES

(Patient should first be placed on a cholesterol-lowering diet)

Hypercholesterolemia

• *Adult:* **PO** 5-40 mg daily; initial dose 10 mg daily, reanalyze lipid levels at 2-4 wk and adjust dosage accordingly

Homozygous FH

• *Adult:* **PO** 20 mg daily, max 40 mg

Dose in patients taking cyclosporine

• *Adult:* **PO** 5 mg daily

Dose when taken with gemfibrozil

• *Adult:* **PO** Max 10 mg daily

Asian patients/predisposition for myopathy

• *Adult:* **PO** 5 mg daily

Renal dose

• *Adult:* **PO** CCr <30 ml/min 5 mg daily; max 10 mg daily

Available forms: Tabs 5, 10, 20, 40 mg

SIDE EFFECTS

CNS: Headache, dizziness, insomnia, paresthesia

GI: Nausea, constipation, abdominal pain, flatus, diarrhea, dyspepsia, heartburn, **kidney failure, liver dysfunction,** vomiting

HEMA: **Thrombocytopenia, hemolytic anemia, leucopenia**

INTEG: Rash, pruritus, photosensitivity

MS: Asthenia, muscle cramps, arthritis, arthralgia, myalgia, **myositis, rhabdomyolysis,** leg, shoulder or localized pain

RESP: Rhinitis, sinusitis, *pharyngitis,* bronchitis, increased cough

Contraindications: Pregnancy (X), hypersensitivity, lactation, active hepatic disease

Precautions: Past hepatic disease, alcoholism, severe acute infections, trauma, hypotension, uncontrolled seizure disorders, severe metabolic disorders, electrolyte imbalances, children, severe renal impairment, geriatric, hypothyroidism

PHARMACOKINETICS

PO: Peak 3-5 hr; minimal live metabolism (about 10%); 88% protein bound; excreted primarily in feces (90%); crosses placenta; half-life 19 hr; not dialyzable

INTERACTIONS

Increase: effects of rosuvastatin—bile acid sequestrants

Increase: myalgia, myositis—cyclo-SPORINE, gemfibrozil, niacin, clofibrate, azole antifungals

Increase: bleeding—warfarin

Drug/Herb

Decrease: rosuvastatin effect—St. John's wort

Drug/Food

• Possible toxicity: grapefruit juice

Drug/Lab Test

Increase: CPK, LFTs

NURSING CONSIDERATIONS

Assess:

• Diet, obtain diet history including fat, cholesterol in diet

• Fasting cholesterol, LDL, HDL, triglycerides periodically during treatment

• LFTs q1-2mo during the first 1½ yr of treatment; AST, ALT, LFTs may increase

• Renal function in patients with compromised renal system: BUN, creatinine, I&O ratio

⚠ For muscle pain, tenderness, obtain CPK; if these occur, drug may need to be discontinued

Administer:

• May be taken at any time of day, with or without food

Perform/provide:

• Storage in cool environment in airtight, light-resistant container

Evaluate:

• Therapeutic response: cholesterol at desired level after 8 wk

Teach patient/family:

• To report suspected pregnancy

• That blood work and ophthalmic exam will be necessary during treatment

• To report blurred vision, severe GI symptoms, dizziness, headache, muscle pain, weakness

• To use sunscreen or stay out of the sun to prevent photosensitivity

• That previously prescribed regimen will continue: low-cholesterol diet, exercise program, smoking cessation

---

salmeterol (℞)
(sal-met′er-ole)
Serevent
Func. class.: β_2-Adrenergic agonist, bronchodilator

Action: Causes bronchodilation by action on β_2 (pulmonary) receptors by increasing levels of cAMP, which relaxes smooth muscle with very little effect on heart rate, maintains improvement in FEV from 3 to 12 hr; prevents nocturnal asthma symptoms

---

⚠ Safety alert   *"Tall Man" lettering

Uses: Prevention of exercise-induced asthma, bronchospasm, COPD

DOSAGE AND ROUTES

• *Adult:* **INH** 50 mcg (one inhalation as dry powder); exercise-induced bronchospasm: 50 mcg (2 inh) ½-1 hr prior to exercise

• *Child 4-12 yr:* **INH** 50 mcg as dry powder bid; exercise-induced bronchospasm 50 mcg as dry powder ½-1 hr prior to exercise

Available forms: Inhalation powder 50 mcg/blister

SIDE EFFECTS

CNS: Tremors, anxiety, insomnia, headache, dizziness, stimulation, restlessness, hallucinations, flushing, irritability

CV: Palpitations, tachycardia, hypertension, angina, hypotension, dysrhythmias

EENT: Dry nose, irritation of nose and throat

GI: Heartburn, nausea, vomiting

MS: Muscle cramps

RESP: **Bronchospasm**

Contraindications: Hypersensitivity to sympathomimetics, tachydysrhythmias, severe cardiac disease

Precautions: Pregnancy (C), lactation, cardiac disorders, hyperthyroidism, diabetes mellitus, hypertension, prostatic hypertrophy, narrow-angle glaucoma, seizures, acute asthma, as a substitute to corticosteroids

PHARMACOKINETICS

INH: Onset 30-50 min; peak 4 hr; duration 12 hr; metabolized in liver; excreted in urine, breast milk; crosses placenta; blood-brain barrier; protein binding 94%-98%; terminal half-life 3-5 hr

INTERACTIONS

Increase: action of aerosol bronchodilators

Increase: action of salmeterol—tricyclics, MAOIs

Decrease: salmeterol action—other β-blockers

Drug/Herb

Increase: stimulation—betel palm, butterbur, coffee, cola nut, figwort, fumitory, guarana, hawthorn, lily of the valley, motherwort, plantain, tea (black/green), yerba maté

NURSING CONSIDERATIONS

Assess:

• Respiratory function: vital capacity, forced expiratory volume, ABGs, lung sounds, heart rate and rhythm

Administer:

• Gum, sips of water for dry mouth

Perform/provide:

• Storage in foil pouch; do not expose to temperatures over 86° F (30° C); discard 6 wk after removal from foil pouch

Evaluate:

• Therapeutic response: absence of dyspnea, wheezing

Teach patient/family:

• Not to use OTC medications; extra stimulation may occur

• Review package insert with patient

• To avoid getting powder in eyes

• To avoid smoking, smoke-filled rooms, persons with respiratory infections

• Not for treatment of acute exacerbation

Treatment of overdose: β₂-Adrenergic blocker

---

salsalate (℞)

(sal'sah-late)
Amigesic, Anaflex, Disalcid, Marthritic, Mono-Gesic, Salflex, salsalate, Salgesic, Salsitab

Func. class.: Nonopioid analgesic, nonsteroidal antiinflammatory

Chem. class.: Salicylate

Action: Blocks formation of peripheral prostaglandins, which cause pain and inflammation; antipyretic action results from inhibition of hypothalamic heat-regulating center; does not inhibit platelet aggregation

Uses: Mild to moderate pain or fever, including arthritis, juvenile rheumatoid arthritis

DOSAGE AND ROUTES
• *Adult:* **PO** 3 g/day in divided doses
Available forms: Caps 500 mg; tabs 500, 750 mg

SIDE EFFECTS
CNS: Stimulation, drowsiness, dizziness, confusion, **seizures**, headache, flushing, hallucinations, **coma**
CV: Rapid pulse, **pulmonary edema**
EENT: Tinnitus, hearing loss
ENDO: Hypoglycemia, hyponatremia, hypokalemia, alteration in acid-base balance
GI: Nausea, vomiting, GI bleeding, diarrhea, heartburn, anorexia, **hepatotoxicity**
HEMA: **Thrombocytopenia, agranulocytosis, leukopenia, neutropenia, hemolytic anemia,** increased protime
INTEG: Rash, urticaria, bruising
RESP: Wheezing, hyperpnea
Contraindications: Hypersensitivity to salicylates, NSAIDs, GI bleeding, bleeding disorders, children <3 yr, vit K deficiency
Precautions: Pregnancy (C) 1st trimester, anemia, renal/hepatic disease, Hodgkin's disease, lactation, geriatric

PHARMACOKINETICS
Metabolized by liver; excreted by kidneys; half-life 1 hr; highly protein bound; crosses blood-brain barrier and placenta slowly

INTERACTIONS
• Toxic effects: PABA
Increase: blood loss—alcohol, heparin, NSAIDs, warfarin
Increase: effects of anticoagulants, insulin, methotrexate, probenecid, penicillins, phenytoin

Decrease: effects of spironolactone, sulfinpyrazone, sulfonamides, loop diuretics
Decrease: effects of salsalate—antacids, steroids, urinary alkalizers
Decrease: blood glucose levels—salicylates

Drug/Food
• Foods that cause acidic urine, may increase salsalate levels

Drug/Lab Test
Increase: Coagulation studies, hepatic studies, serum uric acid, amylase, CO_2, urinary protein
Decrease: Serum potassium, PBI, cholesterol, blood glucose
Interference: Urine catecholamines, pregnancy test

NURSING CONSIDERATIONS
Assess:
• Pain: frequency, intensity, characteristics; relief of pain after medication
⚠ For asthma, aspirin hypersensitivity, nasal polyps; may develop hypersensitivity to this product
• Hepatic studies: AST, ALT, bilirubin (long-term therapy)
• Renal studies: BUN, urine creatinine (long-term therapy)
• Blood studies: CBC, Hct, Hgb, PT (long-term therapy)
• I&O ratio; decreasing output may indicate renal failure (long-term therapy)
• Hepatotoxicity: dark urine, clay-colored stools; jaundiced skin, sclera; itching, abdominal pain, fever, diarrhea (long-term therapy)
• Allergic reactions: rash, urticaria; drug may have to be discontinued
• Ototoxicity: tinnitus, ringing, roaring in ears; audiometric testing is needed before, after long-term therapy
• Visual changes: blurring, halos, corneal and retinal damage
• Edema in feet, ankles, legs
• Drug history; many interactions

⚠ Safety alert   *"Tall Man" lettering

Administer:
• To patient crushed or whole; chewable tablets may be chewed
• With food or milk to decrease gastric symptoms
Evaluate:
• Therapeutic response: decreased pain, fever
Teach patient/family:
• To report any symptoms of hepatotoxicity, renal toxicity, visual changes, ototoxicity, allergic reactions (long-term therapy)
• Not to exceed recommended dosage; acute poisoning may result
• To read label on other OTC drugs; many contain aspirin
• That therapeutic response takes 2 wk (arthritis)
• To avoid alcohol ingestion; GI bleeding may occur
• To watch for signs of bleeding: dark stools
Treatment of overdose: Lavage, activated charcoal, monitor electrolytes, VS

---

saquinavir (℞)
(sa-quen'ah-veer)
Fortovase, Invirase
Func. class.: Antiretroviral
Chem. class.: Protease inhibitor

Action: Inhibits human immunodeficiency virus (HIV-1) protease, which prevents maturation of the infectious virus
Uses: HIV-1 in combination with other antiretrovirals

DOSAGE AND ROUTES
• *Adult:* PO 600 mg (hard cap-Invirase) or 1200 mg (soft cap-Fortovase) tid within 2 hr after a full meal
Available forms: Caps (soft) 200 mg; (hard) 200, 500 mg

SIDE EFFECTS
CNS: Paresthesia, headache
GI: Diarrhea, buccal mucosa ulceration, *abdominal pain, nausea,* vomiting
INTEG: Rash

MISC.: Asthenia, hyperglycemia
MS: Pain
Contraindications: Hypersensitivity
Precautions: Pregnancy (B), hepatic disease, lactation, children, diabetes, pancreatitis

PHARMACOKINETICS
Absorption increased with food, protein binding 98%, extensive first-pass metabolism, terminal half-life 12 hr

INTERACTIONS
• Avoid use with HMG-CoA reductase inhibitors
Increase: toxicity—ergots, midazolam, triazolam, dapsone, quinidine, calcium channel blockers, clindamycin
⚠ *Increase:* vasoconstriction—ergots, do not use concurrently
⚠ *Increase:* CNS depression—midazolam, triazolam, do not use concurrently
Increase: saquinavir levels—ketoconazole, indinavir, delavirdine, nelfinavir, ritonavir, clarithromycin
Decrease: saquinavir levels—rifamycins, carbamazepine, phenobarbital, phenytoin, nevirapine, dexamethasone
Drug/Herb
• St. John's wort may decrease saquinavir levels; avoid concurrent use
Drug/Food
Increase: bioavailability after high-fat meal; grapefruit juice increases levels
Drug/Lab Test
• CPK, glucose (low)

NURSING CONSIDERATIONS
Assess:
• Signs of infection, anemia
• Hepatic studies: ALT, AST
• C&S before drug therapy; drug may be taken as soon as culture is taken; repeat C&S after treatment; determine the presence of other sexually transmitted diseases
• Bowel pattern before, during treatment; if severe abdominal pain with bleeding

S

occurs, drug should be discontinued; monitor hydration

• Skin eruptions, rash, urticaria, itching
• Allergies before treatment, reaction of each medication

Administer:
• Within 2 hr of meal

Teach patient/family:
• To take as prescribed within 2 hr of a full meal; if dose is missed, take as soon as remembered up to 1 hr before next dose; do not double dose
• That drug must be taken in equal intervals around the clock to maintain blood levels for duration of therapy
• That Invirase and Fortovase are not interchangeable

---

sargramostim (℞)

(sar-gram′oh-stim)
Leukine, rhu GM-CSF
Func. class.: Biologic modifier: cytokine
Chem. class.: Granulocyte macrophage colony-stimulating factor (GM-CSF)

Do not confuse:
Leukine/leucovorin/Leukeran

Action: Stimulates proliferation and differentiation of hematopoietic progenitor cells (granulocytes, macrophages)

Uses: Acceleration of myeloid recovery in patients with non-Hodgkin's lymphoma, acute lymphoblastic leukemia, autologous bone marrow transplantation in Hodgkin's disease; bone marrow transplantation failure or engraftment delay, mobilization and transplant of peripheral blood progenitor cells (PBPCs)

Unlabeled uses: Aplastic anemia, Crohn's disease, ganciclovir- or zidovudine-induced neutropenia

DOSAGE AND ROUTES

Myeloid reconstitution after autologous bone marrow transplantation
• *Adult:* IV 250 mcg/m^2/day × 3 wk; give over 2 hr, 2-4 hr after autologous bone marrow infusion, not less than 24 hr af-

ter last dose of antineoplastics and 12 hr after last dose of radiotherapy, bone marrow transplantation failure, or engraftment delay

Acceleration of myeloid recovery
• *Adult:* IV 250 mcg/m^2/day × 14 days; give over 2 hr; may repeat in 7 days, may repeat 500 mcg/m^2/day × 14 days after another 7 days if no improvement

Mobilization of PBPCs
• *Adult:* IV/SUBCUT 250 mcg/m^2/day during collection of PBPCs

After PBPC transplantation
• *Adult:* IV/SUBCUT 250 mcg/m^2/day until ANC >1500 cells/mm^3 × 3 days

Available forms: Powder for inj lyophilized 250, 500 mcg

SIDE EFFECTS

CNS: Fever, malaise, CNS disorder, weakness, chills, dizziness, syncope
CV: **Transient supraventricular tachycardia**, peripheral edema, **pericardial effusion**
GI: Nausea, vomiting, diarrhea, anorexia, **GI hemorrhage**, stomatitis, **liver damage**
GU: Urinary tract disorder, abnormal kidney function
HEMA: **Blood dyscrasias, hemorrhage**
INTEG: Alopecia, rash, peripheral edema
RESP: Dyspnea

Contraindications: Hypersensitivity to GM-CSF, benzyl alcohol, yeast products; excessive leukemic myeloid blast in bone marrow, peripheral blood, neonates
Precautions: Pregnancy (C), lactation, child; renal/hepatic/lung/cardiac disease; pleural, pericardial effusions, peripheral edema

PHARMACOKINETICS

Half-life 2 hr, detected within 5 min after administration, peak 2 hr

INTERACTIONS

• Do not use this drug concomitantly with antineoplastics
Increase: myeloproliferation—lithium, corticosteroids

⚠ Safety alert   *"Tall Man" lettering

NURSING CONSIDERATIONS
Assess:
⚠ Blood studies: CBC, differential count before treatment and twice weekly; leukocytosis may occur (WBC >50,000 cells/mm³, ANC >20,000 cells/mm³), platelets; if ANC >20,000/mm³ or 10,000/mm³ after nadir has occurred, or platelets >500,000/mm³ reduce dose by ½ or discontinue; if blast cells occur, discontinue
• Renal, hepatic studies before treatment: BUN, creatinine, urinalysis; AST, ALT, alk phos; twice weekly monitoring is needed in renal, hepatic disease
• For hypersensitivity, rashes, local inj site reactions; usually transient
• For increased fluid retention in cardiac disease
• For myalgia, arthralgia in legs, feet, use analgesics

Administer:
SUBCUT route
• Use reconstituted sol
IV route
• After reconstituting with 1 ml sterile water for inj without preservative; do not re-enter vial; discard unused portion; direct reconstitution sol at side of vial; rotate contents; do not shake
• Dilute in 0.9% NaCl inj to prepare IV inf; if final concentration is <10 mcg/ml, add human albumin to make a final concentration of 0.1% to NaCl before adding sargramostim to prevent adsorption; for a final concentration of 0.1% albumin, add 1 mg human albumin/1 ml 0.9% NaCl inj run over 2 hr (bone marrow transplant or failure of graft); over 4 hr (chemotherapy for AML); over 24 hr as cont inf (PBPCs); give within 6 hr after reconstitution

Y-site compatibilities: Amikacin, aminophylline, aztreonam, bleomycin, butorphanol, calcium gluconate, carboplatin, carmustine, cefazolin, cefepime, cefotaxime, cefotetan, ceftizoxime, ceftriaxone, cefuroxime, cimetidine, cisplatin, clindamycin, cyclophosphamide, cycloSPORINE, cytarabine, dacarbazine, dactinomycin, dexamethasone, diphenhydrAMINE, DO-

Pamine, DOXOrubicin, doxycycline, droperidol, etoposide, famotidine, fentanyl, floxuridine, fluconazole, fluorouracil, furosemide, gentamicin, granisetron, heparin, idarubicin, ifosfamide, immune globulin, magnesium sulfate, mannitol, mechlorethamine, meperidine, mesna, methotrexate, metoclopramide, metronidazole, mezlocillin, miconazole, minocycline, mitoxantrone, netilmicin, pentostatin, piperacillin/tazobactam, potassium chloride, prochlorperazine, promethazine, ranitidine, teniposide, ticarcillin, ticarcillin/clavulanate, trimethoprim-sulfamethoxazole, vinBLAStine, vinCRIStine, zidovudine

Perform/provide:
• Storage in refrigerator; do not freeze
Evaluate:
• Therapeutic response: WBC and differential recovery

---

scopolamine (℞)
(skoe-pol'a-meen)
Scopolamine Hydrobromide Injection
Func. class.: Cholinergic blocker
Chem. class.: Belladonna alkaloid

Action: Inhibits acetylcholine at receptor sites in autonomic nervous system, which controls secretions, free acids in stomach; blocks central muscarinic receptors, which decreases involuntary movements

Uses: Preoperatively to produce amnesia, sedation and to decrease secretions; motion sickness, parkinsonian symptoms

DOSAGE AND ROUTES
Parkinsonian symptoms
• *Adult:* **IM/SUBCUT/IV** 0.3-0.6 mg tid-qid using dilution provided
Preoperatively
• *Adult:* **IM/IV/SUBCUT** 0.3-0.5 mg; may repeat q4-6h

Nausea and vomiting
- *Child:* **SUBCUT** 0.006 mg/kg or 0.2 mg/m^2; max 0.3 mg/dose

Available forms: Inj 0.3, 0.4, 0.86, 1 mg/ml

SIDE EFFECTS

CNS: Confusion, anxiety, restlessness, irritability, delusions, hallucinations, headache, sedation, depression, incoherence, dizziness, excitement, delirium, flushing, weakness, fatigue, loss of memory

CV: Palpitations, tachycardia, postural hypotension, paradoxic bradycardia

EENT: Blurred vision, photophobia, dilated pupils, difficulty swallowing, mydriasis, cycloplegia

GI: Dryness of mouth, constipation, nausea, vomiting, abdominal distress, **paralytic ileus**

GU: Urinary hesitancy, retention

INTEG: Urticaria, dry skin

MISC: Suppression of lactation, nasal congestion, decreased sweating

Contraindications: Hypersensitivity, narrow-angle glaucoma, myasthenia gravis, GI/GU obstruction, hypersensitivity to belladonna, barbiturates

Precautions: Pregnancy (C), geriatric, lactation, prostatic hypertrophy, CHF, hypertension, dysrhythmia, children, gastric ulcer, renal/hepatic disease, hiatal hernia, GERD, ulcerative colitis, hyperthyroidism

PHARMACOKINETICS

SUBCUT/IM: Peak 30-60 min, duration 7 hr

IV: Peak 10-15 min, duration 2 hr Excreted in urine, bile, feces (unchanged)

INTERACTIONS

Increase: anticholinergic effect—alcohol, opioids, antihistamines, phenothiazines, tricyclics

Drug/Herb

Increase: anticholinergic effects—henbane, jimsonweed, scopolia

NURSING CONSIDERATIONS

Assess:
- VS periodically
- I&O ratio; retention commonly causes decreased urinary output
- Parkinsonism, EPS: shuffling gait, muscle rigidity, involuntary movements if using for Parkinson symptoms
- Urinary hesitancy, retention; palpate bladder if retention occurs
- Constipation; increase fluids, bulk, exercise if this occurs
- For tolerance over long-term therapy; dose may have to be increased or changed
- Mental status: affect, mood, CNS depression, worsening of mental symptoms during early therapy if using for Parkinson symptoms

Administer:
- Parenteral dose with patient recumbent to prevent postural hypotension
- Parenteral dose slowly; keep in bed for at least 1 hr after dose
- With or after meals for GI upset; may give with fluids other than H_2O
- At bedtime to avoid daytime drowsiness in patient with parkinsonism
- With analgesic to avoid behavioral changes when given as a preop

IV route
- Give over 2-3 min, 30-60 min prior to anesthesia

Additive compatibilities: Floxacillin, furosemide, meperidine, succinylcholine

Syringe compatibilities: Atropine, benzquinamide, butorphanol, chlorproMAZINE, cimetidine, diamorphine, dimenhyDRINATE, diphenhydrAMINE, droperidol, fentanyl, glycopyrrolate, hydromorphone, hydrOXYzine, meperidine, metoclopramide, midazolam, morphine, nalbuphine, pentazocine, pentobarbital, perphenazine, prochlorperazine, proMAZINE, promethazine, ranitidine, sufentanil, thiopental

Y-site compatibilities: Heparin, hydrocortisone, potassium chloride, propofol, sufentanil, vit B/C

⚠ Safety alert   *"Tall Man" lettering

Perform/provide:
• Storage at room temperature in light-resistant container
• Hard candy, frequent drinks, sugarless gum to relieve dry mouth

Evaluate:
• Therapeutic response: decreased secretions

Teach patient/family:
• Not to discontinue this drug abruptly; to taper off over 1 wk
• To avoid driving, other hazardous activities; drowsiness may occur
• To avoid OTC medication: cough, cold preparations with alcohol, antihistamines unless directed by prescriber

---

scopolamine ophthalmic
See Appendix C

---

scopolamine (℞) (transdermal)
(skoe-pol'-a-meen)
Transderm-Scop, Transderm-V
Func. class.: Antiemetic, anticholinergic
Chem. class.: Belladonna alkaloid

Action: Competitive antagonism of acetylcholine at receptor site in eye, smooth muscle, cardiac muscle, glandular cells; inhibition of vestibular input to the CNS, resulting in inhibition of vomiting reflex
Uses: Prevention of motion sickness
Unlabeled uses: Drooling

DOSAGE AND ROUTES
• *Adult:* **PATCH** 1 placed behind ear 4-5 hr before travel, reapply q3d, alternate ears
• Not recommended for children
Drooling (unlabeled)
• *Adult:* **TD** 1.5 mg patch q3d
Available forms: Patch, 0.5, 1 mg delivered in 72 hr

SIDE EFFECTS
CNS: Dizziness, drowsiness, confusion, disorientation, memory disturbances, hallucinations
EENT: Blurred vision, altered depth perception, *dilated pupils,* photophobia, *dry mouth;* dry, itchy, red eyes; acute narrow-angle glaucoma
GU: Difficult urination
INTEG: Rash, erythema

Contraindications: Hypersensitivity, glaucoma
Precautions: Pregnancy (C), children, geriatric; pyloric, urinary, bladder neck, intestinal obstruction; renal/hepatic disease

PHARMACOKINETICS
Patch: Onset 4-5 hr, duration 72 hr

INTERACTIONS
Increase: anticholinergic effects—antihistamines, antidepressants

NURSING CONSIDERATIONS
Administer:
• With clean, dry hands; wash, dry hands before and after applying to surface behind ear

Teach patient/family:
• To avoid hazardous activities, activities requiring alertness; dizziness may occur
• To change patch q72h
• To apply at least 4 hr before traveling
• If blurred vision, severe dizziness, drowsiness occurs, to discontinue use, use another type of antiemetic or rotate the patch to other ear
• To read label of all OTC medications; if any scopolamine is found in product, avoid use
• To keep out of children's reach

Rarely Used ⚠ High Alert

secobarbital (℞)
(see-koe-bar'bi-tal)
Seconal
Func. class.: Sedative/hypnotic-
barbiturate

**Controlled Substance Schedule II
(USA), Schedule G (CDSA IV)
(Canada)**
Uses: Insomnia, sedation, preoperative
medication, status epilepticus, acute teta-
nus convulsions

DOSAGE AND ROUTES
Insomnia
• *Adult:* **PO/IM** 100-200 mg at bedtime
• *Child:* **IM** 3-5 mg/kg, not to exceed
100 mg, not to inject >5 ml in one site
Sedation/preoperatively
• *Adult:* **PO** 200-300 mg 1-2 hr preoper-
atively
• *Child:* **PO** 50-100 mg 1-2 hr preoper-
atively
Status epilepticus
• *Adult and child:* **IM/IV** 250-350 mg
Acute psychotic agitation
• *Adult and child:* **IM/IV** 5.5 mg/kg
q3-4h

SIDE EFFECTS
CNS: Complex sleep related reactions:
sleep driving, sleep eating
SYST: **Severe allergic reactions**
Contraindications: Pregnancy (D),
hypersensitivity to barbiturates, respiratory depression, addiction to barbiturates,
severe liver impairment, porphyria, uncontrolled severe pain

selegiline (℞)
(se-le'ji-leen)
Carbex, Eldepryl, Emsam,
Novo-Selegiline ✦ Zelapar
Func. class.: Antiparkinson agent
Chem. class.: MAOI, type B

Do not confuse:
Eldepryl/enalapril
Action: Increased dopaminergic activity
by inhibition of MAO type B activity; not
fully understood
Uses: Adjunct management of Parkinson's disease in patients being treated with
levodopa/carbidopa who had poor response to therapy
Unlabeled uses: Alzheimer's disease,
depression

DOSAGE AND ROUTES
• *Adult:* **PO** 10 mg/day given with
levodopa/carbidopa in divided doses 5 mg
at breakfast and lunch; after 2-3 days begin to reduce dose of levodopa/carbidopa
10%-30%; (oral disintegrating tab) 2.50
mg (2 tabs) initially, then 1.25 (1 tab)
dissolved on tongue daily before breakfast × 6 wk or more; max 2.5 mg daily;
TRANSDERMAL 6 mg/24 hr initially, increase by 3 mg/24 hr at ≥2wk, up to 12
mg/24 hr if needed
Alzheimer's disease (unlabeled)
• *Adult:* **PO** 5 mg bid AM, PM
Available forms: Tabs 5 mg; caps
5 mg; oral disintegrating tabs 1.25 mg;
transdermal 6 mg/24 hr (20 mg/20 cm²),
9 mg/24 hr (30 mg/30 cm²), 12 mg/24
hr (40 mg/40 cm²)

SIDE EFFECTS
CNS: Increased tremors, chorea, restlessness, blepharospasm, increased bradykinesia, grimacing, tardive dyskinesia, dystonic symptoms, involuntary movements,
increased apraxia, hallucinations, *dizziness,* mood changes, nightmares, delusions, lethargy, apathy, overstimulation,
sleep disturbances, headache, migraine,
numbness, muscle cramps, confusion,

⚠ Safety alert   *"Tall Man" lettering

anxiety, tiredness, vertigo, personality change, back/leg pain, **suicide in children/adolescents**

CV: Orthostatic hypotension, hypertension, dysrhythmia, palpitations, angina pectoris, hypotension, **tachycardia**, edema, **sinus bradycardia**, syncope, **hypertensive crisis**

EENT: Diplopia, dry mouth, blurred vision, tinnitus

GI: Nausea, vomiting, constipation, weight loss, anorexia, diarrhea, heartburn, rectal bleeding, poor appetite, dysphagia, xerostomia

GU: Slow urination, nocturia, prostatic hypertrophy, urinary hesitation, retention, frequency, sexual dysfunction

INTEG: Increased sweating, alopecia, hematoma, rash, photosensitivity, facial hair

RESP: Asthma, shortness of breath

Contraindications: Children/adolescents, hypersensitivity

Precautions: Pregnancy (C), lactation

PHARMACOKINETICS

Absorption (tab) 40-90 min (oral disintegrating tab), 10-15 min; peak ½-2 hr; rapidly metabolized (active metabolites: *N*-desmethyldeprenyl, amphetamine, methamphetamine); metabolites excreted in urine; half-life 10 hr; protein binding up to 85%

INTERACTIONS

⚠ Fatal interaction: opioids (especially meperidine); do not administer together

⚠ Serotonin syndrome (confusion, seizures, fever, hypertension, agitation); death—fluoxetine, paroxetine, sertraline, fluvoxamine (discontinue 5 wk prior to selegiline); do not use together

⚠ Fatal interaction: Do not use with tricyclics

Increase: side effects of levodopa/carbidopa

Increase: unusual behavior, psychosis —dextromethorphan

Drug/Herb
Decrease: selegiline action—chaste tree fruit, kava

Drug/Lab Test
Decrease: VMA

False positive: Urine ketones, urine glucose

False negative: Urine glucose (glucose oxidase)

False increase: Uric acid, urine protein

NURSING CONSIDERATIONS

Assess:
• Decreased parkinsonian symptoms: rigidity, unsteady gait, weakness, tremors
• B/P, respiration throughout treatment
• Mental status: affect, mood behavioral changes, depression; perform suicide assessment

Administer:
PO route
• Drug until NPO before surgery
• Adjusting dosage to response
• With meals; limit protein taken with drug
• At doses <10 mg/day, because of risks associated with nonselective inhibition of MAO
• Oral disintegrating tab: peel back foil; remove tab, do not push through foil; place tab on tongue; allow to dissolve, swallow with saliva

Transdermal route
• Apply to dry, intact skin on upper torso, upper thigh, or outer surface of upper arm q12h

Perform/provide:
• Assistance with ambulation during beginning therapy

Evaluate:
• Therapeutic response: decrease in akathisia, improved mood

Teach patient/family:
• To change positions slowly to prevent orthostatic hypotension
• To report side effects: twitching, eye spasms; indicate overdose
• To use drug exactly as prescribed; if discontinued abruptly, parkinsonian crisis may occur
• To avoid foods high in tyramine:

S

Side effects: *italics* = common; **bold** = life-threatening

cheese, pickled products, wine, beer, large amounts of caffeine
• Not to exceed recommended dose of 10 mg (PO); might precipitate hypertensive crisis; report severe headache, other unusual symptoms
Treatment of overdose: IV fluids for hypertension, IV dilute pressure agent for B/P titration

---

selenium topical
See Appendix C

---

senna, sennosides
(otc)
(sen'na)
Black Draught, Dr. Caldwell Dosalax, Ex-Lax Gentle, Fletcher's Castoria, Gentlax, Senexon, Senna-Gen, Senokot, Senokotxtra, Senolax
Func. class.: Laxative-stimulant
Chem. class.: Anthraquinone

Action: Stimulates peristalsis by action on Auerbach's plexus; softens feces by increasing water, electrolytes in large intestine
Uses: Acute constipation; bowel preparation for surgery or examination

DOSAGE AND ROUTES
• *Adult:* **PO** (Senokot) 1-8 tabs/day or ½ to 4 tsp of granules (1 tsp-4 ml) added to water or juice; **RECT SUPP** 1-2 at bedtime; **SYR** 1-4 tsp at bedtime, 7.5-15 ml (Black Draught) ¾ oz dissolved in 2.5 oz liquid given between 2-4 PM the day before procedure (X-Prep)
• *Child >27 kg:* **PO** ½ adult dose; do not use Black Draught for children
• *Child 1 mo-1 yr:* **SYR** (Senokot) 1.25-2.5 ml at bedtime
Available forms: Tabs 6, 8.6, 15, 25 mg; granules 15, 20 mg/5 ml; syrup 8.8 mg/5 ml; liquid 33.3 mg/ml

SIDE EFFECTS
GI: Nausea, vomiting, anorexia, cramps, diarrhea, flatulence
GU: Pink, red or brown, black urine
META: Hypocalcemia, enteropathy, alkalosis, hypokalemia, **tetany**
Contraindications: Hypersensitivity, GI bleeding, obstruction, CHF, lactation, abdominal pain, nausea/vomiting, appendicitis, acute surgical abdomen
Precautions: Pregnancy (C)

PHARMACOKINETICS
PO: Onset 6-24 hr; metabolized by liver, excreted in feces

INTERACTIONS
• Do not use with disulfiram (Antabuse)
Drug/Herb
Increase: laxative effect—flax, senna

NURSING CONSIDERATIONS
Assess:
• Stool: color, consistency, amount
• Blood, urine electrolytes if drug is used often
• I&O ratio to identify fluid loss
• Cause of constipation; fluids, bulk, exercise missing, constipating drugs
• Cramping, rectal bleeding, nausea, vomiting; drug should be discontinued
Administer:
• In morning or evening (oral dose) with full glass of water
• Dissolve granules in water or juice before administration
• On empty stomach for more rapid results
• Shake oral sol before giving
Evaluate:
• Therapeutic response: decrease in constipation
Teach patient/family:
• That urine, feces may turn yellow-brown to red
• Not to use laxatives for long-term therapy; bowel tone will be lost
• That normal bowel movements do not always occur daily

⚠ Safety alert   *"Tall Man" lettering

- Not to use in presence of abdominal pain, nausea, vomiting
- To notify prescriber if constipation unrelieved or of symptoms of electrolyte imbalance: muscle cramps, pain, weakness, dizziness, excessive thirst

sertraline (℞)
(ser'tra-leen)
Zoloft
Func. class.: Antidepressant
Chem. class.: SSRI

Do not confuse:
Zoloft/Zocor
Action: Inhibits serotonin reuptake in CNS; increases action of serotonin; does not affect dopamine, norepinephrine
Uses: Major depressive disorder, obsessive-compulsive disorder (OCD), post-traumatic stress disorder (PTSD), panic disorder, social anxiety disorder, premenstrual disphoric disorder (PMDD)

DOSAGE AND ROUTES

- *Adult:* **PO** 50 mg daily; may increase to max of 200 mg/day; do not change dose at intervals of <1 wk; administer daily in AM or PM; or 100 mg 3 ×/wk (off-label)
- *Geriatric:* **PO** 25 mg daily, increase by 25 mg q3 days to desired dose
- *Child 6-12 yr:* **PO** 25 mg daily
- *Child 13-17 yr:* **PO** 50 mg daily
Premenstrual disorders
- *Adult:* PO 50-150 mg nightly
Available forms: Tabs 25, 50, 100 mg; oral conc 20 mg/ml

SIDE EFFECTS

CNS: Insomnia, agitation, somnolence, dizziness, headache, tremor, fatigue, paresthesia, twitching, confusion, ataxia, gait abnormality (geriatric)
CV: Palpitations, chest pain
EENT: Vision abnormalities
ENDO: SIADH (geriatric)
GI: Diarrhea, nausea, constipation, anorexia, dry mouth, dyspepsia, *vomiting, flatulence*
GU: Male sexual dysfunction, micturition disorder
INTEG: Increased sweating, rash, hot flashes
Contraindications: Hypersensitivity to this drug or SSRIs
Precautions: Pregnancy (B), lactation, geriatric, renal/hepatic disease, epilepsy, recent MI; latex sensitivity (dropper of oral conc)

PHARMACOKINETICS

PO: Peak 4.5-8.4 hr; steady state 1 wk; plasma protein binding 99%, elimination half-life 1-4 days, extensively metabolized, metabolite excreted in urine, bile

INTERACTIONS

- Altered lithium levels: lithium
- Sertraline is contraindicated with pimozide
- Disulfiram reaction: disulfiram and oral conc due to alcohol content
⚠ Fatal reactions: MAOIs
Increase: sertraline levels—cimetidine, warfarin, other highly protein-bound drugs
Increase: effects of antidepressants (tricyclics), diazepam, TOLBUTamide, warfarin, benzodiazepines, sumatriptan
Drug/Herb
- Hypertensive crisis: ephedra
Increase: of SSRI, serotonin syndrome—St. John's wort, SAM-e; do not use together
Increase: anticholinergic effect—corkwood, jimsonweed
Increase: CNS effect—hops, lavender
Drug/Lab Test
Increase: AST, ALT

NURSING CONSIDERATIONS
Assess:
- Mental status: mood, sensorium, affect, suicidal tendencies, increase in psychiatric symptoms, depression, panic
- B/P (lying/standing), pulse q4h; if systolic B/P drops 20 mm Hg, hold drug,

notify prescriber; VS q4h in patients with CV disease
• Weight qwk; appetite may decrease with drug
• Urinary retention, constipation, especially in geriatric
• Alcohol consumption; hold dose until morning

Administer:
• Increased fluids, bulk in diet for constipation, urinary retention
• With food, milk for GI symptoms
• Crushed if patient is unable to swallow medication whole
• Sugarless gum, hard candy, frequent sips of water for dry mouth
• Oral conc: dilute prior to use with 4 oz (½ cup) of water, orange juice, ginger ale or lemon/lime soda; do not mix with other liquids
• Avoid use with other CNS depressants

Perform/provide:
• Storage at room temperature; do not freeze
• Assistance with ambulation during therapy, since drowsiness, dizziness occur
• Safety measures, including side rails, primarily for geriatric
• Checking to see that PO medication is swallowed

Evaluate:
• Therapeutic response: significant improvement in depression, OCS

Teach patient/family:
• That therapeutic effect may take 1 wk or longer
• To use caution in driving, other activities requiring alertness; drowsiness, dizziness, blurred vision may occur
• Not to discontinue medication quickly after long-term use; may cause nausea, headache, malaise
• To avoid alcohol
• To notify prescriber if pregnant or plan to become pregnant or breastfeed

Rarely Used

sevelamer (℞)
(seh-vel'ah-mer)
Renagel
Func. class.: Polymeric phosphate binder

Uses: End-stage renal disease (ESRD)

DOSAGE AND ROUTES

Reduction of serum phosphorus in adults not taking phosphate binders
• *Adult:* **PO** initially 800-1600 mg tid with meals based on serum phosphorus level (see below); adjust dose gradually at 2-wk intervals until serum phosphorus 6 mg/dl
• *Adult, serum phosphorus ≥9 mg/dl:* 1600 mg tid with meals
• *Adult, serum phosphorus ≥7.5 and <9 mg/dl:* 1200-1600 mg tid with meals
• *Adult, serum phosphorus >6 and <7.5 mg/dl:* 800 mg tid with meals
Contraindications: Hypophosphatemia, bowel obstruction, hypersensitivity

Rarely Used

sibutramine (℞)
(si-byoo'tra-meen)
Meridia
Func. class.: Appetite suppressant

Controlled Substance Schedule IV
Uses: Obesity in conjunction with other treatments

DOSAGE AND ROUTES

• *Adult:* **PO** 10 mg daily; may be increased to 15 mg daily after 4 wk, or lowered to 5 mg daily depending on response
Contraindications: Hypersensitivity, hypothyroidism, anorexia nervosa, severe hepatic/renal disease, uncontrolled hypertension, history of CAD, CHF, dysrhythmias, lactation, CVA

A Safety alert   *"Tall Man" lettering

sildenafil (℞)

(sil-den′a-fill)
Revatio, Viagra
Func. class.: Erectile agent, antihypertensive, peripheral vasodilator
Chem. class.: Selective inhibitor of cGMP-PDE5

Action: Enhances the effect of nitric oxide (NO) by inhibiting phosphodiesterase type 5 (PDE5), which is necessary for degrading cGMP in the corpus cavernosum

Uses: Treatment of erectile dysfunction, pulmonary hypertension

Unlabeled uses: Sexual dysfunction (women)

DOSAGE AND ROUTES

Erectile dysfunction (Viagra only)
• *Adult:* PO 50 mg 1 hr before sexual activity, may be taken ½-4 hr before sexual activity; may be increased to 100 mg or decreased to 25 mg; max once/day

Renal/hepatic dose
• *Adult:* PO 25 mg, take 1 hr before sexual activity; do not use more than 1 ×/day

Pulmonary hypertension (Revatio only)
• *Adult:* PO 20 mg tid; take 4-6 hr apart
Available forms: Tabs 20, 25, 50, 100 mg

SIDE EFFECTS

CNS: Headache, flushing, dizziness
CV: **MI, sudden death, CV collapse**
MISC.: Dyspepsia, nasal congestion, UTI, abnormal vision, diarrhea, rash, **NAION (nonarteritic ischemic optic neuropathy)**

Contraindication: Hypersensitivity to this product or nitrates

Precautions: Pregnancy (B), anatomical penile deformities, sickle cell anemia, leukemia, multiple myeloma, retinitis pigmentosa, bleeding disorders, active peptic ulceration, CV/liver/renal disease, multidrug antihypertensive regimens

PHARMACOKINETICS

Rapidly absorbed; bioavailability 40%; metabolized by P45 CYP3A4, 2C9 in the liver (active metabolites); terminal half-life 4 hr, peak ½-1½ hr; reduced absorption with high-fat meal; excreted feces, urine

INTERACTIONS

⚠ Do not use with nitrates; fatal fall in B/P

Increase: sildenafil levels—cimetidine, erythromycin, ketoconazole, itraconazole, antiretroviral protease inhibitors

Decrease: sildenafil levels—rifampin, barbiturates, antacids, bosentan

Decrease: B/P—α-blockers, alcohol, amlodipine, angiotensin II receptor blockers

NURSING CONSIDERATIONS

Assess:
• For any severe loss of vision while taking this or any similar products; these products should not be used
• Use of organic nitrates that should not be used with this drug
• Cardiac status in pulmonary hypertension: B/P, pulse

Administer:
• Approximately 1 hr before sexual activity; do not use more than once a day

Teach patient/family:
• That drug does not protect against sexually transmitted diseases, including HIV
• That drug absorption is reduced with a high-fat meal
• That drug should not be used with nitrates in any form
• That tabs may be split
• To notify prescriber immediately and stop taking product if vision loss occurs

silver nitrate (℞)
Func. class.: Keratolytic

Action: Antiinfective, astringent, caustic
Uses: Cauterization of lesions, warts, burns (low concentrations)

DOSAGE AND ROUTES
• *Adult and child:* **TOP** apply to area to be treated
Available forms: Sticks, sol 10%, 25%, 50%

SIDE EFFECTS
INTEG: Skin discoloration
Contraindications: Hypersensitivity

INTERACTIONS
• Not to be used with alkalines, phosphates, thimerosal, benzalkonium chloride, halogenated acids

NURSING CONSIDERATIONS
Administer:
• After moistening stick with water
• To burns using a wet dressing (low concentrations 0.125%)
Perform/provide:
• Storage in cool area
Evaluate:
• Therapeutic response: absence of lesions, healing of burned areas
Teach patient/family:
• To avoid contact with clothing, unaffected areas; discoloration may occur

---

silver nitrate 1%
See Appendix C

---

silver nitrate sulfacetamide sodium ophthalmic
See Appendix C

---

silver protein, mild
(℞, otc)
Argyrol S.S. 10%, Argyrol S.S. 20%
Func. class.: Disinfectant
Chem. class.: Silver colloidal compound

Action: Destroys gram-positive, gram-negative organisms
Uses: Eye, nose, throat, swelling, infection

DOSAGE AND ROUTES
• *Adult and child:* **TOP** sol use as needed
Available forms: Top sol 5%, 10%, 25%; eyedrops 20%

SIDE EFFECTS
INTEG: Irritation, discolored tissue
Contraindications: Hypersensitivity
Precautions: Pregnancy (C)

NURSING CONSIDERATIONS
Administer:
• To area to be treated only; do not apply to healthy skin
Perform/provide:
• Storage in tight container
Evaluate:
• Area of body involved: irritation, rash, breaks, dryness, scales

---

silver sulfADIAZINE topical
See Appendix C

---

simethicone (otc, ℞)
(si-meth'i-kone)
Extra Strength Gas-X, Extra Strength Maalox Anti-Gas, Extra Stength Maalox GRF Gas Relief Formula ♣, Flatulex, Gas-Relief, Gas-X, Genasyme, Maalox Anti-Gas, Maalox GRF Gas Relief Formula ♣, Maximum Strength Gas Relief, Maximum Strength Mylanta Gas Relief, Maximum Strength Phazyme, Mylanta Gas, Mylicon, Ovol ♣, Phazyme, Phazyme 95, Phazyme 125
Func. class.: Antiflatulent

Do not confuse:
Mylicon/Mylanta Gas
Action: Disperses, prevents gas pockets in GI system; does not decrease gas production
Uses: Flatulence
Unlabeled uses: Dyspepsia

DOSAGE AND ROUTES

• *Adult and child >12 yr:* **PO** 40-100 mg after meals at bedtime
• *Child <2 yr:* **PO** 20 mg qid
Available forms: Chew tabs 40, 80, 125 mg; tabs 60, 80, 95 mg; drops 40 mg/0.6 ml, 40 mg/ml, 95 mg/1.425 ml; caps 95, 125 mg; soft gel caps 125 mg

SIDE EFFECTS

GI: Belching, rectal flatus
Contraindications: Hypersensitivity, GI obstruction/perforation
Precautions: Pregnancy (C), abdominal pain, fistula, hiatal hernia

NURSING CONSIDERATIONS
Assess:
• Reason for excess gas production, decreased bowel sounds, recent surgery, other GI conditions

Administer:
• After meals, at bedtime; shake susp well before giving; chew tabs should be chewed
Evaluate:
• Therapeutic response: absence of flatulence
Teach patient/family:
• That tablets must be chewed
• To shake suspension well before pouring

simvastatin (℞)
(sim-va-sta'tin)
Zocor
Func. class.: Antilipidemic
Chem. class.: HMG-CoA reductase inhibitor

Do not confuse:
Zocor/Cozaar/Zoloft
Action: Inhibits HMG-CoA reductase enzyme, which reduces cholesterol synthesis
Uses: As an adjunct in primary hypercholesterolemia (types IIa, IIb), isolated hypertriglyceridemia (Frederickson type IV) and type III hyperlipoproteinemia, CAD

DOSAGE AND ROUTES

• *Adult:* **PO** 20 mg daily in PM initially; usual range 5-40 mg/day in PM, not to exceed 80 mg/day; dosage adjustments may be made in 4-wk intervals or more; those taking verapamil and amiodarone max 20 mg/day
Renal disease/those taking cycloSPORINE
• *Geriatric:* **PO** 5 mg/day, initially
Cardiac/renal transplantation
• *Adult:* **PO** 5 mg daily; max 10 mg daily
With amiodarone or verapamil
• *Adult:* **PO** max 20 mg daily
With fibrates or niacin
• *Adult:* **PO** max 10 mg daily
Available forms: Tabs 5, 10, 20, 40, 80 mg

S

SIDE EFFECTS

CNS: Headache
EENT: Lens opacities
GI: Nausea, constipation, diarrhea, dyspepsia, flatus, abdominal pain, **liver dysfunction,** pancreatitis
INTEG: Rash, pruritus, photosensitivity
MS: Muscle cramps, myalgia, **myositis, rhabdomyolysis**
RESP: Upper respiratory tract infection
Contraindications: Pregnancy (X), hypersensitivity, lactation, active hepatic disease
Precautions: Past hepatic disease, alcoholism, severe acute infections, trauma, severe metabolic disorders, electrolyte imbalances

PHARMACOKINETICS

Metabolized in liver (active metabolites); highly protein bound; excreted primarily in bile, feces (60%); kidneys (15%)

INTERACTIONS

Increase: effects of warfarin
Increase: myalgia, myositis—cyclo-SPORINE, gemfibrozil, niacin, erythromycin, clofibrate, clarithromycin, ketoconazole, itraconazole, protease inhibitors
Increase: serum level of digoxin
Drug/Herb
Increase: effect—glucomannan
Decrease: effect—gotu kola, St. John's wort
Drug/Lab Test
Increase: CPK, LFTs

NURSING CONSIDERATIONS

Assess:
• 12-hr fasting lipid profile: LDL, HDL, TG, cholesterol at 6-8 wk, and q6mo
• Hepatic studies q1-2mo during the first 1½ yr of treatment; AST, ALT, LFTs may increase
⚠ For rhabdomyolysis: muscle tenderness, increased CPK levels; therapy should be discontinued

• Renal studies in patients with compromised renal system: BUN, I&O ratio, creatinine
Administer:
• Total daily dose in evening
Perform/provide:
• Storage in cool environment in tight container protected from light
Evaluate:
• Therapeutic response: decrease in cholesterol to desired level after 8 wk
Teach patient/family:
• That blood work and eye exam will be necessary during treatment
• To report blurred vision, severe GI symptoms, dizziness, headache
• That previously prescribed regimen will continue: low-cholesterol diet, exercise program

---

sirolimus (Ŗ)
(seer-oh-lie'mus)
Rapamune
Func. class.: Immunosuppressant
Chem. class.: Macrolide

Action: Produces immunosuppression by inhibiting T-lymphocyte activation and proliferation
Uses: Organ transplants to prevent rejection, recommended use is with cyclo-SPORINE and corticosteroids
Unlabeled uses: Psoriasis

DOSAGE AND ROUTES

• *Adult:* PO 2 mg daily with a 6 mg loading dose, may use 5 mg daily with a 15 mg loading dose
• *Child >13 yr weighing <40 kg (88 lb):* to 1 mg/m²/day, 3 mg/m² loading dose
Hepatic dose
• *Adult and child ≥13 yr/<40 kg:* PO Reduce by 33% in maintenance dose
Available forms: Oral sol 1 mg/ml

SIDE EFFECTS

CNS: Tremors, headache, insomnia, paresthesia, chills, fever

CV: Hypertension, *atrial fibrillation, CHF, hypotension, palpitation, tachycardia*
EENT: Blurred vision, photophobia
GI: Nausea, vomiting, diarrhea, constipation
GU: UTIs, **albuminuria, hematuria, proteinuria, renal failure**
HEMA: **Anemia, leukopenia, thrombocytopenia, purpura**
INTEG: *Rash, acne,* photosensitivity
META: Hyperglycemia, increased creatinine, edema, hypercholesterolemia, *hyperlipemia,* hypophosphatemia, weight gain, hyperkalemia, hyperuricemia, hypokalemia, hypomagnesemia
RESP: **Pleural effusion, atelectasis,** *dyspnea*
SYST: **Lymphoma**

Contraindications: Hypersensitivity to this drug or to components of the drug, lactation

Precautions: Pregnancy (C), severe renal/hepatic disease; diabetes mellitus, hyperkalemia, hyperuricemia, lymphomas, infection, other malignancies, children <13 yr, hypertension

PHARMACOKINETICS

Rapidly absorbed, peak 1 hr single dose, 2 hr multiple dosing, protein binding 92%; extensively metabolized by CYP3A4 enzyme system

INTERACTIONS

Increase: blood levels—antifungals, calcium channel blockers, cimetidine, danazol, erythromycin, cycloSPORINE, metoclopramide, bromocriptine, HIV-protease inhibitors
Decrease: blood levels—carbamazepine, phenobarbital, phenytoin, rifamycin, rifapentine
Decrease: effect of vaccines

Drug/Herb
• St. John's wort: may decrease the effect of sirolimus
Increase: effect—ginseng, maitake, mistletoe
Decrease: immunosuppression—astragalus, echinacea, melatonin

Drug/Food
• Alters bioavailability; use consistently with or without food; do not use with grapefruit juice

NURSING CONSIDERATIONS
Assess:
• Blood levels in those that may have altered metabolism, trough level ≥15 ng/ml are associated with increased adverse reactions
• Lipid profile: cholesterol, triglycerides, a lipid-lowering agent may be needed
⚠ For infection and development of lymphoma
⚠ Blood studies: Hgb, WBC, platelets during treatment qmo; if leukocytes <3000/mm³ or platelets <100,000/mm³, drug should be discontinued or reduced; decreased hemoglobulin level may indicate bone marrow suppression
• Hepatic studies: alk phos, AST, ALT, amylase, bilirubin, and for hepatotoxicity: dark urine, jaundice, itching, light-colored stools; drug should be discontinued

Administer:
• Prophylaxis for *Pneumocystis jiroveci* pneumonia for 1 yr after transplantation; prophylaxis for cytomegalovirus (CMV) is recommended for 90 days after transplantation in those at increased risk for CMV
• All medications PO if possible, avoiding IM inj; bleeding may occur
• For 3 days before transplant surgery; patients should be placed in protective isolation
• Use amber oral dose syringe and withdraw amount oral sol needed from the bottle, empty correct dose into plastic/glass container holding 60 ml of water/orange juice, stir vigorously and have patient drink at once, refill container with additional 120 ml water/orange juice, stir vigorously and drink at once, if using a pouch squeeze entire contents into container and follow above directions

S

Side effects: *italics* = common; **bold** = life-threatening

- Store protected from light, refrigerate, stable for 24 mo

Evaluate:

- Therapeutic response: absence of graft rejection; immunosuppression in autoimmune disorders

Teach patient/family:

- To report fever, rash, severe diarrhea, chills, sore throat, fatigue; serious infections may occur; clay-colored stools, cramping (hepatotoxicity)
- To avoid crowds, persons with known infections to reduce risk of infection
- To use contraception before, during and 12 wk after drug has been discontinued, avoid breastfeeding
- Use sunscreen, protective clothing to prevent burns

---

sitagliptin
See Appendix A—Selected New Drugs

---

sodium bicarbonate (℞, OTC)
Baking Soda, Bellans, Citrocarbonate, Neut, Soda Mint
Func. class.: Alkalinizer
Chem. class.: NaHCO$_3$

Action: Orally neutralizes gastric acid, which forms water, NaCl, CO_2; increases plasma bicarbonate, which buffers H^+ ion concentration; reverses acidosis IV

Uses: Acidosis (metabolic), cardiac arrest, alkalinization (systemic/urinary) antacid

DOSAGE AND ROUTES

Acidosis, metabolic

- *Adult and child:* **IV INF** 2-5 mEq/kg over 4-8 hr depending on CO_2, pH

Cardiac arrest

- *Adult and child:* **IV BOL** 1 mEq/kg of 7.5% or 8.4% sol, then 0.5 mEq/kg q10 min, then doses based on ABGs

- *Infant:* **IV INF** not to exceed 8 mEq/kg/day based on ABGs (4.2% sol)

Alkalinization of urine

- *Adult:* **PO** 325 mg-2 g qid or 48 mEq (4g), then 12-24 mEq q4h
- *Child:* **PO** 12-120 mg/kg/day (1-10 mEq/kg)

Antacid

- *Adult:* **PO** 300 mg-2 g chewed, taken with H_2O daily-qid

Available forms: Tabs 300, 325, 600, 650 mg; inj 4.2%, 5%, 7.5%, 8.4%

SIDE EFFECTS

CNS: Irritability, headache, confusion, stimulation, tremors, *twitching, hyperreflexia,* **tetany,** weakness, **seizures** of alkalosis

CV: Irregular pulse, **cardiac arrest,** water retention, edema, weight gain

GI: Flatulence, *belching, distention,* **paralytic ileus,** acid rebound

GU: Calculi

META: Alkalosis

RESP: Shallow, slow respirations; cyanosis, **apnea**

Contraindications: Hypertension, peptic ulcer, renal disease, hypocalcemia

Precautions: Pregnancy (C), CHF, cirrhosis, toxemia, renal disease

PHARMACOKINETICS

PO: Onset 2 min, duration 10 min
IV: Onset 15 min, duration 1-2 hr, excreted in urine

INTERACTIONS

Increase: effects—amphetamines, mecamylamine, quinine, quinidine, pseudoephedrine, flecainide, anorexiants

Increase: sodium and decrease potassium—corticosteroids

Decrease: effects—lithium, chlorpropamide, barbiturates, salicylates, benzodiazepines

Drug/Herb

Decrease: action of sodium bicarbonate—oak bark

Drug/Lab Test

Increase: Urinary urobilinogen

⚠ Safety alert   *"Tall Man" lettering

False positive: Urinary protein, blood lactate

NURSING CONSIDERATIONS
Assess:
• Respiratory and pulse rate, rhythm, depth, lung sounds; notify prescriber of abnormalities
• Fluid balance (I&O, weight daily, edema); notify prescriber of fluid overload
• Electrolytes, blood pH, PO_2, HCO_3^-, during treatment; ABGs frequently during emergencies
• Urine pH, urinary output, during beginning treatment
• Extravasation with IV administration (tissue sloughing, ulceration, and necrosis)
• Weight daily with initial therapy
• Alkalosis: irritability, confusion, twitching, hyperreflexia stimulation, slow respirations, cyanosis, irregular pulse
• Milk-alkali syndrome: confusion, headache, nausea, vomiting, anorexia, urinary stones, hypercalcemia
• For GI perforation secondary to CO_2 in GI tract; may lead to perforation if ulcer is severe enough
Administer:
• Chew antacid tablets and drink 8 oz water
• Do not take antacid with milk or milk-alkali syndrome may result
IV route
• In prepared sol or diluted in an equal amount of compatible sol given 2-5 mEq/kg over 4-8 hr, not to exceed 50 mEq/hr; slower rate in children
Additive compatibilities: Amikacin, aminophylline, amobarbital, amphotericin B, atropine, bretylium, calcium gluceptate, cefoxitin, ceftazidime, cephalothin, cephapirin, chloramphenicol, chlorothiazide, cimetidine, clindamycin, cytarabine, droperidol/fentanyl, ergonovine, erythromycin, esmolol, floxacillin, furosemide, heparin, hyaluronidase, hydrocortisone, kanamycin, lidocaine, mannitol, metaraminol, methotrexate, methyldopate, multivitamins, nafcillin, nal-

mefene, netilmicin, nizatidine, ofloxacin, oxacillin, oxytocin, phenobarbital, phenylephrine, phenytoin, phytonadione, potassium chloride, prochlorperazine, thiopental, verapamil
Syringe compatibilities: Milrinone, pentobarbital
Y-site compatibilities: Acyclovir, amifostine, asparaginase, aztreonam, cefepime, cefmetazole, ceftriaxone, cladribine, cyclophosphamide, cytarabine, DAUNOrubicin, dexamethasone, dexchlorpheniramine, DOXOrubicin, etoposide, famotidine, filgrastim, fludarabine, gallium, granisetron, heparin, ifosfamide, indomethacin sodium trihydrate, insulin, melphalan, mesna, methylPREDNISolone, morphine, paclitaxel, piperacillin/tazobactam, potassium chloride, propofol, remifentanil, tacrolimus, teniposide, thiotepa, tolazoline, vancomycin, vit B/C
Evaluate:
• Therapeutic response: ABGs, electrolytes, blood pH, HCO_3^- WNL
Teach patient/family:
• Not to take antacid with milk, or milk-alkali syndrome may result
• Not to use antacid for more than 2 wk
• To notify prescriber if indigestion is accompanied by chest pain, dyspnea, diarrhea, dark, tarry stools
• About sodium-restricted diet; to avoid use of baking soda for indigestion

---

sodium biphosphate/ sodium phosphate
(otc)
Fleet Enema, Phospho-Soda
Func. class.: Laxative, saline

Action: Increases water absorption in the small intestine by osmotic action, laxative effect occurs by increased peristalsis and water retention
Uses: Constipation, bowel or rectal preparation for surgery, exam

DOSAGE AND ROUTES
• *Adult:* **PO** 20-30 ml (Phospho-Soda)
• *Child:* **PO** 5-15 ml (Phospho-Soda)

- *Adult and child >12 yr:* **RECT** 1 enema (118 ml)
- *Child 2-12 yr:* **RECT** ½ enema (59 ml)

Available forms: Enema 7 g phosphate/19 g biphosphate/118 ml; oral sol 18 g phosphate/48 g biphosphate/100 ml

SIDE EFFECTS

CV: **Dysrhythmias, cardiac arrest,** hypotension, widening QRS complex
GI: Nausea, cramps, diarrhea
META: Electrolyte, fluid imbalances

Contraindications: Hypersensitivity, rectal fissures, abdominal pain, nausea/vomiting, appendicitis, acute surgical abdomen, ulcerated hemorrhoids, sodium-restricted diets, renal failure, hyperphosphatemia, hypocalcemia, hypokalemia, hypernatremia, Addison's disease, CHF, ascites, bowel perforation, megacolon, imperforate anus

Precautions: Pregnancy (C)

PHARMACOKINETICS

Onset 30 min-3 hr, excreted in feces

NURSING CONSIDERATIONS

Assess:

- Stools: color, amount, consistency
- Bowel pattern, bowel sounds, flatulence, distention, fever, dietary patterns, exercise
- Blood, urine electrolytes if drug is used often by patient
- Cramping, rectal bleeding, nausea, vomiting; if these symptoms occur, drug should be discontinued

Administer:

- Alone for better absorption; do not take within 1-2 hr of other drugs

Evaluate:

- Therapeutic response: decrease in constipation

Teach patient/family:

- Not to use laxatives for long-term therapy; bowel tone will be lost
- That normal bowel movements do not always occur daily

- Not to use in presence of abdominal pain, nausea, vomiting
- To notify prescriber if constipation unrelieved or if symptoms of electrolyte imbalance occur: muscle cramps, pain, weakness, dizziness, excessive thirst
- To maintain fluid consumption

---

sodium polystyrene sulfonate (Rx)
(po-lee-stye'reen)
Kayexalate, K-Exit ✦, Kionex, PMS Sodium Polystyrene Sulfonate ✦, SPS
Func. class.: Potassium-removing resin
Chem. class.: Cation exchange resin

Action: Removes potassium by exchanging sodium for potassium in body primarily in large intestine
Uses: Hyperkalemia in conjunction with other measures

DOSAGE AND ROUTES

- *Adult:* **PO** 15 g daily-qid; **RECT** enema 30-50 g/100 ml of sorbitol warmed to body temp q6h
- *Child:* **PO/RECT** 1 mEq of potassium exchanged/g of resin, approximate dose 1 g/kg q6h

Available forms: Susp 15 g polystyrene sulfonate, 21.5 ml sorbitol, 15 g (65 mEq) Na/60 ml; powder 15 g/4 level tsp

SIDE EFFECTS

GI: Constipation, anorexia, nausea, vomiting, diarrhea (sorbitol), fecal impaction, gastric irritation
META: Hypocalcemia, hypokalemia, hypomagnesemia, sodium retention

Contraindications: Hypersensitivity to saccharin or parabens that may be in some products, ileus
Precautions: Pregnancy (C), renal failure, CHF, severe edema, severe hypertension, geriatric, sodium restriction, constipation

---

⚠ Safety alert   *"Tall Man" lettering

INTERACTIONS
Increase: hypokalemia—loop diuretics
Decrease: effect of sodium polysty-rene—antacids, laxatives

NURSING CONSIDERATIONS
Assess:
• Hyperkalemia: confusion, dyspnea, weakness, dysrhythmias
• ECG for spiked T waves, depressed ST segments, prolonged QT and widening QRS complex
• Bowel function daily, note consistency of stools, times/day
• Hypotension: confusion, irritability, muscular pain, weakness
• Serum K, Ca, Mg, Na, acid-base balance
• I&O ratio, weight daily
• For digoxin; toxicity in those receiving digoxin
Administer:
• Oral dose as susp mixed with H_2O or syr (20-100 ml)
• Mild laxative as ordered to prevent constipation, fecal impaction
• Sorbitol as ordered to prevent constipation
• Retention enema after mixing with warm water; introduce by gravity, continue stirring, flush with 100 ml of fluid, clamp, and leave in place
Perform/provide:
• Retention of enema for at least ½-1 hr
• Irrigation of colon after enema with 1-2 qt nonsodium sol, drain
• Storage of freshly prepared sol 24 hr at room temperature
Evaluate:
• Therapeutic response: potassium level 3.5-5 mg/dl
Teach patient/family:
• Reason for medication and expected results

solifenacin (Rx)
(sol-i-fen′a-sin)
VESIcare
Func. class.: Overactive bladder product, anticholinergic
Chem. class.: Muscarinic receptor antagonist

Action: Relaxes smooth muscles in urinary tract by inhibiting acetylcholine at postganglionic sites
Uses: Overactive bladder (urinary frequency, urgency, incontinence)

DOSAGE AND ROUTES
• *Adult:* **PO** 5 mg daily, max 10 mg daily
Renal/hepatic dose
• *Adult:* **PO** CCr <30 ml/min 5 mg daily
Available forms: Tabs 5, 10 mg

SIDE EFFECTS
CNS: Anxiety, paresthesia, fatigue, *dizziness,* headache
CV: Chest pain, hypertension, **QTc prolongation,** edema
EENT: Vision abnormalities, xerophthalmia, nasal dryness
GI: Nausea, vomiting, anorexia, abdominal pain, *constipation, dry mouth,* dyspepsia
GU: Dysuria, urinary retention, frequency, UTI
INTEG: Rash, pruritus
RESP: Bronchitis, cough, pharyngitis, upper respiratory tract infection
Contraindications: Hypersensitivity, uncontrolled narrow-angle glaucoma, urinary retention, gastric retention
Precautions: Pregnancy (C), lactation, children, renal/hepatic disease, controlled narrow-angle glaucoma, bladder outflow obstruction, GI obstruction, decreased GI motility, history of QT prolongation

PHARMACOKINETICS
Rapidly absorbed, 98% highly protein bound, extensively metabolized by CYP3A4, excreted in urine/feces, terminal half-life 45-68 hr

INTERACTIONS

Increase: effects—CYP3A4 inhibitors (ketoconazole, clarithromycin, diclofenac, doxycycline, erythromycin, isoniazid, nefazodone, propofol, protease inhibitors, verapamil), with max dose 5 mg

Decrease: effects—CYP3A4 inducers (carbamazepine, nevirapine, phenobarbital, phenytoin)

Drug/Herb
Increase: effects—henbane, jimsonweed, scopolia
Decrease: effects—St. John's wort

Drug/Food
Increase: effect—grapefruit juice

NURSING CONSIDERATIONS

Assess:
• Urinary patterns: distention, nocturia, frequency, urgency, incontinence
• Allergic reactions: rash; if this occurs, drug should be discontinued

Evaluate:
• Urinary status: dysuria, frequency, nocturia, incontinence

Teach patient/family:
• To avoid hazardous activities; dizziness may occur
• Constipation, blurred vision may occur
• Call prescriber if severe abdominal pain or constipation lasts for 3 or more days
• Heat prostration may occur if used in a hot environment

---

somatropin (℞)
(soe-ma-troe′pin)
Genotropin, Humatrope, Norditropin, Nutropin, Nutropin Depot, Nutropin AQ, Saizen, Serostim
Func. class.: Pituitary hormone
Chem. class.: Growth hormone

Action: Stimulates growth; somatropin similar to natural growth hormone; both preparations developed by recombinant DNA

Uses: Pituitary growth hormone deficiency (hypopituitary dwarfism), children with human growth hormone deficiency, AIDS wasting syndrome, cachexia, adults with somatropin deficiency syndrome (SDS)

DOSAGE AND ROUTES

Genotropin
• *Child:* SUBCUT 0.16-0.24 mg/kg/wk divided into 6 or 7 inj, give in abdomen, thigh, buttocks
• *Adult:* SUBCUT 0.4-0.8 mg/kg/wk divided in 6-7 daily doses

Humatrope
Child: SUBCUT/IM 0.18 mg/kg divided into equal doses either on 3 alternate days or 6 ×/wk, max wk dose is 0.3 mg/kg
• *Adult:* IM 0.018 units/kg/day, max 0.0375 U/kg/day

Nutropin/Nutropin AQ (growth hormone deficiency)
• *Child:* SUBCUT 0.3 mg/kg/wk

Serostim
• *Adult:* SUBCUT at bedtime >55 kg, 6 mg; 45-55 kg, 5 mg; 35-45 kg, 4 mg

Norditropin
• *Child:* SUBCUT 0.024-0.034 mg/kg 6-7 ×/wk

Replacement of GH in GH deficiency
• *Adult:* SUBCUT (Saizen) 0.005 mg/kg/day; may increase after 4 wk to max 0.01 mg/kg/day

Available forms: Powder for inj (lyophilized) 1.5 mg (4 international units/ml), 4 mg (12 international units/vial), 5 mg (13 international units/vial), 5 mg (15 international units/vial), 5 mg (15 international units/vial) rDNA origin, 5.8 mg (15 international units/ml), 6 mg (18 international units/ml), 8 mg (24 international units/vial), 10 mg (26 international units/vial); inj 10 mg (30 international units/vial), 5 mg/1.5 ml, 10 mg/1.5 ml, 15 mg/1.5 ml

SIDE EFFECTS

CNS: Headache, growth of intracranial tumor
ENDO: **Hyperglycemia, ketosis, hypothyroidism**

GU: Hypercalciuria

INTEG: Rash, urticaria, pain; inflammation at inj site

MS: Tissue swelling, joint and muscle pain

SYST: **Antibodies to growth hormone**

Contraindications: Hypersensitivity to benzyl alcohol, closed epiphyses, intracranial lesions

Precautions: Pregnancy (C), lactation, diabetes mellitus, hypothyroidism

PHARMACOKINETICS

Half-life 15-60 min, duration 7 days; metabolized in liver

INTERACTIONS

• Epiphyseal closure: androgens, thyroid hormones

Decrease: growth—glucocorticosteroids

NURSING CONSIDERATIONS

Assess:

• Growth hormone antibodies if patient fails to respond to therapy

• Thyroid function tests: T_3, T_4, T_7, TSH to identify hypothyroidism

• Allergic reaction: rash, itching, fever, nausea, wheezing

• Hypercalciuria: urinary stones; groin, flank pain; nausea, vomiting, urinary frequency, hematuria, chills

• Growth rate of child at intervals during treatment

Administer:

IM route

• Rotate inj site

• Norditropin: after reconstituting 4 or 8 mg/2 ml diluent

• Humatrope: 5 mg/1.5-5 ml diluent, do not shake

• Nutropin/Nutropin AQ: reconstitute 5 mg/1-5 ml or 10 mg/1-10 ml bacteriostatic water for inj (benzyl alcohol preserved)

Perform/provide:

• Storage in refrigerator for <1 mo, if reconstituted <1 wk; do not use discolored or cloudy sol

Evaluate:

• Therapeutic response: growth in children

Teach patient/family:

• That treatment may continue for years; regular assessments are required

• Maintain a growth record, report knee, hip pain or limping

• That treatment is very expensive

---

sorafenib (℞)

(sore-ah-fen'ib)

Nexavar

Func. class.: Antineoplastic—miscellaneous

Chem. class.: Multikinase inhibitor, signal transduction inhibitor

---

Action: Multikinase inhibitor that decreases tumor cell proliferation

Uses: Advanced/metastatic murine renal cell carcinoma

DOSAGE AND ROUTES

• *Adult:* **PO** 400 mg bid without food, continue until no longer benefiting or until unacceptable toxicity occurs

Available forms: Tabs 200 mg

SIDE EFFECTS

CNS: Fatigue, weight loss, headache

CV: **Hypertension, cardiac ischemia, infarction**

GI: Nausea, diarrhea, vomiting, anorexia, **pancreatitis,** mouth ulceration, abdominal pain, constipation

HEMA: **Hemorrhage, leukopenia, lymphopenia, anemia, neutropenia, thrombocytopenia**

INTEG: Rash, pruritus, *dry skin,* erythema, hand-foot rash, **exfoliative dermatitis,** acne, flushing, alopecia

META: Hypophosphatemia

MS: Arthralgia, myalgia

RESP: Hoarseness

Contraindications: Pregnancy (D), hypersensitivity

Precautions: Lactation, children, geriatric, hepatic disease

Side effects: *italics* = common; **bold** = life-threatening

PHARMACOKINETICS

Bioavailability 38%-49%, elimination half-life 25-48 hr, peak 3 hr, high-fat meal decreases bioavailability, plasma protein binding 99.5%, metabolized in the liver, oxidative metabolism by CYP3A4, glucuronidation by UGT1A9, 77% excreted in feces

INTERACTIONS

• May decrease sorafenib levels: phenytoin, rifampin, cimetidine, ranitidine, sodium bicarbonate, carbamazepine, dexamethasone, phenobarbital

Increase: effect of UGT1A1 (irinotecan, DOXOrubicin, gemcitabine, oxaliplatin)

Drug/Lab Test

Increase: lipase, amylase

NURSING CONSIDERATIONS

Assess:

• For skin toxicities: grade 1, continue therapy, topical treatment for relief; grade 2 (1st episode), continue therapy, if no improvement after 7 days, delay treatment until resolved to grade ≤1, resume dose by one dose level; grade 2 (2nd or 3rd episode), delay treatment until resolved to grade ≤1, resume dose by one dose level; grade 2 (4th episode), discontinue therapy; grade 3 (1st or 2nd episode), delay treatment until resolved to grade ≤1, resume dose by one dose level; grade 3 (3rd episode), discontinue therapy

Administer:

• Swallow tab whole; do not break, crush, or chew

• On empty stomach 1 hr before or 2 hr after meal

Perform/provide:

• Storage in room temp, in dry place

Evaluate:

• Therapeutic response: decrease in renal cell carcinoma progression

Teach patient/family:

⚠ To report adverse reactions immediately

• Reason for treatment, expected results

• Use contraception during treatment, birth defects may occur, avoid breastfeeding

• To not double dose if missed

---

sotalol (℞)

(sot'ah-lahl)

Betapace, Betapace AF, Sotocar ✦

Func. class.: Antidysrhythmic group III

Chem. class.: Nonselective β-blocker

Action: Blockade of β_1- and β_2-receptors leads to antidysrhythmic effect, prolongs action potential in myocardial fibers without affecting conduction, prolongs QT interval, no effect on QRS duration

Uses: Life-threatening ventricular dysrhythmias; Betapace AF: to maintain sinus rhythm in symptomatic atrial fibrillation/flutter

DOSAGE AND ROUTES

• *Adult:* **PO** initial 80 mg bid, may increase to 240-320 mg/day

Renal dose

• *Adult:* **PO** CCr 30-60 ml/min, give q24h; CCr 10-29 ml/min, give q36-48h; CCr <10 ml/min, individualize dose

Betapace AF

• *Adult:* **PO** initial 80 mg bid, titrate upward to 120 mg bid during initial hospitalization

Renal dose (Betapace AF)

• *Adult:* **PO** CCr >60 ml/min, give q12h; CCr 40-60 ml/min, give q24h; CCr <40 ml/min, do not use

Available forms: Tabs 80, 120, 160, 240 mg; (Betapace AF) 80, 120, 160 mg

SIDE EFFECTS

CNS: Dizziness, mental changes, drowsiness, fatigue, headache, catatonia, depression, anxiety, nightmares, paresthesia, lethargy, insomnia, decreased concentration

---

⚠ Safety alert   *"Tall Man" lettering

CV: **Prodysrhythmia,** orthostatic hypotension, bradycardia, **CHF,** chest pain, ventricular dysrhythmias, AV block, peripheral vascular insufficiency, palpitations, torsades de pointes; **life-threatening ventricular dysrhythmias (Betapace AF)**

EENT: Tinnitus, visual changes, sore throat, double vision; dry, burning eyes

GI: Nausea, vomiting, diarrhea, dry mouth, flatulence, constipation, anorexia

GU: Impotence, dysuria, ejaculatory failure, urinary retention

HEMA: **Agranulocytosis, thrombocytopenic purpura** (rare), **thrombocytopenia, leukopenia**

INTEG: Rash, alopecia, urticaria, pruritus, fever

MISC: Facial swelling, decreased exercise tolerance, weight change, Raynaud's disease

MS: Joint pain, arthralgia, muscle cramps, pain

RESP: **Bronchospasm,** dyspnea, wheezing, nasal stuffiness, pharyngitis

Contraindications: Hypersensitivity to β-blockers, cardiogenic shock, heart block (2nd or 3rd degree), sinus bradycardia, CHF, bronchial asthma, congenital or acquired long QT syndrome, CCr <40 ml/min

Precautions: Pregnancy (B), major surgery, lactation, diabetes mellitus, renal disease, thyroid disease, COPD, well-compensated heart failure, CAD, nonallergic bronchospasm, electrolyte disturbances, bradycardia, cardiac dysrhythmias, peripheral vascular disease

PHARMACOKINETICS

PO: Onset 1-2 hr, peak 2-4 hr, duration 8-12 hr, half-life 12 hr; excreted unchanged in urine, crosses placenta, excreted in breast milk, protein binding 0%

INTERACTIONS

Increase: hypoglycemia effect—insulin
Increase: effects of lidocaine

Increase: hypotension—diuretics, other antihypertensives, nitroglycerin

Decrease: β-blocker effects—sympathomimetics

Decrease: bronchodilating effects of theophylline, β$_2$-agonists

Decrease: hypoglycemic effects of sulfonylureas

Drug/Herb

• Hypokalemia, increased antidysrhythmic effect: aloe, buckthorn, cascara sagrada, senna

Increase: toxicity, death—aconite

Increase: effect—aloe, broom, chronic buckthorn use, cascara sagrada (chronic use), Chinese rhubarb, figwort, fumitory, goldenseal, kudzu, licorice

Increase: serotonin effect—horehound

Decrease: effect—coltsfoot

Drug/Lab Test

False increase: Urinary catecholamines
Interference: Glucose, insulin tolerance tests

NURSING CONSIDERATIONS

Assess:

• I&O, weight daily; edema in feet, legs daily

• B/P, pulse q4h; note rate, rhythm, quality

⚠ Apical/radial pulse before administration: notify prescriber of any significant changes; monitor ECG continuously (Betapace AF); use QT interval to determine patient eligibility; baseline QT must be ≤450 msec

• Baselines in renal studies before therapy begins

• Skin turgor, dryness of mucous membranes for hydration status

Administer:

• PO before, at bedtime; tablet may be crushed or swallowed whole, give 1 hr before or 2 hr after meals

• Reduced dosage in renal dysfunction

• Betapace and Betapace AF are not interchangeable

Perform/provide:

• Storage in dry area at room temperature; do not freeze

Evaluate:
• Therapeutic response: absence of life-threatening dysrhythmias

Teach patient/family:
• Not to discontinue drug abruptly; taper over 2 wk or may precipitate angina, take exactly as prescribed
• Not to use OTC products containing α-adrenergic stimulants (nasal decongestants, OTC cold preparations) unless directed by prescriber
• To report bradycardia, dizziness, confusion, depression, fever
• To take pulse at home; advise when to notify prescriber
• To avoid alcohol, smoking, sodium intake
• To carry emergency ID to identify drug being taken, allergies
• To avoid hazardous activities if dizziness is present
• To report symptoms of CHF including: difficulty in breathing, especially on exertion or when lying down; night cough, swelling of extremities
• To wear support hose to minimize effects of orthostatic hypotension

Treatment of overdose: Lavage, IV atropine for bradycardia, IV theophylline for bronchospasm, digitalis, O_2, diuretic for cardiac failure; hemodialysis is useful for removal; administer vasopressor (norepinephrine) for hypotension, isoproterenol for heart block

---

spironolactone (℞)
(speer'on-oh-lak'tone)
Aldactone, Novo-Spiroton ✦
Func. class.: Potassium-sparing diuretic
Chem. class.: Aldosterone antagonist

Action: Competes with aldosterone at receptor sites in distal tubule, resulting in excretion of sodium chloride, water, retention of potassium, phosphate

Uses: Edema of CHF, hypertension, diuretic-induced hypokalemia, primary hyperaldosteronism (diagnosis, short-term treatment, long-term treatment), edema of nephrotic syndrome, cirrhosis of the liver with ascites

Unlabeled uses: CHF, acne, hirsutism in women

DOSAGE AND ROUTES
Edema/hypertension
• *Adult:* **PO** 25-200 mg/day in 1-2 divided doses

CHF
• *Adult:* **PO** 12.5-25 mg/day; max 50 mg/day

Edema
• *Child:* **PO** 3.3 mg/kg/day in single or divided doses

Hypertension
• *Child:* **PO** 1-2 mg/kg/day in divided doses

Hypokalemia
• *Adult:* **PO** 25-100 mg/day; if **PO,** potassium supplements must not be used

Primary hyperaldosteronism diagnosis
• *Adult:* **PO** 400 mg/day × 4 days or 4 wk depending on test, then 100-400 mg/day maintenance

Hirsutism in women (unlabeled)
• *Adult:* **PO** 50-200 mg in 1-2 divided doses

Acne in women (unlabeled)
• *Adult:* **PO** 25-200 mg in 1-2 divided doses

Renal dose
• *Adult:* **PO** CCr 10-50 mg/min; give dose q12-24h; CCr <10 mg/min, avoid use

Available forms: Tabs 25, 50, 100 mg

SIDE EFFECTS
CNS: Headache, confusion, drowsiness, lethargy, ataxia
ELECT: Hyperchloremic metabolic acidosis, **hyperkalemia,** hyponatremia
ENDO: Impotence, gynecomastia, irregular menses, amenorrhea, postmenopausal bleeding, hirsutism, deepening voice, breast pain
GI: Diarrhea, cramps, **bleeding,** gastritis, *vomiting,* anorexia, nausea, **hepatocellular toxicity**

HEMA: **Agranulocytosis**

INTEG: Rash, pruritus, urticaria

Contraindications: Pregnancy (D), hypersensitivity, anuria, severe renal disease, hyperkalemia

Precautions: Dehydration, hepatic disease, lactation, renal impairment, electrolyte imbalances, metabolic acidosis, gynecomastia

PHARMACOKINETICS

PO: Onset 24-48 hr, peak 48-72 hr; metabolized in liver, excreted in urine, crosses placenta

INTERACTIONS

Increase: action of antihypertensives, digoxin, lithium

Increase: hyperchloremic acidosis in cirrhosis—cholestyramine

Increase: hyperkalemia—potassium-sparing diuretics, potassium products, ACE inhibitors, salt substitutes

Decrease: effect of anticoagulants

Decrease: effect of spironolactone—ASA, NSAIDs

Drug/Herb

⚠ Fatal hypokalemia: arginine

Increase: hypokalemia—bearberry, gossypol

Increase: severe photosensitivity—St. John's wort

Increase: effect—cucumber, dandelion, horsetail, licorice, nettle, pumpkin, Queen Anne's lace

Increase: hypotension—khella

Drug/Lab Test

Interference: 17-OHCS, 17-KS, radioimmunoassay, digoxin assay

NURSING CONSIDERATIONS

Assess:

• Electrolytes: Na, Cl, K, BUN, serum creatinine, ABGs, CBC, signs of hyperkalemia

• Weight, I&O daily to determine fluid loss; effect of drug may be decreased if used daily; ECG periodically (long-term therapy)

• Signs of metabolic acidosis: drowsiness, restlessness

• Rashes, temp daily

• Confusion, especially in geriatric; take safety precautions if needed

• Hydration: skin turgor, thirst, dry mucous membranes

Administer:

• In AM to avoid interference with sleep

• With food; if nausea occurs, absorption may be decreased slightly

Evaluate:

• Therapeutic response: improvement in edema of feet, legs, sacral area daily if medication is being used in CHF

Teach patient/family:

• To avoid foods with high potassium content: oranges, bananas, salt substitutes, dried apricots, dates; avoid potassium salt substitutes

• That drowsiness, ataxia, mental confusion may occur; observe caution in driving

• To notify prescriber of cramps, diarrhea, lethargy, thirst, headache, skin rash, menstrual abnormalities, deepening voice, breast enlargement

Treatment of overdose: Lavage if taken orally; monitor electrolytes, administer IV fluids, monitor hydration, renal, CV status

---

stavudine (℞)

(sta'vyoo-deen)

d4T, Zerit

Func. class.: Antiretroviral

Chem. class.: Nucleoside reverse transcriptase inihibitor

Action: Prevents replication of HIV by the inhibition of the enzyme reverse transcriptase, causes DNA chain termination

Uses: Treatment of HIV-1 in combination with other antiretrovirals

DOSAGE AND ROUTES

• *Adult >60 kg:* **PO** 40 mg q12h

• *Adult <60 kg:* **PO** 30 mg q12h

• *Child <30 kg:* **PO** 1 mg/kg q12h

Side effects: *italics* = common; **bold** = life-threatening

- *Child ≥30 kg ≤60 kg:* **PO** 30 mg q12h
- *Child >60 kg:* **PO** 40 mg q12h

Renal dose
- *Adult: >60 kg:* **PO** CCr 26-50 ml/min 20 mg q12h; CCr 10-25 ml/min 20 mg q24h
- *Adult: <60 kg:* **PO** CCr 26-50 ml/min 15 mg q12h; CCr 10-25 ml/min 15 mg q24h

Available forms: Caps 15, 20, 30, 40 mg; powder for oral sol 1 mg/ml

SIDE EFFECTS

CNS: *Peripheral neuropathy,* insomnia, anxiety, neuropathy, depression, dizziness, confusion, headache, chills/fever, malaise

CV: Chest pain, vasodilation, hypertension

EENT: Conjunctivitis, abnormal vision

GI: **Hepatotoxicity,** diarrhea, nausea, vomiting, anorexia, dyspepsia, constipation, stomatitis, **pancreatitis**

HEMA: **Bone marrow suppression**

INTEG: Rash, sweating, pruritus, benign neoplasms

MISC: **Lactic acidosis,** asthenia, lipodystrophy

MS: Myalgia, arthralgia

RESP: Dyspnea, pneumonia, asthma

Contraindications: Hypersensitivity to this drug or zidovudine, didanosine, zalcitabine; severe peripheral neuropathy

Precautions: Pregnancy (C), advanced HIV infection, lactation, bone marrow suppression, renal/hepatic disease, peripheral neuropathy, osteoporosis

PHARMACOKINETICS

Excreted in urine, breast milk; peak 1 hr; half-life: elimination: 1-1.6 hr, intracellular: 3-3.5 hr

INTERACTIONS

Increase: myelosuppression—other myelosuppressants

Increase: peripheral neuropathy—lithium, dapsone, chloramphenicol

didanosine, ethambutol, hydrALAZINE, phenytoin, vinCRIStine, zalcitabine

Decrease: stavudine effect—methadone

NURSING CONSIDERATIONS

Assess:

A For lactic acidosis and severe hepatomegaly with steatosis, death may result

- Blood studies: WBC, differential, RBC, Hct, Hgb, platelets
- Renal tests: urinalysis, protein, blood
- C&S before drug therapy; drug may be given as soon as culture is taken
- Bowel pattern before, during treatment
- Weakness, tremors, confusion, dizziness; drug may have to be decreased or discontinued
- Viral load and CD4 counts baseline and throughout treatment
- For peripheral neuropathy: tingling, pain, in extremities; discontinue drug

A For pancreatitis: severe upper abdominal pain, nausea, vomiting throughout treatment, discontinue drug

Administer:
- With or without meals; absorption does not appear to be lowered when taken with food
- Every 12 hr around the clock

Teach patient/family:
- The signs of peripheral neuropathy: burning, weakness, pain, prickling feeling in the extremities
- That drug should not be given with antineoplastics
- That drug is not a cure for AIDS, but will control symptoms
- To call prescriber if sore throat, swollen lymph nodes, malaise, fever occur; other drugs may be needed to prevent other infections
- That even with this drug, patient may pass AIDS virus to others
- That follow-up visits are necessary; serious toxicity may occur; blood counts must be done q2wk
- That serious drug interactions may occur if other medications are ingested; see prescriber before taking chloramphenicol, dapsone, cisplatin, didanosine, eth-

ambutol, lithium, antifungals, antineoplastics
• That drug may cause fainting or dizziness
Evaluate:
• Therapeutic response: decreased symptoms of HIV

⚠ High Alert

streptokinase (℞)
(strep-toe-kye′nase)
Streptase
Func. class.: Thrombolytic enzyme
Chem. class.: β-Hemolytic streptococcus filtrate (purified)

Action: Activates conversion of plasminogen to plasmin (fibrinolysin): plasmin breaks down clots (fibrin), fibrinogen, factors V, VII; occlusion of venous access lines

Uses: Deep vein thrombosis, pulmonary embolism, arterial thrombosis, arterial embolism, lysis of coronary artery thrombi after MI, acute evolving transmural MI

Unlabeled uses: Arteriovenous cannula occlusion

DOSAGE AND ROUTES
Lysis of coronary artery thrombi
• *Adult:* **IC** 20,000 international units, then 2000 international units/min over 1 hr as **IV INF**
Arteriovenous cannula occlusion (unlabeled)
• *Adult:* **IV INF** 250,000 international units/2 ml sol into occluded limb of cannula run over ½ hr; clamp for 2 hr; aspirate contents; flush with NaCl sol and reconnect
Thrombosis/embolism/DVT/ pulmonary embolism
• *Adult:* **IV INF** 250,000 international units over ½ hr, then 100,000 international units/hr for 72 hr for deep vein thrombosis; 100,000 international units/hr

over 24-72 hr for pulmonary embolism; 100,000 international units/hr × 24-72 hr for arterial thrombosis or embolism
Acute evolving transmural MI
• *Adult:* **IV INF** 1,500,000 international units diluted to a volume of 45 ml; give within 1 hr; intracoronary **INF** 20,000 international units by **BOL**, then 2000 international units/min × 1 hr, total dose 140,000 international units
Available forms: Powder for inj, lyophilized, 250,000, 600,000, 750,000, 1,500,000 international units/vial

SIDE EFFECTS
CNS: Headache, fever
CV: Dysrhythmias, hypotension, noncardiogenic pulmonary edema, **pulmonary embolism**
EENT: Periorbital edema
GI: Nausea
HEMA: Decreased Hct, **bleeding**
INTEG: Rash, urticaria, phlebitis at IV inf site, itching, flushing
MS: Low back pain
RESP: Altered respirations, SOB, **bronchospasm**
SYST: **GI, GU, intracranial, retroperitoneal bleeding, surface bleeding, anaphylaxis**
Contraindications: Hypersensitivity, active internal bleeding, recent CVA, intracranial, intrapleural surgery, intraspinal surgery, CNS neoplasms, uncontrolled severe hypertension, lactation, children
Precautions: Pregnancy (C), arterial emboli from left side of heart, ulcerative colitis, enteritis, severe renal disease, hepatic disease, hypocoagulation, COPD, subacute bacterial endocarditis, rheumatic valvular disease, cerebral embolism/thrombosis/hemorrhage, intraarterial diagnostic procedure or surgery (10 days), recent major surgery

PHARMACOKINETICS
IV: Onset immediate, duration <12 hr; half-life <20 min; excreted in bile, urine

INTERACTIONS

• Bleeding potential: aspirin, indomethacin, phenylbutazone, anticoagulants, other NSAIDs, abciximab, eptifibatide, tirofiban, clopidogrel, ticlopidine, some cephalosporins, plicamycin, valproic acid, dipyridamole, GP IIb, IIIa inhibitors

Drug/Lab Test

Increase: PT, aPTT, TT
Decrease: Plasminogen, fibrinogen

NURSING CONSIDERATIONS

Assess:

• Allergy: fever, rash, itching, chills; mild reaction may be treated with antihistamines

⚠ For bleeding during 1st hr of treatment; hematuria, hematemesis, bleeding from mucous membranes, epistaxis, ecchymosis; may require tranfusion (rare), continue to assess for bleeding for 24 hr

• Blood studies (Hct, platelets, PTT, PT, TT, aPTT) before starting therapy; PT or aPTT must be less than 2× control before starting therapy; PTT or PT q3-4h during treatment

⚠ For hypersensitive reactions: fever, rash, dyspnea, facial swelling; drug should be discontinued; for streptokinase reactions previously; notify prescriber immediately, stop drug, keep resuscitative equipment nearby

• VS, B/P, pulse, respirations, neurologic signs, temp at least q4h; temp >104° F (40° C) indicates internal bleeding; systolic pressure increase >25 mm Hg should be reported to prescriber; assess neurologic status, neurologic change may indicate intracranial bleeding

⚠ For neurologic changes that may indicate intracranial bleeding

⚠ Retroperitoneal bleeding: back pain, leg weakness, diminished pulses

• For Guillain-Barré syndrome that may occur after treatment with this drug

• ECG continuously, cardiac enzymes, radionuclide myocardial scanning/coronary angiography

• For respiratory depression

Administer:

IV route

• As soon as thrombi identified; not useful for thrombi over 1 wk old

• Cryoprecipitate or fresh frozen plasma if bleeding occurs

• Loading dose at beginning of therapy; may require increased loading doses

• Heparin after fibrinogen level >100 mg/dl; heparin infusion to increase PTT to 1.5-2 × baseline for 3-7 days; IV heparin with loading dose is recommended after discontinuing streptokinase to prevent redevelopment of thrombi

• After reconstituting with 5 ml NS or D_5W; do not shake; further dilute to total volume of 45 ml; may be diluted to 500 ml in 45 ml increments; may dilute vial in 15 ml NS, further dilute 750,000 international units/50 ml NS or D_5W; further dilute 1,500,000 international units dose/100 ml or more

• About 10% patients have high streptococcal antibody titers requiring increased loading doses

• IV therapy using 0.8-μm filter

Y-site compatibilities: DOBUTamine, DOPamine, heparin, lidocaine, nitroglycerin

Perform/provide:

• Storage of reconstituted sol in refrigerator; discard after 24 hr

• Bed rest during entire course of treatment

• Avoid venous or arterial puncture, inj, rectal temp; any invasive treatment

• Treatment of fever with acetaminophen or aspirin

• Pressure for 30 sec to minor bleeding sites; inform prescriber if this does not attain hemostasis; apply pressure dressing

Evaluate:

• Therapeutic response: resolution of thrombosis, embolism

Teach patient/family:

• Reason for medication and expected results

⚠ Safety alert   *"Tall Man" lettering

streptomycin (℞)
(strep-toe-mye′sin)
Func. class.: Antiinfective/antitubercular
Chem. class.: Aminoglycoside

Action: Interferes with protein synthesis in bacterial cell by binding to ribosomal 30 S, causing inaccurate peptide sequence to form in protein chain, causing bacterial death

Uses: Sensitive strains of *Mycobacterium tuberculosis,* nontuberculous infections caused by sensitive strains of *Yersinia pestis, Brucella, Haemophilus influenzae, Klebsiella pneumoniae, Escherichia coli, Enterobacter aerogenes, Streptococcus viridans, Francisella tularensis, Proteus*

DOSAGE AND ROUTES
Tuberculosis
• *Adult:* **IM** 15 mg/kg (max 1 g) daily × 2-3 mo, then 1 g 2-3 ×/week with other antitubercular drugs
• *Child:* **IM** 20-40 mg/kg/day in divided doses with other antitubercular drugs; max 15 mg/kg/day
Streptococcal endocarditis
• *Adult:* **IM** 1 g q12h × 1 wk with penicillin, then 500 mg bid × 1 wk
Enterococcal endocarditis
• *Adult:* **IM** 1 g q12h × 2 wk, then 500 mg q12h × 4 wk with penicillin, max 15 mg/kg/day
Available forms: Inj 500 mg ✤, 1 g/ml

SIDE EFFECTS

CNS: Confusion, depression, numbness, tremors, **seizures,** muscle twitching, **neurotoxicity,** dizziness
CV: Hypotension, myocarditis, palpitations
EENT: **Ototoxicity,** deafness, visual disturbances, tinnitus
GI: Nausea, vomiting, anorexia, increased ALT, AST, bilirubin; hepatomegaly, **hepatic necrosis,** splenomegaly
GU: **Oliguria, hematuria, renal damage, azotemia, renal failure, nephrotoxicity**
HEMA: **Agranulocytosis, thrombocytopenia, leukopenia, eosinophilia, anemia**
INTEG: Rash, burning, urticaria, dermatitis, alopecia

Contraindications: Pregnancy (D), severe renal disease, hypersensitivity

Precautions: Neonates, mild renal disease, myasthenia gravis, lactation, hearing deficit, geriatric, Parkinson's disease, hepatic disease

PHARMACOKINETICS

IM: Onset rapid, peak 1-2 hr; plasma half-life 2-2½ hr; not metabolized, excreted unchanged in urine, crosses placental barrier, poor penetration into CSF, small amounts enter breast milk

INTERACTIONS

Increase: ototoxicity, neurotoxicity, nephrotoxicity—other aminoglycosides, amphotericin B, polymyxin, vancomycin, ethacrynic acid, furosemide, mannitol, methoxyflurane, cisplatin, cephalosporins, cidofovir
Increase: streptomycin effects—nondepolarizing muscle relaxants, succinylcholine, warfarin, NSAIDs
Drug/Herb
• Do not use acidophilus with antiinfectives; separate by several hours
Increase: toxicity—lysine (large amounts)

NURSING CONSIDERATIONS
Assess:
• Weight before treatment; calculation of dosage is usually based on ideal body weight, but may be calculated on actual body weight
• I&O ratio, urinalysis daily for proteinuria, cells, casts; report sudden change in urine output
• Serum peak 20-30 min after IM inj, trough level drawn 8 hr; acceptable levels—peak 5-25 mcg/ml, trough should not be >5 mcg/ml

S

Side effects: *italics* = common; **bold** = life-threatening

- Renal impairment by collecting urine for CCr testing, BUN, serum creatinine; lower dosage should be given in renal impairment (CCr <80 ml/min), monitor electrolytes: K, Na, Cl, Mg
- Deafness by audiometric testing, ringing, roaring in ears, vertigo; assess hearing before, during, after treatment
- Dehydration: high specific gravity, decrease in skin turgor, dry mucous membranes, dark urine
- Overgrowth of infection: fever, malaise, redness, pain, swelling, perineal itching, diarrhea, stomatitis, change in cough, sputum
- C&S before starting treatment to identify infecting organism
- Vestibular dysfunction: nausea, vomiting, dizziness, headache; drug should be discontinued if severe
- Inj sites for redness, swelling, abscesses; use warm compresses at site

Administer:
- IM inj in large muscle mass; rotate inj sites
- Drug in evenly spaced doses to maintain blood level

Additive compatibilities: Bleomycin
Syringe compatibilities: Penicillin G sodium
Y-site compatibilities: Esmolol
Perform/provide:
- Adequate fluids of 2-3 L/day unless contraindicated to prevent irritation of tubules
- Supervised ambulation, other safety measures with vestibular dysfunction

Evaluate:
- Therapeutic effect: absence of fever, draining wounds, negative C&S after treatment

Teach patient/family:
- To report headache, dizziness, symptoms of overgrowth of infection, renal impairment
- To report loss of hearing, ringing, roaring in ears, fullness in head

Treatment of overdose: Hemodialysis; monitor serum levels of drug

succimer (Ŗ)
(sux′i-mer)
Chemet
Func. class.: Heavy metal chelator antagonist
Chem. class.: Chelating agent

Action: Binds with ions of lead to form a water-soluble complex excreted by kidneys

Uses: Lead poisoning in children with lead levels above 45 mcg/dl; may be beneficial in mercury, arsenic poisoning

DOSAGE AND ROUTES
- *Adult:* **PO** 10-30 mg/kg/day × 5 days
- *Child with lead level >45 mcg/dl:* **PO** 10 mg/kg or 350 mg/m^2 q8h × 5 days, then 10 mg/kg or 350 mg/m^2 q12h × 2 wk; another course may be required depending on lead levels; allow 2 wk between courses

Available forms: Caps 100 mg

SIDE EFFECTS
CNS: Drowsiness, dizziness, paresthesia, sensorimotor neuropathy
EENT: Otitis media, watery eyes, film in eyes, plugged ears
GI: Nausea, vomiting, diarrhea, metallic taste, anorexia
GU: **Proteinuria,** decreased urination, voiding difficulties
HEMA: **Increased platelets, intermittent eosinophilia**
INTEG: Rash, urticaria, pruritus
META: Increased AST, ALT, alk phos, cholesterol
RESP: Sore throat, rhinorrhea, nasal congestion, cough
SYST: Back, stomach, head, rib, flank pain; abdominal cramps, chills, fever, flulike symptoms, head cold, headache

Contraindications: Hypersensitivity
Precautions: Pregnancy (C), lactation, children <1 yr, renal/hepatic disease

---

⚠ Safety alert   *"Tall Man" lettering

PHARMACOKINETICS

PO: Peak 1-2 hr, 49% excreted (39% in feces, 9% urine, 1% as CO_2 from lungs)

INTERACTIONS

• Not recommended concurrently with other chelating agents

NURSING CONSIDERATIONS
Assess:
• Renal, hepatic studies: ALT, AST, alk phos, BUN, creatinine, serum lead level
• I&O
• For lead sources in home, school
• Allergic reactions: rash, pruritus, urticaria; drug should be discontinued if antihistamines fail to help

Administer:
• To children who cannot swallow capsule by separating the capsule and sprinkling content on food or in a spoon followed by a drink; administer immediately after preparation

Perform/provide:
• Adequate fluids; check hydration status daily

Evaluate:
• Therapeutic response: decrease in serum lead level

Teach patient/family:
• That therapeutic effect may take 1-3 mo
• To report urticaria, rash
• To increase fluid intake

⚠ High Alert

succinylcholine (℞)
(suk-sin-ill-koe′leen)
Anectine, Anectine Flo-Pack, Quelicin, succinylcholine chloride, Sucostrin, Suxamethonium
Func. class.: Neuromuscular blocker (depolarizing–ultra short)

Action: Inhibits transmission of nerve impulses by binding with cholinergic receptor sites, antagonizing action of acetylcholine; causes release of histamine

Uses: Facilitation of endotracheal intubation, skeletal muscle relaxation during orthopedic manipulations

DOSAGE AND ROUTES
• *Adult:* IV 0.3-1.1 mg/kg, then 0.5-10 kg/min; IM 3-4 mg/kg
• *Child:* IV/IM 1-4 mg/kg
Available forms: Inj 20, 50, 100 mg/ml; powder for inj 100, 500 mg/vial, 1 g/vial

SIDE EFFECTS
CV: Bradycardia, tachycardia; increased, decreased B/P; **sinus arrest, dysrhythmias**
EENT: Increased secretions, increased intraocular pressure
HEMA: **Myoglobulinemia**
INTEG: Rash, flushing, pruritus, urticaria
MS: Weakness, muscle pain, fasciculations, prolonged relaxation
RESP: **Prolonged apnea, bronchospasm, cyanosis, respiratory depression,** wheezing

Contraindications: Hypersensitivity, malignant hyperthermia, decreased plasma pseudocholinesterase, penetrating eye injuries, acute narrow-angle glaucoma

Precautions: Pregnancy (C), cardiac disease, severe burns, fractures—fasciculations may increase damage—lactation, children <2 yr, electrolyte imbalances, dehydration, renal/hepatic/cardiac/neuromuscular disease, respiratory disease, collagen diseases, glaucoma, eye surgery, geriatric or debilitated patients

PHARMACOKINETICS
IV: Onset 1 min, peak 2-3 min, duration 6-10 min
IM: Onset 2-3 min
Hydrolyzed in blood, excreted in urine (active/inactive metabolites)

INTERACTIONS
• Dysrhythmias: theophylline
Increase: neuromuscular blockade—

aminoglycosides, β-blockers, cardiac glycosides, clindamycin, lincomycin, procainamide, quinidine, local anesthetics, polymyxin antibiotics, lithium, opioids, thiazides, enflurane, isoflurane, magnesium salts, oxytocin

Drug/Herb

• Blocks succinylcholine: melatonin

NURSING CONSIDERATIONS

Assess:

• For electrolyte imbalances (K, Mg); may lead to increased action of this drug
• VS (B/P, pulse, respirations, airway) until fully recovered; rate, depth, pattern of respirations, strength of hand grip
• I&O ratio; check for urinary retention, frequency, hesitancy
• Recovery: decreased paralysis of face, diaphragm, leg, arm, rest of body
• Allergic reactions: rash, fever, respiratory distress, pruritus; drug should be discontinued

Administer:

• Deep IM inj, preferably high in deltoid muscle

IV route

• Using nerve stimulator by anesthesiologist to determine neuromuscular blockade
• Anticholinesterase to reverse neuromuscular blockade
• IV inf: dilute 1-2 mg/ml in D₅, isotonic saline sol; give 0.5-10 mg/min; titrate to response; may be given directly over 1 min

Additive compatibilities: Amikacin, cephapirin, isoproterenol, meperidine, methyldopa, morphine, norepinephrine, scopolamine

Syringe compatibilities: Heparin

Y-site compatibilities: Etomidate, heparin, potassium chloride, propofol, vit B/C

Perform/provide:

• Storage in refrigerator, powder at room temperature; close tightly
• Reassurance if communication is difficult during recovery from neuromuscular blockade; postoperative stiffness is normal, soon subsides

Evaluate:

• Therapeutic response: paralysis of jaw, eyelid, head, neck, rest of body

Treatment of overdose: Edrophonium or neostigmine, atropine, monitor VS; may require mechanical ventilation

---

sucralfate ($\mathbb{R}$)
(soo-kral'fate)
Carafate, Sulcrate ✦
Func. class.: Protectant, antiulcer
Chem. class.: Aluminum hydroxide, sulfated sucrose

Do not confuse:

Carafate/Cafergot

Action: Forms a complex that adheres to ulcer site, adsorbs pepsin

Uses: Duodenal ulcer, oral mucositis, stomatitis after radiation of head and neck

Unlabeled uses: Gastric ulcers, gastroesophageal reflux

DOSAGE AND ROUTES

Duodenal ulcers

• *Adult:* **PO** 1 g qid 1 hr before meals, at bedtime
• *Child:* **PO** 40-80 mg/kg/day

GERD

• *Adult:* **PO** 1 g qid 1 hr before meals and at bedtime
• *Child:* **PO** 500 mg-1 g qid, 1 hr before meals and at bedtime

Available forms: Tabs 1 g; oral susp 1 g/10 ml

SIDE EFFECTS

CNS: Drowsiness, dizziness
GI: Dry mouth, constipation, nausea, gastric pain, vomiting
INTEG: Urticaria, rash, pruritus

Contraindications: Hypersensitivity

Precautions: Pregnancy (B), lactation, children, renal failure

PHARMACOKINETICS

PO: Duration up to 6 hr

⚠ Safety alert   *"Tall Man" lettering

INTERACTIONS

Decrease: action of tetracyclines, phenytoin, fat-soluble vitamins, cimetidine, digoxin, ketoconazole, ranitidine, theophylline

Decrease: absorption of fluoroquinolones

Decrease: absorption of sucralfate—antacids

NURSING CONSIDERATIONS

Assess:
• Gastric pH (>5 should be maintained); blood in stools

Administer:

PO route
• Do not crush or chew tabs; tabs may be broken or dissolved in water
• Do not take antacids 30 min before or after sucralfate
• On an empty stomach, 1 hr before meals and at bedtime

Perform/provide:
• Storage at room temperature

Evaluate:
• Therapeutic response: absence of pain, GI complaints

Teach patient/family:
• To take on empty stomach
• To take full course of therapy, not to use over 8 wk, to avoid smoking
• To avoid antacids within ½ hr of drug

---

*sulfADIAZINE (R)

(sul-fa-dye'a-zeen)
Coptin, sulfADIAZINE
Func. class.: Antiinfective
Chem. class.: Sulfonamide, intermediate acting

Do not confuse:
sulfADIAZINE/sulfiSOXAZOLE
Action: Inhibits folic acid synthesis
Uses: UTIs, rheumatic fever prophylaxis, with pyrimethamine for *Toxoplasma gondii* encephalitis, chancroid, inclusion conjunctivitis, malaria, meningitis, *Haemophilus influenzae,* meningococeal meningitis, nocardiosis, acute otitis media, trachoma, chloroquine-resistant malaria

DOSAGE AND ROUTES

Meningococcal carriers (asymptomatic)
• *Adult:* **PO** 1 g q12h × 2 days
• *Child 1-12 yr:* **PO** 500 mg q12h × 2 days
• *Child 2-12 mo:* **PO** 500 mg daily × 2 days

Rheumatic fever prophylaxis
• *Adult and child >30 kg:* **PO** 1 g daily
• *Child <30 kg:* **PO** 500 mg daily

Available forms: Tabs 500 mg, 7.7 g

SIDE EFFECTS

CNS: Headache, insomnia, hallucinations, depression, vertigo, fatigue, anxiety, **seizures,** drug fever, chills, drowsiness
CV: **Allergic myocarditis**
GI: Nausea, vomiting, abdominal pain, stomatitis, **hepatitis,** glossitis, pancreatitis, diarrhea, **enterocolitis,** anorexia
GU: **Renal failure, toxic nephrosis,** increased BUN, creatinine, crystalluria, hematuria, proteinuria
HEMA: **Leukopenia, thrombocytopenia, agranulocytosis, hemolytic anemia, aplastic anemia**
INTEG: Rash, dermatitis, urticaria, **Stevens-Johnson syndrome,** erythema, photosensitivity, alopecia
SYST: **Anaphylaxis**

Contraindications: Hypersensitivity to sulfonamides, sulfonylureas, thiazide and loop diuretics, salicylates, sunscreens with PABA, lactation, infants <2 mo (except congenital toxoplasmosis), pregnancy at term, porphyria
Precautions: Pregnancy (C), impaired hepatic function, severe allergy, bronchial asthma, renal dysfunction, G6PD deficiency, UV exposure

PHARMACOKINETICS

PO: Rapidly absorbed, onset ½ hr; peak 3-6 hr, 30%-50% bound to plasma proteins, half-life 8-10 hr; excreted in urine, breast milk; crosses placenta, metabolized in liver

Side effects: *italics* = common; **bold** = life-threatening

INTERACTIONS

Increase: hypoglycemic response—sulfonylurea agents

Increase: anticoagulant effects—warfarin

Increase: effects of barbiturates, TOLBUTamide, uricosurics

Increase: free-drug concentrations—indomethacin, probenecid, salicylates

Increase: thrombocytopenia—thiazide diuretics

Increase: nephrotoxicity—cycloSPORINE

Decrease: renal excretion of methotrexate, risk of bone marrow suppression

Decrease: hepatic clearance of phenytoin

Drug/Herb
• Do not use acidophilus with antiinfectives; separate by several hours

Drug/Lab Test
False positive: Urinary glucose test (Benedict's method, Chemstrip uG)

NURSING CONSIDERATIONS

Assess:
• I&O ratio; note color, character, pH of urine if drug administered for UTIs; output should be 800 ml less than intake; if urine is highly acidic, alkalization may be needed
• Renal studies: BUN, creatinine, urinalysis (long-term therapy)
• Blood dyscrasias: skin rash, fever, sore throat, bruising, bleeding, fatigue, joint pain, monitor CBC before and periodically
• Allergic reaction: rash, dermatitis, urticaria, pruritus, dyspnea, bronchospasm

Administer:
• On an empty stomach
• With full glass of H_2O to maintain adequate hydration; increase fluids to 2 L/day to decrease crystallization in kidneys
• Medication after C&S; repeat C&S after full course of medication

Perform/provide:
• Storage in tight, light-resistant container at room temperature

Evaluate:
• Therapeutic response: absence of pain, fever, C&S negative

Teach patient/family:
• To take each oral dose with full glass of water to prevent crystalluria
• To complete full course of treatment to prevent superinfection
• To avoid sunlight or use sunscreen to prevent burns
• To avoid OTC medication (aspirin, vit C) unless directed by prescriber
• To notify prescriber of skin rash, sore throat, fever, mouth sores, unusual bruising, bleeding

---

sulfamethoxazole (℞)
(sul-fa-meth-ox′a-zole)
Apo-Sulfamethoxazole ✦,
Gantanol, Urobak
Func. class.: Antiinfective
Chem. class.: Sulfonamide, intermediate acting

Action: Inhibits folic acid synthesis

Uses: UTIs, chancroid, inclusion conjunctivitis, malaria, meningococcal meningitis, nocardiosis, acute otitis media, toxoplasmosis, trachoma

DOSAGE AND ROUTES

• *Adult:* **PO** 2 g, then 1 g bid or tid for 7-10 days
• *Child >2 mo:* **PO** 50-60 mg/kg × 1 dose then 25-30 mg/kg bid; max 2 g/day

Renal dose
• *Adult:* **PO** CCr <10-30 ml/min give 50% of dose; CCr <10 ml/min give 25% of dose or extend interval

Available forms: Tabs 500 mg; oral susp 500 mg/5 ml

SIDE EFFECTS

CNS: Headache, insomnia, hallucinations, depression, vertigo, fatigue, anxiety, **seizures, drug fever,** chills, drowsiness

CV: **Allergic myocarditis**

GI: *Nausea, vomiting, abdominal pain,* stomatitis, **hepatitis,** glossitis, pancreatitis, diarrhea, **enterocolitis,** anorexia

---

⚠ Safety alert   ✦"Tall Man" lettering

GU: **Renal failure, toxic nephrosis,** increased BUN, creatinine, crystalluria, hematuria, proteinuria

HEMA: **Leukopenia, thrombocytopenia, agranulocytosis, hemolytic anemia, aplastic anemia**

INTEG: Rash, dermatitis, urticaria, **Stevens-Johnson syndrome,** erythema, photosensitivity, alopecia

SYST: **Anaphylaxis**

Contraindications: Hypersensitivity to sulfonamides, sulfonylureas, thiazide and loop diuretics, salicylates, sunscreens with PABA, infants <2 mo (except congenital toxoplasmosis), pregnancy at term, porphyria, lactation, G6PD deficiency

Precautions: Pregnancy (C), impaired renal/hepatic function, severe allergy, bronchial asthma, UV exposure, geriatric

PHARMACOKINETICS

PO: Poorly absorbed, peak 3-4 hr, 50%-70% bound to plasma proteins, half-life 7-12 hr; excreted in urine (unchanged 90%), breast milk; crosses placenta

INTERACTIONS

Increase: effects of barbiturates, uricosurics

Increase: drug-free concentrations—indomethacin, probenecid, salicylates

Increase: thrombocytopenia—thiazide diuretics

Increase: nephrotoxicity—cycloSPORINE

Increase: hypoglycemic response—sulfonylurea agents

Increase: anticoagulant effects—warfarin

Increase: crystalluria—methenamine

Decrease: renal excretion of methotrexate

Decrease: hepatic clearance of phenytoin

Drug/Herb

• Do not use acidophilus with antiinfectives; separate by several hours

Drug/Lab Test

False positive: Urinary glucose test (Benedict's method)

NURSING CONSIDERATIONS

Assess:

• I&O ratio; note color, character, pH of urine if drug administered for UTIs; output should be 800 ml less than intake; if urine is highly acidic, alkalization may be needed

• Renal studies: BUN, creatinine, urinalysis (long-term therapy)

• Blood dyscrasias: skin rash, fever, sore throat, bruising, bleeding, fatigue, joint pain, monitor CBC before and periodically

⚠ Allergic reaction: rash, dermatitis, urticaria, pruritus, dyspnea, bronchospasm

Administer:

PO route

• On empty stomach

• With full glass of H_2O to maintain adequate hydration; increase fluids to 2 L/day to decrease crystallization in kidneys

• Medication after C&S; repeat C&S after full course of medication

Perform/provide:

• Storage in tight, light-resistant container at room temperature

Evaluate:

• Therapeutic response: absence of pain, fever, C&S negative

Teach patient/family:

• To take each oral dose with full glass of H_2O to prevent crystalluria

• To complete full course of treatment to prevent superinfection

• To avoid sunlight or use sunscreen to prevent burns

• To avoid OTC medication (aspirin, vit C) unless directed by prescriber

⚠ To notify prescriber of skin rash, sore throat, fever, mouth sores, unusual bruising, bleeding, crystals in urine

S

sulfasalazine (Ⴗ)

(sul-fa-sal′a-zeen)
Azulfidine, Azulfidine EN-
tabs, PMS-Sulfasalazine ✿,
S.A.S. ✿, Salazopyrin ✿,
sulfasalazine
Func. class.: GI antiinflammatory,
antirheumatic (DMARD)
Chem. class.: Sulfonamide

Do not confuse:

sulfasalazine/sulfiSOXAZOLE

Action: Prodrug to deliver sulfapyridine
and 5-aminosalicylic acid to colon; antiinflammatory in connective tissue also

Uses: Ulcerative colitis; rheumatoid arthritis; juvenile, rheumatoid arthritis
(Azulfidine EN-tabs)

Unlabeled uses: Ankylosing spondylitis, Crohn's disease, granulomatous colitis, regional enteritis

DOSAGE AND ROUTES

Bowel disease

• *Adult:* PO 3-4 g/day in divided doses;
maintenance 2 g/day in divided doses q6h
• *Child ≥6 yr:* PO 40-60 mg/kg/day in
4-6 divided doses, then 30 mg/kg/day in
4 doses, max 2 g/day

Rheumatoid arthritis

• *Adult:* PO 2 g/day in evenly divided
doses, initiate treatment with a lower dose
of enteric-coated tab

Juvenile rheumatoid arthritis

• *Child ≥6 yr:* PO 30-50 mg/kg/24 hr,
divided into 2 doses

Renal dose

• *Adult:* PO CCr 10-30 ml/min give bid;
CCr <10 ml/min give daily

Available forms: Tabs 500 mg; oral
susp 250 mg/5 ml; del rel tabs 500 mg

SIDE EFFECTS

CNS: Headache, confusion, insomnia, hallucinations, depression, vertigo, fatigue,
anxiety, **seizures,** drug fever, chills
CV: **Allergic myocarditis**

GI: Nausea, vomiting, abdominal pain,
stomatitis, **hepatitis,** glossitis, pancreatitis, diarrhea
GU: **Renal failure, toxic nephrosis,** increased BUN, creatinine, crystalluria
HEMA: **Leukopenia, neutropenia,
thrombocytopenia, agranulocytosis,
hemolytic anemia**
INTEG: Rash, dermatitis, urticaria,
Stevens-Johnson syndrome, erythema, photosensitivity
SYST: **Anaphylaxis**

Contraindications: Hypersensitivity to
sulfonamides or salicylates, pregnancy at
term, child <2 yr, intestinal, urinary obstruction, porphyria

Precautions: Pregnancy (B), lactation,
impaired renal/hepatic function, severe
allergy, bronchial asthma, megaloblastic
anemia

PHARMACOKINETICS

PO: Partially absorbed, peak 1½-6 hr,
duration 6-12 hr, half-life 6 hr, excreted
in urine as sulfasalazine (15%), sulfapyridine (60%), 5-aminosalicylic acid and
metabolites (20%-33%), in breast milk;
crosses placenta

INTERACTIONS

Increase: leukopenia risk—thiopurines
(azathioprine, mercaptopurine)
Increase: hypoglycemic response—oral
hypoglycemics
Increase: anticoagulant effects—oral an-
ticoagulants
Decrease: effect of cycloSPORINE, di-
goxin, folic acid
Decrease: renal excretion of metho-
trexate
Drug/Food
Decrease: iron/folic acid absorption
Drug/Lab Test
False positive: Urinary glucose test

NURSING CONSIDERATIONS

Assess:

• Renal studies: BUN, creatinine, urinalysis (long-term therapy)
⚠ Blood dyscrasias: skin rash, fever, sore

throat, bruising, bleeding, fatigue, joint pain; monitor CBC before and q3mo

A Allergic reaction: rash, dermatitis, urticaria, pruritus, dyspnea, bronchospasm

Administer:
• Do not break, crush, or chew delayed rel tabs
• With full glass of H_2O to maintain adequate hydration; increase fluids to 2 L/day to decrease crystallization in kidneys
• Total daily dose in evenly spaced doses and after meals to help minimize GI intolerance

Perform/provide:
• Storage in tight, light-resistant container at room temperature

Evaluate:
• Therapeutic response: absence of fever, mucus in stools, pain in joints

Teach patient/family:
• To take each oral dose with full glass of H_2O to prevent crystalluria
• That contact lens, urine/skin may be yellow-orange
• To avoid sunlight or use sunscreen to prevent burns
• To notify prescriber of skin rash, sore throat, fever, mouth sores, unusual bruising, bleeding

---

sulfinpyrazone (℞)
(sul-fin-peer′a-zone)
Anturan ✦, Anturane,
sulfinpyrazone
Func. class.: Uricosuric
Chem. class.: Pyrazolone

Action: Inhibits tubular reabsorption of urates, with increased excretion of uric acid; inhibits prostaglandin synthesis, which decreases platelet aggregation
Uses: Gout, gouty arthritis

DOSAGE AND ROUTES
Gout/gouty arthritis
• *Adult:* **PO** 100-200 mg bid × 1 wk, then 200-400 mg bid, not to exceed 800 mg/day
• *Child:* **PO** 10 mg/kg/day in 3-4 divided doses

Renal dose
• CCr <50 ml/min; avoid use
Available forms: Tabs 100 mg; caps 200 mg

SIDE EFFECTS
CNS: Dizziness, **seizures, coma**
EENT: Tinnitus
GI: Gastric irritation, nausea, vomiting, anorexia, **hepatic necrosis, GI bleeding**
GU: Renal calculi, hypoglycemia
HEMA: **Agranulocytosis** (rare)
INTEG: Rash, dermatitis, pruritus, fever, photosensitivity
RESP: **Apnea,** irregular respirations
Contraindications: Hypersensitivity to pyrazolone derivatives, salicylates, blood dyscrasias, CCr <50 ml/min, active peptic ulcer, GI inflammation, nephrolithiasis
Precautions: Pregnancy (C), renal disease, NSAIDs hypersensitivity

PHARMACOKINETICS
PO: Peak 1-2 hr, duration 4-6 hr, half-life 4 hr; metabolized by liver, excreted in urine

INTERACTIONS
Increase: toxicity—acetaminophen
Increase: effects of warfarin, TOLBUTamide
Increase: bleeding risk—NSAIDs
Decrease: effects of verapamil, theophylline
Decrease: effects of sulfinpyrazone—salicylates, niacin
Drug/Lab Test
Increase: PSP, aminohippuric acid
False positive: Clinitest

NURSING CONSIDERATIONS
Assess:
• Uric acid levels (3-7 mg/dl); joint mobility, pain, swelling
• Respiratory rate, rhythm, depth; notify prescriber of abnormalities
• Renal function
• Bleeding tendencies, RBC, Hct
• I&O

Side effects: *italics* = common; **bold** = life-threatening

• Electrolytes, CO_2 before, during treatment
• Urine pH, output, glucose during beginning treatment

Administer:
• With glass of milk
• With food for GI symptoms
• Increased fluids to prevent calculi; alkalinization of urine may be required

Evaluate:
• Therapeutic response: absence of pain, stiffness in joints

Teach patient/family:
• To avoid aspirin, NSAIDs, alcohol, high-purine diet

---

*sulfiSOXAZOLE (℞)
(sul-fi-sox'a-zole)
Gantrisin, Novo-Soxazole ✦,
sulfiSOXAZOLE, Gantrisin
Pediatric
Func. class.: Antiinfective
Chem. class.: Sulfonamide, short
acting

Do not confuse:
sulfiSOXAZOLE/sulfasalazine/
sulfADIAZINE
Action: Inhibits folic acid synthesis
Uses: Urinary tract, systemic infections; chancroid; trachoma; toxoplasmosis; acute otitis media, malaria, *Haemophilus influenzae* meningitis, meningococcal meningitis, nocardiosis, eye infections

DOSAGE AND ROUTES

UTIs, other systemic infections
• *Adult:* PO 2-4 g loading dose, then 1-2 g qid × 7-10 days; max 12 g/day
• *Child >2 mo:* PO 75 mg/kg or 2 g/m² loading dose, then 120-150 mg/kg/day or 4 g/m²/day in divided doses q6h, not to exceed 6 g/day

Chlamydia trachomatis
• *Adult:* PO 500 mg-1 g qid × 3 wk

Renal dose
• *Adult:* PO CCr 10-50 ml/min give q8-12h; CCr <10 ml/min give q12-24h

---

Available forms: Tabs 500 mg; *sulfiSOXAZOLE acetyl*: liquid 500 mg/5 ml

SIDE EFFECTS

CNS: Headache, insomnia, hallucinations, depression, vertigo, fatigue, anxiety, **seizures,** drug fever, chills, drowsiness
CV: **Allergic myocarditis, tachycardia**
GI: Nausea, vomiting, abdominal pain, stomatitis, **hepatitis,** glossitis, pancreatitis, diarrhea, **enterocolitis,** anorexia, **pseudomembranous colitis**
GU: **Renal failure, toxic nephrosis,** increased BUN, creatinine, crystalluria, hematuria, proteinuria, urinary retention
HEMA: **Leukopenia, thrombocytopenia, agranulocytosis, hemolytic anemia, aplastic anemia**
INTEG: Rash, dermatitis, urticaria, **Stevens-Johnson syndrome,** erythema, photosensitivity, alopecia
SYST: **Anaphylaxis**
Contraindications: Hypersensitivity to sulfonamides and sulfonylureas, thiazide and loop diuretics, salicylates; sunscreen with PABA, lactation, infants <2 mo (except congenital toxoplasmosis), pregnancy at term, porphyria, G6PD deficiency
Precautions: Pregnancy (C), lactation, impaired renal/hepatic function, severe allergy, bronchial asthma, geriatric, UV exposure

PHARMACOKINETICS

PO: Rapidly absorbed, peak 2-4 hr, 85% protein bound; half-life 4-7 hr, excreted in urine, crosses placenta

INTERACTIONS

Increase: effects of barbiturates, TOLBUTamide, uricosurics
Increase: crystalluria risk—methenamine
Increase: free-drug concentrations—indomethacin, probenecid, salicylates
Increase: thrombocytopenia—thiazides
Increase: nephrotoxicity—cycloSPORINE
Increase: hypoglycemic response—sulfonylurea agents
Increase: anticoagulant effect—warfarin

⚠ Safety alert   *"Tall Man" lettering

Decrease: renal excretion of methotrexate

Decrease: hepatic clearance of phenytoin

Drug/Herb

• Do not use acidophilus with antiinfectives; separate by several hours

Drug/Lab Test

False positive: Urinary glucose test

NURSING CONSIDERATIONS

Assess:

• I&O ratio; note color, character, pH of urine if drug administered for UTIs; output should be 800 ml less than intake; if urine is highly acidic, alkalization may be needed

• Renal studies: BUN, creatinine, urinalysis (long-term therapy); monitor for crystalluria

⚠ Blood dyscrasias: skin rash, fever, sore throat, bruising, bleeding, fatigue, joint pain, monitor CBC before and periodically

⚠ Allergic reaction: rash, dermatitis, urticaria, pruritus, dyspnea, bronchospasm

Administer:

• On an empty stomach

• With full glass of H_2O to maintain adequate hydration; increase fluids to 2 L/day to decrease crystallization in kidneys

• Medication after C&S; repeat C&S after full course of medication

Perform/provide:

• Storage in tight, light-resistant container at room temperature

Evaluate:

• Therapeutic response: absence of pain, fever, C&S negative

Teach patient/family:

• To take each oral dose with full glass of H_2O to prevent crystalluria

• To complete full course of treatment to prevent superinfection

• To avoid sunlight or use sunscreen to prevent burns; avoid hazardous activities if dizziness occurs

• To avoid OTC medication (aspirin, vit C) unless directed by prescriber

• To notify prescriber of skin rash, sore throat, fever, mouth sores, unusual bruising, bleeding

---

sulindac (R)

(sul-in'dak)

Apo-Sulin ✦, Clinoril, NovoSundac ✦, sulindac

Func. class.: Nonsteroidal antiinflammatory, antirheumatic

Chem. class.: Indeneacetic acid derivative

Do not confuse:

Clinoril/Clozaril/Oruvail

Action: Inhibits prostaglandin synthesis by decreasing an enzyme needed for biosynthesis; analgesic, antiinflammatory, antipyretic

Uses: Mild to moderate pain, osteoarthritis; rheumatoid, gouty arthritis; ankylosing spondylitis, bursitis, juvenile arthritis

DOSAGE AND ROUTES

Arthritis

• *Adult:* **PO** 150 mg bid, may increase to 200 mg bid

• *Child:* **PO** 2-4 mg/kg/day in divided doses, max 6 mg/kg/day or 200 mg bid whichever is less (safe and effective dose not established)

Bursitis/acute arthritis

• *Adult:* **PO** 200 mg bid × 1-2 wk, then reduce dose

Available forms: Tabs 150, 200 mg

SIDE EFFECTS

CNS: Dizziness, drowsiness, fatigue, tremors, confusion, insomnia, anxiety, depression, headache

CV: Tachycardia, peripheral edema, palpitations, dysrhythmias, **MI, stroke**

EENT: Tinnitus, hearing loss, blurred vision

GI: Nausea, anorexia, vomiting, diarrhea, jaundice, **cholestatic hepatitis,**

S

constipation, flatulence, cramps, dry mouth, peptic ulcer, **bleeding, ulceration, perforation**

GU: **Nephrotoxicity: dysuria, hematuria, oliguria, azotemia**

HEMA: **Blood dyscrasias** with prolonged use

INTEG: Purpura, *rash, pruritus,* sweating, photosensitivity

Contraindications: Hypersensitivity, asthma, severe renal/hepatic disease, active ulcers, perioperative pain

Precautions: Pregnancy (C) 1st trimester, lactation, children, bleeding disorders, GI disorders, cardiac disorders, hypersensitivity to other antiinflammatory agents, renal disease

PHARMACOKINETICS

PO: Peak 2 hr; half-life 3-3½ hr; metabolized in liver; excreted in urine (metabolites), breast milk; 93% protein binding

INTERACTIONS

• GI side effects: aspirin, corticosteroids, other NSAIDs

Increase: bleeding risk—anticoagulants, thrombolytics, plicamycin, tirofiban, eptifibatide, clopidogrel, ticlopidine, valproic acid, some cephalosporins

Increase: nephrotoxicity—cycloSPORINE

Increase: toxicity—methotrexate, sulfonamides, sulfonylureas, probenecid

Decrease: sulindac effect—diflunisal, do not use together

Drug/Herb

Increase: gastric irritation—arginine, gossypol

Increase: NSAIDs effect—bearberry, bilberry

Increase: bleeding risk—bogbean, chondroitin

NURSING CONSIDERATIONS

Assess:

⚠ Cardiac status: CV thrombotic events, MI, stroke; may be fatal

⚠ GI status: ulceration, bleeding, perforation; may be fatal

• Pain: frequency, intensity, characteristics, relief after med

⚠ Asthma, aspirin hypersensitivity, nasal polyps; increased hypersensitivity

• Renal, hepatic studies: BUN, creatinine, AST, ALT, Hgb, before treatment, periodically thereafter

• Have B/P checked qmo; drug causes sodium retention

• Audiometric, ophthalmic exam before, during, after treatment

• For eye, ear problems: blurred vision, tinnitus may indicate toxicity

Administer:

• With food to decrease GI symptoms; take on empty stomach to facilitate absorption; tablet may be crushed

• With a full glass of water

Perform/provide:

• Storage at room temperature

Evaluate:

• Therapeutic response: decreased pain, stiffness, swelling in joints, ability to move more easily

Teach patient/family:

• To report blurred vision or ringing, roaring in ears (may indicate toxicity)

• To avoid driving, other hazardous activities if dizzy or drowsy

• To report change in urine pattern, weight increase, edema, pain increase in joints, fever, blood in urine (indicates nephrotoxicity)

• That therapeutic effects may take up to 1 mo

• To avoid alcohol and aspirin

• To take with full glass of water

• To use sunscreen

---

sumatriptan (℞)
(soo-ma-trip′tan)
Imitrex
Func. class.: Antimigraine agent
Chem. class.: 5-HT$_{1P}$ receptor agonist, abortive agent, triptan

---

Action: Binds selectively to the vascular 5-HT$_{1D}$ receptor subtype, exerts antimigraine effect; causes vasoconstriction in cranial arteries

---

⚠ Safety alert *"Tall Man" lettering

Uses: Acute treatment of migraine with or without aura and cluster headache

DOSAGE AND ROUTES

• *Adult:* SUBCUT 6 mg or less; may repeat in 1 hr; not to exceed 12 mg/24 hr; **PO** 25 mg with fluids, if no relief in 2 hr, give another dose, max 200 mg/day; **NASAL** one dose of 5, 10, or 20 mg in one nostril, may repeat in 2 hr, max 40 mg/24 hr; 1 puff each nostril q2h

Hepatic dose

• *Adult:* **PO** 25 mg, if no response after 2 hr, give up to 50 mg

Available forms: Inj 12 mg/ml; tabs 25, 50, 100 mg; nasal spray 5 mg/100 mcl-U; dose spray device 20 mg/100 mcl-U

SIDE EFFECTS

CNS: Tingling, hot sensation, burning, feeling of pressure, tightness, numbness, dizziness, sedation, headache, anxiety, fatigue, cold sensation
CV: Flushing, **MI**
EENT: Throat, mouth, nasal discomfort; vision changes
GI: Abdominal discomfort
INTEG: Inj site reaction, sweating
MS: Weakness, neck stiffness, myalgia
RESP: Chest tightness, pressure

Contraindications: Angina pectoris, history of MI, documented silent ischemia, Prinzmetal's angina, ischemic heart disease, IV use, concurrent ergotamine-containing preparations, uncontrolled hypertension, hypersensitivity, basilar or hemiplegic migraine

Precautions: Pregnancy (C), postmenopausal women, men >40 yr, risk factors for CAD, hypercholesterolemia, obesity, diabetes, impaired renal/hepatic function, lactation, children <18 yr, geriatric

PHARMACOKINETICS

Onset of pain relief 10 min-2 hr, peak 10-20 min, 10%-20% plasma protein binding, metabolized in the liver (metabolite), excreted in urine, feces

INTERACTIONS

• Extended vasospastic effects: ergot, ergot derivatives
Increase: sumatriptan effect—MAOIs, SSRIs

Drug/Herb

• Serotonin syndrome: SAM-e, St. John's wort
Increase: effect—butterbur, feverfew

NURSING CONSIDERATIONS

Assess:

• For migraine: type of pain, aura, alleviating, aggravating factors, sensitivity to light, noise
• B/P; signs/symptoms of coronary vasospasms
• Tingling, hot sensation, burning, feeling of pressure, numbness, flushing, inj site reaction
• For stress level, activity, recreation, coping mechanisms
• Neurologic status: LOC, blurring vision, nausea, vomiting, tingling in extremities preceding headache
• Ingestion of tyramine foods (pickled products, beer, wine, aged cheese), food additives, preservatives, colorings, artificial sweeteners, chocolate, caffeine, which may precipitate these types of headaches
• Renal function, urinary output

Administer:

• Swallow tabs whole; do not break, crush, or chew
• SUBCUT only just below the skin; avoid IM or IV administration; use only for actual migraine attack
• Take tabs with fluids as soon as symptoms appear; may take a second dose >4 hr; max 200 mg/24 hr

Perform/provide:

• Quiet, calm environment with decreased stimulation for noise, bright light, excessive talking

Evaluate:

• Therapeutic response: decrease in frequency, severity of migraine

S

Teach patient/family:
• To report chest pain, tightness; sudden, severe abdominal pain to prescriber immediately
• To use contraception while taking drug
• To use nasal spray: one spray in one nostril, may repeat if headache returns, do not repeat if pain continues after 1st dose
• To have dark, quiet environment
• That product does not reduce number of migraines

---

sunitinib (℞)
(soo-nit′-in-ib)
Sutent
Func. class.: Antineoplastic—miscellaneous
Chem. class.: Protein-tyrosine kinase inhibitor

Action: Inhibits multiple receptor tyrosine kinases (RTKs), some are responsible for tumor growth
Uses: Gastrointesitnal stromal tumors (GIST) after disease progression or intolerance to imatinib; advanced renal carcinoma

DOSAGE AND ROUTES
• *Adult:* **PO** 50 mg daily × 4 wk, then 2 wk off; may increase or decrease dose by 12.5 mg; if administered with CYP3A4 inducers, give 87.5 mg daily; if given with CYP3A4 inhibitors give 37.5 mg daily
Available forms: Caps 12.5, 25, 50 mg

SIDE EFFECTS
CNS: **CNS hemorrhage**, headache, dizziness, insomnia, **seizures**, fatigue
CV: Hypertension, **left ventricular dysfunction**
GI: **Nausea, hepatotoxicity, vomiting, dyspepsia**, *anorexia, abdominal pain*, altered taste, constipation, stomatitis, mucositis, **pancreatitis**
HEMA: **Neutropenia, thrombocytopenia**
INTEG: **Rash,** skin discoloration, depigmentation of hair or skin, alopecia

MS: Pain, arthralgia, myalgia
RESP: Cough, dyspnea
SYST: **Bleeding,** electrolyte abnormalities
Contraindications: Pregnancy (D), lactation, hypersensitivity
Precautions: Children, geriatric, active infections

PHARMACOKINETICS
Protein binding 95%; metabolized by CYP3A4; excreted in feces, small amount in urine; peak plasma levels 6-12 hr; terminal half-life 40-60 hr (sunitnib); active metabolite 80-110 hr

INTERACTIONS
Increase: hepatotoxicity—acetaminophen
Increase: sunitinib concentrations—ketoconazole, itraconazole, erythromycin, clarithromycin
Increase: plasma concentrations of simvastatin, calcium channel blockers
Increase: plasma concentration of warfarin; avoid use with warfarin, use low-molecular-weight anticoagulants instead
Decrease: sunitinib concentrations—dexamethasone, phenytoin, carbamazepine, rifampin, phenobarbital
Drug/Herb
Decrease: sunitinib concentration—St. John's wort
Drug/Food
Increase: plasma concentrations—grapefruit juice

NURSING CONSIDERATIONS
Assess:
• ANC and platelets; if ANC $<1 \times 10^9$/L and/or platelets $<50 \times 10^9$/L, stop until ANC $>1.5 \times 10^9$/L and platelets $>75 \times 10^9$/L ; if ANC $<0.5 \times 10^9$/L and/or platelets $<10 \times 10^9$/L, reduce dose by 200 mg, if cytopenia continues, reduce dose by another 100 mg; if cytopenia continues for 4 wk, stop drug until ANC $\geq1 \times 10^9$/L
• CV status: hypertension, QT prolongation can occur; monitor left ventricular

---

ejection fraction (LVEF) baseline periodically

• For renal toxicity: if bilirubin >3 × IULN, withhold sunitinib until bilirubin levels return to <1.5 × IULN

• For hepatotoxicity: monitor LFTs, before treatment and qmo; if liver transaminases >5 × IULN, withhold sunitinib until transaminase levels return to <2.5 × IULN

• CBC, differential, platelet count weekly; withhold drug if WBC is <3500/mm³, or platelet count <100,000/mm³; notify prescriber of these results; drug should be discontinued

• For CHF: adrenal insufficiency in those experiencing trauma

• For bleeding: epistaxis rectal, gingival, upper GI, genital and wound bleeding; tumor-related hemorrhage may occur rapidly

Administer:

• With meal and large glass of water to decrease GI symptoms

Perform/provide:

• Nutritious diet with iron, vitamin supplement, low fiber, few dairy products

• Storage at 25°C (77°F)

Evaluate:

• Therapeutic response: decrease in size of tumor

Teach patient/family:

• To report adverse reactions immediately: SOB, bleeding

• Reason for treatment, expected result

• That many adverse reactions may occur: high B/P, bleeding, mouth swelling, taste change, skin discoloration, depigmentation of hair/skin

• Avoid persons with known upper respiratory infections; immunosuppression is common

---

suprofen ophthalmic
See Appendix C

---

tacrine (R)
(tack′rin)
Cognex
Func. class.: Anti-Alzheimer agent
Chem. class.: Reversible cholinesterase inhibitor

Do not confuse:
Cognex/Corgard

Action: Elevates acetylcholine concentrations (cerebral cortex) by slowing degradation of acetylcholine released in cholinergic neurons; does not alter underlying dementia

Uses: Treatment of mild to moderate dementia in Alzheimer's disease

DOSAGE AND ROUTES

• *Adult:* **PO** 10 mg qid × 4 wk, then 20 mg qid × 4 wk, increase at 4-wk intervals if patient tolerating drug well and if transaminase is WNL, then titrate to higher doses (30-40 mg qid) at 4-wk intervals

Available forms: Caps 10, 20, 30, 40 mg

SIDE EFFECTS

CNS: Dizziness, confusion, insomnia, tremor, *ataxia, somnolence, anxiety, agitation, depression, hallucinations, hostility, abnormal thinking,* chills, fever, headache, **seizures**

CV: Hypotension or hypertension, **bradycardia, heart block**

GI: Nausea, vomiting, anorexia, abdominal pain, constipation, dyspepsia, flatulence, **hepatotoxicity, GI bleeding,** diarrhea

GU: Urinary frequency, UTI, incontinence

INTEG: Rash, flushing

OTHER: Myalgia

RESP: Rhinitis, URI, cough, pharyngitis

Contraindications: Hypersensitivity to this drug or acridine derivatives, patients treated with this drug who developed jaundice with a total bilirubin of >3 mg/dl

Precautions: Pregnancy (C), sick sinus syndrome, history of ulcers, GI bleed-

T

Side effects: *italics* = common; **bold** = life-threatening

ing, hepatic disease, bladder obstruction, asthma, lactation, children, seizure disorders, history of bradyarrhythmias

PHARMACOKINETICS

Rapidly absorbed PO, 55% bound to plasma proteins, extensively metabolized to metabolites by CYP450 enzyme system, elimination half-life 2-4 hr

INTERACTIONS

• Synergistic effect: succinylcholine, cholinesterase inhibitors, cholinergic agonists
• Smoking may decrease drug level
Increase: bleeding risk—NSAIDs
Increase: tacrine levels—cimetidine, ciprofloxacin, fluvoxamine, ritonavir
Increase: elimination half-life of theophylline
Decrease: activity of anticholinergics
Drug/Food:
• May delay absorption, give 1 hr before meals

NURSING CONSIDERATIONS

Assess:
• B/P: hypotension, hypertension
• Mental status: affect, mood, behavioral changes, depression; complete suicide assessment; hallucinations, confusion
• GI status: nausea, vomiting, anorexia, constipation, abdominal pain; add bulk, increase fluids for constipation
• GU status: urinary frequency, incontinence
• Jaundice confirmed by significant increase bilirubin (>3 mg/dl) and/or those with hypersensitivity (rash/fever) with increased ALT, should be immediately, permanently discontinued
• Serum ALT every other week, × 4-16 wk, then q3mo
Administer:
• Between meals; may be given with meals for GI symptoms
• Dosage adjusted to response no more than q4wk

Perform/provide:
• Assistance with ambulation during beginning therapy; dizziness, ataxia may occur
Evaluate:
• Therapeutic response: decrease in confusion, improved mood
Teach patient/family:
• To report side effects; severe nausea, vomiting, sweating, salivation, bradycardia, hypotension, collapse, seizures; indicates overdose
• To use drug exactly as prescribed: at regular intervals, preferably between meals; may be taken with meals for GI upset; drug is not a cure
• To notify prescriber of nausea, vomiting, diarrhea (dose increase or beginning treatment), or rash; very dark or very light stools, jaundice (delayed onset)
• Not to increase or abruptly decrease dose; serious consequences may result
Treatment of overdose: Withdraw drug, administer tertiary anticholinergics, provide supportive care

tacrolimus (Rx)
(tak-roe-li′mus)
Prograf
tacrolimus topical
Protopic
Func. class.: Immunosuppressant
Chem. class.: Macrolide

Action: Produces immunosuppression by inhibiting T-lymphocytes
Uses: Organ transplants to prevent rejection; topical: atopic dermatitis
Unlabeled uses: Autoimmune diseases, severe recalcitrant psoriasis

DOSAGE AND ROUTES

• *Adult and child:* IV 0.03-0.05 mg/kg/day × 3 days then PO 0.15 mg/kg bid; adjust dose in renal impairment
• *Adult:* TOP use 0.03% or 0.1% ointment; apply bid × 7 days
• *Child ≥2-15 yr:* TOP use 0.03% ointment; apply bid × 7 days

Available forms: Inj 5 mg/ml; caps 0.5, 1, 5 mg; ointment 0.03%, 0.1%

SIDE EFFECTS

CNS: Tremors, headache, insomnia, paresthesia, chills, fever, **seizures**
CV: Hypertension, myocardial hypertrophy
EENT: Blurred vision, photophobia
GI: Nausea, vomiting, diarrhea, constipation, **GI bleeding**
GU: UTIs, **albuminuria, hematuria, proteinuria, renal failure**
HEMA: **Anemia, leukocytosis, thrombocytopenia, purpura**
INTEG: Rash, flushing, itching, alopecia
META: Hirsutism, hyperglycemia, hyperkalemia, hyperuricemia, hypokalemia, hypomagnesemia
MS: Back pain, muscle spasms
RESP: **Pleural effusion, atelectasis,** dyspnea
SYST: **Anaphylaxis**
Contraindications: Hypersensitivity to this drug or to some kinds of castor oil; long-term use (TOP); child <2 yr (TOP)
Precautions: Pregnancy (C), severe renal, hepatic disease; diabetes mellitus, hyperkalemia, hyperuricemia, lymphomas, lactation, children <12, hypertension

PHARMACOKINETICS

PO: Extensively metabolized, half-life 10 hr, 75% protein binding

INTERACTIONS

Increase: toxicity—aminoglycosides, cisplatin, cycloSPORINE
Increase: blood levels—antifungals, calcium channel blockers, cimetidine, danazol, erythromycin, mycophenolate, mofetil
Decrease: blood levels—carbamazepine, phenobarbital, phenytoin, rifamycin
Decrease: effect of vaccines
Drug/Herb
Decrease: immunosuppression—astragalus, echinacea, melatonin
Decrease: effect—ginseng, maitake, mistletoe

NURSING CONSIDERATIONS
Assess:
• Blood studies: Hgb, WBC, platelets during treatment qmo; if leukocytes <3000/mm^3 or platelets <100,000/mm^3, drug should be discontinued or reduced; decreased hemoglobulin level may indicate bone marrow suppression
• Hepatic studies: alk phos, AST, ALT, amylase, bilirubin, and for hepatotoxicity: dark urine, jaundice, itching, light-colored stools; drug should be discontinued
Administer:
⚠ Anaphylaxis: rash, pruritus, wheezing, laryngeal edema; stop infusion, initiate emergency procedures
PO/IV route
• All medications PO if possible, avoiding IM inj; bleeding may occur
• With meals to reduce GI upset; nausea is common
• For several days before transplant surgery, patients should be placed in protective isolation
Topical route
• Do not use occlusive dressings
IV route
• After diluting in 0.9% NaCl or D$_5$W to 0.004 to 0.02 mg/ml as a continuous infusion
Additive compatibilities: Cimetidine
Y-site compatibilities: Acyclovir, aminophylline, amphotericin B, ampicillin, ampicillin/sulbactam, benztropine, calcium gluconate, cefazolin, cefotetan, ceftazidime, ceftriaxone, cefuroxime, chloramphenicol, cimetidine, ciprofloxacin, clindamycin, dexamethasone, digoxin, diphenhydrAMINE, DOBUTamine, DOPamine, doxycycline, erythromycin, esmolol, fluconazole, furosemide, ganciclovir, gentamicin, haloperidol, heparin, hydrocortisone, imipenem/cilastatin, insulin (regular), isoproterenol, leucovorin, lorazepam, methylPREDNISolone, metoclopramide, metronidazole, mezlocillin, multivitamins, nitroglycerin, oxacillin, penicillin G potassium, perphenazine, phenytoin, piperacillin, potassium chlo-

ride, propranolol, ranitidine, sodium bicarbonate, sodium nitroprusside, trimethoprim-sulfamethoxazole, vancomycin

Evaluate:

• Therapeutic response: absence of graft rejection; immunosuppression in autoimmune disorders

Teach patient/family:

PO route

• To report fever, rash, severe diarrhea, chills, sore throat, fatigue; serious infections may occur; clay-colored stools, cramping (hepatotoxicity)

• To avoid crowds, persons with known infections to reduce risk of infection

• To avoid exposure to natural or artificial sunlight

• Not to breastfeed while taking this medication

• That repeated lab tests will be needed during treatment

---

tadalafil (℞)

(tah-dal′a-fil)

Cialis

Func. class.: Impotence agent

Chem. class.: Phosphodiesterase type 5 inhibitor

Action: Inhibits phosphodiesterase type 5 (PDE5); enhances erectile function by increasing the amount of cGMP, which causes smooth muscle relaxation and increased blood flow into the corpus cavernosum; improves erectile function for up to 36 hr

Uses: Treatment of erectile dysfunction

DOSAGE AND ROUTES

• *Adult:* PO 10 mg, taken prior to sexual activity, dose may be reduced to 5 mg or increased to a max of 20 mg; usual max dosing frequency is once per day

Renal dose

• *Adult:* PO CCr 31-50 ml/min, 5 mg/ daily, max 10 mg q 48 hr; CCr <30 ml/ min, max 5 mg

Hepatic dose

• *Adult:* PO (Child-Pugh class A, B) max 10 mg daily; (Child-Pugh class C) not recommended

Concomitant medications

• Ketoconazole, itraconazole, ritonavir, max 10 mg q72h

Available forms: Tabs 5, 10, 20 mg

SIDE EFFECTS

CNS: Headache, flushing, dizziness

CV: **MI, sudden death, CV collapse,** hypertension, hypotension, tachycardia

MISC: Back pain/myalgia, *dyspepsia, nasal congestion, UTI,* blurred vision, changes in color vision, *diarrhea,* pruritus, priapism, **NAION (nonarteritic ischemic optic neuropathy),** flushing

Contraindications: Hypersensitivity, patients taking organic nitrates either regularly and/or intermittently, patients taking any α-adrenergic antagonist other than 0.4 mg once daily tamsulosin; newborns, children, women

Precautions: Anatomical penile deformities, sickle cell anemia, leukemia, multiple myeloma renal/hepatic/CV disease, bleeding disorders, active peptic ulcer, prolonged erection

PHARMACOKINETICS

Rapidly absorbed; metabolized by liver; terminal half-life 17.5 hr, peak ½-6 hr; excreted primarily as metabolites in feces, urine; plasma concentration 61% in feces, 36% in urine; 94% protein bound; rate and extent of absorption of tadalafil are not influenced by food

INTERACTIONS

⚠ Do not use with nitrates because of unsafe drop in B/P, which could result in MI or stroke

Increase: tadalafil levels—itraconazole, ketoconazole, ritonavir (although not studied, may also include other HIV protease inhibitors)

Decrease: B/P—alcohol, α-blockers,

---

amlodipine, angiotensin II receptor blockers, enalapril
Decrease: effects of tadalafil—bosentan, antacids

NURSING CONSIDERATIONS
Assess:
- Use of organic nitrates that should not be used with this drug
- For any severe loss of vision, while taking this or any similar products

Administer:
- Give prior to sexual activity; do not use more than once a day
- That drug should not be used with nitrates in any form

Teach patient/family:
- That drug does not protect against sexually transmitted diseases, including HIV
- To tell physician if patient has a bleeding problem
- That drug has no effect in the absence of sexual stimulation
- To seek medical help if an erection lasts more than 4 hours
- To tell physician of all medicines, vitamins, and herbs patient is taking, especially ritonavir, indinavir, ketoconozole, itraconazole, erythromycin, nitrates, α-blockers
- That tadalafil is contraindicated for use with α-blockers except 0.4 mg/daily tamsulosin
- To notify prescriber immediately, and stop taking product if vision loss occurs

---

tamoxifen (R)
(ta-mox'i-fen)
Alpha-Tamoxifen ✤, Med Tamoxifen ✤, Nolvadex, Nolvadex-D ✤, Novo-Tamoxifen ✤, Tamofen ✤, Tamone ✤, Tamoplex ✤
Func. class.: Antineoplastic
Chem. class.: Antiestrogen hormone

Action: Inhibits cell division by binding to cytoplasmic estrogen receptors; resembles normal cell complex but inhibits DNA synthesis and estrogen response of target tissue

Uses: Advanced breast carcinoma not responsive to other therapy in estrogen-receptor-positive patients (usually postmenopausal), prevention of breast cancer, following breast surgery/radiation in ductal carcinoma in situ

Unlabeled uses: Mastalgia, to reduce pain/size of gynecomastia, ovulation stimulation, malignant carcinoid tumor, carcinoid syndrome, metastatic melanoma, desmoid tumors, McCune-Albright syndrome (female pediatric patients)

DOSAGE AND ROUTES
Breast cancer
- *Adult:* **PO** 20-40 mg daily; doses >20 mg/day, divide AM/PM
High risk for breast cancer
- *Adult:* **PO** 20 mg daily × 5 yr
DCIS
- *Adult:* **PO** 20 mg daily × 5 yr
McCune-Albright syndrome (unlabeled)
- *Child 2-10 yr (girls):* **PO** 20 mg daily for up to 1 yr
Available forms: Tabs 10, 20 mg; oral sol 10 mg/5 ml

SIDE EFFECTS
CNS: Hot flashes, headache, lightheadedness, depression
CV: Chest pain, **stroke**
EENT: Ocular lesions, retinopathy, corneal opacity, blurred vision (high doses)
GI: Nausea, vomiting, altered taste (anorexia)
GU: Vaginal bleeding, pruritus vulvae, **uterine malignancies**
HEMA: **Thrombocytopenia, leukopenia,** DVT, PE
INTEG: Rash, alopecia
META: Hypercalcemia
RESP: **Pulmonary embolism**
Contraindications: Pregnancy (D), hypersensitivity, lactation
Precautions: Leukopenia, thrombocytopenia, cataracts, women of childbearing age

PHARMACOKINETICS

PO: Peak 4-7 hr, half-life 7 days (1 wk terminal), excreted primarily in feces

INTERACTIONS

Increase: bleeding—anticoagulants
Increase: tamoxifen levels—bromocriptine
Increase: thromboembolic events—cytotoxics
Decrease: tamoxifen levels—aminoglutethimide, medroxyprogesterone, rifamycin
Decrease: letrozole levels—letrozole
Drug/Lab Test
Increase: serum calcium, T_4, AST, ALT, cholesterol, triglycerides

NURSING CONSIDERATIONS

Assess:
• CBC, differential, platelet count qwk; withhold drug if WBC is <3500 or platelet count is <100,000; notify prescriber
• Bleeding q8h: hematuria, guaiac, bruising, petechiae, mucosa or orifices
• Effects of alopecia on body image; discuss feelings about body changes
🅰 For uterine malignancies, symptoms of stroke, pulmonary embolism that may occur in women with ductal carcinoma in situ (DCIS) and women at high risk for breast cancer
🅰 Symptoms indicating severe allergic reactions: rash, pruritus, urticaria, purpuric skin lesions, itching, flushing
• For bone pain; may give analgesics; pain is usually transient
Administer:
• Do not break, crush, or chew tabs
• Antacid before oral agent; give drug after evening meal, before bedtime; give with food or fluids for GI symptoms
• Antiemetic 30-60 min before giving drug to prevent vomiting
Perform/provide:
• Liquid diet, if needed, including cola, Jell-O; dry toast or crackers may be added if patient is not nauseated or vomiting
• Increase fluid intake to 2-3 L/day to prevent dehydration

• Nutritious diet with iron, vitamin supplements as ordered
• Storage in light-resistant container at room temperature
Evaluate:
• Therapeutic response: decreased tumor size, spread of malignancy
Teach patient/family:
• To report any complaints, side effects to prescriber
• To increase fluids to 2 L/day unless contraindicated
• To wear sunscreen, protective clothing, sunglasses
• That vaginal bleeding, pruritus, hot flashes are reversible after discontinuing treatment
• To report immediately decreased visual acuity, which may be irreversible; stress need for routine eye exams; care providers should be told about tamoxifen therapy
• To report vaginal bleeding immediately
• That tumor flare—increase in size of tumor, increased bone pain—may occur and will subside rapidly; may take analgesics for pain
• That premenopausal women must use mechanical birth control because ovulation may be induced
• That hair may be lost during treatment; a wig or hairpiece may make patient feel better; new hair may be different in color, texture

---

tamsulosin (℞)

(tam-sue-lo′sen)

Flomax

Func. class.: Selective α_1-peripheral adrenergic blocker
Chem. class.: Sulfamoylphenethylamine derivative

Do not confuse:
Flomax/Fosamax/Volmax
Action: Binds preferentially to α_{1A}-adrenoceptor subtype located mainly in the prostate
Uses: Symptoms of benign prostatic hyperplasia (BPH)

DOSAGE AND ROUTES
• *Adult:* **PO** 0.4 mg daily, increasing up to 0.8 mg daily if required
Available forms: Caps 0.4 mg

SIDE EFFECTS
CNS: Dizziness, headache, asthenia, insomnia
CV: Chest pain
EENT: Amblyopia, floppy iris syndrome
GI: Nausea, diarrhea, dysgeusia
GU: Decreased libido, abnormal ejaculation
MS: Back pain
RESP: Rhinitis, pharyngitis, cough
Contraindications: Hypersensitivity
Precautions: Pregnancy (B), children, lactation, hepatic disease, coronary artery disease, severe renal disease

PHARMACOKINETICS
PO: Unknown, peak 4-5 hr, duration 9-15 hr; half-life 14 hr; metabolized in liver; excreted via urine; extensively protein bound (98%)

INTERACTIONS
• Not to be taken with: prazosin, terazosin, doxazosin, β-blockers, vardenafil
Increase: toxicity—cimetidine
Drug/Food
Decrease: absorption with food

NURSING CONSIDERATIONS
Assess:
• Prostatic hyperplasia: change in urinary patterns, baseline and throughout treatment
• CBC with diff and LFTs; B/P and heart rate
• BUN, uric acid, urodynamic studies (urinary flow rates, residual volume)
• I&O ratios, weight daily, edema, report weight gain or edema
Administer:
• Swallow caps whole; do not break, crush, or chew
• Give ½ hr after same meal each day

Perform/provide:
• Storage in tight container in cool environment
Evaluate:
• Therapeutic response: decreased symptoms of benign prostatic hyperplasia
Teach patient/family:
• Not to drive or operate machinery for 4 hr after first dose or after dosage increase

---
telbivudine (℞)
(tel-bi′vyoo-deen)
Tyzeka
Func. class.: Antiretroviral
Chem. class.: Nucleoside reverse transcriptase inhibitor (NRTI)

Action: Inhibits replication of HBV DNA polymerase, which inhibits HBV replication
Uses: Hepatitis B

DOSAGE AND ROUTES
• *Adult and adolescent >16 yr:* **PO** 600 mg daily; max 600 mg daily
Available forms: Tabs 600 mg

SIDE EFFECTS
CNS: Fever, headache, malaise, weakness, *dizziness, insomnia*
EENT: Taste change, hearing loss, photophobia
GI: Nausea, vomiting, diarrhea, anorexia, abdominal pain, hepatomegaly
INTEG: Rash
MISC: Lactic acidosis
MS: Myalgia, arthralgia, muscle cramps
RESP: Cough
Contraindications: Hypersensitivity, lactation
Precautions: Pregnancy (B), lactation, children, severe renal disease, impaired hepatic function, anemia, organ transplant, dialysis, HIV, lactic acidosis, obesity, alcoholism

PHARMACOKINETICS

Excreted by kidneys (unchanged), steady state 5-7 days, protein binding 3.3%, terminal half-life 40-49 hr

INTERACTIONS

• Altered telbivudine levels: any agent altering renal function

Increase: myopathy risk—HMG-CoA reductase inhibitors, fibric acid derivatives, penicillamine, zidovudine, ZDV, cyclo-SPORINE, erythromycin, niacin, azole antifungals, corticosteroids, hydrochloroquine

NURSING CONSIDERATIONS

Assess:

• Liver function tests, hepatitis B serology, creatine kinase, periodically

Administer:

• With or without food with a full glass of water

Perform/provide:

• Storage at room temperature

Evaluate:

• Therapeutic response: decreasing hepatitis B serology

Teach patient/family:

• That GI complaints and insomnia may resolve after 3-4 wk of treatment

• That drug does not cure hepatitis B and does not stop the spread to others

• That follow-up visits must be continued

• That serious drug interactions may occur if OTC products are ingested; check with prescriber before taking

• That drug may cause dizziness; avoid hazardous activities until response is known

• To report symptoms of cough, difficulty sleeping, or excessive headache

telithromycin (Ŗ)
(teh-lih-throw-my'sin)
Ketek
Func. class.: Antiinfective
Chem. class.: Ketolides

Action: Binds to 50S ribosomal subunits of susceptible bacteria and suppresses protein synthesis

Uses: Acute bacterial exacerbation of chronic bronchitis caused by *Streptococcus pneumoniae, Haemophilus influenzae, Moraxella catarrhalis*; acute bacterial sinusitis caused by *S. pneumoniae, H. influenzae, M. catarrhalis, Staphylococcus aureus*, community-acquired pneumonia

Unlabeled uses: Acute tonsillitis/pharyngitis

DOSAGE AND ROUTES

Acute bacterial exacerbation of bronchitis

• *Adult:* **PO** 800 mg daily × 5 days

Acute bacterial sinusitis

• *Adult:* **PO** 800 mg daily × 5 days

Community-acquired pneumonia

• *Adult:* **PO** 800 mg daily × 7-10 days

Available forms: Tabs 300, 400 mg

SIDE EFFECTS

CNS: Dizziness, headache, insomnia, increased sweating

EENT: Blurred vision, diplopia, difficulty focusing

GI: Nausea, vomiting, diarrhea, hepatitis, abdominal pain/distention, stomatitis, anorexia, **pseudomembranous colitis, pancreatitis**

GU: Vaginitis, moniliasis

INTEG: Rash, urticaria

MISC: **Atrial dysrhythmias, QT prolongation,** blurred vision

MS: Muscle cramps

SYST: **Anaphylaxis, superinfection**

Contraindications: Hypersensitivity to this product or macrolide antibiotics, myasthenia gravis

Precautions: Pregnancy (C), lactation,

---

children, geriatric, ongoing prodysrhythmias, hepatic/GI disease, QT prolongation

PHARMACOKINETICS

Peak 1 hr; metabolized in liver (CYP450 enzyme system); excreted in bile, feces; protein binding 60%-70%

INTERACTIONS

⚠ Increase: serious dysrhythmias—pimozide, antidysrhythmics (amiodarone, bretylium, disopyramide, dofetilide, procainamide, quinidine, sotalol); do not use together

Increase: action of atorvastatin, digoxin, ergots, lovastatin, metoprolol, midazolam, simvastatin, theophylline, carbamazepine, cycloSPORINE, tacrolimus, sirolimus, phenobarbital, phenytoin

Increase: telithromycin—itraconazole, ketoconazole

Increase: QT interval—antidysrhythmics (class IA, III); do not use together

Increase: cardiotoxicity—verapamil

Decrease: action of telithromycin—rifampin, phenytoin, carbamazepine, phenobarbital

Decrease: action of sotalol

Drug/Herb
• Do not use acidophilus with antiinfectives; separate by several hours

Drug/Lab Test

Increase: AST/ALT

NURSING CONSIDERATIONS

Assess:
• For infection: temp, sputum, WBCs, baseline and periodically

⚠ Cardiac status: ECG for QT prolongation

⚠ GI status: increasing diarrhea, pseudomembranous colitis may occur

⚠ Anaphylaxis: itching, skin rash, inability to breathe; have emergency equipment available

• Oliguria in renal disease

• Hepatic studies: AST, ALT, if patient is on long-term therapy

• C&S before drug therapy; drug may be given as soon as culture is taken; C&S may be repeated after treatment

Administer:
• May take without regard to food
• Do not use this drug if using class IA or III antidysrhythmics

Perform/provide:
• Storage at room temperature
• Adequate intake of fluids (2 L) during diarrhea episodes

Evaluate:
• Therapeutic response: decreased symptoms of infection

Teach patient/family:
• To report sore throat, fever, fatigue (could indicate superinfection)
• To notify nurse of diarrhea stools, dark urine, pale stools, jaundice of eyes or skin, and severe abdominal pain
• To report blurred vision, if interfering with daily activities
• To inform prescriber of all medications, herbs taking
• To avoid driving, hazardous activities if blurred vision occurs
• To take as prescribed, do not double or skip doses
• To report fainting; not to take if using class IA, III antidysrhythmics, simvastatin, lovastatin, or atorvastatin
• May take without regard to meals

Treatment of hypersensitivity:
• Withdraw drug; maintain airway; administer epINEPHrine, aminophylline, O_2, IV corticosteroids

---

telmisartan (℞)

(tel-mih-sar′tan)
Micardis
Func. class.: Antihypertensive
Chem. class.: Angiotensin II receptor (Type AT_1)

T

Action: Blocks the vasoconstrictor and aldosterone-secreting effects of angiotensin II; selectively blocks the binding of angiotensin II to the AT_1 receptor found in tissues

Uses: Hypertension, alone or in combination

Unlabeled uses: Heart failure

Side effects: *italics* = common; **bold** = life-threatening

DOSAGE AND ROUTES

• *Adult:* **PO** 40 mg daily; range 20-80 mg

Available forms: Tabs 20, 40, 80 mg

SIDE EFFECTS

CNS: Dizziness, insomnia, *anxiety,* headache, fatigue

GI: Diarrhea, dyspepsia, *anorexia, vomiting*

MS: Myalgia, pain

RESP: Cough, *upper respiratory infection,* sinusitis, pharyngitis

Contraindications: Pregnancy (D) 2nd/3rd trimesters, hypersensitivity

Precautions: Pregnancy (C) 1st trimester, hypersensitivity to ACE inhibitors; lactation, children, geriatric, renal/hepatic disease, renal artery stenosis, dialysis, CHF

PHARMACOKINETICS

Onset 3 hr, peak 0.5-1 hr, extensively metabolized, terminal half-life 24 hr, protein binding 99.5%, excreted in feces >97%

INTERACTIONS

Increase: digoxin peak/trough concentrations—digoxin

Increase: antihypertensive action—diuretics, other antihypertensives

Increase: hyperkalemia—potassium-sparing diuretics, potassium salt substitutes

Decrease: antihypertensive effect—NSAIDs, salicylates

Drug/Herb

Increase: toxicity, death—aconite

Increase: antihypertensive effect—barberry, betony, black catechu, black cohosh, bloodroot, broom, burdock, cat's claw, dandelion, goldenseal, hawthorn, Irish moss, Jamaican dogwood, kelp, khella, mistletoe, parsley

Increase or decrease: antihypertensive effect—astragalus, cola tree

Decrease: antihypertensive effect—coltsfoot, guarana, khat, licorice, yohimbine

NURSING CONSIDERATIONS

Assess:

• B/P, pulse q4h; note rate, rhythm, quality

• Electrolytes: K, Na, Cl

• Baselines in renal, hepatic studies before therapy begins

• Edema in feet, legs daily

• Skin turgor, dryness of mucous membranes for hydration status

Administer:

• Without regard to meals

• Increased dose to African-American patients; B/P response may be reduced

Evaluate:

• Therapeutic response: decreased B/P

Teach patient/family:

• To comply with dosage schedule, even if feeling better

• To notify prescriber of mouth sores, fever, swelling of hands or feet, irregular heartbeat, chest pain

• That excessive perspiration, dehydration, vomiting, diarrhea may lead to fall in blood pressure; consult prescriber if these occur

• That drug may cause dizziness, fainting; light-headedness may occur

• To use contraception while taking this drug

• To notify prescriber of all prescriptions, OTC, and supplements taken

temazepam (℞)

(te-maz′e-pam)

Razepam, Restoril, temazepam

Func. class.: Sedative-hypnotic

Chem. class.: Benzodiazepine

Controlled Substance Schedule IV (USA), Schedule F (Canada)

Action: Produces CNS depression at limbic, thalamic, hypothalamic levels of the CNS; may be mediated by neurotransmitter γ-aminobutyric acid (GABA); results are sedation, hypnosis, skeletal muscle relaxation, anticonvulsant activity, anxiolytic action

Uses: Insomnia

DOSAGE AND ROUTES
- *Adult:* **PO** 15-30 mg at bedtime
- *Geriatric:* **PO** 7.5 mg at bedtime

Available forms: Caps 7.5, 15, 30 mg

SIDE EFFECTS
CNS: Lethargy, drowsiness, daytime sedation, dizziness, confusion, lightheadedness, headache, anxiety, irritability, complex sleep related reactions: sleep driving, sleep eating
CV: Chest pain, pulse changes
GI: Nausea, vomiting, diarrhea, heartburn, abdominal pain, constipation, anorexia
HEMA: **Leukopenia, granulocytopenia (rare)**
SYST: **Severe allergic reactions**

Contraindications: Pregnancy (X), hypersensitivity to benzodiazepines, lactation, intermittent porphyria

Precautions: Anemia, renal/hepatic disease, suicidal individuals, drug abuse, geriatric, psychosis, children <15 yr, acute narrow-angle glaucoma, seizure disorders

PHARMACOKINETICS
PO: Onset 30-45 min, duration 6-8 hr, half-life 10-20 hr; metabolized by liver, excreted by kidneys, crosses placenta, excreted in breast milk

INTERACTIONS
Increase: effects of cimetidine, disulfiram, oral contraceptives
Increase: action of both drugs—alcohol, CNS depressants
Decrease: effect of antacids, theophylline, rifampin
Drug/Herb
Increase: CNS depression—catnip, chamomile, clary, cowslip, hops, kava, lavender, mistletoe, nettle, pokeweed, poppy, Queen Anne's lace, senega, skullcap, valerian
Increase: hypotension—black cohosh
Drug/Lab Test
Increase: ALT, AST, serum bilirubin

Decrease: RAI uptake
False increase: Urinary 17-OHCS

NURSING CONSIDERATIONS
Assess:
- Blood studies: Hct, Hgb, RBCs (long-term therapy)
- Hepatic studies: AST, ALT, bilirubin (long-term therapy)
- Mental status: mood, sensorium, affect, memory (long, short)
- ⚠ Blood dyscrasias: fever, sore throat, bruising, rash, jaundice, epistaxis (rare)
- Type of sleep problem: falling asleep, staying asleep
Administer:
- After removal of cigarettes to prevent fires
- After trying conservative measures for insomnia
- ½-1 hr before bedtime for sleeplessness
- On empty stomach for fast onset, but may be taken with food if GI symptoms occur
- Avoid use with CNS depressants; serious CNS depression may result
Perform/provide:
- Assistance with ambulation after receiving dose
- Safety measures: night-light, call bell within easy reach
- Checking to see if PO medication has been swallowed
- Storage in tight container in cool environment
Evaluate:
- Therapeutic response: ability to sleep at night, decreased early morning awakening if taking drug for insomnia
Teach patient/family:
- To avoid driving, other activities requiring alertness until stabilized
- To avoid alcohol ingestion
- That effects may take 2 nights for benefits to be noticed
- Alternative measures to improve sleep: reading, exercise several hours before bedtime, warm bath, warm milk, TV, self-hypnosis, deep breathing
- That hangover, memory impairment are

common in geriatric but less common than with barbiturates

• To use contraception while taking this product

Treatment of overdose: Lavage, activated charcoal; monitor electrolytes, VS

---

temozolomide (Ⓡ)
(tem-oh-zole'oh-mide)
Temodar
Func. class.: Antineoplastic-alkylating agent
Chem. class.: Imidazotetrazine derivative

Action: A prodrug that undergoes conversion to MTIC; MTIC action prevents DNA transcription
Uses: Anaplastic astrocytoma with relapse, glioblastoma multiforme
Unlabeled uses: Metastatic melanoma

DOSAGE AND ROUTES

Anaplastic astrocytoma
• *Adult:* **PO** Adjust dose based on nadir neutrophil and platelet counts 150 mg/m^2/day × 5 days during a 28-day cycle
Glioblastoma multiforme
• *Adult:* **PO** 75 mg/m^2/day × 42 days with focal radiotherapy; then maintenance of 6 cycles
Available forms: Caps 5, 20, 100, 250 mg

SIDE EFFECTS

CNS: **Seizures,** *hemiparesis, dizziness, poor coordination, amnesia, insomnia, paresthesia, somnolence, paresis, ataxia, anxiety, dysphagia, depression, confusion*
GI: Nausea, anorexia, vomiting
GU: Urinary incontinence, UTI, frequency
HEMA: **Thrombocytopenia, leukopenia,** anemia
INTEG: *Rash, pruritus*
MISC: Headache, fatigue, asthenia, fever, edema, back pain, weight increase, diplopia
RESP: URI, pharyngitis, sinusitis, coughing

Contraindications: Pregnancy (D), hypersensitivity to this drug or carbazine, lactation
Precautions: Radiation therapy, renal/hepatic disease

PHARMACOKINETICS

Absorption complete, rapid; crosses blood-brain barrier, excreted in urine/feces, half-life 1.8 hr, peak 1 hr

INTERACTIONS

Increase: myelosuppression—radiation, other antineoplastics
Decrease: antibody reaction—live virus vaccines

NURSING CONSIDERATIONS
Assess:
• CBC on day 22 (21 days after 1st dose), CBC weekly until recovery if ANC is <1.5 × 10^9/L and platelets <100 × 10^9/L, do not administer to patients that do not tolerate 100 mg/m^2, myelosuppression usually occurs late in the treatment cycle
• For seizures throughout treatment
• Monitor temp q4h (may indicate beginning infection)
• Hepatic studies before, during therapy (bilirubin, AST, ALT, LDH), as needed or monthly
• Bleeding: hematuria, guaiac, bruising or petechiae, mucosa or orifices q8h
Administer:
• Do not break, crush, chew, or open caps
• Antiemetic 30-60 min before giving drug to prevent vomiting
• Caps one at a time with 8 oz of water at same time of day
• Fluids IV or PO before chemotherapy to hydrate patient
• If caps accidentally damaged, do not allow contact with skin, or inhale
• Give on empty stomach to prevent nausea/vomiting
Perform/provide:
• Storage in light-resistant container, dry area

Evaluate:
• Therapeutic response: decreased tumor size, spread of malignancy

Teach patient/family:
• To report signs of infection: fever, sore throat, flulike symptoms
• To report signs of anemia: fatigue, headache, faintness, shortness of breath, irritability
• To report bleeding; avoid use of razors, commercial mouthwash
• To avoid use of aspirin products or ibuprofen

⚠ High Alert

tenecteplase (℞)
(ten-ek′ta-place)
TNKase
Func. class.: Thrombolytic enzyme
Chem. class.: Tissue plasminogen activator

Action: Activates conversion of plasminogen to plasmin (fibrinolysin): plasmin breaks down clots (fibrin), fibrinogen, factors V, VII; occlusion of venous access lines

Uses: Acute myocardial infarction

DOSAGE AND ROUTES
• *Adult <60 kg:* **IV BOL** 30 mg, give over 5 sec
• *Adult ≥60-<70 kg:* **IV BOL** 35 mg, give over 5 sec
• *Adult ≥70-<80 kg:* **IV BOL** 40 mg, give over 5 sec
• *Adult ≥80-<90 kg:* **IV BOL** 45 mg, give over 5 sec
• *Adult ≥90 kg:* **IV BOL** 50 mg, give over 5 sec

Available forms: Powder for inj, lyophilized 50 mg

SIDE EFFECTS

CV: Dysrhythmias, hypotension, pulmonary edema, **pulmonary embolism, cardiogenic shock, cardiac arrest, heart failure, myocardial reinfarction, myocardial rupture, tamponade, pericarditis, pericardial effusion, thrombosis**

HEMA: Decreased Hct, **bleeding**

INTEG: Rash, urticaria, phlebitis at IV inf site, itching, flushing

SYST: **GI, GU, intracranial, retroperitoneal bleeding, surface bleeding, anaphylaxis**

Contraindications: Hypersensitivity, arteriovenous malformation, aneurysm, active bleeding, intracranial, intraspinal surgery, CNS neoplasms, severe hypertension, severe renal disease, hepatic disease, history of CVA

Precautions: Pregnancy (C), arterial emboli from left side of heart, lactation, children, hypocoagulation, COPD, subacute bacterial endocarditis, rheumatic valvular disease, cerebral embolism/thrombosis/hemorrhage, intraarterial diagnostic procedure or surgery (10 days), recent major surgery, ulcerative colitis, enteritis, geriatric

PHARMACOKINETICS
IV: Onset immediate, half-life 20-24 min; metabolized by the liver

INTERACTIONS
• Bleeding potential: aspirin, indomethacin, phenylbutazone, anticoagulants, antithrombolytics, glycoprotein IIb, IIIa inhibitors, dipyridamole

Drug/Herb
Increase: risk of bleeding—agrimony, alfalfa, angelica, anise, basil, bay, bilberry, black haw, bogbean, bromelain, buchu, chondroitin, cinchona bark, dong quai, fenugreek, feverfew, garlic, ginger, ginkgo, ginseng, horse chestnut, Irish moss, kelp, kelpware, khella, lovage, lungwort, meadowsweet, motherwort, mugwort, nettle, papaya, parsley (large amts), pau d'arco, pineapple, poplar, prickly ash, safflower, saw palmetto, tonka bean, turmeric, wintergreen, yarrow

Decrease: anticoagulant effect—chamomile, coenzyme Q10, flax, glucomannan, goldenseal, guar gum

Drug/Lab Test
Increase: PT, aPTT, TT
Decrease: Plasminogen, fibrinogen

NURSING CONSIDERATIONS
Assess:
• Allergy: fever, rash, itching, chills; mild reaction may be treated with antihistamines

⚠ For bleeding during 1st hr of treatment; hematuria, hematemesis, bleeding from mucous membranes, epistaxis, ecchymosis; may require tranfusion (rare), continue to assess for bleeding for 24 hr

• Blood studies (Hct, platelets, PTT, PT, TT, aPTT) before starting therapy; PT or aPTT must be less than 2× control before starting therapy; PTT or PT q3-4h during treatment

• For hypersensitive reactions: fever, rash, dyspnea; drug should be discontinued

• VS, B/P, pulse, respirations, neurologic signs, temp at least q4h; temp >104° F (40° C) indicates internal bleeding; systolic pressure increase >25 mm Hg should be reported to prescriber

⚠ For neurologic changes that may indicate intracranial bleeding

⚠ Retroperitoneal bleeding: back pain, leg weakness, diminished pulses

Administer:
IV route
• As soon as thrombi identified; not useful for thrombi over 1 wk old
• Cryoprecipitate or fresh frozen plasma if bleeding occurs
• Heparin after fibrinogen level >100 mg/dl; heparin infusion to increase PTT to 1.5-2 × baseline for 3-7 days; IV heparin with loading dose is recommended
• Aseptically withdraw 10 ml of sterile H₂O for inj from diluent vial, use red cannula syringe-filling device, inject all contents of syringe into drug vial, direct into powder, swirl, withdraw correct dose, discard any unused solution; stand the shield with dose vertically on flat surface and passively recap the red cannula, remove entire shield assembly by twisting counterclockwise, give by IV BOL

• IV therapy: use upper extremity vessel that is accessible to manual compression
Perform/provide:
• Bed rest during entire course of treatment
• Avoidance of venous or arterial puncture, inj, rectal temp; any invasive treatment
• Treatment of fever with acetaminophen or aspirin
• Pressure for 30 sec to minor bleeding sites; inform prescriber if this does not attain hemostasis; apply pressure dressing
Evaluate:
• Therapeutic response: resolution of myocardial infarction
Teach patient/family:
• Proper tooth brushing to avoid bleeding
• Notify prescriber immediately of sudden severe headache
• Notify prescriber of bleeding, hypersensitivity

Rarely Used

teniposide (℞)
(ten-i-poe'side)
Vumon, VM 26
Func. class.: Antineoplastic

Uses: Childhood acute lymphoblastic leukemia (ALL), refractory childhood acute lymphocytic leukemia

DOSAGE AND ROUTES
• *Child:* **IV INF** combo teniposide 165 mg/m² and cytarabine 300 mg/m² 2 ×/wk × 8-9 doses or combo teniposide 250 mg/m² and vinCRIStine 1.5 mg/m² qwk × 4-8 wk and predniSONE 40 mg/m² **PO** × 28 days

Contraindications: Pregnancy (D), hypersensitivity, bone marrow depression, severe renal/hepatic disease, bacterial infection

---

⚠ Safety alert   *"Tall Man" lettering

tenofovir (℞)
(ten-oh-foh'veer)
Viread
Func. class.: Antiretroviral
Chem. class.: Nucleoside analog reverse transcriptase inhibitor

Action: Inhibits replication of HIV virus by competing with the natural substrate and then incorporating into cellular DNA by viral reverse transcriptase, thereby terminating cellular DNA chain

Uses: HIV-1 infection with other antiretrovirals

DOSAGE AND ROUTES
• *Adult:* **PO** 300 mg with meal; if used with didanosine, give tenofovir 2 hr before or 1 hr after didanosine

Renal dose
• CCr 30-49 ml/min 300 mg q48h
• CCr 10-29 ml/min 300 mg 2 ×/wk
• CCr <10 ml/min not recommended

Available forms: Tabs 300 mg (300 mg of fumarate salt equivalent to 245 mg tenofovir disoproxil)

SIDE EFFECTS
CNS: Headache
GI: Nausea, vomiting, diarrhea, anorexia, *flatulence, abdominal pain*
SYST: Change in body fat distribution

Contraindications: Hypersensitivity
Precautions: Pregnancy (B), lactation, children, geriatric, renal disease, hepatic insufficiency, CCr <60 ml/min, osteoporosis

PHARMACOKINETICS
Rapidly absorbed, distributed to extravascular space, excreted unchanged in urine, 70%-80%; terminal half-life 17 hr

INTERACTIONS
Increase: tenofovir level—cidofovir, acyclovir, valacyclovir, ganciclovir, valganciclovir

Increase: level of didanosine when given with tenofovir
Increase: tenofovir level—any drug that decreases renal function

NURSING CONSIDERATIONS
Assess:
• Hepatic studies: AST, ALT, bilirubin; amylase, lipase, triglycerides periodically during treatment
• For bone, renal toxicity: if bone abnormalities are suspected, obtain tests; serum phosphorus, creatinine
⚠ For lactic acidosis, severe hepatomegaly with steatosis

Administer:
• PO daily with meal
• This drug 2 hr before or 1 hr after taking didanosine (if used)

Perform/provide:
• Storage at 25° C (77° F)

Evaluate:
• Therapeutic response: Decrease in signs/symptoms of HIV

Teach patient/family:
• To take with meal
• That GI complaints resolve after 3-4 wk of treatment
• Not to breastfeed while taking this drug
• That drug must be taken daily even if patient feels better
• That follow-up visits must be continued because serious toxicity may occur; blood counts must be done q2wk
• That drug will control symptoms but is not a cure for HIV; patient is still infectious, may pass HIV virus on to others
• That other drugs may be necessary to prevent other infections
• That changes in body fat distribution may occur

terazosin (℞)
(ter-ay'zoe-sin)
Hytrin
Func. class.: Antihypertensive
Chem. class.: α-Adrenergic blocker

Action: Decreases total vascular resistance, which is responsible for a decrease in B/P; this occurs by blockade of α_1-adrenoreceptors

Uses: Hypertension, as a single agent or in combination with diuretics or β-blockers, BPH

DOSAGE AND ROUTES
Hypertension
• *Adult:* **PO** 1 mg at bedtime, may increase dose slowly to desired response; not to exceed 20 mg/day

Benign prostatic hyperplasia
• *Adult:* **PO** 1 mg at bedtime, gradually increase up to 5-10 mg; max 20 mg

Available forms: Tabs 1, 2, 5, 10 mg

SIDE EFFECTS

CNS: Dizziness, headache, drowsiness, anxiety, depression, vertigo, weakness, fatigue

CV: Palpitations, orthostatic hypotension, tachycardia, edema, rebound hypertension

EENT: Blurred vision, epistaxis, tinnitus, dry mouth, red sclera, nasal congestion, sinusitis

GI: Nausea, vomiting, diarrhea, constipation, abdominal pain

GU: Urinary frequency, incontinence, impotence, priapism

RESP: Dyspnea, cough, pharyngitis

Contraindications: Hypersensitivity

Precautions: Pregnancy (C), children, lactation, prostate cancer

PHARMACOKINETICS

Peak 1 hr; half-life 9-12 hr; protein binding 90%-94%; metabolized in liver; excreted in urine, feces

INTERACTIONS

Increase: hypotensive effects—β-blockers, nitroglycerin, verapamil, other antihypertensives, alcohol

Decrease: hypotensive effects—estrogens, NSAIDs, sympathomimetics, salicylates

Drug/Herb

Increase: toxicity, death—aconite

Increase: antihypertensive effect—barberry, betony, black catechu, black cohosh, bloodroot, broom, burdock, cat's claw, dandelion, goldenseal, hawthorn, Irish moss, Jamaican dogwood, kelp, khella, mistletoe, parsley

Increase or decrease: antihypertensive effect—astragalus, cola tree

Decrease: antihypertensive effect—coltsfoot, guarana, khat, licorice, yohimbine

NURSING CONSIDERATIONS
Assess:
• Urinary symptoms associated with BPH
• Orthostatic B/P, pulse, jugular venous distention q4h
• BUN, uric acid if on long-term therapy
• Weight daily, I&O
• Skin turgor, dryness of mucous membranes for hydration status
• Crackles, dyspnea, orthopnea q30min

Administer
• Dose at bedtime or do not operate machinery; fainting may occur

Perform/provide:
• Cool storage in tight container

Evaluate:
• Therapeutic response: decreased B/P, edema in feet, legs, decreased symptoms of BPH

Teach patient/family:
• That fainting occasionally occurs after first dose; not to drive or operate machinery for 4 hr after first dose or after an increase in dose; or take first dose at bedtime
• To rise slowly from sitting/lying position

---

terbinafine (℞)
(ter-bin′a-feen)
Lamisil
Func. class.: Antifungal
Chem. class.: Synthetic allylamine derivative

Action: Interferes with cell membrane permeability in fungi such as *Trichophyton rubrum, Trichophyton mentagrophytes, Trichophyton tonsurans, Epi-*

---

dermophyton floccosum, Microsporum canis, Microsporum audouinii, Microsporum gypseum, Candida, broad-spectrum antifungal
Uses: (TOP) Tinea cruris, tinea corporis, tinea pedis; (oral) onychomycosis of the toenail or fingernail due to dermatophytes
Unlabeled uses: Cutaneous candidiasis, tinea versicolor

DOSAGE AND ROUTES
• *Fingernail:* **PO** 250 mg/day × 6 wk
• *Toenail:* **PO** 250 mg/day × 12 wk
Available forms: Tabs 250 mg

SIDE EFFECTS
GI: Diarrhea, dyspepsia, abdominal pain, nausea, hepatitis
HEMA: **Neutropenia**
INTEG: Rash, pruritus, urticaria, **Stevens-Johnson syndrome**
MISC: Headache, hepatic enzyme changes, taste, visual disturbance
Contraindications: Hypersensitivity, chronic/active hepatic disease, renal disease GFR ≤50 ml/min
Precautions: Pregnancy (B), lactation, children, renal disease

PHARMACOKINETICS
Peak 1-2 hr

INTERACTIONS
Increase: levels of dextromethorphan
Increase: terbinafine clearance—rifampin
Increase: clearance of cycloSPORINE
Decrease: terbinafine clearance—cimetidine
Drug/Herb
• Side effects: cola nut, guarana, yerba maté, tea (black, green), coffee

NURSING CONSIDERATIONS
Assess:
• Hepatic studies (ALT, AST) prior to beginning treatment; do not use in presence of hepatic disease
• CBC in treatment >6 wk

• For continuing infection: increased size, number of lesions
Perform/provide:
• Storage below 25° C (77° F)
Evaluate:
• Therapeutic response: decrease in size, number of lesions
Teach patient/family:
• To notify prescriber of nausea, vomiting, fatigue, jaundice, dark urine, clay-colored stool, RUQ pain, that may indicate hepatic dysfunction

terbinafine topical
See Appendix C

terbutaline (R)
(ter-byoo'te-leen)
Brethine, Bricanyl
Func. class.: Selective β₂-agonist; bronchodilator
Chem. class.: Catecholamine

Action: Relaxes bronchial smooth muscle by direct action on β₂-adrenergic receptors through accumulation of cAMP at β-adrenergic receptor sites; bronchodilation, diuresis, CNS, cardiac stimulation occur; relaxes uterine smooth muscle
Uses: Bronchospasm, hyperkalemia
Unlabeled uses: Premature labor

DOSAGE AND ROUTES
Bronchodilation
• *Adult and child >15 yr:* **PO** 2.5-5 mg q6h during the day, max 15 mg/24 hr
• *Child 12-15 yr:* **PO** 2.5 mg tid q6h
Bronchospasm
• *Adult and child >12 yr:* **PO** 2.5-5 mg q8h; **SUBCUT** 0.25 mg q15-30min, max 0.5 mg in 4 hr
Tocolytic (preterm labor) (unlabeled)
• *Adult:* **PO** 2.5 mg q4-6h until delivery
Renal dose
• *Adult:* **PO** GFR 10-50 ml/min 50% of dose

Severe renal failure
• **Adult:** Avoid GFR if <10 ml/min
Available forms: Tabs 2.5, 5 mg; inj 1 mg/ml

SIDE EFFECTS

CNS: Tremors, anxiety, insomnia, headache, dizziness, stimulation
CV: Palpitations, tachycardia, hypertension, dysrhythmias, **cardiac arrest**
GI: Nausea, vomiting
Contraindications: Hypersensitivity to sympathomimetics, narrow-angle glaucoma, tachydysrhythmias
Precautions: Pregnancy (B), cardiac disorders, hyperthyroidism, diabetes mellitus, prostatic hypertension, lactation, geriatric, hypertension, seizure disorder

PHARMACOKINETICS

PO: Onset ½ hr, peak 1-2 hr, duration 4-8 hr
SUBCUT: Onset 6-15 min, peak ½-1 hr, duration 1½-4 hr

INTERACTIONS

• Incompatible with bleomycin
• Hypertensive crisis: MAOIs
Increase: effects of both drugs—other sympathomimetics
Decrease: action—β-blockers
Drug/Herb
Increase: effect—green tea (large amounts), guarana

NURSING CONSIDERATIONS

Assess:
• Respiratory function: vital capacity, forced expiratory volume, ABGs, B/P, pulse, respiratory pattern, lung sounds, sputum before and after treatment
• Tolerance over long-term therapy; dose may have to be changed; monitor for rebound bronchospasm
⚠ Paradoxical bronchospasm: dyspnea, wheezing, keep emergency equipment nearby
• Labor: maternal heart rate, B/P, contraction, fetal heart rate

Administer:
• With food; may be crushed
• 2 hr before bedtime to avoid sleeplessness
IV route
• IV after diluting each 5 mg/1 L D$_5$W for inf
• IV, run 5 mcg/min; may increase 5 mcg q10min, titrate to response; after ½-1 hr taper dose by 5 mcg; switch to PO as soon as possible
Additive compatibilities: Aminophylline
Syringe compatibilities: Doxapram
Y-site compatibilities: Insulin (regular)
Perform/provide:
• Storage at room temperature; do not use discolored sol
• An increase in fluids of >2 L/day
Evaluate:
• Therapeutic response: absence of dyspnea, wheezing
Teach patient/family:
• Not to use OTC medications; extra stimulation may occur
• All aspects of drug; avoid smoking, smoke-filled rooms, persons with respiratory infections
• To increase fluids >2 L/day; allow 15 min between inhalation of this drug and inhaler containing steroid
• To take on time; if missed, do not make up after 1 hr; wait until next dose
Treatment of overdose: Administer an α-blocker, then norepinephrine for severe hypotension

---

terconazole vaginal antifungal
See Appendix C

⚠ Safety alert   *"Tall Man" lettering

NURSING CONSIDERATIONS
Assess:
- Uric acid, chloride, magnesium, electrolytes, urine pH, vit D, phosphate for normal serum levels; serum calcium may be transiently increased after dosing (max at 4-6 hr post-dose)
- For bone pain, headache, fatigue, changes in LOC, leg cramps
- For signs of persistent hypercalcemia: nausea, vomiting, constipation, lethargy, muscle weakness
- Nutritional status: diet for sources of vit D (milk, some seafood); calcium (dairy products, dark green vegetables), phosphates (dairy products)

Administer:
SUBCUT route
- Give by SUBCUT only, rotate inj sites

Perform/provide:
- Store refrigerated, do not freeze

Evaluate:
- Therapeutic response: increased bone mineral density

Teach patient/family:
- The symptoms of hypercalcemia
- About foods rich in calcium
- How to use delivery device, dispose of needles, not to share pen with others
- To sit or lie down if dizziness or fast heartbeat occurs after the first few doses
- To rotate administration sites

---

teriparatide (℞)
(tah-ree-par'ah-tide)
Forteo
Func. class.: Parathyroid hormone (rDNA)

Action: Contains human recombinant parathyroid hormone, to stimulate new bone growth
Uses: Postmenopausal women with osteoporosis, men with primary or hypogonadal osteoporosis who are at high risk for fracture

DOSAGE AND ROUTES
- *Adult:* **SUBCUT** 20 mcg daily × 29 mo
Available forms: Prefilled pen delivery device (delivers 20 mcg/day)

SIDE EFFECTS
CNS: Dizziness, headache, insomnia, depression, vertigo
CV: Hypertension, angina, syncope
GI: Nausea, diarrhea, dyspepsia, vomiting, constipation
INTEG: Rash, sweating
MISC: Pain, asthenia
MS: Arthralgia, leg cramps
RESP: Rhinitis, cough, pharyngitis, pneumonia, dyspnea
Contraindications: Hypersensitivity, increased baseline risk of osteosarcoma (Paget's disease, open epiphyses; previous bone radiation), bone metastases, history of skeletal malignancies, other metabolic bone diseases, preexisting hypercalcemia
Precautions: Pregnancy (C), lactation, urolithiasis, hypotension, use >2 yr

PHARMACOKINETICS
SUBCUT: Extensively and rapidly absorbed, metabolized by liver, excreted by kidneys

INTERACTIONS
Increase: digoxin toxicity: digoxin
Drug/Lab Test
Increase: Calcium

---

testolactone (℞)
(tess-toe-lak'tone)
Teslac
Func. class.: Antineoplastic
Chem. class.: Androgen hormone

Controlled Substance Schedule III
Action: Acts on adrenal cortex to suppress activity; reduces estrone synthesis
Uses: Advanced breast carcinoma in postmenopausal women; prostatic cancer

DOSAGE AND ROUTES
- *Adult:* **PO** 250 mg qid
Available forms: Tabs 50 mg

SIDE EFFECTS

CNS: Paresthesias, dizziness
CV: Orthostatic hypertension, edema
EENT: Deepening voice
GI: Nausea, vomiting, anorexia, glossitis
GU: Urinary retention, **renal failure**
INTEG: Rash, nail changes, facial hair growth
META: Hypercalcemia

Contraindications: Hypersensitivity, premenopausal women, carcinoma of male breast, lactation
Precautions: Pregnancy (C), renal/cardiac disease, hypercalcemia

PHARMACOKINETICS

None known

INTERACTIONS

• Enhanced effects of oral anticoagulants
Drug/Lab Test
Increase: Urinary 17-OHCS
Decrease: Estradiol

NURSING CONSIDERATIONS

Assess:
• Calcium levels
• B/P q4h; tell patient to rise slowly from sitting or lying down
• Food preferences; list likes, dislikes
• Edema in feet; joint, stomach pain; shaking
⚠ Symptoms indicating severe allergic reaction: rash, pruritus, urticaria, purpuric skin lesions, itching, flushing
• Anorexia, nausea, vomiting, constipation, weakness, loss of muscle tone (indicating hypercalcemia)
Administer:
• For 3 mo or longer for desired response
Evaluate:
• Therapeutic response: decreased tumor size, spread of malignancy
Teach patient/family:
• To recognize and report signs of hepatotoxicity, hypercalcemia, virilization (in females), bleeding if on anticoagulants

---

testosterone cypionate (℞)
Andro-Cyp, Andronate, depAndro, Depotest, Depo-Testosterone, Dura-test, T-Cypionate, Testa-C, Testred, Testoject-LA, Virilon IM
testosterone enanthate (℞)
Andro LA, Andropository, Andryl, Delatest, Delatestryl, Everone, Malog-x ✦, Testone LA, Testrin-PA
testosterone gel (℞)
AndroGel 1%, Testim
testosterone, long-acting (℞)
testosterone pellets (℞)
Testopel
testosterone transdermal (℞)
Androderm, Testoderm, Testoderm TTS, Testoderm with Adhesive
testosterone buccal (℞)
Striant
Func. class.: Androgenic anabolic steroid
Chem. class.: Halogenated testosterone derivative

Controlled Substance Schedule III
Action: Increases weight by building body tissue, increases potassium, phosphorus, chloride, nitrogen levels, bone development
Uses: Female breast cancer, eunuchoidism, male climacteric, oligospermia, impotence, osteoporosis, weight loss in AIDS patients, vulvar dystrophies, low testosterone levels, delayed male puberty (inj)

⚠ Safety alert   *"Tall Man" lettering

DOSAGE AND ROUTES
Replacement
• *Adult:* **IM** 25-50 mg 2-3 ×/wk (base or propionate) or 50-400 mg q2-4wk (enanthate or cypionate)
• *Adult:* **TRANSDERMAL** (Testoderm) 4-6 mg applied q24h; (Androderm) 5 mg applied q24h; **GEL** (AndroGel) 5 mg applied q24h, once daily; **BUCCAL** 1 buccal system (30 mg) to the gum region q12h before meals/PM
Breast cancer
• *Adult:* **IM** 50-100 mg 3 ×/wk (propionate) or 200-400 mg q2-4wk (cypionate or enanthate)
Delayed male puberty
• *Child >12 yr:* **IM** up to 100 mg/mo for up to 6 mo
Available forms: *Enanthate:* inj 200 mg/ml; *cypionate:* inj 100, 200 mg/ml; pellets 75 mg; transdermal 2.5, 4, 5, 6 mg/24 hr; gel 1%; buccal system 30 mg

SIDE EFFECTS
CNS: Dizziness, headache, fatigue, tremors, paresthesias, flushing, sweating, anxiety, lability, insomnia, carpal tunnel syndrome
CV: Increased B/P
EENT: Conjunctival edema, nasal congestion
ENDO: Abnormal GTT
GI: Nausea, vomiting, constipation, weight gain, **cholestatic jaundice**
GU: Hematuria, amenorrhea, vaginitis, decreased libido, decreased breast size, clitoral hypertrophy, testicular atrophy
INTEG: Rash, acneiform lesions, oily hair and skin, flushing, sweating, acne vulgaris, alopecia, hirsutism
MS: Cramps, spasms
Contraindications: Pregnancy (X), severe renal/hepatic/cardiac disease, hypersensitivity, lactation, genital bleeding (rare)
Precautions: Diabetes mellitus, CV disease, MI

PHARMACOKINETICS
PO: Metabolized in liver, excreted in urine, breast milk; crosses placenta

INTERACTIONS
• Edema: ACTH, adrenal steroids
Increase: effects of oxyphenbutazone
Increase: PT—anticoagulants
Decrease: glucose levels may alter need for oral antidiabetics, insulin
Drug/Lab Test
Increase: Serum cholesterol, blood glucose, urine glucose
Decrease: Serum calcium, serum potassium, T_4, T_3, thyroid ^{131}I uptake test, urine 17-OHCS, 17-KS, PBI

NURSING CONSIDERATIONS
Assess:
• Weight daily; notify prescriber if weekly weight gain is >5 lb
• B/P q4h
• I&O ratio; be alert for decreasing urinary output, increasing edema
• Growth rate in children; growth rate may be uneven (linear/bone growth) with extended use
• Electrolytes: K, Na, Cl, Ca; cholesterol
• Hepatic studies: ALT, AST, bilirubin
• Edema, hypertension, cardiac symptoms, jaundice
• Mental status: affect, mood, behavioral changes, aggression
• Signs of masculinization in female: increased libido, deepening of voice, decreased breast tissue, enlarged clitoris, menstrual irregularities; male: gynecomastia, impotence, testicular atrophy
• Hypercalcemia: lethargy, polyuria, polydipsia, nausea, vomiting, constipation; drug may have to be decreased
• Hypoglycemia in diabetics; oral antidiabetic action is increased
Administer:
• Titrated dose; use lowest effective dose
• IM inj deep into upper outer quadrant of gluteal muscle
• Transdermal patches: Testoderm to skin of scrotum; Androderm to skin of back, upper arms, thighs, abdomen; area must be dry-shaved; may be reapplied after bathing, swimming
• Gel: apply daily to clean, dry area on shoulders, upper arms or abdomen

Side effects: *italics* = common; **bold** = life-threatening

Buccal system route
- Do not chew or swallow buccal system
- Rotate sites; place above incisor tooth on either side of mouth
- Open packet; place rounded side of surface against the gum and hold firmly in place with finger over lip for 30 sec; if it falls off, replace with new system; discard in trash can away from children or pets

Perform/provide:
- Diet with increased calories, protein; decrease sodium if edema occurs

Evaluate:
- Therapeutic response: 4-6 wk in osteoporosis

Teach patient/family:
- That drug must be combined with complete health plan: diet, rest, exercise
- To notify prescriber if therapeutic response decreases; if edema occurs
- About changes in sex characteristics
- That women should report menstrual irregularities, voice changes, acne, facial hair growth, if pregnancy is planned or suspected
- That 1-3-mo course is necessary for response in breast cancer
- The proper application of patches

---

tetracaine (Ŗ)
(tet′ra-kane)
Pontocaine
Func. class.: Local anesthetic
Chem. class.: Ester

Action: Competes with calcium for binding sites in nerve membrane that control sodium transport across cell membrane; decreases rise of depolarization phase of action potential
Uses: Spinal anesthesia, epidural and peripheral nerve block, perineum, lower extremities

DOSAGE AND ROUTES
Varies with route of anesthesia
Available forms: Inj 0.2%, 0.3%, 1%; powder

SIDE EFFECTS
CNS: Anxiety, restlessness, **seizures, LOC,** drowsiness, disorientation, tremors, shivering
CV: **Myocardial depression, cardiac arrest, dysrhythmias,** bradycardia, hypo/hypertension, fetal bradycardia
EENT: Blurred vision, tinnitus, pupil constriction
GI: Nausea, vomiting
INTEG: Rash, urticaria, allergic reactions, edema, burning, skin discoloration at inj site, tissue necrosis
RESP: **Status asthmaticus, respiratory arrest, anaphylaxis**
Contraindications: Hypersensitivity, sulfite allergy, severe hepatic disease, heart block
Precautions: Pregnancy (C), geriatric, severe drug allergies, lactation, children <12 yr

PHARMACOKINETICS
Onset MS 3 min; spinal 3-8 min; duration 1.5-3 hr; metabolized by liver, excreted in urine (metabolites)

INTERACTIONS
- Dysrhythmias: epINEPHrine, halothane, enflurane
- Hypertension: MAOIs, tricyclics, phenothiazines
Decrease: action of tetracaine—chloroprocaine
Decrease: action of sulfonamides

NURSING CONSIDERATIONS
Assess:
- B/P, pulse, respiration during treatment
- Fetal heart tones during labor
- Allergic reactions: rash, urticaria, itching
- Cardiac status: ECG for dysrhythmias, pulse, B/P, during anesthesia

Administer:
- Only if not cloudy, does not contain precipitate
- Only with crash cart, resuscitative equipment nearby

⚠ Safety alert   *"Tall Man" lettering

• Only without preservatives for epidural or caudal anesthesia

Perform/provide:
• Use of new sol, discard unused portions, store in refrigerator, avoid freezing

Evaluate:
• Therapeutic response: anesthesia necessary for procedure

Treatment of overdose: Maintain adequate airway, O_2, vasopressor, IV fluids, anticonvulsants for seizures

---

tetracaine ophthalmic
See Appendix C

---

tetracaine topical
See Appendix C

---

tetracycline (Ŗ)
(tet-ra-sye'kleen)
Achromycin V, Actisite (dental product), Apo-Tetra ✦, Novotetra ✦, Nu-Tetra ✦, Panmycin, Robitet, Sumycin, Teline, Tetracap, tetracycline HCl, Tetracyn, Tetralan, Tetram
Func. class.: Broad-spectrum antiinfective
Chem. class.: Tetracycline

Action: Inhibits protein synthesis and phosphorylation in microorganisms; bacteriostatic

Uses: Syphilis, *Chlamydia trachomatis,* gonorrhea, lymphogranuloma venereum; uncommon gram-positive, gram-negative organisms; rickettsial infections

DOSAGE AND ROUTES

Susceptible gram-positive/gram-negative infections
• *Adult:* **PO** 250-500 mg q6h
• *Child >8 yr:* **PO** 25-50 mg/kg/day in divided doses q6h

Chlamydia trachomatis
• *Adult:* **PO** 500 mg qid × 7 days

Syphilis
• *Adult and adolescent:* **PO** 500 mg qid × 2 wk; if syphilis duration >1 yr, must treat 30 days

Brucellosis
• *Adult:* **PO** 500 mg q6h × 3 wk with 1 g streptomycin **IM** q12h × 1 wk, and 1 ×/ day the 2nd wk

***Urethral, endocervical, rectal infections* (C. trachomatis)**
• *Adult:* **PO** 500 mg qid × 7 days

Acne
• *Adult and adolescent:* **PO** 250 mg q6h, then 125-500 mg daily or every other day

Available forms: Oral susp 125 mg/5 ml; caps 250, 500 mg

SIDE EFFECTS

CNS: Fever, headache, paresthesia
CV: Pericarditis
EENT: Dysphagia, glossitis, decreased calcification, discoloration of deciduous teeth, oral candidiasis, oral ulcers
GI: Nausea, abdominal pain, *vomiting, diarrhea,* anorexia, enterocolitis, **hepatotoxicity,** flatulence, abdominal cramps, epigastric burning, stomatitis, **hepatitis**
GU: Increased BUN
HEMA: **Eosinophilia, neutropenia, thrombocytopenia, leukocytosis, hemolytic anemia**
INTEG: Rash, urticaria, photosensitivity, increased pigmentation, **exfoliative dermatitis,** pruritus, **angioedema, Stevens-Johnson syndrome**
MISC: Increased intracranial pressure, candidiasis

Contraindications: Pregnancy (D), hypersensitivity to tetracyclines, children <8 yr, lactation

Precautions: Renal/hepatic disease, UV exposure

PHARMACOKINETICS

PO: Peak 2-3 hr, duration 6 hr, half-life 6-10 hr; excreted in urine, breast milk; crosses placenta; 20%-60% protein bound

---

INTERACTIONS
• Nephrotoxicity: methoxyflurane
Increase: effect of warfarin, digoxin
Decrease: effect of tetracycline—
antacids, NaHCO$_3$, dairy products, alkali
products, iron, cimetidine
Decrease: effect of penicillins, oral con-
traceptives

Drug/Herb
• Do not use acidophilus with antiinfec-
tives; separate by several hours
• Photosensitivity: dong quai

Drug/Lab Test
False increase: Urinary catecholamines

NURSING CONSIDERATIONS
Assess:
• Signs of anemia: Hct, Hgb, fatigue
• I&O ratio
• Blood studies: PT, CBC, AST, ALT, BUN,
creatinine
• Allergic reactions: rash, itching, pruri-
tus, angioedema
• Nausea, vomiting, diarrhea; administer
antiemetic, antacids as ordered
• Overgrowth of infection: fever, malaise,
redness, pain, swelling, drainage, peri-
neal itching, diarrhea, changes in cough
or sputum

Administer:
• After C&S obtained
• 2 hr before or after iron products; 3
hr after antacid products
• Should be given on an empty stomach

Perform/provide:
• Storage in tight, light-resistant container
at room temperature

Evaluate:
• Therapeutic response: decreased temp,
absence of lesions, negative C&S

Teach patient/family:
• To avoid sun exposure; sunscreen does
not seem to decrease photosensitivity
• That all prescribed medication must be
taken to prevent superinfection
• To avoid milk products, antacids, or
separate by 2 hr; take with a full glass of
water

tetrahydrozoline nasal agent
See Appendix C

tetrahydrozoline ophthalmic
See Appendix C

theophylline (℞)
(thee-off'i-lin)
Accurbron, Aquaphyllin, As-
malix, Bronkodyl, Elixomin,
Elixophyllin, Lanophyllin, Qui-
bron-T Dividose, Quibron-T/SR
Dividose, Respbid, Slo-bid
Gyrocaps, Slo-Phyllin, Sustaire,
Theo-24, Theobid Duracaps,
Theochron, Theoclear-80,
Theoclear L.A., Theo-Dur,
Theolair-SR, Theo-Sav,
Theospan-SR, Theostat 80,
Theovent, Theo-X, T-Phyl, Uni-
Dur, Uniphyl
Func. class.: Bronchodilator
Chem. class.: Methylxanthine

Action: Relaxes smooth muscle of respiratory system by blocking phosphodiesterase, which increases cAMP, exact action
unknown
Uses: Bronchial asthma, bronchospasm
of COPD, chronic bronchitis, emphysema

DOSAGE AND ROUTES
Hepatic dose
• *Adult:* **PO** 6 mg/kg loading dose, then
2 mg/kg q8h × 2 doses, then 1-2 mg/kg
q12h; **IV** 4.7 mg/kg, then 0.39 mg/kg/hr
for 12 hr, then 0.08-0.16 mg/kg/hr maintenance
Bronchospasm, bronchial asthma
• *Adult:* **PO** 100-200 mg q6h; dosage
must be individualized; max 800 mg/day
• *Child:* **PO** 50-100 mg q6h, not to exceed 12 mg/kg/24 hr

A Safety alert   *"Tall Man" lettering

COPD, chronic bronchitis
- *Adult:* **PO** 300-800 mg q6-8h after meals
- *Child 1-9 yr:* **PO** 5 mg/kg loading dose, then 4 mg/kg q6h
- *Child 9-16 yr:* **PO** 5 mg/kg loading dose, then 4 mg/kg q6h

Apnea of prematurity
- *Neonate:* 2-10 mg/kg/day divided q8-12h (usual loading dose is 4 mg/kg **PO**)

Available forms: Caps 50, 100, 200, 250 mg; tabs 100, 125, 200, 225, 250, 300 mg; time rel tabs 100, 200, 250, 300, 400, 500 mg; time rel caps 50, 65, 100, 125, 130, 200, 250, 260, 300, 400, 500 mg; elix 80, 11.25 mg/15 ml; sol 80 mg/15 ml; liquid 80, 150, 160 mg/15 ml; susp 300 mg/15 ml

SIDE EFFECTS
CNS: Anxiety, restlessness, insomnia, dizziness, **seizures,** headache, lightheadedness, muscle twitching, tremors
CV: Palpitations, sinus tachycardia, hypotension, **dysrhythmias,** fluid retention with tachycardia
ENDO: Hyperglycemia
GI: Nausea, vomiting, anorexia, diarrhea, bitter taste, dyspepsia, gastric distress
INTEG: Flushing, urticaria
MISC: SIADH, urinary frequency
RESP: Increased rate, tachypnea
Contraindications: Hypersensitivity to xanthines, tachydysrhythmias
Precautions: Pregnancy (C), geriatric, CHF, cor pulmonale, hepatic disease, active peptic ulcer disease, diabetes mellitus, hyperthyroidism, hypertension, children, seizure disorder

PHARMACOKINETICS
PO: Peak 1-2 hr
SOL: Peak 1 hr
Metabolized in liver, excreted in urine and breast milk, crosses placenta, protein binding 40%, terminal half-life 6.5-10.5 hr

INTERACTIONS
- Cardiotoxicity: β-blockers
Increase: theophylline action—cimetidine, propranolol, erythromycin, oral contraceptives, influenza vaccine, fluoroquinolones, mexiletine, corticosteroids, disulfiram, fluvoxamine, interferons
Increase: effects of anticoagulants
Decrease: theophylline level—phenytoin, phenobarbital, carbamazepine, rifampin, smoking
Decrease: effect of lithium

Drug/Herb
- Toxicity: ephedra (ma huang), cola nut, guarana, yerba maté, tea (black, green), coffee
Decrease: theophylline levels—St. John's wort

NURSING CONSIDERATIONS
Assess:
⚠ Theophylline blood levels (therapeutic level is 5-15 mcg/ml); toxicity may occur with small increase above 20 mcg/ml
- Monitor I&O; diuresis occurs; geriatric or child may be dehydrated
- Signs of toxicity: irritability, insomnia, restlessness, tremors, nausea, vomiting
- Respiratory rate, rhythm, depth; auscultate lung fields bilaterally; notify prescriber of abnormalities
- Allergic reactions: rash, urticaria; drug should be discontinued

Administer:
- Do not break, crush, chew or dissolve time-release products
- PO with 8 oz of water for GI symptoms; avoid food; absorption may be affected; take dose consistently; do not take Theo-24 with meals
- Contents of bead-filled capsule sprinkled over food for children's use
- Check OTC medications, current prescriptions for epHEDrine, which will increase stimulation

IV route
- Loading dose over 20-30 min, max 20-25 mg/min; do not give by rapid IV, use only cont inf

Additive compatibilities: Cefepime, chlorproMAZINE, fluconazole, furosemide, hydrocortisone, lidocaine, methylprednisolone, verapamil

Y-site compatibilities: Acyclovir, ampicillin, ampicillin/sulbactam, aztreonam, cefazolin, cefotetan, ceftazidime, ceftriaxone, cimetidine, cisatracurium, clindamycin, dexamethasone, diltiazem, DOBUTamine, DOPamine, doxycycline, erythromycin, famotidine, fluconazole, gentamicin, haloperidol, heparin, hydrocortisone, lidocaine, methyldopate, methylPREDNISolone, metronidazole, midazolam, nafcillin, nitroglycerin, penicillin G potassium, piperacillin, potassium chloride, ranitidine, remifentanil, sodium nitroprusside, ticarcillin, ticarcillin/clavulanate, tobramycin, vancomycin

Evaluate:

• Therapeutic response: ability to breathe more easily

Teach patient/family:

• To check OTC medications, current prescription medications for epHEDrine, which will increase stimulation; to avoid alcohol, caffeine

• To avoid hazardous activities; dizziness may occur

• That if GI upset occurs, to take drug with 8 oz H_2O; avoid food; absorption may be decreased

• To notify prescriber of toxicity: nausea, vomiting, anxiety, insomnia, seizures

• To notify prescriber of change in smoking habit; dosage may have to be changed

---

thiamine (vit B₁)

(po-otc, iv, im-℞)

Betalin S, Betaxin ✦, Biamine, Revitonus, Thiamilate, thiamine HCl

Func. class.: Vit B₁

Chem. class.: Water soluble

Do not confuse:

thiamine/Tenormin

Action: Needed for pyruvate metabolism, carbohydrate metabolism

Uses: Vit B₁ deficiency or polyneuritis, cheilosis adjunct with thiamine beriberi, Wernicke-Korsakoff syndrome, pellagra, metabolic disorders

DOSAGE AND ROUTES

RDA

• *Adult:* **PO** Males 1.2-1.5 mg; females 1.1 mg; pregnancy 1.5 mg; lactation 1.6 mg

• *Child 7-10 yr:* **PO** 1.3 mg

• *Child 4-6 yr:* **PO** 0.9 mg

• *Child 1-3 yr:* **PO** 0.7 mg

• *Infant 6 mo-1 yr:* **PO** 0.4 mg

• *Neonate and infant to 6 mo:* **PO** 0.3 mg

Beriberi

• *Adult:* **IM** 10-20 mg tid × 2 wk, then 5-10 mg daily × 1 mo

Beriberi with cardiac failure

• *Adult and child:* **IV** 10-30 mg tid

Available forms: Tabs 50, 100, 250, 500 mg; inj 100 mg/ml; enteric coated tabs 20 mg

SIDE EFFECTS

CNS: Weakness, restlessness

CV: **Collapse, pulmonary edema,** hypotension

EENT: Tightness of throat

GI: Hemorrhage, *nausea, diarrhea*

INTEG: **Angioneurotic edema,** cyanosis, sweating, warmth

SYST: **Anaphylaxis**

Contraindications: Hypersensitivity

Precautions: Pregnancy (A)

PHARMACOKINETICS

PO/INJ: Unused amounts excreted in urine (unchanged)

NURSING CONSIDERATIONS

Assess:

• Nutritional status: yeast, beef, liver, whole or enriched grains, legumes

Administer:

IM route

• By IM inj; rotate sites if pain and inflammation occur; do not mix with alkaline sols; Z-track to minimize pain

---

⚠ Safety alert   ✦ "Tall Man" lettering

IV route
• Undiluted over 5 min or diluted with IV sol and given as an inf at 100 mg or less/5 min or more
Syringe compatibilities: Doxapram
Y-site compatibilities: Famotidine
Perform/provide:
• Storage in tight, light-resistant container
• Application of cold to help decrease pain
Evaluate:
• Therapeutic response: absence of nausea, vomiting, anorexia, insomnia, tachycardia, paresthesias, depression, muscle weakness
Teach patient/family:
• The necessary foods to be included in diet: yeast, beef, liver, legumes, whole grain

---

thiethylperazine (℞)
(thye-eth-il-per′a-zeen)
Norzine, Torecan
Func. class.: Antiemetic
Chem. class.: Phenothiazine, piperazine derivative

Do not confuse:
Torecan/Toradol
Action: Acts centrally by blocking chemoreceptor trigger zone, which in turn acts on vomiting center; dopamine blocker
Uses: Nausea, vomiting

DOSAGE AND ROUTES
• *Adult:* **PO/IM** 10 mg/daily-tid
Available forms: Tabs 10 mg; inj 5 mg/ml

SIDE EFFECTS
CNS: Euphoria, depression, restlessness, tremor, EPS, **seizures,** drowsiness, confusion, **neuroleptic malignant syndrome**
CV: **Circulatory failure, tachycardia,** postural hypotension, ECG changes
GI: Nausea, vomiting, anorexia, dry mouth, diarrhea, constipation, weight loss, metallic taste, cramps

GU: Urinary retention, dark urine
HEMA: **Agranulocytosis, leukopenia**
RESP: **Respiratory depression**
Contraindications: Pregnancy (X), hypersensitivity to phenothiazines, coma, seizure, encephalopathy, bone marrow depression
Precautions: Children <2 yr, geriatric, lactation, Parkinson's disease

PHARMACOKINETICS
PO: Onset 45-60 min
RECT: Onset 45-60 min, metabolized by liver, crosses placenta, excreted in urine, breast milk

INTERACTIONS
• Avoid use with phenothiazines; seizures may occur
Increase: anticholinergic action—anticholinergics, antiparkinson drugs, tricyclic antidepressants
Increase: sedation—barbiturates, general anesthetics, ethanol, anxiolytics, sedatives, hypnotics, benzodiazepines, opiate agonists
Decrease: effect of thiethylperazine—barbiturates, antacids

NURSING CONSIDERATIONS
Assess:
• VS, B/P; check patients with cardiac disease more often
⚠ For neuroleptic malignant syndrome: dyspnea, fever, seizures, diaphoresis, fatigue, loss of urinary control, tachycardia; have emergency equipment nearby
• Respiratory status before, during, after administration of emetic; check rate, rhythm, character; respiratory depression can occur rapidly with geriatric or debilitated patients
Administer:
• IM inj in large muscle mass; aspirate to avoid IV administration; patient should remain recumbent 1 hr after inj
Syringe compatibilities: Butorphanol, hydromorphone, midazolam, ranitidine
Y-site compatibilities: Aldesleukin

Side effects: *italics* = common; **bold** = life-threatening

Evaluate:
• Therapeutic response: absence of nausea, vomiting

Teach patient/family:
• To avoid hazardous activities, activities requiring alertness; dizziness may occur

Rarely Used

thioguanine (6-TG) (℞)
(thye-oh-gwah'neen)
thioguanine, Lanvis ✦
Func. class.: Antineoplastic-antimetabolite

Uses: Acute leukemias, chronic granulocytic leukemia, lymphomas, multiple myeloma, solid tumors

DOSAGE AND ROUTES
• *Adult and child:* **PO** 2 mg/kg/day, then increase slowly to 3 mg/kg/day after 4 wk
Contraindications: Pregnancy (D), prior drug resistance, leukopenia (<2500/mm³), thrombocytopenia (<100,000/mm³), anemia

⚠ High Alert

thiopental (℞)
(thye-oh-pen'tal)
Pentothal, thiopental sodium
Func. class.: General anesthetic
Chem. class.: Barbiturate

Controlled Substance Schedule III
Action: Acts in reticular-activating system to produce anesthesia, raises seizure threshold
Uses: Short, general anesthesia; narcoanalysis, induction anesthesia before other anesthetics
Unlabeled uses: Increased intracranial pressure

DOSAGE AND ROUTES
Induction and anesthesia
• *Adult:* **IV** 25-75 mg test dose, observe for 60 min; initial dose 50-70 mg given at 20-40 sec interval; additional 25-50 mg as needed

Rapid induction
• *Adult:* **IV** 210-280 mg or 3-5 mg/kg in 2-4 divided doses
• *Child:* **IV** 3-5 mg/kg over 20-30 sec, then 1 mg/kg as needed

Narcoanalysis
• *Adult:* **IV** 100 mg/min, not to exceed 50 ml/min

Sedation or narcosis
• *Adult:* **RECT** 12-20 mg/lb
Available forms: Powder for inj 2%, 2.5% (20 mg/ml, 25 mg/ml)

SIDE EFFECTS
CNS: Retrograde amnesia, prolonged somnolence
CV: Tachycardia, hypotension, **myocardial depression, dysrhythmias**
EENT: Sneezing, coughing
INTEG: Chills, *shivering,* necrosis, pain at inj site
MS: Muscle irritability
RESP: **Respiratory depression, bronchospasm**
Contraindications: Hypersensitivity, status asthmaticus, porphyrias
Precautions: Pregnancy (C), severe CV disease, renal/hepatic disease, hypotension, myxedema, myasthenia gravis, asthma, increased intracranial pressure

PHARMACOKINETICS
IV: Onset 30-60 sec; duration 4-15 min; half-life 11½ hr; crosses placenta

INTERACTIONS
Increase: action—CNS depressants
Drug/Herb
Increase: CNS depression—kava

NURSING CONSIDERATIONS
Assess:
• VS q3-5min during IV administration, after dose, q4h postoperatively
• Extravasation; if it occurs, apply moist heat and 1% procaine to affected area
• Dysrhythmias or myocardial depression

⚠ Safety alert   *"Tall Man" lettering

Administer:
• Only with crash cart, resuscitative equipment nearby

Intermittent IV route
• Dilute to 20-50 mg/ml; give by slow injection over 20-30 sec; max 25 mg/min

CONT INF route
• Dilute to 2-4 mg/ml

Additive compatibilities: Chloramphenicol, hydrocortisone sodium succinate, oxytocin, pentobarbital, phenobarbital, potassium chloride, sodium bicarbonate

Solution compatibilities: D₅/0.45% NaCl, D₅W, multiple electrolyte sol, 0.45% NaCl, 0.9% NaCl, 1/6 M sodium lactate

Syringe compatibilities: Aminophylline, hyaluronidase, hydrocortisone sodium succinate, neostigmine, pentobarbital, propofol, scopolamine, tubocurarine

Y-site compatibilities: Doxacurium, fentanyl, heparin, milrinone, mivacurium, nitroglycerin, ranitidine, remifentanil

Evaluate:
• Therapeutic response: maintenance of anesthesia

---

thioridazine (℞)

(thye-or-rid′a-zeen)
Apo-Thioridazine ✦, Mellaril,
Mellaril Concentrate,
Mellaril-5, Novo-Ridazine ✦,
PMS-Thioridazine ✦,
thioridazine HCl
Func. class.: Antipsychotic, neuroleptic
Chem. class.: Phenothiazine piperidine

Do not confuse:
Mellaril/Elavil

Action: Depresses cerebral cortex, hypothalamus, limbic system, which control activity, aggression; blocks neurotransmission produced by dopamine at synapse; exhibits strong α-adrenergic, anticholinergic blocking action; mechanism for antipsychotic effects is unclear

Uses: Psychotic disorders, schizophrenia, behavioral problems in children, anxiety, major depressive disorders, organic brain syndrome, dementia in geriatric

DOSAGE AND ROUTES

Psychosis
• *Adult:* PO 25-100 mg tid, max dose 800 mg/day; dose is gradually increased to desired response, then reduced to minimum maintenance

Depression/behavioral problems/organic brain syndrome
• *Adult:* PO 25 mg tid, range from 10 mg bid-qid to 50 mg tid-qid
• *Geriatric:* PO 10-25 mg daily-bid, increase 4-7 days by 10-25 mg to desired dose
• *Child 2-12 yr:* PO 0.5-3 mg/kg/day in divided doses

Available forms: Tabs 10, 15, 25, 50, 100, 150, 200 mg; conc 30, 100 mg/ml; susp 25, 100 mg/5 ml; syr 10 mg/15 ml

SIDE EFFECTS

CNS: EPS (rare): pseudoparkinsonism, akathisia, dystonia, tardive dyskinesia, **seizures,** *headache,* confusion, **neuroleptic malignant syndrome,** dizziness

CV: Orthostatic hypotension, **cardiac arrest,** ECG changes, **tachycardia**

EENT: Blurred vision, glaucoma, dry eyes

GI: Dry mouth, nausea, vomiting, anorexia, constipation, diarrhea, jaundice, weight gain

GU: Urinary retention, urinary frequency, enuresis, impotence, amenorrhea, gynecomastia

HEMA: Anemia, **leukopenia, leukocytosis, agranulocytosis**

INTEG: Rash, photosensitivity, dermatitis

RESP: **Laryngospasm,** dyspnea, **respiratory depression**

Contraindications: Hypersensitivity, blood dyscrasias, coma, children <2 yr, brain damage, bone marrow depression

Precautions: Pregnancy (C), lactation, seizure disorders, hypertension, hepatic/cardiac disease

T

PHARMACOKINETICS

PO: Onset erratic, peak 2-4 hr; metabolized by liver, excreted in urine, breast milk; crosses placenta, half-life 26-36 hr

INTERACTIONS

• Oversedation: other CNS depressants, alcohol, barbiturate anesthetics

Increase: anticholinergic effects—anticholinergics

Decrease: thioridazine effect—lithium, barbiturates

Decrease: antihypertensive effect—centrally acting antihypertensives

Decrease: absorption—aluminum hydroxide, magnesium hydroxide antacids

Drug/Herb

Increase: CNS depression—kava

Increase: EPS—betel palm, kava

Increase: effect—cola tree, hops, nettle, nutmeg

Drug/Lab Test

Increase: LFTs, cardiac enzymes, cholesterol, blood glucose, prolactin, bilirubin, PBI, cholinesterase, ^{131}I

Decrease: Hormones (blood, urine)

False positive: Pregnancy test, PKU

False negative: Urinary steroid, pregnancy test

NURSING CONSIDERATIONS

Assess:

• Mental status before first dose

• Swallowing of PO medication; check for hoarding or giving of medication to other patients

• I&O ratio; palpate bladder if low urinary output occurs, urinary retention may be the cause

• Bilirubin, CBC, LFTs qmo

• Urinalysis is recommended before and during prolonged therapy

• Affect, orientation, LOC, reflexes, gait, coordination, sleep pattern disturbances

• B/P standing and lying; also include pulse and respirations q4h during initial treatment; establish baseline before starting treatment; report drops of 30 mm Hg

• Dizziness, faintness, palpitations, tachycardia on rising

• EPS including akathisia (inability to sit still, no pattern to movements), tardive dyskinesia (bizarre movements of jaw, mouth, tongue, extremities), pseudoparkinsonism (rigidity, tremors, pill rolling, shuffling gait)

⚠ For neuroleptic malignant syndrome: altered mental status, muscle rigidity, increased CPK, hyperthermia, dyspnea, fatigue

• Skin turgor daily

• Constipation, urinary retention daily; increase bulk, water in diet

Administer:

• Antiparkinsonian agent on order from prescriber for EPS

• Concentrate mixed in citrus juices or distilled or acidified tap water

• Decreased dose in geriatric

• Remain lying down after IM inj for at least 30 min

• Avoid use with CNS depressants

Perform/provide:

• Decreased sensory input by dimming lights, avoiding loud noises

• Supervised ambulation until stabilized on medication if needed; do not involve in strenuous exercise program because fainting is possible; patient should not stand still for long periods

• Increased fluids to prevent constipation

• Sips of water, candy, gum for dry mouth

• Storage in tight, light-resistant container; avoid contact with skin

Evaluate:

• Therapeutic response: decrease in emotional excitement, hallucinations, delusions, paranoia, reorganization of patterns of thought, speech

Teach patient/family:

• That orthostatic hypotension occurs frequently, to rise from sitting or lying position gradually; to avoid hazardous activities until stabilized on medication

• To avoid hot tubs, hot showers, tub baths; hypotension may occur

• To avoid abrupt withdrawal of thioridazine, or EPS may result; drug should be withdrawn slowly

• To avoid OTC preparations (cough, hay fever, cold) unless approved by prescriber; serious drug interactions may occur; avoid use with alcohol; increased drowsiness may occur

• To use sunscreen to prevent burns

• About compliance with drug regimen

• About the necessity for meticulous oral hygiene, since oral candidiasis may occur

• To report sore throat, malaise, fever, bleeding, mouth sores; if these occur, CBC should be drawn and drug discontinued; may cause vision impairment, report to prescriber

• That in hot weather, heat stroke may occur; take extra precautions to stay cool

• May cause discoloration of urine

Treatment of overdose: Lavage if orally ingested, provide an airway; do not induce vomiting, CV monitoring, continuous EKG

Rarely Used

thiotepa (℞)
(thye-oh-tep′a)
Thioplex
Func. class.: Antineoplastic

Uses: Hodgkin's disease, lymphomas; breast, ovarian, lung, bladder cancer; neoplastic effusions

DOSAGE AND ROUTES

• *Adult:* **IV** 0.3-0.4 mg/kg at 1-4 wk intervals

Neoplastic effusions

• *Adult:* **INTRACAVITY** 0.6-0.8 mg/kg

Bladder cancer

• *Adult:* **INSTILL** 60 mg/30-60 ml water for inj instilled in bladder for 2 hr once weekly × 4 wk

Contraindications: Pregnancy (D), hypersensitivity

Rarely Used

thiothixene (℞)
(thye-oh-thix′een)
Navane, thiothixene
Func. class.: Antipsychotic, neuroleptic

Do not confuse:
Navane/Norvasc

Uses: Psychotic disorders, schizophrenia, acute agitation

DOSAGE AND ROUTES

• *Adult:* **PO** 2-5 mg bid-qid depending on severity of condition; dose gradually increased to 15-30 mg if needed; **IM** 4 mg bid-qid; max dose 30 mg daily; administer **PO** dose as soon as possible

• *Geriatric:* **PO** 1-2 mg daily-bid, increase by 1-2 mg q4-7d to desired dose

Contraindications: Hypersensitivity, blood dyscrasias, child <12 yr, bone marrow depression, circulatory collapse, CNS depression, coma, alcoholism, hepatic/CV disease, Reye's syndrome, narrow-angle glaucoma

---

thyroid USP (desiccated) (℞)
(thye′roid)
Armour Thyroid, Thyrar, Thyroid Strong, Westhroid
Func. class.: Thyroid hormone
Chem. class.: Active thyroid hormone in natural state and ratio

Do not confuse:
Thyrar/Thyrolar

Action: Increases metabolic rates, increases cardiac output, O_2 consumption, body temp, blood volume, growth, development at cellular level

Uses: Hypothyroidism, cretinism (juvenile hypothyroidism), myxedema

---

DOSAGE AND ROUTES

Hypothyroidism
• *Adult:* **PO** 65 mg daily, increased by 65 mg q6-8wk until desired response; maintenance dose 65-195 mg daily
• *Geriatric:* **PO** 7.5-15 mg daily, increase dose q6-8wk until desired response

Cretinism/juvenile hypothyroidism
• *Child over 1 yr:* **PO** up to 180 mg daily titrated to response
• *Child 4-12 mo:* **PO** 30-60 mg daily
• *Child 1-4 mo:* **PO** 15-30 mg daily; may increase q2wk; titrated to response; maintenance dose 30-45 mg daily

Myxedema
• *Adult:* **PO** 16 mg daily, double dose q2wk, maintenance 65-195 mg/day

Available forms: Tabs 16, 32, 65, 98, 130, 195, 260, 325 mg; enteric coated tabs 32, 65, 130 mg; sugarcoated tabs 32, 65, 130, 195 mg; caps 65, 130, 195, 325 mg

SIDE EFFECTS

CNS: Insomnia, tremors, headache, **thyroid storm**

CV: Tachycardia, palpitations, angina, dysrhythmias, hypertension, **cardiac arrest**

GI: Nausea, diarrhea, increased or decreased appetite, cramps

MISC: Menstrual irregularities, weight loss, sweating, heat intolerance, fever

Contraindications: Adrenal insufficiency, MI, thyrotoxicosis

Precautions: Pregnancy (A), geriatric, angina pectoris, hypertension, ischemia, cardiac disease, lactation

PHARMACOKINETICS

PO: Peak 12-48 hr, half-life 6-7 days

INTERACTIONS

Increase: effects of anticoagulants, sympathomimetics, tricyclics, catecholamines

Decrease: thyroid absorption—bile acid sequestrants

Decrease: effects of digoxin, insulin, hypoglycemics

Decrease: thyroid effects—estrogens

Drug/Herb

Decrease: thyroid effect—agar, bugleweed, carnitine, kelpware, soy, spirulina

Drug/Lab Test

Increase: CPK, LDH, AST, PBI, blood glucose

Decrease: Thyroid function tests

NURSING CONSIDERATIONS

Assess:
• B/P, pulse before each dose
• I&O ratio
• Weight daily in same clothing, using same scale, at same time of day
• Height, growth rate of child
• T_3, T_4, which are decreased; radioimmunoassay of TSH, which is increased; radio uptake, which is decreased if dosage is too low
• PT may require decreased anticoagulant; check for bleeding, bruising
• Increased nervousness, excitability, irritability; may indicate too high dose of medication, usually after 1-3 wk of treatment
• Cardiac status: angina, palpitation, chest pain, change in VS

Administer:
• In AM if possible as a single dose to decrease sleepiness
• At same time each day to maintain drug level
• Only for hormone imbalances; not to be used for obesity, male infertility, menstrual disorders, lethargy
• Lowest dose that relieves symptoms

Perform/provide:
• Removal of medication 4 wk before RAIU test

Evaluate:
• Therapeutic response: absence of depression; increased weight loss, diuresis, pulse, appetite; absence of constipation, peripheral edema, cold intolerance; pale, cool, dry skin; brittle nails, alopecia, coarse hair, menorrhagia, night blindness, paresthesias, syncope, stupor, coma, rosy cheeks

---

A Safety alert   *"Tall Man" lettering

Teach patient/family:
• That hair loss will occur in child, is temporary
• To report excitability, irritability, anxiety; indicates overdose
• Not to switch brands unless directed by prescriber
• That hypothyroid child will show almost immediate behavior/personality change
• That treatment drug is not to be taken to reduce weight
• To avoid OTC preparations with iodine; read labels
• To avoid iodine food, iodized salt, soybeans, tofu, turnips, some seafood, some bread

---

tiagabine (℞)
(tie-ah-ga'been)
Gabitril
Func. class.: Anticonvulsant

Action: Mechanism unknown; may increase seizure threshold; structurally similar to GABA; tiagabine binding sites in neocortex, hippocampus
Uses: Adjunct treatment of partial seizures

DOSAGE AND ROUTES

• *Adult:* **PO** 4 mg daily, may increase by 4-8 mg qwk until desired response, max 56 mg/day
• *Child 12-18 yr:* **PO** 4 mg daily, may increase by 4 mg at beginning of wk 2; may increase by 4-8 mg qwk until desired response; max 32 mg/day
Available forms: Tabs 2, 4, 12, 16 mg

SIDE EFFECTS

CNS: Dizziness, anxiety, somnolence, ataxia, confusion, *asthenia,* unsteady gait, depression
CV: Vasodilation
GI: Nausea, vomiting, diarrhea
INTEG: Pruritus, rash
RESP: Pharyngitis, coughing
Contraindications: Hypersensitivity to this drug

Precautions: Pregnancy (C), renal/hepatic disease, lactation, children <12 yr, geriatric

PHARMACOKINETICS

Absorption >95%, half-life 7-9 hr

INTERACTIONS

• Lower doses may be needed when used with valproate
Increase: CNS depression—CNS depressants
Decrease: effect—carbamazepine, phenobarbital, phenytoin, primidone
Drug/Food
• High-fat meal decreases rate of absorption

NURSING CONSIDERATIONS
Assess:
• Renal studies: urinalysis, BUN, urine creatinine q3mo
• Hepatic studies: ALT, AST, bilirubin
• Description of seizures: location, duration, presence of aura
• Mental status: mood, sensorium, affect, behavioral changes; if mental status changes, notify prescriber
Administer:
• With food
Perform/provide:
• Storage at room temperature away from heat and light
• Assistance with ambulation during early part of treatment; dizziness occurs
• Seizure precautions: padded side rails; move objects that may harm patient
Evaluate:
• Therapeutic response: decreased seizure activity; document on patient's chart
Teach patient/family:
• To carry emergency ID stating patient's name, drugs taken, condition, prescriber's name and phone number
• To avoid driving, other activities that require alertness
• Not to discontinue medication quickly after long-term use
• To take with food
Treatment of overdose: Lavage, VS

T

Side effects: *italics* = common; **bold** = life-threatening

ticarcillin (℞)

(tye-kar-sill'in)
Ticar
Func. class.: Broad-spectrum antiinfective
Chem. class.: Extended-spectrum penicillin

Action: Cell wall lysis mediated by cell wall autolytic enzymes

Uses: Respiratory, soft tissue, urinary tract infections, bacterial septicemia; effective for gram-positive cocci *(Staphylococcus aureus, Streptococcus faecalis, Streptococcus pneumoniae)*, gram-negative cocci *(Neisseria gonorrhoeae)*, gram-positive bacilli *(Clostridium perfringens, Clostridium tetani)*, gram-negative bacilli *(Bacteroides, Fusobacterium nucleatum, Escherichia coli, Proteus mirabilis, Salmonella, Morganella morganii, Proteus rettgeri, Enterobacter, Pseudomonas aeruginosa, Serratia)*; and *Peptococcus, Peptostreptococcus, Eubacterium*

DOSAGE AND ROUTES

Bacterial septicemia, respiratory, skin, soft tissue, intraabdominal, reproductive infections
• *Adult:* IV INF 200-300 mg/kg/day in divided doses q4-6h
• *Child <40 kg:* IV INF 33.3-50 mg/kg q4h or 50-75 mg/kg q6h
Urinary tract complicated infections
• *Adult and child:* IV INF 150-200 mg/kg/day in divided doses q4-6h
Uncomplicated urinary infections
• *Adult:* IV Direct/IM 1 g q6h
• *Child <40 kg:* IV Direct/IM 50-100 mg/kg/day q6-8h
Severe infections
(Pseudomonas, Proteus, E. coli)
• *Neonate:* IM/IV <2 kg: 75 mg/kg q8-12h; IM/IV >2 kg: 75-100 mg/kg q8h
Renal dose/hepatic dose
• CCr >60 ml/min 3 g q4h; CCr 30-60 ml/min 2 g q4h; CCr 10-30 ml/min 2 g q8h; CCr <10 ml/min 2 g q12h or 1 g q6h; CCr <10 ml/min and hepatic dysfunction 2 g q24h or 1 g q12h
Available forms: Inj 1, 3, 6, 20, 30 g

SIDE EFFECTS

CNS: Lethargy, hallucinations, anxiety, depression, twitching, **coma, seizures**
GI: Nausea, vomiting, diarrhea; increased AST, ALT; abdominal pain, glossitis, colitis, **pseudomembranous colitis**
GU: Oliguria, proteinuria, hematuria, *vaginitis, moniliasis,* **glomerulonephritis**
HEMA: Anemia, increased bleeding time, **bone marrow depression, granulocytopenia**
INTEG: Rash, **Stevens-Johnson syndrome**
META: Hypokalemia
SYST: **Anaphylaxis**
Contraindications: Hypersensitivity to penicillins
Precautions: Pregnancy (B), hypersensitivity to cephalosporins, lactation, renal/GI disease, diabetes, electrolyte imbalances

PHARMACOKINETICS

IM: Peak 1 hr, duration 4-6 hr
IV: Peak 30-45 min, duration 4 hr, half-life 70 min; small amount metabolized in liver; excreted in urine, breast milk

INTERACTIONS

Increase: effect of neuromuscular blockers, anticoagulants, methotrexate
Increase: ticarcillin concentrations—aspirin, probenecid
Decrease: effect—oral contraceptives, erythromycins
Decrease: antimicrobial effect of ticarcillin—tetracyclines, aminoglycosides IV
Drug/Herb
• Do not use acidophilus with antiinfectives; separate by several hours
Drug/Lab Test
False positive: Urine glucose, urine protein

⚠ Safety alert   *"Tall Man" lettering

NURSING CONSIDERATIONS
Assess:
• I&O ratio; report hematuria, oliguria, since penicillin in high doses is nephrotoxic

⚠ Any patient with compromised renal system, since drug is excreted slowly in poor renal system function; toxicity may occur rapidly

⚠ For anaphylaxis: wheezing, rash, pruritus, laryngeal edema, keep emergency equipment nearby

• Hepatic studies: AST, ALT
• Blood studies: WBC, RBC, Hgb, Hct, bleeding time
• Renal tests: urinalysis, protein, blood, BUN, creatinine
• C&S before drug therapy; drug may be given as soon as culture is taken
• Bowel pattern before, during treatment
• Skin eruptions after administration of penicillin to 1 wk after discontinuing drug
• Allergies before initiation of treatment, reaction of each medication

Administer:
• Drug after C&S has been completed
IM route
• Inject into well-developed muscle
• Reconstitute ticarcillin 1 g/2 ml sterile water for inj, NaCl inj, 1% lidocaine HCl without epINEPHrine (385 mg/ml)
IV route
• After diluting 1 g or less/4 ml sterile H$_2$O for inj; dilute further with 10-20 ml or more D$_5$W, NS, or sterile H$_2$O for inj sol; give 1 g or less/5 min or more or by intermittent inf over ½-2 hr or by continuous inf at prescribed rate
Y-site compatibilities: Acyclovir, allopurinol, amifostine, aztreonam, cisatracurium, cyclophosphamide, diltiazem, DOXOrubicin, famotidine, filgrastim, fludarabine, granisetron, heparin, hydromorphone, IL-2, insulin (regular), magnesium sulfate, melphalan, meperidine, morphine, ondansetron, perphenazine, propofol, remifentanil, sargramostim, teniposide, theophylline, thiotepa, verapamil, vinorelbine

Perform/provide:
• EpINEPHrine, suction, tracheostomy set, endotracheal intubation equipment
• Adequate fluid intake (2 L) during diarrhea episodes
• Scratch test to assess allergy on order from prescriber; done when penicillin is only drug of choice
• Storage at room temperature, reconstituted sol 72 hr at room temperature
Evaluate:
• Therapeutic response: absence of fever, purulent drainage, redness, inflammation
Teach patient/family:
• That culture may be taken after completed course of medication
• To report sore throat, fever, fatigue (may indicate superinfection)
• To wear or carry emergency ID if allergic to penicillins
• To notify nurse of diarrhea
Treatment of overdose: Withdraw drug, maintain airway, administer epINEPHrine, aminophylline, O$_2$, IV corticosteroids for anaphylaxis

---

ticarcillin/ clavulanate (℞)

Timentin
Func. class.: Broad-spectrum antiinfective
Chem. class.: Extended-spectrum penicillin

Action: Interferes with cell wall replication of susceptible organisms; osmotically unstable cell wall swells, bursts from osmotic pressure; clavulanate inhibits β-lactamase and protects against enzymatic degradation of ticarcillin
Uses: Respiratory, soft tissue, and urinary tract infections, bacterial septicemia; effective for gram-positive cocci (*Staphylococcus aureus, Streptococcus faecalis, Streptococcus pneumoniae*), gram-negative cocci (*Neisseria gonorrhoeae*), gram-positive bacilli (*Clostridium perfringens, Clostridium tetani*),

---

gram-negative bacilli *(Bacteroides, Fusobacterium nucleatum, Escherichia coli, Proteus mirabilis, Salmonella, Morganella morganii, Proteus rettgeri, Enterobacter, Pseudomonas aeruginosa, Serratia);* and *Peptococcus, Peptostreptococcus, Eubacterium*

DOSAGE AND ROUTES

Systemic/urinary tract infections, serious infections
- *Adult ≥60 kg:* **IV INF** 3.1 g q4-6h
- *Adult <60 kg:* **IV INF** 200-300 mg/kg/day q4-6h
- *Child >60 kg:* **IV INF** 3.1 g q4h
- *Child <60 kg:* **IV INF** 300 mg/kg/day q4h

Mild/moderate infections
- *Child ≥60 kg:* **IV INF** 3.1 g q6h
- *Child <60 kg:* **IV INF** 200 mg/kg/day q6h

Renal dose
- *Adult:* **IV INF** loading dose 3.1 g; CCr 60 ml/min 3.1 g q4h; CCr 30-60 ml/min 2 g q4h; CCr 10-30 ml/min 2 g q8h; CCr <10 ml/min 2 g q12h; CCr <10 ml/min with hepatic dysfunction 2 g q24h

Available forms: Inj 3 g ticarcillin, 0.1 g clavulanate; IV inf 3 g ticarcillin, 0.1 g clavulanate; powder for inj 3 g ticarcillin, 0.1 g clavulanate

SIDE EFFECTS

CNS: Lethargy, hallucinations, anxiety, depression, twitching, **coma, seizures**
GI: Nausea, vomiting, diarrhea; increased AST, ALT; abdominal pain, glossitis, colitis, **pseudomembranous colitis**
GU: Oliguria, proteinuria, hematuria, *vaginitis, moniliasis,* **glomerulonephritis**
HEMA: Anemia, increased bleeding time, **bone marrow depression, granulocytopenia**
META: Hyperkalemia, hypokalemia, alkalosis, hypernatremia
SYST: **Anaphylaxis, Stevens-Johnson syndrome**
Contraindications: Hypersensitivity to penicillins; neonates

Precautions: Pregnancy (B), hypersensitivity to cephalosporins, renal disease

PHARMACOKINETICS

IV: Peak 30-45 min, duration 4 hr, half-life 64-68 min; excreted in urine

INTERACTIONS

Increase: bleeding—anticoagulants
Increase: methotrexate level—methotrexate
Increase: effect of neuromuscular blockers, heparin
Increase: ticarcillin concentrations—aspirin, probenecid
Decrease: antimicrobial effect of ticarcillin—tetracyclines, aminoglycosides IV
Decrease: effect—oral contraceptives, erythromycin
Drug/Herb
- Do not use acidophilus with antiinfectives; separate by several hours
Drug/Lab Test
False positive: Urine glucose, urine protein, Coombs' test

NURSING CONSIDERATIONS

Assess:
- I&O ratio; report hematuria, oliguria, since penicillin in high doses is nephrotoxic
- ⚠ For pseudomembranous colitis; Stevens-Johnson syndrome
- ⚠ Any patient with compromised renal system, since drug is excreted slowly in poor renal system function; toxicity may occur rapidly
- ⚠ For anaphylaxis: wheezing, rash, laryngeal edema; have emergency equipment nearby
- Hepatic studies: AST, ALT
- Blood studies: WBC, RBC, Hct, Hgb, bleeding time
- Renal studies: urinalysis, protein, blood, BUN, creatinine
- C&S before drug therapy; drug may be given as soon as culture is taken
- Bowel pattern before, during treatment
- Skin eruptions after administration of penicillin to 1 wk after discontinuing drug

⚠ Safety alert   *"Tall Man" lettering

- Allergies before initiation of treatment, reaction of each medication

Administer:

- Drug after C&S

IV route

- After diluting 3.1 g or less/13 ml of sterile H_2O or NaCl (200 mg/ml), shake; may further dilute in 50-100 ml or more NS, D_5W, or LR sol and run over ½ hr

Y-site compatibilities: Allopurinol, amifostine, aztreonam, cefepime, cyclophosphamide, diltiazem, DOXOrubicin liposome, famotidine, filgrastim, fluconazole, fludarabine, foscarnet, gallium, granisetron, heparin, insulin (regular), melphalan, meperidine, morphine, ondansetron, perphenazine, propofol, remifentanil, sargramostim, teniposide, theophylline, thiotepa, vinorelbine

Perform/provide:

- EpINEPHrine, suction, tracheostomy set, endotracheal intubation equipment
- Adequate fluid intake (2 L) during diarrhea episodes
- Scratch test to assess allergy on order from prescriber; usually done when penicillin is only drug of choice
- Storage of reconstituted sol 12-24 hr at room temperature, or 3-7 days refrigerated

Evaluate:

- Therapeutic response: absence of fever, purulent drainage, redness, inflammation

Teach patient/family:

- To report persistent diarrhea
- That culture may be taken after completed course of medication
- To report sore throat, fever, fatigue (may indicate superinfection)
- To wear or carry emergency ID if allergic to penicillins

Treatment of overdose: Withdraw drug, maintain airway, administer epINEPHrine, O_2, IV corticosteroids for anaphylaxis

ticlopidine (R)

(tye-cloe'pi-deen)
Ticlid
Func. class.: Platelet aggregation inhibitor
Chem. class.: Thienopyridine compound

Action: Irreversible inhibition of platelet aggregation through antagonism of ADP

Uses: Reducing the risk of stroke in high-risk patients

Unlabeled uses: Intermittent claudication, chronic arterial occlusion, subarachnoid hemorrhage, uremic patients with AV shunts/fistulas, open heart surgery, coronary artery bypass grafts, primary glomerulonephritis, sickle cell disease, diabetic retinopathy

DOSAGE AND ROUTES

- *Adult:* **PO** 250 mg bid with food

Available forms: Tabs 250 mg

SIDE EFFECTS

CNS: Dizziness
GI: Nausea, vomiting, *diarrhea*, GI discomfort, **cholestatic jaundice, hepatitis,** increased cholesterol, LDL, VLDL, triglycerides
HEMA: **Bleeding (epistaxis, hematuria, conjunctival hemorrhage, GI bleeding), agranulocytosis, neutropenia, thrombocytopenia, thrombotic thombocytopenic purpura**
INTEG: **Rash,** pruritus

Contraindications: Hypersensitivity, severe hepatic disease, blood dyscrasias, active bleeding, coagulopathy

Precautions: Pregnancy (B), past hepatic disease, renal disease, geriatric, lactation, children, increased bleeding risk, anemia, peptic ulcer disease, surgery

PHARMACOKINETICS

Peak 1-3 hr, metabolized by liver, excreted in urine, feces; half-life increases with repeated dosing, initially 12-36 hr, antiplatelet effect 2-5 days, 98% protein binding

INTERACTIONS

Increase: levels of phenytoin

Increase: bleeding tendencies—anticoagulants, salicylates, thrombolytics, NSAIDs, abciximab, eptifibatide, tirofiban, ticlopidine

Increase: effects of ticlopidine—cimetidine

Increase: effects of theophylline

Decrease: plasma levels of ticlopidine—antacids

Decrease: plasma levels of digoxin

NURSING CONSIDERATIONS

Assess:
• Hepatic studies: AST, ALT, bilirubin, creatinine (long-term therapy)
⚠ Blood studies: CBC; CBC q2wk × 3 mo, Hct, Hgb, PT (long-term therapy)
⚠ Bleed time baseline and throughout, levels may be 2-5 × normal limit

Administer:
• With food to decrease gastric symptoms

Evaluate:
• Therapeutic response: absence of stroke

Teach patient/family:
• That blood work will be necessary during treatment
• To report any unusual bleeding to prescriber
• To report side effects such as diarrhea, skin rashes, subcutaneous bleeding, signs of cholestasis (jaundiced skin and sclera, dark urine, light-colored stools)

---

tigecycline (℞)
(tye-ge-sye′kleen)
Tygacil
Func. class.: Broad-spectrum antiinfective
Chem. class.: Glycylcyclines

Action: Inhibits protein synthesis and phosphorylation in microorganisms; bacteriostatic structurally similar to the tetracyclines

Uses: Complicated skin/skin structure infections (*Escherichia coli, Enterococcus faecalis* (vancomycin-susceptible only) *Staphylococcus aureus, Streptococcus agalactiae, S. anginosus* group, *S. pyogenes, Bacteroides fragilis;* complicated intraabdominal infections *(Citrobacter freundii) Enterobacter cloacae, E. coli, Klebsiella oxytoca, K. pneumoniae, E. faecalis* (vancomycin-susceptible only), *S. aureus* (methicillin-susceptible only), *S. anginosus* group, *B. fragilis, Bacteroides thetaiotaomicron, B. uniformis, B. vulgatus, Clostridium perfringens, Peptostreptococcus micros*

DOSAGE AND ROUTES

• *Adult:* **IV** 100 mg, then 50 mg q12h, **IV INF** is given over 30-60 min q12h; given for 5-14 days depending on infection

Hepatic dose (Child-Pugh C)
• *Adult:* **IV** 100 mg, then 25 mg q12h

Available forms: Powder for inj, lyophilized 50 mg

SIDE EFFECTS

CNS: Headache, dizziness, insomnia
CV: Hyper/hypotension, phlebitis
GI: Nausea, vomiting, diarrhea, anorexia, constipation, dyspepsia
HEMA: **Anemia, leukocytosis, thrombocytopenia**
INTEG: Rash, pruritus, sweating, photosensitivity
META: Increased ALT, AST, BUN, lactic acid, alk phos, amylase, hyperglycemia, hypokalemia, hypoproteinemia, bilirubinemia

---

MISC: Back pain, fever, abnormal healing, abdominal pain, abscess, asthenia, infection, pain, peripheral edema, local reactions

RESP: Cough, dyspnea

Contraindications: Pregnancy (D), hypersensitivity to tigecycline, children <18 yr, lactation

Precautions: Renal/hepatic disease, hypersensitivity to tetracyclines

PHARMACOKINETICS

Not extensively metabolized, 22% of unchanged drug is excretion in urine, terminal half-life 42 hr, primarily biliary excreted

INTERACTIONS

Increase: effect of warfarin
Decrease: effect of oral contraceptives

NURSING CONSIDERATIONS

Assess:

⚠ For pseudomembranous colitis
• Signs of anemia: Hct, Hgb, fatigue
• Blood studies: PT, CBC, AST, ALT, BUN creatinine
• Allergic reactions: rash, itching, pruritus, angioedema
• Nausea, vomiting, diarrhea; administer antiemetic, antacids as ordered
• Overgrowth of infection: fever, malaise, redness, pain, swelling, drainage, perineal itching, diarrhea, changes in cough or sputum

Administer:
• After C&S obtained

IV route
• Reconstitute each vial with 5.3 ml of 0.9% NaCl, or D_5 (10 mg/ml); swirl to dissolve; immediately withdraw 5 ml of the reconstituted sol and add to a 100-ml IV bag for inf (1 mg/ml); may be yellow or orange, if not, sol should be discarded; do not give if particulate matter is present

Perform/provide:
• Storage in tight, light-resistant container at room temperature

Evaluate:
• Therapeutic response: decreased temp, absence of lesions, negative C&S

Teach patient/family:
• To avoid sun exposure; sunscreen does not seem to decrease photosensitivity
• To avoid pregnancy while taking this product; fetal harm may occur

---

tiludronate (℞)

(till-oo′droe-nate)
Skelid
Func. class.: Bone resorption inhibitor
Chem. class.: Bisphosphonate

Action: Decreases bone resorption and new bone development

Uses: Paget's disease in those with alk phos at 2× upper limit, patients at risk for future complications of Paget's disease

DOSAGE AND ROUTES

• *Adult:* **PO** 400 mg daily, with 8 oz water × 3 mo

Available forms: Tabs 240 mg (equivalent to 200 mg tiludronic acid)

SIDE EFFECTS

CNS: Headache, somnolence, dizziness, anxiety, vertigo, nervousness, involuntary movements

CV: Chest pain, edema, hypertension, peripheral edema

ENDO: Hyperparathyroidism

GI: Nausea, diarrhea, dry mouth, gastritis, vomiting, flatulence, gastric ulcers, gastritis, dyspepsia

GU: **Nephrotoxicity,** UTI

INTEG: Rash, epidermal necrosis, pruritus, sweating

MS: Bone pain, decreased mineralization of nonaffected bones, pathologic fractures

RESP: Rhinitis, bronchitis, crackles, sinusitis, URI

Contraindications: Hypersensitivity to bisphosphonates, severe renal disease with creatinine >5 mg/dl

T

Precautions: Pregnancy (C), renal/GI disease, lactation, restricted vit D/calcium

PHARMACOKINETICS

Onset up to several wk, protein binding 90%, excreted by kidneys; half-life 150 hr

INTERACTIONS

Increase: tiludronate effect—indomethacin

Decrease: tiludronate absorption—antacids, mineral supplements with magnesium, calcium, aluminum, aspirin, separate by ≥2 hr

NURSING CONSIDERATIONS

Assess:

• GI symptoms, polyuria, flushing, head swelling, tingling, headache—may indicate hypercalcemia; nervousness, irritability, twitching, seizures, spasm, paresthesia indicates hypocalcemia at start of treatment

• Nutritional status; evaluate diet for sources of vit D (milk, some seafood), calcium (dairy products, dark green vegetables), phosphates

• BUN, creatinine, uric acid, chloride, electrolytes, urine pH, urinary calcium, magnesium, phosphate, urinalysis (calcium should be kept at 9-10 mg/dl), albumin, alk phos baseline and q3-6mo; check urine sediment for casts throughout treatment

• For increased drug level—toxic reactions occur rapidly; have calcium chloride or gluconate on hand if calcium level drops too low; check for tetany

Administer:

• On empty stomach to improve absorption (2 hr before meals), with 6-8 oz water

• Take calcium or mineral supplements 2 hr before or 2 hr after tiludronate

• Take aluminum or magnesium antacids ≥2 hr after tiludronate

• Do not take indomethacin within 2 hr

• Tabs from foil strip immediately before use

Evaluate:

• Therapeutic response: calcium levels 9-10 mg/dl; decreasing symptoms of Paget's disease

Teach patient/family:

• To notify prescriber of hypercalcemic relapse: renal calculi, nausea, vomiting, thirst, lethargy, deep bone or flank pain

• To follow a low-calcium diet as prescribed (Paget's disease, hypercalcemia)

• To notify prescriber of diarrhea, nausea; dose may be divided to lessen these symptoms

---

timolol (℞)

(tye'moe-lole)

Apo-Timol ✦, Blocadren, Novo-Timol ✦, timolol maleate

Func. class.: Antihypertensive

Chem. class.: Nonselective β-blocker

Do not confuse:

Timoptic/Viroptic

Action: Competitively blocks stimulation of β-adrenergic receptor within vascular smooth muscle (decreases rate of SA node discharge, increases recovery time), slows conduction of AV node, decreases heart rate, which decreases O_2 consumption in myocardium; also decreases renin-aldosterone-angiotensin system, at high doses inhibits $β_2$-receptors in bronchial system

Uses: Mild to moderate hypertension, migraine prophylaxis

Unlabeled uses: Mitral valve prolapse, hypertrophic cardiomyopathy, thyrotoxicosis, tremors, anxiety, pheochromocytoma, tachydysrhythmias, angina pectoris

DOSAGE AND ROUTES

Hypertension

• *Adult:* **PO** 10 mg bid, or 20 mg daily, may increase by 10 mg q7d, not to exceed 60 mg/day

Myocardial infarction

• *Adult:* **PO** 10 mg bid beginning 1-4 wk after MI

Migraine headache prevention
• *Adult:* **PO** 10 mg bid or 20 mg daily; may increase to 30 mg/day, 20 mg in AM, 10 mg in PM, discontinue if not effective after 8 wk

Available forms: Tabs 5, 10, 20 mg

SIDE EFFECTS

CNS: Insomnia, dizziness, hallucinations, anxiety, fatigue, depression, headache

CV: Hypotension, bradycardia, **CHF,** edema, chest pain, claudication, angina, AV block, ventricular dysrhythmias

EENT: Visual changes, sore throat, *double vision,* dry burning eyes

GI: Nausea, vomiting, **ischemic colitis,** diarrhea, *abdominal pain,* **mesenteric arterial thrombosis,** flatulence, constipation

GU: Impotence, urinary frequency

HEMA: **Agranulocytosis, thrombocytopenia, purpura**

INTEG: Rash, alopecia, pruritus, fever

META: Hypoglycemia

MUSC: Joint pain, muscle pain

RESP: **Bronchospasm,** *dyspnea,* cough, crackles, nasal stuffiness

Contraindications: Hypersensitivity to β-blockers, cardiogenic shock, heart block (2nd or 3rd degree), sinus bradycardia, CHF, cardiac failure, severe COPD, asthma

Precautions: Pregnancy (C), major surgery, lactation, diabetes mellitus, COPD, well-compensated heart failure, CAD, non-allergic bronchospasm, peripheral vascular disease, hepatic/renal/thyroid disease

PHARMACOKINETICS

PO: Peak 1-2 hr; half-life 4 hr; metabolized by liver; excreted in urine, breast milk, protein binding <10%

INTERACTIONS

Increase: hypotension, bradycardia—reserpine, hydrALAZINE, methyldopa, prazosin, anticholinergics, alcohol, reserpine, nitrates

Increase: effects of β-blockers, calcium channel blockers

Decrease: antihypertensive effects—NSAIDs, sympathomimetics, thyroid, salicylates

Decrease: hypoglycemic effects—insulin, sulfonylureas

Decrease: bronchodilation—theophyllines

Drug/Herb

Increase: toxicity, death—aconite

Increase: antihypertensive effect—barberry, betony, black catechu, black cohosh, bloodroot, broom, burdock, cat's claw, dandelion, goldenseal, hawthorn, Irish moss, Jamaican dogwood, kelp, khella, mistletoe, parsley

Increase or decrease: antihypertensive effect—astragalus, cola tree

Decrease: antihypertensive effect—coltsfoot, guarana, khat, licorice, yohimbine

Drug/Lab Test

Increase: Renal, hepatic studies, potassium, uric acid

Decrease: Hct, Hgb, HDL

Interference: Glucose, insulin tolerance test

NURSING CONSIDERATIONS

Assess:

• Headaches: location, severity, duration, frequency baseline and throughout treatment

• I&O, weight daily

• B/P during initial treatment, periodically thereafter, pulse q4h; note rate, rhythm, quality

• Apical/radial pulse before administration; notify prescriber of any significant changes

• Baselines in renal, hepatic studies before therapy begins

• Edema in feet, legs daily

• Skin turgor, dryness of mucous membranes for hydration status

Administer:

• PO before or immediately after meals, at bedtime; tablet may be crushed or swallowed whole

• Reduced dosage in renal dysfunction

T

Perform/provide:

• Dry storage at room temperature; do not freeze

Evaluate:

• Therapeutic response: decreased B/P after 1-2 wk

Teach patient/family:

• To take before or immediately after meals

• Not to discontinue drug abruptly; taper over 2 wk; may cause precipitate angina

• Not to use OTC products containing α-adrenergic stimulants (nasal decongestants, cold preparations) unless directed by prescriber

• To report bradycardia, dizziness, confusion, depression, fever, sore throat, shortness of breath to prescriber

• To take pulse at home; advise when to notify prescriber

• To avoid alcohol, smoking, sodium intake

• To comply with weight control, dietary adjustments, modified exercise program

• To carry emergency ID to identify drug, allergies

• To avoid hazardous activities if dizziness is present

• To report symptoms of CHF: difficulty breathing, especially on exertion or when lying down; night cough; swelling of extremities

• To take medication at bedtime and wear support hose to minimize effect of orthostatic hypotension

Treatment of overdose: Lavage, IV atropine for bradycardia, IV theophylline for bronchospasm, digoxin, O_2, diuretic for cardiac failure, hemodialysis; administer vasopressor (norepinephrine)

---

timolol ophthalmic
See Appendix C

---

tinidazole (Ⓡ)
(tye-ni′da-zole)
Tindamax
Func. class.: Antiprotozoal
Chem. class.: Nitroimidazole derivative

Action: Interferes with DNA/RNA synthesis in protozoa

Uses: Amebiasis, giardiasis, trichomoniasis

DOSAGE AND ROUTES

Amebiasis

• *Adult:* **PO** 2 g/day × 3-5 days

• *Child >3 yr:* **PO** 50 mg/kg/day × 3-5 days, max 2 g

Giardiasis

• *Adult:* **PO** 2 g as a single dose

• *Child >3 yr:* **PO** 50 mg/kg as a single dose, max 2 g

Trichomoniasis

• *Adult:* **PO** 2 g as a single dose

Available forms: Tabs 250, 500 mg

SIDE EFFECTS

CNS: Dizziness, headache, **seizures,** *peripheral neuropathy*

GI: Nausea, vomiting, anorexia, increased AST and ALT, constipation, abdominal pain

HEMA: **Leukopenia,** neutropenia

INTEG: Pruritus, urticaria, *rash,* oral monilia

SYST: **Angioedema**

Contraindications: Hypersensitivity to this product or nitroimidazole derivative, pregnancy 1st trimester

Precautions: Pregnancy (C), hepatic disease, lactation, children, geriatric, CNS depression

PHARMACOKINETICS

Metabolized extensively in the liver; excreted unchanged (20%-25%) in urine, (12%) feces; half-life 12-14 hr; crosses blood-brain barrier

---

INTERACTIONS

• Do not use within 2 wk of taking disulfiram
• CYP3A4 inducers (phenobarbital, rifampin, phenytoin); cholestyramine, oxytetracycline: decrease action of tinidazole
• CYP3A4 inhibitors (cimetidine, ketoconazole): increase action of tinidazole
Increase: action of anticoagulants, cycloSPORINE, tacrolimus, fluorouracil, hydantoins, lithium

NURSING CONSIDERATIONS
Assess:
• Signs of infection, anemia
• Bowel pattern before, during treatment
Administer:
• To those over 3 yr old
• With food to increase plasma concentrations, minimize epigastric distress and other GI effects
Evaluate:
• Therapeutic response: decreased in infection as evidenced by negative culture
Teach patient/family:
• To take with food to increase plasma concentrations, minimize epigastric distress and other GI effects; not to use alcoholic beverages during or for 3 days afterward
• Trichomoniasis: both partners should be treated

⚠ High Alert

tinzaparin (℞)
(tin-zay-par'in)
Innohep
Func. class.: Anticoagulant
Chem. class.: Unfractionated porcine heparin

Action: Increases the inhibitory effect of antithrombin factor Xa, thrombin
Uses: Treatment of deep vein thrombosis, pulmonary emboli after abdominal, knee, hip surgery or knee, hip replacement

DOSAGE AND ROUTES
Treatment of deep vein thrombosis
• *Adult:* SUBCUT 175 anti-Xa international units/kg daily ≥6 days and until adequate anticoagulation with warfarin (therapeutic INR ≥2 for 2 consecutive days)
Prophylaxis of deep vein thrombosis
• *Adult:* 3500 anti-Xa units (50 anti-Xa units/kg) daily beginning 1-2 hr prior to surgery and continued for 5-10 days
Prophylaxis of deep vein thrombosis in orthopedic procedures
• *Adult:* 75 anti-Xa units/kg/day started 12-24 hr after surgery
Available forms: Inj 20,000 international units/1 ml

SIDE EFFECTS
CNS: Fever, confusion, dizziness, insomnia
CV: Angina, dysrhythmias, peripheral edema, tachycardia, hyper/hypotension
GI: Nausea, constipation, flatulence, dyspepsia, **hepatitis**
GU: UTI, hematuria, urinary retention, dysuria
HEMA: Hemorrhage, **anemia, thrombocytopenia,** bleeding
INTEG: Ecchymosis, inj site reaction
MISC: Headache, chest pain, hypersensitivity

Contraindications: Hypersensitivity to this drug, heparin, pork or benzyl alcohol, sulfites; hemophilia, leukemia with bleeding, peptic ulcer disease, thrombocytopenic purpura, heparin-induced thrombocytopenia
Precautions: Pregnancy (B), alcoholism, geriatric, hepatic disease (severe), renal disease (severe), blood dyscrasias, severe, uncontrolled hypertension, subacute bacterial endocarditis, acute nephritis, lactation, children

PHARMACOKINETICS
Maximum antithrombin activity (3-5 hr), elimination half-life 4.5 hr

INTERACTIONS

• Do not mix with other drugs or infusion fluids

Increase: action of tinzaparin—oral anticoagulants, salicylates, thrombolytics, NSAIDs, platelet inhibitors, ticlopidine

Drug/Herb

Increase: risk of bleeding—agrimony, alfalfa, angelica, anise, basil, bay, bilberry, black haw, bogbean, bromelain, buchu, chondroitin, cinchona bark, dong quai, fenugreek, feverfew, garlic, ginger, ginkgo, ginseng, horse chestnut, Irish moss, kelp, kelpware, khella, lovage, lungwort, meadowsweet, motherwort, mugwort, nettle, papaya, parsley (large amts), pau d'arco, pineapple, poplar, prickly ash, safflower, saw palmetto, tonka bean, turmeric, wintergreen, yarrow

Decrease: anticoagulant effect—chamomile, coenzyme Q10, flax, glucomannan, goldenseal, guar gum

NURSING CONSIDERATIONS

Assess:

• Blood studies (Hct, platelets, occult blood in stools), anti-Xa; thrombocytopenia may occur

• Bleeding gums, petechiae, ecchymosis, black tarry stools, hematuria, decreased Hct, Hgb

• For hypersensitivity (fever, urticaria, chills) report to prescriber

• For inj site reactions and neurologic changes in epidural catheters

Administer:

• Only after screening patient for bleeding disorders

• SUBCUT only; do not give IM

• To recumbent patient; give SUBCUT; rotate inj sites (left/right anterolateral, left-right posterolateral abdominal wall)

• Insert whole length of needle into skin fold held with thumb and forefinger

⚠ Only this drug when ordered; not interchangeable with heparin or LMWHs

• At same time each day to maintain steady blood levels

• Do not massage area or aspirate when giving SUBCUT inj

• Avoiding all IM inj that may cause bleeding

Perform/provide:

• Storage at 77° F (25° C); do not freeze

Evaluate:

• Therapeutic response: resolution of deep vein thrombosis

Teach patient/family:

• To use soft-bristle toothbrush to avoid bleeding gums, to use electric razor

• To report any signs of bleeding: gums, under skin, urine, stools

Treatment of overdose: Protamine 1 mg/100 anti-Xa international units of tinzaparin

---

tioconazole vaginal antifungal
See Appendix C

---

tiotropium (Rx)
(ty-oh'tro-pee-um)
Spiriva
Func. class.: Anticholinergic, bronchodilator
Chem. class.: Synthetic quaternary ammonium compound

Action: Inhibits interaction of acetylcholine at receptor sites on the bronchial smooth muscle, resulting in decreased cGMP and bronchodilation

Uses: COPD, for long-term treatment, once-daily maintenance of bronchospasm, associated with COPD, including chronic bronchitis and emphysema

DOSAGE AND ROUTES

• *Adult:* **INH** content of 1 cap daily using HandiHaler inhalation device

Available forms: Powder for inhalation 18 mcg in blister packs containing 6 caps with inhaler; 30 caps with inhaler

SIDE EFFECTS

CNS: Depression, paresthesia
CV: Chest pain, increased heart rate

⚠ Safety alert   *"Tall Man" lettering

EENT: Dry mouth, blurred vision, glaucoma

GI: Vomiting, abdominal pain, constipation, dyspepsia

INTEG: Rash

MISC: Urinary difficulty, urinary retention

RESP: Cough, worsening of symptoms, sinusitis, upper respiratory tract infection, epistaxis, pharyngitis

Contraindications: Hypersensitivity to this drug, atropine or its derivatives

Precautions: Pregnancy (C), lactation, children, narrow-angle glaucoma, prostatic hypertrophy, bladder neck obstruction, geriatric, renal disease

PHARMACOKINETICS

Half-life 5-6 days in animals; does not cross blood-brain barrier, very little metabolized in the liver, excreted in urine

INTERACTIONS

• Anticholinergics: avoid use with other anticholinergics

Drug/Herb

Increase: constipation—black catechu

Increase: anticholinergic effect—butterbur, jimsonweed

Increase: bronchodilator effect—green tea (large amounts), guarana

Decrease: anticholinergic effect—jaborandi tree, pill-bearing spurge

NURSING CONSIDERATIONS

Assess:

• For tolerance over long-term therapy; dose may have to be increased or changed

• For patient's ability to use HandiHaler

Administer:

• Caps are for INH only; do not swallow

• Immediately before administration, peel back foil until cap is visible and until "stop" line; remove cap from blister cavity; open dust cap of HandiHaler by pulling upward, then open mouthpiece; place cap in center chamber; firmly close mouthpiece until it clicks, leaving dust cap open

• When finished taking dose, remove used capsule and dispose; close the mouthpiece and dust cap; store

Evaluate:

• Therapeutic response: ability to breathe easier

Teach patient/family:

• Signs of narrow-angle glaucoma

• That drug is used for long-term maintenance, not for immediate relief of breathing problems

• To avoid getting the powder in the eyes; may cause blurred vision and pupil dilation

• Hold HandiHaler with mouthpiece upward; press button in once, completely, and release; this allows for medication to be released

• Breathe out completely; do not breathe into mouthpiece at any time

• Raise device to mouth and close lips tightly around mouthpiece

• With head upright, breathe in slowly/deeply, but allow the cap to vibrate; breathe until lungs fill; hold breath and remove mouthpiece; resume normal breathing

• Repeat

---

tipranavir (℞)
(ti-pran'a-veer)
Aptivus
Func. class.: Antiretroviral
Chem. class.: Protease inhibitor

Action: Inhibits human immunodeficiency virus (HIV) protease; this prevents the maturation of virus

Uses: HIV in combination with other antiretrovirals

DOSAGE AND ROUTES

• Reduce dose in mild/moderate hepatic impairment and ketoconazole coadministration

• *Adult:* **PO** 500 mg coadministered with ritonavir 200 mg bid with food

Available forms: Caps 250 mg

SIDE EFFECTS

CNS: Headache, insomnia, dizziness, somnolence, fatigue

GI: Diarrhea, abdominal pain, nausea, vomiting, anorexia, dry mouth, **hepatitis B or C, fatalities when given with ritonavir**

GU: Nephrolithiasis

INTEG: Rash

MS: Pain

OTHER: Asthenia, **insulin-resistant hyperglycemia,** hyperlipidemia, **ketoacidosis**

Contraindications: Hypersensitivity, hepatic disease (Child-Pugh B to C)

Precautions: Pregnancy (C), lactation, children, renal disease, history of renal stones, sulfa allergy, hemophilia, diabetes mellitus

PHARMACOKINETICS

Terminal half-life 6 hr, plasma protein binding 99.9%, steady state 7-10 days, metabolism CYP3A4, 80% fecal excretion

INTERACTIONS

⚠ Life-threatening dysrhythmias: ergots, midazolam, rifampin, triazolam

Increase: myopathy—lovastatin, simvastatin

Increase: tipranavir levels—ketoconazole, delavirdine, itraconazole

Increase: levels of both drugs—clarithromycin, zidovudine

Increase: levels of isoniazid—oral contraception

Decrease: tipranavir levels—rifamycins, fluconazole, nevirapine, efavirenz

Drug/Herb

Decrease: tipranavir levels—St. John's wort; avoid concurrent use

Drug/Food

Decrease: tipranavir absorption—grapefruit juice, high-fat, high-protein foods

NURSING CONSIDERATIONS

Assess:

• For complaints of lower back, flank pain, indicates kidney stones

• Signs of infection, anemia, the presence of other sexually transmitted diseases

• Hepatic studies: ALT, AST; total bilirubin, amylase, all may be elevated

• Viral load, CD4 during treatment

• Bowel pattern before, during treatment; if severe abdominal pain with bleeding occurs, drug should be discontinued; monitor hydration

• Skin eruptions; rash, urticaria, itching

• Allergies before treatment, reaction of each medication; place allergies on chart

Administer:

• Swallow cap whole; do not break, crush, or chew

• After meals

• In equal intervals around the clock to maintain blood levels

Teach patient/family:

• To take as prescribed; if dose is missed, take as soon as remembered up to 1 hr before next dose; do not double dose

• That drug must be taken in equal intervals around the clock to maintain blood levels for duration of therapy

⚠ That hyperglycemia may occur; watch for increased thirst, weight loss, hunger, dry, itchy skin; notify prescriber

• To increase fluids to prevent kidney stones, if stone formation occurs, treatment may need to be interrupted

• That drug does not cure AIDS, only controls symptoms; not to donate blood

---

⚠ High Alert

tirofiban (℞)

(tie-roh-fee'ban)

Aggrastat

Func. class.: Antiplatelet

Chem. class.: Glycoprotein IIb/IIIa inhibitor

Action: Antagonist of platelet glycoprotein (GP) IIb/IIIa receptor that leads to binding of fibrinogen and von Willebrand's factor, which inhibits platelet aggregation

Uses: Acute coronary syndrome in combination with heparin

DOSAGE AND ROUTES

• *Adult:* **IV** 0.4 mcg/kg/min × 30 min, then 0.1 mcg/kg/min for 12-24 hr after angioplasty or atherectomy

Renal dose

• *Adult:* **IV** CCr <30 ml/min 0.2 mcg/kg/min × 30 min, then 0.05 mcg/kg/min, during angiography and for up to 24 hr after angioplasty

Available forms: Inj for sol 250 mcg/ml, inj 50 mcg/ml

SIDE EFFECTS

CNS: Dizziness, headache

CV: Bradycardia, hypotension

GI: Nausea, vomiting

HEMA: **Bleeding, thrombocytopenia**

INTEG: Rash

OTHER: Dissection, coronary artery edema, pain in legs/pelvis, sweating

Contraindications: Hypersensitivity, active internal bleeding, stroke, major surgery, severe trauma, intracranial neoplasm, aneurysm, hemorrhage, acute pericarditis, platelets <100,000/mm³, history of thrombocytopenia, coagulopathy

Precautions: Pregnancy (B), lactation, geriatric, renal disease, bleeding tendencies, children, hypertension

Pharmocokinetics: Half-life 2 hr, excretion via urine/feces; plasma clearance 20%-25% lower in geriatric with coronary artery disease; renal insufficiency decreases plasma clearance

INTERACTIONS

Increase: bleeding—aspirin, heparin, NSAIDs, abciximab, eptifibatide, clopidogrel, ticlopidine, dipyridamole, cefamandole, cefotetan, cefoperazone, valproic acid

Drug/Herb

Increase: risk of bleeding—agrimony, alfalfa, angelica, anise, basil, bay, bilberry, black haw, bogbean, bromelain, buchu, chondroitin, cinchona bark, dong quai, fenugreek, feverfew, garlic, ginger, ginkgo, ginseng, green tea, horse chestnut, Irish moss, kelp, kelpware, khella, lovage, lungwort, meadowsweet, motherwort, mugwort, nettle, papaya, parsley (large amts), pau d'arco, pineapple, poplar, prickly ash, safflower, saw palmetto, tonka bean, turmeric, wintergreen, yarrow

Decrease: anticoagulant effect—chamomile, coenzyme Q10, flax, glucomannan, goldenseal, guar gum

NURSING CONSIDERATIONS

Assess:

⚠ Platelet counts, Hct, Hgb, prior to treatment, within 6 hr of loading dose and at least daily thereafter; watch for bleeding from puncture sites, catheters or in stools, urine

Administer:

IV route

• Dilute inj: withdraw and discard 100 ml from a 500-ml bag of sterile 0.9% NaCl or D₅W and replace this vol with 100 ml of tirofiban inj from two vials

• Tirofiban inj for sol is premixed in containers of 500-ml 0.9% NaCl (50 mg/ml)

• Minimize other arterial/venous punctures; IM inj, catheter use, intubation, to reduce bleeding risks

Y-site compatibility: Heparin

Evaluate:

• Therapeutic response: treatment of acute coronary syndrome

Teach patient/family:

• That it is necessary to quit smoking to prevent excessive vasoconstriction

T

---

tizanidine

(ti-za′nih-deen)

Zanaflex

Func. class.: Skeletal muscle relaxant, α₂-adrenergic agonist

Chem. class.: Imidazoline

Action: Increases presynaptic inhibition of motor neurons and reduces spasticity by α₂-adrenergic agonism

Uses: Acute/intermittent management of increased muscle tone associated with spasticity

DOSAGE AND ROUTES

• *Adult:* **PO** 4 mg q6-8h, increase gradually by 2-4 mg increments q6-8h, may repeat dose q6-8h, max 36 mg/24 hr
Available forms: Tabs 2, 4 mg; caps 2, 4, 6 mg

SIDE EFFECTS

CNS: Somnolence, dizziness, speech disorder, dyskinesia, nervousness, hallucination, psychosis
CV: Hypotension, bradycardia
GI: Dry mouth, vomiting, increased ALT, abnormal LFTs, constipation
OTHER: Blurred vision, urinary frequency, pharyngitis, rhinitis, tremor, rash, muscle weakness

Contraindications: Hypersensitivity
Precautions: Pregnancy (C), hypotension, lactation, geriatric, children, renal/hepatic disease

PHARMACOKINETICS

Completely absorbed, widely distributed, peak 1-2 hr; duration 3-6 hr; half-life 2.5 hr; protein binding 30%; metabolized by liver, excreted in urine, feces

INTERACTIONS

Increase: CNS depression—alcohol, other CNS depressants
Decrease: clearance of tizanidine—oral contraceptives
Drug/Lab Test
Increase: Alk phos, AST, ALT, serum glucose

NURSING CONSIDERATIONS

Assess:
• For muscle spasticity baseline and throughout treatment
• For hypotension, gradual dosage increase should lessen hypotensive effects; have patient rise slowly from supine to upright; watch those patients receiving antihypertensives for increased effects

• For increased sedation, dizziness, hallucinations, psychosis; drug may need to be discontinued
• Vision by ophthalmic exam, corneal opacities may occur
• Hepatic studies: 1, 3, 6 mo during treatment and periodically thereafter
Administer
• Consistently either with or without food; food may affect absorption
• Titrate doses carefully
• Avoid use with other CNS depressants
Teach patient/family:
• To rise slowly from lying or sitting to upright position
• To ask for assistance if dizziness, sedation occur; to avoid drinking alcohol, to avoid operating machinery or driving until effects are known
• To avoid use of alcohol
• Discontinue gradually

---

tobramycin (℞)
(toe-bra-mye'sin)
Nebcin, TOBI, tobramycin sulfate
Func. class.: Antiinfective
Chem. class.: Aminoglycoside

Action: Interferes with protein synthesis in bacterial cell by binding to ribosomal subunit, causing inaccurate peptide sequence to form in protein chain, causing bacterial death
Uses: Severe systemic infections of CNS, respiratory, GI, urinary tract, bone, skin, soft tissues caused by *Pseudomonas aeruginosa, Escherichia coli, Enterobacter, Providencia, Citrobacter, Staphylococcus, Proteus, Klebsiella, Serratia;* cystic fibrosis (nebulizer) for *Pseudomonas aeruginosa*

DOSAGE AND ROUTES

• *Adult:* **IM/IV** 3 mg/kg/day in divided doses q8h; may give up to 5 mg/kg/day in divided doses q6-8h; once daily dosing is an option
• *Child:* **IM/IV** 6-7.5 mg/kg/day in 3-4 equal divided doses

---

• *Child ≥6 yr:* **NEB** 300 mg bid in repeating cycles of 28 days on/28 days off of drug; give **INH** over 10-15 min using a handheld PARI LC PLUS reusable nebulizer with a DeVilbiss Pulmo-Aid compressor
• *Neonate <1 wk:* **IM** up to 4 mg/kg/day in divided doses q12h; **IV** up to 4 mg/kg/day in divided doses q12h diluted in 50-100 mg NS or D$_5$W; give over 30-60 min

Renal dose
• *Adult:* **IM/IV** 1 mg/kg, then dose determined by blood levels

Available forms: Inj 10, 40 mg/ml; powder for inj 1.2 g; neb sol 300 mg/5 ml

SIDE EFFECTS

CNS: Confusion, depression, numbness, tremors, **convulsions,** muscle twitching, **neurotoxicity,** dizziness, vertigo
CV: Hypo/hypertension, palpitation
EENT: **Ototoxicity,** deafness, visual disturbances, tinnitus
GI: Nausea, vomiting, anorexia; increased ALT, AST, bilirubin, hepatomegaly, **hepatic necrosis,** splenomegaly
GU: **Oliguria, hematuria, renal damage, azotemia, renal failure, nephrotoxicity**
HEMA: **Agranulocytosis, thrombocytopenia, leukopenia, eosinophilia,** anemia
INTEG: Rash, burning, urticaria, dermatitis, alopecia

Contraindications: Pregnancy (D), severe renal disease, hypersensitivity to aminoglycosides
Precautions: Neonates, mild renal disease, myasthenia gravis, lactation, hearing deficits, Parkinson's disease, geriatric

PHARMACOKINETICS

IM: Onset rapid, peak 1 hr
IV: Onset immediate, peak 1 hr
Plasma half-life 2-3 hr prolonged in neonates; not metabolized, excreted unchanged in urine, crosses placental barrier, poor penetration into CSF

INTERACTIONS

Increase: ototoxicity, neurotoxicity, nephrotoxicity—other aminoglycosides, amphotericin B, polymyxin, vancomycin, ethacrynic acid, furosemide, mannitol, methoxyflurane, cisplatin, cephalosporins, bacitracin, acyclovir, penicillins, cidofovir

Drug/Herb
• Do not use acidophilus with antiinfectives; separate by several hours
• Toxicity: lysine (large amounts)

NURSING CONSIDERATIONS

Assess:
• Weight before treatment; dosage is usually based on ideal body weight, but may be calculated on actual body weight
• I&O ratio, urinalysis daily for proteinuria, cells, casts; report sudden change in urine output
• VS during infusion; watch for hypotension, change in pulse
• IV site for thrombophlebitis, including pain, redness, swelling q30min; change site if needed; apply warm compresses to discontinued site
• Serum peak, drawn at 30-60 min after IV infusion or 60 min after IM inj, trough drawn just before next dose, peak 4-12 mcg/ml, trough 1-2 mcg/ml
• Renal impairment by securing urine for CCr testing, BUN, serum creatinine; lower dosage should be given in renal impairment (CCr <80 ml/min); monitor electrolytes: potassium, sodium, chloride, magnesium monthly, if patient is on long-term therapy
• Deafness by audiometric testing; ringing, roaring in ears; vertigo; assess hearing before, during, after treatment
• Dehydration: high specific gravity, decrease in skin turgor, dry mucous membranes, dark urine
• Overgrowth of infection: fever, malaise, redness, pain, swelling, perineal itching, diarrhea, stomatitis, change in cough, sputum
• C&S before starting treatment to identify infecting organism

T

Side effects: *italics* = common; **bold** = life-threatening

• Vestibular dysfunction: nausea, vomiting, dizziness, headache; drug should be discontinued if severe
• Inj sites for redness, swelling, abscesses; use warm compresses at site

Administer:
• Drug in evenly spaced doses to maintain blood level; separate aminoglycosides and penicillins by ≥1 hr

IM route
• IM inj in large muscle mass; rotate inj sites

Nebulizer route
• Give as close to q12hr apart as possible; do not use <6 hr apart
• Do not mix with dornase alfa in the nebulizer
• Have patient inhale sitting or standing, breathe normally through mouthpiece; may use noseclips

IV route
• Diluted in 50-100 ml 0.9% NaCl or D$_5$W (adult), infuse over 20-60 min
• Do not admix

Syringe compatibilities: Doxapram
Y-site compatibilities: Acyclovir, amifostine, amiodarone, amsacrine, aztreonam, ciprofloxacin, cisatracurium, cyclophosphamide, diltiazem, doxorubicin liposome, enalaprilat, esmolol, filgrastim, fluconazole, fludarabine, foscarnet, furosemide, granisetron, hydromorphone, IL-2, insulin (regular), labetalol, magnesium sulfate, melphalan, meperidine, midazolam, morphine, perphenazine, remifentanil, tacrolimus, teniposide, theophylline, thiotepa, tolazoline, vinorelbine, zidovudine

Perform/provide:
• Adequate fluids of 2-3 L/day unless contraindicated to prevent irritation of tubules
• Flush of IV line with NS or D$_5$W after infusion
• Supervised ambulation, other safety measures with vestibular dysfunction

Evaluate:
• Therapeutic response: absence of fever, draining wounds, negative C&S after treatment

Teach patient/family:
• To report headache, dizziness, symptoms of overgrowth of infection, renal impairment
• To report loss of hearing; ringing, roaring in ears; feeling of fullness in head

Nebulizer
• To use multiple therapies first, then tobramycin

Treatment of overdose: Hemodialysis; monitor serum levels of drug

---

tobramycin ophthalmic
See Appendix C

---

tocainide (℞)
(toe-kay′nide)
Tonocard
Func. class.: Antidysrhythmic (Class Ib)
Chem. class.: Lidocaine analog

Action: Produces dose-dependent decreases in sodium and potassium conduction, thereby decreasing the excitability of myocardial cells; does not affect heart rate or B/P

Uses: Life-threatening ventricular dysrhythmias (multifocal/unifocal PVCs), ventricular tachycardia

DOSAGE AND ROUTES
• *Adult:* **PO** 400 mg q8h, may increase to 1.2-1.8 g/day in divided doses q8-12h
Available forms: Tabs 400, 600 mg

SIDE EFFECTS
CNS: Headache, dizziness, involuntary movement, confusion, psychosis, restlessness, irritability, paresthesias, tremors, **seizures**
CV: Hypotension, bradycardia, angina, PVCs, **heart block, cardiovascular collapse, sinus arrest, CHF,** chest pain, tachycardia, prodysrhythmia
EENT: Tinnitus, blurred vision, hearing loss
GI: Nausea, vomiting, anorexia, diarrhea, hepatitis

A Safety alert   *"Tall Man" lettering

HEMA: **Blood dyscrasias: leukopenia, agranulocytosis, hypoplastic anemia, thrombocytopenia, bone marrow depression**

INTEG: Rash, urticaria, lupus, alopecia, sweating

RESP: Dyspnea, **respiratory depression, pulmonary fibrosis,** pulmonary edema, interstitial pneumonitis pneumonia

Contraindications: Hypersensitivity to amides, severe heart block

Precautions: Pregnancy (C), lactation, children, renal/hepatic disease, CHF, pulmonary depression, myasthenia gravis, blood dyscrasias, hypokalemia, atrial flutter/fibrillation, geriatric

PHARMACOKINETICS

PO: Peak 0.5-3 hr; half-life 10-17 hr; metabolized by liver, excreted in urine, 40% unchanged

INTERACTIONS

Increase: tocainide effects—metoprolol
Decrease: tocainide effects—cimetidine, rifampin
Drug/Herb
Increase: toxicity, death—aconite
Increase: effect—aloe, broom, chronic buckthorn use, cascara sagrada (chronic use), Chinese rhubarb, figwort, fumitory, goldenseal, kudzu, licorice
Increase: serotonin effect—horehound
Decrease: effect—coltsfoot
Drug/Lab Test
Increase: CPK
False positive: ANA titer

NURSING CONSIDERATIONS

Assess:
⚠ Chest x-ray film, pulmonary function tests, hepatic enzymes during treatment, monitor for lung sounds, sputum, SOB after 3-18 wk
• CBC, with differential and platelet count during beginning treatment and q3mo
• I&O ratio; check for decreasing output
• Blood levels (therapeutic level 4-10 mcg/ml)
• B/P continuously for fluctuations

• Lung fields; bilateral crackles may occur in CHF patient
• Increased respiration, increased pulse; drug should be discontinued
• Toxicity: fine tremors, dizziness
• Blood dyscrasias: fatigue, sore throat, fever, bruising
• Cardiac status, respiration: rate, rhythm, character
Administer:
• With meals to decrease GI symptoms
Evaluate:
• Therapeutic response: decreased dysrhythmia
Teach patient/family:
• Of reason for medication and expected results
• Method for taking pulse at home and what to report to prescriber
• To avoid hazardous activities until drug response is known; dizziness, confusion, sedation may occur
• To use a bracelet or other emergency ID indicating medications taken, condition, and prescriber's name and phone number
• To report bleeding, bruising, respiratory symptoms, chills, fever, sore throat to prescriber
Treatment of overdose: O$_2$, artificial ventilation, ECG; administer DOPamine for circulatory depression, diazepam or thiopental for seizures

tolcapone (℞)
(toll'cah'pone)
Tasmar
Func. class.: Antiparkinson agent
Chem. class.: Catecholamine inhibitor (comt)

Action: Selective, reversible inhibitor of catecholamine; used as adjunct to levodopa/carbidopa therapy
Uses: Parkinson's disease

DOSAGE AND ROUTES
• *Adult:* **PO** 100-200 mg tid, with levodopa/carbidopa therapy; max 600 mg/day, discontinue if no benefit in 3 wk

Renal dose
• *Adult:* **PO** Use 100 mg tid or less
Available forms: Tabs 100, 200 mg

SIDE EFFECTS

CNS: Dystonia, dyskinesia, dreaming, *fatigue, headache, confusion,* psychosis, hallucination, dizziness
CV: Orthostatic hypotension, chest pain, hypotension
EENT: Cataract, eye inflammation
GI: Nausea, vomiting, anorexia, abdominal distress, diarrhea, constipation, **fatal hepatic failure,** increased LFTs
GU: UTI, urine discoloration, uterine tumor, micturition disorder, hematuria
HEMA: **Hemolytic anemia, leukopenia, agranulocytosis**
INTEG: Sweating, alopecia
Contraindications: Hypersensitivity
Precautions: Pregnancy (C), renal/hepatic/cardiac disease, hypertension, asthma, lactation

PHARMACOKINETICS

Rapidly absorbed, peak 2 hr, protein binding 99%, extensively metabolized, half-life 2-3 hr, excreted in urine (60%), feces (40%)

INTERACTIONS

• May influence pharmacokinetics of α-methyldopa, DOBUTamine, apomorphine, isoproterenol
• Inhibition of normal catecholamine metabolism: MAOIs, MAO-B inhibitor may be used
Drug/Herb
Decrease: effect—kava

NURSING CONSIDERATIONS

Assess:
⚠ Hepatic studies: AST, ALT, alk phos, LDH, bilirubin, CBC, monitor ALT, AST q2wk × 1 yr, then q4wk × 6 mo, and q8wk thereafter; if LFTs are elevated, this drug should not be used
• Involuntary movements in parkinsonism: akinesia, tremors, staggering gait, muscle rigidity, drooling

• B/P, respiration during initial treatment; hypo/hypertension should be reported
• Mental status: affect, mood, behavioral changes
Administer:
• Only to be used if levodopa/carbidopa does not provide satisfactory result
Evaluate:
• Therapeutic response: decrease in akathisia, increased mood
Teach patient/family:
• To change positions slowly to prevent orthostatic hypotension
• That urine, sweat may change color
• That food taken within 1 hr before meals or 2 hr after meals decreases action of drug by 20%
⚠ To report signs of hepatic injury: clay-colored stools, jaundice, fatigue, appetite loss, lethargy
• To report nausea, vomiting, anorexia; nausea may occur in the beginning of treatment

tolnaftate topical
See Appendix C

tolterodine (℞)
(toll-tehr'oh-deen)
Detrol, Detrol LA
Func. class.: Overactive bladder product
Chem. class.: Muscarinic receptor antagonist

Action: Relaxes smooth muscles in urinary tract by inhibiting acetylcholine at postganglionic sites
Uses: Overactive bladder (urinary frequency, urgency), urinary incontinence

DOSAGE AND ROUTES
• *Adult and geriatric:* **PO** 2 mg bid, hepatic disease 1 mg bid; 4 mg daily, may decrease to 2 mg if needed, max 4 mg/day

Renal dose
• **Adult:** **PO** CCr ≤30 ml/min reduce by 50%
Available forms: Tabs 1, 2 mg; ext rel caps 2, 4 mg

SIDE EFFECTS

CNS: Anxiety, paresthesia, fatigue, *dizziness,* headache
CV: Chest pain, hypertension
EENT: Vision abnormalities, xerophthalmia
GI: Nausea, vomiting, anorexia, abdominal pain, constipation, dry mouth, dyspepsia
GU: Dysuria, urinary retention, frequency, UTI
INTEG: Rash, pruritus
RESP: Bronchitis, cough, pharyngitis, URI
Contraindications: Hypersensitivity, uncontrolled narrow-angle glaucoma, urinary retention, gastric retention
Precautions: Pregnancy (C), lactation, children, renal/hepatic disease, controlled narrow-angle glaucoma

PHARMACOKINETICS

Rapidly absorbed, highly protein bound, extensively metabolized, excreted in urine/feces

INTERACTIONS

Increase: action of tolterodine—antiretroviral protease inhibitors, macrolide antiinfectives, azole antifungals
Increase: anticholinergic effect—antimuscarinics
Increase: urinary frequency—diuretics
Drug/Food
• Food increases the bioavailability of tolterodine

NURSING CONSIDERATIONS
Assess:
• Urinary patterns: distention, nocturia, frequency, urgency, incontinence
• Allergic reactions: rash; if this occurs, drug should be discontinued

Evaluate:
• Urinary status: dysuria, frequency, nocturia, incontinence
Teach patient/family:
• To avoid hazardous activities; dizziness may occur

topiramate (℞)
(toh-pire'ah-mate)
Topamax
Func. class.: Anticonvulsant—miscellaneous
Chem. class.: Monosaccharide derivative

Action: Mechanism of action unknown; may prevent seizure spread as opposed to an elevation of seizure threshold
Uses: Partial seizures in adults and children 2-16 yr old; tonic-clonic seizures; seizures in Lennox-Gastaut syndrome, migraine prophylaxis
Unlabeled uses: Cluster headache, infantile spasms, bipolar disorder, alcohol/cocaine dependence, binge eating disorder, bulimia nervosa, smoking, weight loss in obesity

DOSAGE AND ROUTES
Adjunctive therapy in seizures
• *Adult:* **PO** 25-50 mg/day initially, titrate by 25-50 mg/wk, up to 400 mg/day in 2 divided doses
Renal dose
• *Adult:* **PO** CCr <70 ml/min give ½ dose
Migraine prophylaxis
• *Adult:* **PO** 100 mg/day in divided doses
Available forms: Tabs 25, 50, 100, 200 mg; sprinkle caps 15, 25 mg

SIDE EFFECTS

CNS: Dizziness, fatigue, cognitive disorder, insomnia, *anxiety,* depression, paresthesia, *memory loss, tremor*
EENT: Diplopia, *vision abnormality*
GI: Diarrhea, *anorexia, nausea, dyspepsia,* abdominal pain, constipation, dry mouth
GU: Breast pain, dysmenorrhea, menstrual disorder

INTEG: Rash
MISC: Weight loss, leukopenia
RESP: URI, pharyngitis, sinusitis
Contraindications: Hypersensitivity
Precautions: Pregnancy (C), renal/hepatic disease, acute myopia, secondary angle closure glaucoma, lactation, children

PHARMACOKINETICS

Well absorbed, terminal half-life 19-25 hr; excreted in urine (55%-97% unchanged), crosses placenta, excreted in breast milk, protein binding (9%-17%); steady state 4 days

INTERACTIONS

Increase: renal stones—carbonic anhydrase inhibitors
Increase: effect of amitriptyline
Increase: CNS depression—alcohol, CNS depressants
Increase: topiramate levels—metformin, hydrochlorothiazide, lamotrigine
Decrease: levels of oral contraceptives, estrogen, digoxin, valproic acid, lithium, risperidone
Decrease: topiramate levels—phenytoin, carbamazepine, valproic acid
Drug/Herb
Increase: effect—ginkgo
Decrease: effect—ginseng, santonica

NURSING CONSIDERATIONS

Assess:
• Renal studies: urinalysis, BUN, urine creatinine q3mo; symptoms of renal colic
• Hepatic studies: ALT, AST, bilirubin if on long-term treatment
• CBC during long-term therapy
• Description of seizures: location, type, duration, aura
• Mental status: mood, sensorium, affect, behavioral changes; if mental status changes, notify prescriber
• Body weight, evidence of cognitive disorder

Administer:
• Swallow tabs whole; do not break, crush, or chew tabs; very bitter
• May take without regard to meals
• Sprinkle cap can be given whole or opened and sprinkled on soft food; do not chew
Perform/provide:
• Storage at room temperature away from heat and light
• Assistance with ambulation during early part of treatment; dizziness occurs
• Seizure precautions: padded side rails, move objects that may harm patient
Evaluate:
• Therapeutic response: decreased seizure activity
Teach patient/family:
• To carry emergency ID stating patient's name, drugs taken, condition, prescriber's name, phone number
• To avoid driving, other activities that require alertness
• Not to discontinue medication quickly after long-term use
• To notify prescriber immediately of blurred vision, periorbital pain
• To maintain adequate fluid intake
• To use nonhormonal contraceptive; effect of oral contraceptives is decreased

---

⚠ High Alert

topotecan
(toh-poh-tee'kan)
Hycamtin
Func. class.: Antineoplastic hormone
Chem. class.: Semisynthetic derivative of camptothecin (topoisomerase inhibitor)

Action: Antitumor drug with topoisomerase I–inhibitory activity topoisomerase I relieves torsional strain in DNA by causing single-strand breaks; causes double-strand DNA damage
Uses: Metastatic carcinoma of the ovary after failure of traditional chemotherapy, relapsed small cell lung cancer

---

⚠ Safety alert   *"Tall Man" lettering

DOSAGE AND ROUTES

• *Adult:* **IV INF** 1.5 mg/m² over 30 min daily × 5 days starting on day 1 of a 21-day course × 4 courses; may be reduced to 0.25 mg/m² for subsequent courses if severe neutropenia occurs

Renal dose

• *Adult:* **IV** CCr 20-39 ml/min 0.75 mg/m²/day × 5 days starting on day 1 of a 21-day course

Available forms: Lyophilized powder for inj 4 mg

SIDE EFFECTS

CNS: Arthralgia, asthenia, headache, myalgia, pain

GI: Abdominal pain, constipation, diarrhea, obstruction, nausea, stomatitis, vomiting; increased ALT, AST; anorexia

HEMA: **Neutropenia, leukopenia, thrombocytopenia, anemia, sepsis**

INTEG: Total alopecia

RESP: Dyspnea

Contraindications: Pregnancy (D), hypersensitivity, lactation, severe bone marrow depression

Precautions: Children

PHARMACOKINETICS

Rapidly and completely absorbed; excreted in urine and feces as metabolites; half-life 6 hr, geriatric half-life 8 hr; 94% bound to plasma proteins

INTERACTIONS

Increase: duration of neutropenia when used with G-CSF

Increase: myelosuppression when used with cisplatin

NURSING CONSIDERATIONS

Assess:

• Hepatic studies: AST, ALT, alk phos, which may be elevated

• For CNS symptoms: drowsiness, confusion, depression, anxiety

• CBC, differential, platelet count weekly; withhold drug if WBC is <3500/mm³ or platelet count is <100,000/mm³; notify

prescriber of these results; drug should be discontinued

• Buccal cavity q8h for dryness, sores or ulceration, white patches, oral pain, bleeding, dysphagia

• GI symptoms: frequency of stools, cramping

• Signs of dehydration: rapid respiration, poor skin turgor, decreased urine output, dry skin, restlessness, weakness

Administer:

• Changing of IV site q48h

Perform/provide:

• Increased fluid intake to 2-3 L/day to prevent dehydration, unless contraindicated

• Rinsing of mouth tid-qid with water, club soda; brushing of teeth bid-tid with soft brush or cotton-tipped applicator for stomatitis; use unwaxed dental floss

• Nutritious diet with iron, vit K supplements, low fiber, few dairy products

Evaluate:

• Therapeutic response: decreased tumor size, spread of malignancy

Teach patient/family:

• That total alopecia may occur; hair grows back, but is different in color and texture

• To avoid foods with citric acid or hot or rough texture if stomatitis is present; to drink adequate fluids

• To report stomatitis; any bleeding, white spots, ulcerations in mouth; tell patient to examine mouth daily; report symptoms

• To report signs of anemia: fatigue, headache, faintness, shortness of breath, irritability

• To use effective contraception during treatment, avoid breastfeeding

T

toremifene (℞)
(tor-em'ih-feen)
Fareston
Func. class.: Antineoplastic
Chem. class.: Antiestrogen hormone

Action: Inhibits cell division by binding to cytoplasmic estrogen receptors; resembles normal cell complex but inhibits

---

1014 toremifene

DNA synthesis and estrogen response of target tissue

Uses: Advanced breast carcinoma not responsive to other therapy in estrogen-receptor-positive patients (usually postmenopausal)

DOSAGE AND ROUTES
• *Adult:* **PO** 60 mg daily
Available forms: Tabs 60 mg

SIDE EFFECTS
CNS: Hot flashes, headache, light-headedness, depression
CV: **CHF, MI, pulmonary embolism,** chest pain
EENT: Ocular lesions, retinopathy, corneal opacity, blurred vision (high doses)
GI: Nausea, vomiting, altered taste (anorexia)
GU: Vaginal bleeding, pruritus vulvae
HEMA: **Thrombocytopenia, leukopenia**
INTEG: Rash, alopecia
META: Hypercalcemia

Contraindications: Pregnancy (D), hypersensitivity, history of thromboembolism

Precautions: Leukopenia, thrombocytopenia, lactation, cataracts

PHARMACOKINETICS
PO: Peak 3 hr, excreted primarily in feces

INTERACTIONS
• May increase the effect of warfarin
Drug/Lab Test
Increase: serum calcium

NURSING CONSIDERATIONS
Assess:
• CBC, differential, platelet count qwk; withhold drug if WBC is <3500/mm³ or platelet count is <100,000/mm³; notify prescriber
• Bleeding: hematuria, guaiac, bruising, petechiae, mucosa or orifices q8h
• Effects of alopecia on body image; discuss feelings about body changes

⚠ Symptoms indicating severe allergic reactions: rash, pruritus, urticaria, purpuric skin lesions, itching, flushing

Administer:
• Antacid before oral agent; give drug after evening meal, before bedtime
• Antiemetic 30-60 min before giving drug to prevent vomiting

Perform/provide:
• Liquid diet, if needed, including cola, Jell-O; dry toast or crackers may be added if patient is not nauseated or vomiting
• Increase fluid intake to 2-3 L/day to prevent dehydration
• Nutritious diet with iron, vitamin supplements as ordered
• Storage in light-resistant container at room temperature

Evaluate:
• Therapeutic response: decreased tumor size, spread of malignancy

Teach patient/family:
• To report any complaints, side effects to prescriber
• That vaginal bleeding, pruritus, hot flashes are reversible after discontinuing treatment
• To report immediately decreased visual acuity, which may be irreversible; stress need for routine eye exams; care providers should be told about tamoxifen therapy
• To report vaginal bleeding immediately
• That tumor flare—increase in size of tumor, increased bone pain—may occur and will subside rapidly; may take analgesics for pain
• That premenopausal women must use mechanical birth control because ovulation may be induced
• That hair may be lost during treatment; a wig or hairpiece may make patient feel better; new hair may be different in color, texture

torsemide (℞)
(tor'suh-mide)
Demadex
Func. class.: Loop diuretic
Chem. class.: Sulfonamide derivative

Action: Acts on loop of Henle, proximal, distal tubule by inhibiting absorption of chloride, sodium, water
Uses: Treatment of hypertension and edema in CHF, renal/hepatic disease

DOSAGE AND ROUTES
CHF
• *Adult:* **PO/IV** 10-20 mg/day, may increase as needed up to 200 mg/day
Chronic renal failure
• *Adult:* **PO/IV** 20 mg/day, may increase up to 200 mg/day
Hepatic cirrhosis in combination with aldosterone antagonist/ potassium-sparing diuretic
• *Adult:* **PO/IV** 5-10 mg/day may increase as needed up to 40 mg/day
Hypertension
• *Adult:* **PO** 5 mg/day may increase to 10 mg/day
Available forms: Tabs 5, 10, 20, 100 mg; inj 10 mg/ml

SIDE EFFECTS
CNS: Headache, dizziness, asthenia, insomnia, nervousness
CV: Orthostatic hypotension, chest pain, ECG changes, **circulatory collapse,** ventricular tachycardia, edema
EENT: Loss of hearing, ear pain, tinnitus, blurred vision
ELECT: Hypokalemia, hypochloremic alkalosis, hyponatremia, metabolic alkalosis
ENDO: Hyperglycemia, hyperuricemia
GI: Nausea, diarrhea, dyspepsia, cramps, constipation
GU: Polyuria, **renal failure,** glycosuria
INTEG: Rash, photosensitivity, pruritus
MS: Cramps, stiffness
RESP: Rhinitis, cough increase

Contraindications: Hypersensitivity to sulfonamides, anuria, hypovolemia, infants
Precautions: Pregnancy (B), diabetes mellitus, dehydration, severe renal disease, lactation, electrolyte depletion

PHARMACOKINETICS
PO: Rapidly absorbed; duration 6 hr; excreted in urine, feces, breast milk; crosses placenta; half-life 2-4 hr, plasma protein binding 97%-99%

INTERACTIONS
• Incompatible with any drug in syringe
Increase: toxicity—lithium, nondepolarizing skeletal muscle relaxants, digoxin
Increase: action of antihypertensives, oral anticoagulants, nitrates
Increase: ototoxicity—aminoglycosides, cisplatin, vancomycin
Decrease: antihypertensive effect of torsemide—indomethacin, carbamazepine, phenobarbital, phenytoin, rifampin, NSAIDs
Drug/Herb
• Severe photosensitivity: St. John's wort
Increase: effect—aloe, cucumber, dandelion, horsetail, pumpkin, Queen Anne's lace
Increase: hypotension khella
Drug/Lab Test
Interference: GTT

NURSING CONSIDERATIONS
Assess:
• Hearing when giving high doses
• Weight, I&O daily to determine fluid loss; effect of drug may be decreased if used daily
• Rate, depth, rhythm of respiration, effect of exertion
• B/P lying, standing; postural hypotension may occur
• Electrolytes: K, Na, Cl; include BUN, blood glucose, CBC, serum creatinine, blood pH, ABGs, uric acid, Ca, Mg
• Glucose in urine of diabetic
• Signs and symptoms of metabolic alkalosis: drowsiness, restlessness

Side effects: *italics* = common; **bold** = life-threatening

- Signs and symptoms of hypokalemia: postural hypotension, malaise, fatigue, tachycardia, leg cramps, weakness
- Rashes, temp elevation daily
- Confusion, especially in geriatric; take safety precautions if needed

Administer:
- In AM to avoid interference with sleep if using drug as a diuretic
- Potassium replacement if potassium <3 mg/dl
- With food or milk if nausea occurs; absorption may be decreased slightly

Evaluate:
- Therapeutic response: improvement in edema of feet, legs, sacral area daily if medication is being used in CHF

Teach patient/family:
- To rise slowly from lying, sitting position
- To recognize adverse reactions: muscle cramps, weakness, nausea, dizziness, tinnitus
- To take with food or milk for GI symptoms; to limit alcohol use
- To take early in day to prevent nocturia

Treatment of overdose: Lavage if taken orally; monitor electrolytes, administer dextrose in saline; monitor hydration, CV, renal status

---

trace elements (R)

Concentrated Multiple Trace Elements, ConTE-PAK-4, M.T.E.-4, M.T.E.-4 Concentrated, M.T.E.-5, M.T.E.-5 Concentrated, M.T.E.-6, M.T.E.-6 Concentrated, M.T.E.-7, MulTE-PAK-4, MulTE-PAK-5, Multiple Trace Element, Multiple Trace Element Neonatal, Multiple Trace Element Pediatric, Neotrace 4, PedTE-PAK-4, Pedtrace-4, P.T.E.-4, P.T.E.-5

Func. class.: Mineral supplements

Action: Needed for adequate absorption and synthesis of amino acids

Uses: Prevention of trace element deficiency

DOSAGE AND ROUTES
Usual dosage may be given in TPN sol
Chromium
- *Adult:* IV 10-15 mcg daily
- *Child:* IV 0.14-0.20 mcg/kg/day

Copper
- *Adult:* IV 0.5-1.5 mg/day
- *Child:* IV 0.05-0.2 mg/kg/day

Iodine
- *Adult:* IV 1 mcg/kg/day

Manganese
- *Adult:* IV 1-3 mg/day

Selenium
- *Adult:* 40-120 mcg/day
- *Child:* 3 mcg/kg/day

Zinc
- *Adult:* IV 2-4 mg/day
- *Child:* IV 0.05 mg/kg/day

Available forms: Many forms available—see particular elements

SIDE EFFECTS
CHROMIUM: **Seizures, coma,** nausea, vomiting, ulcers, renal/hepatic toxicity
COPPER: Personality changes, diarrhea, weakness, photophobia, muscle weakness
IODINE: Headache, edema of eyelids, acne, metallic taste, sore mouth, running nose
MANGANESE: Incoordination, headache, irritability, lability, slurred speech, impotence
SELENIUM: Alopecia, depression, vomiting, GI cramping, nervousness, garlic smell
ZINC: Vomiting, oliguria, hypothermia, vision changes, tachycardia, jaundice, **coma**

Precautions: Pregnancy (C), hepatic/biliary disease, lactation, vomiting, diarrhea

NURSING CONSIDERATIONS
Assess:
- Trace element levels; notify prescriber if low; copper 0.07-0.15 mg/ml, zinc 0.05-0.15 mg/100 ml, manganese 4-20 mcg/100 ml, selenium 0.1-0.19 mcg/ml

- Trace element deficiency of patient receiving TPN for extended period

Administer:
- By IV infusion, often mixed with TPN solution

Evaluate:
- Therapeutic response: absence of element deficiency

---

tramadol (℞)
(tram'a-dole)
Ultram
Func. class.: Central analgesic

Do not confuse:
tramadol/Toradol

Action: Not completely understood, binds to opioid receptors, inhibits reuptake of norepinephrine, serotonin; does not cause histamine release or affect heart rate

Uses: Management of moderate to severe pain

DOSAGE AND ROUTES
- *Adult:* **PO** 50-100 mg prn q4-6h; not to exceed 400 mg/day
- *Geriatric >75 years:* **PO** <300 mg/day in divided doses

Renal dose
- CCr <30 ml/min give q12h, max 200 mg/day

Hepatic impairment
- **PO** 50 mg q12h

Available forms: Tabs 50 mg

SIDE EFFECTS

CNS: Dizziness, CNS stimulation, somnolence, headache, anxiety, confusion, euphoria, **seizures,** hallucinations

CV: Vasodilation, orthostatic hypotension, tachycardia, hypertension, abnormal ECG

GI: Nausea, constipation, vomiting, dry mouth, diarrhea, abdominal pain, anorexia, flatulence, *GI bleeding*

GU: Urinary retention/frequency, menopausal symptoms, dysuria, menstrual disorder

INTEG: Pruritus, rash, urticaria, vesicles

Contraindications: Hypersensitivity, acute intoxication with any CNS depressant

Precautions: Pregnancy (C), seizure disorder, lactation, children, geriatric, renal/hepatic disease, respiratory depression, head trauma, increased intracranial pressure, acute abdominal condition, drug abuse

PHARMACOKINETICS
Rapidly and almost completely absorbed, steady state 2 days, may cross blood-brain barrier, extensively metabolized, 30% excreted in the urine as unchanged drug

INTERACTIONS
- Inhibition of norepinephrine and serotonin reuptake: MAO inhibitors, use together with caution

Increase: CNS depression—alcohol, sedatives, hypnotics, opiates
Increase: serotonin syndrome—SSRIs
Decrease: levels of tramadol—carbamazepine

Drug/Herb
Increase: CNS depression—chamomile, hops, kava, skullcap, valerian

Drug/Lab Test
Increase: Creatinine, hepatic enzymes
Decrease: Hgb

NURSING CONSIDERATIONS
Assess:
- Pain: location, type, character, give before pain becomes extreme
- I&O ratio: check for decreasing output; may indicate urinary retention
- Need for drug
- Bowel pattern; for constipation increase fluids, bulk in diet
- CNS changes: dizziness, drowsiness, hallucinations, euphoria, LOC, pupil reaction
- Allergic reactions: rash, urticaria
- For increased side effects in renal/hepatic disease

Administer:
- With antiemetic for nausea, vomiting
- When pain is beginning to return; determine dosage interval by patient response

Perform/provide:
- Storage in cool environment, protected from sunlight
- Assistance with ambulation
- Safety measures: side rails, night-light, call bell within easy reach

Evaluate:
- Therapeutic response: decrease in pain

Teach patient/family:
- To report any symptoms of CNS changes, allergic reactions
- That drowsiness, dizziness, and confusion may occur, to call for assistance
- To make position changes slowly, orthostatic hypotension may occur
- To avoid OTC medications and alcohol unless approved by prescriber

---

trandolapril (℞)

(tran-doe′la-prill)
Mavik
Func. class.: Antihypertensive
Chem. class.: Angiotension-converting enzyme inhibitor

Action: Selectively suppresses renin-angiotensin-aldosterone system; inhibits ACE; prevents conversion of angiotensin I to angiotensin II, dilates arterial and venous vessels, lowers B/P

Uses: Hypertension, heart failure, post-MI/left ventricular dysfunction post MI

DOSAGE AND ROUTES

Hypertension
- *Adult:* PO 1 mg/day, 2 mg/day in African-Americans, make dosage adjustment ≥wk; up to 8 mg/day

Heart failure post-MI/left ventricular dysfunction post MI
- *Adult:* PO 1 mg/day, titrate upward to 4 mg/day if tolerated

Renal/hepatic dose
- CCr <30 ml/min give 0.5 mg/day, may increase gradually up to 4 mg/day

Available forms: Tabs 1, 2, 4 mg

SIDE EFFECTS

CNS: Dizziness, syncope, paresthesias, headache, fatigue, drowsiness, depression, sleep disturbances, anxiety
CV: Hypotension, MI, palpitations, angina, TIAs, **stroke,** *bradycardia,* dysrhythmias
GI: Nausea, vomiting, cramps, diarrhea, constipation, pancreatitis, *dyspepsia*
GU: **Proteinuria, renal failure**
HEMA: **Agranulocytosis, neutropenia, leukopenia, anemia**
INTEG: Rash, purpura, pruritus
MISC: Hyperkalemia, hyponatremia, impotence, *myalgia,* **angioedema,** muscle cramps, *asthenia,* hypocalcemia, gout
RESP: Dyspnea, *cough*

Contraindications: Pregnancy (D) 2nd/3rd trimester, hypersensitivity, history of angioedema

Precautions: Pregnancy (C) 1st trimester, hyperkalemia, hepatic disease, bilateral renal stenosis, post–kidney transplant, aorta/mitral valve stenosis, cirrhosis, severe renal disease, untreated CHF, autoimmune disease, cough, geriatric

PHARMACOKINETICS

PO: Peak 4-10 hr, duration 24 hr, half-life 6-10 h, metabolized by liver (active metabolite trandolaprilat), excreted in urine, protein binding 65%-94%

INTERACTIONS

Increase: effects—phenothiazines, diuretics
Increase: severe hypotension—diuretics, other antihypertensives
Increase: potassium levels—salt substitutes, potassium-sparing diuretics, potassium supplements
Increase: effects of ergots, neuromuscular blocking agents, antihypertensives, hypoglycemics, barbiturates, reserpine, levodopa, lithium

---

▲ Safety alert   *"Tall Man" lettering

Decrease: effects of trandolapril—antacids, NSAIDs, salicylates

Drug/Herb

Increase: toxicity, death—aconite

Increase: antihypertensive effect—barberry, betony, black catechu, black cohosh, bloodroot, broom, burdock, cat's claw, dandelion, goldenseal, hawthorn, Irish moss, Jamaican dogwood, kelp, khella, mistletoe, parsley

Increase or decrease: antihypertensive effect—astragalus, cola tree

Decrease: antihypertensive effect—coltsfoot, guarana, khat, licorice, yohimbine

NURSING CONSIDERATIONS

Assess:

• B/P, pulse q4h; note rate, rhythm, quality

• Electrolytes: K, Na, Cl

• Baselines in renal, hepatic studies before therapy begins

• Edema in feet, legs daily

• Skin turgor, dryness of mucous membranes for hydration status

• Symptoms of CHF: edema, dyspnea, wet crackles

Evaluate:

• Therapeutic response: decreased B/P

Teach patient/family:

• Not to use OTC (cough, cold, or allergy) products unless directed by prescriber

• To avoid sunlight or wear sunscreen for photosensitivity

• To comply with dosage schedule, even if feeling better

• To notify prescriber of mouth sores, sore throat, fever, swelling of hands or feet, irregular heartbeat, chest pain, signs of angioedema

• That excessive perspiration, dehydration, vomiting, diarrhea may lead to fall in blood pressure; consult prescriber if these occur

• That drug may cause dizziness, fainting; light-headedness may occur during 1st few days of therapy

• That drug may cause skin rash or impaired perspiration

• Not to discontinue drug abruptly

• To rise slowly to sitting or standing position to minimize orthostatic hypotension

---

tranylcypromine (R)
(tran-ill-sip′roe-meen)
Parnate
Func. class.: Antidepressant-MAOI
Chem. class.: Nonhydrazine

Action: Increases concentrations of endogenous epinephrine, norepinephrine, serotonin, dopamine in storage sites in CNS by inhibition of MAO; increased concentration reduces depression

Uses: Depression, when uncontrolled by other means

Unlabeled uses: Bulimia, cocaine addiction, migraines, seasonal affective disorder, panic disorder

DOSAGE AND ROUTES

• *Adult:* **PO** 10 mg bid; may increase to 30 mg/day after 2 wk; up to 60 mg/day

Available forms: Tabs 10 mg

SIDE EFFECTS

CNS: Dizziness, drowsiness, confusion, headache, anxiety, tremors, stimulation, weakness, hyperreflexia, mania, insomnia, fatigue

CV: Orthostatic hypotension, hypertension, dysrhythmias, **hypertensive crisis**

EENT: Blurred vision

ENDO: **SIADH-like syndrome**

GI: Constipation, dry mouth, nausea, vomiting, *anorexia,* diarrhea, weight gain

GU: Change in libido, urinary frequency

HEMA: Anemia

INTEG: Rash, flushing, increased perspiration

Contraindications: Hypersensitivity to MAOIs, geriatric, uncontrolled hypertension, CHF, severe hepatic disease, pheochromocytoma, severe renal/hepatic/cardiac disease, suicidal patients

Precautions: Pregnancy (C), seizure disorders, severe depression, schizophrenia, hyperactivity, diabetes mellitus, lactation, child <16 yr, suicidal ideation in children/adolescents

PHARMACOKINETICS

Metabolized by liver, excreted by kidneys, crosses placenta, excreted in breast milk

INTERACTIONS

⚠ Serotonin-syndrome: fluoxetine, fluvoxamine, sertraline, paroxetine

⚠ Hypertensive crisis: tricyclics, meperidine, dibenzazepine agents, methylphenidate, dextromethorphan, nasal decongestants, sinus medications, appetite suppressants, asthma inhalants

Increase: pressor effects—guanethidine, clonidine, indirect-acting sympathomimetics (epHEDrine), busPIRone

Increase: effects of direct-acting sympathomimetics (epINEPHrine), alcohol, barbiturates, benzodiazepines, CNS depressants, levodopa, β-blockers, antidiabetics, sulfonamide, rauwolfia alkaloids, methyldopa, thiazide diuretics, sumatriptan

Drug/Herb

• Hypertensive crisis: betel palm, butcher's broom, capsicum peppers, galanthamine, green tea (large amounts), guarana (large amounts), night-blooming cereus

• Mania: ginseng

• Serotonin syndrome: parsley

Drug/Food

• Tyramine foods; avoid all

NURSING CONSIDERATIONS

Assess:

• B/P (lying, standing), pulse; if systolic B/P drops 20 mm Hg, stop drug, notify prescriber

• Blood studies: CBC, leukocytes, cardiac enzymes (long-term therapy)

• Hepatic studies: ALT, AST, bilirubin; hepatotoxicity may occur

⚠ Toxicity: increased headache, palpitation; discontinue drug immediately; prodromal signs of hypertensive crisis

• Mental status changes: mood, sensorium, affect, memory (long, short), increase in psychiatric symptoms; suicidal ideation in children/adolescents

• Urinary retention, constipation, edema: take weight weekly

• Withdrawal symptoms: headache, nausea, vomiting, muscle pain, weakness

Administer:

• Increased fluids, bulk in diet if constipation occurs

• With food or milk for GI symptoms

• Crushed if patient is unable to swallow medication whole

• Dosage at bedtime if oversedation occurs during day

• Gum, hard candy, frequent sips of water for dry mouth

• Phentolamine for severe hypertension

• Avoid use of CNS depressants

Perform/provide:

• Cool storage in tight container

• Assistance with ambulation during beginning therapy for drowsiness/dizziness

• Safety measures including side rails

• Checking to see if PO medication swallowed

Evaluate:

• Therapeutic response: decreased depression

Teach patient/family:

• That therapeutic effects may take 48 hr-3 wk

• To avoid driving, other activities requiring alertness

• To avoid alcohol ingestion, OTC medications: cold, weight loss, hay fever, cough syrup; increased effects may occur

• Not to discontinue medication quickly after long-term use

⚠ To avoid high-tyramine foods: cheese (aged), sour cream, yogurt, beer, wine, pickled products, liver, raisins, bananas, figs, avocados, meat tenderizers, chocolate, increased caffeine, ginseng; give complete list of tyramine foods

• To report headache, palpitation, neck stiffness

• To rise slowly to prevent postural hypotension

Treatment of overdose: Lavage, activated charcoal; monitor electrolytes, vital signs; diazepam IV, NaHCO$_3$

⚠ High Alert

trastuzumab (R̸)
(tras-tuz'uh-mab)
Herceptin
Func. class.: Antineoplastic—miscellaneous
Chem. class.: Humanized monoclonal antibody

Action: DNA-derived monoclonal antibody selectively binds to extracellular portion of human epidermal growth factor receptor 2; it inhibits proliferation of cancer cells

Uses: Breast cancer; metastatic with overexpression of HER2

DOSAGE AND ROUTES
• *Adult:* IV 4 mg/kg given over 90 min, then maintenance 2 mg/kg given over 30 min; do not give as IV push or BOL
Available forms: Lyophilized powder 440 mg

SIDE EFFECTS

CNS: Dizziness, numbness, paresthesias, depression, insomnia, neuropathy, peripheral neuritis
CV: **Tachycardia, CHF**
GI: Nausea, vomiting, anorexia, diarrhea
HEMA: Anemia, **leukopenia**
INTEG: Rash, acne, herpes simplex
META: Edema, peripheral edema
MISC: Flulike symptoms; fever, headache, chills
MS: Arthralgia, bone pain
RESP: Cough, dyspnea, pharyngitis, rhinitis, sinusitis
SYST: **Anaphylaxis, angioedema**
Contraindications: Hypersensitivity to this drug, Chinese hamster ovary cell protein
Precautions: Pregnancy (B), lactation, children, geriatric, cardiac disease, anemia, leukopenia

PHARMACOKINETICS
Half-life 1.7-12 days

INTERACTIONS
Increase: chance of cardiomyopathy—anthracyclines, cyclophosphamide, avoid use

NURSING CONSIDERATIONS
Assess:
⚠ CHF and other cardiac symptoms: dyspnea, coughing; gallop; obtain a full cardiac workup including ECG, echo, MUGA
• For symptoms of infection; may be masked by drug
• CNS reaction: LOC, mental status, dizziness, confusion
⚠ For hypersensitive reactions, anaphylaxis
⚠ For infusion reactions that may be fatal: fever, chills, nausea, vomiting, pain, headache, dizziness, hypotension, discontinue drug
Administer:
• Acetaminophen as ordered to alleviate fever and headache
IV route
• After reconstituting vial with 20 ml bacteriostatic water for inj, 1.1% benzyl alcohol preserved (supplied) to yield 21 mg/ml, mark date on vial 28 days from reconstitution date, if patient is allergic to benzyl alcohol, reconstitute with sterile water for inj—use immediately
• Do not mix or dilute with other drugs or dextrose sol
Perform/provide:
• Increased fluid intake to 2-3 L/day
Evaluate:
• Therapeutic response: decrease in size of tumors
Teach patient/family:
• To take acetaminophen for fever
• To avoid hazardous tasks, since confusion, dizziness may occur
• To report signs of infection: sore throat, fever, diarrhea, vomiting
• Emotional lability is common; notify prescriber if severe or incapacitating

T

---

travoprost ophthalmic
See Appendix C

trazodone (Ṛ)
(tray′zoe-done)
Desyrel, Desyrel Dividose,
trazodone HCl
Func. class.: Antidepressant—
miscellaneous
Chem. class.: Triazolopyridine

Action: Selectively inhibits serotonin, norepinephrine uptake by brain, potentiates behavorial changes

Uses: Depression

Unlabeled uses: Chronic pain, aggressive behavior, cocaine withdrawal

DOSAGE AND ROUTES

- *Adult:* **PO** 150 mg/day in divided doses; may increase by 50 mg/day q3-4d, not to exceed 600 mg/day
- *Child 6-18 yr:* **PO** 1.5-2 mg/kg/day in divided dose, may increase q3-4d, up to 6 mg/kg/day
- *Geriatric:* **PO** 25-50 mg at bedtime, increase by 25-50 mg q3-7d to desired dose, usual 75-150 mg/day

Available forms: Tabs 50, 100, 150, 300 mg

SIDE EFFECTS

CNS: Dizziness, drowsiness, confusion, headache, anxiety, tremors, stimulation, weakness, insomnia, nightmares, EPS (geriatric), increase in psychiatric symptoms, **suicide in children/adolescents**

CV: Orthostatic hypotension, ECG changes, tachycardia, **hypertension,** palpitations

EENT: Blurred vision, tinnitus, mydriasis

GI: Diarrhea, dry mouth, nausea, vomiting, **paralytic ileus,** increased appetite, cramps, epigastric distress, jaundice, **hepatitis,** stomatitis, constipation

GU: Urinary retention, **acute renal failure,** priapism

HEMA: **Agranulocytosis, thrombocytopenia, eosinophilia, leukopenia**

INTEG: Rash, urticaria, sweating, pruritus, photosensitivity

Contraindications: Hypersensitivity to tricyclics, recovery phase of MI, convulsive disorders, prostatic hypertrophy

Precautions: Pregnancy (C), suicidal patients, severe depression, increased intraocular pressure, narrow-angle glaucoma, urinary retention, hepatic/cardiac disease, hyperthyroidism, electroshock therapy, elective surgery, children/adolescents

PHARMACOKINETICS

Peak 1 hr; metabolized by liver (CYP3A4); excreted by kidneys, feces; half-life 4.4-7.5 hr

INTERACTIONS

⚠ Hyperpyretic crisis, seizures, hypertensive episode: MAOIs

Increase: toxicity, serotonin syndrome—fluoxetine, other SSRIs

Increase: effects of direct-acting sympathomimetics (epINEPHrine), alcohol, barbiturates, benzodiazepines, CNS depressants, digoxin, phenytoin, carbamazepine

Increase: effects of trazodone—phenothiazines, protease inhibitors, azole antifungals

Increase or decrease: effects of warfarin

Decrease: effects of guanethidine, clonidine, indirect-acting sympathomimetics (epHEDrine)

Drug/Herb

Increase: serotonin syndrome—SAM-e, St. John's wort

Increase: CNS depression—chamomile, hops, kava, lavender, skullcap, valerian

Increase: anticholinergic effect—corkwood, jimsonweed

Drug/Lab Test

Increase: Serum bilirubin, blood glucose, alk phos

Decrease: VMA, 5-HIAA

False increase: Urinary catecholamines

⚠ Safety alert   *"Tall Man" lettering

NURSING CONSIDERATIONS
Assess:

• Pain: location, duration, intensity before and 1-2 hr after medication

• B/P (lying, standing), pulse q4h; if systolic B/P drops 20 mm Hg, hold drug, notify prescriber; take vital signs q4h in patients with CV disease

• Blood studies: CBC, leukocytes, differential, cardiac enzymes if patient is receiving long-term therapy

• Hepatic studies: AST, ALT, bilirubin

• Weight qwk; appetite may increase with drug

• ECG for flattening of T wave, bundle branch block, AV block, dysrhythmias in cardiac patients

• EPS, primarily in geriatric: rigidity, dystonia, akathisia

⚠ Mental status changes: mood, sensorium, affect, suicidal tendencies, increase in psychiatric symptoms, depression, panic; observe for suicidal behaviors in children/adolescents

• Urinary retention, constipation; constipation most likely in children

• Withdrawal symptoms: headache, nausea, vomiting, muscle pain, weakness; not usual unless drug discontinued abruptly

• Alcohol consumption; hold dose until morning

Administer:

• Increased fluids, bulk in diet if constipation occurs, especially in geriatric

• With food, milk for GI symptoms

• Dosage at bedtime for oversedation during day; may take entire dose at bedtime; geriatric may not tolerate daily dosing

• Gum, hard candy, frequent sips of water for dry mouth

• Avoid use of CNS depressants

Perform/provide:

• Storage in tight, light-resistant container at room temperature

• Assistance with ambulation during beginning therapy for drowsiness/dizziness

• Safety measures, including side rails, primarily for geriatric

• Checking to see if PO medication swallowed

Evaluate:

• Therapeutic response: decreased depression

Teach patient/family:

• That therapeutic effects may take 2-3 wk

• To use caution in driving, other activities requiring alertness because of drowsiness, dizziness, blurred vision

• To avoid alcohol ingestion

• Not to discontinue medication quickly after long-term use; may cause nausea, headache, malaise

• To report urinary retention immediately

• To wear sunscreen or large hat, since photosensitivity occurs

• Signs of suicidal ideation

Treatment of overdose: ECG monitoring; induce emesis; lavage, activated charcoal; administer anticonvulsant

---

treprostinil (Ⓡ)
(treh-prah′stin-ill)
Remodulin
Func. class.: Antiplatelet agent
Chem. class.: Tricyclic benzidine prostacyclin analog

Action: Direct vasodilation of pulmonary, systemic arterial vascular beds, inhibition of platelet aggregation

Uses: Pulmonary arterial hypertension (PAH) NYHA class II through IV

DOSAGE AND ROUTES

• *Adult:* SUBCUT INF 1.25 ng/kg/min by **CONT INF**, may reduce to 0.625 mg if not tolerated; may increase by 1.25 ng/kg/min qwk for first 4 wk, then 2.5 ng/kg/min/wk for remainder of infusion

Hepatic dose

• *Adult:* SUBCUT INF 0.625 ng/kg ideal body weight/min and increase cautiously

Available forms: Inj 1, 2.5, 5, 10 mg/ml

T

Side effects: *italics* = common; **bold** = life-threatening

SIDE EFFECTS

CNS: Dizziness, headache
CV: Vasodilation, hypotension, edema
GI: Nausea, *diarrhea*
INTEG: Rash, pruritus
OTHER: Jaw pain
SYST: Infusion site reactions, infusion site pain

Contraindications: Hypersensitivity
Precautions: Pregnancy (B), past renal/hepatic disease, geriatric, lactation, children, thromboembolic disease

PHARMACOKINETICS

Metabolized by liver, excreted in urine, feces; terminal half-life 2-4 hr, 90% protein binding

INTERACTIONS

• Excessive hypotension: diuretics, antihypertensives, vasodilators
Increase: bleeding tendencies—anticoagulants, aspirin

NURSING CONSIDERATIONS

Assess:
• Hepatic studies: AST, ALT, bilirubin, creatinine (long-term therapy)
⚠ Blood studies: CBC; CBC q2wk × 3 mo, Hct, Hgb, PT (long-term therapy)
⚠ Bleed time baseline and throughout; levels may be 2-5 × normal limit
Administer:
• By continuous infusion, SUBCUT or surgically placed indwelling central venous catheter using infusion pump
Evaluate:
• Therapeutic response: decreased pulmonary arterial hypertension (PAH)
Teach patient/family:
• That blood work will be necessary during treatment
• To report side effects such as diarrhea, skin rashes
• That therapy will be needed for prolonged periods of time, sometimes years
• To prevent infection, aseptic technique must be used in preparing and administration of treprostinil

---

tretinoin (vit A acid, retinoic acid) (℞)
(tret′i-noyn)
Avita, Renova, Retin-A, Retin-A Micro, Stieva-A ✤
Func. class.: Vit A acid, acne product; antineoplastic (miscellaneous)
Chem. class.: Tretinoin derivative

Action: Decreases cohesiveness of follicular epithelium, decreases microcomedone formation (TOP); induces maturation of acute promyelocytic leukemia, exact action is unknown (PO)
Uses: Acne vulgaris (grades 1-3) (TOP); (PO) acute promyelocytic leukemia, facial wrinkles, photoaging
Unlabeled uses: Acne rosacea, actinic keratosis, ichthyosis, Kaposi's sarcoma, keloids, keratosis follicularis, melasma

DOSAGE AND ROUTES

• *Adult and child:* **TOP** cleanse area, apply 0.025%-0.1% cream or 0.05% liquid at bedtime; cover lightly
Promyelocytic leukemia
• *Adult:* **PO** 45 mg/m²/day given as 2 evenly divided doses until remission, discontinue treatment 30 days after remission or 90 days of treatment, whichever is first
Available forms: Cream 0.01%, 0.02%, 0.025%, 0.05%, 0.1%; gel 0.01%, 0.025%, 0.04%, 0.1%; liquid 0.05%; caps 10 mg

SIDE EFFECTS

Oral

CNS: Headache, fever, sweating, fatigue
CV: Cardiac dysrhythmias, pericardial effusion
GI: Nausea, vomiting, **hemorrhage,** *abdominal pain, diarrhea, constipation, dyspepsia, distention, hepatitis*
INTEG: (TOP) Rash, stinging, warmth, redness, erythema, blistering, crusting, peeling, contact dermatitis, hypopigmentation,

---

⚠ Safety alert   *"Tall Man" lettering

hyperpigmentation, dry skin, pruritus, scaly skin

META: Hypercholesterolemia, hypertriglyceridemia

RESP: Pneumonia, upper respiratory disease

Contraindications: Pregnancy (D) (PO), hypersensitivity to retinoids or sensitivity to parabens

Precautions: Pregnancy (C) (TOP), lactation, eczema, sunburn, sun exposure, rapid-evolving leukocytosis, respiratory compromise

PHARMACOKINETICS

TOP: Poor systemic absorption

INTERACTIONS

• Use with caution: medicated, abrasive soaps, cleansers that have drying effect, products with high concentrations of alcohol astringents (TOP)

Increase: peeling—medication containing agents such as sulfur, benzoyl peroxide, resorcinol, salicylic acid (TOP)

Increase: plasma concentrations of tretinoin—ketoconazole (oral)

Increase: ICP, risk of pseudotumor cerebri—tetracyclines, do not use together

Increase: photosensitivity—retinoids, quinolones, phenothiazines, sulfonamides, sulfonylureas, thiazide diuretics

Increase: thrombotic complications—aninocaproic acid, aprotinin, tranexamic acid

Drug/Lab Test

Increase: AST, ALT

NURSING CONSIDERATIONS

Assess:

Topical

• Area of body involved, what helps or aggravates condition; cysts, dryness, itching; lesions may worsen at beginning of treatment

Oral

• Hepatic function, coagulation, hematologic parameters, also cholesterol, triglyceride

Administer:

Topical

• Once daily before bedtime; cover area lightly using gauze; use gloves to apply

Perform/provide:

Topical

• Storage at room temperature
• Hand washing after application

Evaluate:

• Therapeutic response: decrease in size and number of lesions

Teach patient/family:

Topical

• To avoid application on normal skin, getting cream in eyes, nose, other mucous membranes; do not use product on areas with cuts, scrapes

• To use cream/gel by applying a thin layer to affected skin; rub gently; to use liquid, apply with fingertip or cotton swab

• To avoid sunlight, sunlamps, or use protective clothing, sunscreen

• That treatment may cause warmth, stinging, dryness, peeling will occur

• That cosmetics may be used over drug; not to use shaving lotions

• That rash may occur during first 1-3 wk of therapy

• That drug does not cure condition; only relieves symptoms

• That therapeutic results may be seen in 2-3 wk but may not be optimal until after 6 wk

T

triamcinolone (℞)
(trye-am-sin'oh-lone)
Amcort, Aristocort, Aristocort
Forte, Aristocort Intralesional,
Aristospan Intra-Articular,
Aristospan Intralesional,
Articulose L.A., Atolone,
Azmacort, Cenocort A-40,
Cenocort Forte, Kenacort,
Kenaject-40, Kenalog,
Kenalog-10, Kenalog-40,
Tac-3, Tac-40, Triam-A,
triamcinolone, triamcinolone
acetonide, Triam Forte,
Triamolone 40, Triamonide
40, Tri-Kort, Trilog, Trilone,
Trisoject
Func. class.: Corticosteroid, synthetic
Chem. class.: Glucocorticoid, intermediate-acting

Action: Decreases inflammation by suppression of migration of polymorphonuclear leukocytes, fibroblasts, reversal of increased capillary permeability and lysosomal stabilization
Uses: Severe inflammation, immunosuppression, neoplasms, asthma (steroid dependent), collagen, respiratory, dermatologic disorders

DOSAGE AND ROUTES
• *Adult:* PO 4-12 mg/day in divided doses daily-qid; IM 40 mg qwk (acetonide, or diacetate), 5-48 mg into neoplasms (diacetate, acetonide), 2-40 mg into joint or soft tissue (diacetate, acetonide), 0.5 mg/in² of affected intralesional skin (hexacetonide), 2-20 mg into joint or soft tissue (hexacetonide)
• *Child:* PO 117 mcg/kg/day in divided doses
Asthma
• *Adult:* INH 2 tid-qid, not to exceed 16 **INH**/day
• *Child 6-12 yr:* INH 1-2 tid-qid, not to exceed 12 **INH**/day

Available forms: Tabs 1, 2, 4, 8 mg; syr 2 mg/5 ml, 4.85 mg/5 ml; inj 25, 40 mg/ml diacetate; inj 3, 10, 40 mg/ml acetonide; inj 20, 5 mg/ml hexacetonide; aerosol actuation/100 mcg (acetonide)

SIDE EFFECTS
CNS: Depression, flushing, sweating, headache, mood changes
CV: Hypertension, **circulatory collapse, thrombophlebitis, embolism,** tachycardia, edema
EENT: Fungal infections, increased intraocular pressure, blurred vision
GI: Diarrhea, nausea, abdominal distention, **GI hemorrhage,** increased appetite, **pancreatitis**
HEMA: **Thrombocytopenia**
INTEG: Acne, poor wound healing, ecchymosis, petechiae
MS: Fractures, osteoporosis, weakness
Contraindications: Psychosis, hypersensitivity, idiopathic thrombocytopenia, acute glomerulonephritis, amebiasis, fungal infections, nonasthmatic bronchial disease, child <2 yr, AIDS, TB, adrenal insufficiency
Precautions: Pregnancy (C), diabetes mellitus, glaucoma, osteoporosis, seizure disorders, ulcerative colitis, CHF, myasthenia gravis, renal disease, esophagitis, peptic ulcer, lactation, acne, cataracts, coagulopathy

PHARMACOKINETICS
PO/IM: Peak 1-2 hr, half-life 2-5 hr

INTERACTIONS
Increase: side effects—alcohol, salicylates, indomethacin, amphotericin B, digoxin, cycloSPORINE, diuretics
Increase: action of triamcinolone—salicylates, estrogens, indomethacin, oral contraceptives, ketoconazole, macrolide antiinfectives
Decrease: action of triamcinolone—cholestyramine, colestipol, barbiturates, rifampin, epHEDrine, phenytoin, theophylline

Decrease: effects of anticoagulants, anticonvulsants, antidiabetics, ambenonium, neostigmine, isoniazid, toxoids, vaccines, anticholinesterases, salicylates, somatrem

Drug/Herb

• Hypokalemia: aloe, buckthorn, cascara, Chinese rhubarb, senna

Drug/Lab Test

Increase: Cholesterol, sodium, blood glucose, uric acid, calcium, urine glucose

Decrease: Ca, K, T_4, T_3, thyroid ^{131}I uptake test, urine 17-OHCS, 17-KS, PBI

False negative: Skin allergy tests

NURSING CONSIDERATIONS

Assess:

• Potassium, blood glucose, urine glucose while on long-term therapy; hypokalemia and hyperglycemia

• Weight daily; notify prescriber if weekly gain >5 lb

• B/P q4h, pulse; notify prescriber if chest pain occurs

• I&O ratio; be alert for decreasing urinary output, increasing edema

• Plasma cortisol levels during long-term therapy (normal level: 138-635 nmol/L SI units when drawn at 8 AM)

• Infection: increased temp, WBC, even after withdrawal of medication; drug masks infection

• Potassium depletion: paresthesias, fatigue, nausea, vomiting, depression, polyuria, dysrhythmias, weakness

• Edema, hypertension, cardiac symptoms

• Mental status: affect, mood, behavioral changes, aggression

Administer:

• After shaking susp (parenteral)

• Titrated dose; use lowest effective dose

• IM inj deep in large muscle mass; rotate sites; avoid deltoid; use 21G needle

• In one dose in AM to prevent adrenal suppression; avoid SUBCUT administration; may damage tissue

• With food or milk to decrease GI symptoms, tablet may be crushed

Perform/provide:

• Assistance with ambulation for patient with bone tissue disease to prevent fractures

• Use of spacer device for geriatric patients with inhaler

Evaluate:

• Therapeutic response: ease of respirations, decreased inflammation

Teach patient/family:

• That emergency ID as steroid user should be carried

• To notify prescriber if therapeutic response decreases; dosage adjustment may be needed

• Not to discontinue abruptly; adrenal crisis can result

• To avoid OTC products: salicylates, alcohol in cough products, cold preparations unless directed by prescriber

• About cushingoid symptoms

• The symptoms of adrenal insufficiency: nausea, anorexia, fatigue, dizziness, dyspnea, weakness, joint pain

---

triamcinolone nasal agent
See Appendix C

---

triamcinolone topical
See Appendix C

---

triamcinolone (topical-oral) (OTC)
(trye-am-sin'oh-lone)
Kenalog in Orabase, Oralone Dental
Func. class.: Topical anesthetic
Chem. class.: Synthetic fluorinated adrenal corticosteroid

Action: Binds with steroid receptors, decreases inflammation
Uses: Oral pain

DOSAGE AND ROUTES

• *Adult and child:* **TOP** press ¼ inch into affected area until film appears, repeat bid-tid
Available forms: Paste 0.1%

SIDE EFFECTS

INTEG: Rash, irritation, sensitization
Contraindications: Hypersensitivity, infants <1 yr, application to large areas, presence of fungal, viral, or bacterial infections of mouth or throat
Precautions: Pregnancy (C), child <6 yr, sepsis, denuded skin

NURSING CONSIDERATIONS

Assess:
• Allergy: rash, irritation, reddening, swelling
• Infection: if affected area is infected, do not apply
Administer:
• After cleansing oral cavity after meals
Evaluate:
• Therapeutic response: absence of pain in affected area
Teach patient/family:
• To report rash, irritation, redness, swelling
• How to apply paste

---

triamterene (℞)

(trye-am′ter-een)
Dyrenium
Func. class.: Potassium-sparing diuretic
Chem. class.: Pteridine derivative

Action: Acts on distal tubule to inhibit reabsorption of sodium, chloride; increase potassium retention
Uses: Edema, may be used with other diuretics; hypertension

DOSAGE AND ROUTES

• *Adult:* **PO** 100 mg bid after meals, not to exceed 300 mg/day
• *Geriatric:* **PO** 50 mg daily, max 100 mg/day

Renal dose
• Do not use in CCr <10 ml/min
Available forms: Caps 50, 100 mg

SIDE EFFECTS

CNS: Weakness, headache, dizziness, fatigue
CV: Hypotension, edema, CHF, bradycardia
ELECT: Hyperkalemia, hyponatremia, hypochloremia
GI: Nausea, diarrhea, vomiting, dry mouth, jaundice, constipation
GU: **Azotemia, interstitial nephritis,** increased BUN, creatinine, renal stones, bluish discoloration of urine, **nephrotoxicity**
HEMA: **Thrombocytopenia, megaloblastic anemia, agranulocytosis**
INTEG: Photosensitivity, rash
RESP: Dyspnea
Contraindications: Hypersensitivity, anuria, severe renal/hepatic disease, hyperkalemia, lactation
Precautions: Pregnancy (B), dehydration, renal/hepatic disease, cirrhosis, renal stenosis, hyperuricemia, electrolyte abnormalities

PHARMACOKINETICS

PO: Onset 2 hr, duration 7-9 hr, half-life 3 hr, metabolized in liver, excreted in bile and urine

INTERACTIONS

Increase: effects of antihypertensives
Increase: hyperkalemia—other potassium-sparing diuretics, potassium products, ACE inhibitors, salt substitutes
Drug/Herb
Increase: fatal hypokalemia—arginine
Increase: hypokalemia—bearberry, gossypol
Increase: severe photosensitivity—St. John's wort
Increase: diuretic—cucumber, dandelion, horsetail, licorice, nettle, pumpkin, Queen Anne's lace
Drug/Lab Test
Interference: LDH

NURSING CONSIDERATIONS

Assess:

• Weight, I&O daily to determine fluid loss; effect of drug may be decreased if used daily

• Electrolytes: K, Na, Cl; include BUN, blood glucose, CBC, serum creatinine, blood pH, ABGs, LFTs

• Improvement in CVP q8h

• Signs of metabolic acidosis: drowsiness, restlessness

• Rashes, temp daily

• Confusion, especially in geriatric; take safety precautions if needed

• Hydration: skin turgor, thirst, dry mucous membranes

Administer:

• In AM to avoid interference with sleep

• After meals if nausea occurs; absorption may be decreased slightly

Evaluate:

• Therapeutic response: improvement in edema of feet, legs, sacral area daily if medication is being used in CHF

Teach patient/family:

• To take medication after meals for GI upset

• To avoid prolonged exposure to sunlight; photosensitivity may occur; may turn urine blue

• To avoid foods high in potassium: oranges, bananas, salt substitutes, dried apricots, dates

• To notify prescriber of weakness, headache, nausea, vomiting, dry mouth, fever, sore throat, mouth sores, unusual bleeding or bruising

Treatment of overdose: Lavage if taken orally; monitor electrolytes; administer IV fluids, dialysis; monitor hydration, CV, renal status

---

triazolam (R)

(trye-ay′zoe-lam)
Apo-Triazo ✤, Gen-Triazolam ✤,
Halcion, Novo-Triolam ✤,
Nu-Triazol ✤
Func. class.: Sedative-hypnotic, antianxiety
Chem. class.: Benzodiazepine

Controlled Substance Schedule IV (USA), Targeted (CDSA IV) (Canada)

Action: Produces CNS depression at limbic, thalamic, hypothalamic levels of CNS; may be mediated by neurotransmitter γ-aminobutyric acid (GABA); results are sedation, hypnosis, skeletal muscle relaxation, anticonvulsant activity, anxiolytic action

Uses: Insomnia, sedative, hypnotic

DOSAGE AND ROUTES

• *Adult:* **PO** 0.125-0.5 mg at bedtime

• *Geriatric:* **PO** 0.625-0.125 mg at bedtime

Available forms: Tabs 0.125, 0.25 mg

SIDE EFFECTS

CNS: Headache, lethargy, drowsiness, daytime sedation, dizziness, confusion, light-headedness, anxiety, irritability, amnesia, poor coordination, complex sleep related reactions: sleep driving, sleep eating

CV: Chest pain, pulse changes

GI: Nausea, vomiting, diarrhea, heartburn, abdominal pain, constipation

HEMA: **Leukopenia, granulocytopenia** (rare)

SYST: **Severe allergic reactions**

Contraindications: Pregnancy (X), hypersensitivity to benzodiazepines, lactation, intermittent porphyria

Precautions: Anemia, renal/hepatic disease, suicidal individuals, drug abuse, geriatric, psychosis, child <15 yr, acute narrow-angle glaucoma, seizure disorders

---

Side effects: *italics* = common; **bold** = life-threatening

PHARMACOKINETICS

PO: Onset 30-45 min, duration 6-8 hr; metabolized by liver, excreted by kidneys (inactive metabolites), crosses placenta, excreted in breast milk; half-life 2-3 hr

INTERACTIONS

• Smoking may decrease hypnotic effect

⚠ Increase: effects of cimetidine, disulfiram, erythromycin, macrolides, probenecid, isoniazid, oral contraceptives; do not use concurrently

Increase: action of both drugs—alcohol, CNS depressants

Decrease: effect of antacids, theophylline, rifampin, smoking

Drug/Herb

Increase: CNS depression—catnip, chamomile, clary, cowslip, hops, kava, lavender, mistletoe, nettle, pokeweed, poppy, Queen Anne's lace, senega, skullcap, valerian

Increase: hypotension—black cohosh

Drug/Lab Test

Increase: ALT, AST, serum bilirubin

Decrease: RAI uptake

False increase: Urinary 17-OHCS

NURSING CONSIDERATIONS

Assess:

• Blood studies: Hct, Hgb, RBC if blood dyscrasias suspected (rare)

• Hepatic studies: AST, ALT, bilirubin if hepatic damage has occurred

• Mental status: mood, sensorium, affect, memory (long, short)

• Blood dyscrasias: fever, sore throat, bruising, rash, jaundice, epistaxis (rare)

• Type of sleep problem: falling asleep, staying asleep

Administer:

• After removal of cigarettes to prevent fires

• After trying conservative measures for insomnia

• ½ hr before bedtime for sleeplessness

• On empty stomach for fast onset, but may be taken with food if GI symptoms occur

• Avoid use with CNS depressants; serious CNS depression may result

Perform/provide:

• Assistance with ambulation after receiving dose

• Safety measures: side rails, night-light, call bell within easy reach

• Checking to see if PO medication has been swallowed

• Cool storage in tight container

Evaluate:

• Therapeutic response: ability to sleep at night, decreased amount of early morning awakening if taking drug for insomnia

Teach patient/family:

• That dependence is possible after long-term use

• To avoid driving, other activities requiring alertness until drug is stabilized

• To avoid alcohol ingestion

• That effects may take 2 nights for benefits to be noticed; for short-term use only

• Alternative measures to improve sleep: reading, exercise several hours before bedtime, warm bath, warm milk, TV, self-hypnosis, deep breathing

• That hangover is common in geriatric but less common than with barbiturates; rebound insomnia may occur for 1-2 nights after discontinuing drug

Treatment of overdose: Lavage, activated charcoal; monitor electrolytes, VS

---

trifluoperazine (℞)
(trye-floo-oh-per'a-zeen)
Apo-Trifluoperazine ✦,
Novoflurazine ✦, Solazine ✦,
Suprazine, Terfluzine,
trifluoperazine HCl, Triflurin
Func. class.: Antipsychotic, neuroleptic
Chem. class.: Phenothiazine, piperazine

Do not confuse:

trifluoperazine/trihexyphenidyl

Action: Depresses cerebral cortex, hypothalamus, limbic system, which control activity, aggression; blocks neurotransmission produced by dopamine at synapse; exhibits strong α-adrenergic, anticholinergic blocking action; mechanism for antipsychotic effects is unclear

Uses: Psychotic disorders, nonpsychotic anxiety, schizophrenia

DOSAGE AND ROUTES
Psychotic disorders
• *Adult:* **PO** 2-5 mg bid, usual range 15-20 mg/day, may require 40 mg/day or more; **IM** 1-2 mg q4-6h
• *Geriatric:* **PO** 0.5-1 mg daily-bid, increase q4-7d by 0.5-1 mg/day to desired dose
• *Child >6 yr:* **PO** 1 mg daily or bid; **IM** not recommended for children, but 1 mg may be given daily or bid
Nonpsychotic anxiety
• *Adult:* **PO** 1-2 mg bid, not to exceed 6 mg/day; do not give longer than 12 wk
Available forms: Tabs 1, 2, 5, 10 mg; conc 10 mg/ml; inj 2 mg/ml

SIDE EFFECTS
CNS: EPS: pseudoparkinsonism, akathisia, dystonia, tardive dyskinesia, **seizures,** *headache,* **neuroleptic malignant syndrome,** dizziness
CV: Orthostatic hypotension, hypertension, **cardiac arrest,** ECG changes, **tachycardia**
EENT: Blurred vision, glaucoma, dry eyes
GI: Dry mouth, nausea, vomiting, anorexia, constipation, diarrhea, jaundice, weight gain
GU: Urinary retention, urinary frequency, enuresis, impotence, amenorrhea, gynecomastia
HEMA: Anemia, **leukopenia, leukocytosis, agranulocytosis**
INTEG: Rash, photosensitivity, dermatitis
RESP: **Laryngospasm,** dyspnea, **respiratory depression**
Contraindications: Hypersensitivity, CV disease, coma, blood dyscrasias, severe hepatic disease, child <6 yr, narrow-angle glaucoma

Precautions: Pregnancy (C), breast cancer, seizure disorders, lactation, diabetes mellitus, respiratory conditions, prostatic hypertrophy, geriatric

PHARMACOKINETICS
PO: Onset rapid, peak 2-3 hr, duration 12 hr
IM: Onset immediate, peak 1 hr, duration 12 hr
Metabolized by liver, excreted in urine, breast milk; crosses placenta

INTERACTIONS
• Oversedation: other CNS depressants, alcohol, barbiturate anesthetics
Increase: effects of both drugs—β-adrenergic blockers, alcohol
Increase: anticholinergic effects—anticholinergics
Decrease: absorption—aluminum hydroxide, magnesium hydroxide antacids
Decrease: effects of lithium, levodopa, anticonvulsants
Drug/Herb
Increase: EPS—betel palm, kava
Increase: action—cola tree, hops, nettle, nutmeg
Increase: CNS depression—chamomile, hops, kava, skullcap, valerian
Drug/Lab Test
Increase: LFTs, cardiac enzymes, cholesterol, blood glucose, prolactin, bilirubin, PBI, cholinesterase, ^{131}I
Decrease: Hormones (blood, urine)
False positive: Pregnancy tests, PKU
False negative: Urinary steroids, 17-OHCS, pregnancy tests

NURSING CONSIDERATIONS
Assess:
⚠ For neuroleptic malignant syndrome: seizures, hyper/hypotension, dyspnea, diaphoresis, fatigue, muscle stiffness; notify prescriber immediately
• Mental status before initial administration
• Swallowing of PO medication; check for hoarding or giving of medication to other patients

- I&O ratio; palpate bladder if low urinary output occurs, urinary retention may be the cause
- Bilirubin, CBC, LFTs qmo
- Urinalysis is recommended before and during prolonged therapy
- Affect, orientation, LOC, reflexes, gait, coordination, sleep pattern disturbances
- For hypo/hyperglycemia; appetite patterns
- B/P standing and lying; also include pulse, respirations q4h during initial treatment; establish baseline before starting treatment; report drops of 30 mm Hg
- Dizziness, faintness, palpitations, tachycardia on rising
- EPS including akathisia (inability to sit still, no pattern to movements), tardive dyskinesia (bizarre movements of jaw, mouth, tongue, extremities), pseudoparkinsonism (rigidity, tremors, pill rolling, shuffling gait)
- Skin turgor daily
- Constipation, urinary retention daily; if these occur increase bulk, water in diet

Administer:
- Reduced dose in geriatric
- Antiparkinsonian agent on order from prescriber for EPS
- Lying down after IM inj for at least 30 min
- Avoid use with CNS depressants

PO route
- Conc in 60 ml of tomato or fruit juice, milk, carbonated beverage, coffee, tea, water, or semisolid foods (soup, pudding)

Perform/provide:
- Decreased stimulus by dimming lights, avoiding loud noises
- Supervised ambulation until stabilized on medication if needed; do not involve in strenuous exercise program because fainting is possible; patient should not stand still for long periods
- Increased fluids and bulk in diet to prevent constipation
- Sips of water, candy, gum for dry mouth
- Storage in tight, light-resistant container, oral sol in amber bottles; slight yellowing of inj or conc is common, does not affect potency

Evaluate:
- Therapeutic response: decrease in emotional excitement, hallucinations, delusions, paranoia, reorganization of patterns of thought, speech

Teach patient/family:
- That orthostatic hypotension occurs frequently, and to rise from sitting or lying position gradually; avoid hazardous activities until stabilized on medication
- To avoid hot tubs, hot showers, tub baths; hypotension may occur
- To avoid abrupt withdrawal of this drug or EPS may result; drug should be withdrawn slowly
- To avoid OTC preparations (cough, hay fever, cold) unless approved by prescriber, since serious drug interactions may occur; avoid use with alcohol; increased drowsiness may occur
- To use sunscreen
- About compliance with drug regimen
- About the necessity for meticulous oral hygiene; oral candidiasis may occur
- To report sore throat, malaise, fever, bleeding, mouth sores; CBC should be drawn and drug discontinued
- ⚠ That in hot weather, heat stroke may occur; take extra precautions to stay cool

Treatment of overdose: Lavage if orally ingested; provide an airway; do not induce vomiting

---

trifluridine ophthalmic
See Appendix C

---

trihexyphenidyl (℞)

(trye-hex-ee-fen'i-dill)
Apo-Trihex ♣, Artane, Artane
Sequels, Novohexidyl ♣,
PMS-Trihexyphenidyl ♣,
Trihexane, Trihexy-2,
Trihexy-5, trihexyphenidyl HCl
Func. class.: Cholinergic blocker
Chem. class.: Synthetic tertiary
amine

Do not confuse:
trihexyphenidyl/trifluoperazine
Artane/Altace

Action: Directly inhibits the parasympathetic nervous system; result is relaxation of smooth muscle by direct action on the muscle itself and indirectly via the parasympathetic nervous system

Uses: Parkinson's symptoms, drug-induced EPS

Unlabeled uses: Hypersalivation

DOSAGE AND ROUTES

Parkinson symptoms
• *Adult:* **PO** 1 mg, increased by 2 mg q3-5d to a total of 5-15 mg/day, given in 3-4 divided doses

Drug-induced EPS
• *Adult:* **PO** 1 mg/day; usual dose 5-15 mg/day, in 3-4 divided doses

Available forms: Tabs 2, 5 mg; elix 2 mg/5 ml

SIDE EFFECTS

CNS: Confusion, anxiety, restlessness, irritability, delusions, hallucinations, headache, sedation, depression, incoherence, *dizziness*, flushing, weakness

CV: Palpitations, tachycardia, postural hypotension

EENT: Blurred vision, photophobia, dilated pupils, difficulty swallowing, dry eyes, increased intraocular tension, narrow-angle glaucoma

GI: *Dryness of mouth, constipation,* nausea, vomiting, abdominal distress, **paralytic ileus**

GU: Urinary hesitancy, retention, dysuria

INTEG: Urticaria, rash, dry skin, photosensitivity

MISC: Suppression of lactation, nasal congestion, decreased sweating, hyperthermia, heat stroke, numbness of fingers

MS: Weakness, cramping

Contraindications: Hypersensitivity, tardive dyskinesia, narrow-angle glaucoma, myasthenia gravis, GI/GU obstruction

Precautions: Pregnancy (C), geriatric, lactation, tachycardia, abdominal obstruction, infection, children, gastric ulcer, myocardial ischemia, unstable CV disease, prostatic hypertrophy

PHARMACOKINETICS

PO: Onset 1 hr, peak 2-3 hr, duration 6-12 hr, excreted in urine, half-life 3-4 hr

INTERACTIONS

Increase: anticholinergic effects—antihistamines, phenothiazines, amantadine, tricyclics

Increase: CNS depression—analgesics, alcohol, sedatives/hypnotics, antihistamines, opioids

Increase: levels of digoxin

Decrease: action of haloperidol, levodopa

Decrease: anticholinergic effect—donepezil, rivastigmine, galantamine

Drug/Herb

Increase: henbane, jimsonweed, scopolia

NURSING CONSIDERATIONS

Assess:
• For Parkinson's and EPS baseline and throughout treatment
• I&O ratio; retention commonly causes decreased urinary output
• B/P, pulse frequently while dose is being determined
• Constipation; increase fluids, bulk, exercise
• For tolerance over long-term therapy;

T

dosage may have to be increased or medication changed
• Mental status: affect, mood, CNS depression, worsening of mental symptoms during early therapy

Administer:
• With or after meals for GI upset; may give with fluids other than water
• At bedtime to avoid daytime drowsiness in patient with parkinsonism

Perform/provide:
• Storage at room temperature in light-resistant container
• Hard candy, frequent drinks, sugarless gum to relieve dry mouth

Evaluate:
• Therapeutic response: parkinsonism: shuffling gait, muscle rigidity, involuntary movements

Teach patient/family:
• Not to discontinue this drug abruptly; to taper off over 1 wk
• To avoid driving, other hazardous activities; drowsiness may occur
• To avoid OTC medications: cough, cold preparations with alcohol, antihistamines unless directed by prescriber
• To avoid sudden position changes
• To avoid hot climates; overheating may occur

---

trimethobenzamide (℞)
(trye-meth-oh-ben′za-mide)
Arrestin, Benzacot, Brogan, Stemetic, Ticon, Tiject-20, Triban, Trimethobenzamide, trimethobenzamide HCl
Func. class.: Antiemetic, anticholinergic
Chem. class.: Ethanolamine derivative

Action: Acts centrally by blocking chemoreceptor trigger zone, which in turn acts on vomiting center
Uses: Nausea, vomiting

DOSAGE AND ROUTES
Nausea/vomiting
• *Adult:* IM 200 mg 3-4 × /day; **PO** 300 mg 3-4 × /day
Postoperative
• *Adult:* IM 200 mg followed by a second dose 1 hr later
Available forms: Caps 300 mg; inj 100 mg/ml

SIDE EFFECTS
CNS: **Drowsiness,** headache, dizziness, confusion, disorientation, **coma, seizures,** depression, *vertigo,* EPS
CV: Hypertension, hypotension, palpitation, **cardiac dysrhythmias**
EENT: Dry mouth, blurred vision, photosensitivity
GI: Nausea, diarrhea, vomiting, difficulty swallowing
INTEG: Rash, urticaria, fever, chills, flushing, hyperpyrexia
Contraindications: Hypersensitivity to opioids, shock, children (parenterally)
Precautions: Pregnancy (C), children, cardiac dysrhythmias, geriatric, acute febrile illness, encephalitis, gastroenteritis, dehydration, electrolyte imbalances, Reye's syndrome

PHARMACOKINETICS
PO: Onset 20-40 min, duration 3-4 hr
IM: Onset 15-35 min, duration 2-3 hr
Metabolized by liver, excreted by kidneys

INTERACTIONS
Increase: effect—CNS depressants, alcohol

NURSING CONSIDERATIONS
Assess:
• For nausea, vomiting before, after treatment
• VS, B/P; check patients with cardiac disease more often

• Signs of toxicity of other drugs or masking of symptoms of disease: brain tumor, intestinal obstruction
• Observe for drowsiness, dizziness

Administer:
PO route
• Capsules may be swallowed whole, chewed, allowed to dissolve

IM route
• Inj in large muscle mass; aspirate to avoid IV administration; inj is not to be used in children or infants

Syringe compatibilities: Butorphanol, glycopyrrolate, hydromorphone, midazolam, nalbuphine

Y-site compatibilities: Heparin, hydrocortisone, potassium chloride, vit B/C

Evaluate:
• Therapeutic response: decreased nausea, vomiting

Teach patient/family:
• To avoid hazardous activities, activities requiring alertness; dizziness may occur; to request assistance with ambulation
• To avoid alcohol, other depressants
• To keep out of children's reach

---

trimethoprim (℞)
(trye-meth'oh-prim)
Primsol, Proloprim,
trimethoprim, Trimpex
Func. class.: Urinary antiinfective
Chem. class.: Folate antagonist

Action: Prevents bacterial synthesis by blocking enzyme reduction of dihydrofolic acid

Uses: *Escherichia coli, Proteus mirabilis, Klebsiella, Enterobacter* UTIs, *Haemophilus influenzae*

DOSAGE AND ROUTES
Urinary tract infection
• *Adult:* **PO** 100 mg q12h × 10 days
Otitis media
• *Child >6 mo:* **PO** 5 mg/kg q12h × 10 days

Pneumocystis jiroveci *pneumonia*
• *Adult:* **PO** 20 mg/kg/day with 100 mg dapsone × 21 days
Renal dose
• *Adult:* **PO** CCr 15-30 ml/min 50 mg q12h; CCr <15 ml/min avoid use
Available forms: Tabs 100 mg

SIDE EFFECTS
CNS: Fever
GI: Nausea, vomiting, abdominal pain, abnormal taste, increased AST, ALT, bilirubin, creatinine
HEMA: **Thrombocytopenia, leukopenia, neutropenia, megaloblastic anemia** (rare)
INTEG: **Exfoliative dermatitis, Stevens-Johnson syndrome,** pruritus, rash, candidiasis

Contraindications: Hypersensitivity, CCr <15 ml/min, megaloblastic anemia, hyperkalemia
Precautions: Pregnancy (C), folate deficiency, lactation, fragile X chromosome, child <12 yr old, renal/hepatic disease, geriatric

PHARMACOKINETICS
PO: Peak 1-4 hr; half-life 8-11 hr; metabolized in liver; excreted in urine (unchanged 60%), breast milk; crosses placenta

INTERACTIONS
Increase: action of phenytoin, warfarin, dofetilide
Increase: potassium levels—potassium-sparing diuretics; potassium salts, supplements
Drug/Herb
• Do not use acidophilus with antiinfectives; separate by several hours

NURSING CONSIDERATIONS
Assess:
• For symptoms of UTI: fever, frequency, burning or pain when urinating; baseline and throughout

- Nocturia; may indicate drug resistance
- Signs of infection, anemia
- AST, ALT, BUN, bilirubin, creatinine, urine cultures
- C&S; drug may be given as soon as culture is obtained
- Skin eruptions

Administer:
- With full glass of water
- Drug in equal intervals around clock to maintain blood levels

Perform/provide:
- Storage in tight, light-resistant container
- Adequate intake of fluids (2 L) to decrease bacteria in bladder

Evaluate:
- Therapeutic response: absence of pain in bladder area, negative C&S

Teach patient/family:
- All aspects of drug therapy: need to complete entire course of medication to ensure organism death (10-14 days); culture may be taken after completed course of medication
- That drug must be taken in equal intervals around clock to maintain blood levels
- To notify nurse of nausea, vomiting, rash, severe fatigue, sore throat

trimethoprim-sulfamethoxazole (Rx)
(trye-meth'oh-prim–sul-fa-meth-ox'a-zole)
Apo-Sulfatrim ✦, Apo-Sulfatrim DS ✦, Bactrim, Bactrim IV, Bethaprim, Cotrim, Novo-Trimel ✦, Novo-Trimel DS ✦, Nu-Cotrimox ✦, Nu-Cotrimox DS ✦, Roubac ✦, Septra, Septra DS, SMZ/TMP, Sulfatrim
Func. class.: Antiinfective
Chem. class.: Sulfonamide—miscellaneous

Action: Sulfamethoxazole (SMZ) interferes with bacterial biosynthesis of proteins by competitive antagonism of PABA when adequate levels are maintained; trimethoprim (TMP) blocks synthesis of tetrahydrofolic acid; combination blocks 2 consecutive steps in bacterial synthesis of essential nucleic acids, protein

Uses: UTI, otitis media, acute and chronic prostatitis, shigellosis, *Pneumocystis jiroveci* pneumonitis, chronic bronchitis, chancroid, traveler's diarrhea

DOSAGE AND ROUTES
Based on TMP content
UTI
- *Adult:* **PO** 160 mg TMP q12h × 10-14 days
- *Child:* **PO** 8 mg/kg TMP daily in 2 divided doses q12h

Otitis media
- *Child:* **PO** 8 mg/kg TMP daily in 2 divided doses q12h × 10 days

Chronic bronchitis
- *Adult:* **PO** 160 mg TMP q12h × 14 days

Pneumocystis jiroveci *pneumonitis*
- *Adult and child:* **PO** 20 mg/kg TMP daily in 4 divided doses q6h × 14 days; **IV** 15-20 mg/kg/day (based on TMP) in 3-4 divided doses for up to 14 days
- Dosage reduction necessary in moder-

ate to severe renal impairment (CCr <30 ml/min)

Available forms: Tabs 80 mg trimethoprim/400 mg sulfamethoxazole, 160 mg trimethoprim/800 mg sulfamethoxazole; susp 40 mg/200 mg/5 ml; IV 16 mg/80 mg/ml

SIDE EFFECTS

CNS: Headache, insomnia, hallucinations, depression, vertigo, fatigue, anxiety, **convulsions, drug fever,** chills, **aseptic meningitis**
CV: **Allergic myocarditis**
GI: *Nausea, vomiting, abdominal pain,* stomatitis, **hepatitis,** glossitis, pancreatitis, diarrhea, **enterocolitis,** anorexia, **pseudomembranous colitis**
GU: **Renal failure, toxic nephrosis;** increased BUN, creatinine; crystalluria
HEMA: **Leukopenia, neutropenia, thrombocytopenia, agranulocytosis, hemolytic anemia, hypoprothrombinemia, Henoch-Schönlein purpura, methemoglobinemia, eosinophilia I**
INTEG: Rash, dermatitis, urticaria, **Stevens-Johnson syndrome,** erythema, photosensitivity, pain, inflammation at inj site, **toxic epidermal necrolysis, erythema multiforme**
RESP: Cough, shortness of breath
SYST: **Anaphylaxis, SLE**

Contraindications: Hypersensitivity to trimethoprim or sulfonamides, pregnancy at term, megaloblastic anemia, infants <2 mo, CCr <15 ml/min, lactation, porphyria, hyperkalemia

Precautions: Pregnancy (C), renal disease, geriatric, G6PD deficiency, impaired hepatic/renal function, possible folate deficiency, severe allergy, bronchial asthma, lactation, infants, folate deficiency, UV exposure

PHARMACOKINETICS

PO: Rapidly absorbed, peak 1-4 hr; half-life 8-13 hr, excreted in urine (metabolites and unchanged), breast milk; crosses placenta; 68% bound to plasma proteins; TMP achieves high levels in prostatic tissue and fluid

INTERACTIONS

Increase: thrombocytopenia—thiazide diuretics
Increase: potassium levels—potassium-sparing diuretics, potassium supplements
Increase: hypoglycemic response—sulfonylurea agents
Increase: anticoagulant effects—oral anticoagulants
Increase: levels of dofetilide
Increase: crystalluria—methenamine
Increase: bone marrow depressant effects—methotrexate
Decrease: hepatic clearance of phenytoin
Decrease: response—cycloSPORINE
Drug/Herb
• Do not use acidophilus with antiinfectives; separate by several hours
Drug/Lab Test
Increase: Alk phos, creatinine, bilirubin, AST, ALT

NURSING CONSIDERATIONS

Assess:
• Allergic reactions: rash, fever (AIDS patients more susceptible)
• I&O ratio; note color, character, pH of urine if drug administered for UTI; output should be 800 ml less than intake; if urine is highly acidic, alkalization may be needed
• Renal studies: BUN, creatinine, urinalysis (long-term therapy)
• Type of infection; obtain C&S before starting therapy
• Blood dyscrasias, skin rash, fever, sore throat, bruising, bleeding, fatigue, joint pain
• Allergic reaction: rash, dermatitis, urticaria, pruritus, dyspnea, bronchospasm
Administer:
PO route
• Medication after C&S; repeat C&S after full course of medication
• With resuscitative equipment, epINEPHrine available; severe allergic reactions may occur

T

• On an empty stomach 1 hr before or 2 hr after meals
• With full glass of water to maintain adequate hydration; increase fluids to 2 L/day to decrease crystallization in kidneys

IV route
• After diluting 5 ml of drug/125 ml D$_5$W, run over 1-1½ hr

Syringe compatibilities: Heparin

Y-site compatibilities: Acyclovir, aldesleukin, allopurinol, amifostine, amphotericin B cholesteryl, atracurium, aztreonam, cefepime, cyclophosphamide, diltiazem, DOXOrubicin liposome, enalaprilat, esmolol, filgrastim, fludarabine, gallium, granisetron, hydromorphone, labetalol, lorazepam, magnesium sulfate, melphalan, meperidine, morphine, pancuronium, perphenazine, piperacillin/tazobactam, remifentanil, sargramostim, tacrolimus, teniposide, thiotepa, vecuronium, zidovudine

Perform/provide:

• Storage in tight, light-resistant container at room temperature

Evaluate:

• Therapeutic response: absence of pain, fever, C&S negative

Teach patient/family:

• To take each oral dose with full glass of water to prevent crystalluria; drink 8-10 glasses of water/day; to take on an empty stomach 1 hr before meals, 2 hr after meals
• To complete full course of treatment to prevent superinfection
• To avoid sunlight or use sunscreen to prevent burns
• To avoid OTC medications (aspirin, vit C) unless directed by prescriber
• To use alternative contraceptive measures; decreased effectiveness of oral contraceptives may result
• To notify prescriber if skin rash, sore throat, fever, mouth sores, unusual bruising, bleeding occur

---

trimipramine (℞)
(tri-mip′ra-meen)
Apo-Trimip ✦,
Novo-Tripramine ✦,
Rhotrimine, Surmontil
Func. class.: Antidepressant—tricyclic
Chem. class.: Tertiary amine

Action: Selectively inhibits serotonin uptake by brain; potentiates behavioral changes

Uses: Depression, enuresis in children

DOSAGE AND ROUTES

• *Adult:* **PO** 50-150 mg/day in divided doses, may be increased to 200 mg/day
• *Geriatric:* **PO** 25 mg at bedtime, increase by 25 mg q3-7d, max 100 mg/day
• *Child >6 yr:* 25 mg at bedtime, may increase to 50 mg in child <12 yr or 75 mg in child >12 yr

Available forms: Caps 25, 50, 100 mg

SIDE EFFECTS

CNS: *Dizziness, drowsiness,* confusion, headache, anxiety, tremors, stimulation, weakness, insomnia, nightmares, EPS (geriatric), increase in psychiatric symptoms

CV: *Orthostatic hypotension, ECG changes, tachycardia,* **hypertension,** palpitations

EENT: Blurred vision, tinnitus, mydriasis

GI: Diarrhea, *dry mouth,* nausea, vomiting, **paralytic ileus,** increased appetite, cramps, epigastric distress, jaundice, **hepatitis,** stomatitis, *constipation,* taste change

GU: *Urinary retention,* **acute renal failure**

HEMA: **Agranulocytosis, thrombocytopenia, eosinophilia, leukopenia**

INTEG: Rash, urticaria, sweating, pruritus, photosensitivity

Contraindications: Hypersensitivity to tricyclics, recovery phase of MI, convulsive disorders, prostatic hypertrophy

Precautions: Pregnancy (C), suicidal patients, severe depression, increased in-

---

⚠ Safety alert   *"Tall Man" lettering

traocular pressure, narrow-angle glaucoma, urinary retention, hepatic/cardiac disease, renal disorders, hyperthyroidism, electroshock therapy, elective surgery, geriatric

PHARMACOKINETICS

Metabolized by liver, excreted by kidneys, steady state 2-6 days; half-life 20-26 hr

INTERACTIONS

⚠ Hyperpyretic crisis, convulsions, hypertensive episode: MAOIs

Increase: effects of direct-acting sympathomimetics (epINEPHrine), alcohol, barbiturates, benzodiazepines, CNS depressants, cimetidine, methylphenidate

Decrease: effects of guanethidine, clonidine, indirect-acting sympathomimetics (epHEDrine)

Drug/Herb

• Serotonin syndrome: SAM-e, St. John's wort

Increase: anticholinergic effect—belladonna, corkwood, henbane, jimsonweed

Increase: hypertension—yohimbe

Increase: antidepressant action—scopolia

Drug/Lab Test

Increase: Serum bilirubin, blood glucose, alk phos

Decrease: VMA, 5-HIAA

False increase: Urinary catecholamines

NURSING CONSIDERATIONS

Assess:

• B/P (lying, standing), pulse q4h; if systolic B/P drops 20 mm Hg, hold drug, notify prescriber; take VS q4h in patients with cardiovascular disease

• Blood studies: CBC, leukocytes, differential, cardiac enzymes if patient is receiving long-term therapy

• Hepatic studies: AST, ALT, bilirubin, creatinine

• Weight qwk; appetite may increase with drug

• ECG for flattening of T wave, bundle branch block, AV block, dysrhythmias in cardiac patients

• EPS primarily in geriatric: rigidity, dystonia, akathisia

• Mental status changes: mood, sensorium, affect, suicidal tendencies, increase in psychiatric symptoms, depression, panic

• Urinary retention, constipation; constipation is more likely to occur in children, geriatric

• Withdrawal symptoms: headache, nausea, vomiting, muscle pain, weakness; not usual unless drug is discontinued abruptly

• Alcohol consumption; hold dose until morning

Administer:

• Increased fluids, bulk in diet for constipation, urinary retention

• With food, milk for GI symptoms

• Dosage at bedtime for oversedation during day; may take entire dose at bedtime; geriatric may not tolerate once/day dosing

• Gum, hard candy, or frequent sips of water for dry mouth

• Avoid use with CNS depressants

Perform/provide:

• Storage in tight, light-resistant container at room temperature

• Assistance with ambulation during beginning therapy for drowsiness/dizziness

• Safety measures, including side rails, primarily for geriatric

• Checking to see if PO medication swallowed

Evaluate:

• Therapeutic response: decreased depression or enuresis

Teach patient/family:

• That therapeutic effects may take 2-3 wk

• To use caution in driving, other activities requiring alertness because of drowsiness, dizziness, blurred vision

• That appetite and weight may increase

• That urine may turn blue-green; to report urinary retention

• To avoid alcohol ingestion

• Not to discontinue medication quickly

T

after long-term use; may cause nausea, headache, malaise
• To wear sunscreen or large hat, since photosensitivity occurs
Treatment of overdose: ECG monitoring; induce emesis; lavage, activated charcoal; administer anticonvulsant

---

triptorelin (R)
(trip-toe′rel-in)
Trelstar Depot
Func. class.: Gonadotropin-releasing hormone
Chem. class.: Synthetic decapeptide analog of LHRH

Action: Inhibitor of pituitary gonadotropin secretion; initially increases LH and FSH, with increases in testosterone, reduction in sex steroid levels
Uses: Advanced prostate cancer

DOSAGE AND ROUTES
• *Adult:* **IM** 3.75 mg qmo
Available forms: Microgranules, depot inj 3.75 mg

SIDE EFFECTS
CNS: Headache, insomnia, dizziness, lability, fatigue
CV: Hypertension
ENDO: Gynecomastia, breast tenderness, hot flashes
GI: Nausea, vomiting, diarrhea
GU: Impotence, urinary retention, UTI
INTEG: Rash, pain on inj, pruritus, hypersensitivity
MISC: **Anaphylaxis, angioedema**
MS: Osteoneuralgia
Contraindications: Pregnancy (X), hypersensitivity to this product or other LHRH agonists or LHRH, lactation

PHARMACOKINETICS
Metabolism may be by CYP450, eliminated by liver, kidneys; terminal half-life is 3 hr in healthy males

INTERACTIONS
Drug/Lab Test
Increase: Alk phos, estradiol, FSH, LH, testosterone levels
Decrease: Testosterone levels, progesterone

NURSING CONSIDERATIONS
Assess:
• Severe hypersensitivity: discontinue drug and give antihistamines, have emergency equipment nearby
• I&O ratios; palpate bladder for distention in urinary obstruction
• For relief of bone pain (back pain)
• Assess levels of testosterone and PSA
Administer:
• IM using implant, inserted by qualified person
• Using syringe with 20G needle, withdraw 2 ml sterile water for inj, inject into vial, shake well, withdraw vial contents, inject immediately
Evaluate:
• Therapeutic response: more normal levels of prostate-specific antigen, acid phosphatase, alk phos; testosterone level of <25 ng/dl
Teach patient/family:
• That postmenopausal symptoms may occur but will decrease after treatment is discontinued
• That disease flare may occur at beginning of therapy
• To report allergic reaction immediately

---

tromethamine (R)
(troe-meth′a-meen)
Tham
Func. class.: Alkalinizer
Chem. class.: Amine

Action: Proton acceptor that corrects acidosis by combining with hydrogen ions to form bicarbonate and buffer; acts as diuretic (osmotic)
Uses: Acidosis (metabolic) associated with cardiac disease, COPD, cardiac

bypass surgery, neonatal respiratory distress syndrome (RDS)

DOSAGE AND ROUTES
• *Adult:* **IV** 0.3 M required = kg of weight × HCO_3^- deficit (mEq/L)
• *Child:* **IV** same as above given over 3-6 hr, not to exceed 40 ml/kg
Available forms: Inj 18 g/500 ml

SIDE EFFECTS
CV: Irregular pulse, **cardiac arrest**
GI: **Hepatic necrosis**
INTEG: Infection at inj site, extravasation, phlebitis
META: Alkalosis, hypoglycemia, **hyperkalemia with oliguria**
RESP: Shallow, slow respirations, cyanosis, **apnea**
Contraindications: Hypersensitivity, anuria, uremia
Precautions: Pregnancy (C), severe respiratory disease/respiratory depression, cardiac edema, renal disease, infants

PHARMACOKINETICS
IV: Excreted in urine

INTERACTIONS
Drug/Herb
Decrease: alkaline effect—oak bark

NURSING CONSIDERATIONS
Assess:
• Respiratory rate, rhythm, depth; notify prescriber of abnormalities that may indicate acidosis
• Electrolytes, blood glucose, chloride; CO_2, before, during treatment
• Urine pH, urinary output, urine glucose during beginning treatment
• I&O ratio, report large increase or decrease
• IV site for extravasation, phlebitis, thrombosis
• For signs of potassium depletion
Administer:
• IV slowly to avoid pain at infusion site and toxicity

• IV undiluted as inf or added to priming fluid or ACD blood; give 5 ml or less/min
Evaluate:
• Therapeutic response: decreased metabolic acidosis
Teach patient/family:
• To increase potassium in diet: bananas, oranges, cantaloupe, honeydew, spinach, potatoes, dried fruit

---
tropicamide ophthalmic
See Appendix C

---
trospium (℞)
(trose′pee-um)
Sanctura
Func. class.: Anticholinergic
Chem. class.: Muscarinic receptor antagonist

Action: Relaxes smooth muscles in bladder by inhibiting acetylcholine effect on muscarinic receptors
Uses: Overactive bladder (urinary frequency, urgency)

DOSAGE AND ROUTES
• *Adult:* **PO** 20 mg bid 1 hr before meals or on empty stomach
Renal dose
• *Adult:* **PO** CCr <30 ml/min 20 mg daily at bedtime
• *Geriatric ≥75 yr:* **PO** titrate down to 20 mg daily based on response and tolerance
Available forms: Tabs 20 mg

SIDE EFFECTS
CNS: Fatigue, dizziness, headache
CV: Tachycardia
EENT: Dry eyes, vision abnormalities
GI: Flatulence, abdominal pain, *constipation, dry mouth,* dyspepsia
GU: Urinary retention
INTEG: Dry skin

Contraindications: Hypersensitivity, uncontrolled narrow-angle glaucoma, urinary retention, gastric retention, myasthenia gravis

Precautions: Pregnancy (C), lactation, children, renal/hepatic disease, controlled narrow-angle glaucoma, ulcerative colitis, intestinal atony, bladder outflow obstruction

PHARMACOKINETICS

Rapidly absorbed (10%), protein bound (50%-85%), metabolism in humans not fully understood, extensively metabolized, excreted in urine (6%), feces (85%), excreted in urine by active tubular secretion

INTERACTIONS

Increase: drowsiness—alcohol
Increase or decrease: drugs excreted by active renal secretion (amiloride, digoxin, morphine), metformin, quinidine, procainamide, ranitidine, tenofovir, triamterene, vancomycin

Drug/Herb
Increase: henbane, jimsonweed, scopolia

Drug/Food
Decrease: absorption—high-fat meal

NURSING CONSIDERATIONS

Assess:
• Urinary patterns: distention, nocturia, frequency, urgency, incontinence

Administer:
• 1 hr before meals or on empty stomach

Evaluate:
• Therapeutic response: correction of urinary status: absence of dysuria, frequency, nocturia, incontinence

Teach patient/family:
• To avoid hazardous activities; dizziness may occur
• Alcohol may increase drowsiness
• Define anticholinergic effects that may occur

⚠ High Alert

tubocurarine (℞)
(too-boe-kyoor-ar′een)
Tubarine ✦, Tubocuraine
Func. class.: Neuromuscular blocker, nondepolarizing
Chem. class.: Curare alkaloid

Action: Inhibits transmission of nerve impulses by binding with cholinergic receptor sites, antagonizing action of acetylcholine

Uses: Facilitation of endotracheal intubation, skeletal muscle relaxation during mechanical ventilation, surgery, or general anesthesia

DOSAGE AND ROUTES

• *Adult:* **IV BOL** 0.2-0.6 mg/kg, then 0.04-0.1 mg/kg 20-45 min after 1st dose if needed for long procedures

Available forms: Inj 3 mg/ml, 20 units/ml

SIDE EFFECTS

CV: Bradycardia, tachycardia, increased, decreased B/P
EENT: Increased secretions
INTEG: Rash, flushing, pruritus, urticaria
RESP: **Prolonged apnea, bronchospasm, cyanosis, respiratory depression,** wheezing

Contraindications: Hypersensitivity
Precautions: Pregnancy (C), lactation, children <2 yr, electrolyte imbalances, dehydration, renal/hepatic/cardiac/respiratory/neuromuscular disease

PHARMACOKINETICS

IV: Onset 3-5 min, dose dependent, peak 2-3 min, duration ½-1½ hr; half-life 1-3 hr; degraded in liver, kidney (minimally); excreted in urine (unchanged) crosses placenta

INTERACTIONS

• Dysrhythmias: theophylline
Increase: neuromuscular blockade—aminoglycosides, amphotericin B, clinda-

---

⚠ Safety alert   *"Tall Man" lettering

mycin, loop diuretics, lincomycin, quinidine, local anesthetics, polymyxin antiinfectives, lithium, opioid analgesics, thiazides, enflurane, isoflurane, trimethaphan, magnesium salts, verapamil

NURSING CONSIDERATIONS

Assess:

• For electrolyte imbalances (K, Mg); may lead to increased action of this drug

• VS (B/P, pulse, respirations, airway) q15min until fully recovered; rate, depth, pattern of respirations, strength of hand grip

• I&O ratio; check for urinary retention, frequency, hesitancy

• Recovery: decreased paralysis of face, diaphragm, leg, arm, rest of body; allow to recover fully before completing neurologic assessment

• Allergic reactions: rash, fever, respiratory distress, pruritus; drug should be discontinued

Administer:

• With diazepam or morphine when used for therapeutic paralysis; provides no sedation alone

• Using nerve stimulator by anesthesiologist to determine neuromuscular blockade

• Anticholinesterase to reverse neuromuscular blockade

• IV undiluted 3 mg/ml; give single dose over 1-1½ sec by qualified person; diluted to 4 ml in NS given 0.5 ml/2 min for myasthenia testing

Solution compatibilities: D_5, $D_{10}W$, 0.9% NaCl, 0.45% NaCl, Ringer's, LR, dextrose/Ringer's or dextrose/LR combinations

Syringe compatibilities: Pentobarbital, thiopental

Perform/provide:

• Storage in light-resistant area; use only fresh sol

• Reassurance if communication is difficult during recovery from neuromuscular blockade

Evaluate:

• Therapeutic response: paralysis of jaw, eyelid, head, neck, rest of body

Treatment of overdose: Edrophonium or neostigmine, atropine, monitor VS; may require mechanical ventilation

---

undecylenic acid topical
See Appendix C

---

unoprostone ophthalmic
See Appendix C

Rarely Used

urea (℞)
(yoor-ee'a)
Ureaphil
Func. class.: Diuretic, osmotic

Uses: To decrease intracranial pressure, intraocular pressure

DOSAGE AND ROUTES

• *Adult:* **IV** 1-1.5 g/kg of 30% sol over 1-3 hr, not to exceed 4 ml/min; do not exceed 120 g/day

• *Child >2 yr:* **IV** 0.5-1.5 g/kg, not to exceed 4 ml/min

• *Child <2 yr:* **IV** 0.1 g/kg, not to exceed 4 ml/min

Contraindications: Severe renal disease, active intracranial bleeding, marked dehydration, liver failure, sickle cell disease with CNS involvement

U

⚠ High Alert

urokinase (℞)
(yoor-oh-kin′ase)
Abbokinase, Abbokinase
Open-Cath
Func. class.: Thrombolytic enzyme
Chem. class.: β-Hemolytic strepto-
coccus filtrate (purified)

Action: Promotes thrombolysis by directly converting plasminogen to plasmin
Uses: Venous thrombosis, pulmonary
embolism, arterial thrombosis, arterial
embolism, arteriovenous cannula occlusion, lysis of coronary artery thrombi after MI

DOSAGE AND ROUTES
Lysis of pulmonary emboli
• *Adult and child:* **IV** 4400 international
units/kg/hr over 10 min (90 ml/hr);
CONT IV INF 4400 international units/
kg/hr × 12 hr (15 ml/hr); flush line at
end of INF
Coronary artery thrombosis (MI)
• *Adult:* **INSTILL** 6000 international
units/min into occluded artery for 1-2 hr
after giving **IV BOL** of heparin 2500-
10,000 units
• May also give as **IV INF** 2 million-3
million units over 45-90 min
Venous catheter occlusion
• *Adult and child:* **INSTILL** 5000 international units into line, wait 5 min, then
aspirate, repeat aspiration attempts q5min
× ½ hr; if occlusion has not been removed, cap line and wait ½-1 hr, then
aspirate; may need 2nd dose if still occluded
Available forms: Powder for inj, lyophilized 250,000 international units/vial;
powder for catheter clearance

SIDE EFFECTS
CNS: Headache, fever
CV: Hypotension, dysrhythmias
GI: Nausea, vomiting
HEMA: Decreased Hct, **bleeding**

INTEG: Rash, urticaria, phlebitis at IV inf
site, itching, flushing
MS: Low back pain
RESP: Altered respirations, SOB, **bronchospasm,** cyanosis
SYST: **GI, GU, intracranial, retroperitoneal bleeding,** surface bleeding, **anaphylaxis** (rare)

Contraindications: Hypersensitivity,
internal active bleeding, intraspinal
surgery, neoplasms of CNS, ulcerative
colitis/enteritis, severe uncontrolled hypertension, renal/hepatic disease, hypocoagulation, COPD, subacute bacterial
endocarditis, rheumatic valvular disease,
cerebral embolism/thrombosis/hemor-
rhage, intraarterial diagnostic procedure
or surgery (10 days), recent major
surgery/trauma, aneurysm AV malformation

Precautions: Pregnancy (B), arterial
emboli from left side of heart, hepatic disease

PHARMACOKINETICS

IV: Half-life 10-20 min; small amounts
excreted in urine

INTERACTIONS

• Bleeding potential: aspirin, indomethacin, phenylbutazone, anticoagulants, other
NSAIDs, abciximab, eptifibatide, tirofiban,
clopidogrel, ticlopidine, some cephalosporins, plicamycin, valproic acid, dipyridamole, glycoprotein IIb, IIIa inhibitors
Drug/Lab Test
Increase: PT, APTT, TT

NURSING CONSIDERATIONS
Assess:
• VS, B/P, pulse, resp, neurologic signs,
temp at least q4h; temp >104° F (40° C)
is an indicator of internal bleeding; cardiac rhythm following intracoronary administration
• For neurologic changes that may indicate intracranial bleeding
• Retroperitoneal bleeding: back pain,
leg weakness, diminished pulses

⚠ Safety alert   *"Tall Man" lettering

• Peripheral pulses, lung sounds, respiratory function
• Hypersensitivity: fever, rash, itching, chills, facial swelling, dyspnea; mild reaction may be treated with antihistamines; notify prescriber if severe reactions, stop drug, keep resuscitative equipment nearby
• Bleeding during 1st hr of treatment (hematuria, hematemesis, bleeding from mucous membranes, epistaxis, ecchymosis)
• Blood studies (Hct, platelets, PTT, PT, TT, APTT) before starting therapy; PT or APTT must be less than 2 × control before starting therapy TT; or PT q3-4h during treatment
• ECG continuously, cardiac enzymes, radionuclide myocardial scanning/coronary angiography

Administer:

IV route
• Using infusion pump, terminal filter (0.45 μm or smaller)
• Reconstituting only with 5.2 ml sterile water for inj (not bacteriostatic water), and roll (not shake) to enhance reconstitution; further dilute with 190 ml; give as intermittent inf or give to clear cannula by using 1 ml of diluted drug; inject into cannula slowly, clamp 5 min, aspirate clot; avoid excessive pressure when urokinase is injected into catheter; force could rupture catheter or expel clot into circulation
• As soon as thrombi identified; not useful for thrombi over 1 wk old
• Cryoprecipitate or fresh frozen plasma if bleeding occurs
• Loading dose at beginning of therapy; may require increased loading doses
• Heparin therapy after thrombolytic therapy is discontinued, TT or APTT less than 2 × control (about 3-4 hr)

Y-site compatibilities: TPN 55, 56

Perform/provide:
• Storage in refrigerator; use immediately after reconstitution
• Bed rest during entire course of treatment; use caution in handling patients
• Avoidance of venous, arterial puncture procedures, inj, rectal temp

• Treatment of fever with acetaminophen or aspirin
• Placement of sign above patient's bed stating urokinase therapy
• Pressure for 30 sec to minor bleeding sites; 30 min to sites of arterial puncture followed by pressure dressing; inform prescriber if hemostasis not attained, apply pressure dressing

Evaluate:
• Therapeutic response: decreased clotting, thrombosis, embolism

Teach patient/family:
• To report immediately any sign of bleeding
• That bed rest is needed during treatment
• Reasons for treatment and expected results

---

ursodiol (Rx)
(ur-soh-die'-ohl)
Actigall, Urso
Func. class.: Gallstone solubilizing agent
Chem. class.: Ursodeoxycholic acid

Action: Suppresses hepatic synthesis, secretion of cholesterol; inhibits intestinal absorption of cholesterol

Uses: Dissolution of radiolucent, noncalcified gallbladder stones (less than 20 mm in diameter) in which surgery is not indicated, biliary cirrhosis, gallstone prophylaxis

Unlabeled uses: Severe pruritus, cystic fibrosis, intrahepatic cholestasis of pregnancy (ICP), nonalcoholic steatosis-hepatitis (NASH)

DOSAGE AND ROUTES
• *Adult:* **PO** 8-10 mg/kg/day in 2-3 divided doses using gallbladder ultrasound q6mo; determine if stones have dissolved; if so, continue therapy, repeat ultrasound within 1-3 mo

Gallstone prophylaxis in rapid weight loss
• *Adult:* **PO** 300 mg bid morning and bedtime with food

Available forms: Caps 300 mg; tabs 250, 500 mg

SIDE EFFECTS

CNS: Headache, anxiety, depression, insomnia, fatigue
GI: Diarrhea, nausea, vomiting, abdominal pain, constipation, stomatitis, flatulence, dyspepsia, biliary pain
INTEG: Pruritus, rash, urticaria, dry skin, sweating, alopecia
MS: Arthralgia, myalgia, back pain
OTHER: Cough, rhinitis

Contraindications: Calcified cholesterol stones, radiopaque stones, radiolucent bile pigment stones, chronic hepatic disease, hypersensitivity, biliary obstruction, pancreatitis, compelling for cholecystectomy
Precautions: Pregnancy (B), lactation, children

PHARMACOKINETICS

80% excreted in feces, 20% metabolized, excreted into bile, lost in feces

INTERACTIONS

Increase: risk of stone formation—clofibrate, gemfibrozil, estrogens, oral contraceptives
Decrease: action of ursodiol—cholestyramine, colestipol, aluminum-based antacids

NURSING CONSIDERATIONS

Assess:
• GI status: diarrhea, abdominal pain, nausea, vomiting; drug may have to be discontinued if side effects are severe
• Skin for pruritus, rash, urticaria, dry skin; provide soothing lotion to lesions
• Musculoskeletal status: aches or stiffness in joints
Administer:
• For up to 6-24 mo; if no improvement is seen, discontinue drug; dosing depends on size and composition of stones
Evaluate:
• Therapeutic response: decreasing size of stones on ultrasound

Teach patient/family:
• That anxiety, depression, insomnia are side effects and are reversible after discontinuing drug

---

valacyclovir (℞)
(val-a-sye'kloh-vir)
Valtrex
Func. class.: Antiviral
Chem. class.: Acyclic purine nucleoside analog

Do not confuse:
valacyclovir/valganciclovir
Valtrex/Valcyte
Action: Interferes with DNA synthesis by conversion to acyclovir, causing decreased viral replication, time of lesional healing
Uses: Treatment or suppression of herpes zoster, genital herpes, herpes labialis (cold sores)
Unlabeled uses: Prevention of CMV in advanced HIV, posttransplant patients

DOSAGE AND ROUTES

Herpes zoster
• *Adult:* **PO** 1 g tid × 1 wk
Genital herpes (suppressive, initial)
• *Adult:* **PO** 1 g bid × 10 days initially
Genital herpes (recurrent episodes)
• *Adult:* **PO** 500 mg bid × 3 days
Genital herpes (suppressive therapy)
• *Adult:* **PO** 1 g daily with normal immune function; 500 mg daily for those with ≤9 recurrences/yr; 500 mg bid in HIV-infected patients with CD4 ≥100
Herpes labialis
• *Adult:* **PO** 2 g bid × 1 day
Renal dose
• *Adult:* **PO** CCr 30-49 ml/min 1 g q12h (herpes zoster); 1 g q12h × 1 day (herpes labialis); CCr 10-29 ml/min 1 g q24h (genital herpes/herpes zoster); 500 mg q24h (recurrent genital herpes); CCr <10 ml/min 500 mg q24h (genital herpes/ herpes zoster), 500 mg q24h (recurrent genital herpes)
Available forms: Tabs 500 mg, 1 g

🅰 Safety alert   *"Tall Man" lettering

SIDE EFFECTS

CNS: Tremors, lethargy, *dizziness, headache,* weakness, *depression*
ENDO: Dysmenorrhea
GI: Nausea, vomiting, diarrhea, abdominal pain, constipation, *increased AST*
HEMA: **Thrombocytopenic purpura, hemolytic uremic syndrome**
INTEG: Rash

Contraindications: Hypersensitivity to this drug or acyclovir

Precautions: Pregnancy (B), lactation, hepatic/renal disease, electrolyte imbalance, dehydration, geriatric, thrombotic thrombocytopenic purpura/hemolytic uremic syndrome (TTP/HUS)

PHARMACOKINETICS

PO: Onset unknown, terminal half-life 2½-3½ hr; converted to acyclovir that crosses placenta and enters breast milk, excreted in urine primarily as acyclovir

INTERACTIONS

Increase: blood levels of valacyclovir—cimetidine, probenecid

NURSING CONSIDERATIONS
Assess:
• Signs of infection; characteristics of lesions; therapy should be started at first sign or symptom of herpes and is most effective within 72 hr of outbreak
⚠ For thrombocytopenic purpura, hemolytic uremic syndrome; may be fatal
• C&S before drug therapy; drug may be taken as soon as culture is taken; repeat C&S after treatment; determine the presence of other sexually transmitted diseases
• Bowel pattern before, during treatment
• Skin eruptions: rash
• Allergies before treatment, reaction of each medication
Administer:
• Within 72 hr of outbreak
• Orally before infection occurs

Evaluate:
• Therapeutic response: absence of itching, painful lesions; crusting and healed lesions
Teach patient/family:
• To take as prescribed; if dose is missed, take as soon as remembered up to 2 hr before next dose; do not double dose
• That drug may be taken orally before infection occurs; drug should be taken when itching or pain occurs, usually before eruptions
• That partners need to be told that patient has herpes; they can become infected; condoms must be worn to prevent reinfections
• That drug does not cure infection, just controls symptoms and does not prevent infection of others
Treatment of overdose: Discontinue drug, hemodialysis, resuscitate if needed

---

valganciclovir (℞)
(val-gan-sy′kloh-veer)
Valcyte
Func. class.: Antiviral
Chem. class.: Synthetic nucleoside analog

Do not confuse:
valganciclovir/valacyclovir
Valcyte/Valtrex
Action: Valganciclovir is metabolized to ganciclovir; inhibits replication of human cytomegalovirus in vivo and in vitro by selective inhibition of viral DNA synthesis
Uses: Cytomegalovirus (CMV) retinitis in immunocompromised persons, including those with AIDS, after indirect ophthalmoscopy confirms diagnosis, prevention of CMV in transplantation

DOSAGE AND ROUTES
Treatment of CMV
• *Adult:* **PO** induction 900 mg bid × 21 days with food; maintenance 900 mg daily with food

---

1048 valganciclovir

Transplant
• *Adult:* PO 900 mg daily with food starting within 10 days of transplantation until day 100 of posttransplantation
Renal dose
• *Adult:* PO CCr ≥60 ml/min same as above; CCr 40-59 ml/min 450 mg bid, then 450 mg daily; CCr 25-39 ml/min 450 mg daily, then 450 mg q2 days; CCr 10-24 ml/min 450 mg q2 days, then 450 mg 2×/ week

Available form: Tabs 450 mg

SIDE EFFECTS

CNS: Fever, chills, **coma**, *confusion*, abnormal thoughts, dizziness, bizarre dreams, *headache*, psychosis, tremors, somnolence, *paresthesia, weakness,* **seizures**
EENT: Retinal detachment in CMV retinitis
GI: Abnormal LFTs, nausea, vomiting, anorexia, diarrhea, abdominal pain, **hemorrhage**
GU: **Hematuria**, increased creatinine, BUN
HEMA: **Granulocytopenia, thrombocytopenia, irreversible neutropenia, anemia, eosinophilia**
INTEG: Rash, alopecia, *pruritus,* urticaria, pain at site, phlebitis, **Stevens-Johnson syndrome**
MISC: Local and systemic infections and sepsis

Contraindications: Hypersensitivity to acyclovir or ganciclovir, absolute neutrophil count <500, platelet count <25,000, hemodialysis
Precautions: Pregnancy (C), preexisting cytopenias, renal function impairment, lactation, children <6 mo, geriatric

PHARMACOKINETICS

Metabolized to ganciclovir, which has a half-life of 3-4½ hr, excreted by kidneys (unchanged); crosses blood-brain barrier, CSF

INTERACTIONS
• Severe granulocytopenia: zidovudine, antineoplastics, radiation; do not give together

Increase: toxicity—dapsone, pentamidine, flucytosine, vinCRIStine, vinBLAStine, adriamycin, DOXOrubicin, amphotericin B, trimethoprim-sulfamethoxazole combinations or other nucleoside analogs, cycloSPORINE
Increase: seizures—imipenem/cilastatin
Decrease: effect of didanosine
Decrease: renal clearance of valganciclovir—probenecid

NURSING CONSIDERATIONS
Assess:
• For leukopenia/neutropenia/thrombocytopenia: WBCs, platelets q2d during 2 ×/day dosing and then q1wk
• For leukopenia with daily WBC count in patients with prior leukopenia with other nucleoside analogs or for whom leukopenia counts are <1000 cells/mm^3 at start of treatment
• Serum creatinine or CCr ≥q2wk
Administer:
• With food
Evaluate:
• Therapeutic response: decreased symptoms of CMV
Teach patient/family:
• That drug does not cure condition; regular ophthalmologic and blood tests are necessary
• That major toxicities may necessitate discontinuing drug
• To use contraception during treatment and that infertility may occur; men should use barrier contraception for 90 days after treatment
• To take with food
⚠ To report infection: fever, chills, sore throat; blood dyscrasias: bruising, bleeding, petechiae
• To avoid crowds, persons with respiratory infections
• To use sunscreen to prevent burns

⚠ Safety alert   *"Tall Man" lettering

valproate
(val′proh-ate)
Depacon

valproic acid
(val′proh-ik)
Depakene, Myproic acid

divalproex sodium
(dye-val′proh-ex)
Depakote, Depakote ER,
Epival ✦
Func. class.: Anticonvulsant
Chem. class.: Carboxylic acid derivative

Action: Increases levels of γ-aminobutyric acid (GABA) in brain, which decreases seizure activity

Uses: Simple (petit mal), complex (petit mal) absence, mixed, manic episodes associated with bipolar disorder, prophylaxis of migraine, adjunct in schizophrenia, tardive dyskinesia, aggression in children with ADHD, organic brain syndrome mania, migraines

Unlabeled uses: Tonic-clonic (grand mal), myoclonic seizures; rectal (valproic acid)

DOSAGE AND ROUTES

Epilepsy
• *Adult and child:* **PO** 10-15 mg/kg/day divided in 2-3 doses, may increase by 5-10 mg/kg/day qwk, not to exceed 60 mg/kg/day in 2-3 divided doses; **IV** ≤20 mg/min over 1 hr

Mania (divalproex sodium)
• *Adult:* **PO** 750 mg daily in divided doses, max 60 mg/kg/day

Migraine (divalproex sodium)
• *Adult:* **PO** 250 mg bid, may increase to 1000 mg/day if needed or 500 mg (Depakote ER) daily × 7 days, then 1000 mg daily

Available forms: *Valproate:* inj 100 mg/ml; syr 250 mg/5 ml; *valproic acid:* caps 250 mg; *divalproex:* delayed rel tabs 125, 250, 500 mg; ext rel tabs 250, 500 mg; sprinkle cap 125 mg

SIDE EFFECTS

CNS: Sedation, drowsiness, dizziness, headache, incoordination, depression, hallucinations, behavioral changes, tremors, aggression, weakness

EENT: Visual disturbances, taste perversion

GI: Nausea, vomiting, constipation, diarrhea, dyspepsia, anorexia, cramps, **hepatic failure, pancreatitis, toxic hepatitis,** stomatitis

GU: Enuresis, irregular menses

HEMA: **Thrombocytopenia, leukopenia, lymphocytosis,** increased PT, bruising, epistaxis

INTEG: Rash, alopecia, photosensitivity, dry skin

Contraindications: Pregnancy (D), hypersensitivity, hepatic disease

Precautions: Lactation, child <2 yr, geriatric

PHARMACOKINETICS

PO: Onset 15-30 min, peak 1-4 hr, duration 4-6 hr

Metabolized by liver; excreted by kidneys, breast milk; crosses placenta; half-life 9-16 hr

INTERACTIONS

Increase: valproic acid level—erythromycin, felbamate

Increase: CNS depression—alcohol, opioids, barbiturates, antihistamines, MAOIs, sedative/hypnotics

Increase: toxicity of valproic acid—salicylates

Increase: action of phenytoin, tricyclic antidepressants, carbamazepine, ethosuximide, barbiturates, zidovudine

Increase: bleeding—antiplatelets, NSAIDs, tirofiban, eptifibatide, abciximab, cefoperazone, cefotetan, heparin, thrombolytics

Increase: toxicity of carbamazepine ethosuximide, lamotrigine, zidovudine

Decrease: metabolism of valproic acid—cimetidine

Decrease: valproic acid level—rifampin carbamazepine, lamotrigine

---

Drug/Lab Test
False positive: Ketones, urine
Interference: Thyroid function tests

NURSING CONSIDERATIONS
Assess:
- Seizure disorder: location, aura, activity, duration; seizure precautions should be in place
- Bipolar disorder: mood, activity, sleeping/eating, behavior
- Migraines: frequency, intensity, alleviating factor
- Blood studies: Hct, Hgb, RBC, serum folate, PT, platelets, vit D if on long-term therapy
- Hepatic studies: AST, ALT, bilirubin, hepatic failure
- Blood levels: therapeutic level 50-100 mcg/ml, in seizures
- Respiratory dysfunction: respiratory depression, character, rate, rhythm; hold drug if respirations are <12/min or if pupils are dilated

Administer:
PO route
- Swallow tabs or caps whole; do not break, crush, or chew ER tabs
- Elixir alone; do not dilute with carbonated beverage; do not give syrup to patients on sodium restriction
- Give with food or milk to decrease GI symptoms

Evaluate:
- Therapeutic response: decreased seizures

Teach patient/family:
- That physical dependency may result from extended use
- To avoid driving, other activities that require alertness
- Not to discontinue medication quickly after long-term use; convulsions may result
- To report visual disturbances, rash, diarrhea, abdominal pain, light-colored stools, jaundice, protracted vomiting to prescriber

valsartan (℞)
(val'sahr-tan)
Diovan
Func. class.: Antihypertensive
Chem. class.: Angiotensin II receptor antagonist (Type AT_1)

Action: Blocks the vasoconstrictor and aldosterone-secreting effects of angiotensin II; selectively blocks the binding of angiotensin II to the AT_1 receptor found in tissues
Uses: Hypertension, alone or in combination, CHF

DOSAGE AND ROUTES
Hypertension
- *Adult:* **PO** 80-160 mg daily alone or in combination with other antihypertensives, may increase to 320 mg
CHF
- *Adult:* **PO** 40 mg bid, up to 160 mg bid
Available forms: Tabs 80, 160, 320 mg

SIDE EFFECTS
CNS: Dizziness, insomnia, drowsiness, vertigo, headache, fatigue
CV: Angina pectoris, 2nd-degree AV block, **cerebrovascular accident,** hypotension, **myocardial infarction,** *dysrhythmias*
EENT: Conjunctivitis
GI: Diarrhea, abdominal pain, nausea, **hepatotoxicity**
GU: Impotence, **nephrotoxicity**
HEMA: Anemia, neutropenia
META: Hyperkalemia
MS: Cramps, myalgia, pain, stiffness
RESP: Cough
Contraindications: Pregnancy (D) 2nd/3rd trimester, hypersensitivity, severe hepatic disease, bilateral renal artery stenosis
Precautions: Hypersensitivity to ACE inhibitors; CHF, hypertrophic cardiomyopathy aortic/mitral valve stenosis, CAD, lac-

tation, children, geriatric, angioedema, renal/hepatic disease

PHARMACOKINETICS

Peak 2-4 hr; duration >24 hr; extensively metabolized; protein binding 95%; half-life 6 hr; excreted in feces, urine, breast milk

INTERACTIONS

Increase: effects of lithium
Increase: hyperkalemia—potassium-sparing diuretics, potassium supplements, ACE inhibitors
Decrease: antihypertensive effects—NSAIDs, salicylates
Drug/Herb
Increase: toxicity, death—aconite
Increase: antihypertensive effect—barberry, betony, black catechu, black cohosh, bloodroot, broom, burdock, cat's claw, dandelion, goldenseal, hawthorn, Irish moss, Jamaican dogwood, kelp, khella, mistletoe, parsley
Increase or decrease: antihypertensive effect—astragalus, cola tree
Decrease: antihypertensive effect—coltsfoot, guarana, khat, licorice, yohimbine

NURSING CONSIDERATIONS

Assess:
• B/P, pulse q4h; note rate, rhythm, quality
• Blood studies; BUN, creatinine, LFTs before treatment
• Electrolytes: K, Na, Cl, total CO_2
• Baselines in renal, hepatic studies before therapy begins
• Edema in feet, legs daily
• Skin turgor, dryness of mucous membranes for hydration status
Administer:
• Without regard to meals
Evaluate:
• Therapeutic response: decreased B/P
Teach patient/family:
• To comply with dosage schedule, even if feeling better

• To notify prescriber of fever, swelling of hands or feet, irregular heartbeat, chest pain
• That excessive perspiration, dehydration, diarrhea may lead to fall in blood pressure; consult prescriber if these occur
• That drug may cause dizziness, fainting; light-headedness may occur
• To rise slowly to sitting or standing position to minimize orthostatic hypotension
• Not to take this medication if pregnant or breastfeeding, or have had an allergic reaction to this drug
• That if a dose is missed, to take it as soon as possible, unless it is within an hour before next dose

---

vancomycin (℞)

(van-koe-mye'sin)
Lyphocin, Vancocin,
Vancoled, vancomycin HCl
Func. class.: Antiinfective—miscellaneous
Chem. class.: Tricyclic glycopeptide

Action: Inhibits bacterial cell wall synthesis
Uses: Resistant staphylococcal infections, pseudomembranous colitis, staphylococcal enterocolitis, endocarditis prophylaxis for dental procedures, diphtheroid endocarditis

DOSAGE AND ROUTES

Serious staphylococcal infections
• *Adult:* IV 500 mg q6-8h or 1 g q12h
• *Child:* IV 40 mg/kg/day divided q6-8h
• *Neonate:* IV 15 mg/kg initially followed by 10 mg/kg q8-24h
Pseudomembranous/staphylococcal enterocolitis
• *Adult:* PO 500 mg/day in divided doses for 7-10 days
• *Child:* PO 40 mg/kg/day divided q6h, not to exceed 2 g/day

Endocarditis prophylaxis
- *Adult:* IV 1 g over 1 hr, 1 hr before procedure
- *Child:* IV 20 mg/kg over 1 hr, 1 hr prior to procedure

Available forms: Pulvules 125, 250 mg; powder for oral sol 1, 10 g; powder for inj 500 mg, 1, 5, 10 g

SIDE EFFECTS

CV: **Cardiac arrest, vascular collapse (rare),** hypotension

EENT: Ototoxicity, permanent deafness, tinnitus, nystagmus

GI: **Nausea, pseudomembranous colitis**

GU: **Nephrotoxicity,** *increased BUN, creatinine, albumin,* **fatal uremia**

HEMA: **Leukopenia, eosinophilia, neutropenia**

INTEG: Chills, fever, rash, thrombophlebitis at inj site, urticaria, pruritus, necrosis (Red man syndrome)

RESP: Wheezing, dyspnea

SYST: **Anaphylaxis, superinfection**

Contraindications: Hypersensitivity, previous hearing loss

Precautions: Pregnancy (C), renal disease, lactation, geriatric, neonates

PHARMACOKINETICS

IV: Peak 5 min; half-life 4-8 hr; excreted in urine (active form)
PO: Absorption: poor

INTERACTIONS

Increase: ototoxicity or nephrotoxicity—aminoglycosides, cephalosporins, colistin, polymyxin, bacitracin, cisplatin, amphotericin B, nondepolarizing muscle relaxants, cidofovir, polymyxin B

Drug/Herb
- Do not use acidophilus with antiinfectives; separate by several hours

NURSING CONSIDERATIONS

Assess:
- I&O ratio; report hematuria, oliguria; nephrotoxicity may occur

⚠ Any patient with compromised renal system; drug is excreted slowly in poor renal system function; toxicity may occur rapidly; BUN, creatinine
- Blood studies: WBC
- Serum levels: peak 1 hr after 1 hr inf 25-40 mg/ml; trough prior to next dose 5-10 mg/ml
- C&S; drug may be given as soon as culture is taken
- Auditory function during, after treatment
- B/P during administration; sudden drop may indicate Red man syndrome
- Signs of infection
- Hearing loss, ringing, roaring in ears; drug should be discontinued
- Skin eruptions
- Respiratory status: rate, character, wheezing, tightness in chest
- Allergies before treatment, reaction of each medication

Administer:
- Antihistamine if Red man syndrome occurs: decreased B/P, flushing of neck, face
- Dose based on serum concentration

IV route
- After reconstitution with 10 ml sterile water for injection (500 mg/10 ml); further dilution is needed for IV, 500 mg/100 ml 0.9% NaCl, D_5W given as int inf over 1 hr; decrease rate of infusion if Red man syndrome occurs

Y-site compatibilities: Acyclovir, allopurinol, amifostine, amiodarone, amsacrine, atracurium, cisatracurium, cyclophosphamide, diltiazem, DOXOrubicin liposome, enalaprilat, esmolol, filgrastim, fluconazole, fludarabine, gallium, granisetron, hydromorphone, insulin (regular), labetalol, lorazepam, magnesium sulfate, melphalan, meperidine, meropenem, midazolam, morphine, ondansetron, paclitaxel, pancuronium, perphenazine, propofol, remifentanil, sodium bicarbonate, tacrolimus, teniposide, theophylline, thiotepa, tolazoline, vecuronium, vinorelbine, warfarin, zidovudine

Perform/provide:
- Storage at room temperature for up to 2 wk after reconstitution

---

⚠ Safety alert   *"Tall Man" lettering

• EpINEPHrine, suction, tracheostomy set, endotracheal intubation equipment on unit; anaphylaxis may occur
• Adequate intake of fluids (2 L/day) to prevent nephrotoxicity

Evaluate:
• Therapeutic response: absence of fever, sore throat; negative culture

Teach patient/family:
• All aspects of drug therapy: need to complete entire course of medication to ensure organism death (7-10 days); culture may be taken after completed course of medication
• To report sore throat, fever, fatigue; could indicate superinfection
• That drug must be taken in equal intervals around clock to maintain blood levels

vardenafil (Rx)

(var-den'a-fil)
Levitra
Func. class.: Impotence agent
Chem. class.: Phosphodiesterase type 5 inhibitor

Action: Inhibits phosphodiesterase type 5 (PDE5), enhances erectile function by increasing the amount of cGMP, which in turn causes smooth muscle relaxation and increased blood flow into the corpus cavernosum

Uses: Treatment of erectile dysfunction

DOSAGE AND ROUTES

• *Adult:* **PO** 10 mg, taken 1 hr before sexual activity, dose may be reduced to 5 mg or increased to a max of 20 mg; max dosing frequency is once daily
• *Geriatric >65 yr:* **PO** 5 mg initially

Hepatic dose (Child-Pugh B)
• *Adult:* **PO** 5 mg, max 10 mg daily

Concomitant medications
• Ritonavir, max 2.5 mg q72hr; for indinavir, ketoconazole 400 mg/day and itraconazole 400 mg/day, max 2.5 mg/day; for ketoconazole 200 mg/day, itraconazole 200 mg/day and erythromycin max 5 mg/day

Available forms: Tabs 2.5, 5, 10, 20 mg

SIDE EFFECTS

CNS: Headache, flushing, dizziness, insomnia
CV: Hypertension, **MI, CV collapse,** chest pain
EENT: Conjunctivitis, tinnitus, photophobia, diminished vision, glaucoma
GU: Abnormal ejaculation, priapism
MISC: Rash, GERD, GGTP increased, **NAION (nonarteritic ischemic optic neuropathy),** dyspepsia
MS: Myalgia, arthralgia, neck pain
RESP: Rhinitis, sinusitis, dyspnea, pharyngitis, epistaxis

Contraindications: Hypersensitivity, coadministration of α-blockers or nitrates, renal failure

Precautions: Pregnancy (B), hepatic impairment, retinis pigmentosa, CV disease including congenital or acquired QT prolongation, anatomical penile deformities, sickle cell anemia, leukemia, multiple myeloma, bleeding disorders, active peptic ulceration, renal disease; not indicated for women, children, or newborns

PHARMACOKINETICS

Rapidly absorbed; bioavailability 15%; protein binding 95%; metabolized by liver; terminal half-life 4-5 hr, onset 20 min, peak ½-1½ hr, duration <5 hr, reduced absorption with high-fat meal; primarily excreted in feces (91-95%)

INTERACTIONS

⚠ Do not use with nitrates because of unsafe decrease in B/P, which could result in MI or stroke
Increase: hypotension—α-blockers, protease inhibitors, metoprolol, nifedipine, alcohol, amlodipine, angiotensin II receptor blockers; do not use concurrently
Increase: vardenafil levels—erythromycin, azole antifungals (ketoconazole, intraconazole), cimetidine, antiretroviral protease inhibitors

NURSING CONSIDERATIONS

Assess:
- If any severe loss of vision occurs while taking this or any similar products, these products should not be used
- Use of organic nitrates that should not be used with this drug

Administer:
- Approximately 1 hr before sexual activity; do not use more than once a day
- Do not use with nitrates in any form

Teach patient/family:
- That drug does not protect against sexually transmitted diseases, including HIV
- That drug absorption is reduced with a high-fat meal
- That drug should not be used with nitrates in any form
- That drug has no effect in the absence of sexual stimulation
- That patient should seek immediate medical attention if erections last for more than 4 hr
- To inform physician of all medications being taken
- To notify prescriber immediately and stop taking product if vision loss occurs

---

varenicline
See Appendix A—Selected New Drugs

---

vasopressin (℞)
(vay-soe-press'in)
Pitressin Synthetic
Func. class.: Pituitary hormone
Chem. class.: Lysine vasopressin

Action: Promotes reabsorption of water by action on renal tubular epithelium; causes vasoconstriction

Uses: Diabetes insipidus (nonnephrogenic/nonpsychogenic), abdominal distention postoperatively, bleeding esophageal varices

DOSAGE AND ROUTES

Diabetes insipidus
- *Adult:* **IM/SUBCUT** 5-10 units bid-qid as needed; **IM/SUBCUT** 2.5-5 units q2-3d (Pitressin Tannate) for chronic therapy
- *Child:* **IM/SUBCUT** 2.5-10 units bid-qid as needed; **IM/SUBCUT** 1.25-2.5 units q2-3d (Pitressin Tannate) for chronic therapy

Abdominal distention
- *Adult:* **IM** 5 units, then q3-4h, increasing to 10 units if needed (aqueous)

Available forms: Inj 20, 5 units/ml (tannate), spray, cotton pledgets

SIDE EFFECTS

CNS: Drowsiness, headache, lethargy, flushing
CV: Increased B/P
EENT: Nasal irritation, congestion, rhinitis
GI: Nausea, heartburn, cramps
GU: Vulval pain, uterine cramping
MISC: Tremor, sweating, vertigo, urticaria, bronchial constriction

Contraindications: Hypersensitivity, chronic nephritis

Precautions: Pregnancy (C), lactation, CAD

PHARMACOKINETICS

Nasal: Onset 1 hr, duration 3-8 hr, half-life 15 min; metabolized in liver, kidneys; excreted in urine

NURSING CONSIDERATIONS

Assess:
- Nasal mucosa if given by intranasal spray; for irritation
- Pulse, B/P, when giving drug IV or IM
- I&O ratio, weight daily; check for edema in extremities; if water retention is severe, diuretic may be prescribed
- H_2O intoxication: lethargy, behavioral changes, disorientation, neuromuscular excitability

Evaluate:
- Therapeutic response: absence of severe thirst, decreased urine output, osmolality

---

Teach patient/family:
- To measure and record I&O
- To avoid alcohol, all OTC medications unless approved by prescriber

⚠ High Alert

vecuronium (℞)
(vek-yoo-roe'nee-um)
Norcuron
Func. class.: Neuromuscular blocker, nondepolarizing
Chem. class.: Monoquaternary analog of pancuronium

Do not confuse:
Norcuron/narcan

Action: Inhibits transmission of nerve impulses by binding with cholinergic receptor sites, antagonizing action of acetylcholine

Uses: Facilitation of endotracheal intubation, skeletal muscle relaxation during mechanical ventilation, surgery, general anesthesia

DOSAGE AND ROUTES
- *Adult and child >9 yr:* **IV BOL** 0.08-0.10 mg/kg, then 0.01-0.015 mg/kg for prolonged procedures
Available forms: 10 mg/5 ml vial

SIDE EFFECTS
CNS: Skeletal muscle weakness or paralysis (rare)
INTEG: Urticaria
RESP: **Prolonged apnea, possible respiratory paralysis,** bronchospasm, tachycardia, flushing, wheezing
SYST: **Anaphylaxis**
Contraindications: Hypersensitivity
Precautions: Pregnancy (C), lactation, children <2 yr, electrolyte imbalances, dehydration, hepatic/cardiac/respiratory/neuromuscular disease

PHARMACOKINETICS
IV: Onset 2-3 min, peak 3-5 min, duration 15-25 (recovery index) min; half-life 65-75 min; not metabolized; excreted in urine/feces; crosses placenta

INTERACTIONS
- Dysrhythmias: theophylline
Increase: neuromuscular blockade—aminoglycosides, amphotericin B, clindamycin, lincomycin, quinidine, local anesthetics, polymyxin antibiotics, lithium, opioid analgesics, phenytoin, piperacillin, thiazides, enflurane, isoflurane, succinylcholine, verapamil

NURSING CONSIDERATIONS
Assess:
- VS (B/P, pulse, respirations, airway) q15min until fully recovered; rate, depth, pattern of respirations, strength of hand grip
- I&O ratio; check for urinary retention, frequency, hesitancy
- Recovery: decreased paralysis of face, diaphragm, leg, arm, rest of body; allow to recover fully before completing neurologic assessment
- Allergic reactions: rash, fever, respiratory distress, pruritus; drug should be discontinued
Administer:
- With diazepam or morphine when used for therapeutic paralysis; provides no sedation alone
- Using nerve stimulator by anesthesiologist to determine neuromuscular blockade
- Anticholinesterase to reverse neuromuscular blockade
- IV after diluting with diluent provided; give by direct IV over 1 min; may give as continuous inf 10-20 mg/100 ml; titrate to patient response (only by qualified person)
Y-site compatibilities: Aminophylline, cefazolin, cefuroxime, cimetidine, diltiazem, DOBUTamine, DOPamine, epiNEPHrine, esmolol, fentanyl, fluconazole, gentamicin, heparin, hydrocortisone, hydromorphone, isoproterenol, labetalol, lorazepam, midazolam, milrinone, morphine, niCARdipine, nitroglycerin, norepinephrine, propofol, ranitidine, sodium nitroprusside, trimethoprim-sulfamethoxazole, vancomycin

V

Perform/provide:
• Storage in refrigerator; discard in 24 hr
• Reassurance if communication is difficult during recovery from neuromuscular blockade

Evaluate:
• Therapeutic response: paralysis of jaw, eyelid, head, neck, rest of body

Treatment of overdose: Edrophonium or neostigmine, atropine, monitor VS; may require mechanical ventilation

venlafaxine (R)
(ven-la-fax′een)
Effexor, Effexor-XR
Func. class.: Antidepressant—miscellaneous

Action: Potent inhibitor of neuronal serotonin and norepinephrine uptake, weak inhibitor of DOPamine; no muscarinic, histaminergic, or α-adrenergic receptors in vitro

Uses: Prevention/treatment of major depression, to treat depression at end of life, long-term treatment of general anxiety disorder; social anxiety disorder

Unlabeled uses: Hot flashes, obsessive-compulsive disorder (OCD), premenstrual dysphoric disorder (PMDD), posttraumatic stress disorder (PTSD)

DOSAGE AND ROUTES

Renal dose
• Mild-moderate impairment, 75% of dose

Hepatic dose
• Moderate impairment, 50% of dose

Depression
• *Adult:* PO 75 mg/day in 2 or 3 divided doses; taken with food, may be increased to 150 mg/day; if needed, may be further increased to 225 mg/day; increments of 75 mg/day at intervals of no less than 4 days; some hospitalized patients may require up to 375 mg/day in 3 divided doses; **EXT REL** 37.5-75 mg PO daily, max 225 mg/day; give XR daily

Hot flashes (unlabeled)
• *Adult:* PO 12.5 mg bid × 4 wk or **EXT REL** 37.5 mg × 4 wk

Available forms: Tabs scored (Effexor) 25, 37.5, 50, 75, 100 mg; ext rel cap (Effexor-XR) 37.5, 75, 150 mg

SIDE EFFECTS

CNS: Emotional lability, vertigo, apathy, ataxia, CNS stimulation, euphoria, hallucinations, hostility, increased libido, hypertonia, hypotonia, psychosis, insomnia, anxiety, **suicidal ideation in children/adolescents, seizures**

CV: Migraine, angina pectoris, hypertension, extrasystoles, postural hypotension, syncope, thrombophlebitis

EENT: Abnormal vision, taste, *ear pain,* cataract, conjunctivitis, corneal lesions, dry eyes, otitis media, photophobia

GI: Dysphagia, eructation, nausea, anorexia, dry mouth, colitis, gastritis, gingivitis, **rectal hemorrhage,** stomatitis, stomach and mouth ulceration

GU: Anorgasmia, abnormal ejaculation, *dysuria, hematuria, metrorrhagia, vaginitis, impaired urination,* albuminuria, amenorrhea, kidney calculus, cystitis, nocturia, breast and bladder pain, polyuria, **uterine hemorrhage, vaginal hemorrhage,** moniliasis

HEMA: **Agranulocytosis, aplastic anemia, neutropenia, pancytopenia**

INTEG: Ecchymosis, acne, alopecia, brittle nails, dry skin, photosensitivity

META: Peripheral edema, weight loss or gain, diabetes mellitus, edema, glycosuria, hyperlipemia, hypokalemia

MS: Arthritis, bone pain, bursitis, myasthenia tenosynovitis, arthralgia

RESP: Bronchitis, dyspnea, asthma, chest congestion, epistaxis, hyperventilation, laryngitis

SYST: Malaise, neck pain, enlarged abdomen, cyst, facial edema, hangover, hernia

Contraindications: Hypersensitivity, bipolar disorder

Precautions: Pregnancy (C), mania, lactation, children, geriatric, hypertension, seizure disorder, recent MI, cardiac disease

PHARMACOKINETICS

Well absorbed, extensively metabolized in the liver to an active metabolite; 87% of drug recovered in urine; 27% protein binding; half-life 5-7, 11-13 hr (active metabolite) respectively

INTERACTIONS

A Hyperthermia, rigidity, rapid fluctuations of vital signs, mental status changes, neuroleptic malignant syndrome: MAOIs
Increase: venlafaxine effect—cimetidine
Increase: CNS depression—alcohol, opioids, antihistamines, sedative/hypnotics
Increase: levels of clozapine, desipramine, haloperidol, warfarin
Increase: serotonin syndrome—sibutramine, sumatriptan, trazadone
Decrease: effect of indinavir
Decrease: venlafaxine effect—cyproheptadine

Drug/Herb
• Serotonin syndrome: SAM-e, St. John's wort
Increase: CNS depression—chamomile, hops, kava, lavender, skullcap, valerian
Increase: anticholinergic effect—corkwood, jimsonweed
Increase: hypertension—yohimbe

Drug/Lab Test
Increase: Alk phos, bilirubin, AST, ALT, BUN, creatinine, serum cholesterol, CPK, LDH

NURSING CONSIDERATIONS

Assess:
• B/P lying, standing; pulse q4h; if systolic B/P drops 20 mm Hg, hold drug, notify prescriber; take VS q4h in patients with CV disease
• Electrolytes: Hypo/hyperkalemia, hypo/hyperphosphatemia, hyponatremia, hyperuricemia, hypo/hyperglycemia can occur
• Blood studies: CBC, leukocytes, differential cardiac enzymes if patient is receiving long-term therapy
• Hepatic studies: AST, ALT, bilirubin
• Weight qwk; weight loss or gain; appetite may increase; peripheral edema may occur

• With food, milk for GI symptoms
• Sugarless gum, hard candy, frequent sips of water for dry mouth
• Mental status: mood, sensorium, affect, increase in psychiatric symptoms; depression, panic; assess for suicidal ideation in children/adolescents
• Withdrawal symptoms: headache, nausea, vomiting, muscle pain, weakness; not usual unless drug is discontinued abruptly

Administer:
• Avoid use with CNS depressants
• In small amounts because of suicide potential, especially in the beginning of therapy

Perform/provide:
• Storage in tight container at room temperature; do not freeze
• Assistance with ambulation during beginning therapy, since drowsiness, dizziness occur
• Checking to see if PO medication swallowed

Evaluate:
• Therapeutic response; decreased depression

Teach patient/family:
• To notify prescriber of rash, hives or allergic reactions
• To use with caution when driving or other activities requiring alertness because of drowsiness, dizziness, blurred vision
• To avoid alcohol ingestion
• Not to discontinue medication quickly after long-term use; may cause nausea, headache, malaise
• To wear sunscreen or large hat, since photosensitivity occurs
• To avoid pregnancy or lactation while taking this product

Treatment of overdose: ECG monitoring; induce emesis; lavage, activated charcoal; administer anticonvulsant

V

verapamil (Ᵽ)

(ver-ap'a-mill)

Apo-Verap ✦, Calan, Calan SR, Covera-HS, Isoptin, Isoptin SR, verapamil HCl, verapamil HCl SR, Verelan PM

Func. class.: Calcium channel blocker; antihypertensive; antianginal

Chem. class.: Diphenylalkylamine

Action: Inhibits calcium ion influx across cell membrane during cardiac depolarization; produces relaxation of coronary vascular smooth muscle; dilates coronary arteries; decreases SA/AV node conduction; dilates peripheral arteries

Uses: Chronic stable, vasospastic, unstable angina; dysrhythmias; hypertension, supraventricular tachycardia, atrial flutter or fibrillation

Unlabeled uses: Prevention of migraine headaches, ventricular outflow obstruction in hypertrophic cardiomyopathy, recumbent nocturnal leg cramps

DOSAGE AND ROUTES

Angina
• *Adult:* PO 80-120 mg tid, increase qwk
Dysrhythmias
• *Adult:* PO 240-320 mg/day in 3-4 divided doses in digitalized patients
• *Adult:* IV **BOL** 5-10 mg (0.075-0.15 mg/kg) over 2 min, may repeat 10 mg (0.15 mg/kg) ½ hr after 1st dose
• *Child 1-15 yr:* IV **BOL** 0.1-0.3 mg/kg over 2 min or more, repeat in 30 min, not to exceed 5 mg in a single dose
• *Child 0-1 yr:* IV **BOL** 0.1-0.2 mg/kg over ≥2 min, may repeat after 30 min
Hypertension
• *Adult:* PO 80 mg tid, may titrate upward; **EXT REL** 120-240 mg/day as a single dose, may increase to 240-480 mg/day
Available forms: Tabs 40, 80, 120 mg; ext rel tabs 120, 180, 240 mg; inj 2.5 mg/ml; ext rel caps 100, 200, 240, 300 mg

SIDE EFFECTS

CNS: Headache, drowsiness, dizziness, anxiety, depression, weakness, insomnia, confusion, light-headedness, asthenia, fatigue
CV: Edema, **CHF,** bradycardia, hypotension, palpitations, AV block
GI: Nausea, diarrhea, gastric upset, *constipation,* increased LFTs
GU: Impotence, gynecomastia, nocturia, polyuria
INTEG: Rash, bruising
MISC: Gingival hyperplasia
SYST: **Stevens-Johnson syndrome**
Contraindications: Sick sinus syndrome, 2nd- or 3rd-degree heart block, hypotension <90 mm Hg systolic, cardiogenic shock, severe CHF
Precautions: Pregnancy (C), CHF, hypotension, hepatic injury, lactation, children, renal disease, concomitant β-blocker therapy, geriatric

PHARMACOKINETICS

IV: Onset 3 min, peak 3-5 min, duration 10-20 min
PO: Onset variable, peak 3-4 hr, duration 17-24 hr, half-life (biphasic) 4 min, 3-7 hr (terminal)
Metabolized by liver, excreted in urine (70% as metabolites)

INTERACTIONS

Increase: hypotension—prazosin, quinidine, fentanyl, other antihypertensives, nitrates
Increase: effects of verapamil—β-blockers, cimetidine
Increase: levels of digoxin, theophylline, cycloSPORINE, carbamazepine, nondepolarizing muscle relaxants
Decrease: effects of lithium
Decrease: antihypertensive effects—NSAIDs
Drug/Herb
Increase: effect—barberry, betel palm, burdock, goldenseal, khat, lily of the valley, plantain
Decrease: effect—yohimbe

⚠ Safety alert   *"Tall Man" lettering

Drug/Food
Increase: hypotensive effects—grapefruit juice
Drug/Lab Test
Increase: AST, ALT, alk phos, BUN, creatinine, serum cholesterol

NURSING CONSIDERATIONS
Assess:
• Cardiac status: B/P, pulse, respiration, ECG intervals (PR, QRS, QT)
⚠ I&O ratios, weight daily; CHF: crackles, weight gain, dyspnea, jugular vein distention
• Renal, hepatic studies during long-term treatment, serum potassium periodically
Administer:
PO route
• Do not crush or chew ext rel products; caps may be opened and contents sprinkled on food; do not dissolve chew cap contents
• Before meals, at bedtime; give ext rel with food
IV route
• Undiluted through Y-tube or 3-way stopcock of compatible sol; give over 2 min, or 3 min geriatric, discard unused solution
Additive compatibilities: Amikacin, amiodarone, ascorbic acid, atropine, bretylium, calcium chloride, calcium gluconate, cefazolin, cefotaxime, cefoxitin, cephapirin, chloramphenicol, cimetidine, clindamycin, dexamethasone, diazepam, digoxin, DOPamine, epINEPHrine, erythromycin, gentamicin, heparin, hydrocortisone sodium phosphate, hydrocortisone, hydromorphone, insulin (regular), isoproterenol, lidocaine, magnesium sulfate, mannitol, meperidine, metaraminol, methicillin, methyldopate, methylPREDNISolone, metoclopramide, mezlocillin, morphine, moxalactam, multivitamins, naloxone, nitroglycerin, norepinephrine, oxytocin, pancuronium, penicillin G potassium, penicillin G sodium, pentobarbital, phenobarbital, phentolamine, phenytoin, piperacillin, potassium chloride, potassium phosphates, procainamide, propranolol, protamine, quinidine, so-

dium bicarbonate, sodium nitroprusside, theophylline, ticarcillin, tobramycin, tolazoline, vancomycin, vasopressin, vit B/C
Syringe compatibilities: Amrinone, heparin, milrinone
Y-site compatibilities: Amrinone, ciprofloxacin, DOBUTamine, DOPamine, famotidine, hydrALAZINE, meperidine, methicillin, milrinone, penicillin G potassium, piperacillin, propofol, ticarcillin
Evaluate:
• Therapeutic response: decreased anginal pain, decreased B/P, dysrhythmias
Teach patient/family:
• To increase fluids/fiber to counteract constipation
• How to take pulse before taking drug; to keep record or graph
• To avoid hazardous activities until stabilized on drug, dizziness no longer a problem
• To limit caffeine consumption; no alcohol products
• To avoid OTC drugs unless directed by prescriber
• To comply with all areas of medical regimen: diet, exercise, stress reduction, drug therapy
• To change positions slowly to prevent syncope
Treatment of overdose: Defibrillation, atropine for AV block, vasopressor for hypotension, IV calcium

---

vidarabine ophthalmic
See Appendix C

⚠ High Alert

vinBLAStine (VLB) (℞)
(vin-blast'een)
Velban, Velbe ✳, vinblastine
sulfate
Func. class.: Antineoplastic
Chem. class.: Vinca rosea alkaloid

Do not confuse:
vinBLAStine/vinCRIStine

Action: Inhibits mitotic activity, arrests cell cycle at metaphase; inhibits RNA synthesis, blocks cellular use of glutamic acid needed for purine synthesis; a vesicant

Uses: Breast, testicular cancer, lymphomas, neuroblastoma; Hodgkin's, non-Hodgkin's lymphomas; mycosis fungoides, histiocytosis, Kaposi's sarcoma

DOSAGE AND ROUTES

• *Adult:* IV 0.1 mg/kg or 3.7 mg/m² qwk or q2wk, not to exceed 0.5 mg/kg or 18.5 mg/m² qwk
• *Child:* 2.5 mg/m² then 3.75, 5, 6.25, 7.5 at 7-day intervals

Available forms: Inj, powder 10 mg for 10 ml IV

SIDE EFFECTS

CNS: Paresthesias, peripheral neuropathy, depression, headache, **seizures**
CV: Tachycardia, orthostatic hypotension
GI: Nausea, vomiting, ileus, *anorexia, stomatitis,* constipation, abdominal pain, **GI, rectal bleeding, hepatotoxicity,** pharyngitis
GU: Urinary retention, **renal failure**
HEMA: **Thrombocytopenia, leukopenia, myelosuppression**
HEMA: Agranulocytosis, granulocytosis, aplastic anemia, neutropenia, pancytopenia
INTEG: Rash, alopecia, photosensitivity
META: SIADH
RESP: **Fibrosis, pulmonary infiltrate, bronchospasm**

Contraindications: Pregnancy (D), hypersensitivity, infants, leukopenia, granulocytopenia, lactation
Precautions: Renal/hepatic disease

PHARMACOKINETICS

Half-life (triphasic) 35 min, 53 min, 19 hr; metabolized in liver, excreted in urine, feces; crosses blood-brain barrier

INTERACTIONS

• Synergism: bleomycin
• Bronchospasm: mitomycin
• Do not use with radiation
Increase: toxicity, bone marrow suppression—antineoplastics
Increase: action of methotrexate
Increase: adverse reactions—live virus vaccines
Decrease: phenytoin level—phenytoin

NURSING CONSIDERATIONS

Assess:
⚠ CBC, differential, platelet count qwk; withhold drug if WBC is <2000/mm³ or platelet count is <75,000/mm³; notify prescriber
• Pulmonary function tests, chest x-ray studies before, during therapy; chest x-ray film should be obtained q2wk during treatment
• Neurologic status: sensory-vibratory evaluation if side effects occur
• Renal studies: BUN, serum uric acid, urine CCr, electrolytes before, during therapy
• I&O ratio; report fall in urine output of 30 ml/hr
• Monitor temp q4h; may indicate beginning infection
• Hepatic studies before, during therapy (bilirubin, AST, ALT, LDH) as needed or qmo
• RBC, Hct, Hgb, since these may be decreased
• Bleeding: hematuria, guaiac, bruising or petechiae, mucosa of orifices q8h

---

⚠ Safety alert   *"Tall Man" lettering

- Dyspnea, crackles, unproductive cough, chest pain, tachypnea, fatigue, increased pulse, pallor, lethargy
- Effects of alopecia on body image; discuss feelings about body changes
- Sensitivity of feet/hands, which precedes neuropathy
- Jaundiced skin, sclera; dark urine, clay-colored stools, itchy skin, abdominal pain, fever, diarrhea
- Buccal cavity q8h for dryness, sores or ulceration, white patches, oral pain, bleeding, dysphagia
- Local irritation, pain, burning, discoloration at inj site
- Symptoms indicating severe allergic reaction: rash, pruritus, urticaria, purpuric skin lesions, itching, flushing
- Frequency of stools and characteristics: cramping; acidosis; signs of dehydration: rapid respirations, poor skin turgor, decreased urine output, dry skin, restlessness, weakness

Administer:
- Antiemetic 30-60 min before giving drug and prn to prevent vomiting
- Transfusion for anemia

IV route
- After diluting 10 mg/10 ml NaCl; give through Y-tube or 3-way stopcock or directly over 1 min
- Hyaluronidase 150 units/ml in 1 ml NaCl, warm compress for extravasation for vesicant activity treatment

Additive compatibilities: Bleomycin
Syringe compatibilities: Bleomycin, cisplatin, cyclophosphamide, droperidol, fluorouracil, leucovorin, methotrexate, metoclopramide, mitomycin, vinCRIStine
Y-site compatibilities: Allopurinol, amifostine, amphotericin B cholesteryl, aztreonam, bleomycin, cisplatin, cyclophosphamide, DOXOrubicin, DOXOrubicin liposome, droperidol, filgrastim, fludarabine, fluorouracil, granisetron, heparin, leucovorin, melphalan, methotrexate, metoclopramide, mitomycin, ondansetron, paclitaxel, piperacillin/tazobactam, sargramostim, teniposide, thiotepa, vinCRIStine, vinorelbine

Perform/provide:
- Deep-breathing exercises with patient 3-4 ×/day; place in semi-Fowler's position
- Liquid diet: cola, Jell-O; dry toast or crackers may be added if patient is not nauseated or vomiting
- Increase fluid intake to 2-3 L/day to prevent urate deposits, calculi formation
- Rinsing of mouth tid-qid with water
- Brushing of teeth bid-tid with soft brush or cotton-tipped applicators for stomatitis; use unwaxed dental floss
- Nutritious diet with iron, vitamin supplements
- HOB raised to facilitate breathing

Evaluate:
- Therapeutic response: decreased tumor size, spread of malignancy

Teach patient/family:
- To report any complaints or side effects to nurse or prescriber
- To report any changes in breathing or coughing; to avoid exposure to persons with infection
- That hair may be lost during treatment, a wig or hairpiece may make patient feel better; tell patient that new hair may be different in color, texture
- To report change in gait or numbness in extremities; may indicate neuropathy
- To avoid foods with citric acid, hot or rough texture
- To report any bleeding, white spots or ulcerations in mouth to prescriber; to examine mouth daily
- To wear sunscreen, protective clothing, sunglasses
- To avoid receiving vaccinations
- To use effective contraception, avoid breastfeeding

Side effects: *italics* = common; **bold** = life-threatening

> ⚠ **High Alert**

vinCRIStine (VCR) (℞)
(vin-kris'teen)
Oncovin, Vincasar PFS, vincristine sulfate
Func. class.: Antineoplastic—miscellaneous
Chem. class.: Vinca alkaloid

Do not confuse:
vinCRIStine/vinBLAStine

Action: Inhibits mitotic activity, arrests cell cycle at metaphase; inhibits RNA synthesis, blocks cellular use of glutamic acid needed for purine synthesis; a vesicant

Uses: Breast, lung cancer, lymphomas, neuroblastoma, Hodgkin's disease, acute lymphoblastic and other leukemias, rhabdomyosarcoma, Wilms' tumor, osteogenic and other sarcomas

DOSAGE AND ROUTES
• *Adult:* IV 1-2 mg/m²/wk, not to exceed 2 mg
• *Child:* IV 1.5-2 mg/m²/wk, not to exceed 2 mg
Available forms: Inj 1 mg/ml; powder for inj 5 mg/vial

SIDE EFFECTS
CNS: Decreased reflexes, numbness, weakness, motor difficulties, CNS depression, cranial nerve paralysis, **seizures**
CV: Orthostatic hypotension
GI: Nausea, vomiting, anorexia, stomatitis, constipation, **paralytic ileus,** *abdominal pain,* **hepatotoxicity**
HEMA: **Thrombocytopenia, leukopenia, myelosuppression, anemia**
INTEG: Alopecia
Contraindications: Pregnancy (D), hypersensitivity, infants, radiation therapy, lactation
Precautions: Renal/hepatic disease, hypertension, neuromuscular disease

PHARMACOKINETICS
Half-life (triphasic) 0.85 min, 7.4 min, 164 min; metabolized in liver; excreted in bile, feces; crosses placental barrier, blood-brain barrier

INTERACTIONS
• Neurotoxicity: peripheral nervous system drugs
• Do not use with radiation
• Acute pulmonary reactions: mitomycin-c
Increase: action of methotrexate, anticoagulants
Decrease: digoxin level—digoxin
Decrease: action of vinCRIStine—L-asparaginase

NURSING CONSIDERATIONS
Assess:
• CBC, differential, platelet count qwk; withhold drug if WBC is <4000/mm³ or platelet count is <75,000/mm³; notify prescriber
• Renal studies: BUN, serum uric acid, urine CCr, electrolytes before, during therapy
• I&O ratio, report fall in urine output of 30 ml/hr
• Monitor temp q4h; may indicate beginning infection
• Hepatic studies before, during therapy (bilirubin, AST, ALT, LDH) as needed or monthly
• RBC, Hct, Hgb; may be decreased
• Deep tendon reflexes; drug is neurotoxic
• Sensitivity of feet/hands, which precedes neuropathy
• Bleeding: hematuria, guaiac, bruising or petechiae, mucosa of orifices q8h
• Effects of alopecia on body image, discuss feelings about body changes
• Jaundiced skin, sclera; dark urine, clay-colored stools, itchy skin, abdominal pain, fever, diarrhea
• Buccal cavity q8h for dryness, sores or ulceration, white patches, oral pain, bleeding, dysphagia

• Symptoms indicating severe allergic reaction: rash, pruritus, urticaria, purpuric skin lesions, itching, flushing

• Frequency of stools, characteristics: cramping, acidosis; signs of dehydration: rapid respirations, poor skin turgor, decreased urine output, dry skin, restlessness, weakness

Administer:

• Agents to prevent constipation

• Antiemetic 30-60 min before giving drug and prn

• Transfusion for anemia

• Antispasmodic for GI symptoms

IV route

• After diluting with diluent provided or 1 mg/10 ml of sterile H_2O or NaCl; give through Y-tube or 3-way stopcock or directly over 1 min

• Hyaluronidase 150 units/ml in 1 ml NaCl; apply warm compress for extravasation

Additive compatibilities: Bleomycin, cytarabine, fluorouracil, methotrexate

Syringe compatibilities: Bleomycin, cisplatin, cyclophosphamide, doxapram, DOXOrubicin, droperidol, fluorouracil, heparin, leucovorin, methotrexate, metoclopramide, mitomycin, vinBLAStine

Y-site compatibilities: Allopurinol, amifostine, amphotericin B cholesteryl, aztreonam, bleomycin, cisplatin, cladribine, cyclophosphamide, DOXOrubicin, DOXOrubicin liposome, droperidol, filgrastim, fludarabine, fluorouracil, granisetron, heparin, leucovorin, melphalan, methotrexate, metoclopramide, mitomycin, ondansetron, paclitaxel, piperacillin/tazobactam, sargramostim, teniposide, thiotepa, vinBLAStine, vinorelbine

Perform/provide:

• Liquid diet: cola, Jell-O; dry toast or crackers may be added if patient is not nauseated or vomiting

• Rinsing of mouth tid-qid with water

• Brushing of teeth bid-tid with soft brush or cotton-tipped applicators for stomatitis; use unwaxed dental floss

• Nutritious diet with iron, vitamin supplements

Evaluate:

• Therapeutic response: decreased tumor size, spread of malignancy

Teach patient/family:

• To report change in gait or numbness in extremities; may indicate neuropathy

• To report any complaints or side effects to nurse or prescriber

• To report any bleeding, white spots or ulcerations in mouth to prescriber; to examine mouth daily

• To increase bulk, fluids, exercise to prevent constipation

• To avoid persons with infections

• To avoid vaccinations

• That hair may be lost; hair will grow back but different texture, color

• To use effective contraception, avoid breastfeeding

> ⚠ **High Alert**
>
> **vinorelbine** (Ⓡ)
> (vi-nor′el-bine)
> Navelbine
> *Func. class.:* Antineoplastic—miscellaneous
> *Chem. class.:* Semisynthetic vinca alkaloid

Action: Inhibits mitotic activity, arrests cell cycle at metaphase; inhibits RNA synthesis, blocks cellular use of glutamic acid needed for purine synthesis; a vesicant

Uses: Unresectable advanced non–small cell lung cancer (NSCLC) stage IV; may be used alone or in combination with cisplatin for stage III or IV NSCLC breast cancer

DOSAGE AND ROUTES

• *Adult:* IV 30 mg/m² qwk

Hepatic dose

• *Adult:* IV total bilirubin 2.1-3 mg/dl 15 mg/m² qwk; total bilirubin ≥3 mg/dl 7.5 mg/m² daily

Available forms: Inj 10 mg/ml

SIDE EFFECTS

CNS: Paresthesias, peripheral neuropathy, depression, headache, **seizures,** weakness, jaw pain

CV: Chest pain

GI: Nausea, vomiting, ileus, *anorexia, stomatitis,* constipation, abdominal pain, diarrhea, **hepatotoxicity**

HEMA: **Neutropenia, anemia, thrombocytopenia, granulocytopenia**

INTEG: Rash, alopecia, photosensitivity

META: SIADH

MS: Myalgia

RESP: Shortness of breath

Contraindications: Pregnancy (D), hypersensitivity, infants, granulocyte count <1000 cells/mm^3 pretreatment, lactation

Precautions: Renal/hepatic disease, geriatric, children

PHARMACOKINETICS

Half-life 27-43 hr, peak 1-2 hr

INTERACTIONS

• Possible increased toxicity: fluorouracil

NURSING CONSIDERATIONS

Assess:

• B/P (baseline and q15min) during administration

• CBC, differential, platelet count weekly; withhold drug if WBC is <4000/mm^3 or platelet count is <75,000/mm^3; notify prescriber of results, recovery will take 3 wk

• For dyspnea, crackles, unproductive cough, chest pain, tachypnea

• Renal studies: BUN, serum uric acid, urine CCr before, during therapy; I&O ratio; report fall in urine output to <30 ml/hr; for decreased hyperuricemia

• For cold, fever, sore throat (may indicate beginning infection); notify prescriber if these occur; effects of alopecia on body image

• For bleeding: hematuria, guaiac, bruising or petechiae, mucosa or orifices q8h, no rectal temps; avoid IM inj; use pressure to venipuncture sites

• Nutritional status: an antiemetic may be needed

⚠ For symptoms of severe allergic reactions: rash, pruritus, urticaria, itching, flushing, bronchospasm, hypotension, epINEPHrine and crash cart should be nearby

Administer:

• Antiemetic 30-60 min before giving drug and prn to prevent vomiting

IV route

• Hyaluronidase 150 units/ml in 1 ml NaCl, warm compress for extravasation for vesicant activity treatment

• By cont inf: 40 mg/m^2 q3wk after an IV bol of 8 mg/m^2; may be given in combination with DOXOrubicin, fluorouracil, cisplatin

Y-site compatibilities: Amikacin, aztreonam, bleomycin, bumetanide, buprenorphine, butorphanol, calcium gluconate, carboplatin, carmustine, cefotaxime, ceftazidime, ceftizoxime, chlorproMAZINE, cimetidine, cisplatin, clindamycin, cyclophosphamide, cytarabine, dacarbazine, dactinomycin, DAUNOrubicin, dexamethasone, diphenhydrAMINE, DOXOrubicin, DOXOrubicin liposome, doxycycline, droperidol, enalaprilat, etoposide, famotidine, filgrastim, floxuridine, fluconazole, fludarabine, gallium, gentamicin, granisetron, haloperidol, heparin, hydrocortisone, hydromorphone, hydrOXYzine, idarubicin, ifosfamide, imipenem-cilastatin, lorazepam, mannitol, mechlorethamine, melphalan, meperidine, mesna, methotrexate, metoclopramide, metronidazole, minocycline, mitoxantrone, morphine, nalbuphine, netilmicin, ondansetron, plicamycin, streptozocin, teniposide, ticarcillin, ticarcillin/clavulanate, tobramycin, vancomycin, vinBLAStine, vinCRIStine, zidovudine

Perform/provide:

• Liquid diet: cola, Jell-O; dry toast or crackers if patient not nauseated or vomiting

• Brushing of teeth bid-tid with soft brush or cotton-tipped applicators for stomatitis; unwaxed dental floss

---

⚠ Safety alert   *"Tall Man" lettering

• Nutritious diet with iron, vitamin supplements

Evaluate:

• Therapeutic response: decreased tumor size, spread of malignancy

Teach patient/family:

• To report change in gait or numbness in extremities; may indicate neuropathy

• To report any complaints or side effects to nurse or prescriber

• To examine mouth daily for bleeding, white spots, ulcerations; notify prescriber

• To avoid crowds, people with infections, vaccinations

• To use effective contraception, avoid breastfeeding

• That hair may be lost; hair will grow back, but different texture, color

---

vitamin A (℞, otc)

Aquasol A, Del-Vi-A, Vitamin A
Func. class.: Vitamin, fat soluble
Chem. class.: Retinol

Action: Needed for normal bone, tooth development, visual dark adaptation, skin disease, mucosa tissue repair, assists in production of adrenal steroids, cholesterol, RNA

Uses: Vit A deficiency

DOSAGE AND ROUTES

• *Adult and child >8 yr:* **PO** 100,000-500,000 international units daily × 3 days, then 50,000 daily × 2 wk; dose based on severity of deficiency; maintenance 10,000-20,000 international units for 2 mo

• *Child 1-8 yr:* **IM** 5000-15,000 international units daily × 10 days

• *Infant <1 yr:* **IM** 5000-15,000 international units × 10 days

Maintenance

• *Child 4-8 yr:* **IM** 15,000 international units daily × 2 mo

• *Child <4 yr:* **IM** 10,000 international units daily × 2 mo

Available forms: Caps 10,000, 25,000, 50,000 international units; drops 5000 in-

ternational units; inj 50,000 international units/ml; tabs 10,000, 25,000, 50,000 international units

SIDE EFFECTS

CNS: Headache, **increased intracranial pressure, intracranial hypertension,** lethargy, malaise

EENT: Gingivitis, papilledema, exophthalmos, inflammation of tongue and lips

GI: Nausea, vomiting, anorexia, abdominal pain, **jaundice**

INTEG: Drying of skin, pruritus, increased pigmentation, night sweats, alopecia

META: Hypomenorrhea, hypercalcemia

MS: Arthralgia, retarded growth, hard areas on bone

Contraindications: Hypersensitivity to vit A, malabsorption syndrome (PO)

Precautions: Pregnancy (C), lactation, impaired renal function

PHARMACOKINETICS

Stored in liver, kidneys, fat; excreted (metabolites) in urine, feces

INTERACTIONS

Increase: levels of vit A—corticosteroids, oral contraceptives

Decrease: absorption of vit A—mineral oil, cholestyramine, colestipol

Drug/Lab Test

False increase: Bilirubin, serum cholesterol

NURSING CONSIDERATIONS

Assess:

• Nutritional status: yellow and dark green vegetables, yellow/orange fruits, vit A–fortified foods, liver, egg yolks

• Vit A deficiency: decreased growth, night blindness, dry, brittle nails; hair loss; urinary stones; increased infection, hyperkeratosis of skin; drying of cornea

Administer:

PO route

• With food (PO) for better absorption

• Do not administer IV because of risk of anaphylactic shock; IM only

• Oral preparations are not indicated for

vitamin A deficiency in those with malabsorption syndrome

Perform/provide:
• Storage in tight, light-resistant container

Evaluate:
• Therapeutic response: increased growth rate, weight; absence of dry skin and mucous membranes, night blindness

Teach patient/family:
• That if dose is missed, it should be omitted
• That ophthalmic exams may be required periodically throughout therapy
• Not to use mineral oil while taking this drug
• To notify prescriber of nausea, vomiting, lip cracking, loss of hair, headache
• Not to take more than the prescribed amount

Treatment of overdose: Discontinue drug

**vitamin D (chole-
calciferol, vitamin D₃ or
ergocalciferol, vitamin
D₂)** (℞, otc)

Calciferol, Delta-D, Drisdol,
Radiostol ✿, Radiostol Forte ✿,
Vitamin D, Vitamin D₃
Func. class.: Vit D
Chem. class.: Fat soluble

Do not confuse:
Calciferol/calcitriol

Action: Needed for regulation of calcium, phosphate levels, normal bone development, parathyroid activity, neuromuscular functioning

Uses: Vit D deficiency, rickets, renal osteodystrophy, hypoparathyroidism, hypophosphatemia, psoriasis, rheumatoid arthritis

DOSAGE AND ROUTES

Deficiency
• *Adult:* **PO/IM** 12,000 international units daily, then increased to 500,000 international units/day
• *Child:* **PO/IM** 1500-5000 international

units daily × 2-4 wk, may repeat after 2 wk or 600,000 international units as single dose

Hypoparathyroidism
• *Adult and child:* **PO/IM** 200,000 international units given with 4 g calcium tab

Available forms: Tabs 400, 1000, 50,000 international units; caps 25,000, 50,000 international units; liq 8000 international units/ml; inj 500,000 international units/ml, 500,000 international units/5 ml

SIDE EFFECTS

CNS: Fatigue, weakness, drowsiness, **seizures,** headache, psychosis
CV: Hypertension, dysrhythmias
GI: Nausea, vomiting, anorexia, cramps, diarrhea, constipation, metallic taste, dry mouth
GU: Polyuria, nocturia, **hematuria, albuminuria, renal failure,** decreased libido
INTEG: Pruritus, photophobia
MS: Decreased bone growth, early joint pain, early muscle pain

Contraindications: Hypersensitivity, hypercalcemia, renal dysfunction, hyperphosphatemia

Precautions: Pregnancy (C), CV disease, renal calculi

PHARMACOKINETICS

Half-life 12-22 hr; stored in liver, duration 2 mo; excreted in bile (metabolites) and urine

INTERACTIONS

Increase: toxicity—diuretics (thiazides), antacids, verapamil
Decrease: effects of vit D—cholestyramine, colestipol, phenobarbital, phenytoin

NURSING CONSIDERATIONS

Assess:
• Vit D levels q2wk during treatment
• Calcium, PO₄, magnesium, BUN, alk phos, urine Ca, creatinine
• In children, monitor height and weight

• Nutritional status: egg yolk, fortified dairy products, cod, halibut, salmon, sardines

Administer:
• IM inj deep in large muscle mass; administer slowly; aspirate carefully; rotate inj sites; avoid IV administration
• A decrease of antacids and laxatives containing magnesium

Evaluate:
• Therapeutic response: absence of rickets/osteomalacia, adequate calcium/phosphate levels, decrease in bone pain

Teach patient/family:
• That if dose is missed, to omit
• The necessary foods in diet
• To avoid vitamin supplements unless directed by prescriber
• To keep appointments with health care providers; line between therapeutic and toxic doses is narrow
• To report weakness, lethargy, headache, anorexia, loss of weight
• To report nausea, vomiting, abdominal cramps, diarrhea, constipation, excessive thirst, polyuria, muscle and bone pain
• To decrease intake of antacids and laxatives containing magnesium

---

vitamin E (otc)

Amino-Opti-E, Aquasol E, Daltose ♣, E-Complex-600, E-Ferol, E-Vitamin Succinate, E-200 I.U. Softgels, Gordo-Vite E, Tocopherol, Vitamin E, Vita-Plus E Softgels, Vitec
Func. class.: Vit E
Chem. class.: Fat soluble

Action: Needed for digestion and metabolism of polyunsaturated fats, decreases platelet aggregation, decreases blood clot formation, promotes normal growth and development of muscle tissue, prostaglandin synthesis
Uses: Vit E deficiency, impaired fat absorption, hemolytic anemia in premature neonates, prevention of retrolental fibro-

plasia, sickle cell anemia, supplement in malabsorption syndrome

DOSAGE AND ROUTES
Deficiency
• *Adult:* **PO** 60-75 international units daily
• *Child:* **PO** 1 mg/0.6 g of dietary fat
Prevention of deficiency
• *Adult:* **PO** 30 international units/day; **TOP** apply to affected areas
• *Infant:* **PO** 5 international units/day
Available forms: Caps 100, 200, 400, 500, 600, 1000 international units; tabs 100, 200, 400 international units; drops 50 mg/ml; chew tabs 400 units; ointment; cream; lotion; oil

SIDE EFFECTS
CNS: Headache, fatigue
CV: Increased risk of thrombophlebitis
EENT: Blurred vision
GI: Nausea, cramps, diarrhea
GU: Gonadal dysfunction
INTEG: Sterile abscess, contact dermatitis
META: Altered metabolism of hormones: thyroid, pituitary, adrenal; altered immunity
MS: Weakness
Contraindications: IV use in infants
Precautions: Pregnancy (A)

PHARMACOKINETICS
PO: Metabolized in liver, excreted in bile

INTERACTIONS
Increase: action of oral anticoagulants
Decrease: absorption—cholestyramine, colestipol, mineral oil, sucralfate

NURSING CONSIDERATIONS
Assess:
• Nutritional status: wheat germ, dark green leafy vegetables, nuts, eggs, liver, vegetable oils, dairy products, cereals
Administer:
PO route
• Administer with or after meals
• Chew chewable tabs well

V

- Sol may be dropped in mouth or mixed with food

Topical route
- To moisturize dry skin

Perform/provide:
- Storage in tight, light-resistant container

Evaluate:
- Therapeutic response: absence of hemolytic anemia, adequate vit E levels, improvement in skin lesions, decreased edema

Teach patient/family:
- The necessary foods in diet
- To omit if dose is missed
- To avoid vitamin supplements unless directed by prescriber

---

voriconazole (℞)

(vohr-i-kahn'a-zol)
Vfend
Func. class.: Antifungal, systemic
Chem. class.: Triazole derivative

Action: Inhibits fungal CYP 450-mediation demethylation, needed for biosynthesis

Uses: Invasive aspergillosis, serious fungal infections (*Scedosporium apiospermum, Fusarium* sp, *Monosporium, Apiospermum*)

DOSAGE AND ROUTES

- *Adult:* **PO** Give 1 hr before or after meals; ≥40 kg: 200 mg q12h; ≤40 kg: 100 mg q12h
- *Adult:* **IV** Loading dose 6 mg/kg q12h × 2 dose, then 4 mg/kg q12h; may switch to oral dosing

Renal dose
- *Adult:* **PO** CCr <50 ml/min; use only orally

Hepatic dose
- *Adult:* **PO** 6 mg/kg q12h × 2 doses, then 2 mg/kg q12h or 100 mg q12h if >40 kg; 50 mg q12h if <40 kg

Available forms: Tabs 50, 200 mg; powder for inj, lyophilized 200 mg voriconazole, powder for oral susp 45 g (40 mg/ml after reconstitution)

SIDE EFFECTS

CNS: Headache, paresthesias, peripheral neuropathy, hallucinations, psychosis, EPS, depression, Guillain-Barré syndrome, insomnia, suicidal ideation, dizziness

CV: **Tachycardia,** hyper/hypotension, vasodilation, **atrial arrhythmias, atrial fibrillation, AV block, bradycardia, CHF, MI**

EENT: Blurred vision, eye hemorrhage

GI: Nausea, vomiting, anorexia, diarrhea, cramps, **hemorrhagic gastroenteritis, acute hepatic failure, hepatitis, intestinal perforation, pancreatitis**

GU: Hypokalemia, azotemia, **renal tubular necrosis, permanent renal impairment, anuria, oliguria**

HEMA: Anemia, **eosinophilia,** hypomagnesemia, **thrombocytopenia, leukopenia, pancytopenia**

INTEG: Burning, irritation, pain, necrosis at inj site with extravasation, dermatitis, rash, photosensitivity

MISC: Respiratory disorder

SYST: **Stevens-Johnson syndrome, toxic epidermal necrolysis, sepsis**

Contraindications: Pregnancy (D), hypersensitivity, severe bone marrow depression, lactation, children, severe hepatic disease

Precautions: Renal disease (IV)

PHARMACOKINETICS

By CYP450 enzymes, protein binding 58%; max serum conc 1-2 hr after dosing; eliminated via hepatic metabolism

INTERACTIONS

Increase: effects of benzodiazepines, calcium channel blockers, cycloSPORINE, ergots, HMG-CoA reductase inhibitors, pimozide, quinidine, prednisoLONE, sirolimus, sulfonylureas, tacrolimus, vinca alkaloids, warfarin, rifabutin, proton pump inhibitors, NNRTIs, protease inhibitors, phenytoin

Increase: nephrotoxicity—other nephrotoxic antibiotics (aminoglycosides, cis-

---

platin, vancomycin, cycloSPORINE, polymyxin B)

Increase: hypokalemia—corticosteroids, digoxin, skeletal muscle relaxants, thiazides

Drug/Herb
Increase: possibility of nephrotoxicity—gossypol

Drug/Food
• Avoid use with high-fat meals

NURSING CONSIDERATIONS
Assess:
• VS q15-30min during first infusion; note changes in pulse, B/P
• I&O ratio; watch for decreasing urinary output, change in specific gravity; discontinue drug to prevent permanent damage to renal tubules
• Blood studies: CBC, K, Na, Ca, Mg q2wk, BUN, creatinine weekly
• Weight weekly; if weight increases over 2 lb/wk, edema is present; renal damage should be considered
⚠ For renal toxicity: increasing BUN, serum creatinine; if BUN is >40 mg/dl or if serum creatinine >3 mg/dl, drug may be discontinued or dosage reduced
⚠ For hepatotoxicity: increasing AST, ALT, alk phos, bilirubin
• For allergic reaction: dermatitis, rash; drug should be discontinued, antihistamines (mild reaction) or epINEPHrine (severe reaction) administered
• For hypokalemia: anorexia, drowsiness, weakness, decreased reflexes, dizziness, increased urinary output, increased thirst, paresthesias
• For ototoxicity: tinnitus (ringing, roaring in ears), vertigo, loss of hearing (rare); visual disturbance

Administer:
PO route
• Oral susp: tap bottle; add 46 ml of water to bottle; shake well; remove cap; push bottle adaptor into neck of bottle; replace cap; write expiration date (14 days); shake well before each use; administer using only oral dispenser supplied
• 1 hr before or after meals

IV route
• Drug only after C&S confirms organism, drug needed to treat condition; make sure drug is used in life-threatening infections
• Reconstitute powder with 19 ml water for inj to 10 mg/ml, shake until dissolved; infuse over 1-2 hr at a conc of 5 mg/ml or less; do not admix with other drugs, 4.2% sodium bicarbonate inf
• Store at room temp (powder, tabs)

Evaluate:
• Therapeutic response: decreased fever, malaise, rash, negative C&S for infecting organism

Teach patient/family:
• That long-term therapy may be needed to clear infection (2 wk–3 mo depending on type of infection)
• To notify prescriber of bleeding, bruising, or soft tissue swelling
• Take 1 hr before or after meal
• Do not drive at night because of vision changes
• Avoid strong, direct sunlight
• Women of childbearing age should use effective contraceptive

---

⚠ High Alert

warfarin (℞)
(war′far-in)
Coumadin, warfarin sodium, Warfilone ✦
Func. class.: Anticoagulant

Do not confuse:
Coumadin/Cardura/Compazine

Action: Interferes with blood clotting by indirect means; depresses hepatic synthesis of vit K–dependent coagulation factors (II, VII, IX, X)

Uses: Pulmonary emboli, deep vein thrombosis; prevention or treatment of venous thrombosis, pulmonary embolism, thromboembolic complications associated with atrial fibrillation, or cardiac valve replacement; after MI to reduce risk of death

W

Side effects: *italics* = common; **bold** = life-threatening

DOSAGE AND ROUTES

- *Adult:* **PO/IV** 2.5-10 mg/day × 3 days, then titrated to INR
- *Geriatric:* **PO/IV** 2-10 mg/day
- *Child:* 0.1 mg/kg/day titrated to INR

Available forms: Tabs 1, 2, 2.5, 3, 4, 5, 6, 7.5, 10 mg; inj 5.4 mg powder for inj

SIDE EFFECTS

CNS: Fever

GI: Diarrhea, nausea, vomiting, anorexia, stomatitis, cramps, **hepatitis**

GU: **Hematuria**

HEMA: **Hemorrhage, agranulocytosis, leukopenia, eosinophilia,** anemia

INTEG: Rash, dermatitis, urticaria, alopecia, pruritus

MISC: Purple toe syndrome, epistaxis, hemoptysis

Contraindications: Pregnancy (X), hypersensitivity, hemophilia, leukemia with bleeding, peptic ulcer disease, thrombocytopenic purpura, hepatic disease (severe), malignant hypertension, subacute bacterial endocarditis, acute nephritis, blood dyscrasias, eclampsia, preeclampsia, lactation, hemorrhagic tendencies; surgery of CNS, eye; traumatric surgery with large open surface, bleeding tendencies of GI/GU/respiratory, stroke, aneurysms, pericardial effusion, spinal puncture, major regional/lumbar block anesthesia

Precautions: Alcoholism, geriatric, CHF, debilitated patients, trauma, indwelling catheters, severe hypertension, active infections, protein C deficiency, polycythemia vera, vasculitis, severe diabetes

PHARMACOKINETICS

PO: Onset 12-24 hr, peak 1½-4 days, duration 3-5 days, effective half-life 20-60 hr; metabolized in liver, excreted in urine/feces (active/inactive metabolites), crosses placenta, 99% bound to plasma proteins

INTERACTIONS

Increase: warfarin action—allopurinol, chloramphenicol, furosemide, HMG-CoA reductase inhibitors, SSRIs, amiodarone, diflunisal, heparin, steroids, cimetidine, disulfiram, thyroid, glucagon, metronidazole, quinidine, sulindac, sulfinpyrazone, sulfonamides, clofibrate, salicylates, ethacrynic acids, indomethacin, mefenamic acid, oxyphenbutazones, phenylbutazone, penicillins, chloral hydrate, cotrimoxazole, erythromycin, quinolone antiinfectives, isoniazid, thrombolytic agents, tricyclics, NSAIDs, COX-2 selective inhibitors

Increase: toxicity—oral sulfonylureas, phenytoin

Decrease: warfarin action—aprepitant, azathioprine, barbiturates, bile acid sequestrants, bosentan, carbamazepine, dicloxacillin, estrogens, ethchlorvynol, griseofulvin, nafcillin, oral contraceptives, phenytoin, rifampin, sucralfate, sulfasalazine, thyroid, vit K, vit K foods

Drug/Herb

Increase: risk of bleeding—agrimony, angelica, anise, basil, bay, bilberry, black currant, black haw, bogbean, bromelain, buchu, cat's claw, chamomile, chondroitin, cinchona bark, cranberry, devil's claw, dong quai, evening primrose, fenugreek, feverfew, garlic, ginger, ginkgo, ginseng, horse chestnut, Irish moss, kava, kelp, kelpware, khella, licorice, lovage, lungwort, meadowsweet, melatonin, motherwort, mugwort, nettle, papaya, parsley (large amts), pau d'arco, pineapple, poplar, prickly ash, red clover, safflower, saw palmetto, skullcap, tonka bean, turmeric, wintergreen, yarrow

Decrease: anticoagulant effect—alfalfa, coenzyme Q10, flax, glucomannan, goldenseal, guar gum, St. John's wort

Drug/Lab Test

Increase: T_3 uptake

Decrease: Uric acid

⚠ Safety alert   *"Tall Man" lettering

NURSING CONSIDERATIONS
Assess:
• Blood studies (Hct, platelets, occult blood in stools) q3mo
• INR: In hospital daily after 2nd or 3rd dose; once in therapeutic range for 2 consecutive days, monitor 2-3 × wk for 1-2 wk, them less frequently depending on stability of INR results; Outpatient: monitor every few days until stable dose, then periodically thereafter depending on stability of INR results
• Bleeding gums, petechiae, ecchymosis, black tarry stools, hematuria
⚠ Fever, skin rash, urticaria
• Needed dosage change q1-2wk; when stable, PT q3wk
Administer:
• At same time each day to maintain steady blood levels
• Tabs whole or crushed
• Avoiding all IM inj that may cause bleeding
IV route
• Reconstitute with 2.7 ml of sterile water for inj; do not use solution that is discolored or has particulates
• Give over 1-2 min into peripheral vein
Y-site compatibilities: Amikacin, cefazolin, ceftriaxone, DOPamine, heparin, lidocaine, morphine, nitroglycerin, potassium chloride, ranitidine
Perform/provide:
• Storage in tight container
Evaluate:
• Therapeutic response: decrease of deep vein thrombosis
Teach patient/family:
• To avoid OTC preparations that may cause serious drug interactions unless directed by prescriber
• To use soft-bristle toothbrush to avoid bleeding gums, and to use electric razor
• To carry emergency ID identifying drug taken
• The importance of compliance
• To report any signs of bleeding: gums, under skin, urine, stools

• To avoid hazardous activities (football, hockey, skiing), dangerous work
• The importance of avoiding unusual changes in vitamin intake, diet, or lifestyle
• To inform dentists and other physicians of anticoagulant intake
Treatment of overdose: Administer vit K

xylometazoline nasal agent
See Appendix C

zafirlukast (℞)
(za-feer′loo-cast)
Accolate
Func. class.: Bronchodilator
Chem. class.: Leukotriene receptor antagonist

Action: Antagonizes the contractile action of leukotrienes (LTC_4, LTD_4, LTE_4) in airway smooth muscle; inhibits bronchoconstriction caused by antigens
Uses: Prophylaxis and chronic treatment of asthma in adults/children >5 yr
Unlabeled uses: Chronic urticaria

DOSAGE AND ROUTES
• *Adult and child ≥12 yr:* **PO** 20 mg bid, take 1 hr before meals or 2 hr after meals
• *Child 5-11 yr:* **PO** 10 mg bid
Available forms: Tabs 10, 20 mg

SIDE EFFECTS
CNS: Headache, dizziness
GI: Nausea, diarrhea, abdominal pain, vomiting, dyspepsia
OTHER: Infections, pain, asthenia, myalgia, fever, increased ALT, urticaria, rash, **angioedema**
Contraindications: Hypersensitivity
Precautions: Pregnancy (B), geriatric, lactation, children, hepatic disease

PHARMACOKINETICS

Rapidly absorbed, peak 3 hr, 99% protein binding (albumin), extensively metabolized; inhibits CYP4502C9 and 3A4 enzyme systems; excreted in feces, clearance is reduced in the geriatric, hepatic impairment, half-life 10 hr

INTERACTIONS

Increase: plasma levels of zafirlukast—aspirin
Increase: PT—warfarin
Decrease: plasma levels of zafirlukast—erythromycin, theophylline
Drug/Herb
Increase: effect—green tea (large amounts), guarana
Drug/Food
Decrease: bioavailability

NURSING CONSIDERATIONS

Assess:
⚠ Adult patients carefully for symptoms of Churg-Strauss syndrome (rare), including eosinophilia, vasculitic rash, worsening pulmonary symptoms, cardiac complications, and/or neuropathy
• Respiratory rate, rhythm, depth; auscultate lung fields bilaterally; notify prescriber of abnormalities
Administer:
• 1 hr before or 2 hr after meals; absorption may be decreased if given with food
• With water if GI upset occurs
Evaluate:
• Therapeutic response: ability to breathe more easily
Teach patient/family:
• To check OTC medications, current prescription medications, which will increase stimulation
• To avoid hazardous activities; dizziness may occur
• That if GI upset occurs, to take drug with 8 oz water; avoid food if possible, absorption may be decreased
• To notify prescriber of nausea, vomiting, diarrhea, abdominal pain, fatigue, jaundice, anorexia, flulike symptoms (hepatic dysfunction)

• Not to use for acute asthma episodes
• Not to take if breastfeeding
• To take even if symptom free

---

zalcitabine (R̵)
(zal-sit′a-bin)
ddC, dideoxycytidine, HIVID
Func. class.: Antiretroviral
Chem. class.: Nucleoside reverse transcriptase inhibitor (NRTI)

Action: Inhibits HIV-1 replication by the conversion of this drug by cellular enzymes to an active antiviral metabolite, a chain terminator
Uses: HIV-1 infections in combination in adults, children >13 yr

DOSAGE AND ROUTES

• *Adult:* PO 0.75 mg q8h in combination with other antiretrovirals, in presence of peripheral neuropathy initiate dose at 0.375 mg q8h of zalcitabine
Renal dose
• *Adult:* PO CCr 10-40 ml/min 0.75 mg q12h; CCr <10 ml/min 0.75 mg q24h
Available forms: Tabs 0.375, 0.75 mg

SIDE EFFECTS

CNS: Headache, *peripheral neuropathy,* **seizures,** confusion, anxiety, hypertonia, abnormal thinking, asthenia, insomnia, CNS depression, pain, *dizziness,* chills, *fever*
CV: Hypertension, vasodilation, dysrhythmia, syncope, palpitation, tachycardia, **cardiomyopathy, CHF**
EENT: Ear pain, otitis, photophobia, visual impairment
ENDO: Hypoglycemia, hyponatremia, hyperbilirubinemia, hyperglycemia
GI: **Pancreatitis,** *diarrhea, nausea, vomiting,* abdominal pain, constipation, stomatitis, dysplasia, hepatic abnormalities, *oral ulcers,* flatulence, taste perversion, dry mouth, oral thrush, melena, *increased ALT, AST, alk phos, amylase*
GU: Uric acid, **toxic nephropathy,** polyuria

⚠ Safety alert   *"Tall Man" lettering

HEMA: **Leukopenia, granulocytopenia, thrombocytopenia,** anemia

INTEG: Rash, pruritus, alopecia, sweating, acne

MS: Myalgia, arthritis, myopathy, muscular atrophy

RESP: Cough, pneumonia, dyspnea, asthma, hypoventilation

SYST: **Lactic acidosis**

Contraindications: Hypersensitivity

Precautions: Pregnancy (C), renal/hepatic disease, lactation, child <13 yr, peripheral neuropathy, heart failure

PHARMACOKINETICS

PO: Peak 0.5-2 hr, elimination half-life 1-3 hr; elimination via kidneys

INTERACTIONS

Increase: risk of pancreatitis with agents that can cause pancreatitis (ddI, d4T)

Increase: risk of peripheral neuropathy with other agents that can cause peripheral neuropathy—aminoglycosides, amphotericin B, chloramphenicol, cimetidine, cisplatin, dapsone, disulfiram, ethionamide, foscarnet, glutethimide, gold, hydrALAZINE, iodoquinol, isoniazid, metronidazole, nitrofurantoin, phenytoin, probenecid, ribavirin, vinCRIStine, other nucleoside analogs

Decrease: absorption—ketoconazole, dapsone, food, antacids, metoclopramide

NURSING CONSIDERATIONS

Assess:

• Neuropathy: tingling or pain in hands and feet, distal numbness

⚠ Pancreatitis: abdominal pain, nausea, vomiting, elevated hepatic enzymes; drug should be discontinued, since condition can be fatal

⚠ For lactic acidosis, severe hepatomegaly with steatosis that can be fatal, drug should be discontinued

• Children by dilated retinal exam q6mo to rule out retinal depigmentation

• Viral load CD4 baseline and throughout treatment

• CBC, differential, platelet count qwk; withhold drug if WBC is <4000/mm^3 or platelet count is <75,000/mm^3; notify prescriber

• Renal studies: BUN, serum uric acid, urine CCr before, during therapy

• Temp q4h; may indicate beginning infection

• Hepatic studies before, during therapy (bilirubin, AST, ALT), triglycerides, amylase prn or qmo

Administer:

• 1 hr before or 2 hr after meals

Perform/provide:

• Strict medical asepsis, protective isolation if WBC levels are low

Evaluate:

• Therapeutic response: absence of infection; symptoms of HIV

Teach patient/family:

• To report signs of infection: fever, sore throat, flulike symptoms

• To report signs of anemia: fatigue, headache, faintness, shortness of breath, irritability

• To report bleeding; avoid use of razors, commercial mouthwash

• That hair may be lost during therapy; a wig or hairpiece may make patient feel better

zaleplon (℞)

(zal'eh-plon)

Sonata

Func. class.: Sedative/hypnotic, antianxiety

Chem. class.: Pyrazolopyrimidine

Controlled Substance Schedule IV

Action: Binds selectively to omega-1 receptor of the GABA$_A$ receptor complex; results are sedation, hypnosis, skeletal muscle relaxation, anticonvulsant activity, anxiolytic action

Uses: Insomnia

DOSAGE AND ROUTES

• *Adult:* **PO** 10 mg at bedtime; may increase dose to 20 mg at bedtime if needed; 5 mg may be used in low-weight persons

Side effects: *italics* = common; **bold** = life-threatening

• *Geriatric:* **PO** 15 mg at bedtime; may increase if needed
Available forms: Caps 5, 10 mg

SIDE EFFECTS

CNS: Lethargy, drowsiness, daytime sedation, dizziness, confusion, anxiety, amnesia, depersonalization, hallucinations, hyperesthesia, paresthesia, somnolence, tremor, vertigo, complex sleep related reactions: sleep driving, sleep eating
EENT: Vision change, ear/eye pain, hyperacusis, parosmia
GI: Nausea, abdominal pain, constipation, anorexia, colitis, dyspepsia, dry mouth
MISC: Asthenia, fever, headache, myalgia, dysmenorrhea
SYST: **Severe allergic reactions**
Contraindications: Hypersensitivity
Precautions: Pregnancy (C), renal/hepatic disease, geriatric, psychosis, child <15 yr, lactation

PHARMACOKINETICS

PO: Rapid onset, metabolized by liver extensively; excreted by kidneys (inactive metabolites); half-life 1 hr

INTERACTIONS

Increase: effects of zaleplon—cimetidine
Decrease: effect of zaleplon—rifampin
Drug/Herb
Increase: CNS depression—catnip, chamomile, clary, cowslip, hops, kava, lavender, mistletoe, nettle, pokeweed, poppy, Queen Anne's lace, senega, skullcap, valerian
Increase: hypotension—black cohosh
Drug/Food
• Prolonged absorption, sleep onset reduced: high-fat/heavy meal

NURSING CONSIDERATIONS
Assess:
• Mental status: mood, sensorium, affect, memory (long, short)
• Type of sleep problem: falling asleep, staying asleep

Administer:
• After removal of cigarettes to prevent fires
• After trying conservative measures for insomnia
• Immediately before bedtime for sleeplessness
• On empty stomach for fast onset
• Avoid use with CNS depressants
Perform/provide:
• Assistance with ambulation after receiving dose
• Safety measure: night-light, call bell within easy reach
• Checking to see if PO medication has been swallowed
• Storage in tight container in cool environment
Evaluate:
• Therapeutic response: ability to sleep at night, decreased amount of early morning awakening
Teach patient/family:
• To avoid driving or other activities requiring alertness until drug is stabilized
• To avoid alcohol ingestion
• Alternative measures to improve sleep: reading, exercise several hr before bedtime, warm bath, warm milk, TV, self-hypnosis, deep breathing
• That drug may cause memory problems, dependence (if used for longer periods of time), changes in behavior/thinking
• That drug is for short-term use only
• To take immediately before going to bed
• Not to ingest a high-fat/heavy meal before taking

zanamivir (R)
(zan'ah-mih-veer)
Relenza
Func. class.: Antiviral
Chem. class.: Neuramidase inhibitor

Action: Inhibits neuramidase enzyme needed for influenza virus replication
Uses: Treatment of influenza types A and B for those that have been symptomatic for no more than 2 days

Unlabeled uses: Prophylaxis against influenza and biinfections; avian flu (H3N1)

DOSAGE AND ROUTES

• *Adult and child >7 yr:* **INH** 2 inhalations (two 5 mg blisters) q12h × 5 days, on the 1st day 2 doses should be taken with at least 2 hr between doses

Available forms: Blisters of powder for inhalation: 5 mg

SIDE EFFECTS

CNS: Headache, dizziness, fatigue
EENT: Ear, nose, throat infections
GI: Nausea, vomiting, diarrhea
RESP: Nasal symptoms, cough, sinusitis, bronchitis

Contraindications: Hypersensitivity
Precautions: Pregnancy (C), lactation, children <7 yr, respiratory disease, geriatric

PHARMACOKINETICS

Half-life 2½-5 hr, not metabolized, excreted in urine unchanged

INTERACTIONS

• None known

NURSING CONSIDERATIONS

Assess:
• Bowel pattern before, during treatment
• Skin eruptions, photosensitivity after administration of drug
• Respiratory status: rate, character, wheezing, tightness in chest
• Allergies before initiation of treatment, reaction of each medication
• Signs of infection

Administer:
• Within 2 days of symptoms of influenza; continue for 5 days
• Give patient "Patient's Instruction for Use" and review all points before using delivery system

Perform/provide:
• Storage in tight, dry container

Evaluate:
• Therapeutic response: absence of fever, malaise, cough, dyspnea in infection

Teach patient/family:
• That this drug does not reduce transmission risk of influenza to others
• Patients with asthma or COPD to carry a fast-acting inhaled bronchodilator since bronchospasm may occur; to use scheduled inhaled bronchodilators before using this drug
• To avoid hazardous activities if dizziness occurs
• To take drug exactly as prescribed

---

zidovudine (R)

(zye-doe′-vue-deen)
Apo-Zidovudine ✤,
Azidothymidine, AZT,
Novo-AZT ✤, Retrovir
Func. class.: Antiretroviral
Chem. class.: Nucleoside reverse transcriptase inhibitor (NRTI)

Action: Inhibits replication of HIV-1 virus by incorporating into cellular DNA by viral reverse transcriptase, thereby terminating the cellular DNA chain

Uses: Used in combination with other antiretrovirals for HIV-1 infection

DOSAGE AND ROUTES

• *Adult:* **PO** 600 mg daily in divided doses, either 200 mg tid or 300 mg bid in combination with other antiretrovirals; **IV** 1-2 mg/kg q4h, initiate **PO** as soon as possible up to 1000 mg
• *Child 6 wk-12 yr:* **PO** 160 mg/m² q8h (480 mg/m²/day, max 200 mg q8h) in combination with other antiretrovirals; **IV** same as adult
• *Neonate:* **PO** 2-3 mg/kg/dose q6h; **IV** 1.5 mg/kg infused over 30 min q6h

Prevention of maternal-fetal HIV transmission
• *Neonatal:* **PO** 2 mg/kg/dose q6h × 6 wk beginning 8-12 hr after birth; **IV** 1.5 mg/kg/dose over 30 min q6h until able to take **PO**
• *Maternal (>14 wk gestation):* **PO** 100

Side effects: *italics* = common; **bold** = life-threatening

Z

mg 5 ×/day until start of labor, then during labor/delivery **IV** 2 mg/kg over 1 hr followed by **IV INF** 1 mg/kg/hr until umbilical cord clamped

Symptomatic HIV infection
• *Adult:* **PO** 100 mg q4h; **IV** 1-2 mg/kg over 1 hr q4h
• *Child 3 mo to 12 yr:* **PO** 90-180 mg/m² q6h (max 200 mg q6h); **IV** 1-2 mg/kg over 1 hr q4h

Prevention of HIV following needle-stick
• *Adult:* **PO** 200 mg tid plus lamivudine 150 mg bid, plus a protease inhibitor for high-risk exposure; begin within 2 hr of exposure

Available forms: Caps 100; tabs 300 mg; inj 200 mg/20 ml; oral syr 50 mg/5 ml

SIDE EFFECTS

CNS: Fever, headache, malaise, diaphoresis, dizziness, insomnia, paresthesia, somnolence, chills, tremor, twitching, anxiety, confusion, depression, lability, vertigo, loss of mental acuity, **seizures**
EENT: Taste change, hearing loss, photophobia
GI: Nausea, vomiting, diarrhea, anorexia, cramps, dyspepsia, constipation, dysphagia, flatulence, rectal bleeding, mouth ulcer, abdominal pain
GU: Dysuria, polyuria, urinary frequency, hesitancy
HEMA: **Granulocytopenia, anemia**
INTEG: Rash, acne, pruritus, urticaria
MS: Myalgia, arthralgia, muscle spasm
RESP: Dyspnea

Contraindications: Hypersensitivity
Precautions: Pregnancy (C), granulocyte count <1000/mm³ or Hgb <9.5 g/dl, lactation, child, severe renal disease, impaired hepatic function, anemia

PHARMACOKINETICS

PO: Rapidly absorbed from GI tract, peak ½-1½ hr, metabolized in liver (inactive metabolites), excreted by kidneys, protein binding 38%, terminal half-life ½-3 hr

INTERACTIONS
• Toxicity: probenecid, fluconazole
Increase: bone marrow depression—antineoplastics, radiation, ganciclovir, valganciclovir, trimethoprim sulfamethoxazole
Increase: zidovudine level—methadone

NURSING CONSIDERATIONS
Assess:
• Blood counts q2wk; watch for decreasing granulocytes, Hgb; if low, therapy may have to be discontinued and restarted after hematologic recovery; blood transfusions may be required; viral load, CD4 counts baseline and throughout

Administer:
• By mouth; capsules should be swallowed whole
• Bid or tid
• Trimethoprim-sulfamethoxazole, pyrimethamine, or acyclovir as ordered to prevent opportunistic infections; if these drugs are given, watch for neurotoxicity
IV route
• After diluting each 1 mg/0.25 ml or more D₅W to 4 mg/ml or less; give over 1 hr

Y-site compatibilities: Acyclovir, allopurinol, amifostine, amikacin, amphotericin B, amphotericin B cholesteryl, aztreonam, cefepime, ceftazidime, ceftriaxone, cimetidine, cisatracurium, clindamycin, dexamethasone, DOBUTamine, DOPamine, DOXOrubicin liposome, erythromycin, filgrastim, fluconazole, fludarabine, gentamicin, granisetron, heparin, imipenem/cilastatin, lorazepam, melphalan, metoclopramide, morphine, nafcillin, ondansetron, oxacillin, paclitaxel, pentamidine, phenylephrine, piperacillin, piperacillin/tazobactam, potassium chloride, ranitidine, remifentanil, sargramostim, teniposide, thiotepa, tobramycin, trimethoprim-sulfamethoxazole, trimetrexate, vancomycin, vinorelbine
Perform/provide:
• Storage in cool environment; protect from light

Evaluate:

• Blood dyscrasias (anemia, granulocytopenia): bruising, fatigue, bleeding, poor healing

Teach patient/family:

• That GI complaints and insomnia resolve after 3-4 wk of treatment

• That drug is not cure for AIDS but will control symptoms

• To notify prescriber of sore throat, swollen lymph nodes, malaise, fever; other infections may occur

• That patient is still infective, may pass AIDS virus on to others

• That follow-up visits must be continued since serious toxicity may occur; blood counts must be done q2wk

• That drug must be taken bid or tid

• That serious drug interactions may occur if OTC products are ingested; check with prescriber before taking aspirin, acetaminophen, indomethacin

• That other drugs may be necessary to prevent other infections

• That drug may cause fainting or dizziness

---

zinc (℞, OTC)

Orazinc, PMS Egozinc ✦, Verazinc, Zinca-Pak, Zincate, Zinc 15, Zinc-220, zinc sulfate
Func. class.: Trace element; nutritional supplement

Action: Needed for adequate healing, bone and joint development (23% zinc)
Uses: Prevention of zinc deficiency, adjunct to vit A therapy
Unlabeled uses: Wound healing

DOSAGE AND ROUTES

Dietary supplement
• *Adult:* PO 25-50 mg/day
Nutritional supplement (IV)
• *Adult:* IV 2.5-4 mg/day; may increase by 2 mg/day if needed
• *Child 1-5 yr:* IV 100 mcg/kg/day
• *Infant <1.5-3 kg:* IV 300 mcg/kg/day

Wound healing
Adult: PO 50 mg daily × 1-2 mo
Available forms: Tabs 66, 110 mg; caps 220 mg; inj 1 mg, 5 mg/ml

SIDE EFFECTS

GI: Nausea, vomiting, cramps, heartburn, ulcer formation
OVERDOSE: Diarrhea, rash, dehydration, restlessness
Precautions: Pregnancy (A)

INTERACTIONS

Decrease: absorption of fluoroquinolones tetracyclines

NURSING CONSIDERATIONS
Assess:
• Zinc levels during treatment
Administer:
• With meals to decrease gastric upset; avoid dairy products
Evaluate:
• Therapeutic response: absence of zinc deficiency
Teach patient/family:
• That element must be taken for 2-3 mo to be effective
• To report immediately nausea, diarrhea, rash, severe vomiting, restlessness, abdominal pain, tarry stools

---

ziprasidone (℞)
(zi-praz'ih-dohn)
Geodon
Func. class.: Antipsychotic/neuroleptic
Chem. class.: Benzisoxazole derivative

Action: Unknown; may be mediated through both DOPamine type 2 (D_2) and serotonin type 2 (5-HT_2) antagonism
Uses: Schizophrenia, acute agitation

DOSAGE AND ROUTES
• *Adult:* PO 20 mg bid with food, adjust dosage every 2 days upward to max of 80 mg bid; IM 10-20 mg; may give 10 mg

q2h; doses of 20 mg may be given q4h; max 40 mg/day

Available forms: Caps 20, 40, 60, 80 mg; inj 20 mg/ml

SIDE EFFECTS

CNS: EPS, pseudoparkinsonism, akathisia, dystonia, tardive dyskinesia; drowsiness, insomnia, agitation, anxiety, headache, **seizures, neuroleptic malignant syndrome,** dizziness, tremor

CV: Orthostatic hypotension, **tachycardia, prolonged QT/QTc,** hypertension; **sudden death, heart failure (geriatric)**

EENT: Blurred vision

GI: Nausea, vomiting, *anorexia, constipation,* jaundice, weight gain, diarrhea, dry mouth, abdominal pain

RESP: Rhinitis, dyspnea

Contraindications: Hypersensitivity, lactation, seizure disorders

Precautions: Pregnancy (C), children, renal/hepatic disease, geriatric, breast cancer

PHARMACOKINETICS

PO: Extensively metabolized by liver to a major active metabolite, plasma protein binding 90%

INTERACTIONS

Increase: sedation—other CNS depressants, alcohol

Increase: EPS—other antipsychotics, lithium

Increase: ziprasidone excretion—carbamazepine

Increase: ziprasidone level—ketoconazole

Increase: hypotension—antihypertensives

Drug/Herb

Increase: CNS depression—chamomile, hops, kava, skullcap, valerian

Increase: EPS—betel palm, kava

Increase: action—cola tree, hops, nettle, nutmeg

NURSING CONSIDERATIONS

Assess:

• Mental status before initial administration

⚠ Geriatric closely; heart failure, sudden death have occured

• Swallowing of PO medication; check for hoarding or giving of medication to other patients

• I&O ratio; palpate bladder if urinary output is low

• Bilirubin, CBC, LFTs qmo

• Urinalysis before, during prolonged therapy

• Affect, orientation, LOC, reflexes, gait, coordination, sleep pattern disturbances

• B/P standing and lying; also pulse, respirations; take these q4h during initial treatment; establish baseline before starting treatment; report drops of 30 mm Hg; watch for ECG changes

• Dizziness, faintness, palpitations, tachycardia on rising

• EPS, including akathisia (inability to sit still, no pattern to movements), tardive dyskinesia (bizarre movements of the jaw, mouth, tongue, extremities), pseudoparkinsonism (rigidity, tremors, pill rolling, shuffling gait)

⚠ For neuroleptic malignant syndrome: hyperthermia, increased CPK, altered mental status, muscle rigidity

• Skin turgor daily

• Constipation, urinary retention daily; if these occur, increase bulk and water in diet

Administer:

PO route

• Reduced dose in geriatric

• Antiparkinsonian agent on order from prescriber, to be used for EPS

• Avoid use with CNS depressants

IM route

• Add 1.2 ml sterile water for inj to vial; shake vigorously until drug is dissolved; do not admix; give only IM

Perform/provide:

• Decreased stimulus by dimming lights, avoiding loud noises

• Supervised ambulation until patient is

⚠ Safety alert   *"Tall Man" lettering

stabilized on medication; do not involve in strenuous exercise program because fainting is possible; patient should not stand still for a long time

• Increased fluids to prevent constipation

• Sips of water, candy, gum for dry mouth

• Storage in tight, light-resistant container

Evaluate:

• Therapeutic response: decrease in emotional excitement, hallucinations, delusions, paranoia; reorganization of patterns of thought, speech

Teach patient/family:

• That orthostatic hypotension may occur and to rise from sitting or lying position gradually

• To avoid hot tubs, hot showers, tub baths; hypotension may occur

• To avoid abrupt withdrawal of this drug; EPS may result; drug should be withdrawn slowly

• To avoid OTC preparations (cough, hay fever, cold) unless approved by prescriber, since serious drug interactions may occur; avoid use with alcohol; increased drowsiness may occur

• To avoid hazardous activities if drowsy or dizzy

• Compliance with drug regimen

• To report impaired vision, tremors, muscle twitching

• In hot weather, that heat stroke may occur; take extra precautions to stay cool

Treatment of overdose: Lavage if orally ingested; provide airway; *do not induce vomiting*

---

zoledronic acid (℞)

(zoh'leh-drah'nick ass'id)
Zometa
Func. class.: Bone-resorption inhibitor
Chem. class.: Bisphosphonate

Action: Inhibits normal and abnormal bone resorption, potent inhibitor of osteoclastic bone resorption; inhibits osteoclastic activity, inhibits skeletal calcium release caused by stimulating factors re-

leased by tumors; reduction of abnormal bone resorption is responsible for therapeutic effect in hypercalcemia; may directly block dissolution of hydroxyapatite bone crystals

Uses: Moderate to severe hypercalcemia associated with malignancy; multiple myeloma; bone metastases from solid tumors (used with antineoplastics)

DOSAGE AND ROUTES

Hypercalcemia of malignancy

• *Adult:* **IV INF** 4 mg, given as a single infusion over ≥15 min; may re-treat with 4 mg if serum calcium does not return to normal within 1 wk

Multiple myeloma/metastatic bone lesions

• *Adult:* **IV INF** 4 mg, give over 15 min q3-4wk; may continue treatment for 9-15 months, depending on condition

Available form: Powder for inj 4 mg

SIDE EFFECTS

CNS: Dizziness, headache, anxiety, confusion, insomnia, agitation

CV: Hypotension, leg edema

GI: Abdominal pain, anorexia, constipation, nausea, diarrhea, vomiting, mucositis

GU: UTI, possible reduced renal function

META: Anemia, hypokalemia, hypomagnesemia, hypophosphatemia, hypocalcemia, increased serum creatinine

MISC: Fever, chills, flulike symptoms

MS: Bone pain, *arthralgias, myalgias*

Contraindications: Pregnancy (D), hypersensitivity to this drug or bisphosphonates

Precautions: Children, nursing mothers, renal dysfunction, aspirin sensitive asthmatic patients

PHARMACOKINETICS

Rapidly cleared from circulation and taken up mainly by bones, not metabolized, eliminated primarily by kidneys; approximately 50% is eliminated in urine within 24 hr of administration; max effect 7 days

Z

INTERACTIONS

• Hypomagnesemia, hypokalemia: digoxin

• Do not mix with calcium-containing infusion sol such as lactated Ringer's sol

Decrease: effect of zoledronic acid—calcium, vit D

Decrease: serum calcium, aminoglycosides, loop diuretics

NURSING CONSIDERATIONS

Assess:

• Renal tests and Ca, P, Mg, K; creatinine, if creatinine is elevated hold treatment

• For hypercalcemia: paresthesia, twitching, laryngospasm; Chvostek's, Trousseau's signs

Administer:

• Saline hydration must be performed before administration; urine output should be 2 L/day during treatment, do not overhydrate

IV route

• Administer after reconstituting by adding 5 ml of sterile water for inj to each vial, then add to ≥100 ml of sterile 0.9% NaCl, D₅W; run over ≥15 min

• Administer in separate IV line from all other drugs

Perform/provide:

• Sol reconstituted with sterile water may be stored under refrigeration for up to 24 hr

Evaluate:

• Therapeutic response: decreased calcium levels

Teach patient/family:

• To report hypercalcemic relapse: nausea, vomiting, bone pain, thirst

• To continue with dietary recommendations including calcium and vit D; take a multiple vitamin daily, 500 mg of calcium, 400 international units vit D in multiple myeloma

• If nausea/vomiting occur, eat small frequent meals, use lozenges or chewing gum

• If bone pain occurs, notify prescriber to obtain analgesics

• Avoid use in pregnancy

---

zolmitriptan (℞)
(zole-mih-trip′tan)
Zomig, Zomig-ZMT
Func. class.: Migraine agent, abortive
Chem. class.: 5-HT₁B/5HT₁D receptor agonist (triptan)

Action: Binds selectively to the vascular 5-HT₁B/5HT₁D receptor subtype, exerts antimigraine effect; causes vasoconstriction in cranial arteries

Uses: Acute treatment of migraine with or without aura

DOSAGE AND ROUTES

• *Adult:* **PO** Start on 2.5 mg or lower (tab may be broken), may repeat after 2 hr, max 10 mg/24 hr; **NASAL** 1 spray in each nostril at onset of migraine, repeat in 2 hr, if no relief

Available forms: Tabs 2.5, 5 mg; orally disintegrating tabs 2.5, 5 mg; nasal spray 5 mg

SIDE EFFECTS

CNS: Tingling, hot sensation, burning, feeling of pressure, tightness, numbness, dizziness, sedation
CV: Palpitations, chest pain
GI: Abdominal discomfort, nausea, dry mouth, dyspepsia, dysphagia
MISC: Odd taste (spray)
MS: Weakness, neck stiffness, myalgia
RESP: Chest tightness, pressure

Contraindications: Angina pectoris, history of MI, documented silent ischemia, ischemic heart disease, concurrent ergotamine-containing preparations, uncontrolled hypertension, hypersensitivity, basilar or hemiplegic migraine, risk of CV events

Precautions: Pregnancy (C), postmenopausal women, men >40 yr, risk factors for CAD, hypercholesterolemia, obesity, diabetes, impaired renal/hepatic function, lactation, children, geriatric

---

⚠ Safety alert   *"Tall Man" lettering

PHARMACOKINETICS

Duration 2-3½ hr; 25% plasma protein binding; half-life 3-3½ hr; metabolized in the liver (metabolite); excreted in urine (60%-80%), feces (20%-40%)

INTERACTIONS

⚠ Extended vasospastic effects: ergot, ergot derivatives

⚠ Do not use within 2 wk of MAOIs

⚠ Weakness, hyperreflexia, incoordination: SSRIs (fluoxetine, fluvoxamine, paroxetine, sertraline)

Increase: half-life of zolmitriptan—cimetidine, oral contraceptives

Increase: zolimitriptan levels—sibutramine

Drug/Herb

• Serotonin syndrome: SAM-e, St. John's wort

Increase: effect—butterbur, feverfew

NURSING CONSIDERATIONS

Assess:

• Tingling, hot sensation, burning, feeling of pressure, numbness, flushing

• For stress level, activity, recreation, coping mechanisms

• Neurologic status: LOC, blurring vision, nausea, vomiting, tingling in extremities preceding headache

• Ingestion of tyramine foods (pickled products, beer, wine, aged cheese), food additives, preservatives, colorings, artifical sweeteners, chocolate, caffeine, which may precipitate these types of headaches

• For serotonin syndrome, if also taking an SSRI

• Kidney function, urine output

Administer:

• Take with fluids as soon as symptoms of migraine occur

Perform/provide:

• Quiet, calm environment with decreased stimulation for noise, bright light, excessive talking

Evaluate:

• Therapeutic response: decrease in frequency, severity of headache

Teach patient/family:

• To report any side effects to prescriber
• To use contraception while taking drug
• That product does not prevent or reduce the number of migraines

---

zolpidem (℞)
(zole'pih-dem)
Ambien, Ambien CR
Func. class.: Sedative-hypnotic
Chem. class.: Nonbenzodiazepine of imidazopyridine class

Controlled Substance Schedule IV
Action: Produces CNS depression at limbic, thalamic, hypothalamic levels of CNS; may be mediated by neurotransmitter γ-aminobutyric acid (GABA); results are sedation, hypnosis, skeletal muscle relaxation, anticonvulsant activity, anxiolytic action

Uses: Insomnia, short-term treatment; insomnia with difficulty of sleep onset/maintenance (ext rel)

DOSAGE AND ROUTES

• *Adult:* **PO** 10 mg at bedtime × 7-10 days only; total max dose 10 mg; **EXT REL** 12.5 mg immediately before bedtime

• *Geriatric:* **PO** 5 mg at bedtime

Available forms: Tabs 5, 10 mg; ext rel tabs 6.25, 12.5 mg

SIDE EFFECTS

CNS: Headache, lethargy, drowsiness, daytime sedation, dizziness, confusion, lightheadedness, anxiety, irritability, amnesia, poor coordination, complex sleep related reactions: sleep driving, sleep eating
CV: Chest pain, palpitation
GI: Nausea, vomiting, diarrhea, heartburn, abdominal pain, constipation
HEMA: **Leukopenia, granulocytopenia (rare)**
SYST: **Severe allergic reactions**
Contraindications: Hypersensitivity to benzodiazepines

Precautions: Pregnancy (B), anemia, renal/hepatic disease, suicidal individuals, drug abuse, geriatric, psychosis, child <18 yr, seizure disorders, lactation

PHARMACOKINETICS

PO: Onset 1.5 hr, metabolized by liver, excreted by kidneys (inactive metabolites), crosses placenta, excreted in breast milk; half-life 2-3 hr

INTERACTIONS

Increase: action of both drugs—alcohol, CNS depressants
Drug/Herb
Increase: CNS depression—chamomile, hops, kava, skullcap, valerian
Drug/Lab Test
Increase: ALT, AST, serum bilirubin
Decrease: RAI uptake
False increase: Urinary 17-OHCS

NURSING CONSIDERATIONS
Assess:
• Blood studies: Hct, Hgb, RBC, if blood dyscrasias are suspected (rare)
• Hepatic studies: AST, ALT, bilirubin if hepatic damage has occurred
• Mental status: mood, sensorium, affect, memory (long, short)
• Blood dyscrasias: fever, sore throat, bruising, rash, jaundice, epistaxis (rare)
• Type of sleep problem: falling asleep, staying asleep
Administer:
• Do not break, crush, or chew ext rel products
• After trying conservative measures for insomnia
• ½-1 hr before bedtime for sleeplessness
• On empty stomach for fast onset but may be taken with food if GI symptoms occur
• Avoid use with CNS depressants; serious CNS depression may result
Perform/provide:
• Assistance with ambulation after receiving dose

• Safety measures: side rails, night-light, call bell within easy reach
• Checking to see if PO medication has been swallowed
• Storage in tight container in cool environment
Evaluate:
• Therapeutic response: ability to sleep at night, decreased amount of early morning awakening if taking drug for insomnia
Teach patient/family:
• That dependence is possible after long-term use
• To avoid driving or other activities requiring alertness until drug is stabilized
• To avoid alcohol ingestion
• That effects may take 2 nights for benefits to be noticed
• Alternative measures to improve sleep: reading, exercise several hours before bedtime, warm bath, warm milk, TV, self-hypnosis, deep breathing
• That hangover is common in geriatric but less common than with barbiturates; rebound insomnia may occur for 1-2 nights after discontinuing drug
Treatment of overdose: Lavage, activated charcoal; monitor electrolytes, VS

zonisamide (R)
(zone-is'a-mide)
Zonegran
Func. class.: Anticonvulsant
Chem. class.: Sulfonamides

Action: May act through action at sodium and calcium channels, but exact action is unknown
Uses: Epilepsy, adjunctive therapy of partial seizures

DOSAGE AND ROUTES
• *Adult and child >16 yr:* 100 mg daily, may increase after 2 wk to 200 mg/day, may increase q2wk, maximum dose 600 mg/day
Available forms: Caps 25, 50, 100 mg

SIDE EFFECTS

CNS: Dizziness, insomnia, paresthesias, depression, fatigue, headache, confusion, somnolence, agitation, irritability

EENT: Diplopia, verbal difficulty, speech abnormalities, taste perversion

GI: Nausea, constipation, anorexia, weight loss, diarrhea, dyspepsia

HEMA: **Aplastic anemia, granulocytopenia** (rare)

INTEG: Rash

SYST: **Stevens-Johnson syndrome**

Contraindications: Hypersensitivity to this drug or sulfonamides, psychiatric condition, hepatic failure

Precautions: Pregnancy (C), allergies, renal/hepatic disease, geriatric, lactation, child <16 yr

PHARMACOKINETICS

Peak 2-6 hr, half-life 63 hr
Metabolized by liver, excreted by kidneys

INTERACTIONS

Decrease: half-life of zonisamide—drugs inducing CYP450 enzymes (carbamazepine, phenytoin, phenobarbital)

NURSING CONSIDERATIONS

Assess:
• For seizures: duration, type, intensity precipitating factors
• Renal function: albumin conc
• Mental status: mood, sensorium, affect, memory (long, short)

Evaluate:
• Therapeutic response; decrease in severity of seizures

Teach patient/family:
• Not to discontinue drug abruptly; seizures may occur
• To avoid hazardous activities until stabilized on drug
• To carry emergency ID stating drug use
• To notify prescriber of rash immediately; also, back pain, abdominal pain, blood in urine, increase fluid intake to reduce risk of kidney stones
• To notify prescriber if pregnancy is planned or suspected

Side effects: *italics* = common; **bold** = life-threatening

Z

Bibliography

Drug information: Bethesda, American Hospital Formulary Service.

Facts and comparisons: St Louis, updated monthly.

Gahart BL: *Intravenous medications,* ed 23, St Louis, 2007, Mosby.

Brunton L, Lazo J, Parker K: *Goodman and Gilman's the pharmacological basis of therapeutics,* ed 11, New York, 2005, McGraw-Hill.

McKenry LM, Tessier E, Hogan MA: *Mosby's pharmacology in nursing,* ed 22, St Louis, 2006, Mosby.

Mediphor Editorial Group: *Drug interaction facts,* Philadelphia, updated quarterly, Lippincott Williams & Wilkins.

Review of natural products: Philadelphia, updated monthly, *Facts and Comparisons.*

Appendixes

Appendix a

Selected new drugs

---

anidulafungin
See page 140

---

arformoterol (℞)
(ar-for-moe'ter-ole)
Brovana
Func. class.: Long–acting adrenergic β$_2$-agonist, sympathomimetic, bronchodilator

Action: Causes bronchodilation by action on β$_2$ (pulmonary) receptors by increasing levels of cAMP, which relaxes smooth muscle; produces bronchodilation and CNS, cardiac stimulation, as well as increased diuresis and gastric acid secretion; longer acting than isoproterenol
Uses: COPD, including chronic bronchitis, emphysema

DOSAGE AND ROUTES
COPD
• *Adult:* NEB 15 mcg, bid, AM, PM
Available forms: Inh sol 15 mcg/2 ml

SIDE EFFECTS

CNS: Tremors, anxiety, insomnia, headache, dizziness, stimulation, *restlessness,* hallucinations, flushing, irritability
CV: Palpitations, tachycardia, hypertension, angina, hypotension, dysrhythmias
EENT: Dry nose, irritation of nose and throat
GI: Heartburn, nausea, vomiting
MISC: Flushing, sweating, anorexia, bad taste/smell changes, hypokalemia, **anaphylaxis**
MS: Muscle cramps

RESP: Cough, wheezing, dyspnea, **bronchospasm,** dry throat
Contraindications: Hypersensitivity to sympathomimetics, this product, or racemic formoterol; tachydysrhyhmias, severe cardiac disease, heart block, children, actively deteriorating COPD
Precautions: Pregnancy (C), lactation, cardiac disorders, hyperthyroidism, diabetes mellitus, hypertension, prostatic hypertrophy, narrow-angle glaucoma, seizures, hypoglycemia

PHARMACOKINETICS
Onset 5 min; peak 1-1½ hr; duration 4-6 hr; terminal half-life (COPD) 26 hr; extensively metabolized by direct conjugation by CYP2D6, CYP2C19; crosses placenta; protein binding 52%-65%; excreted in urine 63%, feces 11%

INTERACTIONS
Increase: severe hypotension—oxytocics
Increase: toxicity—theophylline
Increase: ECG changes/hypokalemia—potassium-losing diuretics
Increase: action of nebulized bronchodilators
Increase: action of arformoterol—tricyclics, MAOIs, other adrenergics; do not use together
Decrease: arformoterol action—other β-blockers
Drug/Herb
Increase: stimulation—caffeine (cola nut, green/black tea, guarana, yerba maté, coffee, chocolate)

NURSING CONSIDERATIONS
Assess:
• Respiratory function: vital capacity, forced expiratory volume, ABGs; lung

---

⚠ Safety alert   *"Tall Man" lettering

sounds, heart rate and rhythm, B/P, sputum (baseline and peak)
• That patient has not received theophylline therapy or other bronchodilators before giving dose
• Patient's ability to self-medicate
• For evidence of allergic reactions; anaphylaxis may occur
• Paradoxical bronchospasm; hold medication, notify prescriber if bronchospasm occurs
Administer:
• Must be used by nebulization
Perform/provide:
• Storage in refrigerator
Evaluate:
• Therapeutic response: absence of dyspnea, wheezing after 1 hr, improved airway exchange, improved ABGs
Teach patient/family:
• To use exactly as prescribed; that death has resulted from asthma with products similar to this one
• Not to use OTC medications; excess stimulation may occur

conivaptan
See page 304

darunavir (℞)
(dar-ue'na-vir)
Prezista
Func. class.: Antiretroviral
Chem. class.: Protease inhibitor

Action: Inhibits human immunodeficiency virus (HIV-1) protease; this prevents maturation of virus
Uses: HIV-1 in combination with ritonavir and other antiretrovirals

DOSAGE AND ROUTES
Reduce dose in mild/moderate hepatic impairment and ketaconazole coadministration
• **Adult: PO** 600 mg bid; if given with ritonavir 100 mg bid with food
Available forms: Tabs 300 mg

SIDE EFFECTS
CNS: Headache, insomnia, dizziness, somnolence
GI: Diarrhea, abdominal pain, nausea, vomiting, anorexia, dry mouth
GU: Nephrolithiasis
INTEG: Rash
MS: Pain
OTHER: Asthenia, **insulin-resistant hyperglycemia,** hyperlipidemia, **ketoacidosis,** lipodystrophy
Contraindications: Hypersensitivity
Precautions: Pregnancy (B), hepatic/renal disease, lacation, children, history of renal stones, diabetes, hypercholesterolemia

PHARMACOKINETICS
95% protein binding; metabolized by CYP3A; peak 2.5-4 hr; terminal half-life 15 hr; excreted in feces 79.5%, urine 13.9%

INTERACTIONS
⚠ Life-threatening dysrhythmias: ergots, midazolam, rifampin, pimozide, triazolam; do not use concurrently
Increase: myopathy—atorvastatin, lovastatin, simvastatin
Increase: darunavir levels—ketoconazole, delavirdine, itraconazole
Increase: levels of both drugs—clarithromycin, zidovudine
Increase: levels of isoniazid, oral contraceptives
Decrease: darunavir levels—rifamycins, fluconazole, nevirapine, efavirenz
Decrease: of both drugs—anticonvulsants
Drug/Herb
Decrease: darunavir levels—St. John's wort; avoid concurrent use
Drug/Food
Increase: darunavir absorption

NURSING CONSIDERATIONS
Assess:
• For complaints of lower back, flank pain; indicates kidney stones

- Signs of infection, anemia, the presence of other sexually transmitted diseases
- Hepatic studies: ALT, AST, bilirubin, amylase; all may be elevated
- Viral load, CD4 during treatment
- Bowel pattern before, during treatment; if severe abdominal pain with bleeding occurs, drug should be discontinued; monitor hydration
- Skin eruptions: rash, urticaria, itching
- Allergies before treatment, reaction of each medication; place allergies on chart

Administer:
- With food and ritonavir
- Water to 1.5 L/day minimum to prevent nephrolithiasis

Evaluate:
- Therapeutic response: decreased viral load and increased CD4 count

Teach patient/family:
- To take as prescribed; if dose is missed, take as soon as remembered up to 1 hr before next dose; do not double dose
- That drug must be taken in equal intervals around the clock to maintain blood levels for duration of therapy
- ⚠ That hyperglycemia may occur; watch for increased thirst, weight loss, hunger, dry, itchy skin; notify prescriber
- To increase fluids to prevent kidney stones; if stone formation occurs, treatment may need to be interrupted
- That drug does not cure AIDS, only controls symptoms; do not donate blood

---

dasatinib (℞)
(da-si'ti-nib)
Sprycel
Func. class.: Antineoplastic—miscellaneous
Chem. class.: Protein-tyrosine kinase inhibitor

Action: Inhibits BCR-ABL, SRC, LCK, YES, FYN, C-KIT, EPHA$_2$, and PDGFR-β tyrosine kinase created in chronic myeloid leukemia (CML)

Uses: Treatment of CML, accelerated blast crisis, or chronic phase or acute lymphoblastic leukemia (ALL)

DOSAGE AND ROUTES
- *Adult:* **PO** 70 mg bid

Available forms: Tabs 20, 50, 70 mg

SIDE EFFECTS
CNS: **CNS hemorrhage,** headache, dizziness, insomnia, neuropathy, asthenia
CV: Dysrhythmias, chest pain, CHF, pericardial effusion
GI: *Nausea,* **vomiting,** *anorexia, abdominal pain,* constipation, diarrhea, GI bleeding, muscositis, stomatitis
HEMA: **Neutropenia, thrombocytopenia, bleeding**
INTEG: *Rash, pruritus*
META: Fluid retention, edema
MISC: Increased/decreased weight
MS: Pain, arthralgia, myalgia
RESP: Cough, dyspnea, pulmonary edema/hypertension, pneumonia, URI

Contraindications: Pregnancy (D), hypersensitivity

Precautions: Lactation, children, geriatric

PHARMACOKINETICS
Metabolized by CYP3A4; 96% protein bound; peak 0.5-6 hr; excreted in feces (85%), small amount in urine (4%); terminal half-life 1.3-5 hr

INTERACTIONS
- Altered action of CYP3A4 substrates: alfentanil, cycloSPORINE, ergots, fentanyl, pimozide, quinidine, sirolimus, tacrolimus

Increase: dasatinib concentrations—ketoconazole, itraconazole, erythromycin, clarithromycin, nefazodine, protease inhibitors, telithromycin

Increase: plasma concentrations of simvastatin

Decrease: dasatinib concentrations—CYP3A4 inducers (dexamethasone, phenytoin, carbamazepine, rifampin, pheno-

---

⚠ Safety alert   *"Tall Man" lettering

barbital), H_2 blockers (famotidine), proton pump inhibitors (omeprazole)

Drug/Herb
Decrease: dasatinib concentration—St. John's wort

NURSING CONSIDERATIONS

Assess:
• ANC and platelets; in chronic phase if ANC <1 × 10^9/L and/or platelets <50 × 10^9/L, stop until ANC >1.5 × 10^9/L and platelets >75 × 10^9/L; in accelerated phase/blast crisis if ANC <0.5 × 10^9/L and/or platelets <10 × 10^9/L, determine whether cytopenia is related to biopsy/aspirate, if not, reduce dose by 200 mg, if cytopenia continues, reduce dose by another 100 mg; if cytopenia continues for 4 wk, stop drug until ANC ≥1 × 10^9/L
• For renal toxicity: if bilirubin >3 × IULN, withhold until bilirubin levels return to <1.5 × IULN
• For hepatotoxicity: monitor LFTs, before treatment and qmo; if liver transaminases >5 × IULN, withhold until transaminase levels return to <2.5 × IULN
• CBC, differential, platelet count weekly; withhold drug if WBC is <3500/mm³, or platelet count <100,000/mm³; notify prescriber of these results; drug should be discontinued
• Signs of fluid retention, edema: weigh, monitor lung sounds, assess for edema, some fluid retention is dose dependent

Administer:
• Do not break, crush, or chew tab
• After meal and with large glass of water

Perform/provide:
• Nutritious diet with iron, vitamin supplement
• Storage at 25° C (77° F)

Evaluate:
• Therapeutic response: decrease in leukemic cells or size of tumor

Teach patient/family:
• To report adverse reactions immediately: SOB, swelling of extremities, bleeding
• Reason for treatment, expected result

decitabine
See page 334

Rarely Used
deferasirox (℞)
(def-a'sir-ox)
Exjade
Func. class.: Heavy metal chelating agent

Uses: Chronic iron overload

DOSAGE AND ROUTES
• *Adult:* **PO** 20-30 mg/kg/day; oral dispersion tablet is dissolved in water <1 g in 3.5 oz; >1 g in 7 oz or more; give on empty stomach at least 30 min before meals

Contraindications: Hypersensitivity, lactation, children, severe hepatic/renal disease

Rarely Used
desonide (℞)
(dess'oh-nide)
Desonate, Verdeso
Func. class.: Topical antiinflammatory

Uses: Atopic dermatitis

DOSAGE AND ROUTES
• *Adult:* **TOP** apply to affected area; do not use more than 4 consecutive weeks
Contraindications: Open wounds, burns

Rarely Used
idursulfase (℞)
(eye-dur-sul'fase)
Elaprase
Func. class.: Enzyme replacement

Uses: Mucopolysaccharidosis II (Hunter's syndrome) (MPS-11)

DOSAGE AND ROUTES

• *Adult:* **IV INF** 0.5 mg/kg/wk; dilute calculated volume of concentrated drug in 100 ml of 0.9% NaCl; use a 0.2 micron filter

• *Child >5 yr:* **IV INF** 0.5 mg/kg/wk given over 1-3 hr

Contraindications: Hypersensitivity, IM/intrathecal administration

---

Rarely Used

kunecatechins (℞)
Veregen
Func. class.: Topical keratolytic

Uses: External genital/perianal warts

DOSAGE AND ROUTES

• *Adult:* **TOP** Apply ointment using a 0.5-cm strand applied to warts tid; continue treatment until complete clearance has occurred, max 16 wk

Contraindications: Hypersensitivity

---

lubiprostone
See page 632

---

micafungin
See page 682

---

nabilone
See page 709

---

natalizumab
See page 723

---

panitumumab
See page 785

---

posaconazole (℞)
(poe′sa-kon′a-zole)
Noxafil
Func. class.: Antifungal—systemic
Chem. class.: Triazole derivative

Action: Inhibits a portion of cell wall synthesis; alters cell membranes and inhibits several fungal enzymes

Uses: Prevention of aspergillus, candida infection, oropharyngeal candidiasis in the immunocompromised

DOSAGE AND ROUTES

• *Adult:* **PO** 800 mg/day in 2-4 divided doses

• *Child:* **PO** 100 mg tid

Available forms: Oral susp 200 mg/5 ml

SIDE EFFECTS

CNS: Headache, dizziness, insomnia, fever, rigors, weakness, anxiety

CV: Hypertension, hypotension, tachycardia, anemia

GI: Nausea, vomiting, anorexia, diarrhea, cramps, abdominal pain, flatulence, **GI bleeding, hepatotoxicity**

GU: Gynecomastia, impotence, decreased libido

INTEG: Pruritus, fever, *rash,* **toxic epidermal necrolysis**

MISC: Edema, fatigue, malaise, hypokalemia, tinnitus, **rhabdomyolysis**

Contraindications: Hypersensitivity to this product or other systemic antifungal or azoles, fungal meningitis, onchomycosis or dermatomycosis in cardiac dysfunction

Precautions: Pregnancy (C), hepatic disease, cardiac disease, children, lactation

PHARMACOKINETICS

Well absorbed, enhanced by food, protein binding 98%-99%, peak 4-11 hr, half-life 19-35 hr, metabolized in liver, excreted in feces (77% unchanged)

⚠ Safety alert   *"Tall Man" lettering

INTERACTIONS

⚠ Life-threatening reactions: pimozide, quinidine, dofetilide, ergots

Increase: tinnitus, hearing loss—quinidine

Increase: hepatotoxicity—other hepatotoxic drugs

Increase: edema—calcium channel blockers

Increase: severe hypoglycemia—oral hypoglycemics

Increase: sedation—triazolam, oral midazolam

Increase: levels, toxicity—busPIRone, busulfan, clarithromycin, cycloSPORINE, diazepam, digoxin, felodipine, indinavir, isradipine, niCARdipine, niFEDipine, nimodipine, phenytoin, quinidine, ritonavir, saquinavir, tacrolimus, warfarin

Decrease: effect of oral contraceptives

Decrease: posaconazole action—antacids, H$_2$-receptor antagonists, rifamycin, didanosine

Drug/Herb
Nephrotoxicity: gossypol

Drug/Food
Food increases absorption

NURSING CONSIDERATIONS

Assess:
• For type of infection; may begin treatment prior to obtaining results
• For infection: temp, WBC, sputum, baseline and periodically
• I&O ratio, potassium levels
• Hepatic studies (ALT, AST, bilirubin) if on long-term therapy
• For allergic reaction: rash, photosensitivity, urticaria, dermatitis
⚠ For hepatotoxicity: nausea, vomiting, jaundice, clay-colored stools, fatigue

Administer:
• Shake well; use calibrated measuring device; take only with a full meal or liquid nutritional supplements such as Ensure; rinse measuring device after each use

Perform/provide:
• Storage in a tight container in refrigerator; do not freeze

Evaluate:
• Therapeutic response: decreased fever, malaise, rash, negative C&S for infecting organism

Teach patient/family:
• That long-term therapy may be needed to clear infection (1 wk-6 mo depending on infection)
• To avoid hazardous activities if dizziness occurs
• To take 2 hr before administration of other drugs that increase gastric pH (antacids, H$_2$-blockers, omeprazole, sucralfate, anticholinergics); to notify health care provider of all medications taken
• The importance of compliance with drug regimen; to use alternative method of contraception
• To notify prescriber of GI symptoms, signs of hepatic dysfunction (fatigue, nausea, anorexia, vomiting, dark urine, pale stools)

---

ranibizumab (R)
(ran-ih-biz'oo-mab)
Lucentis
Func. class.: Ophthalmic
Chem. class.: Selective vascular endothelial growth factor antagonist

Action: Binds to receptor-binding site of active forms of vascular endothelial growth factor A (VEGF-A) that causes angiogenesis and cell proliferation
Uses: Macular degeneration (neovascular) (wet)

DOSAGE AND ROUTES

• *Adult:* **Intravitreal** 0.5 mg (0.05 ml) qmo
Available forms: Sol for inj 0.5 mg/0.05 ml

SIDE EFFECTS

CNS: Dizziness, headache
EENT: Blepharitis, cataract, conjunctival hemorrhage/hyperemia, detachment of the retinal pigment epithelium, dry/irritation/pain in the eye, visual impairment, vitreous floaters, ocular infection

---

Side effects: *italics* = common; **bold** = life-threatening

GI: Constipation, nausea
MISC: Hypertension, UTI, thromboembolism
RESP: Bronchitis, cough, sinusitis, URI
Contraindications: Hypersensitivity, ocular infections
Precautions: Pregnancy (C), lactation, children, retinal detachment, increased intraocular pressure

PHARMACOKINETICS
Elimination half-life 9 days

INTERACTIONS
Increase: severe inflammation—verteporfin photodynamic therapy (PDT)

NURSING CONSIDERATIONS
Assess:
• For eye changes: redness, sensitivity to light, vision change, intraocular pressure change; report to ophthalmologist immediately
Administer:
• By ophthalmologist via intravitreal injection
Perform/provide:
• Storage in refrigerator; do not freeze
• Protect from light
Evaluate:
• Therapeutic response: prevention of increasing macular degeneration
Teach patient/family:
• That if eye becomes red, sensitive to light, painful, or if there is a change in vision, seek immediate care from ophthalmologist
• Reason for treatment, expected results

ranolazine (℞)
(ruh-no′luh-zeen)
Ranexa
Func. class: Antianginal

Action: Antianginal, antiischemic; unknown, may work by inhibiting portal fatty-acid oxidation
Uses: Chronic stable angina pectoris; use in those who have not responded to other treatment options; should be used in combination with other antianginals such as amlodipine, β-blockers, or nitrates

DOSAGE AND ROUTES
• *Adult:* **PO** 500 mg bid and increased to 1000 mg bid based on response; max 1000 mg bid
Available forms: Ext rel tabs 500 mg

SIDE EFFECTS
CNS: Headache, dizziness
CV: Palpitations, **QT prolongation**
GI: Nausea, vomiting, constipation, dry mouth
MISC: Peripheral edema
RESP: Dyspnea
Contraindications: Preexisting QT prolongation, hepatic disease (Child-Pugh class A, B, C), hypersensitivity, hypokalemia, renal failure, torsades de pointes, ventricular dysrhythmia, ventricular tachycardia
Precautions: Pregnancy (C), hypotension, lactation, children, geriatric, renal disease

PHARMACOKINETICS
Absorption varied; peak 2-5 hr; half-life 7 hr; metabolized by CYP3A, and lesser by CYP2D6; excreted in urine (75%), feces (25%); protein binding 62%

INTERACTIONS
Increase: ranolazine action—diltiazem, ketoconazole, macrolide antibiotics, dofetilide, paroxetine, protease inhibitors, quinidine, sotalol, thioridazine, verapamil, ziprasidone
Increase: action of digoxin, simvastatin
Increase: ranolazine action and QT prolongation; do not use concurrently—CYP3A4 inhibitors (ketoconazole, fluconazole, itraconazole, IV miconazole, voriconazole, diltiazem, verapamil)
Increase: QTc interval—macrolides (clarithromycin, erythromycin, troleandomycin)
Increase: ranolazine absorption, toxicity—antiretroviral protease inhibitors

Increase: QT prolongation and torsades de pointes—class IA/III antidysrhythmics, arsenic trioxide, chloroquine, droperidol, grepafloxacin, halofantrine, haloperidol, levomethadyl, methadone, pentamidine, chlorpromazine, mesoridazine, thioridazine, pimozide, probucol, sparfloxacin

Drug/Food

• Do not use with grapefruit or grapefruit juice

NURSING CONSIDERATIONS

Assess:

• Cardiac status: B/P, pulse, respiration, ECG; watch for prolongation of QT

Administer:

• Bid, without regard to meals

Evaluate:

• Therapeutic response: decreased anginal pain

Teach patient/family:

• Do not break, crush, or chew tabs; to take drugs as prescribed; do not double or skip dose

• To avoid hazardous activities until stabilized on drug, dizziness is no longer a problem

• To avoid OTC drugs, grapefruit juice, drugs prolonging QTc (quinidine, dofetilide, sotalol, erythromycin, thioridazine, ziprasidone or protease inhibitors, diltiazem, ketoconazole, macrolide antibiotics, verapamil) unless directed by prescriber

• To comply in all areas of medical regimen

• To notify prescriber of palpitations, fainting

• To notify all health care providers of this drug use

---

rasagiline
See page 888

---

sitagliptin (℞)

(sit-a-glip′tin)
Januvia
Func. class.: Antidiabetic, oral
Chem. class.: Dipeptidyl-peptidase-4 inhibitor (DPP-4 inhibitor)

Action: Slows the inactivation of incretin hormones; improves glucose homeostasis, improves glucose-dependent insulin synthesis, lowers glucagon secretions, and slows gastric emptying time

Uses: Type 2 diabetes mellitus as monotherapy or in combination with other antidiabetic agents

DOSAGE AND ROUTES

• *Adult:* **PO** 100 mg daily; may use with other antidiabetic agents (metformin, pioglitazone, rosiglitazone)

Available forms: Tabs 25, 50, 100 mg

SIDE EFFECTS

CNS: Headache
ENDO: Hypoglycemia
GI: Nausea, vomiting, abdominal pain

Contraindications: Hypersensitivity, diabetic ketoacidosis (DKA)

Precautions: Pregnancy (C), hypersensitivity, geriatric, GI obstruction, thyroid disease, surgery, hepatic/renal disease, trauma

PHARMACOKINETICS

Rapidly absorbed, excreted by the kidneys (unchanged 79%), terminal half-life 12.4 hr, peak 1-4 hr

INTERACTIONS

Increase: sitagliptan level—cimetidine, disopyramide
Increase: levels of digoxin
Increase: hypoglycemia—androgens, insulins, β-blockers, cimetidine, corticosteroids, salicylates, MAOIs, fibric acid derivatives, fluoxetine
Decrease: antidiabetic effect—thiazide diuretics, ACE inhibitors, protease in-

---

hibitors, sympathomimetics, aripiprazole, clozapine, olanzapine, quetiapine, risperidone, ziprasidone, phenytoin, fosphenytoin, phenothiazines, estrogens, progestins, oral contraceptives

Drug/Herb

Increase: hyperglycemia—glucosamine

Increase: hypoglycemia—chromium, coenzyme Q-10, fenugreek

Increase: antidiabetic effect—alfalfa, aloe, basil, bay, bilberry, bitter melon, black catechu, buchu, burdock, coriander, dandelion, eyebright (po), fenugreek, garlic, ginseng, glucomannan, glucosamine, goat's rue, gymnema, horehound, horse chestnut, jambul, myrrh, myrtle

Decrease: antidiabetic effect—bee pollen, blue cohosh, broom, chromium, elecampane, eucalyptus, gotu kola

NURSING CONSIDERATIONS

Assess:
• For hypoglycemic reactions (sweating, weakness, dizziness, anxiety, tremors, hunger), hyperglycemic reactions soon after meals
• CBC (baseline, q3mo) during treatment; check LFTs periodically, AST, LDH, renal studies: BUN, creatinine during treatment; glycosylated hemoglobin A1c
• Monitor blood glucose (BG) as needed

Administer:
• May be taken with or without food
• 100 mg daily

Perform/provide:
• Conversion from other antidiabetic agents; change may be made with gradual dosage change
• Storage in tight container in cool environment

Evaluate:
• Therapeutic response: decrease in polyuria, polydipsia, polyphagia; clear sensorium; absence of dizziness; stable gait, blood glucose at normal level

Teach patient/family:
• To use regular self-monitoring of blood glucose using blood glucose meter
• The symptoms of hypo/hyperglycemia; what to do about each

• That drug must be continued on daily basis; explain consequence of discontinuing drug abruptly
• To avoid OTC medications, alcohol, digoxin, exenatide, insulins, nateglinide, repaglinide and other drugs that lower blood glucose, unless approved by prescriber
• That diabetes is a lifelong illness; that this drug is not a cure, only controls symptoms
• That all food included in diet plan must be eaten to prevent hyper/hypoglycemia
• To carry emergency ID

---

sunitinib
See page 958

---

telbivudine
See page 965

---

varenicline (℞)
(var-e-ni'kleen)
Chantix
Func. class.: Smoking cessation agent

Action: Partial agonist for nicotine receptors; partially activates receptors to help curb cravings; occupies receptors to prevent nicotine binding

Uses: Smoking deterrent

DOSAGE AND ROUTES

• *Adult:* **PO** Therapy should begin 1 week prior to smoking stop date (i.e., take drug plus tobacco for 7 days); titrate for 1 wk, days 1 through 3, 0.5 mg daily; days 4 through 7, 0.5 mg bid; day 8 through end of treatment 1 mg bid; treatment is 12 wk and may repeat for another 12 wk

Available forms: Tabs 0.5, 1 mg

⚠ Safety alert   *"Tall Man" lettering

SIDE EFFECTS

CNS: Headache, agitation, dizziness, insomnia, abnormal dreams, fatigue, malaise

CV: Dysrhythmias, hypertension, palpitations, tachycardia, angina, hypotension, **MI**

EENT: Blurred vision, tinnitus

GI: Nausea, vomiting, anorexia, *dry mouth,* increased/decreased appetite, *constipation,* flatulence, GERD

GU: Erectile dysfunction, urinary frequency, menstrual irregularities

INTEG: Rash, pruritus

MISC: Weight loss or gain

RESP: Dyspnea, rhinorrhea

Contraindications: Hypersensitivity, eating disorders

Precautions: Pregnancy (C), renal disease, recent MI, lactation, children <18 yr, geriatric

PHARMACOKINETICS

Elimination half-life 24 hr; metabolism is minimal, 92% excreted unchanged in urine; steady state 4 days

NURSING CONSIDERATIONS

Assess:
• Renal function in geriatric

• For smoking cessation after 12 wk; if progress has not been made, drug may be used for an additional 12 wk

• Mental status: mood, sensorium, affect

Administer:
• Do not break, crush, or chew tabs
• Increased fluids, bulk in diet if constipation occurs
• After eating with a full glass of water
• Sugarless gum, hard candy, or frequent sips of water for dry mouth

Evaluate:
• Therapeutic response: smoking cessation

Teach patient/family:
• That treatment for smoking cessation lasts 12 wk and another 12 wk may be required
• To use caution in driving, other activities requiring alertness; blurred vision may occur
• To set a date to quit smoking and initiate treatment 1 wk prior to that date
• How to titrate product
• Not to use with nicotine patches unless directed by prescriber; may increase B/P
• To notify prescriber if pregnancy is suspected or planned
• Common side effects to be expected

Appendix b

Recent FDA drug approvals

Generic name	Trade name	Use
aliskiren	Tekturna	Hypertension
eculizumab	Soliris	Paroxysmal nocturnal hemoglobinuria
lisdexamfetamine	Vyvanse	Attention deficit/hyperactivity disorder
paliperidone	Invega	Schizophrenia

Appendix C

Ophthalmic, otic, nasal, and topical products

OPHTHALMIC PRODUCTS

α-ADRENERGIC BLOCKER
dapiprazole (R)
(da-pip′ra-zole)
Rev-Eyes

ANESTHETICS
proparacaine (R)
(proe-par′a-kane)
Alcaine, Diocaine ♣,
Ophthaine, Ophthestic
tetracaine (R)
(tet′ra-kane)
Minims Tetracaine ♣,
Pontocaine, Tetracaine

ANTIHISTAMINES
azelastine (R)
(ay-zell′ah-steen)
Optivar
emedastine (R)
(ee-med′ah-steen)
Emadine
epinastine (R)
(ep-een′as-teen)
Elestat
ketotifen (R)
(kee-toh-tif′en)
Zaditor
levocabastine (R)
(lee-voh-cab′ah-steen)
Livostin
olopatadine (R)
(oh-loh-pat′ah-deen)
Patanol

ANTIINFECTIVES
chloramphenicol (R)
(klor-am-fen′i-kole)
AK-Chlor, Chloramphenicol,
Chloromycetin Ophthalmic,
Chloroptic, Chloroptic S.O.P.,
Fenicol ♣, Isopto Fenicol ♣,
Pentamycin ♣
ciprofloxacin (R)
(sip-ro-floks′a-sin)
Ciloxan
erythromycin (R)
(er-ith-roe-mye′sin)
Erythromycin, Ilotycin
gatifloxacin (R)
(gat-i-flox′a-sin)
Zymar
gentamicin (R)
(jen-ta-mye′sin)
Garamycin Ophthalmic,
Genoptic Ophthalmic,
Genoptic S.O.P., Gentacidin,
Gentamicin Ophthalmic,
Gentak
levofloxacin (R)
(lee-voh-floks′a-sin)
Quixin
moxifloxacin (R)
(mox-i-flox′a-sin)
Vigamox
natamycin (R)
(nat-a-mye′sin)
Natacyn

♣ Canada only   Side effects: *italics* = common; **bold** = life-threatening

norfloxacin (R)
(nor-floks′a-sin)
Chibroxin

ofloxacin (R)
(oh-flox′a-sin)
Ocuflox

silver nitrate 1% (R)
silver nitrate
sulfacetamide
sodium (R)
(sul-fa-seet′a-mide)
AK-Sulf, Bleph-10, Bleph-10
S.O.P., Cetamide, Isopto
Cetamide, Ocusulf-10,
Sodium Sulamyd, Sodium
Sulfacetamide, Storzsulf, Sulf-
10, Sulster

tobramycin (R)
(toe-bra-mye′sin)
AKTob, Defy, Tobrex

trifluridine (R)
(trye-floor′i-deen)
Viroptic

vidarabine (R)
(vye-dare′a-been)
Vira-A

β-ADRENERGIC BLOCKERS
betaxolol (R)
(beh-tax′oh-lole)
Betoptic, Betoptic 5

carteolol (R)
(kar-tee′oh-lole)
Carteolol HCl, Ocupress

levobetaxolol (R)
(lee-voh-beh-tax′oh-lole)
Betaxon

levobunolol (R)
(lee-voe-byoo′no-lole)
AKBeta, Betagen

metipranolol (R)
(met-ee-pran′oh-lole)
OptiPranolol

timolol (R)
(tye′moe-lole)
Apo-Timop ♣, Betimol,
Timoptic, Timoptic-XE

**CARBONIC ANHYDRASE
INHIBITORS**
brinzolamide (R)
(brin-zoh′la-mide)
Azopt

dorzolamide (R)
(dor-zol′a-mide)
Trusopt

CHOLINERGICS
(Direct-acting)
acetylcholine (R)
(ah-see-til-koe′leen)
Miochol-E

carbachol (R)
(kar′ba-kole)
Carbastat, Carboptic, Isopto
Carbachol, Miostat

pilocarpine (R)
(pye-loe-kar′peen)
Adsorbocarpine, Akarpine,
Isopto Carpine,
Ocu-Carpine,
Ocusert Pilo-20, Ocusert
Pilo-40, Pilagan, Pilocar,
pilocarpine, Pilopine HS,
Piloptic-½, Piloptic-1,
Piloptic-2, Piloptic-3,
Piloptic-4, Piloptic-6, Pilostat,
Pilopto-Carpine

**CHOLINESTERASE
INHIBITORS**
demecarium (R)
(dem-e-kare′ee-um)
Humorsol

echothiophate (R)
(ek-oh-thye′eh-fate)
Phospholine Iodide

⚠ Safety alert   *"Tall Man" lettering

isoflurophate (Ŗ)
(i-se'flur-e'fate)
Floropryl
physostigmine (Ŗ)
(fi-zoe-stig'meen)
Eserine Salicylate, Isopto
Eserine

CORTICOSTEROIDS
dexamethasone (Ŗ)
(dex-a-meth'a-sone)
AK-Dex, Decadron
Phosphate, Dexamethasone
Ophthalmic Suspension,
Maxidex
fluorometholone (Ŗ)
(flure-oh-meth'oh-lone)
Flarex, Fluor-Op, FML, FML
Forte, FML S.O.P.
loteprednol (Ŗ)
(loe-tee-pred'nole)
Alrex, Lotemax
medrysone (Ŗ)
(me'dri-sone)
HMS
*prednisoLONE (Ŗ)**
(pred-niss'oh-lone)
Econopred, Econopred Plus,
AK-Pred, Inflamase Forte,
Inflamase Mild, Pred-Forte
rimexolone (Ŗ)
(ri-mex'a-lone)
· Vexol

MYDRIATICS
atropine (Ŗ)
(a'troe-peen)
Atropine-1, Atropine Care,
Atropine Sulfate Ophthalmic,
Atropisol, Isopto Atropine
cyclopentolate (Ŗ)
(sye-kloe-pen'toe-late)
AK-Pentolate, Cyclogyl,
Cyclopentolate HC

homatropine (Ŗ)
(home-a'troe-peen)
Homatrine HBr, Isopto
Homatropine, Minims
Homatropine ♣
phenylephrine (OTC)
(fen-ill-ef'rin)
AK-Dilate, AK-Nefrin, Isopto
Frin, Neo-Synephrine 2.5%,
Neo-Synephrine 10%,
phenylephrine HCl, 2.5%
Mydfrin, Phenoptic Relief,
Prefrin
scopolamine (Ŗ)
(skoe-pol'a-meen)
Isopto Hyoscine
tropicamide (Ŗ)
(troe-pik'a-mide)
Mydriacyl, Opticyl, Tropicacyl,
Tropicamide

**NONSTEROIDAL
ANTIINFLAMMATORIES**
bromfenac (Ŗ)
(brome'fen-ak)
Xibrom
diclofenac (Ŗ)
(dye-kloe'fen-ak)
Voltaren
flurbiprofen (Ŗ)
(flure-bih-proh'fen)
Ocufen
ketorolac (Ŗ)
(kee-toe'role-ak)
Acular
nepafenac (Ŗ)
(ne-pa-fen'ak)
Nevanac
suprofen (Ŗ)
(soo-proe'fen)
Profenal

SYMPATHOMIMETICS
apraclonidine (Ŗ)
(a-pra-klon'i-deen)
Lopidine

brimonidine (℞)

(brih-moh'nih-deen)

Alphagan, Alphagan P

dipivefrin (℞)

(dye-pi'vef-rin)

Propine, AKPro

*epINEPHrine/
epinephryl borate** (℞)

(ep-i-nef'rin)

Epifrin, Glaucon/Epinal, Eppy ✦

**OPHTHALMIC
DECONGESTANTS/
VASOCONSTRICTORS**
lodoxamide

(loe-dox'a-mide)

Alomide

naphazoline (otc, ℞)

(naf-az'oh-leen)

20/20 Eye Drops, Allergy Drops, AK-Con, Albalon, Allerest Eye Drops, Clear Eyes, Clear Eyes ACR, Comfort Eye Drops, Degest 2, Maximum Strength Allergy Drops, Nafazair, naphazoline HCl, Naphcon, Naphcon Forte, Opcon, Vasoclear, Vasocon Regular

oxymetazoline (℞)

(ox-i-meth'oh-lone)

OcuClear, Visine L.R.

tetrahydrozoline (otc)

(tet-ra-hye-dro'zoe-leen)

Collyrium Fresh, Eyesine, Geneye, Geneye Extra, Mallazine Eye Drops, Murine Plus, Optigene 3, tetrahydrozoline HCl, Tetrasine, Tetrasine Extra, Visine Moisturizing

**MISCELLANEOUS
OPHTHALMICS**
bimatoprost (℞)

(by-mat'oh-prahst)

Lumigan

brinzolamide (℞)

(brin-zole'a-mide)

Azopt

dorzolamide (℞)

(dor-zol'a-mide)

Trusopt

latanoprost (℞)

(la-tan'oh-proest)

Xalatan

travoprost (℞)

(trav'oh-prahst)

Travatan

unoprostone (℞)

(un-oh-proe'stone)

Rescula

Pregnancy categories: Demecarium, isoflurophate (X); apraclonidine, cyclopentolate, ecothiophate, glucocorticoids, levobunalol, metipranolol, pilocarpine, proparacaine, suprofen, tetracaine (C); dapiprazole, dipivefrin (B)

β-*Adrenergic blockers*

Action: Reduces production of aqueous humor by unknown mechanism

Uses: Ocular hypertension, chronic open-angle glaucoma

Anesthetics

Action: Decreases ion permeability by stabilizing neuronal membrane

Uses: Cataract extraction, tonometry, gonioscopy, removal of foreign objects, corneal suture removal, glaucoma surgery (ophthalmic); pruritus, sunburn, toothache, sore throat, cold sores, oral pain, rectal pain and irritation, control of gagging (topical)

🅐 Safety alert   *"Tall Man" lettering

Antiinfectives
Action: Inhibits folic acid synthesis by preventing PABA use, which is necessary for bacterial growth
Uses: Conjunctivitis, superficial eye infections, corneal ulcers, prophylaxis against infection after removal of foreign matter from the eye

Antiinflammatories
Action: Decreases inflammation, resulting in decreased pain, photophobia, hyperemia, cellular infiltration
Uses: Inflammation of eye, eyelids, conjunctiva, cornea; uveitis, iridocyclitis, allergic conditions, burns, foreign bodies, postoperatively in cataract

Carbonic anhydrase inhibitor
Action: Converted to epINEPHrine, which decreases aqueous production and increases outflow
Uses: Open-angle glaucoma, ocular hypertension

Direct-acting miotic
Action: Acts directly on cholinergic receptor sites; induces miosis, spasm of accommodation, fall in intraocular pressure, caused by stimulation of ciliary, pupillary sphincter muscles, which leads to pulling away of iris from filtration angle, resulting in increased outflow of aqueous humor
Uses: Primary glaucoma, early stages of wide-angle glaucoma (less useful in advanced stages), chronic open-angle glaucoma, acute narrow-angle glaucoma before emergency surgery; also neutralizes mydriatics used during eye exam; may be used alternately with mydriatics to break adhesions between iris and lens

SIDE EFFECTS

CNS: Headache
CV: Hypertension, tachycardia, dysrhythmias
EENT: Burning, stinging
GI: Bitter taste
Contraindications: Hypersensitivity
Precautions: Pregnancy, lactation, children, aphakia, hypersensitivity to carbonic anhydrase inhibitors, sulfonamides, thia-zide diuretics, ocular inhibitors, hepatic and renal insufficiency

NURSING CONSIDERATIONS
Assess:
• Ophth exams and intraocular pressure readings
• Blood counts; hepatic, renal function tests and serum electrolytes during long-term treatment
Perform/provide:
• Storage at room temperature away from light
Evaluate:
• Positive therapeutic response
• Absence of increased intraocular pressure
Teach patient/family:
• How to instill drops
• That drug may cause burning, itching, blurring, dryness of eye area

NASAL AGENTS

NASAL DECONGESTANTS
azelastine (℞)
(ay-zell'ah-steen)
Astelin
desoxyephedrine (OTC)
(des-oxy-e-fed'rin)
Vicks Vapor Inhaler
*epHEDrine (OTC)
(e-fed'rin)
Pretz-D
*epINEPHrine (OTC)
(ep-i-neff'rin)
Adrenalin
naphazoline (OTC)
(naff-a-zoe'leen)
Privine
oxymetazoline (OTC)
(ox-i-met-az'oh-leen)
12-Hour Nasal, Afrin 12-Hour Original, Afrin 12-Hour Original Pump Mist, Afrin Severe Congestion with Menthol, Afrin Sinus with

---

Vapornase, Afrin No-Drip 12-Hour, Afrin No-Drip 12-Hour Extra Moisturizing, Dristan, Duramist Plus, Duration, Genasal, Nafrine ♣, Nasal Relief, Neo-Synephrine 12-Hour, Nostrilla, oxymetazoline HCl, Nasal Decongestant, Maximum Strength, Vicks Sinex 12-Hour Long-Acting, Vicks Sinex 12-Hour Ultra Fine Mist for Sinus Relief

phenylephrine (OTC)
(fen-ill-eff'rin)
Alconefrin 12, Children's Nostril, Neo-Synephrine, Sinex

propylhexadrine (OTC)
(proe-pil-hex'a-dreen)
Benzedrex Inhaler

pseudoephedrine (R, OTC)
(soo-doe-e-fed'rin)
Cenafed, Decofed, Dimetapp, Genaphed, PediCare Infants' Decongestant Drops, Sudafed, Triaminic

tetrahydrozoline (OTC)
(tet-ra-hye-dro'zoe-leen)
Tyzine, Tyzine Pediatric

xylometazoline (OTC)
(zye-loh-meh-tazz'oh-leen)
Natru-vent, Otrivin, Otrivin Pediatric Nasal

NASAL STEROIDS
beclomethasone (R)
(be-kloe-meth'a-sone)
Beconase AQ Nasal, Beconase Inhalation, Vancenase AQ Nasal, Vancenase Pocket Inhaler

budesonide (R)
(byoo-des'oh-nide)
Rhinocort, Rhinocort Aqua

flunisolide (R)
(floo-niss'oh-lide)
Nasalide, Nasarel

fluticasone (R)
(floo-tic'a-son)
Flonase

triamcinolone (R)
(trye-am-sin'oh-lone)
Nasacort AQ

Pregnancy category: C
Action: Produces vasoconstriction (rapid, long acting) of arterioles, thereby decreasing fluid exudation, mucosal engorgement by stimulation of α-adrenergic receptors in vascular smooth muscle
Uses: Nasal congestion

DOSAGE AND ROUTES
Desoxyephedrine
• *Adult and child >6 yr:* 1-2 **INH** in each nostril q2h or less
EpHEDrine
• *Adult:* Fill dropper to the level marked, then use in each nostril q4h or less
EpINEPHrine
• *Adult and child >6 yr:* Apply with swab, drops, spray prn
Naphazoline
• *Adult and child >6 yr:* 1-2 drops/spray q6h or less
Oxymetazoline
• *Adult and child >6 yr:* **INSTILL** 2-3 gtt or sprays to each nostril bid
• *Child 2-6 yr:* **INSTILL** 2-3 gtt or sprays 0.025 sol bid, not to exceed 3 days
Phenylephrine
• *Adult and child >12 yr:* 2-3 drops/spray (0.25-0.5) in each nostril q3-4h or less; or 2-3 drops/spray (1%) in each nostril q4h or less
• *Child 6-12 yr:* 2-3 drops/spray (0.25%) in each nostril q3-4h
• *Infant >6 mo:* 1-2 drops (0.16%) in each nostril q3h
Propylhexadrine
• *Adult and child >6 yr:* 1-2 **INH** in each nostril q2h or less

▲ Safety alert   *"Tall Man" lettering

Tetrahydrozoline
• *Adult and child >6 yr:* 2-4 drops (0.1%) q3-4h prn or 3-4 sprays in each nostril q4h prn
• *Child 2-6 yr:* 2-3 drops (0.05%) in each nostril q4-6h prn

Xylometazoline
• *Adult and child >12 yr:* 2-3 drops/spray (0.1%) in each nostril q8-10h
• *Child 2-12 yr:* 2-3 drops (0.05%) in each nostril q8-10h
Available forms: Nasal sol 0.025%, 0.05%

SIDE EFFECTS

CNS: Anxiety, restlessness, tremors, weakness, insomnia, dizziness, fever, headache
EENT: Irritation, burning, sneezing, stinging, dryness, rebound congestion
GI: Nausea, vomiting, anorexia
INTEG: Contact dermatitis

Contraindications: Hypersensitivity to sympathomimetic amines
Precautions: Pregnancy (C), children <6 yr, geriatric, diabetes, cardiovascular disease, hypertension, hyperthyroidism, increased intracranial pressure, prostatic hypertrophy, glaucoma

NURSING CONSIDERATIONS

Assess:
• For redness, swelling, pain in nasal passages before and during treatment
• For systemic absorption; hypertension, tachycardia; notify prescriber; systemic absorption occurs at high doses or after prolonged use

Administer:
• Having patient tilt head back, squeeze bulb to create a vacuum, and draw correct amount of sol into dropper; insert 2 gtt of sol into nostril; repeat in other nostril
• Store in light-resistant container; do not expose to high temp or let sol come into contact with aluminum
• For <4 consecutive days
• Environmental humidification to decrease nasal congestion, dryness

Evaluate:
• Therapeutic response: decreased nasal congestion

Teach patient/family:
• That stinging may occur for several applications; drying of mucosa may be decreased by environmental humidification
• To notify prescriber if irregular pulse, insomnia, dizziness, or tremors occur
• Proper administration to avoid systemic absorption
• To rinse dropper with very hot water to prevent contamination

TOPICAL GLUCOCORTICOIDS

betamethasone (℞)
(bay-ta-meth′a-sone)
Alphatrex, Beben ✤, Betacort ✤, Betatrex, Beta-Val, Bethovate ✤, Celestoderm ✤, Diprosone, Ectosone ✤, Luxiq, Maxivate, Metaderm ✤, Psorion, Valisone

betamethasone (augmented) (℞)
(bay-ta-meth′a-sone)
Diprolene, Diprolene AF

clobetasol (℞)
(kloe-bay′ta-sol)
Cormax, Dermovate ✤, Embeline E 0.05%, Temovate

desoximetasone (℞)
(dess-ox-i-met′a-sone)
Topicort, Topicort LP

dexamethasone (℞)
(dex-a-meth′a-sone)
Aeroseb-Dex, Decaspray

fluocinolone (℞)
(floo-oh-sin′oh-lone)
Fluocin, Licon, Lidemol ✤, Lidex, Lyderm ✤, Topsyn ✤, Vasoderm

---

✤ Canada only Side effects: *italics* = common; **bold** = life-threatening

flurandrenolide (℞)

(flure-an-dren'oh-lide)
Cordran, Cordran SP,
Drenison 1/4 ✤, Drenison
Tape ✤

fluticasone (℞)

(floo-tik'a-sone)
Cutivate

halcinonide (℞)

(hal-sin'oh-nide)
Halog, Halog-E

hydrocortisone (℞)

(hye-droe-kor'ti-sone)
Acticort, Aeroseb-HC, Ala-
Cort, Allercort, Alphaderm,
Anusol HC, Bactine,
Barriere-HC ✤, Calde-CORT
Anti-Itch, Carmol HC,
Cetacort, Cortacet ✤,
Cortaid, Cortate ✤, Cort-
Dome, Cortef ✤, Corticaine,
Corticreme ✤, Cortifair, Corti-
zone, Cortoderm ✤, Cortril,
Delcort, Dermacort,
DemiCort, Dermtex HC,
Emo-Cort, Epifoam,
FoilleCort, Gly-Cort,
Gynecort, Hi-Cor, Hycort,
Hyderm ✤, Hydro-Tex,
Hytone, Lacti-Care-HC,
Lanacort, Lemoderm, Locoid,
My Cort, Novohydrocort ✤,
Nutracort Pharm,
Pharmacort, Pentacort,
Rederm, Rhulicort S-T Cort,
Synacort, Sarna HC ✤, Texa-
Cort, Unicort ✤, Westcort

triamcinolone (℞)

(trye-am-sin'oh-lone)
Aristocort, Delta-Tritex, Flutex,
Kenac, Kenalog, Kenonel,
Triaderm, Trianide ✤, Triderm,
Trymex

Pregnancy category: C
Action: Antipruritic, antiinflammatory
Uses: Psoriasis, eczema, contact derma-
titis, pruritus; usually reserved for severe

dermatoses that have not responded to
less potent formulation

DOSAGE AND ROUTES
• *Adult and child:* Apply to affected area

SIDE EFFECTS
INTEG: Acne, atrophy, epidermal thin-
ning, purpura, striae
Contraindications: Hypersensitivity, vi-
ral infections, fungal infections
Precautions: Pregnancy (C)

NURSING CONSIDERATIONS
Assess:
• Temp; if fever develops, drug should
be discontinued
• For systemic absorption, increased
temp, inflammation, irritation
Administer:
• Only to affected areas; do not get in
eyes
• Leaving site uncovered or lightly cov-
ered; occlusive dressing is not
recommended—systemic absorption may
occur
• Use only on dermatoses; do not use on
weeping, denuded, or infected area
• Cleansing before application of drug
• Continuing treatment for a few days af-
ter area has cleared
• Store at room temperature
Evaluate:
• Therapeutic response: absence of se-
vere itching, patches on skin, flaking
Teach patient/family:
• To avoid sunlight on affected area,
burns may occur
• To limit treatment to 14 days

TOPICAL ANTIFUNGALS

clotrimazole (OTC)

(kloe-trye'ma-zole)
Canestew ✤, Clotrimaderm ✤,
Clotrimazole, Cruex, Desenex,
Lotrimin AF, Myclo ✤,
Neozol ✤

⚠ Safety alert   ✤ "Tall Man" lettering

econazole (OTC)
(ee-kon'a-zole)
Spectazole

ketoconazole (OTC)
(kee-toe-kon'a-zole)
Nizoral

miconazole (OTC)
(mye-kon'a-zole)
Absorbine Antifungal Foot
Powder, Breeze Mist
Antifungal, Fungoid Tincture,
Lotrimin AF, Maximum
Strength Desenex Antifungal,
Micatin, Monistat-Derm, Ony-
clear, Tetterine, Zeasorb-AF

nystatin (OTC)
(nye-stat'in)
Mycostatin, Nadostine ✤,
Nilstat, Nyaderm ✤, Nystex

selenium (OTC)
(see-leen'ee-um)
Exsel, Head and Shoulders
Intensive Treatment,
Selenium Sulfide, Selsun,
Selsun Blue

terbinafine (OTC)
(ter-bin'a-feen)
Lamisil

tolnaftate (OTC)
(tole-naf'tate)
Absorbine Athlete's Foot
Cream, Aftate for Athlete's
Foot, Aftate for Jock Itch,
Genaspor, Quinsana Plus,
Tinactin, Ting, tolnaftate

undecylenic acid (OTC)
(un-deh-sih-len'ik)
Blis-To-Sol, Breeze Mist,
Caldesene, Cruex,
Decylenes, Desenex,
Desenex Maximum Strength,
Pedi-Pro, Phicon F, Protectol

Pregnancy category: B
Action: Interferes with fungal cell membrane permeability

Uses: Tinea cruris, tinea pedis, diaper rash, minor skin irritations; amphotericin B is used for candida infections

DOSAGE AND ROUTES
• Massage into affected area, surrounding area daily or bid, continue for 7-14 days, not to exceed 4 wk

SIDE EFFECTS
INTEG: Burning, stinging, dryness, itching, local irritation
Contraindications: Hypersensitivity
Precautions: Pregnancy (B), lactation, children
Interactions: None

NURSING CONSIDERATIONS
Assess:
• Skin for fungal infections; peeling, dryness, itching before and throughout treatment
• For continuing infection; increased size, number of lesions
Administer:
Topical route
• To affected area, surrounding area; do not cover with occlusive dressings
• Store below 30° C (86° F)
Evaluate:
• Therapeutic response: decrease in size, number of lesions
Teach patient/family:
• To apply with glove to prevent further infection; not to cover with occlusive dressings
• That long-term therapy may be needed to clear infection (2 wk-6 mo depending on organism); compliance is needed even after feeling better
• Proper hygiene; hand-washing technique, nail care, use of concomitant top agents if prescribed
• To avoid use of OTC creams, ointments, lotions unless directed by prescriber
• To use medical asepsis (hand washing) before, after each application; to change socks and shoes once a day during treatment of tinea pedis

• To report to healthcare prescriber if infection persists or recurs; if blisters, burning, oozing, swelling occur
• To avoid alcohol because nausea, vomiting, hypertension may occur
• To use sunscreen or avoid direct sunlight to prevent photosensitivity
• To notify healthcare prescriber of sore throat, fever, skin rash, which may indicate overgrowth of organisms

TOPICAL ANTIINFECTIVES

azelaic acid (℞)
(a-zuh-lay'ic)
Azelex, Finacen

bacitracin (otc)
(bass-i-tray'sin)
Bacitin ✦, Bacitracin

clindamycin (℞)
(klin-da-my'sin)
Cleocin T, Clindagel, ClindaMax, Clindets

erythromycin (otc, ℞)
(er-ith-roe-mye'sin)
A/T/S, Akne-Mycin, Eryderm, Erygel, Erythromycin, Staticin, T-Stat

gentamicin (℞)
(jen-ta-mye'sin)
Gentamicin

mafenide (℞)
(ma'fe-nide)
Sulfamylon

metronidazole (℞)
(met-roh-nye'da-zole)
MetroGel, MetroCream, MetroLotion, Noritate

mupirocin (℞)
(myoo-peer'oh-sin)
Bactroban

neomycin (otc)
(nee-oh-mye'sin)
Neomycin Sulfate

nitrofurazone (℞)
(nye-troe-fyoor'a-zone)
Furacin, Nitrofurazone

*silver sulfADIAZINE (℞)
(sul-fa-dye'a-zeen)
Flamazine ✦, Silvadene, SSD, SSD AF, Thermazine

Pregnancy category: C
Action: Interferes with bacterial protein synthesis
Uses: Skin infections, minor burns, wounds, skin grafts, primary pyodermas, otitis externa

SIDE EFFECTS
INTEG: Rash, urticaria, scaling, redness
Contraindications: Hypersensitivity, large areas, burns, ulcerations
Precautions: Pregnancy (C), lactation, impaired renal function, external ear or perforated eardrum

NURSING CONSIDERATIONS
Assess:
• Allergic reaction: burning, stinging, swelling, redness
• For signs of nephrotoxicity or ototoxicity
Administer:
• Enough medication to cover lesions completely
• After cleansing with soap, water before each application; dry well
• To less than 20% of body surface area when patient has impaired renal function
Perform/provide:
• Storage at room temperature in dry place
Evaluate:
• Therapeutic response: decrease in size, number of lesions

TOPICAL ANTIVIRALS

acyclovir (℞)
(ay-sye'kloe-ver)
Zovirax

penciclovir (℞)
(pen-sye'kloe-ver)
Denavir

Pregnancy category: C
Action: Interferes with viral DNA replication
Uses: Simple mucocutaneous herpes simplex, in immunocompromised clients with initial herpes genitalis

SIDE EFFECTS

INTEG: Rash, urticaria, stinging, burning, pruritus, vulvitis
Contraindications: Hypersensitivity
Precautions: Pregnancy (C), lactation

NURSING CONSIDERATIONS

Assess:
• Allergic reaction: burning, stinging, swelling, redness, rash, vulvitis, pruritus
Administer:
• Using finger cot or rubber glove to prevent further infection
• Enough medication to cover lesions completely
• After cleansing with soap, water before each application; dry well
Perform/provide:
• Storage at room temperature in dry place
Evaluate:
• Therapeutic response: decrease in size, number of lesions
Teach patient/family:
• Not to use in eyes or when there is no evidence of infection
• To apply with glove to prevent further infection
• To avoid use of OTC creams, ointments, lotions unless directed by prescriber
• To use medical asepsis (hand washing) before, after each application and avoid contact with eyes
• To adhere strictly to prescribed regimen to maximize successful treatment outcome
• To begin taking drug when symptoms arise

TOPICAL ANESTHETICS

benzocaine (OTC)
(ben'zoe-kane)
Americaine Anesthetic, Anbesol Maximum Strength, Baby Anbesol, Biozene, Boil-Ease, Children's Chloraseptic, Dermoplast, Foille, Foille Plus, Hurricaine, Lanacane, Medamint, Orabase, Oracin, Ora-Jel

dibucaine (OTC)
(dye'byoo-kane)
Dibucaine, Nupercainal

lidocaine (OTC, ℞)
(lye'doe-kane)
Anestacon, Burn-O-Jel, Derma Flex, Dentipatch, ELA-Max, Lidocaine HCl Topical, Lidocaine Viscous, Numby Stuff, Solarcaine Aloe Extra Burn Relief, Xylocaine, Xylocaine 10% oral, Xylocaine Viscous, Zilactin-L

pramoxine (OTC)
(pra-mox'een)
Itch-X, PrameGel, Prax, Tronothane

tetracaine (OTC, ℞)
(tet'ra-cane)
Pontocaine, Viractin

Pregnancy category: C
Action: Inhibits conduction of nerve impulses from sensory nerves
Uses: Oral irritation, sore throat, toothache, cold sore, canker sore, sunburn, minor cuts, insect bites, pain, itching

DOSAGE AND ROUTES

• *Adult and child:* **TOP** apply qid as needed; **RECT** insert tid and after each BM

SIDE EFFECTS

INTEG: Rash, irritation, sensitization
Contraindications: Hypersensitivity, infants <1 yr, application to large areas
Precautions: Pregnancy (C), child <6 yr, sepsis, denuded skin

NURSING CONSIDERATIONS

Assess:
• Pain: location, duration, characteristics before and after administration
• For infection: redness, drainage, inflammation; this drug should not be used until infection is treated
Perform/provide:
• Storage in tight, light-resistant container; do not freeze, puncture, or incinerate aerosol container
Evaluate:
• Therapeutic response: decreased redness, swelling, pain
Teach patient/family:
• To avoid contact with eyes
• Not to use for prolonged periods: use for <1 wk; if condition remains, prescriber should be contacted

TOPICAL MISCELLANEOUS

docosanol (OTC)
(doe-koe'san-ole)
Abreva
pimecrolimus (℞)
(pim-eh-croh'lim-us)
Elidel

VAGINAL ANTIFUNGALS

butoconazole (OTC)
(byoo-toh-kone'ah-zole)
Femstat-3, Gynazol-1, Mycelex-3
clotrimazole (OTC)
(kloe-trye'ma-zole)
Canesten ✿, Clotrimazole, Gyne-Lotrimin 3, Gyne-Lotrimin 7, Mycelex 7, Myclo ✿
miconazole (OTC)
(mye-kon'a-zole)
Femizole-M, Monistat, Monistat 3, Monistat 7, Monistat Dual Pak, M-Zole 7 Dual Pack
nystatin (OTC)
(nye-stat'in)
Nystatin
terconazole (OTC)
(ter-kone'ah-zole)
Terazol 7, Terazol 3
tioconazole (OTC)
(tye-oh-kone'ah-zole)
Gyne-Trosyd ✿, Monistat 1, Vagistat-1

Pregnancy category: Nystatin (A); clotrimazole (B); butoconazole, terconazole, tioconazole (C)
Action: Interferes with fungal DNA replication; binds sterols in fungal cell membranes, which increases permeability, leaking of nutrients
Uses: Vaginal, vulval, vulvovaginal candidiasis (moniliasis)

DOSAGE AND ROUTES

Butoconazole
• *Adult:* **VAG** 5 g (1 applicator) at bedtime × 3-6 days
Clotrimazole
• *Adult:* 100 mg (1 vag tab, 100 mg) at bedtime × 1 wk, or 200 mg (2 vag tab, 100 mg) at bedtime × 3 nights, or 500

mg (1 vag tab, 500 mg); or 5 g (1 applicator) at bedtime × 1-2 wk

Miconazole
• *Adult:* 200 mg supp at bedtime × 3 days or 100 mg supp × 1 wk

Nystatin
• *Adult:* 100,000 units daily × 2 wk

Terconazole
• *Adult:* **VAG** 5 g (1 applicator) at bedtime × 7 days

Tioconazole
• *Adult:* 1 applicator at bedtime × 1 wk

SIDE EFFECTS
GU: Vulvovaginal burning, itching, pelvic cramps
INTEG: Rash, urticaria, stinging, burning
MISC: **Headache**, body pain
Contraindications: Hypersensitivity
Precautions: Children <2 yr, pregnancy, lactation
Interactions: None

NURSING CONSIDERATIONS
Assess:
• For allergic reaction: burning, stinging, itching, discharge, soreness
Administer:
Topical route
• One full applicator every night high into the vagina
• Store at room temperature in dry place
Evaluate:
• Therapeutic outcome: decrease in itching or white discharge (vaginal)
Teach patient/family:
• About asepsis (hand washing) before, after each application
• To apply with applicator only; to avoid use of any other vaginal product unless directed by prescriber; sanitary napkin may prevent soiling of undergarments
• To abstain from sexual intercourse until treatment is completed; reinfection and irritation may occur

• To notify prescriber if symptoms persist

OTIC ANTIINFECTIVES

boric acid (OTC)
Auro-Dri, Dri/Ear, Ear Dry
chloramphenicol (Ŗ)
(klor-am-fen′i-kole)
Chloromycetin Otic

Action: Inhibits protein synthesis in susceptible microorganisms
Uses: Ear infection (external), short-term use

SIDE EFFECTS
EENT: Itching, irritation in ear
INTEG: Rash, urticaria
Contraindications: Hypersensitivity, perforated eardrum
Precautions: Pregnancy (C)

NURSING CONSIDERATIONS
Assess:
• For redness, swelling, fever, pain in ear, which indicates superinfection
Administer:
• After removing impacted cerumen by irrigation
• After cleaning stopper with alcohol
• After restraining child if necessary
• After warming sol to body temp
Evaluate:
• Therapeutic response: decreased ear pain
Teach patient/family:
• The correct method of instillation using aseptic technique, including not touching dropper to ear
• That dizziness may occur after instillation

Appendix d Vaccines and toxoids

GENERIC NAME	TRADE NAME	USES	DOSAGE AND ROUTES	CONTRAINDICATIONS
BCG vaccine	TICE BCG	TB exposure	Adult and child >1 mo: 0.2-0.3 ml Child <1 mo: Reduce dose by 50% using 2 ml of sterile water after reconstituting	Hypersensitivity, hypogammaglobulinemia, positive TB test, burns
cholera vaccine	No trade name	Immunization for cholera in other countries	Adult and child >10 yr: IM/SUBCUT 2× of 0.5 ml, 7-30 days before traveling to cholera areas Booster is used q6mo 0.5 ml prn	Hypersensitivity, acute febrile illness
diphtheria and tetanus toxoids, adsorbed	No trade name	Induces antitoxins to provide immunity to diphtheria and tetanus	Adult and child ≥7 yr: IM (adult strength) 0.5 ml q4-8wk × 2 doses, then 3rd dose 6-12 mo after 2nd dose, booster IM 0.5 ml q10yr Child 1-6 yr: IM (pediatric strength) 0.5 ml q4wk × 2 doses, booster 6-12 mo after 2nd dose Infant 6 wk-1 yr: IM (pediatric strength) 0.5 ml q4wk × 3 doses, booster 6-12 mo after 3rd dose	Hypersensitivity to mercury, thimerosal; immunocompromised patients; radiation; corticosteroids; acute illness
diphtheria and tetanus toxoids and whole-cell pertussis vaccine (DPT, DTP)	DTwP, Tr-Immunol	Prevention of diphtheria, tetanus, pertussis	Adult: Booster dose q10yr Child >6 wk-6 yr: IM 0.5 ml at 2, 4, 6 mo, 1½ yr; booster needed 0.5 ml at age 6	Hypersensitivity, active infection, poliomyelitis outbreak, immunosuppression, febrile illness
diphtheria and tetanus toxoids and acellular pertussis vaccine	Acel-Imune, DTaP, Tripedia			
haemophilus b conjugate vaccine, diphtheria CRM$_{197}$ protein conjugate (HbOC)	HibTITER	Polysaccharide immunization of children 2-6 yr against *H. influenzae* b, conjugate	**HibTITER (IM only)** Child: IM 0.5 ml Child 2-6 mo: 0.5 ml q2mo × 3 inj	Hypersensitivity, febrile illness, active infection

haemophilus b conjugate vaccine, meningococcal protein conjugate (PRP-OMP)	PedvaxHIB	Immunization of child 2, 4, 6 mo	Child 7-11 mo: Previously unvaccinated 0.5 ml inj q2mo inj Child 12-14 mo: Previously unvaccinated 0.5 ml × 1 inj **PedvaxHIB (IM only)** Child 2-14 mo: 0.5 ml × 2 inj at 2, 4 mo of age (6 mo dose not needed), then booster at 12-18 mo against invasive disease Child ≥15 mo: Previously unvaccinated 0.5 ml inj	
hepatitis A vaccine, inactivated	Havrix, Vaqta	Active immunization against hepatitis A virus	Adult: IM 1440 EL units (Havrix) or 50 units (Vaqta) as a single dose; booster dose is the same given at 6, 12 mo Child 2-18 yr: IM 720 EL units (Havrix) or 25 units (Vaqta) as a single dose, booster dose is the same given at 6, 12 mo	Hypersensitivity
hepatitis B vaccine, recombinant	Engerix-B, Recombivax HB	Immunization against all subtypes of hepatitis B virus	Varies widely	Hypersensitivity to this vaccine or yeast
human papillomavirus recombinant vaccine, quadrivalent	Gardasil	Prevention of HPV types 6, 11, 16, 18, cervical cancer, genital warts, precancerous dysplasic lesions	Adult and child >9 yr: IM give as 3 separate doses; 1st dose as elected; 2nd dose 2 mo after 1st dose; 3rd dose 6 mo after 1st dose	Child <9 yr, pregnancy, lactation, geriatric, active disease, hypersensitivity
influenza virus vaccine, trivalent A and B (whole virus/split virus)	Fluogen, Flushield, Fluvial*, Fluvirin, Fluzone, influenza virus vaccine, trivalent	Prevention of Russian, Chilean, Philippine influenza	Adult and child >12 yr: IM 0.5 ml in 1 dose Child 3-12 yr: IM 0.5 ml, repeat in 1 mo (split) unless 1978-1985 vaccine was given Child 6 mo to 3 yr: IM 0.25 ml, repeat in 1 mo (split) unless 1978-1985 vaccine was given	Hypersensitivity, active infection, chicken egg allergy, Guillain-Barré syndrome, active neurologic disorders
Japanese encephalitis virus vaccine, inactivated	JE-VAX	Active immunity against Japanese encephalitis (JE)	Adult and child ≥3 yr: SUBCUT 1 ml, days 0, 7, 30; booster SUBCUT 1 ml 2 yr after last dose Child 1-3 yr: SUBCUT 0.5 ml, days 0, 7, 30; booster SUBCUT 0.5 ml 2 yr after last dose	Hypersensitivity to murine, thimerosal; allergic reactions to previous dose
Lyme disease vaccine (recombinant OspA)	LYMErix	Immunization against Lyme disease	Adult and adolescent 15-70: IM 30 mcg in deltoid, repeat at 1, 12 mo after first dose	Hypersensitivity, antibiotic refactory Lyme arthritis

*Canada only.

Continued

Appendix d Vaccines and toxoids—cont'd

GENERIC NAME	TRADE NAME	USES	DOSAGE AND ROUTES	CONTRAINDICATIONS
measles and rubella virus vaccine, live attenuated	M-R-Vax II	Immunity to measles and rubella by antibody production	Adult and child ≥15 mo: SUBCUT 0.5 ml (1000 units)	Hypersensitivity, immunocompromised patients, active untreated TB, cancer, blood dyscrasias, radiation, corticosteroids, pregnancy; allergic reactions to neomycin, eggs
measles, mumps, and rubella vaccine, live	M-M-R-II	Prevention of measles, mumps, rubella	Adult: SUBCUT 1 vial; 2 vials separated by 1 mo, in person born after 1957 Child >15 mo and adult: SUBCUT 0.5 ml	Hypersensitivity, blood dyscrasias, anemia, active infection, immunosuppression; egg, chicken allergy; pregnancy, febrile illness, neomycin allergy, neoplasms
measles virus vaccine, live attenuated	Attenuvax	Immunity to measles by antibody production	Adult and child ≥15 mo: SUBCUT 0.5 ml (1000 units), 1 dose 15 mo, 2nd dose age 4-6 or 11, or 12	Hypersensitivity to eggs, neomycin; cancer, radiation, corticosteroids, pregnancy, immunocompromised patients, blood dyscrasias, active untreated TB
meningococcal polysaccharide vaccine	Menomune-A/C/Y/W-135	Prophylaxis to meningococcal meningitis	Adult and child >2 yr: SUBCUT 0.5 ml	Hypersensitivity to thimerosal, pregnancy, acute illness
mumps virus vaccine, live	Mumpsvax	Active immunity to mumps	Adult and child ≥1 yr: SUBCUT 0.5 ml (20,000 units)	Hypersensitivity to eggs, neomycin; cancer, radiation, corticosteroids, pregnancy, immunocompromised patients, blood dyscrasias, active untreated TB
plague vaccine	No trade name	Active immunity to *Yersinia pestis* plague	Adult: IM 1 ml, then 0.2 ml in 4-12 wk, then 0.2 ml 5-6 mo after 2nd dose; booster 0.1-0.2 ml q6mo when in plague area	Hypersensitivity to phenol, sulfites, formaldehyde, beef, soy, casein; pregnancy, coagulation disorders

pneumococcal 7-valent conjugate vaccine	Prevnar	Immunity against *Streptococcus pneumoniae*	Child: IM 0.5 ml × 3 doses (7-11 mo); × 2 doses (12-23 mo); × 1 dose >2-9 yr	Hypersensitivity to diphtheria toxoid or this product
pneumococcal vaccine, polyvalent	Pneumovax 23, Pnu-Imune 23	Pneumococcal immunization	Adult and child >2 yr: IM/SUBCUT 0.5 ml	Hypersensitivity, Hodgkin's disease, ARDS
poliovirus vaccine, live, oral, trivalent (TOPV) poliovirus vaccine (IPV)	Orimune, IPOL	Prevention of polio	Adult and child >2 yr: PO 0.5 ml, given q8wk × 2 doses, then 0.5 ml ½-1 yr after dose 2 Infant: PO 0.5 ml at 2, 4, 18 mo; booster at 4-6 yr; may also be given: IPV at 2, 4 mo, then TOPV at 12-18 mo, booster at 4-6 yr	Hypersensitivity, active infection, allergy to neomycin/streptomycin, immunosuppression, vomiting, diarrhea
rabies vaccine, adsorbed	No trade name	Active immunity to rabies	**Preexposure** Adult and child: IM 1 ml day 0, 7, 21, or 28 days (total 3 doses); booster IM 1 ml prn q2-5 yr **Postexposure** Adult and child not vaccinated: IM 20 international units/kg of human rabies immune globulin (HRIG), give 5 total doses of 1-ml inj of rabies vaccine on days 0, 3, 7, 14, 28	Severe hypersensitivity to previous inj of vaccine, thimerosol
rabies vaccine, human diploid cell (HDCV)	Imovax Rabies, Imovax Rabies I.D.	Active immunity to rabies	**Preexposure** Adult and child: IM 1 ml day 0, 7, 21 or 28 (total 4 doses) **Postexposure** Adult and child: IM 1 ml on day 0, 3, 7, 14, 28 (total 5 doses)	No contraindications
rotovirus	RotoTeq	Prevents rotovirus	Infant: PO 3 doses given between 6 and 32 wk of age; 1st dose between 6-12 wk of age; 2nd and 3rd doses q4-10wk	Hypersensitivity, immunocompromised, blood products given within 6 wk of age, lymphatic disorders
rubella and mumps virus vaccine, live	Biavax II	Immunity to rubella and mumps by antibody production	Adult and child ≥1 yr: SUBCUT 0.5 ml	Hypersensitivity to eggs, neomycin; cancer, radiation, corticosteroids, pregnancy, immunocompromised patients, blood dyscrasias, active untreated TB

*Canada only.

Continued

Appendix d Vaccines and toxoids—cont'd

GENERIC NAME	TRADE NAME	USES	DOSAGE AND ROUTES	CONTRAINDICATIONS
rubella virus vaccine, live attenuated (RA 27/3)	Meruvax II	Immunity to rubella by antibody production	Adult and child ≥1 yr: SUBCUT 0.5 ml (1000 units)	Hypersensitivity to eggs, neomycin; cancer, radiation, corticosteroids
tetanus toxoid, adsorbed/tetanus toxoid	No trade name	Tetanus toxoid: Used for prophylactic treatment of wounds	Adult and child: IM 0.5 ml q4-6wk × 2 doses, then 0.5 ml 1 yr after dose 2 (adsorbed); SUBCUT/IM 0.5 ml q4-8wk × 3 doses, then 0.5 ml ½-1 yr after dose 3, booster dose 0.5 ml q10yr	Hypersensitivity, active infection, poliomyelitis outbreak, immunosuppression
typhoid vaccine, parenteral	No trade name	Active immunity to typhoid fever	Adult: PO 1 cap 1 hr before meals × 4 doses, booster q5yr	Parenteral: Systemic or allergic reaction, acute respiratory or other acute infection, intensive physical exercise in high temperatures
typhoid vaccine, oral	Vivotif Berna Vaccine		Adult and child >10 yr: SUBCUT 0.5 ml, repeat in 4 wk, booster q3yr Child 6 mo-10 yr: SUBCUT 0.25 ml, repeat in 4 wk, booster q3yr	Oral: Hypersensitivity, acute febrile illness, suppressive or antibiotic drugs
typhoid Vi polysaccharide vaccine	Typhim Vi	Active immunity to typhoid fever	Adult and child ≥2 yr: IM 0.5 ml as a single dose, reimmunize q2yr 0.5 ml IM, if needed	Hypersensitivity, chronic typhoid carriers
varicella virus vaccine	Varivax	Prevention of varicella-zoster (chickenpox)	Adult and child ≥13 yr: SUBCUT 0.5 ml, 2nd dose SUBCUT 0.5 ml 4-8 wk later	Hypersensitivity to neomycin; blood dyscrasias, immunosuppression, active untreated TB, acute illness, pregnancy, diseases of lymphatic system
yellow fever vaccine	YF-Vax	Active immunity to yellow fever	Adult and child ≥9 mo: SUBCUT 0.5 ml deeply, booster q10yr Child 6-9 mo: same as above if exposed	Hypersensitivity to egg or chicken embryo protein, pregnancy, child <6 mo, immunodeficiency
zoster vaccine, live	Zostavax	Herpes zoster prevention	Reconstitute immediately after removing from freezer; give SUBCUT as a single dose; inject total amount of single-dose vial	Immunosuppression; neomycin, gelatin allergy; children, TB, pregnancy (C)

*Canada only.

Appendix e Antitoxins and antivenins

GENERIC NAME	TRADE NAME	USE	DOSAGE AND ROUTES	CONTRAINDICATIONS
Black widow spider antivenin (*Lactrodectus mactans*)	No trade name	Black widow spider bite	Adult and child: IM 2.5 ml, 2nd dose may be given if severe; give in anterolateral thigh, obtain test for sensitivity before inj	Hypersensitivity to this product or horse serum
Crotalidae antivenom, polyvalent	No trade name	Rattlesnake bite	Adult and child: IV 20-150 ml depending on seriousness of bite, may give additional doses based on response	Hypersensitivity
Diphtheria antitoxin, equine	No trade name	Diphtheria	Adult and child: IM/slow IV 20,000-120,000 units, may give additional doses after 24 hr	Hypersensitivity
Micrurus fulvius antivenin	No trade name	East/Texas coral snake bite	Adult and child: IV 30-50 ml, give through running IV line of normal saline, give 1st 1-2 ml over 4-5 min, watch for allergic reaction	Hypersensitivity

Appendix f Less frequently used antihistamines

GENERIC NAME	TRADE NAME(S)	USES	DOSAGES AND ROUTES	AVAILABLE FORMS	INTERACTIONS	CONTRAINDICATIONS
acrivastine/ pseudoephedrine (B)	Semprex-D	• Rhinitis • Allergy symptoms • Chronic idiopathic urticaria	• Adult and child >12 yr: PO 8 mg q4-6h	• Caps 8 mg/60 mg	• Increased CNS depression: alcohol, opiates, sedatives, hypnotics • Hypertensive crisis: MAOIs • May increase CNS depression: kava • May increase anticholinergic effect: henbane leaf	• Hypersensitivity to this drug or tripolidine • Severe hypertension • Cardiac disease
azatadine (B)	Optimine	• Allergy symptoms • Rhinitis • Chronic urticaria	• Adult: PO 1-2 mg bid, not to exceed 4 mg/day • Geriatric: PO 1 mg daily-bid	• Tabs 1 mg	• Increased CNS depression: barbiturates, opiates, hypnotics, tricyclics, alcohol • Decreased effect of: oral anticoagulants • Increased effect of azatadine: MAOIs • Increased CNS depression: kava • Increased anticholinergic effect: henbane leaf	• Hypersensitivity to H_1-receptor antagonists • Acute asthma attack • Lower respiratory tract disease • Child <12 yr
buclizine (B)	Bucladin-S, Softabs	• Motion sickness • Dizziness • Nausea • Vomiting • Antihistamine	• Adult: PO 25-50 mg prm ½ hr before travel; may be repeated q4-6h prm	• Tabs 50 mg	• Increased anticholinergic effect: henbane leaf • Increased CNS depression: kava	• Hypersensitivity to cyclizines • Shock

Drug	Trade names	Uses	Dosage	Forms	Interactions	Contraindications
clemastine **(B)**	Contac Allergy 12 Hour, Tavist, Antihist-1	• Allergy symptoms • Rhinitis • Angioedema • Urticaria • Common cold	• Adult and child >12 yr: PO 1.34-2.68 mg bid-tid, not to exceed 8.04 mg/day	• Tabs 1.34, 2.68 mg • Syr 0.67 mg/ml	• Increased CNS depression: barbiturates, opiates, hypnotics, tricyclics, alcohol • Increased effect of clemastine: MAOIs • Increased CNS depression: kava • Increased anticholinergic effect: henbane leaf	• Hypersensitivity to H₁-receptor antagonists • Acute asthma attack • Lower respiratory tract disease
cyclizine (otc, **B**)	Marezine	• Motion sickness • Prevention of postoperative vomiting • Antihistamine	*Vomiting* • Adult: IM 25-50 mg ½ hr before termination of surgery, then q4-6h prn (lactate) • Child: IM 3 mg/kg divided in 3 equal doses *Motion sickness* • Adult: PO 50 mg then q4-6h prn, not to exceed 200 mg/day (HCl) • Child: PO 25 mg q4-6h prn	• Tabs 50 mg • Inj 50 mg/ml	• May increase CNS effect: alcohol, tranquilizers, opiates • Increased CNS depression: kava	• Hypersensitivity to cyclizines • Shock
dexchlorpheniramine **(B)**	Dexchlor, dexclorpheniramine maleate, Poladex, Polaramine	• Allergy symptoms • Rhinitis • Pruritus • Contact dermatitis	• Adult: PO 1-2 mg tid-qid; repeat action 4-6 mg bid-tid • Child 6-11 yr: PO 1 mg q4-6h, or timerel 4 mg at bedtime	• Tabs 2 mg • Repeat action tabs 4, 6 mg • Syr 2 mg/5 ml	• Increased CNS depression: barbiturates, opiates, hypnotics, tricyclics, alcohol • Decreased effect: oral	• Hypersensitivity to H₁-receptor antagonists • Acute asthma attack • Lower respiratory tract disease

*Canada only.

Continued

Appendix f Less frequently used antihistamines—cont'd

GENERIC NAME	TRADE NAME(S)	USES	DOSAGES AND ROUTES	AVAILABLE FORMS	INTERACTIONS	CONTRAINDICATIONS
					anticoagulants, heparin • Increased effect of dexchlorpheniramine: MAOIs • Increased anticholinergic effect: henbane leaf	
trimeprazine (B)	Panectyl*, Temaril	• Pruritus	• Adult: PO 2.5 mg qid; time-rel 5 mg bid • Geriatric: PO 2.5 mg bid • Child 3-12 yr: PO 2.5 mg tid or at bedtime • Child 6 mo-1 yr: PO 1.25 mg tid or at bedtime	• Tabs 2.5 mg • Time-rel spanules 5 mg • Syr 2.5 mg/5 ml	• Increased CNS depression: barbiturates, opiates, hypnotics, tricyclics, alcohol • Decreased effect of oral anticoagulants, heparin • Increased effect of trimeprazine: MAOIs • Increased anticholinergic effect: henbane leaf	• Hypersensitivity to H_1-receptor antagonists • Acute asthma attack • Lower respiratory tract disease
tripelennamine (B)	PBZ, PBZ-SR, Pelamine, tripelennamine HCl	• Rhinitis • Allergy symptoms	• Adult: PO 25-50 mg q4-6h, not to exceed 600 mg/day; time-rel 100 mg bid-tid, not to exceed 600 mg/day • Child >5 yr: PO time-rel 50 mg q8-12h, not to exceed 300 mg/day • Child <5 yr: PO 5 mg/kg/day in 4-6 divided doses, not to exceed 300 mg/day	• Tabs 25, 50 mg • Time-rel tabs 100 mg • Elix 37.5 mg/5 ml	• Increased CNS depression: barbiturates, opiates, hypnotics, tricyclics, alcohol • Decreased effect of oral anticoagulants, heparin • Increased effect of tripelennamine: MAOIs • Increased anticholinergic effect: henbane leaf	• Hypersensitivity to H_1-receptor antagonists • Acute asthma attack • Lower respiratory tract disease

*Canada only.

Appendix g

Herbal products

acidophilus

Uses: Diarrhea, vaginal and other candida infections, urinary tract infections, atopic dermatitis (eczema), atopic disease, IBS, respiratory tract infections

alfalfa

Uses:
• *External:* Boils and insect bites
• *Internal:* Constipation, arthritis, increase blood clotting, diuretic, relieve inflammation of the prostate, treat acute or chronic cystitis, nutrient source

aloe

Uses of aloe vera gel: Minor burns, skin irritations, minor wounds, frostbite, radiation-caused injuries

angelica

Uses: Poor blood flow to the extremities, headaches, backaches, osteoporosis, asthma, allergies, skin disorders, diuretic, antispasmodic, cholagogue, stomach cancer, mild antiseptic, expectorant, bronchitis, ease rheumatic pains, stomach cramps, muscle spasms

anise

Uses:
• *External:* Treat catarrhs of respiratory system (asthma, bronchitis), cancer, cholera, colic, dysmenorrheal, epilepsy, indigestion, insomnia, lice, migraine, nausea, neuralgia, rash, scabies; given to children to reduce gas, colic, and respiratory symptoms
• *Internal:* Expectorant, bronchitis, emphysema, whooping cough, antibacterial, antispasmodic, abortifacient (large quantities), diaphoretic, diuretic, stimulant, tonic, flavoring in food

astragalus

Uses: Bronchitis, COPD, colds, flu, gastrointestinal conditions, weakness, fatigue, chronic hepatitis, ulcers, hypertension and viral myocarditis, immune stimulant, aphrodisiac, and improve sperm motility

bilberry

Uses: Improve night vision, prevent cataracts, macular degeneration, glaucoma, varicose veins, hemorrhoids, diabetic retinopathy, myopia, mild diarrhea, dyspepsia in adults or children, controlling insulin levels, diuretic, urinary antiseptic

Adapted from Skidmore-Roth L: *Mosby's Handbook of Herbs & Natural Supplements, ed 3,* St. Louis, 2006, Elsevier.

black cohosh

Uses: Smooth-muscle relaxant, antispasmodic, antitussive, astringent, diuretic, antidiarrheal, antiarthritic, hormone balancer in perimenopausal women, decrease uterine spasms in first trimester of pregnancy, antiabortion agent, dysmenorrheal

buckthorn

Uses: Powerful laxative

capsicum peppers

Uses:
• *External:* Diabetic neuropathy, psoriasis, postmastectomy pain, Raynaud's disease, herpes zoster, arthritic, muscular pain, poor peripheral circulation
• *Internal:* Cardiovascular health, CAD, reduce cholesterol and blood clotting, peptic ulcer disease, cold, flu

cascara

Uses: Laxative

chamomile

Uses:
• *External:* As an antiseptic and soothing agent for inflamed skin and minor wounds
• *Internal:* As an antispasmodic, antianxiety, gas-relieving, and antiinflammatory agent for the treatment of digestive problems; light sleep aid and sedative

chondroitin

Uses: Alone or in combination with glucosamine for joint conditions, as an antithrombotic, extravasation therapy agent, for ischemic heart disease, hyperlipidemia

chromium

Uses: Essential trace mineral required for proper metabolic functioning, decreases glucose tolerance, arteriosclerosis, elevated cholesterol, glaucoma, hypoglycemia, diabetes, obesity

coenzyme Q10

Uses: Ischemic heart disease, congestive heart failure (CHF), angina pectoris, hypertension, arrhythmias, diabetes mellitus, deafness, Bell's palsy, decreased immunity, mitral valve prolapse, periodontal disease, infertility

dong quai

Uses: Menopausal symptoms, menstrual irregularities, headache neuralgia, herpes infections, malaria, vitiligo, anemia

echinacea

Uses:
• *External:* Wound healing, bruises, burns, scratches, leg ulcers
• *Internal:* Immune stimulant, prophylaxis for colds, influenzae, other infections

eyebright

Uses: Internally and externally to relieve eye fatigue, redness, sty and eye infections, nasal catarrh in sinusitis and hay fever

feverfew

Uses: Menstrual irregularities, threatened spontaneous abortion, arthritis, fever

flax

Uses:
- *External*: Inflammatory
- *Internal*: Laxative anticholesteremic

garlic

Uses: Antilipidemic, antimicrobial, antiasthmatic, antiinflammatory, possible antihypertensive, treatment for some heavy metal poisonings

ginger

Uses: Antioxidant, nausea, motion sickness, vomiting, sore throat, migraine headaches

ginkgo

Uses: Poor circulation, age-related decline in cognition, memory; vascular disease, antioxidant, depressive mood disorders, sexual dysfunction, asthma, glaucoma, menopausal symptoms, multiple sclerosis, headaches, tinnitus, dizziness, arthritis, altitude sickness, intermittent claudication

ginseng

Uses: Physical and mental exhaustion, stress, sluggishness, fatigue, weak immunity, as a tonic

goldenseal

Uses: Gastritis, gastrointestinal ulceration, peptic ulcer disease, mouth ulcer, bladder infection, sore throat, postpartum hemorrhage, skin disorders, cancer, tuberculosis, wound healing, antiinflammatory, in combination with echinacea for cold and flu

green tea

Uses: Antioxidant, anticancer agent, diuretic, stimulant, antibacterial, antilipidemic, antiatherosclerotic

hops

Uses: Analgesic, hyperactivity, anthelmintic, mild sedative, insomnia, menopausal symptoms

kava

Uses: Anxiolytic, antiepileptic, antidepressant, antipsychotic, nervous anxiety, hyperactivity, restlessness, sleep disturbances, headache, muscle relaxant, wound healing

Side effects: *italics* = common; **bold** = life-threatening

khat

Uses: Fatigue, obesity, gastric ulcers, depression

lemon balm

Uses:
• *External:* Cold sores
• *Internal:* Insomnia, anxiety, gastric conditions, psychiatric conditions, Graves' disease, attention deficit disorder (ADD)

licorice

Uses: Allergies, arthritis, asthma, constipation, esophagitis, gastritis, hepatitis, inflammatory conditions, peptic ulcers, poor adrenal function, poor appetite

lysine

Uses: Cold sores, herpes infections, Bell's palsy, rheumatoid arthritis, detoxify opiates

maitake

Uses: Diabetes, hypertension, high cholesterol, obesity, cancer

melatonin

Uses: Insomnia, inhibit cataract formation, increase longevity, epilepsy, hypertension, various cancers, jet lag, cancer protection, oral contraceptive

panax ginseng

Uses: Physical and mental exhaustion, stress, sluggishness, fatigue, weak immunity, as a tonic

papaya

Uses:
• *External:* Debridement of worms
• *Internal:* Intestinal worms, gastrointestinal disorders, injection in a herniated lumbar intervertebral disk

raspberry

Uses:
• *External:* Leaves promote diuresis, treat inflammation, cough, wounds
• *Internal:* UTIs, renal calculi, antimicrobial action, morning sickness and speed, ease labor in pregnancy

red clover

Uses: Antispasmodic, expectorant, sedative, psoriasis, eczema, amenorrhea

St. John's wort

Uses:
• *External:* Antiinflammatory, relieve hemorrhoids, treat vitiligo, burns
• *Internal:* Depression, anxiety

⚠ Safety alert   *"Tall Man" lettering

SAM-e

Uses: Depression, Alzheimer's disease, migraine headache, hypersensitivity, chronic liver disease, fibromyalgia pain, inflammation in osteoarthritis

saw palmetto

Uses: Benign prostatic hypertrophy, mild diuretic, chronic and subacute cystitis, increase breast size, sperm count, sexual potency

senna

Uses: Laxative

Siberian ginseng

Uses: Increase immunity, energy and performance, decrease inflammation and insomnia

turmeric

Uses: Menstrual disorders, colic, inflammation, bruising, dyspepsia, hematuria, flatulence

valerian

Uses: Sedative

wintergreen

Uses:
• *External:* Sore, inflamed muscles and joints
• *Internal:* Bladder inflammation, urinary tract diseases, diseases of prostate and kidney

yohimbe

Uses: Aphrodisiac, hallucinogenic

Appendix h

Combination products

A-200 Shampoo:
0.33% pyrethrins
4% piperonyl butoxide
Uses: Scabicide, pediculicide
Accuretic 10/12.5:
quinapril 10 mg
hydrochlorthiazide 12.5 mg
Uses: Antihypertensive
Accuretic 20/12.5:
quinapril 20 mg
hydrochlorthiazide 12.5 mg
Uses: Antihypertensive
Accuretic 20/25:
quinapril 20 mg
hydrochlorthiazide 25 mg
Uses: Antihypertensive
Aceta-Gesic:
acetaminophen 325 mg
phenyltoloxamine 30 mg
Uses: Pain
Actifed:
pseudoephedrine 60 mg
triprolidine 2.5 mg
Uses: Decongestant
Actifed Cold and Allergy:
pseudoephedrine 60 mg
triprolidine 2.5 mg
Uses: Adrenergic, antihistamine
Actifed Cold and Sinus:
chlorpheniramine 2 mg
pseudoephedrine 30 mg
acetaminophen 500 mg
Uses: antihistamine, adrenergic, analgesic
Activella Tablets:
estriol 1 mg
norethindrone 0.5 mg
Uses: Vasomotor symptoms (menopause)

Actoplus Met:
pioglitazone 15 mg
metformin 500 mg
pioglitazone 15 mg
metformin 850 mg
Uses: Type 2 diabetes
Adderall 5 mg:
dextroamphetamine sulfate 1.25 mg
dextroamphetamine saccharate 1.25 mg
amphetamine sulfate 1.25 mg
amphetamine aspartate 1.25 mg
Uses: CNS stimulant
Adderall 7.5 mg:
dextroamphetamine sulfate 1.875 mg
dextroamphetamine saccharate 1.875 mg
dextroamphetamine aspartate 1.875 mg
amphetamine sulfate 1.875 mg
Uses: CNS stimulant
Adderall 10 mg:
dextroamphetamine sulfate 5 mg
dextroamphetamine saccharate 2.5 mg
amphetamine sulfate 2.5 mg
amphetamine aspartate 2.5 mg
Uses: CNS stimulant
Adderall 12.5 mg:
dextroamphetamine sulfate 3.125 mg
dextroamphetamine saccharate 3.125 mg
dextroamphetamine aspartate 3.125 mg
amphetamine sulfate 3.125 mg
Uses: CNS stimulant
Adderall 20 mg:
dextroamphetamine sulfate 5 mg
dextroamphetamine saccharate 5 mg
amphetamine sulfate 5 mg
amphetamine aspartate 5 mg
Uses: CNS stimulant
Adderall 30 mg:
dextroamphetamine sulfate 7.5 mg

⚠ Safety alert   *"Tall Man" lettering

dextroamphetamine saccharate 7.5 mg
amphetamine sulfate 7.5 mg
amphetamine aspartate 7.5 mg
Uses: CNS stimulant
Adderall XR 5 mg:
dextroamphetamine sulfate 1.25 mg
dextroamphetamine saccharate 1.25 mg
amphetamine sulfate 1.25 mg
amphetamine aspartate 1.25 mg
Uses: CNS stimulant
Adderall XR 10 mg:
dextroamphetamine sulfate 2.5 mg
dextroamphetamine saccharate 2.5 mg
amphetamine sulfate 2.5 mg
amphetamine aspartate 2.5 mg
Uses: CNS stimulant
Adderall XR 15 mg:
dextroamphetamine sulfate 3.75 mg
dextroamphetamine saccharate 3.75 mg
amphetamine sulfate 3.75 mg
amphetamine aspartate 3.75 mg
Uses: CNS stimulant
Adderall XR 20 mg:
dextroamphetamine sulfate 5 mg
dextroamphetamine saccharate 5 mg
amphetamine sulfate 5 mg
amphetamine aspartate 5 mg
Uses: CNS stimulant
Adderall XR 25 mg:
dextroamphetamine sulfate 6.25 mg
dextroamphetamine saccharate 6.25 mg
amphetamine sulfate 6.25 mg
Uses: CNS stimulant
Adderall XR 30 mg:
dextroamphetamine sulfate 7.5 mg
dextroamphetamine saccharate 7.5 mg
amphetamine sulfate 7.5 mg
amphetamine aspartate 7.5 mg
Uses: CNS stimulant
Advair Diskus 100:
fluticasone 100 mcg
salmeterol 50 mcg
Uses: Corticosteroid, bronchodilator
Advair Diskus 250:
fluticasone 250 mcg
salmeterol 50 mcg

Uses: Corticosteroid, bronchodilator
Advair Diskus 500:
fluticasone 500 mcg
salmeterol 50 mcg
Uses: Corticosteroid, bronchodilator
Advicor 500:
niacin 500 mg
lovastatin 20 mg
Uses: Antilipidemic
Advicor 750:
niacin 750 mg
lovastatin 20 mg
Uses: Antilipidemic
Advicor 1000:
niacin 1000 mg
lovastatin 20 mg
Uses: Antilipidemic
Advicor 1000:
niacin 1000 mg
lovastatin 40 mg
Uses: Antilipidemic
Advil Cold and Sinus Caplets:
pseudoephedrine 30 mg
ibuprofen 200 mg
Uses: Decongestant
Aggrenox:
200 mg ext rel dipyridamole
25 mg aspirin
Uses: Antiplatelet
AK-Cide Ophthalmic Suspension/ Ointment:
10% sulfacetamide sodium
0.5% prednisoLONE acetate
Uses: Ophthalmic antiinfective, antiinflammatory
Aldactazide 25/25:
spironolactone 25 mg
hydrochlorothiazide 25 mg
Uses: Diuretic
Aldactazide 50/50:
spironolactone 50 mg
hydrochlorothiazide 50 mg
Uses: Diuretic

Side effects: *italics* = common; **bold** = life-threatening

Aldoclor-150:
methyldopa 250 mg
chlorothiazide 150 mg
Uses: Antihypertensive

Aldoclor-250:
methyldopa 250 mg
chlorothiazide 250 mg
Uses: Antihypertensive

Aldoril 15:
methyldopa 250 mg
hydrochlorothiazide 15 mg
Uses: Antihypertensive

Aldoril 25:
methyldopa 250 mg
hydrochlorothiazide 25 mg
Uses: Antihypertensive

Aldoril D30:
methyldopa 500 mg
hydrochlorothiazide 30 mg
Uses: Antihypertensive

Aldoril D50:
methyldopa 500 mg
hydrochlorothiazide 50 mg
Uses: Antihypertensive

Aleve Cold and Sinus:
naproxen 200 mg
ER pseudoephedrine 120 mg
Uses: Analgesic, adrenergic

Aleve Sinus and Headache:
naproxen 220 mg
ER pseudoephedrine 120 mg
Uses: Analgesic, adrenergic

Alka-Seltzer Effervescent, Original:
sodium bicarbonate 1916 mg
citric acid 1000 mg
aspirin 325 mg
Uses: Antacid, adsorbent, antiflatulent

Alka-Seltzer Plus Cold Effervescent Tablets:
acetaminophen 250 mg
chlorpheniramine 2 mg
phenylephrine 5 mg
Uses: Decongestant, analgesic, antihistamine

Alka-Seltzer Plus Night-Time Cold Liqui-Gels:
doxylamine 6.25 mg
dextromethorphan 10 mg
pseudoephedrine 30 mg
acetaminophen 325 mg
Uses: Antiussive, decongestant, antihistamine, analgesic

Alka-Seltzer Plus Ready Relief Tablets:
chlorpheniramine 2 mg
pseudoephedrine 30 mg
Uses: Antihistamine, decongestant

Alka-Seltzer PM Effervescent Tablets:
aspirin 325 mg
diphenhydramine 38 mg
Uses: Analgesic, antihistamine

Allegra-D:
fexofenadine 60 mg
pseudoephedrine 120 mg
Uses: Antihistamine, adrenergic

Allercon Tablets:
triprolidine 2.5 mg
pseudoephedrine 60 mg
Uses: Antihistamine, adrenergic

Allerest Maximum Strength Tablets:
pseudoephedrine 30 mg
chlorpheniramine 2 mg
Uses: Decongestant, antihistamine

Allerest Allergy Sinus Relief Maximum Strength:
pseudoephedrine 30 mg
acetaminophen 325 mg
Uses: Antihistamine, analgesic

Allerfrim Syrup:
Per 5 ml:
triprolidine 1.25 mg
pseudoephedrine 30 mg
Uses: Antihistamine, adrenergic

Allerfrim Tablets:
triprolidine 2.5 mg
pseudoephedrine 60 mg
Uses: Antihistamine, adrenergic

All-Nite Cold Liquid:
Per 15 ml:
pseudoephedrine 30 mg

doxylamine 6.25 mg
dextromethorphan 15 mg
acetaminophen 500 mg
Uses: Decongestant, antihistamine,
  analgesic

Alor 5/500:
hydrocodone 5 mg
aspirin 500 mg
Uses: Analgesic

Amaphen:
acetaminophen 325 mg
butalbital 50 mg
caffeine 40 mg
Uses: analgesic, barbiturates

Ambenyl Cough Syrup:
Per 5 ml:
bromodiphenhydramine 12.5 mg
codeine 10 mg
5% alcohol
Uses: Antihistamine, opioid analgesic

Anacin:
aspirin 400 mg
caffeine 32 mg
Uses: Analgesic

Anacin Maximum Strength:
aspirin 500 mg
caffeine 32 mg
Uses: Analgesic

Anacin PM (Aspirin Free):
diphenhydrAMINE 25 mg
acetaminophen 500 mg
Uses: Analgesic

Anaplex DM:
Per 5 ml:
brompheniramine 4 mg
dextromethorphan 30 mg
pseudoephedrine 60 mg
Uses: Decongestant, antitussive, antihistamine

Anaplex DMX:
Per 5 ml:
brompheniramine 8 mg
dextromethorphan 60 mg
pseudoephedrine 90 mg
Uses: Decongestant, antitussive,
  antihistamine

Anaplex HD Syrup:
Per 5 ml:
hydrocodone 1.7 mg
phenylephrine 5 mg
chlorpheniramine 2 mg
Uses: Analgesic, adrenergic, antihistamine

Anaplex HD Oral Liquid:
Per 5 ml:
hydrocodone 1.7 mg
brompheniramine 2 mg
pseudoephedrine 30 mg
Uses: Antihistamine, decongestant, analgesic

Anatuss LA:
pseudoephedrine 120 mg
guaifenesin 400 mg
Uses: Adrenergic, expectorant

Anexsia 5/500:
hydrocodone 5 mg
acetaminophen 500 mg
Uses: Analgesic

Anexsia 7.5/650:
hydrocodone 7.5 mg
acetaminophen 650 mg
Uses: Analgesic

Angeliq:
drospirenone 0.5 mg
estradiol 1 mg
Uses: Vasomotor symptoms (menopause)

Apresazide 25/25:
hydrALAZINE 25 mg
hydrochlorothiazide 25 mg
Uses: Antihypertensive

Apresazide 50/50:
hydrALAZINE 50 mg
hydrochlorothiazide 50 mg
Uses: Antihypertensive

Apri:
desorgestrel 0.15 mg
ethinyl estradiol 30 mcg
Uses: Estrogen, progestin

Arthritis Pain Formula:
aspirin 500 mg
aluminum hydroxide 27 mg
magnesium hydroxide 100 mg
Uses: Analgesic, antacid

Arthrotec:
diclofenac 50 or 75 mg
misoprostol 200 mcg
Uses: NSAID, gastric protectant

Ascriptin:
aspirin 325 mg
magnesium hydroxide 50 mg
aluminum hydroxide 50 mg
calcium carbonate 50 mg
Uses: Nonopioid analgesic, antipyretic

Ascriptin A/D:
aspirin 325 mg
aluminum hydroxide 75 mg
magnesium hydroxide 75 mg
calcium carbonate 75 mg
Uses: Analgesic

Aspirin-Free Bayer Select Allergy Sinus:
pseudoephedrine 30 mg
chlorpheniramine 2 mg
acetaminophen 500 mg
Uses: Adrenergic, antihistamine, analgesic

Aspirin Free Excedrin:
acetaminophen 500 mg
caffeine 65 mg
Uses: Analgesic

Aspirin Free Excedrin Dual:
acetaminophen 500 mg
calcium carbonate 111 mg
magnesium carbonate 64 mg
magnesium oxide 30 mg
Uses: Analgesic, antacid

Atacand HCT 16:
candesartan 16 mg
hydrochlorthiazide 12.5 mg
Uses: Antihypertensive

Atacand HCT 32:
candesartan 32 mg
hydrochlorthiazide 12.5 mg
Uses: Antihypertensive

Augmentin 250:
amoxicillin 250 mg
clavulanic acid 125 mg
Uses: Antiinfective

Augmentin 500:
amoxicillin 500 mg
clavulanic acid 125 mg
Uses: Antiinfective

Augmentin 875:
amoxicillin 875 mg
clavulanic acid 125 mg
Uses: Antiinfective

Augmentin 125 Chewable:
amoxicillin 125 mg
clavulanic acid 31.25 mg
Uses: Antiinfective

Augmentin 200 Chewable:
amoxicillin 200 mg
clavulanic acid 28.5 mg
Uses: Antiinfective

Augmentin 250 Chewable:
amoxicillin 250 mg
clavulanic acid 62.5 mg
Uses: Antiinfective

Augmentin 400 Chewable:
amoxicillin 400 mg
clavulanic acid 57 mg
Uses: Antiinfective

Augmentin 125 mg/5 ml Suspension:
Per 5 ml:
amoxicillin 125 mg
clavulanic acid 31.25 mg
Uses: Antiinfective

Augmentin 200 mg/5 ml Suspension:
Per 5 ml:
amoxicillin 200 mg
clavulanic acid 28.5 mg
Uses: Antiinfective

Augmentin 250 mg/5 ml Suspension:
Per 5 ml:
amoxicillin 250 mg
clavulanic acid 62.5 mg
Uses: Antiinfective

Augmentin 400 mg/5 ml Suspension:
Per 5 ml:
amoxicillin 400 mg
clavulanic acid 57 mg
Uses: Antiinfective

Auralgan Otic Solution:
5.4% antipyrine
1.4% benzocaine
Uses: Otic analgesic

A Safety alert   *"Tall Man" lettering

Avalide:
hydrochlorthiazide 12.5 mg
irbesartan 150 mg
Uses: Antihypertensive
Avalide 300:
hydrochlorthiazide 12.5 mg
irbesartan 300 mg
Uses: Antihypertensive
Avandamet:
rosiglitazone/metformin
1 mg/500 mg
2 mg/500 mg
2 mg/1000 mg
4 mg/500 mg
4 mg/1000 mg
Uses: Diabetes mellitus
Avandaryl 4/1:
rosiglitazone 4 mg
glimepiride 1 mg
Uses: Antidiabetic
Avandaryl 4/2:
rosiglitazone 4 mg
glimepiride 2 mg
Uses: Antidiabetic
Avandaryl 4/4:
rosiglitazone 4 mg
glimepiride 4 mg
Uses: Antidiabetic
B&O Supprettes No. 15A Supps:
belladonna extract 15 mg
opium 30 mg
Uses: Anticholinergic, opioid analgesic
B&O Supprettes No. 16A Supps:
belladonna extract 16.2 mg
opium 60 mg
Uses: Anticholinergic, opioid analgesic
Bactrim:
trimethoprim 80 mg
sulfamethoxazole 400 mg
Uses: Antiinfective
Bactrim DS:
trimethoprim 160 mg
sulfamethoxazole 800 mg
Uses: Antiinfective
Bactrim I.V.:
Per 5 ml:

trimethoprim 80 mg
sulfamethoxazole 400 mg
Uses: Antiinfective
Bancap HC:
acetaminophen 500 mg
hydrocodone 5 mg
Uses: Analgesic
Bayer Plus, Extra Strength:
aspirin 500 mg
calcium carbonate 250 mg
Uses: Analgesic, antacid
Bayer Select Chest Cold:
dextromethorphan 15 mg
acetaminophen 500 mg
Uses: Antitussive, analgesic
Bayer Select Flu Relief:
acetaminophen 500 mg
pseudoephedrine 30 mg
dextromethorphan 15 mg
chlorpheniramine 2 mg
Uses: Analgesic, adrenergic, antitussive,
  antihistamine
Bayer Select Head Cold:
pseudoephedrine 30 mg
acetaminophen 500 mg
Uses: Adrenergic, analgesic
**Bayer Select Maximum Strength
  Headache:**
acetaminophen 500 mg
caffeine 65 mg
Uses: Nonopioid analgesic
**Bayer Select Maximum Strength
  Menstrual:**
acetaminophen 500 mg
pamabrom 25 mg
Uses: Nonopioid analgesic
**Bayer Select Maximum Strength
  Night-Time Pain Relief:**
acetaminophen 500 mg
diphenhydrAMINE 25 mg
Uses: Analgesic, antihistamine
**Bayer Select Maximum Strength
  Sinus Pain Relief:**
acetaminophen 500 mg
pseudoephedrine 30 mg
Uses: Analgesic, adrenergic

Side effects: *italics* = common; **bold** = life-threatening

Bayer Select Night Time Cold:
acetaminophen 500 mg
pseudoephedrine 30 mg
dextromethorphan 15 mg
triprolidine 1.25 mg
Uses: Analgesic, adrenergic, antitussive, antihistamine

Bellatal:
phenobarbital 16.2 mg
hyoscyamine sulfate 0.1037 mg
atropine sulfate 0.0194 mg
scopolamine hydrobromide 0.0065 mg
Uses: Barbiturate, anticholinergic

Bellergal-S:
ergotamine 0.6 mg
belladonna alkaloids 0.2 mg
phenobarbital 40 mg
Uses: α-Adrenergic blocker, anticholinergic, barbiturate

Bel-Phen-Ergot-SR:
phenobarbital 40 mg
ergotamine tartrate 0.6 mg
belladonna alkaloids 0.2 mg
Uses: α-Adrenergic blocker, anticholinergic, barbiturate

Benadryl Allergy Decongestant Liquid:
Per 5 ml:
diphenhydrAMINE 12.5 mg
pseudoephedrine 30 mg
Uses: Antihistamine, adrenergic

Benadryl Allergy/Sinus Headache Caplets:
diphenhydrAMINE 12.5 mg
pseudoephedrine 30 mg
acetaminophen 500 mg
Uses: Antihistamine, adrenergic, analgesic

Benadryl Decongestant Allergy:
pseudoephedrine 60 mg
diphenhydrAMINE 25 mg
Uses: Adrenergic, antihistamine

Benylin Expectorant Liquid:
Per 5 ml:
dextromethorphan 5 mg
guaifenesin 100 mg
5% alcohol
Uses: Expectorant, antitussive

Benylin Multi-Symptom Liquid:
Per 5 ml:
dextromethorphan 5 mg
pseudoephedrine 15 mg
guaifenesin 100 mg
Uses: Antitussive, adrenergic, expectorant

Benzamycin:
benzoyl peroxide 5%
erythromycin 3%
Uses: Antiinfective

BenzaClin:
clindamycin 10%
benzoyl peroxide 5%
Uses: Antiinfective

Beta Tan Suspension:
Per 5 ml:
carbetapentane 30 mg
brompheniramine 4 mg
phenylephrine 7.5 mg
Uses: Antitussive

BiDil:
isosorbide 20 mg
hydrALAZINE 37.5 mg
Uses: Vasodilator

Blephamide Ophthalmic Suspension/ Ointment:
0.2% prednisoLONE
10% sodium sulfacetamide
Uses: Ophthalmic antiinfective, antiinflammatory

Bromfed Capsules:
pseudoephedrine 120 mg
brompheniramine 12 mg
Uses: Antihistamine, adrenergic

Bromfed-PD Capsules:
pseudoephedrine 60 mg
brompheniramine 6 mg
Uses: Adrenergic, antihistamine

Bromfed Tablets:
pseudoephedrine 60 mg
brompheniramine 4 mg
Uses: Antihistamine, adrenergic

Bromfenex:
brompheniramine 12 mg
pseudoephedrine 120 mg

Uses: Antihistamine, adrenergic
Bromfenex PD:
brompheniramine 6 mg
pseudoephedrine 60 mg
Uses: Antihistamine, adrenergic
Bromfenex PE:
phenylephrine 15 mg
brompheniramine 12 mg
Uses: Antihistamine, adrenergic
Bromfenex PE Pediatric:
phenylephrine 7.5 mg
brompheniramine 6 mg
Uses: Antihistamine adrenergic
Bromo-Seltzer:
sodium bicarbonate 2781 mg
acetaminophen 325 mg
citric acid 2224 mg
Uses: Antacid, analgesic
Bufferin:
aspirin 325 mg
calcium carbonate 158 mg
magnesium oxide 63 mg
magnesium carbonate 34 mg
Uses: Analgesic, antacid
Bufferin AF Nite-Time:
acetaminophen 500 mg
diphenhydrAMINE 38 mg
Uses: Analgesic, antihistamine
Butibel:
belladonna extract 15 mg
butabarbital 15 mg
Uses: Anticholinergic, barbiturate
Cafatine PB:
ergotamine 1 mg
caffeine 100 mg
belladonna alkaloids 0.125 mg
pentobarbital 30 mg
Uses: Migraine agent
Cafergot:
ergotamine 1 mg
caffeine 100 mg
Uses: Adrenergic blocker
Cafergot Suppositories:
ergotamine 2 mg
caffeine 100 mg
Uses: Adrenergic blocker

Caladryl:
8% calamine, camphor
2.2% alcohol
1% pramoxine
Uses: Top antihistamine
Calcet:
calcium 152.8 mg
vitamin D 100 international units
Uses: Supplement
Caltrate 600+D:
vitamin D 200 international units
calcium 600 mg
Uses: Supplement
Cama Arthritis Pain Reliever:
aspirin 500 mg
magnesium oxide 150 mg
aluminum hydroxide 125 mg
Uses: Nonopioid analgesic,
    antacid
Capital w/Codeine:
Per 5 ml:
acetaminophen 120 mg
codeine 12 mg
Uses: Opioid analgesic
Capozide 25/15:
captopril 25 mg
hydrochlorothiazide 15 mg
Uses: Antihypertensive
Capozide 25/25:
captopril 25 mg
hydrochorothiazide 25 mg
Uses: Antihypertensive
Capozide 50/15:
captopril 50 mg
hydrochlorothiazide 15 mg
Uses: Antihypertensive
Capozide 50/25:
captopril 50 mg
hydrochlorothiazide 25 mg
Uses: Antihypertensive
Cardec DM Syrup:
Per 5 ml:
pseudoephedrine 60 mg
carbinoxamine 4 mg
dextromethorphan 15 mg
Uses: Adrenergic, antitussive

Side effects: *italics* = common; **bold** = life-threatening

Cenafed Plus Tablets:
triprolidine 2.5 mg
pseudoephedrine 60 mg
Uses: Antihistamine, adrenergic

Cetapred Ophthalmic Ointment:
0.25% prednisoLONE
10% sodium sulfacetamide
Uses: Ophthalmic antiinfective,
   antiinflammatory

Cheracol Cough Syrup:
Per 5 ml:
codeine 10 mg
guaifenesin 100 mg
Uses: Analgesic, expectorant

Cheracol Syrup:
Per 5 ml:
codeine 10 mg
guaifenesin 100 mg
Uses: Analgesic, expectorant

Children's Cepacol Liquid:
Per 5 ml:
acetaminophen 160 mg
pseudoephedrine 15 mg
Uses: Analgesic, adrenergic

Chlor-Trimeton 4 Hour Relief:
pseudoephedrine 60 mg
chlorpheniramine 4 mg
Uses: Antihistamine, adrenergic

**Chlor-Trimeton 12 Hour Relief
   Tablets:**
pseudoephedrine 120 mg
chlorpheniramine 8 mg
Uses: Antihistamine, adrenergic

Chromagen:
ferrous fumarate 66 mg
vitamin B_{12} 10 mcg
vitamin C 250 mg
intrinsic factor 100 mg
Uses: Supplement

Cipro HC Otic:
Per 1 ml:
ciprofloxacin 2 mg
hydrocortisone 10 mg
Uses: Antiinfective/antiinflammatory

Claritin-D 12 Hour:
loratidine 5 mg

pseudoephedrine 120 mg
Uses: Antihistamine, adrenergic

Claritin-D 24-Hour:
loratidine 10 mg
pseudoephedrine 240 mg
Uses: Antihistamine, adrenergic

Climara Pro (transdermal)
estradiol 0.045 mg
levonorgestrel 0.015 mg
Uses: Vasomotor symptoms (menopause)

Clindex:
chlordiazepoxide 5 mg
clidinium 2.5 mg
Uses: Antianxiety, anticholinergic

Clomycin Ointment:
bacitracin 500 units
neomycin sulfate 3.5 g
polymyxin B sulfate 500 units
lidocaine 40 mg
Uses: Antiinfective, local anesthetic

Co-Apap:
pseudoephedrine 30 mg
chlorpheniramine 2 mg
dextromethorphan 15 mg
acetaminophen 325 mg
Uses: Adrenergic, antihistamine, antitussive,
   analgesic

Co-Gesic:
acetaminophen 500 mg
hydrocodone 5 mg
Uses: Analgesic

**Codeprex Extended Release
   Suspension:**
Per 5 ml:
codeine 20 mg
chlorpheniramine 4 mg
Uses: Cough, rhinitis

Codiclear DH Syrup:
Per 5 ml:
hydrocodone 5 mg
guaifenesin 100 mg
Uses: Analgesic, expectorant

Codimal:
pseudoephedrine 30 mg
chlorpheniramine 2 mg

acetaminophen 500 mg
Uses: Adrenergic, antihistamine, analgesic
Codimal DH Syrup:
Per 5 ml:
hydrocodone 1.66 mg
phenylephrine 5 mg
pyrilamine 8.33 mg
Uses: Analgesic, adrenergic
Codimal DM Syrup:
Per 5 ml:
phenylephrine 5 mg
pyrilamine 8.33 mg
dextromethorphan 10 mg
Uses: Adrenergic, antitussive
Codimal-LA:
chlorpheniramine 8 mg
pseudoephedrine 120 mg
Uses: Antihistamine, adrenergic
Codimal PH Syrup:
Per 5 ml:
codeine 10 mg
phenylephrine 5 mg
pyrilamine 8.33 mg
Uses: Analgesic, adrenergic
ColBenemid:
probenecid 500 mg
colchicine 0.5 mg
Uses: Antigout agent
Coldrine:
pseudoephedrine 30 mg
acetaminophen 500 mg
Uses: Decongestant, nonopioid analgesic
Col-Probenecid:
probenecid 500 mg
colchicine 0.5 mg
Uses: Antigout
Coly-Mycin S Otic Suspension:
1% hydrocortisone
neomycin base 3.3 mg/ml
colistin 3 mg/ml
0.05% thonzonium bromide
Uses: Otic antiinfective
CombiPatch 0.05/0.14:
estradiol 0.05 mg/day
norethindrone 0.14 mg/day
Uses: Hypoestrogenism

CombiPatch 0.05/0.25:
estradiol 0.05 mg/day
norethindrone 0.25 mg/day
Uses: Hypoestrogenism
Combipres 0.1:
chlorthalidone 15 mg
clonidine 0.1 mg
Uses: Antihypertensive
Combipres 0.2:
chlorthalidone 15 mg
clonidine 0.2 mg
Uses: Antihypertensive
Combipres 0.3:
chlorthalidone 15 mg
clonidine 0.3 mg
Uses: Antihypertensive
Combivent:
ipratropium bromide 18 mcg
albuterol 103 mcg/actuation
Uses: Bronchodilator
Combivir:
lamivudine 150 mg
zidovudine 300 mg
Uses: HIV
**Comtrex Acute Head Cold Maximum
    Strength Tablets:**
acetaminophen 500 mg
brompheniramine 2 mg
pseudoephedrine 30 mg
Uses: Antihistamine, analgesic, decongestant
**Comtrex Allergy-Sinus Maximum
    Strength Tablets:**
chlorpheniramine 2 mg
acetaminophen 500 mg
pseudoephedrine 30 mg
Uses: Antihistamine, analgesic, decongestant
**Comtrex Allergy-Sinus Night and Day
    Tablets:**
chlorpheniramine 2 mg
acetaminophen 500 mg
pseudoephedrine 30 mg
Uses: Antihistamine, analgesic, decongestant

Comtrex Cold and Flu Maximum Strength Liquid:
Per 30 ml:
chlorpheniramine 4 mg
acetaminophen 1000 mg
pseudoephedrine 60 mg
dextromethorphan 30 mg
Uses: Antihistamine, analgesic, decongestant, antitussive

Comtrex Day and Night Cold and Cough Maximum Strength Tablets:
chlorpheniramine 2 mg
acetaminophen 500 mg
pseudoephedrine 30 mg
dextromethorphan 15 mg
Uses: Analagesic, decongestant, antitussive

Comtrex Deep Chest Cold Capsules:
acetaminophen 250 mg
dextromethorphan 10 mg
guaifensin 100 mg
pseudoephedrine 30 mg
Uses: Analgesic, antitussive, expectorant, decongestant

Comtrex Liquid:
Per 5 ml:
chlorpheniramine 0.67 mg
acetaminophen 108.3 mg
pseudoephedrine 10 mg
dextromethorphan 3.3 mg
Uses: Antihistamine, analgesic, antitussive, decongestant

Comtrex Maximum Strength Caplets:
chlorpheniramine 2 mg
acetaminophen 500 mg
pseudoephedrine 30 mg
dextromethorphan 15 mg
Uses: Analgesic, decongestant, antihistamine, antitussive

Comtrex Maximum Strength Multi-Symptoms Cold, Flu Relief:
chlorpheniramine 2 mg
acetaminophen 500 mg
pseudoephedrine 30 mg
dextromethorphan 15 mg
Uses: Analgesic, decongestant, antihistamine, antitussive

Congess SR:
guaifenesin 250 mg
pseudoephedrine 120 mg
Uses: Expectorant, decongestant

Congestac:
guaifenesin 400 mg
pseudoephedrine 60 mg
Uses: Expectorant, decongestant

Contac Cough & Chest Cold Liquid:
Per 5 ml:
guaifenesin 50 mg
pseudoephedrine 15 mg
dextromethorphan 5 mg
acetaminophen 125 mg
Uses: Decongestant, antitussive, expectorant, analgesic

Contac Cough & Sore Throat Liquid:
Per 5 ml:
dextromethorphan 5 mg
acetaminophen 125 mg
Uses: Antitussive, analgesic

Contac Day Allergy/Sinus:
pseudoephedrine 60 mg
acetaminophen 650 mg
Uses: Decongestant, analgesic

Contac Day Cold and Flu:
pseudoephedrine 60 mg
dextromethorphan 30 mg
acetaminophen 650 mg
Uses: Decongestant, antitussive, analgesic

Contac Night Allergy Sinus:
pseudoephedrine 60 mg
diphenhydrAMINE 50 mg
acetaminophen 650 mg
Uses: Decongestant, antihistamine, analgesic

Contac Night Cold and Flu Caplets:
pseudoephedrine 60 mg
diphenhydrAMINE 50 mg
acetaminophen 650 mg
Uses: Decongestant, antihistamine, antitussive, analgesic

Contac Non-Drowsy Maximum Strength 12 Hour:
pseudoephedrine 120 mg
Uses: Adrenergic

A Safety alert   *"Tall Man" lettering

Contac Severe Cold & Flu Nighttime Liquid:
Per 5 ml:
chlorpheniramine 0.67 mg
acetaminophen 167 mg
pseudoephedrine 10 mg
dextromethorphan 5 mg
18.5% alcohol
Uses: Decongestant, antihistamine, antitussive, analgesic

Coricidin:
chlorpheniramine 2 mg
acetaminophen 325 mg
Uses: Antihistamine, analgesic

Coricidin D Tablets:
chlorpheniramine 2 mg
acetaminophen 325 mg
Uses: Antihistamine, analgesic

Coricidin D Cold, Flu & Sinus:
chlorpheniramine 2 mg
acetaminophen 325 mg
pseudoephedrine sulfate 30 mg
Uses: Antihistamine, analgesic, decongestant

Coricidin HBP Congestion & Cough Softgels Capsules:
dextromethorphan 10 mg
guaifenesin 200 mg
Uses: Antitussive, expectorant

Corcidin HBP Cough and Cold:
chlorpheniramine 4 mg
dextromethorphan 30 mg
Uses: Antihistamine, expectorant

Corcidin HBP Maximum Strength Flu:
acetaminophen 500 mg
chlorpheniramine 2 mg
dextromethorphan 15 mg
Uses: Analgesic, antihistamine, expectorant

Cortisporin Ophthalmic/Otic Suspension:
0.35% neomycin polymyxin B 10,000 units/ml
1% hydrocortisone
Uses: Ophthalmic antiinfective, antiinflammatory

Cortisporin Topical Cream:
0.5% neomycin sulfate
polymyxin B 10,000 units
0.5% hydrocortisone
Uses: Topical antiinfective

Cortisporin Topical Ointment:
0.5% neomycin sulfate
bacitracin 400 units
polymyxin B 5000 units
1% hydrocortisone
Uses: Topical antiinfective

Corzide 40/5:
nadolol 40 mg
bendroflumethiazide 5 mg
Uses: Antihypertensive

Corzide 80/5:
nadolol 80 mg
bendroflumethiazide 5 mg
Uses: Antihypertensive

Cosopt:
dorzolamide 2%
timolol 0.5%
Uses: Antihypertensive

Cough-X:
dextromethorphan 5 mg
benzocaine 2 mg
Uses: Antitussive, local anesthetic

Creon:
lipase 8000 units
amylase 30,000 units
protease 13,000 units
pancreatin 300 mg
Uses: Digestive enzyme

Cyclomydril Ophthalmic Solution:
0.2% cyclopentolate
1% phenylephrine
Uses: Mydriatic

Dallergy Tablets:
chlorpheniramine 4 mg
phenylephrine 10 mg
methscopolamine 1.25 mg
Uses: Antihistamine, adrenergic

Damason-P:
hydrocodone 5 mg
aspirin 500 mg
Uses: Analgesic

Darvocet-N 100:
propoxyphene-N 100 mg
acetaminophen 650 mg
Uses: Analgesic
Darvon Compound-65:
propoxyphene 65 mg
aspirin 389 mg
caffeine 32.4 mg
Uses: Analgesic
♣ **Darvon-N Compound:**
aspirin 375 mg
propoxyphene 100 mg
caffeine 30 mg
Uses: Analgesic
♣ **Darvon-N w/A.S.A.:**
aspirin 325 mg
propoxyphene 100 mg
Uses: Analgesic
Deconamine:
pseudoephedrine 60 mg
chlorpheniramine 4 mg
Uses: Antihistamine, decongestant
Deconamine SR:
pseudoephedrine 120 mg
chlorpheniramine 8 mg
Uses: Antihistamine, decongestant
Deconamine Syrup:
Per 5 ml:
pseudoephedrine 30 mg
chlorpheniramine 2 mg
Uses: Antihistamine, decongestant
Demi-Regroton:
chlorthalidone 25 mg
reserpine 0.125 mg
Uses: Antihypertensive
Demulen 1/35:
ethinyl estradiol 35 mcg
ethynodiol diacetate 1 mg
Uses: Oral contraceptive
Demulen 1/50:
ethinyl estradiol 50 mcg
ethynodiol diacetate 1 mg
Uses: Oral contraceptive
Desogen:
ethinyl estradiol 30 mcg
desorgestrel 0.15 mg

Uses: Estrogen, progestin
Dexacidin Ophthalmic Ointment/
 Suspension:
Per ml:
0.1% dexamethasone
0.35% neomycin
polymyxin B 10,000 units/g
Uses: Ophthalmic, antiinfective/
 antiinflammatory
Dexasporin Ophthalmic Ointment:
Per gram:
0.1% dexamethasone
0.35% neomycin
polymyxin B 10,000 units
Uses: Ophthalmic, antiinfective/
 antiinflammatory
DHC Plus:
dihydrocodeine 16 mg
acetaminophen 356.4 mg
caffeine 30 mg
Uses: Analgesic
Di-Gel Liquid:
Per 5 ml:
aluminum hydroxide 200 mg
magnesium hydroxide 200 mg
simethicone 20 mg
Uses: Antacid, adsorbent, antiflatulent
Dihistine DH Liquid:
Per 5 ml:
pseudoephedrine 30 mg
chlorpheniramine 2 mg
codeine 10 mg
Uses: Decongestant, antihistamine,
 analgesic
Dilaudid Cough Syrup:
Per 5 ml:
guaifenesin 100 mg
hydromorphone 1 mg
5% alcohol
Uses: Expectorant, analgesic
Dimetapp DM Elixir:
Per 5 ml:
pseudoephedrine 5 mg
brompheniramine 2 mg
dextromethorphan 10 mg

Uses: Antihistamine, adrenergic, expectorant
Dimetapp Sinus:
pseudoephedrine 30 mg
ibuprofen 200 mg
Uses: Decongestant, analgesic
Diovan 80 HCT:
valsartan 80 mg
hydrochlorthiazide 12.5 mg
Uses: Antihypertensive
Diovan 160 HCT:
valsartan 160 mg
hydrochlorthiazide 12.5 mg
Uses: Antihypertensive
Diurigen w/Reserpine:
chlorothiazide 250 mg
reserpine 0.125 mg
Uses: Antihypertensive
Diutensen-R:
methylclothiazide 2.5 mg
reserpine 0.1 mg
Uses: Antihypertensive
Doan's PM Extra Strength:
magnesium salicylate 500 mg
diphenhydrAMINE 25 mg
Uses: Analgesic, antihistamine
Dolacet:
hydrocodone 5 mg
acetaminophen 500 mg
Uses: Analgesic
Donnatal:
phenobarbital 16.2 mg
hyoscyamine 0.1037 mg
atropine 0.0194 mg
scopolamine 0.0065 mg
Uses: Anticholinergic, barbiturate
Donnatal Elixir:
Per 5 ml:
phenobarbital 16.2 mg
hyoscyamine 0.1037 mg
atropine 0.0194 mg
scopolamine 0.0065 mg
23% alcohol
Uses: Anticholinergic, barbiturate
Donnatal Extentabs:
phenobarbital 48.6 mg

hyoscyamine 0.3111 mg
atropine 0.0582 mg
scopolamine 0.0195 mg
Uses: Anticholinergic, barbiturate
Donnazyme:
pancreatin 500 mg
lipase 1000 units
protease 12,500 units
amylase 12,500 units
Uses: Pancreatic enzymes
Dristan Cold:
pseudoephedrine 30 mg
acetaminophen 500 mg
Uses: Decongestant, analgesic
Dristan Cold Maximum Strength Caplets:
pseudoephedrine 30 mg
brompheniramine 2 mg
acetaminophen 500 mg
Uses: Decongestant, antihistamine, analgesic
Dristan Cold Multi-Symptom Formula:
acetaminophen 325 mg
phenylephrine 5 mg
chlorpheniramine 2 mg
Uses: Analgesic, adrenergic, antihistamine
Dristan Sinus:
pseudoephedrine 30 mg
ibuprofen 200 mg
Uses: Decongestant, analgesic
Drixoral Allergy Sinus:
pseudoephedrine 60 mg
dexbrompheniramine 3 mg
acetaminophen 500 mg
Uses: Decongestant, antihistamine, analgesic
Drixoral Cold & Allergy:
pseudoephedrine 120 mg
dexbrompheniramine 6 mg
Uses: Decongestant, antihistamine
Drixoral Cold & Flu:
pseudoephedrine 60 mg
dexbrompheniramine 3 mg
acetaminophen 500 mg
Uses: Decongestant, antihistamine, analgesic

Drixoral Nasal Decongestant:
pseudoephedrine 120 mg
Uses: Decongestant

DT:
Per 5 ml dose:
diphtheria toxoid 2 LfU
tetanus toxoid 5 LfU
Uses: Vaccine

DTP:
Per 0.5 ml dose:
diphtheria toxoid 6.5 LfU
tetanus toxoid 5 LfU
pertussis 4 LfU
Uses: Vaccine

DuoNeb:
Per 3 ml:
albuterol 3 mg
ipratroprium 0.5 mg
Uses: Bronchodilator

Dura-Vent/DA:
phenylephrine 20 mg
chlorpheniramine 8 mg
methscopolamine 2.5 mg
Uses: Adrenergic, antihistamine

Dyazide:
hydrochlorothiazide 25 mg
triamterene 37.5 mg
Uses: Diuretic

Dylline-GG Tablets:
dyphylline 200 mg
guaifenesin 200 mg
Uses: Bronchodilator, expectorant

Dynafed Asthma Relief:
epHEDrine 25 mg
guaifenesin 200 mg
Uses: Adrenergic, expectorant

Dynafed Plus Maximum Strength:
pseudoephedrine 30 mg
acetaminophen 500 mg
Uses: Decongestant, analgesic

Dyphylline-GG Elixir:
Per 5 ml:
dyphylline 100 mg
guaifenesin 100 mg
Uses: Bronchodilator, expectorant

Elase Ointment:
Per gram:
fibrinolysin 1 unit
desoxyribonuclease 666.6 units
Uses: Enzyme

Elixophyllin GG Liquid:
Per 5 ml:
theophylline 100 mg
guaifenesin 100 mg
Uses: Expectorant, bronchodilator

EMLA Cream:
lidocaine 2.5 mg
prilocaine 2.5 mg
Uses: Local anesthetic

Empirin w/Codeine #3:
aspirin 325 mg
codeine phosphate 30 mg
Uses: Analgesic

Empirin w/Codeine #4:
aspirin 325 mg
codeine phosphate 60 mg
Uses: Analgesic

♣ **Empracet-60:**
acetaminophen 300 mg
codeine 60 mg
Uses: Analgesic

Endocet:
acetaminophen 325 mg
oxycodone 5 mg
Uses: Analgesic

♣ **Endodan:**
aspirin 325 mg
oxycodone 5 mg
Uses: Analgesic

Entex PSE:
pseudoephedrine 120 mg
guaifenesin 600 mg
Uses: Adrenergic, expectorant

Epifoam Aerosol Foam:
1% hydrocortisone
1% pramoxine
Uses: Topical corticosteroid

Epzicom:
abacavir 600 mg
lamivudine 300 mg
Uses: HIV infection

Eryzole:
Per 5 ml:
erythromycin 200 mg
sulfisoxazole 600 mg
Uses: Macrolide antiinfective

Esgic-Plus:
butalbital 50 mg
acetaminophen 500 mg
caffeine 40 mg
Uses: Barbiturate, analgesic

Esimil:
guanethidine 10 mg
hydrochlorothiazide 25 mg
Uses: Antihypertensive

Estratest:
esterified estrogens 1.25 mg
methyltestosterone 2.5 mg
Uses: Vasomotor symptoms (menopause)

Estratest HS:
esterified estrogens 1.25 mg
methyltestosterone 2.5 mg
Uses: Vasomotor symptoms (menopause)

Excedrin Migraine:
aspirin 250 mg
acetaminophen 250 mg
caffeine 65 mg
Uses: Migraine agent

Excedrin P.M.:
acetaminophen 500 mg
diphenhydrAMINE citrate 38 mg
Uses: Analgesic, antihistamine

Excedrin P.M. Liquigels:
acetaminophen 500 mg
diphenhydrAMINE 25 mg
Uses: Analgesic, antihistamine

Excedrin Sinus Extra Strength:
pseudoephedrine 30 mg
acetaminophen 500 mg
Uses: Decongestant, analgesic

Fansidar:
sulfidoxine 500 mg
pyrimethamine 25 mg
Uses: Antimalarial

Fedahist:
pseudoephedrine 60 mg
chlorpheniramine 4 mg

Uses: Decongestant, antihistamine

Fedahist Expectorant Syrup:
Per 5 ml:
guaifenesin 200 mg
pseudoephedrine 20 mg
Uses: Expectorant, decongestant

Fedahist Gyrocaps:
pseudoephedrine 65 mg
chlorpheniramine 10 mg
Uses: Decongestant, antihistamine

Fedahist Timecaps:
pseudoephedrine 120 mg
chlorpheniramine 8 mg
Uses: Decongestant, antihistamine

Fem-1:
acetaminophen 500 mg
pamabrom 25 mg
Uses: Nonopioid analgesic

Femhrt 1/5:
norethindrone 1 mg
ethinyl estradiol 5 mcg
norethindrone 1 mg
ethinyl estradiol 5 mcg
Uses: Vasomotor symptoms (menopause)

Ferro-Sequels:
docusate sodium 100 mg
ferrous fumarate 150 mg
Uses: Laxative, hematinic

Fioricet:
acetaminophen 325 mg
caffeine 40 mg
butalbital 50 mg
Uses: Analgesic, barbiturate

Fioricet w/Codeine:
acetaminophen 325 mg
caffeine 40 mg
butalbital 50 mg
codeine 30 mg
Uses: Analgesic, barbiturate

Fiorinal:
aspirin 325 mg
caffeine 40 mg
butalbital 50 mg
Uses: Analgesic, barbiturate

Fiorinal w/Codeine:
aspirin 325 mg

caffeine 40 mg
butalbital 50 mg
codeine 30 mg
Uses: Analgesic, barbiturate

FML-S Ophthalmic Suspension:
0.1% fluorometholone
10% sulfacetamide
Uses: Ophthalmic, antiinfective/
antiinflammatory

Gas-Ban:
calcium carbonate 500 mg
simethicone 40 mg
Uses: Antiflatulent, antacid

Gaviscon:
magnesium trisilicate 20 mg
aluminum hydroxide 80 mg
Uses: Antacid, adsorbent, antiflatulent

Gaviscon Liquid:
Per 5 ml:
aluminum hydroxide 31.7 mg
magnesium carbonate 119.3 mg
Uses: Antacid, adsorbent, antiflatulent

Gelusil:
aluminum hydroxide 200 mg
magnesium hydroxide 200 mg
simethicone 25 mg
Uses: Antacid, adsorbent, antiflatulent

Genac Tablets:
triprolidine 2.5 mg
pseudoephedrine 60 mg
Uses: Antihistamine

Genatuss DM Syrup:
Per 5 ml:
guaifenesin 100 mg
dextromethorphan 10 mg
Uses: Expectorant, antitussive

Glucovance 1.25:
glyBURIDE: 1.25 mg
metformin: 250 mg
Uses: Antidiabetic

Glucovance 2.50:
glyBURIDE: 2.5 mg
metformin: 500 mg
Uses: Antidiabetic

Glucovance 5:
glyBURIDE: 5 mg
metformin: 500 mg
Uses: Antidiabetic

Guaifenex PSE 60:
pseudoephedrine 60 mg
guaifenesin 600 mg
Uses: Decongestant, expectorant

Guaifenex PSE 120:
pseudoephedrine 120 mg
guaifenesin 600 mg
Uses: Decongestant, expectorant

Guiatuss AC:
Per 5 ml:
codeine 10 mg
guafenesin 100 mg
Uses: Analgesic, expectorant

Haley's M-O Liquid:
Per 15 ml:
magnesium hydroxide 900 mg
mineral oil 3.75 ml
Uses: Laxative

Halotussin-DM Sugar Free Liquid:
Per 5 ml:
guaifenesin 100 mg
dextromethorphan 10 mg
Uses: Expectorant, antitussive

Helidac:
In a compliance package:
bismuth subsalicylate 262.4 mg tabs
metronidazole 250 mg tabs
tetracycline 500 mg caps
Uses: Antiinfective

Humalog Mix 50/50:
insulin lispro protamine 50%
insulin lispro (rDNA) 50%
Uses: Antidiabetic

Humalog Mix 75/25:
insulin lispro protamine 75%
insulin lispro (rDNA) 25%
Uses: Antidiabetic

Humibid DM Pediatric:
dextromethorphan 15 mg
guaifenesin 300 mg
Uses: Expectorant, antitussive

Humibid DM Tablets:
dextromethorphan 30 mg
guaifenesin 600 mg

Uses: Expectorant, antitussive

HycoClear Tuss:
Per 5 ml:
hydrocodone 5 mg
guaifenesin 100 mg
Uses: Analgesic, expectorant

Hycodan:
hydrocodone 5 mg
homatropine 1.5 mg
Uses: Analgesic, mydriatic

Hycodan Syrup:
Per 5 ml:
hydrocodone 5 mg
homatropine 1.5 mg
Uses: Analgesic, mydriatic

Hycomine Compound:
chlorpheniramine 2 mg
acetaminophen 250 mg
phenylephrine 10 mg
hydrocodone 5 mg
caffeine 30 mg
Uses: Antihistamine, analgesic,
   adrenergic

Hycotuss Expectorant Syrup:
Per 5 ml:
guaifenesin 100 mg
hydrocodone 5 mg
10% alcohol
Uses: Expectorant

Hydrocet:
hydrocodone 5 mg
acetaminophen 500 mg
Uses: Opioid analgesic

Hydrogesic:
hydrocodone 5 mg
acetaminophen 500 mg
Uses: Opioid analgesic

Hydropres-50:
hydrochlorothiazide 50 mg
reserpine 0.125 mg
Uses: Antihypertensive

Hyzaar:
losartan potassium 50 mg
hydrochlorothiazide 12.5 mg
potassium 4.24 mg
Uses: Antihypertensive

Imodium Advanced:
loperamide 2 mg
simethicone 125 mg
Uses: Antidiarrheal, antiflatulent

Innovar:
Per ml:
droperidol 2.5 mg
fentanyl 0.05 mg
Uses: Opioid analgesic, general anesthetic

Iofed:
brompheniramine 12 mg
pseudoephedrine 120 mg
Uses: Antihistamine, adrenergic

Iofed PD:
brompheniramine 6 mg
pseudoephedrine 60 mg
Uses: Antihistamine, adrenergic

Kaletra Capsules:
lopinavir 133.3 mg
ritonavir 33.3 mg
Uses: HIV

Kaletra Solution:
Per 1 ml:
lopinavir 80 mg
ritonavir 20 mg
Uses: HIV

Kaletra Tablets
lopinavir 200 mg
ritonavir 50 mg
Uses: HIV

Lactinex:
Mixed culture of:
Lactobacillus acidophilus and
Lactobacillus bulgaricus
Uses: Supplement

Levell 12.5 ml Suspension:
carbetapentane 30 mg
phenylephrine 30 mg
Uses: Antitussive

Levlite:
levonorgestrel 0.100 mg
ethinyl estradiol 20 mcg
Uses: Estrogen, progestin

Levsin PB Drops:
Per ml:
hyoscyamine 0.125 mg

Side effects: *italics* = common; **bold** = life-threatening

phenobarbital 15 mg
5% alcohol
Uses: Anticholinergic, barbiturate
Levsin w/Phenobarbital:
hyoscyamine 0.125 mg
phenobarbital 15 mg
Uses: Anticholinergic, barbiturate
Lexxel 1:
enalapril 5 mg
felodipine 5 mg
Uses: Antihypertensive
Lexxel 2:
enalapril 5 mg
felodipine 2.5 mg
Uses: Antihypertensive
Librax:
chlordiazepoxide 5 mg
clidinium 2.5 mg
Uses: Antianxiety, anticholinergic
Lida-Mantel-HC-Cream:
0.5% hydrocortisone
3% lidocaine
Uses: Antiinflammatory, analgesic
Limbitrol DS 10-25:
chlordiazepoxide 10 mg
amitriptyline 25 mg
Uses: Antidepressant, antianxiety
Lobac:
salicylamide 200 mg
phenyltoloxamine 20 mg
acetaminophen 300 mg
Uses: Skeletal muscle relaxant,
  analgesic
Loestrin Fe 1/20:
norethindrone acetate 1 mg/tablet
ethinyl estradiol 20 mcg/tablet
with 7 tablets of ferrous fumarate 75 mg/
  container
Uses: Oral contraceptive
Loestrin Fe 1.5/30:
norethindrone acetate 1.5 mg
ethinyl estradiol 30 mcg
Uses: Oral contraceptive
Lomotil:
diphenoxylate 2.5 mg
atropine 0.025 mg

Uses: Antidiarrheal, anticholinergic
Lomotil Liquid:
Per 5 ml:
diphenoxylate 2.5 mg
atropine 0.025 mg
Uses: Antidiarrheal, anticholinergic
Lo Ovral:
ethinyl estradiol 30 mcg
norgestrel 0.3 mg
Uses: Oral contraceptive
Lopressor HCT 50/25:
metoprolol 50 mg
hydrochlorothiazide 25 mg
Uses: Antihypertensive
Lopressor HCT 100/25:
metoprolol 100 mg
hydrochlorothiazide 25 mg
Uses: Antihypertensive
Lopressor HCT 100/50:
metoprolol 100 mg
hydrochlorothiazide 50 mg
Uses: Antihypertensive
Lorcet 10/650:
acetaminophen 650 mg
hydrocodone 10 mg
Uses: Analgesic
Lorcet-HD:
hydrocodone 10 mg
acetaminophen 300 mg
Uses: Analgesic
Lorcet Plus:
acetaminophen 650 mg
hydrocodone 7.5 mg
Uses: Analgesic
Lortab 2.5/500:
hydrocodone 2.5 mg
acetaminophen 500 mg
Uses: Analgesic
Lortab 5/500:
hydrocodone 5 mg
acetaminophen 500 mg
Uses: Analgesic
Lortab 7.5/500:
hydrocodone 7.5 mg
acetaminophen 500 mg
Uses: Analgesic

Lortab 10/500:
hydrocodone 10 mg
acetaminophen 500 mg
Uses: Analgesic
Lortab ASA:
aspirin 500 mg
hydrocodone 5 mg
Uses: Analgesic
Lortab Elixir:
Per 5 ml:
hydrocodone 2.5 mg
acetaminophen 167 mg
Uses: Analgesic
Losec 1-2-3A ✦:
omeprazole 20 mg
clarithromycin 500 mg
amoxicillin 1 g
Uses: Antiinfective
Losec 1-2-3M ✦:
omeprazole 20 mg
clarithromycin 250 mg
metronidazole 500 mg
Uses: Antiinfective
Lotensin HCT 5/6.25:
benazepril 5 mg
hydrochlorothiazide 6.25 mg
Uses: Antihypertensive
Lotensin HCT 10/12.5:
benazepril 10 mg
hydrochlorothiazide 12.5 mg
Uses: Antihypertensive
Lotensin HCT 20/12.5:
benazepril 20 mg
hydrochlorothiazide 12.5 mg
Uses: Antihypertensive
Lotensin HCT 20/25:
benazepril 20 mg
hydrochlorothiazide 25 mg
Uses: Antihypertensive
Lotrel 2.5/10:
amlopidine 2.5 mg
benazepril 10 mg
Uses: Antihypertensive
Lotrel 5/10:
amlodipine 5 mg
benazepril 10 mg
Uses: Antihypertensive
Lotrel 5/20:
amlodipine 5 mg
benazepril 20 mg
Uses: Antihypertensive
Lotrisone Topical:
0.05% betamethasone
1% clotrimazole
Uses: Local antiinfective, antiinflammatory
Lufyllin-EPG Elixir:
Per 5 ml:
dyphylline 150 mg
epHEDrine 24 mg
guaifenesin 300 mg
phenobarbital 24 mg
Uses: Bronchodilator, expectorant
Lufyllin-GG:
dyphylline 200 mg
guaifenesin 200 mg
Uses: Bronchodilator, expectorant
Lunelle Monthly Contraceptive Injection:
25 mg medroxyprogesterone
5 mg estradiol/0.5 ml
Uses: Contraceptive
M-M-R-II:
measles
mumps
rubella
Uses: Vaccine, toxoid
Maalox:
aluminum hydroxide 200 mg
magnesium hydroxide 200 mg
Uses: Antacid, adsorbent, antiflatulent
Maalox Plus:
aluminum hydroxide 200 mg
magnesium hydroxide 200 mg
simethicone 25 mg
Uses: Antacid, adsorbent, antiflatulent
Maalox Plus Extra Strength Suspension:
Per 5 ml:
aluminum hydroxide 500 mg
magnesium hydroxide 450 mg
simethicone 40 mg
Uses: Antacid, adsorbent, antiflatulent

Side effects: *italics* = common; **bold** = life-threatening

Maalox Suspension:
Per 5 ml:
aluminum hydroxide 225 mg
magnesium hydroxide 200 mg
Uses: Antacid, adsorbent, antiflatulent
Macrobid:
nitrofurantoin macrocrystals 25 mg
nitrofurantoin monohydrate 75 mg
Uses: Antiinfective
Malarone:
250 mg atovaquone
100 mg proguanil
Uses: Malaria
Malarone Pediatric:
62.5 mg atovaquone
25 mg proguanil
Uses: Malaria
Mapap Cold Formula:
acetaminophen 325 mg
chlorpheniramine 2 mg
pseudoephedrine 30 mg
dextromethorphan 15 mg
Uses: Bronchodilator, expectorant
Maxitrol Ophthalmic Suspension/
  Ointment:
Per ml:
0.35% neomycin
0.1% dexamethasone
polymyxin B 10,000 units
Uses: Ophthalmic antiinfective,
  antiinflammatory
Maxzide:
hydrochlorothiazide 50 mg
triamterene 75 mg
Uses: Antihypertensive, diuretic
Maxzide-25 MG:
hydrochlorothiazide 25 mg
triamterene 37.5 mg
Uses: Diuretic
Medi-Flu Liquid:
Per 5 ml:
pseudoephedrine 10 mg
chlorpheniramine 0.67 mg
dextromethorphan 5 mg
acetaminophen 167 mg
18.5% alcohol

Uses: Decongestant, antihistamine,
  antitussive, analgesic
Medigesic:
acetaminophen 325 mg
caffeine 40 mg
butalbital 50 mg
Uses: Nonopioid analgesic
Mepergan Fortis:
meperidine 50 mg
promethazine 25 mg
Uses: Analgesic, antihistamine
Mepergan Injection:
meperidine 25 mg
promethazine 25 mg
Uses: Analgesic
Metaglip 2.5:
glipizide/metformin 2.5 mg/250 mg,
  2.5 mg/500 mg, 5 mg/500 mg
Uses: Diabetes mellitus
Metimyd Ophthalmic Suspension/
  Ointment:
0.5% prednisoLONE
10% sodium sulfacetamide
Uses: Ophthalmic antiinfective,
  antiinflammatory
Micardis HCT 40:
telmesartan 40 mg
hydrochlorthiazide 12.5 mg
Uses: Antihypertensive
Micardis HCT 80:
telmesartan 80 mg
hydrochlorthiazide 12.5 mg
Uses: Antihypertensive
Microgestin Fe 1/20:
norethindrone 1 mg
ethinyl estradiol 20 mcg
ferrous fumarate 75 mg in container
Uses: Estrogen, progestin
Microgestin Fe 1.5/30:
norethindrone 1.5 mg
ethinyl estradiol 30 mcg
ferrous fumarate 75 mg in container
Uses: Estrogen, progestin
Midol Maximum Strength Multi-
  Symptom Menstrual Gelcaps:
acetaminophen 500 mg

A Safety alert   *"Tall Man" lettering

pyrilamine 15 mg
caffeine 60 mg
Uses: Analgesic
Midol PM:
acetaminophen 500 mg
diphenhydrAMINE 25 mg
Uses: Analgesic, antihistamine
Midol PMS Maximum Strength Caplets:
acetaminophen 500 mg
pyrilamine 15 mg
pamabrom 25 mg
Uses: Analgesic
Midol, Teen:
acetaminophen 400 mg
pamabrom 25 mg
Uses: Analgesic
Midrin:
isometheptene 65 mg
acetaminophen 325 mg
dichloralphenazone 100 mg
Uses: Analgesic
Minizide 1:
prazosin 1 mg
polythiazide 0.5 mg
Uses: Antihypertensive
Minizide 2:
prazosin 2 mg
polythiazide 0.5 mg
Uses: Antihypertensive
Minizide 5:
prazosin 5 mg
polythiazide 0.5 mg
Uses: Antihypertensive
Moduretic:
hydrochlorothiazide 50 mg
amiloride 5 mg
Uses: Diuretic
Monopril-HCT 10:
fosinopril 10 mg
hydrochlorthiazide 12.5 mg
Uses: Antihypertensive
Monopril-HCT 20:
fosinopril 20 mg
hydrochlorthiazide 12.5 mg
Uses: Antihypertensive

Motrin Children's Cold Suspension:
Per 5 ml:
ibuprofen 100 mg
pseudoephedrine 15 mg
Uses: Nonopioid analgesic, decongestant
Motrin Sinus Headache:
pseudoephedrine 30 mg
ibuprofen 200 mg
Uses: Adrenergic, analgesic
Mucinex:
guaifenesin 600 mg or 1200 mg
Uses: Cough suppressant, expectorant
Mucinex D:
guaifenesin/pseudoephedrine 1200 mg/ 120 mg, 600 mg/60 mg
Uses: Expectorant, decongestant
Mucinex DM:
dextromethorphan 30 mg
guaifenesin 600 mg
Uses: Antitussive, expectorant
Murocoll-2 Ophthalmic Drops:
0.3% scopolamine
10% phenylephrine
Uses: Ophthalmic anticholinergic, mydriatic
Mycolog II Topical:
Per gram:
0.1% triamcinolone acetonide
nystatin 100,000 units
Uses: Local antiinfective, antiinflammatory
Mylanta:
aluminum hydroxide 200 mg
magnesium hydroxide 200 mg
simethicone 20 mg
Uses: Antacid, adsorbent, antiflatulent
Mylanta Double Strength Liquid:
Per 5 ml:
aluminum hydroxide 400 mg
magnesium hydroxide 400 mg
simethicone 40 mg
Uses: Antacid, adsorbent, antiflatulent
Mylanta Gelcaps:
calcium carbonate 311 mg
magnesium carbonate 232 mg
Uses: Antacid, adsorbent, antiflatulent

Side effects: *italics* = common; **bold** = life-threatening

Naphcon-A Ophthalmic Solution:
0.25% naphazoline
0.3% pheniramine
Uses: Ophthalmic vasoconstrictor

Nasatab LA:
guaifenesin 500 mg
pseudoephedrine 120 mg
Uses: Expectorant, decongestant

NeoDecadron Ophthalmic Ointment:
0.35% neomycin
0.05% dexamethasone
Uses: Ophthalmic antiinfective, antiinflammatory

NeoDecadron Ophthalmic Solution:
0.35% neomycin
0.1% dexamethasone
Uses: Ophthalmic antiinfective, antiinflammatory

Neosporin Cream:
Per gram:
polymyxin B 10,000 units
neomycin 3.5 mg
Uses: Top antiinfective

Neosporin G.U. Irrigant:
Per ml:
neomycin 40 mg
polymyxin B 200,000 units
Uses: Antiinfective

Neosporin Topical Ointment:
Per gram:
polymyxin B 5000 units
bacitracin zinc 400 units
neomycin 3.5 mg
Uses: Top antiinfective

Neosporin Ophthalmic Solution:
Per ml:
neomycin 1.75 mg
polymyxin B 10,000 units
gramicidin 0.025 mg
Uses: Ophthalmic antiinfective

Neosporin Ophthalmic Ointment:
Per gram:
neomycin 3.5 mg
polymyxin B 10,000 units
bacitracin zinc 400 units
Uses: Ophthalmic antiinfective

Neosporin Plus Cream:
polymyxin B 10,000 units
neomycin 3.5 mg
lidocaine 40 mg
Uses: Top antiinfective

Niferex-150 Forte:
ferrous sulfate 150 mg
vitamin B_{12} 25 mcg
folic acid 1 mg
Uses: Supplement

Norco 5/325:
hydrocodone 5 mg
acetaminophen 325 mg
Uses: Analgesic, opioid, nonopioid

Norco:
hydrocodone 10 mg
acetaminophen 325 mg
Uses: Analgesic, opioid, nonopioid

Norgesic:
orphenadrine 25 mg
aspirin 385 mg
caffeine 30 mg
Uses: Skeletal muscle relaxant, analgesic

Norgesic Forte:
orphenadrine 50 mg
aspirin 770 mg
caffeine 60 mg
Uses: Skeletal muscle relaxant, analgesic

Novacet Lotion:
sodium sulfacetamine 10%
sulfur 5%
Uses: Acne agent

Novafed A:
pseudoephedrine 120 mg
chlorpheniramine 8 mg
Uses: Adrenergic, antihistamine

Novo-Gesic ♣C8:
acetaminophen 300 mg
codeine 8 mg
caffeine 15 mg
Uses: Analgesic

NuLytely:
PEG 3350/420 g
sodium bicarbonate 5.72 g
sodium chloride 11.2 g

A Safety alert   *"Tall Man" lettering

potassium chloride 1.48 g
Uses: Laxative

Octicair Otic Suspension:
1% hydrocortisone
neomycin 5 mg/ml
polymyxin B 10,000 units/ml
Uses: Otic antiinflammatory,
   antiinfective

Opcon-A Ophthalmic Solution:
0.027% naphazoline
0.315% pheniramine
Uses: Ophthalmic vasoconstrictor

Ornade Spansules:
phenylpropanolamine 75 mg
chlorpheniramine 12 mg
Uses: Antihistamine, decongestant

Ornex:
pseudoephedrine 30 mg
acetaminophen 500 mg
Uses: Adrenergic, analgesic

Ornex No Drowsiness Caplets:
acetaminophen 325 mg
pseudoephedrine 30 mg
Uses: Adrenergic, analgesic

Orphengesic:
orphenadrine 25 mg
aspirin 385 mg
caffeine 30 mg
Uses: Analgesic

Orphengesic Forte:
orphenadrine 50 mg
aspirin 770 mg
caffeine 60 mg
Uses: Analgesic

Ortho-cept:
ethinyl estradiol 30 mcg
desogestrel 0.15 mg
Uses: Oral contraceptive

Ortho-cyclen:
ethinyl estradiol 35 mcg
norgestimate 0.25 mg
Uses: Oral contraceptive

Ortho-Prefest:
estradiol 1 mg (15)
norgestimate 0.09 mg (15)
Uses: Vasomotor symptoms (menopause)

Ovcon-50:
ethinyl estradiol 50 mcg
norethindrone 1 mg
Uses: Oral contraceptive

♣ **Oxycocet:**
acetaminophen 325 mg
oxycodone 5 mg
Uses: Analgesic

P-A-C Analgesic:
aspirin 400 mg
caffeine 32 mg
Uses: Nonopioid analgesic

Pain-X Topical:
0.05% capsaicin
5% menthol
4% camphor
Uses: Top analgesic

Pamprin Maximum Pain Relief:
acetaminophen 250 mg
pamabrom 25 mg
magnesium salicylate 250 mg
Uses: Analgesic

Pamprin Multi-Symptom:
acetaminophen 500 mg
pamabrom 25 mg
pyrilamine 15 mg
Uses: Analgesic

Panacet 5/500:
hydrocodone 5 mg
acetaminophen 500 mg
Uses: Analgesic

Panasal 5/500:
hydrocodone 5 mg
aspirin 500 mg
Uses: Analgesic

Pancrease Capsules:
amylase 20,000 units
protease 25,000 units
lipase 4500 units (microspheres)
Uses: Digestive enzyme

Pedia Care Cold-Allergy Chewable:
pseudoephedrine 15 mg
chlorpheniramine 1 mg
Uses: Adrenergic, antihistamine

Pedia Care Cough-Cold Liquid:
Per 5 ml:

♣ Canada only

pseudoephedrine 15 mg
chlorpheniramine 1 mg
dextromethorphan 5 mg
Uses: Adrenergic, antihistamine, antitussive
Pedia Care NightRest Cough-Cold Liquid:
Per 5 ml:
pseudoephedrine 15 mg
chlorpheniramine 1 mg
dextromethorphan 7.5 mg
Uses: Adrenergic, antihistamine, antitussive
Pediazole Suspension:
Per 5 ml:
erythromycin 200 mg
sulfiSOXAZOLE 600 mg
Uses: Antiinfective
Pepcid Complete:
calcium carbonate 800 mg
magnesium hydroxide 165 mg
famotidine 10 mg
Uses: Antiulcer agent
Percocet 2.5/325:
oxycodone 2.5 mg
acetaminophen 325 mg
Uses: Analgesic
Percocet 5/325:
oxycodone 5 mg
acetaminophen 325 mg
Uses: Analgesic
Percocet 7.5/500:
oxycodone 7.5 mg
acetaminophen 500 mg
Uses: Analgesic
Percocet 10/650:
oxycodone 10 mg
acetaminophen 650 mg
Uses: Analgesic
Percodan:
oxycodone 4.88 mg
aspirin 325 mg
Uses: Analgesic
Percogesic:
phenyltoloxamine 30 mg
acetaminophen 325 mg
Uses: Analgesic

Perdiem Granules:
Per teaspoon:
senna 0.74 g
psyllium 3.25 g
sodium 1.8 mg
potassium 35.5 mg
Uses: Laxative
Peri-Colace:
docusate sodium 100 mg
casanthranol 30 mg
Uses: Laxative
Peri-Colace Syrup:
Per 15 ml:
docusate sodium 60 mg
casanthranol 30 mg
Uses: Laxative
Phenerbel-S:
ergotamine tartrate 0.6 mg
belladonna alkaloids 0.2 mg
phenobarbital 40 mg
Uses: α-Adrenergic blocker, anticholinergic
Phenergan VC Syrup:
Per 5 ml:
phenylephrine 5 mg
promethazine 6.25 mg
Uses: Adrenergic, antihistamine
Phenergan VC w/Codeine Syrup:
Per 5 ml:
phenylephrine 5 mg
promethazine 6.25 mg
codeine 10 mg
Uses: Adrenergic, antihistamine, opioid analgesic
Phenergan w/Codeine Syrup:
Per 5 ml:
promethazine 6.25 mg
codeine 10 mg
Uses: Antihistamine, analgesic
Polaramine Expectorant Liquid:
Per 5 ml:
guaifenesin 100 mg
dexchlorpheniramine 2 mg
pseudoephedrine 20 mg
7.5% alcohol
Uses: Expectorant

⚠ Safety alert   *"Tall Man" lettering

Polycitra Syrup:
Per 5 ml:
potassium citrate 550 mg
sodium citrate 500 mg
citric acid 334 mg
Uses: Laxative

Poly-Histine Elixir:
Per 5 ml:
pheniramine 4 mg
pyrilamine 4 mg
phenyltoloxamine 4 mg
4% alcohol
Uses: Antihistamine

Polysporin Ophthalmic Ointment:
Per gram:
polymyxin B 10,000 units
bacitracin zinc 500 units
Uses: Ophthalmic antiinfective

Polysporin Topical Ointment:
Per gram:
polymyxin B 10,000 units
bacitracin zinc 500 units
Uses: Top antiinfective

Polytrim Ophthalmic Solution:
Per ml:
trimethoprim 1 mg
polymyxin B 10,000 units
Uses: Ophthalmic antiinfective

Pravigard PAC:
aspirin 81 mg
pravastatin 20, 40, 80 mg
aspirin 325 mg
pravastatin 20, 40, 80 mg
Uses: Antihyperlipidemic, antithrombotic

Prefest:
estradiol 1 mg
norgestimate 0.09 mg
Uses: Vasomotor symptoms (menopause)

Premphase:
In a compliance package:
conjugated estrogens 0.625 mg
medroxyPROGESTERone 5 mg
Uses: Vasomotor symptoms (menopause)

Prempro:
In a compliance package:
conjugated estrogens 0.3 mg

medroxyPROGESTERone 1.5 mg,
conjugated estrogens 0.45 mg
medroxyPROGESTERone 1.5 mg,
conjugated estrogens 0.625 mg
medroxyPROGESTERone 2.5 mg,
conjugated estrogens 0.625 mg
medroxyPROGESTERone 5 mg
Uses: Vasomotor symptoms (menopause)

Premsyn PMS:
acetaminophen 500 mg
pamabrom 25 mg
pyrilamine 15 mg
Uses: Analgesic

Prevpac:
In a compliance package:
amoxicillin 500 mg caps
clarithromycin 500 mg tabs
lansoprazole 30 mg caps
Uses: Antiinfective

Primatene:
theophylline 130 mg
epHEDrine 24 mg
phenobarbital 7.5 mg
Uses: Bronchodilator, barbiturate

Primaxin 250 mg IV for Injection:
imipenem 250 mg
cilastatin sodium 250 mg
Uses: Antiinfective

Primaxin 500 mg IV for Injection:
imipenem 500 mg
cilastatin sodium 500 mg
Uses: Antiinfective

Prinzide 10-12.5:
lisinopril 10 mg
hydrochlorothiazide 12.5 mg
Uses: Antihypertensive

Prinzide 20-12.5:
lisinopril 20 mg
hydrochlorothiazide 12.5 mg
Uses: Antihypertensive

Prinzide 20-25:
lisinopril 20 mg
hydrochlorothiazide 25 mg
Uses: Antihypertensive

Proben-C:
colchicine 0.5 mg

Side effects: *italics* = common; **bold** = life-threatening

probenecid 500 mg
Uses: Antigout agent
Proctofoam-HC Aerosol Foam:
1% hydrocortisone
1% pramoxine
Uses: Topical corticosteroid
Propacet 100:
propoxyphene-N 100 mg
acetaminophen 650 mg
Uses: Analgesic
Pseudo-Chlor:
pseudoephedrine 120 mg
chlorpheniramine 8 mg
Uses: Antihistamine
Pseudo-Gest Plus:
pseudoephedrine 60 mg
chlorpheniramine 4 mg
Uses: Antihistamine
Quadrinal:
epHEDrine 24 mg
theophylline 65 mg
potassium iodide 320 mg
phenobarbital 24 mg
Uses: Adrenergic, bronchodilator,
    barbiturate
Quelidrine Cough Syrup:
Per 5 ml:
dextromethorphan 10 mg
phenylephrine 5 mg
epHEDrine 5 mg
chlorpheniramine 2 mg
ammonium chloride 40 mg
ipecac 0.005 ml
Uses: Expectorant, adrenergic,
    antihistamine
Quibron-300:
theophylline 300 mg
guaifenesin 180 mg
Uses: Bronchodilator, expectorant
R&C Shampoo:
0.3% pyrethrins
3% piperonyl butoxide
Uses: Scabicide, pediculicide
Rauzide:
bendroflumethiazide 4 mg
powdered *Rauwolfia serpentina* 50 mg

Uses: Diuretic, antihypertensive
Rebetron:
interferon alfa-2b 3 million units/0.5 ml
ribavirin, PO 200 mg
Uses: Biologic response modifier, antiviral
Regulace:
docusate sodium 100 mg
casanthranol 30 mg
Uses: Laxative
Renese-R:
polythiazide 2 mg
reserpine 0.25 mg
Uses: Diuretic, antihypertensive
Respahist:
pseudoephedrine 60 mg
brompheniramine 6 mg
Uses: Adrenergic, antihistamine
Respaire-60:
guaifenesin 200 mg
pseudoephedrine 60 mg
Uses: Expectorant, adrenergic
RID Mousse:
pyrethrins 0.33%
piperonyl butoxide 4%
Uses: Scabicide, pediculicide
RID Shampoo:
0.3% pyrethrins
3% piperonyl butoxide
Uses: Scabicide, pediculicide
Rifamate:
isoniazid 150 mg
rifampin 300 mg
Uses: Antitubercular, antileprotic
Rifater:
rifampin 120 mg
isoniazid 50 mg
pyrazinamide 300 mg
Uses: Antitubercular
Riopan Plus Suspension:
Per 5 ml:
magaldrate 540 mg
simethicone 40 mg
Uses: Antacid, adsorbent, antiflatulent
Robaxisal:
methocarbamol 400 mg
aspirin 325 mg

⚠ Safety alert   *"Tall Man" lettering

Uses: Skeletal muscle relaxant, analgesic
Robitussin A/C Syrup:
codeine 10 mg
guaifenesin 100 mg
35% alcohol
Uses: Antitussive, opioid analgesic
Robitussin Cold & Cough Liquigels:
pseudoephedrine 30 mg
guaifenesin 200 mg
dextromethorphan 10 mg
Uses: Antitussive, expectorant, decongestant
Robitussin-DM Liquid:
Per 5 ml:
guaifenesin 100 mg
dextromethorphan 10 mg
Uses: Expectorant, antitussive
Robitussin Honey Flu Multi-Symptom Liquid:
dextromethorphan 6.6 mg
pseudoephedrine 20 mg
acetaminophen 166.7
Uses: Antitussive, decongestant, analgesic
Robitussin Maximum Strength Cough and Cold Syrup:
dextromethorphan 15 mg
pseudoephedrine 30 mg
Uses: Antitussive, adrenergic
Robitussin Night Relief Liquid:
dextromethorphan 5 mg
pyrilamine 8.3 mg
pseudoephedrine 10 mg
acetaminophen 108.3 mg
Uses: Antitussive, adrenergic
Robitussin Pediatric Cough & Cold Liquid:
Per 5 ml:
pseudoephedrine 15 mg
dextromethorphan 7.5 mg
Uses: Antitussive, adrenergic
Rolaids Calcium Rich:
magnesium hydroxide 80 mg
calcium carbonate 412 mg
Uses: Antacid, adsorbent, antiflatulent
Rondec:
pseudoephedrine 60 mg
carbinoxamine 4 mg

Uses: Adrenergic
Rondec DM Drops:
Per ml:
pseudoephedrine 25 mg
carbinoxamine 2 mg
dextromethorphan 4 mg
Uses: Adrenergic, antitussive
Rondec DM Syrup:
Per 5 ml:
pseudoephedrine 60 mg
carbinoxamine 4 mg
dextromethorphan 15 mg
Uses: Adrenergic, antitussive
Rondec Oral Drops:
Per 5 ml:
pseudoephedrine 25 mg
carbinoxamine 2 mg
Uses: Adrenergic
Roxicet:
Per 5 ml:
acetaminophen 325 mg
oxycodone 5 mg
Uses: Opioid analgesic
Roxicet 5/500:
oxycodone 5 mg
acetaminophen 500 mg
Uses: Opioid analgesic
Roxicet Oral Solution:
Per 5 ml:
acetaminophen 325 mg
oxycodone 5 mg
Uses: Analgesic
Roxiprin:
aspirin 325 mg
oxycodone HCl 4.5 mg
oxycodone terephthalate 0.38 mg
Uses: Analgesic
Ru-Tuss DE:
pseudoephedrine 120 mg
guaifenesin 600 mg
Uses: Adrenergic, expectorant
Ru-Tuss Expectorant Liquid:
Per 5 ml:
guaifenesin 100 mg
pseudoephedrine 30 mg
dextromethorphan 10 mg

10% alcohol
Uses: Adrenergic, expectorant, antitussive
Ru-Tuss with Hydrocodone Liquid:
Per 5 ml:
hydrocodone: 1.7 mg
phenylephrine 5 mg
pyrilamine 3.3 mg
pheniramine 3.3 mg
phenylpropanolamine 3.3 mg
5% alcohol
Uses: Antihistamine, analgesic,
  decongestant
Ryna-C Liquid:
Per 5 ml:
pseudoephedrine 30 mg
chlorpheniramine 2 mg
codeine 10 mg
Uses: Adrenergic, antihistamine, analgesic
Ryna Liquid:
Per 5 ml:
pseudoephedrine 30 mg
chlorpheniramine 2 mg
Uses: Adrenergic, antihistamine
Rynatan:
phenylephrine 25 mg
chlorpheniramine 8 mg
pyrilamine 25 mg
Uses: Adrenergic, antihistamine
Rynatan Pediatric Suspension:
Per 5 ml:
phenylephrine 5 mg
chlorpheniramine 2 mg
pyrilamine 12.5 mg
Uses: Adrenergic, antihistamine
Rynatuss:
epHEDrine 10 mg
carbetapentane 60 mg
chlorpheniramine 5 mg
phenylephrine 10 mg
Uses: Adrenergic, antihistamine
Salutensin Demi:
hydroflumethiazide 25 mg
reserpine 0.125 mg
Uses: Antihypertensive
Scot-Tussin DM Liquid:
Per 5 ml:

chlorpheniramine 2 mg
dextromethorphan 15 mg
Uses: Antihistamine, antitussive
**Scot-Tussin Original 5-Action
  Liquid:**
phenylephrine 4.2 mg
pheniramine 13.3 mg
sodium citrate 83.3 mg
sodium salicylate 83.3 mg
caffeine citrate 25 mg
Uses: Adrenergic, analgesic
Sedapap-10:
acetaminophen 650 mg
butalbital 50 mg
Uses: Analgesic, barbiturate
Semprex-D:
acrivastine 8 mg
pseudoephedrine 60 mg
Uses: Adrenergic, bronchodilator
Senokot-S:
docusate 50 mg
senna concentrate 187 mg
Uses: Laxative
Septra:
sulfamethoxazole 400 mg
trimethroprim 80 mg
Uses: Antiinfective
Septra DS:
sulfamethoxazole 800 mg
trimethroprim 160 mg
Uses: Antiinfective
Septra I.V. for Injection:
Per 5 ml:
trimethoprim 80 mg
sulfamethoxazole 400 mg
Uses: Antiinfective
Septra Suspension:
Per 5 ml:
trimethoprim 40 mg
sulfamethoxazole 200 mg
Uses: Antiinfective
Ser-Ap-Es:
hydrochlorothiazide 15 mg
reserpine 0.1 mg
hydrALAZINE 25 mg
Uses: Diuretic, antihypertensive

Silafed Syrup:
Per 5 ml:
pseudoephedrine 30 mg
triprolidine 1.25 mg
Uses: Adrenergic, antihistamine
Silaminic Cold Syrup:
Per 5 ml:
phenylpropanolamine 12.5 mg
chlorpheniramine 2 mg
Uses: Antihistamine, decongestant
Sinarest Extra Strength:
pseudoephedrine 30 mg
chlorpheniramine 2 mg
acetaminophen 500 mg
Uses: Adrenergic, antihistamine, analgesic
Sinarest No Drowsiness:
pseudoephedrine 30 mg
acetaminophen 500 mg
Uses: Adrenergic, analgesic
Sinarest Sinus:
pseudoephedrine 30 mg
chlorpheniramine 2 mg
acetaminophen 325 mg
Uses: Adrenergic, antihistamine, analgesic
Sine-Aid IB:
pseudoephedrine 30 mg
ibuprofen 200 mg
Uses: Adrenergic, analgesic
Sine-Aid Maximum Strength:
pseudoephedrine 30 mg
acetaminophen 500 mg
Uses: Adrenergic, analgesic
Sinemet 10/100:
carbidopa 10 mg
levodopa 100 mg
Uses: Antiparkinsonian
Sinemet 25/100:
carbidopa 25 mg
levodopa 100 mg
Uses: Antiparkinsonian
Sinemet 25/250:
carbidopa 25 mg
levodopa 250 mg
Uses: Antiparkinsonian
Sinemet CR 25-100:
carbidopa 25 mg

levodopa 100 mg
Uses: Antiparkinsonian
Sinemet CR 50-200:
carbidopa 50 mg
levodopa 200 mg
Uses: Antiparkinsonian
**Sine-Off Maximum Strength No
  Drowsiness Formula Caplets:**
pseudoephedrine 30 mg
acetaminophen 500 mg
Uses: Adrenergic, analgesic
Sine-Off Sinus Medicine:
pseudoephedrine 30 mg
chlorpheniramine 2 mg
acetaminophen 500 mg
Uses: Adrenergic, antihistamine, analgesic
Sinus-Relief:
acetaminophen 325 mg
pseudoephedrine 30 mg
Uses: Nonopioid analgesic
Sinutab:
acetaminophen 325 mg
chlorpheniramine 2 mg
pseudoephedrine 30 mg
Uses: Nonopioid analgesic
**Sinutab Maximum Strength Sinus
  Allergy:**
acetaminophen 500 mg
pseudoephedrine 30 mg
chlorpheniramine 2 mg
Uses: Analgesic, adrenergic, antihistamine
**Sinutab Maximum Strength Without
  Drowsiness:**
acetaminophen 500 mg
pseudoephedrine 30 mg
Uses: Analgesic, adrenergic
Sinutab Non-Drying:
pseudoepedrine 30 mg
guaifenesin 200 mg
Uses: Adrenergic, expectorant
Slo-Phyllin GG Syrup:
theophylline 150 mg
guaifenesin 90 mg
Uses: Bronchodilator, expectorant
Slow-Salt-K:
sodium chloride 410 mg

potassium chloride 15 mg
Uses: Potassium, sodium supplement
Solage:
mequinol 2%
tretinoin 0.01%
Uses: Antineoplastic
Soma Compound:
carisoprodol 200 mg
aspirin 325 mg
Uses: Skeletal muscle relaxant
Spec-T Lozenge:
dextromethorphan 10 mg
benzocaine 10 mg
Uses: Antitussive, topical anesthetic
Stalevo 50:
carbidopa 12.5 mg
levodopa 50 mg
entacapone 200 mg
Uses: Parkinsonism
Stalevo 100:
carbidopa 25 mg
levodopa 100 mg
entacapone 200 mg
Uses: Parkinsonism
Stalevo 150:
carbidopa 37.5 mg
levodopa 150 mg
entacapone 200 mg
Uses: Parkinsonism
Sudafed Cold & Allergy:
pseudoephedrine 60 mg
chlorpheniramine 4 mg
Uses: Adrenergic, antihistamine
Sudafed Cold & Cough Liquicaps:
pseudoephedrine 30 mg
dextromethorphan 10 mg
guaifenesin 100 mg
acetaminophen 250 mg
Uses: Adrenergic, antitussive, expectorant, analgesic
Sudafed Cold & Sinus:
pseudoephedrine 30 mg
acetaminophen 325 mg
Uses: Adrenergic, analgesic
Sudafed Plus:
pseudoephedrine 60 mg

chlorpheniramine 4 mg
Uses: Adrenergic, antihistamine
Sudafed Severe Cold:
pseudoephedrine 30 mg
dextromethorphan 15 mg
Uses: Adrenergic, antitussive
Sudafed Sinus Maximum Strength:
pseudoephedrine 30 mg
acetaminophen 500 mg
Uses: Adrenergic, analgesic
Sudal 60/500:
pseudoephedrine 60 mg
guaifenesin 500 mg
Uses: Adrenergic, expectorant
Sudal 120/600:
pseudoephedrine 120 mg
guaifenesin 600 mg
Uses: Adrenergic, expectorant
Sultrin Triple Sulfa Vaginal Cream:
3.42% sulfathiazole
2.86% sulfacetamine
3.7% sulfabenzamide
Uses: Antiinfective
Sultrin Triple Sulfa Vaginal Tablets:
sulfathiazole 172.5 mg
sulfacetamide 143.75
sulfabenzamide 184 mg
Uses: Antiinfective
Symbyax:
olanzapine 6 mg
fluoxetine 25 mg

olanzapine 6 mg
fluoxetine 50 mg

olanzapine 12 mg
fluoxetine 25 mg
olanzapine 12 mg
fluoxetine 50 mg
Uses: Bipolar disorder
Synalgos-DC:
aspirin 356.4 mg
caffeine 30 mg
dihydrocodeine 16 mg
Uses: Analgesic
Synercid:
quinupristin 150 mg

dalfopristin 350 mg
Uses: Antiinfective
Syntest H.S.:
esterified estrogens 0.625 mg
methylTESTOSTERone 1.25 mg
Uses: Vasomotor symptoms (menopause)
Talacen:
acetaminophen 650 mg
pentazocine 25 mg
Uses: Analgesic
Talwin Compound:
aspirin 325 mg
pentazocine 12.5 mg
Uses: Analgesic
Talwin NX:
pentazocine 50 mg
naloxone 0.5 mg
Uses: Analgesic, opioid antagonist
Tarka 182:
trandolapril 2 mg (immed rel)
verapamil 180 mg (sus rel)
Uses: Antihypertensive, calcium channel
blocker
Tarka 241:
trandolapril 1 mg (immed rel)
verapamil 240 mg (sus rel)
Uses: Antihypertensive, calcium channel
blocker
Tarka 242:
trandolapril 2 mg (immed rel)
verapamil 240 mg (sus rel)
Uses: Antihypertensive, calcium channel
blocker
Tarka 244:
trandolapril 4 mg (immed rel)
verapamil 240 mg (sus rel)
Uses: Antihypertensive, calcium channel
blocker
Tavist Allergy/Sinus Headache:
clemastine 0.335 mg
pseudoephedrine 30 mg
acetaminophen 500 mg
Uses: Antihistamine, adrenergic, analgesic
Tavist Sinus:
acetaminophen 500 mg
pseudoephedrine 30 mg

Uses: Analgesic, adrenergic
♣ **Tecnal:**
aspirin 330 mg
caffeine 40 mg
butalbital 50 mg
Uses: Nonopioid analgesic
Teczem:
enalapril 5 mg (extended release)
diltiazem 180 mg (extended release)
Uses: Antihypertensive, calcium channel
blocker
Tegrin-LT Shampoo:
0.33% pyrethrins
3.15% piperonyl butoxide
Uses: Scabicide, pediculicide
Tenoretic 50:
atenolol 50 mg
chlorthalidone 25 mg
Uses: Antihypertensive
Tenoretic 100:
atenolol 100 mg
chlorthalidone 25 mg
Uses: Antihypertensive
Terra-Cortril Ophthalmic Suspension:
1.5% hydrocortisone acetate
0.5% oxytetracycline
Uses: Ophthalmic antiinflammatory, antiinfective
**Terramycin w/Polymycin B Sulfate
Ophthalmic Ointment:**
Per gram:
polymyxin B 10,000 units
oxytetracycline 5 mg
Uses: Ophthalmic antiinfective
T-Gesic:
hydrocodone 5 mg
acetaminophen 500 mg
Uses: Analgesic
Thera-Flu Cold & Cough Powder:
Per packet:
pseudoephedrine 60 mg
chlorpheniramine 4 mg
dextromethorphan 20 mg
acetaminophen 650 mg
Uses: Adrenergic, antihistamine, antitussive,
analgesic

Thera-Flu Flu & Chest Congestion Non-Drowsy Powder:
dextromethorphan 30 mg
guaifenesin 400 mg
pseudoephedrine 60 mg
acetaminophen 1000 mg
Uses: Antitussive, expectorant, decongestant, analgesic

Thera-Flu NightTime Powder:
dextromethorphan 30 mg
chlorpheniramine 4 mg
pseudoephedrine 60 mg
acetaminophen 1000 mg
Uses: Antitussive, antihistamine, decongestant, analgesic

Thera-Flu Maximum Strength Flu, Cold & Cough Powder:
dextromethorphan 30 mg
guaifenesin 400 mg
pseudoephedrine 60 mg
acetaminophen 1000 mg
Uses: Antitussive, expectorant, decongestant, analgesic

Thera-Flu Non-Drowsy Flu, Cold & Cough Maximum Strength Powder:
Per packet:
pseudoephedrine 60 mg
dextromethorphan 30 mg
acetaminophen 1000 mg
Uses: Decongestant, antitussive, analgesic

Thera-Flu Severe Cold & Congestion NightTime Maximum Strength Powder:
Per packet:
pseudoephedrine 60 mg
chlorpheniramine 4 mg
dextromethorphan 30 mg
acetaminophen 1000 mg
Uses: Decongestant, antihistamine, antitussive, analgesic

Thera-Flu Severe Cold & Congestion Non-Drowsy Maximum Strength Powder:
dextromethorphan 30 mg
pseudoephedrine 60 mg
acetaminophen 1000 mg
Uses: Antitussive, decongestant, acetaminophen

Thera-Flu Severe Cold & Cough Powder:
dextromethorphan 30 mg
chlorpheniramine 4 mg
pseudoephedrine 60 mg
acetaminophen 1000 mg
Uses: Antitussive, antihistamine, decongestant, analgesic

Thera-Flu Severe Cold Non-Drowsy Packet:
dextromethorphan 30 mg
pseudoephedrine 60 mg
acetaminophen 1000 mg
Uses: Antitussive, decongestant, acetaminophen

Thera-Flu Severe Cold Non-Drowsy Tablets:
dextromethorphan 15 mg
pseudoephedrine 30 mg
acetaminophen 500 mg
Uses: Antitussive, decongestant, analgesic

Thera-Flu Severe Cold Tablets:
dextromethorphan 15 mg
chlorpheniramine 2 mg
pseudoephedrine 30 mg
acetaminophen 500 mg
Uses: Antitussive, antihistamine, decongestant, analgesic

Timentin for Injection:
Per 3.1-g vial:
ticarcillin 3 g
clavulanic acid 0.1 g
Uses: Antiinfective

Timolide 10/25:
timolol 10 mg
hydrochlorothiazide 25 mg
Uses: Antihypertensive

Titralac Plus:
calcium carbonate 420 mg
simethicone 21 mg
Uses: Antacid, adsorbent, antiflatulent

Tobra Dex Ophthalmic Suspension/Ointment:
tobramycin 0.3%

dexamethasone 0.1%
Uses: Ophthalmic antiinfective,
  antiinflammatory
Triacin-C Cough Syrup:
Per 5 ml:
codeine 10 mg
pseudoephedrine 30 mg
triprolidine 1.25 mg
Uses: Analgesic, adrenergic, antihistamine
Tri-Hydroserpine:
hydrALAZINE 25 mg
hydrochlorothiazide 15 mg
reserpine 0.1 mg
Uses: Antihypertensive
Tri-Levlen:
Phase I:
levonorgestrel 0.05 mg
ethinyl estradiol 30 mcg
Phase II:
levonorgestrel 0.075 mg
ethinyl estradiol 40 mcg;
Phase III:
levonorgestrel 0.125 mg
ethinyl estradiol 30 mcg
Uses: Oral contraceptive
**Triaminic AM Cough & Decongestant
  Formula Liquid:**
Per 5 ml:
pseudoephedrine 15 mg
dextromethorphan 7.5 mg
Uses: Adrenergic, antitussive
Triaminic Nite Light Liquid:
Per 5 ml:
pseudoephedrine 15 mg
chlorpheniramine 1 mg
dextromethorphan 7.5 mg
Uses: Adrenergic, antihistamine, antitussive
**Triaminic Sore Throat Formula
  Liquid:**
Per 5 ml:
pseudoephedrine 15 mg
dextromethorphan 7.5 mg
acetaminophen 160 mg
Uses: Adrenergic, antitussive
Triavil 2-10:
perphenazine 2 mg

amitriptyline 10 mg
Uses: Antipsychotic, antidepressant
Triavil 2-25:
perphenazine 2 mg
amitriptyline 25 mg
Uses: Antipsychotic, antidepressant
Triavil 4-10:
perphenazine 4 mg
amitriptyline 10 mg
Triavil 4-25:
perphenazine 4 mg
amitriptyline 25 mg
Uses: Antipsychotic, antidepressant
Triavil 4-50:
perphenazine 4 mg
amitriptyline 50 mg
Uses: Antipsychotic, antidepressant
Trinalin Repetabs:
azatadine maleate 1 mg
pseudoephedrine 120 mg
Uses: Antihistamine
Triphasil:
Phase I:
levonorgestrel 0.05 mg
ethinyl estradiol 30 mcg
Phase II:
levonorgestrel 0.075 mg
ethinyl estradiol 40 mcg
Phase III:
levonorgestrel 0.125 mg
ethinyl estradiol 30 mcg
Uses: Oral contraceptive
**Triple Antibiotic Ophthalmic
  Ointment:**
Per gram:
polymyxin B 10,000 units
neomycin 3.5 mg
bacitracin 400 units
Uses: Antiinfective
**Triprolidine/Pseudoephedrine Syrup
  (generic):**
Per 5 ml
triprolidine 1.25 mg
pseudoephedrine 50 mg
Uses: Antihistamine, decongestant

Triprolidine/Pseudoephedrine Tablets (generic):
triprolidine 2.5 mg
pseudoephedrine 60 mg
Uses: Antihistamine, decongestant

Trizivir:
300 mg abacavir
150 mg lamivudine
300 mg zidovudine
Uses: HIV

Tuinal 100 mg:
amobarbital 50 mg
secobarbital 50 mg
Uses: Sedative-hypnotic

Tusibron-DM Syrup:
Per 5 ml:
guaifenesin 100 mg
dextromethorphan 15 mg
Uses: Expectorant, antitussive

Tussionex Pennkinetic Suspension:
Per 5 ml:
chlorpheniramine 8 mg
hydrocodone 10 mg
Uses: Antihistamine, analgesic

Tussi-Organidin NR Liquid:
Per 5 ml:
codeine 10 mg
guaifenesin 100 mg
Uses: Analgesic, expectorant

Tussi-Organidin DM NR Liquid:
Per 5 ml:
guaifenesin 100 mg
dextromethorphan 10 mg
Uses: Expectorant, antitussive

Twinrix:
hepatitis A vaccine
hepatitis B vaccine
Uses: Vaccine

Tylenol Allergy Sinus, DayTime Caplet:
acetaminophen 500 mg
chlorpheniramine 2 mg
pseudoephedrine 30 mg
Uses: Antihistamine, adrenergic, analgesic

Tylenol Children's Cold:
acetaminophen 80 mg
chlorpheniramine 0.5 mg

pseudoephedrine 7.5 mg
Uses: Antihistamine, adrenergic, analgesic

Tylenol Children's Cold Multi-Symptom Plus Cough Liquid:
Per 5 ml:
acetaminophen 160 mg
dextromethorphan 5 mg
chlorpheniramine 1 mg
pseudoephedrine 15 mg
Uses: Antihistamine, adrenergic, analgesic

Tylenol Children's Cold Plus Cough Chewable:
acetaminophen 80 mg
pseudoephedrine 7.5 mg
dextromethorphan 2.5 mg
chlorpheniramine 0.5 mg
Uses: Antihistamine, adrenergic, analgesic

Tylenol Cold Multi-Symptom Tablets:
acetaminophen 325 mg
chlorpheniramine 2 mg
pseudoephedrine 30 mg
dextromethorphan 15 mg
Uses: Antihistamine, adrenergic, analgesic

Tylenol Cold & Flu Severe DayTime Liquid:
dextromethorphan 5 mg
pseudoephedrine 10 mg
acetaminophen 166.7 mg
Uses: Antitussive, decongestant, analgesic

Tylenol Cold Severe Congestion Tablets:
dextromethorphan 15 mg
guaifenesin 200 mg
pseudoephedrine 32 mg
acetaminophen 325 mg
Uses: Antitussive, expectorant, decongestant, analgesic

Tylenol Cough & Sore Throat DayTime Liquid:
dextromethorphan 5 mg
acetaminophen 166.7 mg
Uses: Antitussive, analgesic

Tylenol Flu Day Non-Drowsy Gelcaps:
diphenhydramine 25 mg
pseudoephedrine 30 mg
acetaminophen 500 mg

Uses: Analgesic, adrenergic, antitussive

Tylenol Flu NightTime Gelcaps:
diphenhydramine 25 mg
doxylamine 2.1 mg
pseudoephedrine 30 mg
acetaminophen 500 mg
Uses: Antihistamine, decongestant, analgesic

Tylenol PM, Extra Strength:
acetaminophen 500 mg
diphenhydrAMINE 25 mg
Uses: Analgesic, antihistamine

Tylenol Severe Allergy:
diphenhydrAMINE 12.5 mg
acetaminophen 500 mg
Uses: Analgesic, antihistamine

Tylenol w/Codeine Elixir:
Per 5 ml:
acetaminophen 120 mg
codeine 12 mg
Uses: Analgesic

Tylenol w/Codeine No. 1:
acetaminophen 300 mg
codeine 7.5 mg
Uses: Analgesic

Tylenol w/Codeine No. 2:
acetaminophen 300 mg
codeine 15 mg

Tylenol w/Codeine No. 3:
acetaminophen 300 mg
codeine 30 mg
Uses: Analgesic

Tylenol w/Codeine No. 4:
acetaminophen 300 mg
codeine 60 mg
Uses: Analgesic

Tylox:
oxycodone 5 mg
acetaminophen 500 mg
Uses: Analgesic

Tyrodone Liquid:
Per 5 ml:
hydrocodone 5 mg
pseudoephedrine 60 mg
5% alcohol
Uses: Analgesic, adrenergic

Ultracet:
tramadol 37.5 mg
acetaminophen 325 mg
Uses: Analgesic

Unasyn for Injection 3 g:
ampicillin 2 g
sulbactam 1 g
Uses: Antiinfective

Uniretic:
moexipril 7.5 mg
hydrochlorothiazide 12.5 mg
or moexipril 15 mg
hydrochlorothiazide 25 mg
Uses: Antihypertensive, diuretic

Unituss HC Syrup:
hydrocodone 2.5 mg
phenylephrine 5 mg
chlorpheniramine 2 mg
Uses: Analgesic, adrenergic, antihistamine

Urised:
methenamine 40.8 mg
phenylsalicylate 18.1 mg
atropine 0.03 mg
hyoscyamine 0.03 mg
benzoic acid 4.5 mg
methylene blue 5.4 mg
Uses: Antiinfective

Vanquish:
aspirin 227 mg
acetaminophen 194 mg
caffeine 33 mg
aluminum hydroxide 25 mg
magnesium hydroxide 50 mg
Uses: Nonopioid analgesic

Vaseretic 5-12.5:
enalapril 5 mg
hydrochlorthiazide 12.5 mg
Uses: Antihypertensive diuretic

Vaseretic 10-25:
enalapril 10 mg
hydrochlorothiazide 25 mg
Uses: Antihypertensive, diuretic

Vasocidin Ophthalmic Ointment:
sulfacetamide 10%
prednisoLONE 0.5%

Uses: Ophthalmic antiinfective,
antiinflammatory

Vasocidin Ophthalmic Solution:
sulfacetamide 10%
prednisoLONE 0.25%
Uses: Ophthalmic antiinfective,
antiinflammatory

Vasocon-A Ophthalmic Solution:
naphazoline 0.05%
antazoline 0.5%
Uses: Ophthalmic vasoconstrictor

**Vicks 44D Cough & Head Congestion
Liquid:**
Per 5 ml:
dextromethorphan 10 mg
pseudoephedrine 20 mg
Uses: Antitussive, adrenergic

Vicks 44E Liquid:
Per 5 ml:
dextromethorphan 6.7 mg
guaifenesin 66.7 mg
Uses: Antitussive, expectorant

**Vicks 44M Cold, Flu, & Cough
LiquiCaps:**
dextromethorphan 10 mg
pseudoephedrine 30 mg
chlorpheniramine 2 mg
acetaminophen 250 mg
Uses: Antitussive, adrenergic, antihistamine,
analgesic

**Vicks 44 Non-Drowsy Cold & Cough
LiquiCaps:**
dextromethorphan 30 mg
pseudoephedrine 60 mg
Uses: Antitussive, adrenergic

**Vicks Children's NyQuil Nighttime
Cough/Cold Liquid:**
Per 5 ml:
pseudoephedrine 10 mg
chlorpheniramine 0.67 mg
dextromethorphan 5 mg
Uses: Adrenergic, antihistamine,
antitussive

Vicks DayQuil Liquid:
dextromethorphan 3.3 mg
pseudoephedrine 10 mg

acetaminophen 108.3 mg
guaifenesin 33.3 mg
Uses: Antitussive, adrenergic, analgesic,
expectorant

**Vicks DayQuil Multi-Symptom Cold/
Flu Relief Liquid:**
dextromethorphan 33 mg
pseudoephedrine 10 mg
acetaminophen 108.3 mg
Uses: Antitussive, decongestant, analgesic

Vicks DayQuil Pressure & Pain Caplet:
pseudoephedrine 30 mg
ibuprofen 200 mg
Uses: Adrenergic, analgesic

Vicks NyQuil LiquiCaps:
pseudoephedrine 30 mg
doxylamine 6.25 mg
dextromethorphan 10 mg
acetaminophen 250 mg
Uses: Adrenergic, antihistamine, antitussive,
analgesic

**Vicks NyQuil Multi-Symptom Cold Flu
Relief Liquid:**
pseudoephedrine 10 mg
doxylamine 2.1 mg
dextromethorphan 5 mg
acetaminophen 167 mg
Uses: Adrenergic, antihistamine, antitussive,
analgesic

Vicks 44M Pediatric Liquid:
Per 5 ml:
pseudoephedrine 15 mg
chlorpheniramine 1 mg
Uses: Adrenergic, antihistamine, antitussive

Vicodin:
acetaminophen 500 mg
hydrocodone 5 mg
Uses: Analgesic

Vicodin ES:
acetaminophen 750 mg
hydrocodone 7.5 mg
Uses: Analgesic

Vicodin HP:
acetaminophen 660 mg
hydrocodone 10 mg
Uses: Analgesic

A Safety alert   *"Tall Man" lettering

VicodinTuss:
Per 5 ml:
hydrocodone 5 mg
guaifenesin 100 mg
Uses: Analgesic, expectorant
Vicoprofen:
hydrocodone 7.5 mg
ibuprofen 200 mg
Uses: Analgesic
Vytorin:
ezetimibe: 10, 10, 10, 10 mg
simvastatin: 10, 20, 40, 80 mg
Uses: Antihyperlipidemic
Wigraine Suppositories:
ergotamine 2 mg
caffeine 100 mg
Uses: α-Adrenergic blocker
Yasmin 28:
ethinyl estadiol 30 mcg
dropirenone 3 mg
Uses: Oral contraceptive
YAZ:
prospirenone 3 mg
ethinyl estradiol 0.02 mg
Uses: Vasomotor symptoms (menopause)
Zegerid Capsules:
omeprazole 20 mg
sodium bicarbonate 1100 mg,
omeprazole 40 mg
Uses: Gastric ulcer, GERD
Zegerid Powder (Oral Solution):
omeprazole 20 mg
sodium bicarbonate 1680 mg,
omeprazole 40 mg
sodium bicarbonate 1680 mg
Uses: Gastric ulcer, GERD
Zestoretic 10/12.5:
lisinopril 10 mg
hydrochlorothiazide 12.5 mg

Uses: Antihypertensive
Zestoretic 20/12.5:
lisinopril 20 mg
hydrochlorothiazide 12.5 mg
Uses: Antihypertensive
Zestoretic 20/25:
lisinopril 20 mg
hydrochlorothiazide 25 mg
Uses: Antihypertensive
Ziac 2.5:
bisoprolol 2.5 mg
hydrochlorothiazide 6.25 mg
Uses: Antihypertensive
Ziac 5:
bisoprolol 5 mg
hydrochlorothiazide 6.25 mg
Uses: Antihypertensive
Ziac 10:
bisoprolol 10 mg
hydrochlorothiazide 6.25 mg
Uses: Antihypertensive
Ziks Cream:
methyl salicylate 12%
menthol 1%
capsaicin 0.025%
Uses: Analgesic, decongestant
Zotrim
phenazopyridine 200 mg
sulfamethoxazole 160 mg
trimethoprim 800 mg
Uses: Antiinfective
Zydone:
hydrocodone 5 mg
acetaminophen 500 mg
Uses: Analgesic
Zyrtec-D
cetirizine 5 mg
pseudoephedrine 120 mg
Uses: Antihistamine, decongestant

Appendix i

Look-alike/sound-alike drug names

Accolate	Accupril	adenosine	adenosine phosphate
Accolate	Accutane		
Accupril	Accutane	adenosine phosphate	Adenocard
Accupril	Aciphex		
Accupril	Accolate	adenosine phosphate	adenosine
Accupril	Altace	Adipex-P	Aciphex
Accupril	Aricept	Adriamycin	Aredia
Accupril	Monopril	Adriamycin	Idamycin
Accutane	Accolate	Advair	Advicor
Accutane	Accupril	Advicor	Advair
acebutolol	albuterol	Aggrastat	Aggrenox
acetaminophen and codeine	acetaminophen and hydrocodone	Aggrastat	argatroban
		Aggrenox	Aggrastat
acetaminophen and codeine	acetaminophen and oxycodone	Akarpine	atropine
acetaminophen and hydrocodone	acetaminophen and codeine	albuterol	acebutolol
		albuterol	atenolol
acetaminophen and oxycodone	acetaminophen and codeine	Aldara	Alora
		aldesleukin	oprelvekin
acetaZOLAMIDE	acetoHEXAMIDE	Aldomet	Adalat CC
acetaZOLAMIDE	acetylcysteine	Alkeran	Leukeran
acetaZOLAMIDE	acyclovir	Allegra	Adalat CC
acetoHEXAMIDE	acetaZOLAMIDE	Allegra	Allegra-D
acetylcysteine	acetaZOLAMIDE	Allegra	Asacol
Aciphex	Accupril	Allegra	Viagra
Aciphex	Adipex-p	Allegra-D	Allegra
Aciphex	Aricept	Allegra-D	Allerx-D
Activase	Retavase	Allerx-D	Allegra-D
Actonel	Actos	allopurinol	Apresoline
Actos	Actonel	Alora	Aldara
Acular	Ocular lubricants	alprazolam	clonazepam
Acyclovir	acetaZOLAMIDE	alprazolam	diazepam
Acyclovir	famiciclovir	alprazolam	lorazepam
Adalat CC	Aldomat	Altace	Accupril
Adalat CC	Allegra	Altace	alteplase
Adderall	Inderal	Altace	Amaryl
Adenocard	adenosine phosphate	Altace	Amerge
		Altace	Artane
		Altace	Norvasc
		alteplase	Altace

Alupent	Atrovent	Anaprox	Avapro
amantadine	amiodarone	Anaspaz	Antispas
amantadine	ranitidine	Anbesol	Anusol
amantadine	rimantadine	Ansaid	Asacol
Amaryl	Altace	antacid	Atacand
Amaryl	Amerge	Anti-Xa	Arixtra
Amaryl	Avandia	Antispas	Anaspaz
Amaryl	Symmetrel	Anusol	Anbesol
Ambien	Amen	Anusol	Anusol-HC
Ambien	Ativan	Anusol-HC	Anusol
Ambien	Coumadin	Anzemet	Aricept
Amen	Ambien	Apresoline	allopurinol
Amerge	Altace	Apresoline	Priscoline
Amerge	Amaryl	Aredia	Adriamycin
Amicar	Amikin	argatroban	Aggrastat
amikacin	anakinra	argatroban	Orgaran
Amikin	Amicar	Aricept	Accupril
amiloride	amlodipine	Aricept	Aciphex
aminophylline	amitriptyline	Aricept	Anzemet
amiodarone	trazodone	Arixtra	Anti-Xa
amiodarone	amantadine	Artane	Altace
amiodarone	amlodipine	Asacol	Allegra
amiodarone	inamrinone	Asacol	Ansaid
amitriptyline	aminophylline	Asacol	Os-Cal
amitriptyline	imipramine	asparaginase	pegaspargase
amitriptyline	nortriptyline	Atacand	antacid
amlodipine	amiloride	Atacand	Avandia
amlodipine	amiodarone	Atarax	amoxicillin
amlodipine	felodipine	Atarax	Ativan
amoxapine	amoxicillin	atenolol	albuterol
amoxapine	Amoxil	atenolol	metoprolol
amoxicillin	amoxapine	Atgam	ratgam
amoxicillin	Amoxil		(synonym for
amoxicillin	ampicillin		Thymo-globulin)
amoxicillin	Atarax	Ativan	Ambien
amoxicillin	Augmentin	Ativan	Atarax
Amoxil	amoxapine	atorvastatin	pravastatin
Amoxil	amoxicillin	atropine	Akarpine
Amphotericin B, lipid complex	amphotericin B, liposomal	Atrovent	Alupent
Amphotericin B, liposomal	amphotericin B, lipid complex	Atrovent	Azmacort
ampicillin	amoxicillin	Atrovent	Flovent
ampicillin	Augmentin	Atrovent	Natru-Vent
ampicillin	oxacillin	Atrovent	Serevent
Anaflex	Zanaflex	Attenuvax	Meruvax
Anafranil	enalapril	Augmentin	amoxicillin
anakinra	amikacin	Augmentin	ampicillin
		Avandia	Amaryl
		Avandia	Atacand

Avandia	Avelox	bisacodyl	bisoprolol
Avandia	Coumadin	bisacodyl	Visicol
Avandia	Prandin	bisoprolol	bisacodyl
Avapro	Anaprox	bisoprolol	fosinopril
Avapro	Avelox	Boost bar	BuSpar
Avelox	Avandia	Brevibloc	Brevital
Avelox	Avapro	Brevital	Brevibloc
Avelox	Cerebyx	Bumex	Bentyl
Avinza	Invanz	Bumex	Buprenex
Avonex	Lovenox	Bumex	Nimbex
azithromycin	erythromycin	Bumex	Permax
azithromycin	vancomycin	bupivacaine	ropivacaine
azithromycin	aztreonam	Buprenex	Bumex
Azmacort	Atrovent	buPROPion	busPIRone
Azmacort	Nasacort	BuSpar	Boost bar
aztreonam	azithromycin	busPIRone	buPROPion
Bactocill	Pathocil	butalbital,	butalbital, aspirin,
Bactrim	Biaxin	acetaminophen,	and caffeine
Bactrim DS	Bancap HC	and caffeine	
Bancap HC	Bactrim DS	butalbital, aspirin,	butalbital,
Baycol	Bellergal	and caffeine	acetaminophen,
Beclovent	Beconase		and caffeine
Beconase	Beclovent	Cafergot	Carafate
Beconase	Beconase AQ	Calan	Calan SR
Beconase AQ	Beconase	Calan	Colace
Bellergal	Baycol	Calan SR	Calan
Benadryl	benazepril	Calciferol	calcitriol
Benadryl	Bentyl	calcitriol	Calciferol
Benadryl	Benylin	calcium acetate	calcium carbonate
benazepril	Benadryl	calcium carbonate	calcium acetate
benazepril	benzonatate	calcium carbonate	calcium gluconate
benazepril	donepezil	calcium chloride	calcium gluconate
benazepril	lisinopril	calcium gluconate	calcium carbonate
Bentyl	Benadryl	calcium gluconate	calcium chloride
Bentyl	Bumex	Capitrol	captopril
Bentyl	Proventil	Capoten	Catapres
Benylin	Benadryl	captopril	Capitrol
Benylin	Ventolin	captopril	carvedilol
benzonatate	benazepril	Carafate	Cafergot
benzonatate	benztropine	Carbatrol (carba-	Carbrital (pentobar-
benztropine	benzonatate	mezapine in U.S.)	bitone sodium
Betagan	Betoptic		in Australia)
Betapace	Betapace AF	carbidopa	levodopa and
Betapace AF	Betapace		carbidopa
Betoptic	Betagan	carboplatin	cisplatin
Betoptic	Betoptic S	Carbrital (pentobar-	Carbatrol (carba-
Betoptic S	Betoptic	bitone sodium	mezapine in
Biaxin	Bactrim	in Australia)	U.S.)

Cardene	Cardizem
Cardene	Cardura
Cardene	codeine
Cardiem	Cardizem
Cardizem	Cardene
Cardizem	Cardiem
Cardizem	clonidine
Cardura	Cardene
Cardura	Cordarone
Cardura	Coumadin
Cardura	K-Dur
Cardura	Ridaura
Cartia (aspirin in New Zealand)	Cartia XT (diltiazem in U.S.)
Cartia XT	Diltia XT
Cartia XT (diltiazem in U.S.)	Cartia (aspirin in New Zealand)
Cartia XT	Procardia XL
carvedilol	captopril
Cataflam	Catapres
Catapres	Capoten
Catapres	Cataflam
Catapres	Catarase
Catarase	Catapres
Ceclor	Ceclor CD
Ceclor CD	Ceclor
cefaclor	cephalexin
cefazolin	cefepime
cefazolin	cefotaxime
cefazolin	cefotetan
cefazolin	cefoxitin
cefazolin	cefprozil
cefazolin	ceftazidime
cefazolin	ceftizoxime
cefazolin	ceftriaxone
cefazolin	cefuroxime
cefazolin	cephalexin
cefepime	cefazolin
cefepime	cefotetan
cefepime	Cefotan
cefixime	cefpodoxime
Cefobid	celecoxib
Cefobid	Levbid
Cefol	Cefzil
Cefotan	Ceftin
Cefotan	Claforan
Cefotan	cefepime
Cefotan	ceftriaxone
cefotaxime	cefazolin
cefotaxime	cefotetan
cefotaxime	cefoxitin
cefotaxime	ceftazidime
cefotaxime	ceftizoxime
cefotaxime	ceftriaxone
cefotaxime	cefuroxime
cefotetan	cefazolin
cefotetan	cefepime
cefotetan	cefotaxime
cefotetan	cefoxitin
cefotetan	ceftazidime
cefotetan	ceftizoxime
cefotetan	ceftriaxone
cefoxitin	cefazolin
cefoxitin	cefotaxime
cefoxitin	cefotetan
cefoxitin	ceftriaxone
cefoxitin	cefuroxime
cefpodoxime	cefixime
cefprozil	cefazolin
cefprozil	cefuroxime
ceftazidime	cefazolin
ceftazidime	cefotaxime
ceftazidime	cefotetan
ceftazidime	ceftizoxime
ceftazidime	ceftriaxone
ceftazidime	cefuroxime
Ceftin	Cefotan
Ceftin	Cefzil
Ceftin	Cipro
Ceftin	Rocephin
ceftizoxime	cefazolin
ceftizoxime	cefotaxime
ceftizoxime	cefotetan
ceftizoxime	ceftazidime
ceftizoxime	cefuroxime
ceftriaxone	cefazolin
ceftriaxone	cefotaxime
ceftriaxone	cefotetan
ceftriaxone	cefoxitin
ceftriaxone	ceftazidime
ceftriaxone	cefuroxime
ceftriaxone	Cefotan
cefuroxime	cefazolin
cefuroxime	cefotaxime

cefuroxime	cefprozil
cefuroxime	ceftazidime
cefuroxime	ceftizoxime
cefuroxime	ceftriaxone
cefuroxime	cephalexin
cefuroxime	deferoxamine
cefuroxime	cefoxitin
Cefzil	Cefol
Cefzil	Ceftin
Cefzil	Kefzol
Celebrex	Celexa
Celebrex	Cerebra
Celebrex	Cerebyx
celecoxib	Cefobid
Celexa	Celebrex
Celexa	Cerebra
Celexa	Cerebyx
Celexa	Zyprexa
cephalexin	cefaclor
cephalexin	cefazolin
cephalexin	cefuroxime
cephalexin	ciprofloxacin
Cerebra	Celebrex
Cerebra	Celexa
Cerebyx	Avelox
Cerebyx	Celebrex
Cerebyx	Celexa
cetirizine	cyclobenzaprine
chlordiazepoxide	chlorproMAZINE
chlorhexidine	chlorproMAZINE
chlorothiazide	chlorproMAZINE
chlorothiazide	chlorthalidone
chlorothiazide	chlorproPAMIDE
chlorproMAZINE	chlordiazepoxide
chlorproMAZINE	clorhexidine
chlorpromazine	chlorothiazide
chlorproMAZINE	chlorproPAMIDE
chlorproMAZINE	chlorthalidone
chlorproMAZINE	prochlorperazine
chlorproMAZINE	thioridazine
chlorproPAMIDE	chlorothiazide
chlorproPAMIDE	chlorproMAZINE
chlorthalidone	chlorothiazide
chlorthalidone	chlorproMAZINE
Cipro	Ceftin
ciprofloxacin	cephalexin
ciprofloxacin	levofloxacin
ciprofloxacin	ofloxacin
cisplatin	carboplatin
Citracal	Citrucel
Citrucel	Hydrocil
Citrucel	Citracal
Claforan	Cefotan
Claritin	Claritin-D
Claritin-D	Claritin
Clinoril	Clozaril
clomiPHENE	clomiPRAMINE
clomiPRAMINE	clomiPHENE
clomiPRAMINE	desipramine
clomiPRAMINE	Norpramin
Clonapam (clonazepam in Canada)	Corlopam (fenoldopam in U.S.)
clonazepam	alprazolam
clonazepam	clonidine
clonazepam	clorazepate
clonazepam	Klonopin
clonazepam	diazepam
clonazepam	lorazepam
clonidine	colchicine
clonidine	Cardizem
clonidine	clonazepam
clonidine	Klonopin
clorazepate	clonazepam
Clozaril	Clinoril
Clozaril	Colazal
codeine	Cardene
codeine	iodine
Codiclear DH	Codimal DH
Codimal DH	Codiclear DH
Cognex	Corgard
Colace	Calan
Colace	Peri-Colace
Colace (docusate sodium)	Colace (glycerin suppository)
Colace (glycerin suppository)	Colace (docusate sodium)
Colazal	Clozaril
colchicine	clonidine
Combivir	Epivir
Compazine	Coumadin
Cordarone	Cardura
Cordarone	Coumadin
Cordarone	Inocor
Corgard	Cognex
Corgard	Cozaar

Corlopam (fenoldopam in U.S.)	Clonapam (clonazepam in Canada)
Cortane	Cortane-B
Cortane-B	Cortane
Cortef	Lortab
cortisone	hydrocortisone
Cortisporin (ophthalmic)	Cortisporin (otic)
Cortisporin (otic)	Cortisporin (ophthalmic)
Cosopt	Trusopt
Coumadin	Avandia
Coumadin	Cardura
Coumadin	Compazine
Coumadin	Cordarone
Coumadin	Ambien
Covera	Provera
Cozaar	Corgard
Cozaar	Hyzaar
Cozaar	Zocor
cyclobenzaprine	cetirizine
cyclobenzaprine	cyproheptadine
cyclophosphamide	cycloSPORINE
cycloSERINE	cycloSPORINE
cycloSPORINE	cyclophosphamide
cycloSPORINE	cycloSERINE
cyproheptadine	cyclobenzaprine
cytarabine	Cytosar
cytarabine	Cytoxan
CytoGam	Gamimune N
Cytosar	cytarabine
Cytosar	Cytovene
Cytosar	Cytoxan
Cytosar-U	Neosar
Cytotec	Cytoxan
Cytovene	Cytosar
Cytoxan	cytarabine
Cytoxan	Cytosar
Cytoxan	Cytotec
danazol	Dantrium
Danocrine	Dantrium
Dantrium	danazol
Dantrium	Danocrine
Darvocet	Percocet
Darvocet-N	Darvon
Darvocet-N	Darvon-N
Darvon	Darvocet-N
Darvon	Diovan
Darvon-N	Darvocet-N
Datril	Detrol
DAUNOrubicin	DOXOrubicin
Daypro	Diupres
Decadron	Percodan
deferoxamine	cefuroxime
Demadex	Demerol
demeclocycline	dicyclomine
Demerol	Demadex
Demerol	Desyrel
Demerol	Dilaudid
Denavir	indinavir
Depakene	Depakote
Depakote	Depokene
Depakote	Senokot
Depakote	Depakote ER
Depakote ER	Depakote
Depo-Estradiol	Depo-Testadiol
Depo-Medrol	Depo-Provera
Depo-Provera	Depo-Medrol
Depo-Testadiol	Depo-Estradiol
Deseril (methysergide maleate in Australia)	Desyrel (trazodone in U.S.)
Desferal	DexFerrum
desipramine	clomiPRAMINE
desipramine	imipramine
desipramine	nortriptyline
Desyrel	Demerol
Desyrel (trazodone in U.S.)	Deseril (methysergide maleate in Australia)
Detrol	Datril
Detrol	Dextrostat
DexFerrum	Desferal
dextroamphetamine	dextroamphetamine and amphetamine
dextroamphetamine and amphetamine	dextroamphetamine
Dextrostat	Detrol
DiaBeta	Zebeta
DiaBeta	Zetia
Diamox	Dobutrex

Diamox	Trimox
Diamox	Tylox
Diastix	Keto-Diastix
Diatex (diazepam in Mexico)	Diatx (multivitamin in U.S.)
Diatx (multivitamin in U.S.)	Diatex (diazepam in Mexico)
diazepam	alprazolam
diazepam	clonazepam
diazepam	Ditropan
diazepam	Ditropan XL
diazepam	lorazepam
diazepam	midazolam
dicloxacillin	doxycycline
dicyclomine	demeclocycline
dicyclomine	diphenhydrAMINE
dicyclomine	doxycycline
Diflucan	Dilantin
Diflucan	Diprivan
digoxin	doxepin
Dilantin	Diflucan
Dilaudid	Demerol
Diltia XT	Cartia XT
dimenhyDRINATE	diphenhydrAMINE
Dimetapp	Donnatal
Diovan	Darvon
Diovan	Zyban
diphenhydrAMINE	dicyclomine
diphenhydrAMINE	dimenhyDRINATE
diphenhydrAMINE	dipyridamole
diphtheria and tetanus toxoid	tetanus toxoid
Diprivan	Diflucan
Diprivan	Ditropan
dipyridamole	diphenhydrAMINE
Ditropan	diazepam
Ditropan	Diprivan
Ditropan XL	diazepam
Diupres	Daypro
DOBUTamine	DOPamine
Dobutrex	Diamox
Dobutrex	DOPamine
docetaxel	paclitaxel
docusate calcium	docusate sodium
docusate sodium	docusate calcium
Dolobid	Slo-bid
donepezil	benazepril
donepezil	doxazosin
Donnatal	Dimetapp
Donnatal	Donnatal Extentabs
Donnatal Extentabs	Donnatal
DOPamine	Dobutrex
DOPamine	DOBUTamine
doxazosin	terazosin
Doxazosin	donepezil
doxepin	digoxin
doxepin	doxycycline
DOXOrubicin	DAUNOrubicin
DOXOrubicin	DOXOrubicin liposomal
DOXOrubicin	idarubicin
DOXOrubicin	Idamycin
DOXOrubicin liposomal	DOXOrubicin
doxycycline	dicloxacillin
doxycycline	dicyclomine
doxycycline	doxepin
Duratuss	Duratuss-G
Duratuss-G	Duratuss
Dynacin	DynaCirc
DynaCirc	Dynacin
Edecrin	Eulexin
Efavirenz	nelfinavir
Effexor	Effexor XR
Effexor XR	Effexor
Efudex	Eurax
Eldepryl	enalapril
Eldopaque Forte	Eldoquin Forte
Eldoquin Forte	Eldopaque Forte
Elidel	Eligard
Eligard	Elidel
Elmiron	Imuran
enalapril	Eldepryl
enalapril	lisinopril
enalapril	ramipril
enalapril	Anafranil
Enduron	Imuran
Entex LA	Eulexin
Entuss	Entuss-D
Entuss-D	Entuss
epHEDrine	epINEPHrine
epINEPHrine	epHEDrine

epINEPHrine	Neo-Synephrine	felodipine	NIFEdipine
epINEPHrine	norepinephrine	felodipine	ranitidine
Epivir	Combivir	fentanyl	Sufenta
Epogen	Neupogen	fentanyl citrate	sufentanil citrate
Equagesic	EquiGesic	Fer-In-Sol	Poly-Vi-Sol
EquiGesic	Equagesic	Fioricet	Fiorinal
Erex	Urex	Fioricet	Florinef
Erythrocin	Ethmozine	Fiorinal	Fioricet
erythromycin	azithromycin	Fleet Enema	Fleet
Eskalith	Estratest		Phospho-Soda
esmolol	Osmitrol	Fleet	Fleet Enema
esomeprazole	omeprazole	Phospho-Soda	
Estrance	Evista	Flomax	Flonase
Estraderm	Testoderm	Flomax	Flovent
estradiol	ethinyl estradiol	Flomax	Fosamax
estradiol	Risperdal	Flomax	Volmax
estramustine	exemestane	Flonase	Flomax
Estratab	Estratest	Flonase	Flovent
Estratest	Eskalith	Florinef	Fioricet
Estratest	Estratab	Florinef	fluoride
Estratest	Estratest HS	Flovent	Atrovent
Estratest HS	Estratest	Flovent	Flomax
ethambutol	Ethmozine	Flovent	Flonase
Ethinyl estradiol	estradiol	flucytosine	fluorouracil
ethinyl estradiol	ethinyl estradiol	Fludara	FUDR
and	and norgestrel	fludarabine	Flumadine
levonorgestrel		Flumadine	fludarabine
ethinyl estradiol	ethinyl estradiol	fluocinolone	fluocinonide
and norgestrel	and	fluocinonide	fluocinolone
	levonorgestrel	fluocinonide	fluorouracil
Ethmozine	ethambutol	fluoride	Florinef
Ethmozine	Erythrocin	fluorouracil	flucytosine
etidronate	etomidate	fluorouracil	fluocinonide
etidronate	etretinate	fluoxetine	fluphenazine
etomidate	etidronate	fluoxetine	fluvoxamine
etretinate	etidronate	fluoxetine	famotidine
Eulexin	Edecrin	fluoxetine	fluvastatin
Eulexin	Entex LA	fluoxetine	furosemide
Eurax	Efudex	fluoxetine	paroxetine
Evista	Estrace	fluphenazine	fluoxetine
Evista	E-Vista	fluphenazine	perphenazine
E-Vista	Evista	fluphenazine	trifluoperazine
exemestane	estramustine	flurazepam	temazepam
famciclovir	acyclovir	fluvastatin	fluoxetine
famotidine	fluoxetine	fluvoxamine	fluoxetine
famotidine	furosemide	FML Forte	FML S.O.P.
Fam-Pren Forte	Parafon Forte DSC	FML S.O.P.	FML Forte
felodipine	amlodipine	folic acid	folinic acid

folinic acid	folic acid	Haldol	Inderal
Foltex PFS	FOLTX	Haldol	Stadol
FOLTX	Foltex PFS	Haldol Decanoate	Haldol
Foradil	Toradol	haloperidol	Halotestin
Fortovase	Invirase	Halotestin	haloperidol
Fosamax	Flomax	Hemoccult	Seracult
fosinopril	bisoprolol	heparin	Levaquin
fosinopril	furosemide	heparin	Hespan
fosinopril	lisinopril	Herceptin	Perceptin
fosinopril	minoxidil	Hespan	heparin
fosphenytoin	phenytoin	Humalog	Humalog Mix
FUDR	Fludara	Humalog Mix	Humalog
furosemide	famotidine	Humalog, Insulin	Humulin, Insulin
furosemide	fluoxetine	Human	Human
furosemide	fosinopril	Humulin 70/30	Humulin N
furosemide	torsemide	Humulin 70/30	Humulin R
Gamimune N	CytoGam	Humulin L	Humulin N
Garamycin	kanamycin	Humulin L (Lente)	Humulin U
Gamulin Rh	MICRh₀GAM		(Ultralente)
Gemzar	Zinecard	Humulin N	Humulin 70/30
Gengraf	Prograf	Humulin N	Humulin R
gentamicin	tobramycin	Humulin N	Humulin U
gentamicin	vancomycin	Humulin N	Novolin N
glipiZIDE	Glucotrol	Humulin N	Humulin L
glipiZIDE	glyBURIDE	Humulin R	Humulin 70/30
Glucophage	Glucophage XR	Humulin R	Humulin N
Glucophage	Glucotrol	Humulin R	Humulin U
Glucophage	Glutofac	Humulin R	Novolin R
Glucophage XR	Glucotrol XL	Humulin U	Humulin N
Glucophage XR	Glucophage	Humulin U	Humulin R
Glucophage XR	Glucotrol	Humulin U	Humulin L (Lente)
Glucotrol	glipiZIDE	(Ultralente)	
Glucotrol	Glucophage XR	Humulin, Insulin	Humalog, Insulin
Glucotrol	Glucophage	Human	Human
Glucotrol	Glucotrol XL	Hycodan	Vicodin
Glucotrol	glyBURIDE	hydrALAZINE	hydrochlorothiazide
Glucotrol XL	Glucophage XR	hydrALAZINE	hydrocortisone
Glucotrol XL	Glucotrol	hydrALAZINE	hydrOXYzine
Glutofac	Glucophage	hydrochlorothiazide	hydrALAZINE
glyBURIDE	glipiZIDE	hydrochlorothiazide	hydroxychloroquine
glyBURIDE	Glucotrol	Hydrocil	Citrucel
Glycerin	nitroglycerin	hydrocodone	hydrocortisone
Granulex	Regranex	hydrocodone and	oxycodone and
guaifenesin	guanfacine	acetaminophen	acetaminophen
guanfacine	guaifenesin	hydrocodone and	hydromorphone
Halcion	Haldol	acetaminophen	
Haldol	Halcion	hydrocortisone	cortisone
Haldol	Haldol Decanoate	hydrocortisone	hydrALAZINE

hydrocortisone	hydrocodone
hydromorphone	hydrocodone and acetaminophen
hydromorphone	meperidine
hydromorphone	morphine
hydroxychloroquine	hydrochlorothiazide
hydroxyurea	hydrOXYzine
hydrOXYzine	hydrALAZINE
hydrOXYzine	hydroxyurea
Hygroton	Regroton
Hypergel	MPM GelPad Hydrogel Saturated Dressing
Hyzaar	Cozaar
Idamycin	Adriamycin
Idamycin	DOXOrubicin
idarubicin	DOXOrubicin
IMDUR	Imuran
IMDUR	Inderal LA
IMDUR	K-Dur
Imferon	Imuran
Imferon	Roferon-A
imipenem	meropenem
imipenem	Omnipen
imipramine	amitriptyline
imipramine	desipramine
Imodium	Indocin
Imovax	Imovax I.D.
Imovax I.D.	Imovax
Imuran	Elmiron
Imuran	Enduron
Imuran	Imferon
Imuran	IMDUR
Imuran	Tenormin
inamrinone	amiodarone
Inapsine	Lanoxin
Idamycin	DOXOrubicin
Inderal	Adderall
Inderal	Haldol
Inderal	Isordil
Inderal	Toradol
Inderal LA	Imdur
indinavir	Denavir
Indocin	Imodium
infliximab	rituximab
Inocor	Cordarone
insulin	Integrilin

insulin human	lispro, insulin human
insulin human	isophane, insulin human
Integrilin	insulin
Invanz	Avinza
Invirase	Fortovase
iodine	codeine
Ismo	Isordil
isophane, insulin human	insulin human
Isopto Carpine	Propine
Isordil	Inderal
Isordil	Ismo
isosorbide dinitrate	isosorbide mononitrate
isosorbide mononitrate	isosorbide dinitrate
Kaletra	Keppra
kanamycin	Garamycin
Kaopectate	Kayexalate
Kayexalate	Kaopectate
Kayexalate	potassium acetate
K-Dur	Cardura
K-Dur	Imdur
K-Dur	K-Lor
Keflex	Kefzol
Keflex	Norflex
Kefurox	Kefzol
Kefzol	Cefzil
Kefzol	Keflex
Kefzol	Kefurox
Kenalog	Ketalar
Keppra	Kaletra
Ketalar	Kenalog
Keto-Diastix	Diastix
ketorolac	ketotifen
ketotifen	ketorolac
Klonopin	clonazepam
Klonopin	clonidine
K-Lor	K-Dur
K-Lor	K-Lyte
K-Lyte	K-Lor
K Lyte	K-Lyte Cl
K Lyte Cl	K-Lyte
Kogenate	Kogenate-2
Kogenate-2	Kogenate
K-Phos Neutral	Neutra-Phos-K

labetolol	Lamictal
Lacrilube	Surgilube
Lamicel	Lamisil
Lamictal	labetolol
Lamictal	Lamisil
Lamictal	Lomotil
Lamictal	Ludiomil
Lamisil	Lamicel
Lamisil	Lamictal
Lamisil	Lomotil
lamivudine	lamotrigine
lamivudine	zidovudine
lamotrigine	lamivudine
Lanoxin	Inapsine
Lanoxin	Lasix
Lanoxin	levothyroxine
Lanoxin	Levoxine
Lanoxin	Levoxyl
Lanoxin	Lomotil
Lanoxin	Levsin
Lanoxin	Lonox
Lanoxin	Lovenox
Lanoxin	Xanax
Lantus, Insulin Human	Lente, Insulin Human
Lasix	Lanoxin
Lasix	Lomotil
Lasix	Luvox
L-Dopa	levodopa
L-Dopa	methyldopa
Lente, Insulin Human	lipro, insulin human
Lente, Insulin Human	Lantus, Insulin Human
leucovorin	Leukeran
leucovorin	Leukine
leucovorin	levothyroxine
Leukeran	Alkeran
Leukeran	leucovorin
Leukeran	Leukine
Leukeran	Myleran
Leukine	leucovorin
Leukine	Leukeran
Levaquin	heparin
Levaquin	Lovenox
Levaquin	Tequin
Levbid	Cefobid
Levbid	Lithobid
Levbid	Lopid
Levbid	Lorabid
Levlen	Tri-Levlen
levobunolol	levocabastine
levocabastine	levobunolol
levocarnitine	levofloxacin
levodopa	L-Dopa
levodopa	methyldopa
levodopa and carbidopa	carbidopa
levofloxacin	ciprofloxacin
levofloxacin	levocarnitine
levothyroxine	Lanoxin
levothyroxine	leucovorin
levothyroxine	liothyronine
Levoxine	Lanoxin
Levoxyl	Lanoxin
Levoxyl	Luvox
Levsin	Lanoxin
Lexapro	loxapine
Librax	Librium
Librium	Librax
Lioresal	Lotensin
liothyronine	levothyroxine
Lipitor	Zocor
lisinopril	benazepril
lisinopril	enalapril
lisinopril	fosinopril
lisinopril	quinapril
lisinopril	Risperdal
lispro, insulin human	insulin human
lispro, insulin human	Lente, Insulin Human
Lithobid	Levbid
Lithobid	Lithostat
Lithostat	Lithobid
Lomotil	Lamictal
Lomotil	Lamisil
Lomotil	Lanoxin
Lomotil	Lasix
Loniten	Lotensin
Lonox	Lanoxin
loperamide	lorazepam
Lopid	Levbid
Lopid	Lorabid
Lopid	Slo-bid
Lopurin	Lupron

Lorabid	Levbid
Lorabid	Lopid
Lorabid	Lortab
Lorabid	Slo-bid
loratadine	losartan
lorazepam	alprazolam
lorazepam	clonazepam
lorazepam	diazepam
lorazepam	loperamide
lorazepam	midazolam
lorazepam	temazepam
Lorcet	Lortab
Lortab	Cortef
Lortab	Lorabid
Lortab	Lorcet
Lortab	Luride
losartan	loratadine
losartan	valsartan
Lotensin	Lioresal
Lotensin	Loniten
Lotensin	lovastatin
Lotrimin	Lotrisone
Lotrisone	Lotrimin
Lotronex	Lovenox
Lotronex	Protonix
lovastatin	Lotensin
Lovenox	Avonex
Lovenox	Lanoxin
Lovenox	Levaquin
Lovenox	Lotronex
Lovenox	Luvox
loxapine	Lexapro
Loxitane	Soriatane
Ludiomil	Lamictal
Lupron	Lopurin
Lupron	Nuprin
Luride	Lortab
Luvox	Lasix
Luvox	Levoxyl
Luvox	Lovenox
magnesium citrate	magnesium sulfate
magnesium sulfate	magnesium citrate
Maxipime (cefepime hydrochloride in U.S.)	Moxapen (amoxacillin trihydrate in Thailand)

meclofenamate	mycophenolate
Medigesic	Medi-Gesic
Medi-Gesic	Medigesic
medroxyPRO-GESTERone	methylPRED-NISolone
medroxyPRO-GESTERone	metolazone
mefloquine	meloxicam
Megace	Reglan
Mellaril	melphalan
meloxicam	mefloquine
melphalan	Mellaril
melphalan	Myleran
meperidine	hydromorphone
meperidine	meprobamate
meperidine	methadone
meperidine	morphine
meprobamate	meperidine
Mepron (atovaquone in U.S.)	Mepron (meprobamate in Australia)
meropenem	imipenem
Meruvax	Attenuvax
mesalamine	sulfasalazine
Metadate CD	Metadate ER
Metadate ER	Metadate CD
metaxalone	metolazone
metformin	metronidazole
methadone	meperidine
methadone	methylphenidate
methazolamide	methimazole
methazolamide	metronidazole
methimazole	methazolamide
methohexital	methotrexate
methotrexate	methohexital
methotrexate	metolazone
methyldopa	L-Dopa
methyldopa	levodopa
methylphenidate	methadone
methylPRED-NISolone	medroxyPRO-GESTERone
methylPRED-NISolone	methylTESTOS-TERone
methylPRED-NISolone	predniSONE
methylTESTOS-TERone	methylPRED-NISolone
metoclopramide	metolazone

metoclopramide	metoprolol	molindone	midodrine
metoclopramide	metronidazole	Monoket	Monopril
metolazone	medroxyPRO-GESTERone	Monopril	Accupril
metolazone	metaxalone	Monopril	minoxidil
metolazone	methotrexate	Monopril	Monoket
metolazone	metoclopramide	morphine	hydromorphone
metolazone	metoprolol	morphine	meperidine
metoprolol	atenolol	Moxapen (amoxicillin trihydrate in Thailand)	Maxipime (cefepime hydrochloride in U.S.)
metoprolol	metoclopramide		
metoprolol	metolazone		
metoprolol	metronidazole	MPM GelPad Hydrogel Saturated Dressing	Hypergel
metoprolol	misoprostol		
metoprolol succinate	metoprolol tartrate		
metoprolol tartrate	metoprolol succinate	MS Contin	OxyContin
MetroGel	MetroGel-Vaginal	Murocel	Murocoll-2
MetroGel-Vaginal	MetroGel	Murocoll-2	Murocel
metronidazole	metformin	Mycelex	Mycolog
metronidazole	methazolamide	Mycolog	Mycelex
metronidazole	metoclopramide	mycophenolate	meclofenamate
metronidazole	metoprolol	Mylanta	Mylicon
metronidazole	miconazole	Myleran	Leukeran
Miacalcin	Micatin	Myleran	melphalan
Micatin	Miacalcin	Mylicon	Mylanta
miconazole	metronidazole	Naprelan	Naprosyn
MICRhₒGAM	Gamulin Rh	Naprosyn	Naprelan
Micro-K	Micronase	Naprosyn	Niaspan
Micronase	Micro-K	Narcan	Norcuron
Micronase	Microzide	Narcan	Nubain
Microzide	Micronase	Nasacort	Azmacort
midazolam	diazepam	Nasalcrom	Nasalide
midazolam	lorazepam	Nasalide	Nasalcrom
midodrin	Midrin	Nasarel	Nizoral
midodrine	molindone	Natru-Vent	Atrovent
Midrin	midodrin	Navane	Norvasc
mifepristone	misoprostol	Nebcin	Nubain
minoxidil	fosinopril	nefazodone	nelfinavir
minoxidil	Monopril	nelfinavir	efavirenz
MiraLax	Mirapex	nelfinavir	nefazodone
Mirapex	MiraLax	nelfinavir	nevirapine
misoprostol	metoprolol	Neoral	Neurontin
misoprostol	mifepristone	Neoral	Nizoral
mitomycin	mitoxantrone	Neosar	Cytosar-U
mitoxantrone	mitomycin	Neo-Synephrine	epINEPHrine
Moban	Mobic	Neo-Synephrine	Neo-Synephrine 12 Hour
Mobic	Moban	Neo-Synephrine	norepinephrine

Neo-Synephrine	Neo-Synephrine
12 Hour	
Nephrox	Niferex
Neumega	Neupogen
Neupogen	Epogen
Neupogen	Neumega
Neurontin	Neoral
Neurontin	Noroxin
Neutra-Phos	Neutra-Phos-K
Neutra-Phos-K	K-Phos Neutral
Neutra-Phos-K	Neutra-Phos
nevirapine	nelfinavir
niacin	Niaspan
Niaspan	Naprosyn
Niaspan	niacin
niCARdipine	NIFEdipine
niCARdipine	nimodipine
Nicobid	Nitro-Bid
Nicoderm	Nitroderm
NicoDerm CQ	Nitro-Dur
NIFEdipine	felodipine
NIFEdipine	niCARdipine
NIFEdipine	nimodipine
Niferex	Nephrox
Nimbex	Bumex
Nimbex	Revex
nimodipine	niCARdipine
nimodipine	NIFEdipine
Nitro-Bid	Nicobid
Nitro-Bid	Nitro-Dur
Nitroderm	Nicoderm
Nitro-Dur	NicoDerm CQ
Nitro-Dur	Nitro-Bid
Nitro-Dur	NitroQuick
nitroglycerin	glycerin
NitroQuick	Nitro-Dur
nizatidine	tizanidine
Nizoral	Nasarel
Nizoral	Neoral
Nolvadex	Norvasc
Norcuron	Narcan
norepinephrine	epINEPHrine
norepinephrine	Neo-Synephrine
norepinephrine	phenylephrine
Norflex	Keflex
Norflex	norfloxacin
Norflex	Noroxin
Norflex	Norvasc

norfloxacin	Norflex
norfloxacin	Noroxin
Noroxin	Neurontin
Noroxin	Norflex
Noroxin	norfloxacin
Norpramin	clomiPRAMINE
Norpramin	nortriptyline
nortriptyline	amitriptyline
nortriptyline	desipramine
nortriptyline	Norpramin
Norvasc	Altace
Norvasc	Navane
Norvasc	Nolvadex
Norvasc	Norflex
Norvasc	Vasotec
Norvir	Retrovir
Novolin 70/30	Novolin N
Novolin 70/30	Novolin 70/30
Penfill	Prefilled
Novolin L	Novolin N
Novolin N	Humulin N
Novolin N	Novolin 70/30
Novolin N	Novolin L
Novolin N	Novolin R
Novolin R	Humulin R
Novolin R	Novolin N
Nubain	Narcan
Nubain	Nebcin
Nuprin	Lupron
Nutropin	Nutropin AQ
Nutropin AQ	Nutropin
Ocufen	Ocuflox
Ocufen	Ocupress
Ocuflox	Ocufen
ocular lubricants	Acular
Ocumycin	Ocu-Mycin
Ocu-Mycin	Ocumycin
Ocupress	Ocufen
ofloxacin	ciprofloxacin
olanzapine	oxcarbazepine
omeprazole	esomeprazole
Omnipen	imipenem
opium tincture,	opium,
deodorized	camphorated
opium,	opium tincture,
camphorated	deodorized
oprelvekin	aldesleukin
oprelvekin	Proleukin

Orgaran	argatroban
Ortho Tri-Cyclen	Ortho-Cyclen
Ortho Tri-Cyclen	Tri-Levlen
Ortho-Cept	Ortho-Cyclen
Ortho-Cept	Ortho-Est
Ortho-Cyclen	Ortho-Cept
Ortho-Cyclen	Ortho Tri-Cyclen
Ortho-Est	Ortho-Cept
Os-Cal	Asacol
Osmitrol	esmolol
oxacillin	ampicillin
oxazepam	oxycodone
oxazepam	temazepam
oxcarbazepine	olanzapine
oxybutynin	OxyContin
oxycodone	oxazepam
oxycodone	OxyContin
oxycodone and acetaminophen	hydrocodone and acetaminophen
oxycodone and acetaminophen	oxycodone and aspirin
oxycodone and aspirin	oxycodone and acetaminophen
OxyContin	MS Contin
OxyContin	oxybutynin
OxyContin	oxycodone
paclitaxel	docetaxel
paclitaxel	paroxetine
paclitaxel	Paxil
Pamelor	Panlor SS
Panlor SS	Pamelor
papaverine	propafenone
Parafon Forte DSC	Fam-Pren Forte
Parafon Forte DSC	Profen Forte
Paraplatin	Platinol
Parlodel	pindolol
Parlodel	Provera
paroxetine	fluoxetine
paroxetine	paclitaxel
paroxetine	pyridoxine
Pathocil	Bactocil
Paxil	paclitaxel
Paxil	Plavix
Paxil	Taxol
Pediapred	Pediazole
Pediapred	Risperdal
Pediazole	Pediapred
pegaspargase	asparaginase
penicillamine	penicillin
penicillin	penicillamine
penicillin G potassium	penicillin G procaine
penicillin G procaine	penicillin G potassium
pentobarbital	phenobarbital
Pepcid	Prevacid
Perative	Periactin
Perceptin	Herceptin
Percocet	Darvocet
Percocet	Percodan
Percocet	Procet
Percodan	Decadron
Percodan	Percocet
Percodan	Peri-Colace
Percodan	Vicodin
Periactin	Perative
Peri-Colace	Colace
Peri-Colace	Percodan
Peri-Colace	Procardia
Permax	Bumex
Permax	Permitil
permethrin	pyrethrins, piperonyl butoxide
Permitil	Permax
perphenazine	fluphenazine
phenazopyridine	promethazine
Phenergan	Theragran
phenobarbital	pentobarbital
phenylephrine	norepinephrine
phenylephrine	phenytoin
phenytoin	fosphenytoin
phenytoin	phenylephrine
physostigmine	pyridostigmine
Pilocar	Polocaine
pilocarpine	proparacaine
pindolol	Parlodel
pindolol	Plendil
pioglitazone	rosiglitazone
Pitocin	Pitressin
Pitressin	Pitocin
Platinol	Paraplatin
Plavix	Paxil
Plendil	pindolol
Plendil	Pletal
Plendil	Prilosec

Plendil	Prinivil
Pletal	Plendil
pneumococcal vaccine, 23-valent (polyvalent)	pneumococcal vaccine, 7-valent
pneumococcal vaccine, 7-valent	pneumococcal vaccine, 23-valent (polyvalent)
Polocaine	Pilocar
Poly-Vi-Sol	Fer-In-Sol
potassium	predniSONE
potassium acetate	Kayexalate
potassium acetate	potassium chloride
potassium bicarbonate and potassium chloride	potassium bicarbonate and potassium citrate
potassium bicarbonate and potassium citrate	potassium bicarbonate and potassium chloride
potassium chloride	potassium acetate
potassium chloride	potassium citrate
potassium chloride	sodium chloride
potassium citrate	potassium chloride
potassium phosphate	sodium phosphate
Prandin	Avandia
Pravachol	Prevacid
Pravachol	Prinivil
Pravachol	propranolol
pravastatin	atorvastatin
prazosin	terazosin
Precare	Precose
Precose	Precare
prednisoLONE	predniSONE
predniSONE	methylPRED-NISolone
predniSONE	potassium
predniSONE	prednisoLONE
predniSONE	Prilosec
predniSONE	primidone

predniSONE	pseudoephedrine
Premarin	Prempro
Premarin	Prevacid
Premarin	Primaxin
Premarin	Provera
Premphase	Prempro
Premphase	Vancenase
Prempro	Premarin
Prempro	Premphase
Prevacid	Prinivil
Prevacid	Pepcid
Prevacid	Pravachol
Prevacid	Premarin
Prevacid	Prilosec
Preven	Preveon
Preveon	Preven
Prilosec	Plendil
Prilosec	predniSONE
Prilosec	Prevacid
Prilosec	Prinivil
Prilosec	Prozac
Primacor	Primaxin
Primatene	ProAmatine
Primaxin	Premarin
Primaxin	Primacor
primidone	predniSONE
Prinivil	Plendil
Prinivil	Pravachol
Prinivil	Prevacid
Prinivil	Prilosec
Prinivil	Prinzide
Prinivil	Proventil
Prinzide	Prinivil
Priscoline	Apresoline
ProAmatine	Primatene
ProAmatine	Protamine
probenecid	Procanbid
procainamide	prochlorperazine
Procan SR	Proscar
Procanbid	probenecid
Procardia	Peri-Colace
Procardia	Provera
Procardia XL	Cartia XT
Procet	Percocet
prochlorperazine	chlorproMAZINE
prochlorperazine	procainamide
prochlorperazine	promethazine
Proctocort	Proctocream HC

Proctocream HC	Proctocort
Profen	Profen II
Profen	Profen LA
Profen Forte	Parafon Forte DSC
Profen II	Profen
Profen II	Profen LA
Profen LA	Profen
Profen LA	Profen II
Prograf	Gengraf
Prokine	Proleukin
Proleukin	oprelvekin
Proleukin	Prokine
Prolixin	Proloid
Proloid	Prolixin
promethazine	phenazopyridine
promethazine	prochlorperazine
promethazine VC	promethazine w/codeine
promethazine VC w/codeine	promethazine w/codeine
promethazine w/codeine	promethazine VC w/codeine
promethazine w/codeine	promethazine VC
propafenone	papaverine
proparacaine	pilocarpine
Propine	Isopto Carpine
propranolol	Pravachol
propranolol	Propulsid
Propulsid	propranolol
propythiouracil	Purinethol
Proscar	Procan SR
Proscar	ProSom
Proscar	Prozac
Proscar	Provera
ProSom	Proscar
ProSom	Prozac
Protamine	ProAmatine
Protonix	Lotronex
Proventil	Bentyl
Proventil	Prinivil
Provera	Covera
Provera	Parlodel
Provera	Premarin
Provera	Procardia
Provera	Proscar
Prozac	Prilosec
Prozac	Proscar
Prozac	ProSom
pseudoephedrine	predniSONE
Pulmicort	Pulmozyme
Pulmozyme	Pulmicort
Purinethol	propythiouracil
pyrazinamide	pyridostigmine
pyrethrins, piperonyl butoxide	permethrin
Pyridium	pyridoxine
pyridostigmine	physostigmine
pyridostigmine	pyrazinamide
pyridostigmine	pyridoxine
pyridoxine	paroxetine
pyridoxine	Pyridium
pyridoxine	pyridostigmine
pyridoxine	pyrimethamine
pyrimethamine	pyridoxine
Quibron	Quibron-T
Quibron	Quibron-T/SR
Quibron-T	Quibron
Quibron-T	Quibron-T/SR
Quibron-T/SR	Quibron
Quibron-T/SR	Quibron-T
quinacrine	quinidine
quinapril	lisinopril
quinidine	quinacrine
quinidine	quinine
quinine	quinidine
raloxifene	ropinirole
ramipril	enalapril
ramipril	rifampin
ranitidine	amantadine
ranitidine	rimantadine
ranitidine	felodipine
ratgam (synonym for thymoglobulin)	Atgam
ReFresh (breath drops)	Refresh (lubricant eye drops)
Refresh (lubricant eye drops)	ReFresh (breath drops)
Reglan	Megace
Reglan	Renagel
Reglan	Robitussin
Reglan	Zofran
Regranex	Granulex
Regroton	Hygroton

Relafen	Rezulin	Robitussin	Reglan
Remegel	Renagel	Robitussin	Robitussin DM
Remeron	Restoril	Robitussin AC	Robitussin DAC
Remeron	Zemuron	Robitussin AC	Robitussin DM
Renagel	Reglan	Robitussin DAC	Robitussin AC
Renagel	Remegel	Robitussin DM	Robitussin
Reno-60	Renografin-60	Robitussin DM	Robitussin AC
Renografin-60	Reno-60	Robitussin DM	Rondec DM
Reopro	Rheomacrodex	Rocephin	Ceftin
repaglinide	rosiglitazone	Roferon-A	Imferon
Requip	Risperdal	Rondec DM	Robitussin DM
reserpine	Risperdal	ropinirole	raloxifene
reserpine	risperidone	ropinirole	risperidone
Restoril	Remeron	ropivacaine	bupivacaine
Restoril	Risperdal	rosiglitazone	pioglitazone
Restoril	Vistaril	rosiglitazone	repaglinide
Retavase	Activase	Roxanol	Roxicet
Retrovir	Norvir	Roxanol	Roxicodone
Retrovir	ritonavir	Roxanol	Roxicodone Intensol
Revex	Nimbex		
Revex	ReVia	Roxicet	Roxanol
ReVia	Revex	Roxicet	Roxicodone
Rezulin	Relafen	Roxicodone	Roxanol
Rheomacrodex	Reopro	Roxicodone	Roxicet
Ridaura	Cardura	Roxicodone	Roxicodone Intensol
rifabutin	rifampin		
Rifadin	Rifater	Roxicodone Intensol	Roxanol
rifampin	ramipril		
rifampin	rifabutin	Roxicodone Intensol	Roxicodone
Rifater	Rifadin		
rimantadine	amantadine	Rynatan	Rynatuss
rimantadine	ranitidine	Rynatuss	Rynatan
risedronate	risperidone	Salagen	selegiline
Risperdal	estradiol	Salbutamol (albuterol in other countries)	salmeterol
Risperdal	lisinopril		
Risperdal	Pediapred		
Risperdal	Requip		
Risperdal	reserpine	salmeterol	Salbutamol (albuterol in other countries)
Risperdal	risperidone		
Risperdal	Restoril		
risperidone	reserpine		
risperidone	Risperdal	salsalate	sulfasalazine
risperidone	risedronate	Sarafem	Serophene
risperidone	ropinirole	Sarafem	Sinequan
Ritalin	Ritalin SR	selegiline	Salagen
Ritalin SR	Ritalin	selegiline	Serentil
ritonavir	Retrovir	selegiline	sertraline
rituximab	infliximab	selegiline	Serzone

Senna	Soma
Senokot	Depakote
Senokot	Sinemet
Seracult	Hemoccult
Serentil	selegiline
Serentil	Seroquel
Serentil	sertraline
Serentil	Serzone
Serentil	Sinequan
Serevent	Atrovent
Serevent	Serevent Diskus
Serevent Diskus	Serevent
Serophene	Sarafem
Seroquel	Serentil
Seroquel	Serzone
Seroquel	Sinequan
Seroquel	Symmetrel
Seroquel	sertraline
sertraline	selegiline
sertraline	Serentil
sertraline	Serzone
sertraline	Seroquel
Serzone	selegiline
Serzone	Serentil
Serzone	Seroquel
Serzone	sertraline
Serzone	Sinequan
Sinemet	Senokot
Sinemet	Sinemet CR
Sinemet CR	Sinemet
Sinequan	Sarafem
Sinequan	Serentil
Sinequan	Seroquel
Sinequan	Serzone
Sinequan	Singulair
Singulair	Sinequan
Slo-bid	Dolobid
Slo-bid	Lopid
Slo-bid	Lorabid
Slow Fe	Slow-K
Slow-K	Slow Fe
sodium bicarbonate	sodium chloride
sodium chloride	potassium chloride
sodium chloride	sodium bicarbonate
sodium phosphate	potassium phosphate

Solu-Cortef	Solu-Medrol
Solu-Medrol	Depo-Medrol
Solu-Medrol	Solu-Cortef
Soma	Senna
Soma	Soma Compound
Soma Compound	Soma
Soriatane	Loxitane
sotalol	Stadol
sotalol	Subdue
Stadol	Haldol
Stadol	Toradol
Stadol	sotalol
Subdue	sotalol
Sufenta	fentanyl
sufentanil citrate	fentanyl citrate
sulfADIAZINE	sulfasalazine
sulfADIAZINE	sulfiSOXAZOLE
sulfasalazine	mesalamine
sulfasalazine	salsalate
sulfasalazine	sulfADIAZINE
sulfasalazine	sulfiSOXAZOLE
sulfiSOXAZOLE	sulfADIAZINE
sulfiSOXAZOLE	sulfasalazine
sumatriptan	zolmitriptan
Suprax	Surfak
Surfak	Suprax
Surgilube	Lacrilube
Symmetrel	Amaryl
Symmetrel	Seroquel
Symmetrel	Synthroid
Synagis	Synvisc
Synthroid	Symmetrel
Synvisc	Synagis
Tambocor	Temodar
Tamiflu	tamoxifen
Tamiflu	Theraflu
tamoxifen	Tamiflu
tamoxifen	tamsulosin
tamsulosin	tamoxifen
Taxol	Paxil
Taxol	Taxotere
Taxotere	Taxol
Tedral	Teldrin
Tegretol	Toradol
Tegretol	Trental
Tegretol	Trileptal
Tegretol-XR	Toprol-XR
Teldrin	Tedral

temazepam	flurazepam
temazepam	lorazepam
temazepam	oxazepam
Temodar	Tambocor
Tenormin	Imuran
Tenormin	thiamine
Tenormin	Trovan
Tequin	Levaquin
Tequin	Ticlid
terazosin	prazosin
terazosin	doxazosin
Testoderm	Estraderm
tetanus toxoid	diphtheria and tetanus toxoid
tetracycline	tetradecyl sulfate
tetradecyl sulfate	tetracycline
Thalitone	Thalomid
Thalomid	Thalitone
Theraflu	Tamiflu
Theragran	Phenergan
thiamine	Tenormin
thioridazine	chlorproMAZINE
Thorazine	thioridazine
thioridazine	Thorazine
Thyrar	Thyrolar
Thyrolar	Thyrar
tiagabine	tizanidine
Tiazac	Tigan
Tiazac	Ziac
Ticlid	Tequin
Tigan	Tiazac
Timoptic	Timoptic-XE
Timoptic	Viroptic
Timoptic-XE	Timoptic
tizanidine	nizatidine
tizanidine	tiagabine
TNKase	t-PA (synonym for alteplase, recombinant)
Tobradex	Tobrex
tobramycin	gentamicin
Tobrex	Tobradex
TOLAZamide	TOLBUTamide
TOLBUTamide	TOLAZamide
tolcapone	tolterodine
tolterodine	tolcapone
Topamax	Toprol-XL
topiramate	torsemide
Toprol-XL	Tegretol-XR
Toprol-XL	Topamax
Toradol	Foradil
Toradol	Inderal
Toradol	Stadol
Toradol	Tegretol
Toradol	Torecan
Toradol	tramadol
Torecan	Toradol
torsemide	furosemide
torsemide	topiramate
t-PA (synonym for alteplase, recombinant)	TNKase
tramadol	Toradol
tramadol	trandolapril
tramadol	trazodone
tramadol	Voltaren
Trandate	Trental
Trandate	Tridrate
trandolapril	tramadol
trazodone	amiodarone
trazodone	tramadol
Trental	Tegretol
Trental	Trandate
Triad (butalbital, acetaminophen, caffeine)	Triad (topical)
Triad (topical)	Triad (butalbital, acetaminophen, caffeine)
triamterene	trimethoprim
Tridrate	Trandate
trifluoperazine	fluphenazine
trifluoperazine	trihexyphenidyl
trihexyphenidyl	trifluoperazine
Trileptal	Tegretol
Tri-Levlen	Levlen
Tri-Levlen	Ortho Tri-Cyclen
trimethoprim	triamterene
Trimox	Diamox
Trimox	Tylox
Tri-Nasal	Triphasil
Tri-Norinyl	Triphasil
Triphasil	Tri-Nasal
Triphasil	Tri-Norinyl
Trovan	Tenormin
Trusopt	Cosopt

Tylenol	Tylenol w/codeine	Vasocon A	Vasocon
Tylenol Children's	Tylenol w/codeine	Vasotec	Norvasc
Tylenol w/codeine	Tylenol	vecuronium	vancomycin
Tylenol w/codeine	Tylenol Children's	Ventolin	Benylin
Tylox	Diamox	Ventolin	Vantin
Tylox	Trimox	Vepesid	Versed
Tylox	Wymox	verapamil	Verelan
Tylox	Xanax	Verelan	verapamil
Ultane	Ultram	Verelan	Virilon
Ultracef	Ultracet	Versed	Valium
(cefadroxil in	(acetaminophen/	Versed	Vepesid
other	tramadol	Versed	Vistaril
countries)	hydrochloride	Vexol	VoSol
	in U.S.)	Viagra	Allegra
Ultracet	Ultracef	Vibramycin	vancomycin
(acetaminophen/	(cefadroxil	Vicodin	Hycodan
tramadol	in other	Vicodin	Percodan
hydrochloride	countries)	Vicodin	Uridon
in U.S.)		Vicodin	Valium
Ultram	Ultane	Vicodin	Vicodin ES
Ultram	Voltaren	Vicodin ES	Vicodin
Unasyn	Zosyn	vinBLAStine	vinCRIStine
Uniretic	Univasc	vinCRIStine	vinBLAStine
Univasc	Uniretic	Viracept	Viramune
Univasc	Urispas	Viramune	Viracept
Urex	Erex	Virilon	Verelan
Uridon	Vicodin	Viroptic	Timoptic
Urised	Urocit-K	Visicol	bisacodyl
Urispas	Univasc	Vistaril	Restoril
Urispas	Uro-Mag	Vistaril	Versed
valacyclovir	valgancyclovir	Vistaril	Zestril
Valcyte	Valtrex	Vitamin C	Vitamin E
valgancyclovir	valacyclovir	Vitamin D	Vitamin E
Valium	Versed	Vitamin E	Vitamin C
Valium	Vicodin	Vitamin E	Vitamin D
valsartan	losartan	Volmax	Flomax
Valtrex	Valcyte	Voltaren	tramadol
Vancenase	Premphase	Voltaren	Ultram
Vancenase	Vanceril	VoSol	Vexol
Vancenase AQ	Vanceril DS	Wellbutrin	Wellbutrin SR
Vanceril	Vancenase	Wellbutrin SR	Wellbutrin
Vanceril DS	Vancenase AQ	Wymox	Tylox
vancomycin	azithromycin	Xalatan	Xalcom
vancomycin	gentamicin		(latanoprost,
vancomycin	vecuronium		timolol in other
vancomycin	Vibramycin		countries)
Vantin	Ventolin		
Vasocon	Vasocon A		

Xalcom (latanoprost, timolol in other countries)	Xalatan
Xanax	Lanoxin
Xanax	Tylox
Xanax	Zanaflex
Xanax	Zantac
Xanax	Zyrtec
Xeloda	Xenical
Xenical	Xeloda
Xigris	zydis (dosage form trademark)
Yocon	Zocor
Zagam	Zyban
zaleplon	zolpidem
Zanaflex	Anaflex
Zanaflex	Xanax
Zantac	Xanax
Zantac	Zofran
Zantac	Zyrtec
Zaroxolyn	Zyprexa
Zebeta	DiaBeta
Zebeta	Zetia
Zemuron	Remeron
Zerit	Zestril
Zestril	Vistaril
Zestril	Zerit
Zestril	Zocor
Zestril	Zyrtec
Zetia	DiaBeta
Zetia	Zebeta
Ziac	Tiazac
Ziac	Zocor
zidovudine	lamivudine
zidovudine	zidovudine and lamivudine
zidovudine	ziprasidone
zidovudine and lamivudine	zidovudine

Zinacef	Zithromax
Zinecard	Gemzar
ziprasidone	zidovudine
Zithromax	Zinacef
Zocor	Cozaar
Zocor	Lipitor
Zocor	Yocon
Zocor	Zestril
Zocor	Ziac
Zocor	Zoloft
Zofran	Reglan
Zofran	Zantac
Zofran	Zosyn
zolmitriptan	sumatriptan
Zoloft	Zocor
Zoloft	Zyloprim
zolpidem	zaleplon
Zonalon	Zone A Forte
Zone A Forte	Zonalon
Zosyn	Unasyn
Zosyn	Zofran
Zovirax	Zyvox
Zyban	Diovan
Zyban	Zagam
Zydis (dosage from trademark)	Xigris
Zyloprim	Zoloft
Zyprexa	Celexa
Zyprexa	Zaroxolyn
Zyprexa	Zyprexa Zydis
Zyprexa	Zyrtec
Zyprexa Zydis	Zyprexa
Zyrtec	Xanax
Zyrtec	Zantac
Zyrtec	Zestril
Zyrtec	Zyprexa
Zyvox	Zovirax

Appendix j

Medications that may be inappropriate for geriatric patients

DRUG	CONCERN
Antihistamines Anticholinergic antihistamines: • chlorpheniramine (Chlor-Trimeton) • cyproheptadine (Periactin) • dexchlorpheniramine (Polaramine) • diphenhydramine (Benadryl) • hydrOXYzine (Vistaril, Atarax) • promethazine (Phenergan) • tripelennamine (PBZ)	• Potent anticholinergics • May cause confusion and excessive sedation • Should not be used as a hypnotic • Use nonanticholinergic antihistamines in the geriatric population
Antidepressants Anticholinergic antidepressants: • amitriptyline (Elavil) • doxepin (Sinequan)	• Strong anticholinergic and sedation properties • Rarely the antidepressant of choice for the geriatric population
fluoxetine (Prozac)	• Long half-life with greater risk for CNS stimulation
Antidiabetic Agents chlorpropamide (Diabinese)	• Prolonged half-life in geriatric patients with risk for prolonged hypoglycemia • Risk for SIADH
Antiinfective nitrofurantoin (Macrodantin)	• Not effective with renal impairment
Antipsychotics mesoridazine (Serentil) thioridazine (Mellaril)	• Higher risk CNS and anticholinergic adverse drug effects • Risk for QT interval prolongation and torsades de pointes
Anxiolytics/Sedatives Barbiturates used for sedative/hypnotic (exception: phenobarbital for seizure control)	• Potential for dependence • Greater risk for adverse drug effects than alternative therapies
Benzodiazepines (long acting) • chlordiazepoxide (Librium) • diazepam (Valium) • flurazepam (Dalmane)	• Prolonged half-life in geriatric patients • Prolonged sedation effects • Increased risk for falls

Benzodiazepines (short acting [do not exceed dose in brackets]) • alprazolam (Xanax) [2 mg] • lorazepam (Ativan) [3 mg] • temazepam (Restoril) [15 mg]	• Higher doses do not usually provide additional benefit • Higher doses associated with increased risk of adverse drug effects
meprobamate (Miltown)	• May cause dependence • Excessive sedation
Cardiovascular Agents amiodarone (Cordarone)	• Associated with QT interval prolongation and risk for torsades de pointes • Lack of efficacy in geriatric patients
disopyramide (Norpace, Norpace CR)	• Potent negative inotrope with risk for heart failure • Anticholinergic
guanadrel (Hylorel) guanethidine (Ismelin)	• May cause orthostatic hypotension • Safer alternatives exist
methyldopa (Aldomet)	• Risk for bradycardia • Increased risk for depression in geriatric patients
nifedipine, short acting (Procardia, Adalat)	• Risk for hypotension and constipation
ticlopidine (Ticlid)	• No more effective than aspirin as antiplatelet • Safer alternatives available
Gastrointestinal (GI) Drugs GI antispasmodic agents: • dicyclomine (Bentyl) • hyoscyamine (Levsin, Levsinex) • propantheline (Pro-Banthine) • belladonna alkaloids (Donnatal) • clidinium-chlordiazepoxide (Librax)	• Highly anticholinergic • Of uncertain benefit
trimethobenzamide (Tigan)	• Extrapyramidal effects (EPS) • Among the least effective antiemetics
Hormonal Agents desiccated thyroid	• Risk cardiac adverse effects
methyltestosterone (Android, Virilon, Testrad)	• Potential for prostatic enlargement • Potential for cardiac problems
Laxatives Stimulant laxatives (long term): • bisacodyl (Dulcolax) • cascara sagrada (Neoloid)	• Risk for increased bowel dysfunction considered appropriate in the presence of opiate therapy
mineral oil	• Risk for aspiration pneumonia

Muscle Relaxants and Antispasmodics carisoprodol (Soma) chlorzoxazone (Paraflex) cyclobenzaprine (Flexeril) metaxalone (Skelaxin) methocarbamol (Robaxin) orphenadrine (Norflex) oxybutynin (Ditropan)	• Anticholinergic adverse effects • Excessive sedation and weakness • Often poorly tolerated in older adults
Nonsteroidal Antiinflammatory Drugs (NSAIDs) indomethacin (Indocin and Indocin SR)	• NSAID that produces the most CNS adverse effects
ketorolac (Toradol)	• Significant number of asymptomatic GI pathologic conditions
NSAIDs, long-term use of longer half-life, non–COX-selective • naproxen (Naprosyn, Anaprox, Aleve) • oxaprozin (Daypro) • piroxicam (Feldene)	Greater risk for: • GI bleeding • Renal failure • Hypertension • Heart failure
Opioid Analgesics meperidine (Demerol)	• Not as effective as oral analgesics in commonly prescribed dosages • May cause confusion, seizures
pentazocine (Talwin)	• Cases more CNS adverse effects than other opioid analgesics (e.g., confusion and hallucinations)
Stimulants amphetamines anorexic drugs	• May cause dependence • Cardiovascular risks: hypertension, angina, MI

In McKenry LM, Tessier E, Hogan MA: *Mosby's pharmacology in nursing*, ed 22, St. Louis, 2006, Mosby. Modified from Fick DM, Cooper JW, Wade WE, et al: Updating the Beers criteria for potentially inappropriate medication use in older adults, *Archives of Internal Medicine* 163(22): 2716-2724, 2003.

Appendix k Drugs metabolized by known P450s

SUBSTRATES

1A2	2B6	2C8	2C19	2C9	2D6	2E1	3A4, 5, 7
clozapine	bupropion		**Proton Pump Inhibitors:**	**NSAIDs:**	**Beta-Blockers:**	acetaminophen	**Macrolide antibiotics:**
			omeprazole	diclofenac	S-metoprolol	chlorzoxazone	clarithromycin
cyclobenzaprine	cyclophosphamide		lansoprazole	ibuprofen	propafenone	ethanol	erythromycin
imipramine	efavirenz		pantoprazole	piroxicam	timolol		NOT azithromycin
mexiletine	ifosfamide		rabeprazole	**Oral Hypoglycemic Agents:**	**Antidepressants:**		telithromycin
naproxen	methadone						
				tolbutamide	amitriptyline		**Antiarrhythmics:**
riluzole			**Antiepileptics:**	glipizide	clomipramine		quinidine
tacrine			diazepam	**Angiotensin II Blockers:**	desipramine		**Benzodiazepines:**
theophylline			phenytoin	NOT candesartan	imipramine		alprazolam
			phenobarbitone	irbesartan	paroxetine		diazepam
			amitriptyline	losartan	**Antipsychotics:**		midazolam
			clomipramine	NOT valsartan	haloperidol		triazolam
			cyclophosphamide	celecoxib	risperidone		**Immune Modulators:**
			progesterone				cyclosporine
				fluvastatin	thioridazine		

Continued

Appendix k Drugs metabolized by known P450s—cont'd

1A2	2B6	2C8	2C19	2C9	2D6	2E1	3A4, 5, 7
				naproxen	aripiprazole		tacrolimus (FK506)
							HIV Protease Inhibitors:
				phenytoin	codeine		indinavir
							ritonavir
				sulfamethoxazole	dextromethorphan		saquinavir
				tamoxifen	duloxetine		**Prokinetic:**
				tolbutamide	flecainide		cisapride
				torsemide	mexiletine		**Antihistamines:**
				warfarin	ondansetron		astemizole
					tamoxifen		chlorpheniramine
					tramadol		**Calcium Channel Blockers:**
					venlafaxine		amlodipine
							diltiazem
							felodipine
							nifedipine
							nisoldipine
							nitrendipine
							verapamil

HMG-CoA Reductase Inhibitors:							
atorvastatin							
cerivastatin							
lovastatin							
NOT pravastatin							
simvastatin							
aripiprazole							
buspirone							
gleevec							
haloperidol (in part)							
methadone							
pimozide							
quinine							
NOT rosuvastatin							
sildenafil							
tamoxifen							
trazodone							
vincristine							

Continued

Appendix k Drugs metabolized by known P450s—cont'd

INHIBITORS

1A2	2B6	2C8	2C19	2C9	2D6	2E1	3A4, 5, 7
cimetidine	thiotepa	gemfibrozil	fluoxetine	amiodarone	amiodarone	disulfiram	**HIV Protease Inhibitors:**
fluoroquinolones	ticlopidine	montelukast	fluvoxamine	fluconazole	buproprion		indinavir
fluvoxamine			ketoconazole	isoniazid	chlorpheniramine		nelfinavir
ticlopidine			lansoprazole		cimetidine		ritonavir
			omeprazole		clomipramine		amiodarone
			ticlopidine		duloxetine		NOT azithromycin
					fluoxetine		cimetidine
					haloperidol		clarithromycin
					methadone		diltiazem
					mibefradil		erythromycin
					paroxetine		fluvoxamine
					quinidine		grapefruit juice
					ritonavir		itraconazole
							ketoconazole
							mibefradil
							nefazodone
							troleandomycin
							verapamil

INDUCERS

1A2	2B6	2C8	2C19	2C9	2D6	2E1	3A4, 5, 7
tobacco	phenobarbital		N/A	rifampin	N/A	ethanol	carbamazepine
	phenytoin			secobarbital		isoniazid	phenobarbital
	rifampin						phenytoin
							rifabutin
							rifampin
							St. John's wort
							troglitazone

Copyright 2006, David A. Flockhart, MD, PhD, Indiana University School of Medicine, http://medicine.iupui.edu/flockhart.

Appendix I

Safety in handling chemotherapeutic agents

PREVENTION OF INHALATION OF AEROSOLS

1. Mix all drugs in an approved class II or III vertical airflow biologic safety cabinet (BSC), wearing gloves made of latex or nitrile at all times. Surgical masks do not prevent aerosol inhalation and should not be used. Wear eye and face barriers if splashes are likely to occur or sprays or aerosols are used.
2. Prime all intravenous (IV) bags within the BSC before adding the drug. Use a maintenance bag of normal saline or 5% dextrose in water (D_5W) to prime the tubing and all the chemotherapy bags afterward.
3. Break ampules by wrapping a sterile gauze pad or alcohol wipe around the neck (decreases chance of droplet contamination).
4. Vent vials with only enough air to allow the drug to be aspirated easily using a hydrophobic filter needle.
5. Syringes and needles used in cytotoxic drug preparation should not be crushed, clipped, or recapped. They should immediately be placed in a sharps container labeled "cytotoxic waste" for disposal.
6. Use a gauze pad when removing syringes and needles from IV injection ports or spikes from IV bags.

PREVENTION OF DRUG ABSORPTION THROUGH SKIN

1. Wear latex or nitrile gloves and a gown of nonpermeable fabric with a closed front and cuffed, long sleeves.
2. Change gloves every 60 minutes.
3. Remove gloves immediately after spilling drug solution on them or puncturing or tearing them.
4. Wash hands before putting on gloves and after removing them.
5. Cover the work surface with a plastic-backed absorbent pad; change pad when cabinet is cleaned or after a spill.
6. Clean all surfaces of the BSC before and after drug preparation in accordance with manufacturer's instructions. Discard equipment used in a leakproof, puncture-proof, chemical-waste container.
7. Use syringes and IV sets with Luer-Lok fittings.
8. Place an absorbent pad under injection sites to catch accidental spillage.
9. Label all antineoplastic drugs with a chemotherapy warning label.
10. Wash skin thoroughly with soap and water as soon as possible in the event of skin contact with drugs.
11. Flush eyes with eye solution or clean water in the event of eye contact; seek medical attention.

🅐 Safety alert   *"Tall Man" lettering

PREVENTION OF INGESTION

1. Do not eat, drink, chew gum, apply cosmetics, store food, or smoke in drug preparation areas.
2. Wash hands before and after preparing or giving drugs.
3. Avoid hand-to-mouth or hand-to-eye contact when handling the drugs.

SAFE DISPOSAL

1. Discard nonsharp cytotoxic waste products in a leakproof, puncture-proof, sealable plastic bag of a different color than regular trash bags. Label "cytotoxic waste."
2. Use a leakproof, puncture-proof container labeled "cytotoxic waste" for needles and sharp, breakable items.
3. Keep waste in labeled, covered containers for disposal.
4. Ensure housekeeping personnel are instructed in safe procedures and wear latex or nitrile gloves and gowns of nonpermeable fabric.
5. All waste produced by cytotoxic drug administration in the home should be placed in a sealed receptacle and transported in the nonpassenger area of a vehicle to the home agency for disposal.

PREVENTION OF CONTAMINATION BY BODY FLUIDS

1. Wear latex or nitrile gloves and disposable, nonpermeable fabric when handling any body fluids.
2. Empty waste products into the toilet by pouring close to the water to avoid splashing. Close the lid and flush two or three times (in the home).
3. Wear gloves and gown when handling linen soiled with body fluids; place in isolation linen bag for separate laundry.
4. Place soiled linens in separate, washable pillow cases and wash twice, separately from other household linens (in the home).
5. A standard duration of 48 hours is accepted as the time after which most cytotoxic drugs will have been metabolized or excreted. For most cytotoxic agents, urinary excretion is complete within 48 hours after administration (range of 1 to 6 days) and stool excretion is complete within 7 days (range of 5 to 7 days).

From Monahan FD, et al: *Phipps' medical-surgical nursing,* ed 8, St. Louis, 2007, Mosby.

Appendix m

High-alert drugs

The Institute for Safe Medication Practices (ISMP) recently compiled a list of the medications with the greatest potential for patient harm if they are used in error. These high-alert medications include drugs in the 19 classes listed below, as well as the specific drugs listed below. To help nurses identify these drugs, each specific drug monograph is clearly identified in this book. While care should be taken in giving any medication, nurses are advised to exercise extra precautions when administering these high-risk drugs.

Class/Category of Medications
adrenergic agonists, IV (e.g., epINEPHrine)
adrenergic antagonists, IV (e.g., propranolol)
anesthetic agents, general, inhaled and IV (e.g., propofol)
cardioplegic solutions
chemotherapeutic agents, parenteral and oral
dextrose, hypertonic, 20% or greater
dialysis solutions, peritoneal and hemodialysis
epidural or intrathecal medications
glycoprotein IIb/IIIa inhibitors (e.g., eptifibatide)
hypoglycemics, oral
inotropic medications, IV (e.g., digoxin, milrinone)
liposomal forms of drugs (e.g., liposomal amphotericin B)
moderate sedation agents, IV (e.g., midazolam)
moderate sedation agents, oral, for children (e.g., chloral hydrate)
narcotics/opiates, IV and oral (including liquid concentrates, immediate- and sustained-release) formulations
neuromuscular blocking agents (e.g., succinylcholine)
radiocontrast agents, IV
thrombolytics/fibrinolytics, IV (e.g., tenecteplase)
total parenteral nutrition solutions

Individual Medications

abciximab
adenosine
aldesleukin
alteplase
amiodarone
anistreplase
antihemophilic factor VIII (AHF)
antithrombin III, human
argatroban
arsenic trioxide
asparaginase
atropine

azacitidine
basiliximab
bevacizumab
bivalirudin
bleomycin
busulfan
carboplatin
carmustine
celecoxib
cisplatin
coagulation factor VIIa,
   recombinant

A Safety alert   *"Tall Man" lettering

cyclophosphamide
cytarabine
dacarbazine
daclizumab
dactinomycin
dalteparin
DAUNOrubicin
DAUNOrubicin citrate liposome
digoxin
diltiazem
DOPamine
doxacurium
DOXOrubicin
DOXOrubicin liposome
droperidol
enoxaparin
epHEDrine
epINEPHrine
epirubicin
eptifibatide
etoposide
factor IX complex (human)
fentanyl
fentanyl transdermal
fluorouracil
gemtuzumab
heparin
hydromorphone
ibutilide
idarubicin
ifosfamide
inamrinone
insulins
insulin, inhaled
irinotecan
lepirudin
leuprolide
lidocaine (parenteral)
magnesium sulfate
melphalan
meperidine
methadone

methotrexate (amethopterin, MTX)
milrinone
mitomycin
mitoxantrone
mivacurium
morphine
nalbuphine
nesiritide
nitroprusside
norepinephrine
oxycodone
oxymorphone
oxytocin
pancuronium
pegaspargase
pemetrexed
pentazocine
pentobarbital
pentostatin
phenobarbital
plicamycin
poractant alfa
propofol
propoxyphene
remifentanil
rocuronium
secobarbital
streptokinase
succinylcholine
tenecteplase
thiopental
tinzaparin
tirofiban
topotecan
trastuzumab
tubocurarine
urokinase
vecuronium
vinBLAStine
vinCRIStine
vinorelbine
warfarin

1. Cohen MR, Kilo CM: High-alert medications: safeguarding against errors. In Cohen MR, editor: *Medication errors,* Washington, DC, 1999, American Pharmaceutical Association.
2. High-alert medications and patient safety, *Sentinel Event Alert* 11, Nov 1999.
3. *ISMP's list of high-alert medications,* accessed 1/23/07 at http://www.ismp.org/tools/highalertmedications.pdf.

Appendix n

Controlled substance chart

Drugs	United States*
Heroin, LSD, peyote, marijuana, mescaline	**Schedule I** • High abuse potential • No currently accepted medical use
Opium (morphine), meperidine, amphetamines, cocaine, short-acting barbiturates (secobarbital)	**Schedule II** • High abuse potential; potentially severe psychologic or physical dependence • Currently accepted medical use but may be severely restricted • Telephone orders only in emergencies if written Rx follows promptly • No refills
Glutethimide, paregoric, phendimetrazine	**Schedule III** • Abuse potential less than the drugs/substances in Schedules I and II; potentially moderate or low physical dependence or high psychologic dependence • Currently accepted medical use • Telephone orders permitted • Prescriber may authorize limited refills
Chloral hydrate, chlordiazepoxide, diazepam, mazindol, meprobamate, phenobarbital	**Schedule IV** • Low abuse potential relative to drugs/substances in Schedule III; potentially limited physical or psychologic dependence • Currently accepted medical use • Telephone orders permitted • Prescriber may authorize limited refills
Antidiarrheals with opium, antitussives	**Schedule V** • Lowest abuse potential; potentially very limited physical or psychologic dependence • Currently accepted medical use • Prescriber determines refills • Some products containing limited amounts of Schedule V substances (e.g., cough suppressants) available OTC to patients >18 yr

*See appendix q for Canadian controlled substance chart

Appendix o Recommended childhood and adolescent immunization schedule—United States, 2007

Immunization Schedule for Persons Aged 0–6 Years

Vaccine ▼ Age ►	Birth	1 month	2 months	4 months	6 months	12 months	15 months	18 months	19–23 months	2–3 years	4–6 years
Hepatitis B [*]	HepB	HepB		see footnote1		HepB			HepB Series		
Rotavirus [*]			Rota	Rota	Rota						
Diphtheria, Tetanus, Pertussis [*]			DTaP	DTaP	DTaP		DTaP				DTaP
Haemophilus influenzae type b [*]			Hib	Hib	Hib [4]	Hib		Hib			
Pneumococcal [*]			PCV	PCV	PCV	PCV				PCV / PPV	
Inactivated Poliovirus			IPV	IPV		IPV					IPV
Influenza [*]						Influenza (Y early)					
Measles, Mumps, Rubella [*]						MMR					MMR
Varicella [*]						Varicella					Varicella
Hepatitis A [*]						HepA (2 doses)				HepA Series	
Meningococcal [*]										MPSV4	

Legend:
- Range of recommended ages
- Catch-up immunization
- Certain high-risk groups

This schedule indicates the recommended ages for routine administration of currently licensed childhood vaccines, as of December 1, 2006, for children aged 0–6 years. Any dose not administered at the recommended age should be administered at any subsequent visit, when indicated and feasible. Additional vaccines may be licensed and recommended during the year. Licensed combination vaccines may be used whenever any components of the combination are indicated and other components of the vaccine are not contraindicated and if approved by the Food and Drug Administration for that dose of the series. Providers should consult the respective ACIP statement for detailed recommendations. Clinically significant adverse events that follow immunization should be reported to the Vaccine Adverse Event Reporting System (VAERS). Guidance about how to obtain and complete a VAERS form is available at http://www.vaers.hhs.gov or by telephone, **800-822-7967**.

[*] For complete information go to http://www.cdc.gov/nip/recs/child-schedule.htm#printable.

Immunization Schedule for Persons Aged 7–18 Years

Vaccine ▼	Age ▶	7–10 years	11–12 YEARS	13–14 years	15 years	16–18 years
Tetanus, Diphtheria, Pertussis*		*see website	Tdap		Tdap	
Human Papillomavirus*		*see website	HPV (3 doses)	HPV Series		
Meningococcal*		MPSV4	MCV4		MCV4[3] MCV4	
Pneumococcal*			PPV			
Influenza*			Influenza (Yearly)			
Hepatitis A*			HepA Series			
Hepatitis B*			HepB Series			
Inactivated Poliovirus*			IPV Series			
Measles, Mumps, Rubella*			MMR Series			
Varicella*			Varicella Series			

Legend:
- Range of recommended ages
- Catch-up immunization
- Certain high-risk groups

This schedule indicates the recommended ages for routine administration of currently licensed childhood vaccines, as of December 1, 2006, for children aged 7–18 years. Any dose not administered at the recommended age should be administered at any subsequent visit, when indicated and feasible. Additional vaccines may be licensed and recommended during the year. Licensed combination vaccines may be used whenever any components of the combination are indicated and other components of the vaccine are not contraindicated and if approved by the Food and Drug Administration for that dose of the series. Providers should consult the respective ACIP statement for detailed recommendations. Clinically significant adverse events that follow immunization should be reported to the Vaccine Adverse Event Reporting System (VAERS). Guidance about how to obtain and complete a VAERS form is available at http://www.vaers.hhs.gov or by telephone, **800-822-7967.**

*For complete information go to http://www.cdc.gov/nip/recs/child-schedule.htm#printable.

Appendix p

High-alert Canadian medications

High-alert medications are medications that have a narrow margin of safety and when misused have the greatest potential to cause significant client harm. The Institute for Safe Medication Practices Canada (ISMP Canada) is a national nonprofit organization that independently reviews voluntary reports of medication errors and develops recommendations for safe medication practices throughout Canada to reduce the harm to clients. In 2003, the ISMP compiled a list of high-alert medications that includes medications in the 19 classes listed below, as well as the specific medications listed below. When these drugs appear in this book, each specific drug monograph is highlighted with a light color screen to help nurses identify them. While care should be taken in giving any medication, nurses are advised to exercise extra precautions when administering these high-risk drugs.

Class/Category of Medications
adrenergic agonists, IV (e.g., epINEPHrine)
adrenergic antagonists, IV (e.g., propranolol)
anesthetic agents, general, inhaled and IV (e.g., propofol)
cardioplegic solutions
chemotherapeutic agents, parenteral and oral
dextrose, hypertonic, 20% or greater
dialysis solutions, peritoneal and hemodialysis
epidural or intrathecal medications
glycoprotein IIb/IIIa inhibitors (e.g., eptifibatide)
hypoglycemics, oral
inotropic medications, IV (e.g., digoxin, milrinone)
liposomal forms of drugs (e.g., liposomal amphotericin B)
moderate sedation agents, IV (e.g., midazolam)
moderate sedation agents, oral, for children (e.g., chloral hydrate)
narcotics/opiates, IV and oral (including liquid concentrates, immediate- and sustained-release)
neuromuscular blocking agents (e.g., succinylcholine)
radiocontrast agents, IV
thrombolytics/fibrinolytics, IV (e.g., tenecteplase)
total parenteral nutrition solutions

Individual Medications
amiodarone, IV
colchicine injection
heparin, low molecular weight, injection
heparin, unfractionated, IV
insulin, subcutaneous and IV
lidocaine, IV
magnesium sulfate, injection

Side effects: *italics* = common; **bold** = life-threatening

methotrexate, oral, nononcologic use
nesiritide
nitroprusside, sodium, for injection
potassium chloride, concentrate, for injection
potassium phosphates, injection
sodium chloride, hypertonic, more than 0.9% concentration, injection
warfarin

1. Cohen MR, Kilo CM: High-alert medications: safeguarding against errors. In Cohen MR, editor: *Medication errors,* Washington, DC, 1999, American Pharmaceutical Association.
2. High-alert medications and patient safety, *Sentinel Event Alert* 11, Nov 1999.
3. ISMP's list of high-alert medications, accessed 12/28/04 at http://www.ismp.org/MSAarticles/highalert.htm.
4. ISMP Canada accessed 12/28/04 at http://www.ismp-canada.org/index.htm.

A Safety alert   *"Tall Man" lettering

Appendix q

Canadian controlled substance chart

Drugs	Canada
LSD, mescaline (peyote), harmaline, psilocin & psilocybin (magic mushrooms)	**Part J of the Food and Drug Regulation (FDR)** • Considered "restricted drugs" • High misuse potential • No recognized medical use • Marihuana exemption from FDR if produced for medical reasons
Sedatives such as barbiturates and derivatives (secobarbital), thiobarbiturates (pentothal sodium); anabolic steroids (androstanolone), weight reduction drugs (anorexiants)	**Part G of the FDR** • Controlled drugs • Misuse potential • Verbal and written prescriptions under certain conditions • Only prescribed if required for medical condition • Specified number of refills (conditions apply) • Records must be kept • May be administered under emergency situations (conditions apply)
Amphetamines; benzphetamine; methamphetamine; phenmetrazine; phendimetrazine	**Part G of the FDR** • Designated controlled drug • May be used for designated medical conditions outlined in FDR
Benzodiazepine tranquilizers such as diazepam, lorazepam, flunitrazepam, zolpidem	**Benzodiazepines and Other Targeted Substances Regulations** • Misuse potential • Verbal and written prescriptions under certain conditions • Only prescribed if required for medical condition • Specified number of refills (conditions apply) • Records must be kept • May be administered under emergency situations (conditions apply)
Opiates: heroin, morphine, codeine >8 mg, amidones (methadone), coca and derivatives (cocaine), phencyclidine (PCP), benzazocines (analgesics such as pentazocine), fentanyls	**Narcotic Control Regulation** • High misuse potential • Written prescriptions for specific medical conditions* • Records of opiate prescription file must be kept • No refills (limited amounts in a prescription) • Heroin and methadone are subject to specific controls
Chloral hydrate, chlordiazepoxide	**Schedule F of the FDR** • Low misuse potential

*Verbal prescriptions are permitted for certain opioid preparations (such as Tylenol No. 2 and No. 3), but not for opiate alone, or opiates with 1 other active nonopioid ingredient.

Explanation of Controlled Drugs and Substances Chart for Canada

The *Canadian Controlled Drugs and Substances Act (CDSA)* is a "legislative framework for the control of substances that can alter mental processes and that may produce harm to the health of an individual and to society when diverted or misused" (*Canada Gazette*, 2003, paragraph 5) that is under the jurisdiction of Health Canada. A "controlled substance" means a substance included in Schedules I to VI. Schedules VII and VIII specify amounts of substances in Schedule II (e.g., cannabis and cannabis resin) associated of the FDR or the *Benzodiazepines and Other Targeted Substances Regulations* (Targeted Substances Regulations). Different levels of control measures are found within the various regulations that apply to licensed dealers, pharmacists, practitioners, and hospitals. Part J of the FDR regulates the use of controlled substances with no recognized medical use; substances listed in the schedule to Part J of the FDR are defined as "restricted drugs" and include such substances as LSD and mescaline. Controlled substances included in CDSA Schedules III and IV that have some therapeutic use are regulated under either Part G of the FDR or the Targeted Substances Regulations with the former having more stringent controls over distribution.

Canada Gazette. (2003). Order amending schedule III to the controlled drugs and substances act. Retrieved January 3, 2005 from http://canadagazette.gc.ca/partII/2003/20031231/html/sor412-e.html.

Department of Justice Canada. (2004). *Narcotic Control Regulations.* Retrieved January 6, 2005 from http://laws.justice.gc.ca/en/C-38.8/C.R.C.-c.1041/76122.html.

Department of Justice Canada. (2004). *Controlled Drugs and Substances Act.* Retrieved December 31, 2004 from http://laws.justice.gc.ca/en/C-38.8/.

Health Canada. (2004). *Food and Drugs Act.* Part G–Controlled Drugs. Part J–Restricted Drugs. Schedule F. Retrieved January 6, 2005 from http://www.hc-sc.gc.ca/food-aliment/friia-raaii/food_drugs-aliments_drogues/act-loi/e_index.html.

National Association of Pharmacy Regulatory Authorities (NAPRA). *Controlled Drugs and Substances Act and Regulations.* Retrieved January 6, 2005 from http://www.napra.org/docs/0/93/143.asp.

NAPRA. (2003). *Marihuana Exception (Food and Drugs Act) Regulations.* Retrieved January 6, 2005 from http://www.napra.ca/pdfs/fedleg/0307marihuana exemption.pdf.

NAPRA. *Benzodiazepines and Other Targeted Substances Regulations.* Retrieved January 6, 2005 from http://www.napra.ca/pdfs/fedleg/benzodiaz.pdf.

Appendix r Canadian recommended immunization schedules for infants and children

VACCINE	MONTHS						YEARS	
	2	4	6	12	18	4 TO 6	9 TO 13	14 TO 16
Hepatitis B*	3 doses	3 doses	3 doses	3 doses	3 doses	3 doses	3 doses	
Diphtheria, Pertussis, and Tetanus (DPT)	DPT	DPT	DPT		DPT	DPT		Td
								**
Haemophilus influenzae type b *** (Hib)	Hib	Hib	Hib		Hib			
Polio (inactivated polio vaccine/oral polio vaccine)	Polio	Polio	Polio		Polio	Polio		Polio
			****					****
Measles, Mumps, and Rubella ***** (MMR)				MMR	MMR	MMR		
					*****	*****		

* Adolescents who have not received hepatitis B vaccine in infancy should receive it through school programs according to the provincial and territorial policies.

** Td (tetanus and diphtheria toxoids, adult formulation).

*** Recommended schedule for both Hib-TITER® and AcHIB®.

**** If oral polio vaccine is used exclusively, boosters at 6 months and 14 to 16 years of age may be omitted.

***** The second dose of MMR is routinely recommended at either 18 months or at 4 to 6 years of age. It should be given any time before school entry provided that there is at least a 1-month interval between receipt of the first and second doses.

Appendix s

FDA pregnancy categories

A   No risk demonstrated to the fetus in any trimester

B   No adverse effects in animals, no human studies available

C   Only given after risks to the fetus are considered; animal studies have shown adverse reactions, no human studies available

D   Definite fetal risks, may be given in spite of risks if needed in life-threatening conditions

X   Absolute fetal abnormalities; not to be used anytime during pregnancy

Note: **UK** = Unknown fetal risk (used in this text but not an official FDA pregnancy category).

Appendix t

Weights and equivalents

METRIC SYSTEM

Weight

kilogram	=	kg	=	1000 grams
gram	=	g	=	1 gram
milligram	=	mg	=	0.001 gram
microgram	=	mcg	=	0.001 milligram

Volume

liter	=	L	=	1 L
milliliter	=	ml	=	0.001 L

AVOIRDUPOIS WEIGHT

1 ounce (oz)	=	437.5 grains
1 pound (lb)	=	16 ounces = 7000 grains

METRIC AND APOTHECARY EQUIVALENTS

Exact weight equivalents

Metric	Apothecary
1 mg	1/64.8 grain
64.8 mg	1 grain
324 mg	5 grains
1 g	15.432 grains
31.103 g	1 ounce = 480 grains

Exact volume equivalents

Metric	Apothecary		
1.00 ml	16.23 minims		
3.69 ml	1 fluidram	=	60 minims
29.57 ml	1 fluid ounce	=	480 minims
473.16 ml	1 pint	=	7680 minims
946.33 ml	1 quart	=	15,360 minims

Appendix u

Abbreviations

AAS argininosuccinic acid synthetase
abd abdomen
ABG arterial blood gas
ACE angiotensin-converting enzyme
ADA American Diabetes Association
ADH antidiuretic hormone
ALT alanine aminotransferase
ANA antinuclear antibody
AP anteroposterior
APTT activated partial thromboplastin time
ASA acetylsalicylic acid, aspirin
ASHD arteriosclerotic heart disease
AST aspartate aminotransferase (SGOT)
AV atrioventricular
bid twice a day
BM bowel movement
BMR basal metabolic rate
B/P blood pressure
BPH benign prostatic hypertrophy
BPM beats per minute
BS blood sugar
BUN blood urea nitrogen
C Celsius (centigrade)
Ca cancer
CAD coronary artery disease
cap capsule
Cath catheterization or catheterize
CBC complete blood cell count
CC chief complaint
cc cubic centimeter
CCr creatinine clearance
CHF congestive heart failure
cm centimeter
CNS central nervous system
CO₂ carbon dioxide
CONT continuous
COPD chronic obstructive pulmonary disease
CPAP continuous positive airway pressure
CPK creatine phosphokinase
CPR cardiopulmonary resuscitation
CPS carbamoyl phosphate synthetase

C&S culture and sensitivity
C sect cesarean section
CSF cerebrospinal fluid
CV cardiovascular
CVA cerebrovascular accident
CVP central venous pressure
D&C dilatation and curettage
DIC diffuse intravascular coagulation
DIR INF direct infusion
dr dram
D₅W 5% glucose in distilled water
ECG electrocardiogram (EKG)
EDTA ethylenediamine tetraacetic acid
EEG electroencephalogram
EENT ear, eye, nose, and throat
EPS extrapyramidal symptom
ESR erythrocyte sedimentation rate
EXT-REL extended release
EXTRA-STREN-SUSP extra strength suspension
FBS fasting blood sugar
FHT fetal heart tones
FSH follicle-stimulating hormone
g gram
GABA γ-aminobutyric acid
GI gastrointestinal
gr grain
GT glucose tolerance test
gtt drops
GU genitourinary
H₂ histamine₂
hCG human chorionic gonadotropin
Hct hematocrit
HDCV human diploid cell rabies vaccine
Hgb hemoglobin
H & H hematocrit and hemoglobin
5-HIAA 5-hydroxindoleacetic acid
HIV human immunodeficiency virus (AIDS)
H₂O water

HOB	head of bed	**od**	right eye
HR	heart rate	**OR**	operating room
hr	hour	**os**	left eye
IgG	immunolobulin G	**OTC**	over-the-counter
IM	intramuscular	**OU**	each eye
INF	infusion	**oz**	ounce
INH	inhalation	**p̄**	after
inj	injection	**P56**	plasma-lyte 56
I&O	intake and output	**PaCO₂**	arterial carbon dioxide tension (pressure)
INT	intermittent		
IPPB	intermittent positive-pressure breathing	**PaO₂**	arterial oxygen tension (pressure)
		PAT	paroxysmal atrial tachycardia
ITP	idiopathic thrombocytopenic purpura	**PBI**	protein-bound iodine
		PCWP	pulmonary capillary wedge pressure
IUD	intrauterine device	**PEEP**	positive end-expiratory pressure
IV	intravenous	**PERRLA**	pupils equal, round, react to light and accommodation
IVP	intravenous pyelogram		
K	potassium	**pH**	hydrogen ion concentration
kg	kilogram	**PO**	by mouth
L	liter	**postop**	postoperative
lb	pound	**PP**	postprandial
LDH	lactic dehydrogenase	**preop**	preoperative
LE	lupus erythematosus	**prn**	as required
LFT	liver function test	**PT**	prothrombin time
LH	luteinizing hormone	**PTT**	partial thromboplastin time
LLQ	left lower quadrant	**PVC**	premature ventricular contraction
LMP	last menstrual period	**pwd**	powder
LOC	level of consciousness	**qAM**	every morning
LR	lactated Ringer's solution	**qh**	every hour
LT	leukotriene	**q2h**	every 2 hours
LUQ	left upper quadrant	**q3h**	every 3 hours
M	meter	**q4h**	every 4 hours
m	minim	**q6h**	every 6 hours
m²	square meter	**q12h**	every 12 hours
MAC	monitored anesthesia care	**qid**	four times daily
MAOI	monoamine oxidase inhibitor	**qPM**	every night
mEq	milliequivalent	**qs**	sufficient quantity
mg	milligram	**qt**	quart
MI	myocardial infarction	**R**	right
min	minute	**RAIU**	radioactive iodine uptake
ml	milliliter	**RBC**	red blood cell count or red blood cell
mm	millimeter		
mo	month	**RECT**	rectal
Na	sodium	**RLQ**	right lower quadrant
neg	negative	**ROM**	range of motion
ng	nanogram	**RUQ**	right upper quadrant
NOS	not otherwise specified	**SIMV**	synchronous intermittent mandatory ventilation
NPO	nothing by mouth (Lat. *nulla per os*)		
NS	normal saline	**SL**	sublingual
O₂	oxygen	**SLE**	systemic lupus erythematosus
OBS	organic brain syndrome	**SOB**	shortness of breath

sol	solution	**UTI**	urinary tract infection
ss	one half	**UV**	ultraviolet
SUBCUT	subcutaneous	**vag**	vaginal
suppos	suppository	**VMA**	vanillylmandelic acid
SUS REL	sustained release	**vol**	volume
syr	syrup	**VS**	vital sign
T&A	tonsillectomy and adenoidectomy	**WBC**	white blood cell count
tab	tablet	**wk**	week
tbsp	tablespoon	**wt**	weight
temp	temperature	**yr**	year
tid	three times daily	>	greater than
tinc	tincture	<	less than
TPN	total parenteral nutrition	=	equal
top	topical	°	degree
TRANS	transdermal	%	percent
TSH	thyroid-stimulating hormone	α	alpha
tsp	teaspoon	β	beta
TT	thrombin time	γ	gamma
UA	urinalysis		

- For a list of the Institute for Safe Medicine Practices (ISMP) error-prone abbreviations, symbols and dose designations, please see http://www.ismp.org/tools/errorproneabbreviations.pdf.
- For 2007 National Patient Safety Goals, please visit The Joint Commission website at http://www.jointcommission.org/PatientSafety/NationalPatientSafetyGoals.

Index

Entries can be identified as follows: *Combination Products,* DISEASES/DISORDERS, *DRUG CATEGORIES,* generic names, Trade Names.

Entries can be identified as follows: *Combination Products,* DISEASES/DISORDERS,
DRUG CATEGORIES, generic names, Trade Names.

Entries can be identified as follows: *Combination Products,* DISEASES/DISORDERS,
DRUG CATEGORIES, generic names, Trade Names.

Entries can be identified as follows: *Combination Products,* DISEASES/DISORDERS,
DRUG CATEGORIES, generic names, Trade Names.

Entries can be identified as follows: *Combination Products,* DISEASES/DISORDERS,
DRUG CATEGORIES, generic names, Trade Names.

Entries can be identified as follows: *Combination Products,* DISEASES/DISORDERS,
DRUG CATEGORIES, generic names, Trade Names.

1220 index

Entries can be identified as follows: *Combination Products,* DISEASES/DISORDERS, *DRUG CATEGORIES,* generic names, Trade Names.

Entries can be identified as follows: *Combination Products,* DISEASES/DISORDERS,
DRUG CATEGORIES, generic names, Trade Names.

Entries can be identified as follows: *Combination Products,* DISEASES/DISORDERS,
DRUG CATEGORIES, generic names, Trade Names.

Entries can be identified as follows: *Combination Products,* DISEASES/DISORDERS,
DRUG CATEGORIES, generic names, Trade Names.

Entries can be identified as follows: *Combination Products,* DISEASES/DISORDERS, *DRUG CATEGORIES,* generic names, Trade Names.

Entries can be identified as follows: *Combination Products,* DISEASES/DISORDERS,
DRUG CATEGORIES, generic names, Trade Names.

Entries can be identified as follows: *Combination Products,* DISEASES/DISORDERS, *DRUG CATEGORIES,* generic names, Trade Names.

Entries can be identified as follows: *Combination Products,* DISEASES/DISORDERS, *DRUG CATEGORIES,* generic names, Trade Names.

Entries can be identified as follows: *Combination Products,* DISEASES/DISORDERS, *DRUG CATEGORIES,* generic names, Trade Names.

1242 index

Entries can be identified as follows: *Combination Products,* DISEASES/DISORDERS, *DRUG CATEGORIES,* generic names, Trade Names.

Entries can be identified as follows: *Combination Products,* DISEASES/DISORDERS,
DRUG CATEGORIES, generic names, Trade Names.

Entries can be identified as follows: *Combination Products,* DISEASES/DISORDERS,
DRUG CATEGORIES, generic names, Trade Names.

Entries can be identified as follows: *Combination Products*, DISEASES/DISORDERS, *DRUG CATEGORIES*, generic names, Trade Names.

Kidrolase, 153-154
Kineret, 138-139
Kionex, 934-935
K-Lease, 833-835
KLEPTOMANIA
  fluoxetine for, 457-476
K-Long, 833-835
Klonopin, 288-290, 1168, 1173
K-Lor, 833-835, 1173
Klor-Con, 833-835
Klor-Con EF, 833-835
Klorvess, 833-835
Klorvess Effervescent Granules, 833-835
Klotrix, 833-835
K-Lyte, 833-835, 1173
K-Lyte/Cl, 833-835, 1173
K-Lyte/Cl powder, 833-835
K-Lyte DS, 833-835
K-med, 833-835
K-Norm, 833-835
Koate-DVI, 143-144
Koffex, 352
Kogenate, 143-144, 1173
Kogenate-2, 1173
Kogenate FS, 143-144
Kolyum, 833-835
Konsyl, 869-870
Konsyl Orange, 869-870
Konyne 80, 447-448
K-pek, 187-188
K-Phos Neutral, 1173, 1177
KRAUROSIS VULVAE
  estradiol for, 436-438
Kristalose, 593-595
K-Sol, 833-835
K-tab, 833-835
kunecatechins, 1092
Ku-Zyme HP, 783
K-Vescent, 833-835
Kwell, 613-614
Kytril, 519-520

L
LA-12, 312-313
labetalol, 17, 31, 591-593, 1174
LABOR PAIN
  meperidine for, 650-652
  ropivacaine for, 911-912

Lacrilube, 1174, 1182
Lacti-Care-HC, 1106
Lactinex, 1143
Lactulax, 593-595
lactulose, 43, 593-595
Lactulose PSE, 593-595
Lamicel, 1174
Lamictal, 596-597, 1174, 1175
Lamictal Chewable Dispersible, 596-597
Lamisil, 974-975, 1107-1108, 1174
lamivudine, 594-595, 1174, 1185
lamotrigine, 8, 596-597, 1174
Lamprene, 285
Lanacane, 1109-1110
Lanacort, 1106
Laniazid, 580-581
Lanophyllin, 982-984
Lanoxicaps, 362-365
Lanoxin, 362-365, 1173, 1174, 1175, 1185
lansoprazole, 597-598, 1189, 1192
lanthanum, 598
Lantus, 565-567
Lantus, Insulin Human, 1174
Lanvis, 986
Largactil, 261-264
Larodopa, 607-608
laronidase, 598
LARYNGITIS
  omeprazole for, 761-762
Lasix, 496-498, 1174, 1175
Lasix Special, 496-498
latanoprost, 1102-1103
latanoprost ophthalmic, 598
latanoprost timolol, 1184, 1185
LAXATIVES, 42-43, 1187
Laxit, 186-187
L-Dopa, 607-608, 1174, 1175
LEAD ENCEPHALOPATHY
  edetate calcium disodium for, 402-403

LEAD POISONING
  dimercaprol for, 370
  edetate calcium disodium for, 403
leflunomide, 598-599
LEFT VENTRICULAR DYSFUNCTION
  captopril for, 219-220
  trandolapril for, 1018-1019
LEFT VENTRICULARA HYPERTROPHY
  losartan for, 628-629
LEG CRAMPS
  quinine for, 880
Lemoderm, 1106
lemon balm, 1124
LENNOX-GAUSTAUT SYNDROME
  felbamate for, 452-453
Lente, 564-567
Lente, Insulin Human, 1174
lepirudin, 7, 599-601, 1197
LEPROSY
  clofazimine for, 285
Lescol, 482-483
Lescol XL, 482-483
letrozole, 601-602
leucovorin, 602-603, 1174
leucovorin calcium, 602-603
LEUKEMIA
  busulfan for, 205-206
  cytarabine for, 320-322
  hydroxyurea for, 540-542
  imatinib for, 552-553
  immune globulin for, 556-558
  interferon alfa for, 569-570
  methotrexate for, 663-665
  tretinoin for, 1024-1025
LEUKAPHERESIS
  hetastarch for, 528-529
Leukeran, 252-254, 1164, 1174, 1176
Leukine, 918-919, 1174
leuprolide, 22, 603-604, 1197

Entries can be identified as follows: *Combination Products*, DISEASES/DISORDERS, *DRUG CATEGORIES*, generic names, Trade Names.

Entries can be identified as follows: *Combination Products,* DISEASES/DISORDERS, *DRUG CATEGORIES,* generic names, Trade Names.

Entries can be identified as follows: *Combination Products*, DISEASES/DISORDERS,
DRUG CATEGORIES, generic names, Trade Names.

Entries can be identified as follows: *Combination Products,* DISEASES/DISORDERS,
DRUG CATEGORIES, generic names, Trade Names.

Entries can be identified as follows: *Combination Products,* DISEASES/DISORDERS,
DRUG CATEGORIES, generic names, Trade Names.

Entries can be identified as follows: *Combination Products,* DISEASES/DISORDERS, *DRUG CATEGORIES,* generic names, Trade Names.

Entries can be identified as follows: *Combination Products,* DISEASES/DISORDERS,
DRUG CATEGORIES, generic names, Trade Names.

1260 index

Entries can be identified as follows: *Combination Products,* DISEASES/DISORDERS, *DRUG CATEGORIES,* generic names, Trade Names.

Entries can be identified as follows: *Combination Products,* DISEASES/DISORDERS, *DRUG CATEGORIES,* generic names, Trade Names.

Entries can be identified as follows: *Combination Products,* DISEASES/DISORDERS, *DRUG CATEGORIES,* generic names, Trade Names.

Entries can be identified as follows: *Combination Products,* DISEASES/DISORDERS,
DRUG CATEGORIES, generic names, Trade Names.

Entries can be identified as follows: *Combination Products,* DISEASES/DISORDERS, *DRUG CATEGORIES,* generic names, Trade Names.

Entries can be identified as follows: *Combination Products,* DISEASES/DISORDERS,
DRUG CATEGORIES, generic names, Trade Names.

Entries can be identified as follows: *Combination Products*, DISEASES/DISORDERS, *DRUG CATEGORIES*, generic names, Trade Names.

Entries can be identified as follows: *Combination Products*, DISEASES/DISORDERS, *DRUG CATEGORIES*, generic names, Trade Names.

Entries can be identified as follows: *Combination Products,* DISEASES/DISORDERS, *DRUG CATEGORIES,* generic names, Trade Names.

Entries can be identified as follows: *Combination Products,* DISEASES/DISORDERS, *DRUG CATEGORIES,* generic names, Trade Names.

Entries can be identified as follows: *Combination Products*, DISEASES/DISORDERS, *DRUG CATEGORIES*, generic names, Trade Names.

Entries can be identified as follows: *Combination Products,* DISEASES/DISORDERS,
DRUG CATEGORIES, generic names, Trade Names.

Entries can be identified as follows: *Combination Products,* DISEASES/DISORDERS,
DRUG CATEGORIES, generic names, Trade Names.

Entries can be identified as follows: *Combination Products,* DISEASES/DISORDERS, *DRUG CATEGORIES,* generic names, Trade Names.